Clinical Breast Imaging

THE ESSENTIALS

Clinical Breast Imaging

THE ESSENTIALS

Gilda Cardeñosa, MD, FSBI, FACR

The Veronica Donovan Sweeney
Professor of Breast Imaging
Director of Breast Imaging
Virginia Commonwealth University Medical Center
Richmond, Virginia

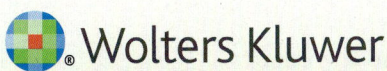 Wolters Kluwer

Philadelphia · Baltimore · New York · London
Buenos Aires · Hong Kong · Sydney · Tokyo

Senior Executive Editor: Jonathan W. Pine, Jr.
Acquisitions Editor: Ryan Shaw
Product Development Editor: Amy G. Dinkel
Production Project Manager: Alicia Jackson
Senior Manufacturing Coordinator: Beth Welsh
Marketing Manager: Dan Dresssler
Senior Designer: Stephen Druding
Production Service: S4Carlisle Publishing Services

© 2015 by Wolters Kluwer

Two Commerce Square
2001 Market Street
Philadelphia, PA 19103, USA

LWW.com

All rights reserved. This book is protected by copyright. No part of this book may be reproduced in any form by any means, including photocopying, or utilized by any information storage and retrieval system without written permission from the copyright owner, except for brief quotations embodied in critical articles and reviews. Materials appearing in this book prepared by individuals as part of their official duties as U.S. government employees are not covered by the above-mentioned copyright.

Printed in China

Library of Congress Cataloging-in-Publication Data

Cardeñosa, Gilda, author.
  Clinical breast imaging : the essentials / Gilda Cardeñosa. -- First edition.
     p. ; cm.
  Includes bibliographical references and index.
     ISBN 978-1-4511-5177-0 (hardback : alk. paper) — ISBN 1-4511-5177-2 (hardback : alk. paper)
  [DNLM: 1. Breast Diseases—diagnosis.   2. Breast Neoplasms—diagnosis.   3. Magnetic Resonance Imaging.   4. Mammography.   5. Ultrasonography, Mammary.   WP 815]
  RG493.5.R33
  618.1'907572—dc23
                                                        2014010149

Care has been taken to confirm the accuracy of the information presented and to describe generally accepted practices. However, the authors, editors, and publisher are not responsible for errors or omissions or for any consequences from application of the information in this book and make no warranty, expressed or implied, with respect to the currency, completeness, or accuracy of the contents of the publication. Application of the information in a particular situation remains the professional responsibility of the practitioner.

The authors, editors, and publisher have exerted every effort to ensure that drug selection and dosage set forth in this text are in accordance with current recommendations and practice at the time of publication. However, in view of ongoing research, changes in government regulations, and the constant flow of information relating to drug therapy and drug reactions, the reader is urged to check the package insert for each drug for any change in indications and dosage and for added warnings and precautions. This is particularly important when the recommended agent is a new or infrequently employed drug.

Some drugs and medical devices presented in the publication have Food and Drug Administration (FDA) clearance for limited use in restricted research settings. It is the responsibility of the health care provider to ascertain the FDA status of each drug or device planned for use in their clinical practice.

To purchase additional copies of this book, call our customer service department at (800) 638-3030 or fax orders to (301) 223-2320. International customers should call (301) 223-2300.

Visit Lippincott Williams & Wilkins on the Internet: at LWW.com. Lippincott Williams & Wilkins customer service representatives are available from 8:30 am to 6 pm, EST.

10 9 8 7 6 5 4 3 2 1

To Kathleen M. Connelly, MBA

With profound, heartfelt thanks . . .

SERIES FOREWORD

The *Essentials* series is a collection of radiology textbooks following a standardized format. Each book in the *Essentials* series is a practical tool for those wanting to quickly acquire a broad base of knowledge in a specialty area. The content is limited to the essentials of that specialty so as not to overwhelm the novice, yet provides enough detail that it can serve as a quick review for residents or practicing radiologists, a guide for those who teach the specialty, and a reference for specialty physicians and other health care professionals whose patients are referred for imaging in that specialty area. What sets *Essentials* texts apart from other similar texts is that they (i) are compact and of practical size for a resident to read during an initial 4-week rotational experience, (ii) include learning objectives at the beginning of each chapter, and (iii) provide an exercise for self-assessment. Each book includes citations from the most recent literature that are called out in the text.

Self-assessment is a key component of the *Essentials* texts. Multiple-choice items are included at the end of every chapter, and a self-assessment examination is included at the end of each text. This should be of particular benefit to those who are preparing for the new image-rich computer-based examinations that are a component of professional certification and maintenance of certification.

The series includes not only texts related to clinical specialties that are rich with radiologic images and illustrations, but also texts related to noninterpretive subjects such as radiologic physics and quality and safety in medical imaging. The goal of the *Essentials* series is to provide a collection of practical references to accompany a well-rounded education in diagnostic imaging and imaging-guided therapy.

JANNETTE COLLINS, MD, MED, FCCP, FACR

PREFACE

As a radiologist, I am incredibly proud of all that our specialty has contributed to medicine. It is the driving force behind incredible advances in patient care. As a breast imager I stand in awe of the path paved by so many colleagues who provided the scientific evidence supporting the use of screening mammography. Several randomized controlled trials have shown that the detection of early breast cancer through screening mammography saves lives. These same individuals now stand steadfast in the ongoing battles to derail the routine use of screening mammography and, with it, the decreases we are seeing in the mortality from breast cancer. Rather than re-litigate the data from randomized controlled trials, our goal at this point should be to aggressively increase compliance with annual screening mammography starting at age 40. Concomitantly, we need to redouble our efforts to train breast imaging clinicians, maximize their interpretative skills and encourage them to exercise sound judgment relative to how best to apply the tools available to them while emphasizing the unique position they are in to transition patients through the process accurately, efficiently and empathetically.

This book is a miniscule contribution in an effort to improve interpretative skills. This book presents a basic, commonsense, practical, and clinically oriented approach to breast imaging—it is **not** a comprehensive scientific review. There are several outstanding books that provide that level of detail and information. As with all of my books, my efforts have been to include as many images as possible to *illustrate* the basic points presented in the text. Inherent in the organization of this book is a certain amount of repetition that has been done purposefully.

This book is intended for residents in radiology, pathology, surgery, plastic surgery, radiation therapy, and medical oncology; radiologists and other clinicians in practice taking care of women with breast related issues; and technologists who want to learn a practical, workable, commonsense approach to breast imaging with useful tips and guidelines. As I have stated before, writing these books is an effort on my part to give back to my patients and honor their courage in battling breast cancer. It is also to share my experiences. It is an attempt to teach others, who are taking care of patients, what I have learned and continue to learn from my patients. Our approach to patient care in breast imaging is based on common sense and a commitment to providing the best possible patient care experience. Clinical breast imaging is an incredibly rewarding subspecialty that, when done with compassion and commitment, provides a needed and invaluable service. It is a subspecialty through which we save women's lives and improve their quality of life.

GILDA CARDEÑOSA

ACKNOWLEDGMENTS

I am privileged to work with Priti A. Shah, MD, and Tiffany M. Tucker, MD. They are gifted breast imaging clinicians focused on the detection, evaluation, and management of patients with breast diseases. We are proudly "infected" with the clinical breast-imaging virus that presents itself as an incurable passion for what we do and manifests itself in everything we do to take care of our patients in a kind, efficient, empathetic, and data-driven manner. Once infected, there is no cure. The three of us are supported by an amazingly professional and dedicated management team, led by Joanne Cousins, RTR(M), and includes Lynda Giardini, RTR(M), Amy Silva, RTR(M), and Diane Cunningham. Every day brings requests for "big favors," which they always get done promptly, professionally, and with unassailable grace, even when it requires them to set aside personal time. For these individuals, there is no task too difficult, no challenge that can't be met and surpassed, and no mountain peak beyond their reach. With our clerical staff (Jennifer Campbell, Rena Davis, Tami Freeman, Nicole Hansom, LaSandia Holmes, Joyce Jackson, Patricia Lacy, Anthony McLauren, Pamela Ramirez, and Raleigh Poindexter) and technical staff, all certified mammography technologists (Courtney Ayala Rivas, Fareeda Connor, Sandra Jessup, Kristin McMahan, Elizabeth Nissly, Rebecca Stuart, and Theresa Taylor), we share an unshakeable, unifying focus: our patients. All of our staff are compassionate, dedicated, and loyal. Whatever is asked of them gets accomplished with enthusiasm and professionalism. They all know that the answer to any request from our patients and referring physicians is "yes, we can do that," and then they make it happen effortlessly. In my work on this book in particular, I would be remiss in not acknowledging Mrs. Nancy Cooper, our administrative assistant. She has been there every step of the way, email after email, phone call after phone call, to assist with all projects related to the Section and take on increasing amounts of responsibility and special projects. For her ability to research things and her skills with the English language, she has earned the nicknames of Sherlock and Mrs. Merriam Webster; her assistance and support are invaluable.

The Department of Radiology at the Virginia Commonwealth University Health System is a special place, providing our clinical breast imaging program and staff the ongoing support and nurturing needed to thrive. For this wonderful home, I am indebted to Ann S. Fulcher, MD, Chair of the Department of Radiology, Mary Ann Turner, MD, Vice Chair of Faculty, Sherry Elliott, MBA, FACMPE, Vice Chair of Administration and Operations, and Sharon Gibbs, MSHA, CRA, CNMT, Director of Radiology. They have embraced the concept of our Section being a clinical service focused not only on interpreting images but enhancing patient care and at every turn have provided the needed impetus to make this happen.

At Lippincott Williams and Wilkins, I feel privileged to have worked with Jonathan Pine. He championed this project. Time and again he provided the guidance and support any author welcomes. His integrity, availability, willingness to listen, and inordinate amount of patience are missed. I am saddened he is not here to see the final product and fervently hope he would be proud. I continue to carry and apply advice and guidance provided by Lisa McAllister and Brian Brown (though not directly involved in this project), who were both incredibly supportive and wise advisors on prior projects. I also extend my sincere thanks to Franny Murphy and Amy Dinkel for their hard work as the development editors as well as Alicia Jackson (production product manager), Beth Welsh (senior manufacturing coordinator), Dan Dressler (marketing manager) and Stephen Druding (senior designer). A big thank you also goes to Shailaja Subramanian and her team at S4Carlisle for their dedication and diligent work on this project; they have made every effort to accommodate my concerns and taught me much in the process.

Lastly, with an immense sense of humility and gratitude, every day brings thoughts of my mother and the realization that none of this would be possible if it were not for her courageous and tenacious efforts to imbue in me the needed freedom of mind and spirit to embrace challenges and work hard for a good, productive life.

CONTENTS

Series Foreword   vii
Preface   ix
Acknowledgments   xi

Chapter 1	Breast Cancer: An Overview	1
Chapter 2	Screening Mammography	13
Chapter 3	Diagnostic Breast Imaging	48
Chapter 4	Breast Ultrasound	80
Chapter 5	Breast Magnetic Resonance Imaging	113
Chapter 6	Breast Calcifications	145
Chapter 7	Evaluation and Imaging Features of Benign Breast Masses	172
Chapter 8	Evaluation and Imaging Features of Malignant Breast Masses	234
Chapter 9	Miscellaneous Mammographic Findings	283
Chapter 10	The Male Breast	316
Chapter 11	The Altered Breast	331
Chapter 12	Interventional Procedures	378
Chapter 13	Communication and Accountability in Breast Imaging	424

Self-Assessment Exam   431
Appendix A   452
Index   455

Breast Cancer: An Overview

LEARNING OBJECTIVES

1. Overview of risk factors associated with breast cancer risk
   - Chemoprevention
2. Screening mammography
   - Randomized controlled trials
   - Controversies
   - Screening guidelines
3. Mammography Quality Standards Act
4. American College of Radiology: Mammography Accreditation Program
5. Overview of treatment options
   - Lumpectomy, mastectomy
   - Sentinel lymph node biopsy versus axillary lymph node dissection
   - Radiation therapy
     Accelerated partial breast radiation
   - Chemotherapy
     Use of Oncotype DX
     Neoadjuvant therapy
   - Chemoprevention
6. Breast cancer staging
   - TNM
   - Genetic profiling of breast tumors
7. Considerations when reviewing patient images in breast imaging

Breast cancer is a common, life-threatening disease. If skin cancers are excluded, breast cancer is the most frequently diagnosed malignancy and the second leading cause of cancer mortality among women second only to lung cancer (1,2). Women have a 12.5% (1 in 8 women) lifetime risk of developing breast cancer by age 85 (3,4). It is estimated that 232,670 women and 2,360 men will be diagnosed with invasive breast cancer in the United States in 2014. An additional 62,570 women are estimated to be diagnosed with in situ breast cancer, 85% of which will be ductal. It is estimated that 40,430 breast cancer–related deaths will occur in the United States in 2014 (40,000 in women, 430 in men) (1,2). Breast cancer–related deaths have been progressively decreasing since 1989 such that approximately 30% fewer women are dying from it annually (5). A close to 7% decrease in the incidence rate of breast cancer reported from 2002 to 2003 is attributed in part to the reduction in the use of hormone replacement therapy. No change in the incidence rate for breast cancer was reported between 2005 and 2009 (1,2).

RISK FACTORS

Many factors are reportedly associated with an increased risk of breast cancer, but only a few are considered significant. Included among these are gender, age, a personal or family history of breast cancer in first-degree relatives, prior breast biopsy with certain histological diagnoses, a history of high-dose radiation to the chest between the ages of 10 and 30, and mutations in *BRCA1* and *BRCA2* genes as well as several other relatively rare breast cancer susceptibility genes (2–4,6). Other factors that have been implicated include: early menarche, late menopause, late first-term pregnancy, nulliparity, and postmenopausal obesity. For these risk factors, prolonged exposure of breast tissue to estrogen is thought to play a role (2–4,6). The density of the breast parenchyma on a mammogram has also been suggested and described as an indicator for increased breast cancer risk (2–4,6–13); the extent to which this is true remains to be defined (see below) (14).

Women are about 100 times more likely to develop breast cancer than men, and the incidence of breast cancer increases as women get older (2). The risk increases rapidly in premenopausal women and more slowly in postmenopausal women. Women with a personal history of breast cancer have a three- to fourfold increase in the risk of developing a new breast cancer compared with women who have never had the disease. The risk of developing breast cancer is doubled in women with one, and increased threefold with two first-degree relatives with breast cancer (mother, sisters, or daughters), particularly if the breast cancer in the relative developed premenopausally and was bilateral or multiple. The associated risk for women who have had a father or brother with breast cancer is increased, but it is not known by exactly how much. It is important to emphasize, however, that approximately 85% of women diagnosed with breast cancer do not have a family history of the disease (3,4,6).

Women who have had a breast biopsy may also be at increased risk for the development of breast cancer (2). Benign breast disease can be subdivided into three general categories: (i) Non-proliferative lesions have little effect on the risk for breast cancer; these include fibrosis and fibrocystic changes, apocrine and squamous metaplasia, mild hyperplasia, adenosis, solitary papillomas, fat necrosis, duct ectasia, lipoma, fibroadenolipoma, neurofibroma, and vascular lesions. (ii) Proliferative lesions with no atypia are reportedly associated with an increased risk of 1.5 to 2 times that of "normal" women. These processes include ductal hyperplasia of the usual type, fibroadenoma, sclerosing adenosis, multiple papillomas, and complex sclerosing lesions. (iii) Proliferative lesions with atypia increase the risk in patients by 3.5 to 5 times that of patients who do not have these processes. Atypical ductal hyperplasia (ADH) and atypical lobular hyperplasia (ALH) are the two primary lesions in this group. The associated risk is even higher for patients with these proliferative processes and a family history of breast cancer. The significance and risk associated with more recently described pathological entities such as flat epithelial atypia, columnar cell change with atypia, and atypical papillomas are not yet adequately defined. Unlike ductal carcinoma in situ (DCIS) that is considered to be a cancer, lobular carcinoma in situ (LCIS) has traditionally been considered a marker lesion of increased risk and not a precursor. Patients with LCIS have a 7- to 11-fold increase in the risk of developing breast cancer. The risk associated with LCIS applies to both breasts, and the patients have an equal likelihood of developing invasive ductal or lobular cancers (3,4,6,15).

Two genes (*BRCA1*, *BRCA2*) have been isolated in some women with breast cancer. It is estimated that 5% to 10% of all breast cancers in the United States are hereditary, related to mutations in the *BRCA1* or *BRCA2* genes; these genes are more common in Jewish people of Ashkenazi descent, but can occur in anyone. Women with mutations in the *BRCA1* gene are also at increased risk for developing ovarian cancer. The risk of developing breast cancer in women who carry mutations in this gene is 85% by age 70 (63% for ovarian cancer by age 70); the average risk for breast cancer in *BRCA1* carriers is 55% to 65%. These patients are likely to be younger and premenopausal with multiple tumors and bilateral synchronous or metachronous lesions. The tumors in these patients are often aggressive and phenotypically triple negative (e.g., estrogen receptor, progesterone receptor, and HER2/neu negative). Women who carry mutations in the *BRCA2* gene have an increased breast cancer risk of approximately 45% but are not at increased risk for ovarian cancer. Breast cancers in patients with this mutation are also more likely to develop in younger women and be bilateral. Hereditary male breast cancer is associated with mutations in the *BRCA2* gene but not with *BRCA1*. There are some genetic diseases (Li-Fraumeni syndrome, Cowden disease, Bannayan–Riley–Ruvalcaba syndrome, and ataxia-telangiectasia) associated with breast cancer susceptibility genes and an increased risk of breast cancer among affected patients (2–4,6). Genetic testing for the *BRCA1* and *BRCA2* mutations as well as other genes (*PTEN* or *TP53*) is available; however, patients are encouraged strongly to consider genetic counseling before being tested.

High-dose radiation to the chest between the ages of 10 and 30 for the treatment of lymphoma, or women who have had radiation therapy for an enlarged thymus, are at increased risk for breast cancer (2–4,6). The breast cancers in these women develop approximately 10 to 15 years following the radiation therapy and tend to be the more aggressive forms of breast cancer.

Early menarche and the establishment of regular menses are risk factors in breast cancer development. It is estimated that the risk for breast cancer decreases by 10% to 15% with each year or two that menarche is delayed (3,4). Late menopause is another factor associated with increased breast cancer risk. The risk for breast cancer can be decreased by 50% with bilateral oophorectomy before age 40, and it is estimated that women undergoing natural menopause before age 45 have half the risk of developing breast cancer compared with women who undergo menopause after age 55 (6). Breast cancer risk is reduced by 50% if the first-term pregnancy occurs before age 20 compared with after age 35 (2–4,6). Nulliparous women, or those who are obese after menopause, are at increased risk compared with women with children or those who are not obese in their postmenopausal years.

In the 1960s and 1970s, Wolfe was the first to suggest a link between parenchymal patterns on mammography and an increased risk for breast cancer (7–9). Parenchymal pattern descriptors included in the American College of Radiology Breast Imaging Reporting and Data Systems, however, were developed in an attempt to alert clinicians regarding the possible decrease in our ability to detect some cancers in women with "dense" tissue, not as indicators for the risk of breast cancer (14,16,17). The use of these descriptors is subjective with high inter- and intraobserver variability. Additionally, as Kopans (14) points out, it is not possible to accurately measure the percentage of tissue by volume when using two-dimensional mammogram images if exposure values, half-value layers, and compression thickness are not known (e.g., three-dimensional information cannot be obtained accurately using two-dimensional images). In support of this, it is interesting to note that in magnetic resonance imaging (MRI), small amounts of glandular tissue may be seen in some women with seemingly dense tissue mammographically. Additional flaws in these studies include failure to take into account the variability in the positioning of patients for mammograms, the exclusive use of the craniocaudal (CC) projection in some studies, and difficulties in defining the exact extent of the breast and breast tissue (14). It is likely that there is some relationship between the risk for breast cancer and the "density" of the parenchyma on mammography; however, additional studies are needed to further elucidate the exact nature and significance of the relationship.

At this time, other factors reportedly associated with increased breast cancer risk are controversial. These include oral contraceptive use, alcohol intake, exogenous estrogen use (after 10 years of use), breast-feeding, physical activity, and dietary fat intake (saturated fats). In fact, lactation, exercise, and monounsaturated fat intake may have protective benefits. Long-term heavy smoking may be a risk factor, particularly in women who started smoking at an early age (2). Even more controversial risk factors include the use of antiperspirants, bras, induced abortions, and breast implants.

Chemoprevention of breast cancer is controversial and receiving much attention. It may be that drugs such as tamoxifen and raloxifene (selective estrogen receptor modulators [SERMs]) as well as aromatase inhibitors can reduce the risk of developing breast cancer in patients at increased risk. Tamoxifen is approved for use as a breast cancer preventive agent in pre- and postmenopausal women with a significantly increased risk of breast cancer (e.g., patients with atypical ductal hyperplasia or lobular carcinoma in situ). Raloxifene is as effective as tamoxifen in reducing the risk of invasive breast cancer and when compared with tamoxifen, is associated with lower risks of thromboembolic events and cataracts. Tamoxifen is also associated with an increased risk of uterine cancer in women over the age of 50.

SCREENING MAMMOGRAPHY AND SCREENING RECOMMENDATIONS

Mammography is the most studied screening test in medicine, and although there is an abundance of data from randomized controlled trials (RCTs) and service screening studies proving the benefit of screening mammography, the annual use of mammography in women starting at age 40 remains controversial in the minds of some (18,19). The goal of screening mammography is to identify breast cancer as early as possible before it becomes apparent clinically as a lump or with skin changes or distant metastases. But how do we know that mammography can show early breast cancers consistently? And if it can, how do we know that finding these early breast cancers is of any benefit to the patient? The ability of mammography to demonstrate small breast cancers consistently and the benefits of detecting these breast cancers through mammography were established through several RCTs.

Specifically, seven RCTs of screening mammography all of which included women in their 40s have shown a benefit (20–27); two of these were done in North America, one in Scotland, and four in Sweden. Fewer women died of breast cancer among the population invited to screening mammography, compared with the control group of women not invited to undergo screening mammography. The reported benefit ranges from a 20% to 40% reduction in breast cancer mortality among the women invited to screening mammography. Breast cancers are consistently identified through the routine use of screening mammography (20–27). The diagnosis and treatment of women with breast cancers identified through mammography saves lives.

The issue of screening women 40 to 49 years of age has been particularly controversial (28). However, a statistically significant benefit has been reported from several of the RCTs, including the Gothenberg and Malmo trials that reported 44% and 36% reductions in breast cancer mortality, respectively. Also, a statistically significant 26% benefit to screening 40- to 49-year-old women is reported from a meta-analysis (a statistical test that combines data reported from multiple trials) that used data from the seven population-based screening trials (27). In determining appropriate screening intervals, it is important to consider tumor sojourn times. Tumor sojourn time, defined as the time taken for cancers to go from mammographic-preclinical to clinical detectability, is 1.7 years in premenopausal women and 3.3 years in postmenopausal women (29). Screening women in their 40s, therefore, is optimally done at annual intervals.

The Canadian National Breast Screening Study-1 (CNBSS-1) was purportedly aimed at evaluating women in the 40 to 49 age range; however, the flaws in the design and execution of this study are such that the data should not be considered in the same light as those of other RCTs (5,30,31). The two most significant flaws in this study include: (i) The lack of power to show anything less than a 40% decrease in mortality; something that is further impacted by noncompliance (e.g., women in the study group not having screening mammograms) and high contamination (e.g., women assigned to the control group availing themselves of the potential benefits of screening mammography) and

(ii) Randomization methodology. The *blind* randomization of patients into study and control groups is a fundamental requirement of RCTs. For reasons that are unclear, this trial was designed such that a clinical breast examination was done before the randomization of patients into study and control groups. The fact that significantly more women with four or more positive nodes were assigned to the study (mammography) group indicates a serious problem with randomization (32). Additionally, if you consider the over-90% 5-year survival reported for women in the control group, it in essence requires that almost no deaths occur in the study group for a benefit to be shown. As a testament to the fatal randomization issues and resulting imbalances in this trial, the reported 90% 5-year survival in the control group needs to be compared with the 75% 5-year survival in 40- to 49-year-old women in Canada at the time of the study (5). The poor quality of the mammography used for this trial should also be considered. One of the study's reference physicists stated that the quality of the mammography was not state of the art and that it was even below the quality of mammography being practiced in Canada at that time (33).

Using the cumulative data from all of the randomized controlled screening trials, the American Cancer Society (ACS) in March of 1997 (34) issued new screening guidelines recommending annual screening mammography for all women starting at age 40. This was followed by an update in 2003 (35) that recommends mammography starting at age 40, and advocates that women should be told about the benefits and limitations of breast self-examination (BSE), but states that it is acceptable for women to choose not to do BSE or to do BSE irregularly. The ACS recommends an annual physical examination by a health care provider every 3 years for 20- to 33-year-old women and annually starting at age 40. Currently, the ACS also recommends annual screening MRI for women at high risk, including (36): women with a *BRCA* mutation and their untested first-degree relatives, women who have had chest wall radiation between the ages of 10 and 30, women with syndromes (Li-Fraumeni, Cowden, and Bannayan–Riley–Ruvalcaba syndromes) associated with an increased breast cancer risk, and those women with a lifetime risk of greater than 20% to 25% (see Fig. 5.36) as determined by risk models (BRCAPRO, Tyrer-Cuzick) (36).

Although there have been no rigorous trials to evaluate the use and benefit of screening mammography in high-risk women, many radiologists recommend starting screening mammography at age 30 for women in a high-risk category including those with a family history of breast cancer (first-degree relative), particularly if the family member developed premenopausal, bilateral, or multiple breast cancers. In a woman whose mother developed breast cancer before the age of 40, mammographic screening should be started 10 years before the age of detection in the mother. So if the mother developed her breast cancer at age 36, mammographic screening in the daughter should be started at age 26.

In 2009, the US Preventive Services Task Force (USPSTF) issued new guidelines (37) for screening mammography every 2 years in 50- to 74-year-old women; they specifically recommended *not* screening 40- to 49-year-old women or those over the age of 74, and abandoned recommendations for breast self-examination and clinical breast examination (37). The impetus for these recommendations remains unclear since only the Age Trial in England (18), also flawed in design, had been reported since the previous USPSTF guidelines in 2002 (38). Additionally, that computer modeling with rather subjective assumptions would be used to replace the results of RCTs is absurd. The widespread application of these recommendations would be a travesty and likely to reverse the decreases in mortality from breast cancer that have been reported with only 50% of eligible women routinely availing themselves of screening mammography (39). Not only should we be screening women starting at age 40 annually, we should redouble our efforts to encourage more women to avail themselves of this potentially life-saving study starting at age 40; our goal should be 100% compliance with screening recommendations. If there are legitimate issues regarding patient anxiety and false-positive studies, these can be effectively tackled with models such as the ones presented in this book: intense training of radiologists can effectively reduce callback rates to well under 10% and "false-positive biopsies" such that positive predictive values for biopsy recommendations can approximate 50% consistently. Indicated biopsies can be done the day of the recommendation, and if collaborative relationships are established with pathologists and surgeons, pathology results can be obtained within 24 hours of a core biopsy and consultation with a surgeon for definitive treatment can be accomplished within 48 hours of a breast cancer diagnosis. Sadly, it seems to me that the USPSTF is all too willing to throw the baby out with the bathwater in an effort to minimize cost. This is shortsighted and likely to result in the opposite effect. Why are we walking away from the data generated by what in medicine has been the gold standard for establishing proof: the RCTs? RCTs have proven that mammography works starting at age 40, and in the trials as well as in practice, we have seen that its widespread implementation leads to significant decreases in mortality from breast cancer.

Mammography provides the ability to diagnose stage I or II breast cancers and in many patients when it is at the noninvasive, intraductal stage (stage 0) (40,41). The diagnosis of early, potentially curable breast cancer increases available treatment options for patients and probably renders treatment more effective. Regardless of the histological grade (aggressiveness) of a tumor, or the status of the axillary lymph nodes, women with breast cancers that are less than 1 cm in size, have a 12-year survival rate of 95% (20). The goal of screening mammography, therefore, becomes the identification of cancers that are less than 1 cm in size. Inclusion of all breast tissue in the images through optimal mammographic positioning, high contrast, high resolution and well-exposed images, and the interpretive skills of the radiologist, becomes pivotal in our ability to identify cancers that are less than 1 cm in size consistently.

Mammography is not a perfect test. In some women with breast cancer, the cancer is not visible on the mammogram, even under the best of circumstances. The false-negative rates for mammography range from 7% to 15% (40–42). The sensitivity of mammography is known to be decreased particularly in women with dense tissue mammographically (43,44). This is why it is important that women recognize the need for breast self-examination and annual breast examinations by a health care provider. Although there are false-negative mammograms, screening mammography is an effective method for finding early, potentially curable breast cancers and saving lives. It is the best, and currently the only, reliable defense women have against breast cancer.

MAMMOGRAPHY QUALITY STANDARDS ACT

In 1992, following reports describing a wide range of problems with mammography in the United States, Congress passed the Mammography Quality Standards Act (MQSA) to establish quality standards for mammography. The legislation, authorized for 5 years, was signed on December 12, 1993, and reauthorized on October 8, 1998, extending it into 2002. MQSA regulates mammographic modalities defined as technologies for radiography of the breast. Stereotactic biopsies, needle localizations, and ductography are procedures currently exempt from the definition of mammographic modality and not regulated under MQSA; ultrasound, MRI, and nuclear medicine studies are nonradiographic procedures and not regulated under MQSA.

Effective October 1, 1994, all mammography facilities (except those of the Department of Veterans Affairs) must: (i) Get accredited by an approved accrediting body every 3 years; (ii) Get certified by the Secretary of Health and Human Services (HHS) every 3 years; (iii) Undergo annual on-site inspection by Food and Drug Administration (FDA)–trained and certified federal or state inspectors on behalf of HHS.

The current FDA-approved accrediting bodies include the American College of Radiology (ACR) and the States of Arkansas, Iowa, and Texas. The last update of MQSA statistics on the FDA website (www.fda.gov) reports 8,698 certified facilities as of November 1, 2013, with 13,053 accredited units; 7,970 facilities are certified with full field digital mammography (FFDM) units representing 12,100 accredited FFDM units. As of the November 1, 2013, update available on the FDA website, 88% of inspected facilities were in compliance; 0.2% of inspected facilities had level I noncompliance violations requiring immediate action for remedy, reinspection, and sanctions if corrective actions are not taken; 10.8% had level II violations requiring a written response with corrective actions required within 30 days, and 1% had level III violations requiring corrective action before the next inspection. As of October 1, 2007, the inspection fee for facilities is $2,150 for the first unit and $250 for each additional unit. The fee for facilities requiring reinspection is $1,140.

Final MQSA regulations are in effect as of April 28, 1999. The *Federal Register* publication of October 28, 1997 (45) provides the final regulations. This law regulates mammographic facilities, including initial and continuing qualification standards for interpreting physicians, radiologic technologists, medical physicists, and mammography facility inspectors. The law spells out quality standards for mammographic equipment and practices, what is needed for the quality assurance (QA)/quality control (QC) program, record keeping, mammography reports, as well as patient and referring physician notification. Familiarity with the details is recommended, particularly for those designated as the lead interpreting physician (please refer to the Federal Register publication for all the nuances of the law—beyond the scope of this book).

AMERICAN COLLEGE OF RADIOLOGY MAMMOGRAPHY ACCREDITATION PROGRAM

Since the late 1980s, the ACR has taken a leadership role in addressing mammographic image quality. The Mammography Accreditation Program (MAP) developed by the ACR is now the oldest and largest accreditation program in the United States. The MAP program accredits units (FDA certifies facilities) every 3 years. For accreditation facilities, submit: (i) Completed form providing information on equipment, personnel qualifications, and test image data; (ii) Phantom image for image quality and dose evaluations, using an approved phantom and thermoluminescent dosimeter; (iii) Two normal mammograms (fatty and dense breasts); (iv) Processor quality control for a 30-day period; and (v) Fee (initial cycle and renewal $1,475 for first unit and $1,300 for each additional unit) (46).

Facilities are also required to provide the ACR with an annual update. This update includes QC documentation, the medical physicist's annual survey for each unit, and an application data update (e.g., changes in personnel). Under MQSA, the ACR is required to perform on-site surveys of at least 5% of the facilities it accredits; 50% of these are selected randomly and the others based on problems identified through FDA inspections, serious consumer complaints, or history of noncompliance. A medical physicist, radiologist, and an ACR staff person make up the survey team. Additionally, at least 3% of accredited facilities are randomly selected to undergo a random clinical image review (46).

The ACR has subsequently developed accreditation programs for stereotactic breast biopsy, diagnostic breast ultrasound,

ultrasound-guided breast biopsy, and breast MRI. The ACR now also provides a "Breast Imaging Center of Excellence designation" to those facilities that are ACR-accredited in mammography, stereotactic breast biopsies, breast ultrasound, ultrasound-guided biopsy, and breast MRI. The readers are strongly encouraged to familiarize themselves with these programs by contacting the ACR or visiting their website (www.ACR.org).

TREATMENT OPTIONS

The treatment of breast cancer usually entails a combination of surgery, radiation therapy, and chemotherapy. Surgical options include mastectomy or lumpectomy. With the exception of some patients with localized DCIS, sampling of the axillary lymph nodes with a sentinel lymph node (SLN) biopsy or axillary lymph node dissection (ALND) is done at the time of the patient's definitive surgery. Immediate or delayed reconstruction with an implant or autologous tissue transplantation is always an option that should be discussed with patients undergoing mastectomy; in these patients, reduction of the contralateral breast may also be appropriate.

Needless to say, mastectomy is always an option for patients; however, depending on the size of the lesion relative to the size of the breast, lumpectomy and radiation therapy (see below) are as effective as mastectomy in treating most patients with localized breast cancer. The goal of lumpectomy is to remove the entire tumor so there is little, if any, cancer left in the breast with, ideally, a cosmetic result that is acceptable to the patient. The margins of the lumpectomy specimen are evaluated histologically, and if disease extends to the margins, re-excision of the tumor bed is usually done as a separate surgical procedure. The goal of re-excision is to get negative margins. If the margins are grossly positive after re-excision, the patient may not be a good candidate for conservative therapy and mastectomy may be more appropriate. The increasing use of breast MRI to delineate the extent of disease at the time of diagnosis may facilitate preoperative surgical decisions since it can help distinguish patients with extensive or multifocal disease needing mastectomy from those with localized lesions who are more amenable to lumpectomy.

Historically, patients with invasive breast cancer had full ALNDs involving the excision of multiple (but a variable number) lymph nodes from the axilla. Complications associated with ALND include lymphedema, arm and shoulder numbness, paresthesias involving the arm and shoulder, loss of range of motion at the shoulder, and the formation of fluid pockets (seromas, hematomas) in the axilla. Many surgeons have adopted SLN biopsies to initially stage patients with clinically node-negative breast cancer. The limited dissections needed for SLN biopsies have minimized the complications associated with ALND and, as such, have made a significant contribution to patient care and overall quality of life for patients.

The concept of the SLN biopsy is fairly simple and first developed in the evaluation of patients with melanoma. If the lymphatic drainage from the breast to the axilla proceeds in an orderly, stepwise manner, one or two lymph nodes in the axilla should receive the lymphatic drainage from the breast first and consistently. If these lymph nodes can be identified reliably, and if they reflect the overall status of the axillary lymph nodes accurately, axillary dissections can be limited to the removal of the SLNs. To identify the SLN, a vital blue dye, technetium-labeled sulfur colloid particles, or both are injected subcutaneously, peri-tumoral or peri-areolar. Visual inspection of the axilla by the surgeon for collection of vital blue dye, or radioactivity detected with a handheld gamma probe, is used to identify one, two, and sometimes three nodes considered the SLN(s) (47–50). The use of both methods increases the likelihood of identifying the SLN in up to 90% of patients with an overall accuracy of 98.2% and a false-negative rate of 5.8% (51). In those patients in whom the SLNs cannot be mapped an ALND is done.

The use of SLN biopsy is indicated in patients with T1- and T2-sized tumors, multicentric disease, DCIS when mastectomy is planned, in older and obese patients and in men with breast cancer. Although not always done, efforts can be made to assess (imprint or touch prep, cytology of cells scraped from the cut surface of node, or frozen section) the sampled lymph node at the time of surgery: if metastatic disease is identified with the patient still in the operating room, the surgeon can do the ALND. If the touch prep is not done at the time of surgery, or if it is interpreted as negative, and metastatic disease is identified on the permanent hematoxylin and eosin (H & E) stained slides of the SLN, the patient is scheduled for a completion ALND since approximately 43% of these patients are found to have additional node disease on the ALND (52).

The significance of isolated tumor cells (ITC) and micrometastases (>0.2 mm but not >2 mm) in axillary lymph nodes remains unclear. Reportedly, metastases are identified in non-sentinel lymph nodes in 10% of patients with ITCs and in 20% to 35% of patients with micrometastatic disease in the SLN (52). Currently, the American Society of Clinical Oncology (ASCO) recommends ALND in patients with micrometastases in the SLN regardless of the method of detection (52).

Patients with large or locally advanced invasive breast cancers, inflammatory carcinoma, or in whom axillary disease is suspected clinically, are not considered good candidates for SLN biopsy and, as such, undergo ALND. In pregnant patients, SLN biopsies are done using the technetium labeled sulfur colloid but not the blue dye. In patients with prior breast surgery and invasive disease, SLN biopsy is attempted, however, if the nodes do not map an ALND is indicated. Several major questions remain unanswered with respect to sentinel node biopsies in women with breast cancer. These include: (i) Which patients with positive SLN biopsies can be treated with breast or axillary radiation, and which patients need completion ALND; (ii) The clinical significance of negative SLN biopsy after neoadjuvant therapy; and (iii) What is the clinical significance of ITCs, and do these patients need an ALND? (52).

Radiation therapy for local control is usually recommended following lumpectomy. In a small number of patients, radiation therapy to the chest wall or axilla is also recommended following mastectomy to reduce the likelihood of chest wall or axillary recurrence. Whole breast irradiation is usually started 2 to 5 weeks after the lumpectomy and is given 5 days a week for 6 weeks (40 to 50 Gy). On the basis of the size of the tumor, patient age, disease-free surgical margins, and in those with negative axillary lymph nodes, accelerated partial breast irradiation (APBI) may be recommended in some patients. This entails high doses of radiation localized to the lumpectomy site commonly given over a 5-day period. APBI methods under investigation include: (i) Intracavitary brachytherapy using an inflatable balloon catheter placed in the lumpectomy bed intraoperatively or percutaneously after the lumpectomy; (ii) Interstitial brachytherapy using multiple afterloading catheters placed around the lumpectomy bed and (iii) Intraoperative radiation therapy.

In thinking about chemotherapy consider three major groups of patients: (i) Those with hormone receptor–positive cancers who can be managed with receptor targeted therapy ± chemotherapy (see discussion on Oncotype); (ii) Those with HER2/neu positive tumors in whom trastuzumab (and Lapatinib approved for patients with HER2/neu positive metastatic disease) can be used in conjunction with chemotherapy; and (iii) Those with estrogen (ER) negative, progesterone (PR) negative, HER2/neu negative tumors (triple negative tumors; TNT) in whom chemotherapy is the only systemic treatment available.

Chemotherapy is usually recommended if there is metastatic disease to the axillary lymph nodes or in patients with distant metastases. In patients with node-negative estrogen receptor–positive tumors, the use of the Oncotype DX assay reportedly provides prognostic information with respect to the likelihood of recurrence and response to chemotherapy (CMF = cyclophosphamide, methotrexate, and fluorouracil) (53). Oncotype DX is a reverse transcriptase/polymerase chain reaction assay based on the analysis of a 21-gene panel. It is used to calculate a recurrence score (RS) of 0 to 100. Patients with a low RS (RS < 18) have indolent tumors that are sensitive to hormonal therapy, and chemotherapy adds little, if any, benefit (53). Patients with a high RS (RS ≥ 31) have aggressive tumors less likely to respond to hormone therapy, and benefit significantly from adjuvant therapy with a decrease in the recurrence rate at 10 years of 27.6% (53). In patients with an intermediate recurrence score (RS ≥18 to 30), it is unclear whether the benefits of chemotherapy exceed the risks (53).

Neoadjuvant therapy is recommended in patients with larger sized tumors, locally advanced breast cancer, or inflammatory carcinoma and is being increasingly used in women with larger lesions in whom lumpectomy may become an option after therapy. Depending on the response of the tumor, neoadjuvant therapy can be followed by mastectomy or, in selected patients, lumpectomy. Radiation therapy and additional chemotherapy may be recommended in these patients after their definitive surgery.

The 5-year relative survival rate for women diagnosed with lymph node–negative invasive lesions is 98%; survival rates decrease to 84% and 24% in patients with metastatic disease to regional lymph nodes and those with distant metastatic disease, respectively. For all breast cancer stages combined, relative survival rates at 10 and 15 years are 83% and 77%, respectively. Five-year relative survival rates for invasive lesions have improved from 75% in the mid-70s to 90% in 2014 (2).

BREAST CANCER STAGING

Women diagnosed with breast cancer are staged based on the size of the tumor (T), the presence or absence of regional lymph node (N) involvement, and the presence or absence of cancer cells at sites distant (M) to the breast. This system is referred to as the TNM system (54). Numbers are assigned to each of these letters to define the characteristics of the cancer found in an individual patient.

Clinical staging (cTNM) is based on information obtained from the clinical evaluation of patients, including a complete physical examination, imaging (except lymphoscintigraphy), biopsy, and surgical exploration before any treatment is given (see Tables 1.1 and 1.2). Pathological staging (pTNM) is based on information from the clinical evaluation and complete removal and evaluation of the primary tumor and regional lymph nodes (see Table 1.3) following surgery but before any treatment is given (20). After each one of these three components (TNM) is classified (see Table 1.4 for classification of "M"), the patient is assigned into one of several stages (see Table 1.5). Recommendations for treatment, and the overall prognosis of a patient, vary depending on the stage of the breast cancer at the time of diagnosis. Post-neoadjuvant therapy TNM findings are designated by the prefix "yc" if clinical (ycTNM) or "yp" if pathological (ypTNM). Currently, no stage is provided for patients who have a complete pathological response following neoadjuvant therapy (ypT0ypN0cM0).

Axillary, internal mammary, and supraclavicular lymph nodes on the side (ipsilateral) of the primary tumor are considered regional lymph nodes in patients with breast cancer. Level I (low axilla) axillary lymph nodes are defined as those lateral to the lateral margin of the pectoralis minor muscle. Level II (mid axilla) axillary lymph nodes are those found between the medial and lateral borders of the pectoralis minor muscle; this includes interpectoral nodes (e.g., Rotter lymph nodes). Level III (apical axilla) axillary lymph nodes are those found medial to the medial margin of the pectoralis minor muscle and

Table 1.1 PRIMARY TUMOR (T) CLASSIFICATION

TX	Primary tumor cannot be assessed
T0	No evidence of primary tumor
Tis	Carcinoma in situ
Tis (DCIS)	
Tis (LCIS)	
Tis (Paget)	Only if NOT associated with DCIS or invasive disease in the breast
T1	Tumor ≤2 cm
T1mi	Tumor ≤0.1 cm
T1a	Tumor >0.1 cm but ≤0.5 cm
T1b	Tumor >0.5 cm but ≤1 cm
T1c	Tumor >1 cm but ≤2 cm
T2	Tumor >2 cm but ≤5 cm
T3	Tumor >5 cm
T4	Tumor of any size extending to chest wall or skin
T4a	Tumor extends to chest wall not including pectoralis muscle
T4b	Edema, ulceration of the skin, or satellite skin nodules confined to same breast
T4c	Both T4a and T4b
T4d	Inflammatory carcinoma

Modified from American Joint Committee on Cancer. *Cancer Staging Manual*. 7th ed. New York, NY: Springer; 2010.

inferior to the clavicle (aka apical or infraclavicular nodes). For the purposes of classification and staging, intramammary lymph nodes are considered axillary lymph nodes. If metastatic disease is identified in cervical, contralateral axillary, or internal mammary lymph nodes, it is considered distant disease (M1).

SLN biopsy (up to six lymph nodes), or ALND, if the SLN is positive, is almost always done in women with invasive breast cancer to stage the cancer pathologically. SLN biopsy or ALND is not usually done in patients with localized DCIS (<2 cm); however, it is considered in: (i) Patients with more extensive DCIS (particularly if high grade) in whom microinvasive disease may go undetected or (ii) Patients with DCIS who are having a mastectomy. SLN biopsies cannot be done after a mastectomy, so if the patient is diagnosed with invasive disease after the mastectomy specimen is evaluated, she would need to have a full ALND done. Internal mammary lymph nodes are not usually sampled because they are difficult to access without extensive surgery; however, our ability to assess internal mammary lymph nodes is improved when breast MRI is used to evaluate newly diagnosed breast cancer patients. Ultrasound-guided fine needle aspiration can be done in some patients with MRI, or chest CT, detected internal mammary adenopathy (see Fig. 12.19).

Changes to the TNM classification system for breast cancer have been incorporated in the seventh edition (54) of the American Joint Commission on Cancer (AJCC) Staging Manual. (The reader is encouraged to consult and review this manual for details beyond the scope of this book.)

Traditionally, the TNM staging system described in combination with the histological features of a tumor and assessment of the tumor for expression of ER, PR and epidermal growth factor receptors (HER2/neu) are used to establish management

Table 1.2 **CLINICAL REGIONAL LYMPH NODE (N) CLASSIFICATION**

NX	Regional lymph nodes (LNs) cannot be assessed (previously removed)
N0	No metastases to the regional LNs
N1	Metastases to movable ipsilateral level I, II axillary LNs
N2	Metastases to ipsilateral level I, II axillary LNs fixed or matted or in clinically (includes imaging other than lymphoscintigraphy) apparent ipsilateral internal mammary nodes in the absence of clinically evident axillary LN mets
N2a	Metastases to ipsilateral level I, II axillary lymph nodes fixed to one another or to other structures
N2b	Metastases only in clinically detected (includes imaging other than lymphoscintigraphy) ipsilateral internal mammary nodes and in the absence of clinically evident axillary lymph node metastasis
N3	Metastases in ipsilateral infraclavicular (level III) LNs with or without level I, II axillary LN involvement or metastases to clinically detected ipsilateral internal mammary lymph nodes with clinically evident level I, II axillary lymph node metastases, or metastases to ipsilateral supraclavicular LNs with or without axillary LN involvement or internal mammary LN involvement
N3a	Metastases in ipsilateral infraclavicular LNs
N3b	Metastases in ipsilateral internal mammary LNs and axillary LNs
N3c	Metastases in ipsilateral supraclavicular LNs

Modified from American Joint Committee on Cancer. *Cancer Staging Manual*. 7th ed. New York, NY: Springer; 2010.

Table 1.3 **PATHOLOGICAL LYMPH NODE (N) CLASSIFICATION**

pNx	Regional LN cannot be assessed
pN0	No regional LN metastases histologically, no study for (ITC)
pN0(i−)	No regional LN metastases histologically, negative immunohistochemical (IHC)
pN0(i+)	Malignant cells in regional LNs (detected by H&E or IHC including ITC)
pN0(mol−)	No regional LN metastases histologically, negative molecular findings (RT-PCR)
pN0(mol+)	Positive molecular findings (RT-PCR) but no regional lymph node metastases detected histologically or with IHC
pN1	Micrometastases or metastases in 1–3 LNs, and/or internal mammary LNs with microscopic disease detected by sentinel LN dissection but not clinically apparent
pN1mi	Micrometastases (>0.2 mm and/or more than 200 cells but none >2.0 mm)
pN1a	Metastases in 1–3 axillary LNs; at least one metastasis >2 mm
pN1b	Metastases in internal mammary LN with micro or macrometastases detected by sentinel LN biopsy but not clinically apparent
pN1c	Metastases in 1–3 axillary LNs and internal mammary LNs with micro or macrometastases detected by sentinel LN biopsy but not clinically apparent
pN2	Metastases in 4–9 axillary LNs or in clinically detected internal mammary LNs in the absence of axillary LN metastases
pN2a	Metastases in 4–9 axillary LNs (at least one tumor deposit >2 mm)
pN2b	Metastases in clinically detected internal mammary LNs in the absence of axillary LNs
pN3	Metastases in 10 or more axillary LNs or in infraclavicular (level III axillary) LNs or in clinically detected ipsilateral internal mammary LNs in the presence of one or more positive level I, II axillary LNs or in more than three axillary LNs and in internal mammary LNs with micro or macrometastases detected by sentinel lymph node biopsy but not clinically detected or in ipsilateral supraclavicular LNs
pN3a	Metastases in 10 or more axillary LNs (at least one tumor deposit >2 mm) or metastasis to infraclavicular (level III axillary) LNs
pN3b	Metastases in clinically detected ipsilateral internal mammary LNs in the presence of one or more positive axillary LNs or in more than 3 axillary LNs and in internal mammary LNs with micro or macrometastases detected by sentinel lymph node biopsy but not clinically apparent
pN3c	Metastases in ipsilateral supraclavicular LNs

Classification based on sentinel lymph node biopsy only is designated as "sn," for example, pN0(sn).
IHC, immunohistochemical; ITC, isolated tumor cells (clusters of cells not >0.2 mm or single tumor cells or a cluster of fewer than 200 cells in a single histologic cross section); RT-PCR, reverse transcriptase/polymerase chain reaction.
Modified from American Joint Committee on Cancer. *Cancer Staging Manual*. 7th ed. New York, NY: Springer; 2010.

Table 1.4	DISTANT (M) METASTASIS
MX	Distant metastases cannot be assessed
M0	No clinical or radiographic evidence of distant metastases
cM0(i+)	No clinical or radiographic evidence of distant metastases, but deposits of molecularly or microscopically detected tumor cells in circulating blood, bone marrow, or other non-regional nodal tissues that are larger than 0.2 mm in a patient without symptoms or signs of metastases
M1	Distant detectable metastases as determined by classic clinical and radiographic means and/or histologically proven larger than 0.2 mm

Modified from American Joint Committee on Cancer. *Cancer Staging Manual*. 7th ed. New York, NY: Springer; 2010.

Table 1.5	BREAST CANCER STAGING		
Stage 0	Tis	N0	M0
Stage IA	T1	N0	M0
Stage IB	T0	N1mi	M0
	T1	N1mi	M0
Stage IIA	T0	N1	M0
	T1	N1	M0
	T2	N0	M0
Stage IIB	T2	N1	M0
	T3	N0	M0
Stage IIIA	T0	N2	M0
	T1	N2	M0
	T2	N2	M0
	T3	N1	M0
	T3	N2	M0
Stage IIIB	T4	N0	M0
	T4	N1	M0
	T4	N2	M0
Stage IIIC	Any T	N3	M0
Stage IV	Any T	Any N	M1

Modified from American Joint Committee on Cancer. *Cancer Staging Manual*. 7th ed. New York, NY: Springer; 2010.

recommendations and prognosis for individual patients. Less commonly used tests to evaluate tumors include p53, tumor ploidy, S-phase, and Ki67 as a marker of cellular proliferation. In general, tumors expressing estrogen receptors may respond to treatment with estrogen receptor modulators (e.g., tamoxifen raloxifene) or aromatase inhibitors and usually have a better prognosis. Tumors that are ER, PR, and HER2/neu receptor negative have higher and quicker recurrence and mortality rates compared with tumors that have ER and PR receptors (3,4,6). Overexpression of *erbB-2* (HER2/neu) is associated with a poor prognosis (3,4,6); however, targeted therapy with trastuzumab is available and effective.

The use of genetic profiling (55–57) has led to the classification of breast cancers into five major biologically distinct profiles that may be of prognostic significance (58): (i) Luminal A, (ii) Luminal B, (iii) HER2/neu positive, (iv) Basal-like, and (v) Normal-like tumors. Given the heterogeneity of breast cancer, it is not surprising that the idea of "one treatment fits all" is far from optimal. Although not currently in use clinically, the ability to genetically profile tumors portends the future direction of breast cancer treatment: the use of targeted therapy to maximize the effectiveness while minimizing (or eliminating) the side effects in patients not likely to respond. In fact, the use of Oncotype DX to establish recurrence scores in patients with node-negative, ER-positive tumors described previously is an effort to target therapy more appropriately. The use of several biomarkers (described below) may be useful in approximating the molecular subtype of breast cancers.

Luminal A tumors are typically ER positive and/or PR positive, HER2 negative and have a low Ki67 (<14%). These are usually lower histological grade tumors with lower proliferation-related genes. Luminal A tumors typically have a good prognosis, respond well to endocrine therapy, are characterized by low recurrence scores on the Oncotype DX assay, and are associated with significantly lower local and regional relapses (59).

Luminal B tumors can be subdivided into: (i) Patients with ER positive and/or PR positive, HER2 negative, and high Ki67 (>14%) tumors or (ii) Those with ER positive and/or PR positive and HER2/neu positive, also called the luminal-HER2 group. Although luminal B tumors are often ER positive, they usually have lower levels of ER expression, may be PR negative, and 30% express HER2/neu. Histologically, they are higher in grade and associated with a higher expression of proliferation-related genes such that Ki67 may be useful in distinguishing these from luminal A tumors. Clinically, these tumors are often more aggressive with a worse prognosis and likely to be lymph node positive. Luminal B tumors may be less responsive to tamoxifen, but are more likely to respond to chemotherapy when added to the endocrine treatment; patients with HER2 positive tumors benefit from targeted therapy with trastuzumab comparable to that seen in patients with HER2 positive/ER negative tumors. Luminal B tumors typically have a high recurrence score on the Oncotype DX assay.

The HER2 tumors are ER negative, PR negative, and HER2/neu positive. They are more likely to have p53 mutations, higher histologic grade, and patients are likely to be of younger age at presentation. They are characterized by an aggressive clinical course and have an overall poor prognosis. These types of tumors are more likely to respond to anthracyclines and in general have a good response to trastuzumab therapy in combination with chemotherapy; complete pathological response is seen following neoadjuvant and trastuzumab therapy.

The basal-like profile is characterized by ER negative, PR negative, and HER2/neu negative tumors. The neoplastic cells in basal-like tumors express genes typically found in normal basal/myoepithelial cells, including the cytokeratins (CK) associated with basal cells: CK5/6, CK14, and CK17, and they are also commonly positive for the epidermal growth factor receptor (EGFR) (60,61). The basal-like profile is found in approximately 15% of breast cancers and is identified more commonly in younger patients (62,63). They are characterized by an aggressive clinical course and poor prognosis with an increased likelihood of early systemic recurrence. Histologically, these are high-grade tumors with a high mitotic index, central areas of necrosis, pushing margins, and a surrounding lymphocytic infiltrate. Metaplastic elements and medullary features are common. The metastatic pattern of these tumors tends to be hematogenous with metastatic deposits in the brain and lungs and less commonly involves axillary lymph nodes and bone (63). The tumors in patients with *BRCA1* mutations are often basal-like (62,63). Compared with luminal tumors, basal-like tumors are more sensitive to anthracyclines and taxanes, and complete pathological response is seen in patients undergoing neoadjuvant therapy.

Currently, not much is known about the normal-like profile, but it clusters with the HER2 positive and basal-like tumors; however, they seem to have a better prognosis than basal-like lesions, may not respond well to neoadjuvant therapy, may have a higher association with hormone replacement therapy, and represent approximately 10% of all breast cancers (62). Although the basal-like profile is characterized by tumors that are ER negative, PR negative, and HER2/neu negative and there is much overlap with TNTs, the basal-like profile and TNT are not synonymous (62,63). Triple negative tumors are also identified more commonly as interval cancers in younger patients and in African American women (62,63), but these are heterogeneous tumors that, in addition to lesions with a basal-like profile, also include normal-like lesions. Reportedly, 56% to 84% of TNTs express basal CKs and EGFR. Triple negative tumors with a basal-like profile have a shorter disease-free survival compared with TNTs that do not have the basal-like markers (62,63). Ongoing research may one day permit the genetic profiling of each individual patient's tumor so that therapy can be individualized to increase effectiveness and minimize side effects.

CONSIDERATIONS WHEN REVIEWING PATIENT IMAGES IN BREAST IMAGING

As an introduction to the remainder of the textbook, consider the following suggestions when reviewing patient images in breast imaging. As you are going through the book and after completing it, you may want to refer back to these suggestions.

- When presented with images on a patient for discussion, consider demographic information, relevant clinical issues, and pertinent imaging findings in formulating a logical and reasonable list of diagnostic considerations. This, in conjunction with an understanding of the manifestations of breast diseases, facilitates narrowing the considerations to one or two most likely etiologies. By adopting a logical approach, and recognizing that "common things are common," justifiable management decisions can be made routinely (and if not, one is usually dealing with an obscure entity that in practice would not be a primary consideration anyway).
- A well-developed, complete, and logical patient ("case") discussion is an art to be mastered. Although getting the "right" answer is often the focus, this is not what counts. The ability to make observations, integrate relevant information in the formulation of appropriate diagnostic considerations, and the approach taken in sorting through the differential is what, in the long run, serves patients and referring physicians.
- Armed with common sense, the best approach in mastering the art of patient discussions is involvement. Review as many images as possible, and discuss patient images whenever there is an opportunity. Unfortunately, the tendency is to take the path of least resistance and make learning a passive experience. Conferences are given priority over active involvement in patient care, and didactic conferences are requested over patient discussion conferences. There seems to be a widely held belief that becoming a good radiologist can be accomplished by passive (non)-participation at conferences and in the daily activities of a section. Reading has taken a secondary role. I urge you to get involved with patient care directly, review as many images as possible, and depend on yourself for teaching by reading critically.
- Develop a systematic approach to reviewing mammographic images.
- Evaluate technique.
  - Is the tissue well exposed?
  - Are the images high-contrast images?
  - Is there blurring? (Specifically look for blurring; otherwise, you will not perceive subtle blurring. Remember that blurring does not always involve the image diffusely; it can be focal.)
  - Are there any artifacts that could interfere with interpretation?
  - Are the films labeled appropriately?
- Evaluate positioning on the mediolateral oblique (MLO) views.
  - Is pectoral muscle thick in the axilla and seen to the level of the nipple?
  - Is the anterior margin of the pectoral muscle convex?
  - Is the breast lifted up and pulled out?
  - Is the inframammary fold open, and is there a small amount of upper abdomen on the image?
  - Is there tissue at the edge of the film inferiorly (between the pectoral muscle and the inframammary fold), suggesting exclusion of posterior tissue from the image?
  - Is there a possibility that tissue, or a lesion, has been excluded from the image?
- Evaluate positioning on the CC views.
  - Is pectoral muscle imaged?
  - If pectoral muscle is not imaged, is cleavage seen?
  - If neither pectoral muscle nor cleavage is imaged, did you measure the posterior nipple line (PNL)?
  - Is there lateral tissue extending to the edge of the film? Should an exaggerated CC (XCCL) view be done?
  - Is there a possibility that tissue, or a lesion, has been excluded from the image?
- With right and left MLO images back to back, evaluate the
  - Upper third of the breasts
  - Middle third of the breasts
  - Lower third of the breasts
  - Usually fatty stripe between pectoral muscle and glandular tissue
  - Uppermost cone of tissue
  - Fat-glandular interfaces
  - Retroareolar area
  - Inframammary fold area
- With right and left CC views back to back, evaluate the
  - Outer third of the breasts
  - Middle third of the breasts
  - Medial third (usually fatty) of the breasts
  - Retroglandular fat and fat-glandular interfaces
  - Subareolar area
- If there is a possible abnormality, undertake additional evaluation before making recommendations or drawing significant conclusions (do whatever it takes to resolve the clinical or mammographic issue).
  - Previous films for comparisons
  - Spot compression views
  - Micro-focus spot compression magnification views
  - Spot tangential views
  - Spot rolled or change-of-angle views
  - Cleavage views
  - 90-degree lateral views: mediolateral (ML) to evaluate medial lesions or lateromedial (LM) to evaluate lateral lesions
  - Correlative physical examination
  - Breast ultrasound
  - Ductography (in patients with spontaneous nipple discharge regardless of character)
  - Cyst aspiration (and possibly pneumocystography)
  - Fine needle aspiration (FNA)
  - Imaging guided needle biopsy
- Before undertaking additional evaluation or recommending any interventional procedure on patients, procure and review prior studies.
- If there is something obvious clinically, or on the images, look away and review remaining tissue before returning to consider obvious findings (otherwise, you may miss additional more subtle lesions).

- If there is nothing obvious, start talking and
  - Systematically go through the images
  - Send your eyes out, and specifically look for microcalcifications, masses, architectural distortion, diffuse changes, and adenopathy
  - In going through the images aloud the abnormality usually becomes apparent
- Learn your blind spots.
  - Areas where you have missed significant findings in the past
- When discussing patients, structure the discussion and progress through the four Ds.
  - *Detection*: Review films systematically, request or inquire about prior studies
  - *Description*: Describe the abnormality, providing relevant positive and negative findings
  - *Differential* diagnosis: On the basis of the description of the finding(s), construct a logical differential in order of likelihood. Start with possible benign lesions, and progress into possible malignant lesions. Try not to go back and forth between benign and malignant lesions, and don't start by saying, "I don't think this is . . . ." Don't discuss what the lesions are not likely to be, but, rather, what are reasonable benign and malignant considerations.
  - *Diagnosis*: End the discussion by suggesting what you think the most likely diagnosis is on the basis of the integration of patient demographics, relevant history, described features of the lesion, and your differential considerations.
- In formulating a differential, consider
  - Gender—don't assume all patients are women
  - Age (i.e., fibroadenomas are unlikely to develop in a 70-year-old woman; mucinous carcinomas are more common in older women.)
  - Type of study: screening or diagnostic (i.e., asymptomatic or symptomatic patient; are there any radiopaque markers or metallic markers on the films and their significance?)
  - Prior studies
  - Medications (estrogen replacement therapy, tamoxifen, chemotherapy)
  - Relevant history: medical and surgical
- If you don't know something, be willing to admit it—don't try to talk yourself out of situations.
- Think critically and be succinct with descriptions—verbosity accomplishes little, obscures the message, and often reflects sloppy, imprecise thinking.
- Be precise with terminology.
  - "There is a large mass . . ."—how is "large" defined? One person's definition of "large" may be someone's definition of "small." Give specific measurements for the lesion.
  - "There appears to be a mass . . ."—what does "appears" mean? Is there a mass or not? Make up your mind, and don't be afraid to call "a spade a spade."
  - "There is fatty replacement . . ."—how do you know that anything has been replaced? You need to have prior films available to state that something has been replaced.
  - Know the ACR's BI-RADS lexicon, and learn how to use it. How is "mass" defined? What information should you provide relative to masses? Relative to calcifications? How are focal and global parenchymal asymmetry defined?
  - Think critically about what you say: "the upper outer right breast"—how many breasts are there? Is there also an upper inner right breast? Should it not be the upper outer quadrant of the right breast?
- Don't just memorize a list of possible lesions—know the different disease processes, and learn how to sort through them on the basis of patient demographics, presentation, and imaging findings.
- Know the limitations of the studies under review and how to overcome them. On screening studies, be careful with characterization. Obtain additional mammographic images, ultrasound, ductography, or needle biopsies for characterization.
- Know what biopsy results need to be discussed with the pathologist directly and under what circumstances the patient should undergo repeat biopsy.

References

1. Siegel R, Ma J, Zou Z, et al. Cancer Statistics, 2014. *CA Cancer J Clin.* 2014;64:9–29.
2. American Cancer Society. *Cancer Facts and Figures 2014.* Atlanta, GA: American Cancer Society; 2014.
3. Bland KI, Copeland EM, eds. *The Breast.* 4th ed. Philadelphia, PA: WB Saunders; 2009.
4. Roses DF. *Breast Cancer.* 2nd ed. Philadelphia, PA: Elsevier Churchill Livingstone; 2005.
5. Kopans DB. The 2009 U.S. preventive services task force guidelines ignore important scientific evidence and should be revised or withdrawn. *Radiology.* 2010;256:15–20.
6. Harris JR, Lippman ME, Morrow M, et al. *Diseases of the Breast.* 4th ed. Philadelphia, PA: Lippincott Williams & Wilkins; 2009.
7. Wolfe JN. A study of breast parenchyma by mammography in the normal woman and those with benign and malignant disease of the breast. *Radiology.* 1967;89:201–205.
8. Wolfe JN. Breast parenchymal patterns: prevalent and incident cancers. *Radiology.* 1979;131:267–268.
9. Wolfe JN. Breast patterns as an index of risk for developing breast cancer. *AJR Am J Roentgenol.* 1976;126:1130–1139.
10. Janzon L, Andersson I, Petersson H. Mammographic patterns as indicators of risk of breast cancer. *Radiology.* 1982;43:417–419.
11. Tabar L, Dean PB. Mammographic parenchymal patterns: risk indicator for breast cancer? *JAMA.* 1982;247:185–189.
12. Harvey JA, Bovbjerg VE. Quantitative assessment of mammographic breast density: relationship with breast cancer risk. *Radiology.* 2004;230:29–41.
13. Boyd NF, Lockwood GA, Byng JW, et al. Mammographic density and the risk and detection of breast cancer. *N Engl J Med.* 2007;356:227–236.
14. Kopans DB. Basic physics and doubts about relationship between mammographically determined tissue density and breast cancer risk. *Radiology.* 2008;246:348–353.
15. Rosen PP. *Rosen's Breast Pathology.* 3rd ed. Philadelphia, PA: Lippincott Williams & Wilkins; 2008.
16. D'Orsi CJ, Bassett LW, Berg WA, et al. BI-RADS: mammography. In: D'Orsi CJ, Mendelson EB, Ikeda DM, et al, eds. *Breast Imaging Reporting and Data System: ACR BI-RADS®—Breast Imaging Atlas.* Reston, VA: American College of Radiology; 2003.
17. Sickles EA. Wolfe mammographic parenchymal patterns and breast cancer risk. *AJR Am J Roentgenol.* 2007;188:301–303.
18. Moss SM, Cuckle H, Evans A, et al. Effect of mammographic screening from age 40 on breast cancer mortality at 10 years' follow up: a randomized controlled trial. *Lancet.* 2006;368:2053–2060.
19. Petitti DB, Calonge N, LeFevre ML, et al. Breast cancer screening: from science to recommendation. *Radiology.* 2010;256:8–14.
20. Tabár L, Fagerberg G, Duffy SW, et al. Update of the Swedish two-county program of mammographic screening for breast cancer. *Radiol Clin North Am.* 1992;30:187–210.
21. Elwood JM, Cox B, Richardson AK. The effectiveness of breast cancer screening by mammography in younger women. *Online J Curr Clin Trials (serial on line).* February 1993:Doc No 32.
22. Kerlikowske K, Grady D, Rubin SM, et al. Efficacy of screening mammography: a meta-analysis. *JAMA.* 1995;273:149–154.
23. Feig S. Determination of mammographic screening intervals with surrogate measures for women aged 40–49 years. *Radiology.* 1994;193:311–314.
24. Shapiro S. Screening: assessment of current studies. *Cancer.* 1994;74:231–238.

25. Tabár L, Vitak B, Chen HH, et al. Beyond randomized controlled trials: organized mammographic screenings substantially reduces breast carcinoma mortality. *Cancer* 2001;91:1724–1731.
26. Duffy SW, Tabár L, Chen HH, et al. The impact of organized mammography service screening on breast carcinoma mortality in seven Swedish counties. *Cancer*. 2002;95:458–469.
27. Hendrick RE, Smith RA, Rutledge JH, et al. Benefit of screening mammography in women aged 40–49: a new meta-analysis of randomized controlled trials. *J Natl Cancer Inst Monogr*. 1997;(22):87–92.
28. *Report of the Consensus Development Conference Panel on Breast Cancer Screening for Women Aged 40–49, January 21–23, 1997*. Bethesda, MD: National Institute of Health, 1997.
29. Tabár L, Fagerberg G, Day NE, et al. Breast cancer treatment and natural history: new insights from result of screening. *Lancet*. 1992;1:412–414.
30. Miller AB, Baines CJ, To T, et al. Canadian National Breast Screening Study-1: breast cancer detection and death rates among women aged 40 to 49 years. *CMAJ*. 1992;147:1459–1476.
31. Kopans DB, Feig SA. The Canadian National Breast Screening Study: a critical review. *AJR Am J Roentgenol*. 1993;161:755–760.
32. Tarone RE. The excess of patients with advanced breast cancer in young women screened with mammography in the Canadian National Breast Screening Study. *Cancer*. 1995;75:997–1003.
33. Yaffe MJ. Correction: Canada study [letter]. *J Natl Cancer Inst*. 1993;85:94.
34. Leitch AM, Dodd GD, Costanza M, et al. American Cancer Society guidelines for the early detection of breast cancer: update 1997. *CA Cancer J Clin*. 1997;47:150–153.
35. Smith RA, Saslow D, Sawyer KA, et al. American Cancer Society guidelines for breast cancer screening: update 2003. *CA Cancer J Clin*. 2003;53:141–169.
36. Saslow D, Boetes C, Burke W, et al. American Cancer Society guidelines for breast screening with MRI as an adjunct to mammography. *CA Cancer J Clin*. 2007;57:75–89.
37. US Preventive Services Task Force. Screening for breast cancer: US Preventive Services Task Force recommendation statement. *Ann Intern Med*. 2009;151:716–726.
38. US Preventive Services Task Force. Screening for breast cancer: recommendations and rationale. *Ann Intern Med*. 2002;137:344–346.
39. Hendrick RE, Helvie MA. United States Preventive Services Task Force screening mammography recommendations: science ignored. *AJR Am J Roentgenol*. 2011;196:W112–W116.
40. Rosenberg RD, Yankaskas BC, Abraham LA, et al. Performance benchmarks for screening mammography. *Radiology*. 2006;241:55–66.
41. Carney PA, Sickles EA, Monsees BS, et al. Identifying minimally acceptable interpretive performance criteria for screening mammography. *Radiology*. 2010;255:354–361.
42. Linver MN, Osuch JR, Brenner RJ, et al. The mammography audit: a primer for the Mammography Quality Standards Act (MQSA). *AJR Am J Roentgenol*. 1995;165:19–25.
43. Kerlikowske K, Grady D, Barclay J, et al. Effect of age, breast density, and family history on the sensitivity of first screening mammography. *JAMA*. 1996;276:33–38.
44. Carney PA, Miglioretti DL, Yankaskas BC, et al. Individual and combined effects of age, breast density and hormone replacement therapy use on the accuracy of mammography. *Ann Intern Med*. 2003;138:168–175.
45. Department of Health and Human Services, Food and Drug Administration. Quality mammography standards; final rule. *Fed Regist*. 1997;62:55852–55993. 21 CFR parts 16 and 900.
46. American College of Radiology. Mammography Accreditation Program requirements. www.acr.org/~/media/ACR/Documents/Accreditation/Mammography/Requirements.pdf.
47. Krag D, Weaver D, Ashikaga T, et al. The sentinel node is breast cancer. *N Engl J Med*. 1998;339:941–946.
48. McIntosh SA, Purushotham AD. Lymphatic mapping and sentinel node biopsy in breast cancer. *Br J Surg*. 1998;85:1347–1356.
49. Liberman L, Cody HS, Hill ADK, et al. Sentinel lymph node biopsy after percutaneous diagnosis of nonpalpable breast cancer. *Radiology*. 1999;211:835–844.
50. DeAngelis GA, Gizienski T, Moore MM. Axillary sentinel node biopsy in breast cancer staging. *Appl Radiol*. June 1999:8–11.
51. Donegan WL, Spratt JS. *Cancer of the Breast*. 5th ed. Philadelphia, PA: WB Saunders; 2002.
52. Lyman GH, Giuliano AE, Somerfeld MR, et al. American Society of Clinical Oncology guideline recommendations for sentinel lymph node biopsy in early stage breast cancer. *J Clin Oncol*. 2005;23:7703–7720.
53. Paik S, Tang G, Shak S, et al. Gene expression and benefit of chemotherapy in women with node-negative, estrogen receptor-positive breast cancer. *J Clin Oncol*. 2006;24:3726–3734.
54. American Joint Committee on Cancer. *Cancer Staging Manual*. 7th ed. New York, NY: Springer; 2010.
55. Perou CM, Sørlie T, Eisen MB, et al. Molecular portraits of human breast cancer tumours. *Nature*. 2000;406:747–752.
56. Sørlie T, Perou CM, Tibshirani R, et al. Gene expression patterns of breast carcinomas distinguish tumor subclass with clinical implications. *Proc Natl Acad Sci U S A*. 2001;98:10869–10874.
57. Sørlie T, Tibshirani R, Parker J, et al. Repeated observation of breast tumor subtypes in independent gene expression data sets. *Proc Natl Acad Sci U S A*. 2003;100:8418–8423.
58. Schnitt S. Classification and prognosis of invasive breast cancer: from morphology to molecular taxonomy. *Mod Pathol*. 2010;23:60–64.
59. Voduc KD, Cheang MCU, Tyldesley S, et al. Breast cancer subtypes and the risk for local and regional relapse. *J Clin Oncol*. 2010;28:1684–1691.
60. Cheang MCU, Voduc KD, Bajdik C, et al. Basal-like cancer defined by five biomarkers has superior prognostic value than triple negative phenotype. *Clin Cancer Res*. 2008;14:1368–1375.
61. Nielsen TO, Hsu FD, Jensen K, et al. Immunohistochemical and clinical characterization of the basal-like subtype of invasive breast carcinoma. *Clin Cancer Res*. 2004;10:5367–5374.
62. Rakha EA, Ellis IO. Triple-negative/basal-like breast cancer: review. *Pathology*. 2009;41:40–47.
63. Reis-Filho JS, Tutt ANJ. Triple negative tumours: a critical review. *Histopathology*. 2008;52:108–118.

CHAPTER SELF-ASSESSMENT QUESTIONS

1. Based on these pre- and postcontrast T1-weighted sagittal reconstructions of the left breast, what is the "T" for this patient's clinical TNM (cTNM) classification?

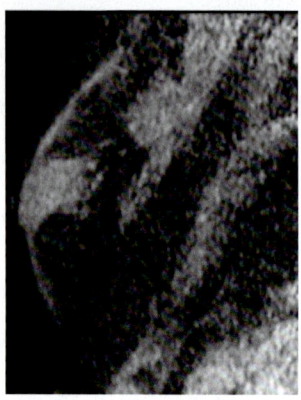
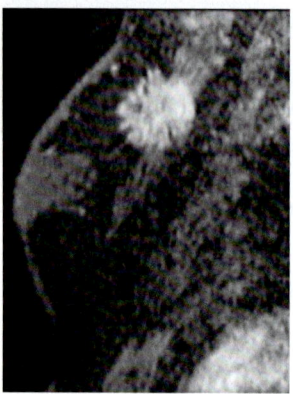

A   T1
B   T2
C   T3
D   T4

2. Based on this postcontrast T1-weighted sagittal reconstruction of the left breast, what is the most likely clinical stage for this patient?

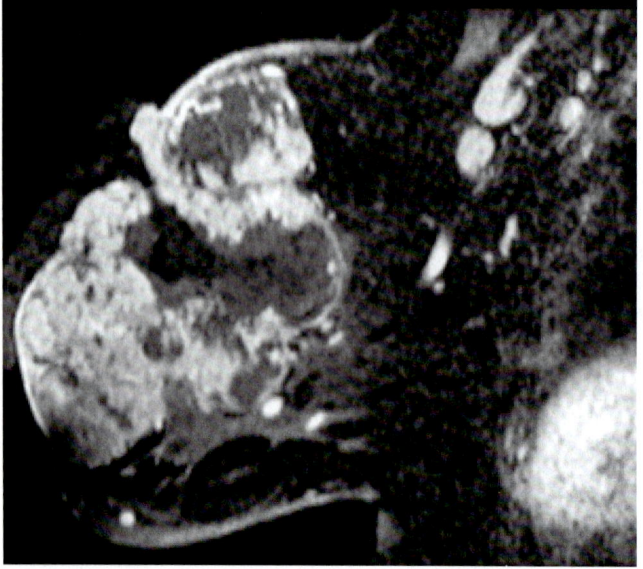

A   Stage IIB
B   Stage IIIA
C   Stage IIIB
D   Stage IV

Answers to Chapter Self-Assessment Questions

1. B   In this patient, a heterogeneously enhancing round mass with spiculated margins invades the pectoral muscle. This mass measures more than 2 cm but less than 5 cm in size. Although T4 tumors are defined as tumors of any size with direct extension to the chest wall and/or to the skin, involvement of the pectoral muscles is *not* considered chest wall. The chest wall includes ribs, intercostal muscles, and serratus anterior muscle. T1 tumors are those that are less than or equal to 2 cm in greatest dimension. On the basis of size, the T1 tumors can be further subdivided into T1mi, T1a, T1b, and T1c (see Table 1.1). Tumors that are greater than 2 cm but less than or equal to 5 cm in greatest dimension are designated as T2 tumors and those that are larger than 5 cm in greatest dimension are T3 tumors.

2. C   In this patient, a 13-cm heterogeneously enhancing mass with smooth lobulated margins and associated ulceration of the skin is present in the left breast. Given the skin ulceration, this is a T4b tumor. T4 tumors with or without nodal disease are considered Stage IIIB. Stage IIB tumors are either T2 tumors with nodal involvement (N1) or T3 tumors with clinically negative lymph nodes. Stage IIIA tumors can include T0, T1, T2, and T3 tumors with nodal involvement (N2). Stage IV tumors are any of the T tumors with either nodal involvement (N3) or any N tumor with distant metastasis (see Table 1.5).

Screening Mammography 2

LEARNING OBJECTIVES

1. Quality assurance and quality control requirements under Mammography Quality Standards Act (MQSA)
   - Tests done by the technologists and the required frequency
     Actions required if tests fail
   - Tests done annually by the physicist
   - Phantom images
   - Films labeling
     Required under MQSA
     Recommended
2. Indicated imaging algorithms in screening
   - Standard views
   - Additional images done in women with implants
   - Exaggerated craniocaudal views laterally
   - Anterior compression views
   - Imaging women with small or large breasts
3. Positioning basics
   - Mediolateral oblique (MLO) views
   - Craniocaudal (CC) views
   - Exaggerated craniocaudal views
4. Assessing adequacy of positioning
   - MLO views
   - CC view
     Posterior nipple line measurement
   - Exaggerated craniocaudal views
5. Assessing images for motion
6. Artifacts related to
   - Equipment
   - Software processing
   - Patients
7. Screening
   - Definition
   - Standard views
   - Viewing conditions
   - Approach to lesion detection
8. Evaluation of images
   - Technical adequacy of images
     Positioning
     Exposure
     Contrast
     Motion (Sharpness)
     Noise
     Compression
     Film labeling
     Artifacts
   - Review images in totality for global changes
     Size asymmetry
     Diffuse trabecular or parenchymal changes
     Technical factors used for exposure
     Focal and global areas of parenchymal asymmetry
   - Review images specifically looking for
     Masses (correlating size and distance from nipple on CC and MLO views)
     Calcifications
     Distortion
   - Review images in thirds
     CC: lateral, retroareolar, medial
     MLO: upper, mid and lower
   - Review specific locations
     CC: medial quadrants, subareolar, retroglandular fat and tissue interface
     MLO: fatty strip between pectoral muscle and tissue, subareolar, upper cone of tissue, tissue immediately superior to inframammary fold (IMF)
     CC and MLO: all fat-glandular tissue interfaces

QUALITY CONTROL TESTS

Under the Mammography Quality Standards Act (MQSA) (1), mammographic facilities are required to have a quality assurance (QA) and quality control (QC) program. For digital systems, facilities need to implement the QA/QC program as specified by the manufacturer of the unit(s) being used (1,2). Weekly quality control tests typically include DICOM printer quality control, detector flat-field calibration to assure the system is calibrated properly, artifact evaluation (for the detector), signal-to-noise and contrast-to-noise measurements to assure consistency of the digital image receptor, phantom image to assure overall image quality, compression thickness indicator to assure indicated compression thickness is accurate to ±0.5 cm from actual thickness, diagnostic review workstation QC, and viewboxes and viewing conditions. The visual checklist, repeat analysis, and compression QC test are done monthly, quarterly, and semiannually, respectively. The annual tests done by physicists typically include mammographic unit assembly evaluation, collimation assessment, artifact evaluation, kVp accuracy and reproducibility, beam quality assessment (half-value layer [HVL] measurement), evaluation of system resolution, automatic exposure control (AEC) function performance, radiation output rate, phantom image quality evaluation, signal-to-noise and contrast-to-noise measurements, diagnostic review workstation QC, breast entrance exposure, AEC reproducibility, and average glandular dose. Evaluation of detector ghosting is optional. The reader is advised to consult the equipment manufacturers' QC manual for details on the specific tests required as well as how each test should be done and interpreted.

For facilities using film-screen systems, QC tests that need to be done by the technologist daily, monthly, quarterly, and semiannually and the annual tests required of the physicist are detailed under the MQSA (1) and the American College of Radiology's (ACR) *Mammography Quality Control Manual* (3). The reader is advised to consult this manual for details on how each test is done and interpreted.

PHANTOM IMAGES

A basic understanding of the phantom image in mammography is important since this is used routinely to ensure the entire imaging system (and the processor if film-screen mammography is in use) is operating optimally with respect to uniformity, lack of artifacts, and overall image quality. As part of the QA/QC program, phantom images are done weekly. These are also done after the equipment is serviced, when film or screen type is changed (for facilities doing film-screen mammography) or as needed when troubleshooting problems with the imaging chain. The reader is encouraged to review and understand how phantom images are obtained, evaluated, and scored (ACR's *Mammography Quality Control Manual*) (3). The phantom (Radiation Measurement, Inc. RMI 156 or Nuclear Associates 18-220) simulates a 4.2-cm-thick compressed breast composed of 50% glandular and 50% fatty tissue. It contains six fibers (range, 1.56 to 0.4 mm), five specks (1.56- to 0.4-mm diameter range), and five masses (2.00- to 0.25-mm diameter range). An acrylic disc (4-mm thick, 1-cm diameter) is placed, or permanently attached to the phantom.

At a minimum, the four largest fibers, three largest speck groups, and three largest masses should be seen (Fig. 2.1). The image is also reviewed for artifacts and these are factored into the scoring. Regions of interest (ROI) are placed one over the disc and the other in an area adjacent to disc so that signal-to-noise ratios (SNR) and contrast-to-noise ratios (CNR) can be calculated. The measured SNR must be equal to or greater than 40 and the CNR must be within ±15% of the value determined by the medical physicists when the image receptor was installed or after any major upgrade. If the criteria specified by the equipment manufacturer are not met, the service engineer needs to be contacted before any further clinical imaging is done.

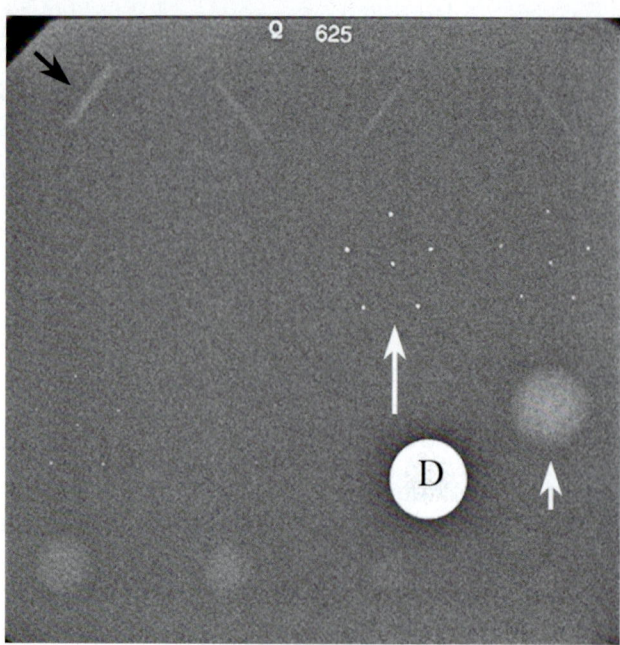

FIG. 2.1 • **Phantom image.** Radiation Measurement, Inc. (RMI 156) phantom. For our system, five fibers (*black arrow*), four speck groups (*long white arrow*), and four masses (*short white arrow*) need to be seen to pass. In addition, the image is reviewed for homogeneity and artifacts. The acrylic disc (*D*) attached to the phantom is used to calculate SNR and CNR. As part of the QA/QC program, phantom images are done weekly, and the images are retained for one full year.

FILM LABELING

Mammography films are legal documents and must be labeled appropriately as required under MQSA (1). The information that must be included on the images is listed in Table 2.1. When printing images from a digital study, please make sure that the required data is not printed over any part of the breasts or pectoral muscles.

Technical factors (kVp, mAs, cm of compression) used for exposure should be available readily so that they can be reviewed in conjunction with the images. As will be discussed and illustrated repeatedly, the technical factors used for exposure (right breast compared with left or from 1 year to another) in some patients provide additional information that can be used in establishing the presence of underlying pathology and formulating differential considerations.

IMAGING ALGORITHM

By definition, screening mammography is done in asymptomatic women (4). We recommend annual screening mammography starting

Table 2.1 REQUIRED INFORMATION ON IMAGES

Patient name
Unique patient identifying number
Date of study
Radiopaque laterality and projection markers placed closest to axilla
Facility name
Facility location (minimum: city, state, and zip code)
Technologist identification
Mammography unit identification number/room number (if more than one unit/facility)

at age 40. In women with a strong family history of breast cancer, we start screening annually at age 30. Additionally, if a patient has two first-degree relatives with breast or ovarian cancer, particularly if the diagnosis of breast cancer in the relative occurred premenopausally, she is referred to a genetic counselor for risk assessment. If the risk assessment yields a 20% or higher lifetime risk for breast cancer, we recommend annual screening with mammography and breast magnetic resonance imaging (5).

Craniocaudal (CC) and mediolateral oblique (MLO) views of each breast are done for screening (4). At the discretion of the technologist, anterior compression and exaggerated craniocaudal (XCCL) views are obtained in a small number of women to adequately compress anterior tissue and image posterolateral tissue in the CC projection, respectively. A metallic BB is used to mark any prominent skin lesions that may be mistaken for a breast mass. Our technologists are required to document the location and reason for using skin markers on the patient's history form. Likewise, they document surgical scars on a diagram of the breast provided on the history form. We do not routinely use radiopaque markers on biopsy scars or the nipples (see excisional biopsy section in Chapter 11 for additional discussion).

In women with implants, we obtain four views of each breast: CC and MLO views with the implants in the field of view and CC and MLO views with displacement of the implants (1,3,4,6). Implant-displaced (ID) views may be difficult (or not possible) to obtain in women with implants that are encapsulated (see Fig. 11.49). If the ID views cannot be done, the technologist documents this in the patient's history form and the radiologist states this in the breast imaging consultation report. We do not obtain any special consent from patients with implants prior to imaging them.

IMAGING WOMEN WITH SMALL BREASTS (OR MEN)

In women with small breasts, for ID views in some women, or in male patients, it can be hard for the technologist to maintain breast positioning, particularly for MLO views, without potentially hurting her hand and scraping the skin over her knuckles as compression is applied. After positioning, the technologist holds the breast in position, and as the paddle comes down on the breast, she needs to pull her hand out from under the paddle. This maneuver can be a challenge when using the standard compression paddle in these groups of patients. To overcome these potential limitations, a compression paddle that is half the width of the standard compression paddle is available (Fig. 2.2A); this paddle is also sometimes helpful in obtaining optimal axillary views.

IMAGING WOMEN WITH LARGE BREASTS

For most digital systems, compression paddles (Fig. 2.2B, C) with resulting collimation are available in two sizes (18 × 24 cm and 24 × 30 cm). The selection of which size to use is made based on the woman's breast size. The large paddle and the resulting larger field of collimation is not used for women with small breasts. Likewise, the small paddle and small field of collimation is not used on a woman with large breasts. Some women with large breasts may need more than two views of each breast to image all the breast tissue adequately in the two standard projections (Fig. 2.3).

MEDIOLATERAL OBLIQUE VIEWS

Factors to be considered in obtaining optimal positioning of the breasts on MLO views are listed in Table 2.2. If these simple concepts

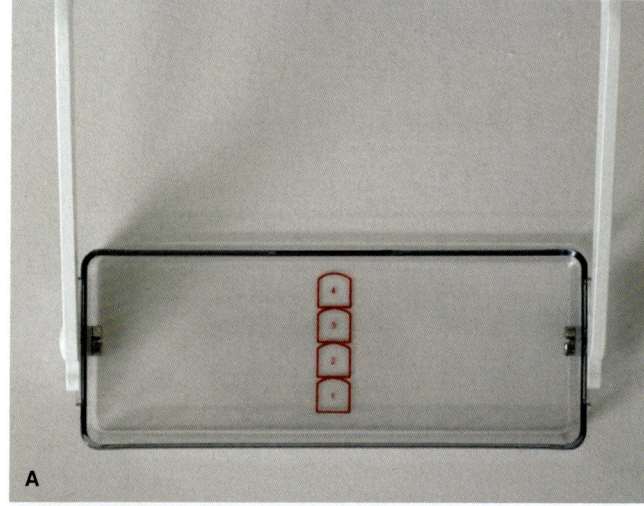
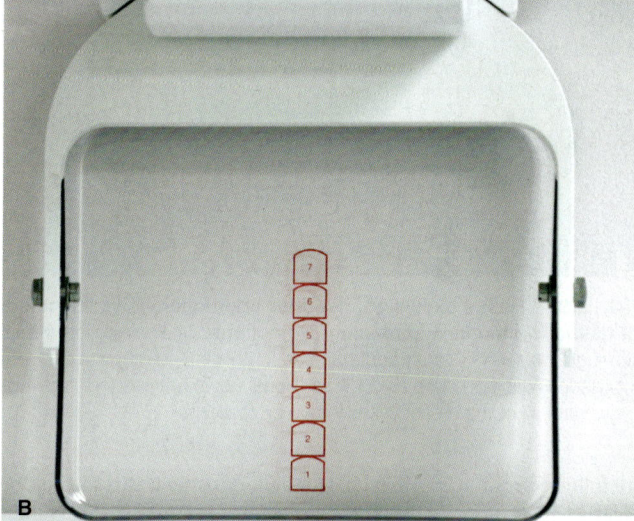
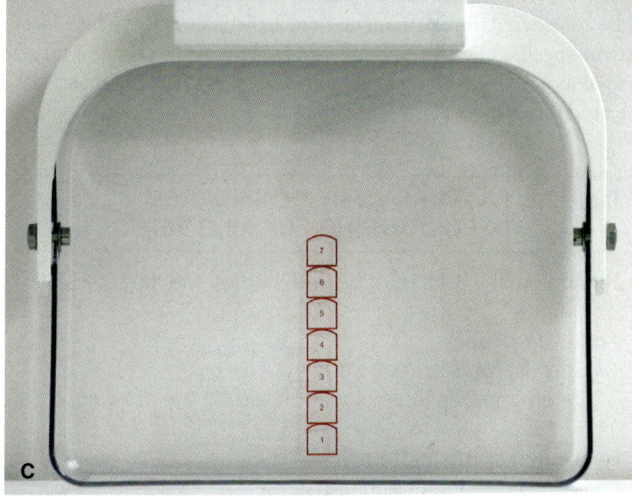

FIG. 2.2 • **Compression paddles, screening. A:** This compression paddle is half the width of the standard 18 × 24 cm paddle. It is particularly helpful in imaging women with small breasts, men, and for ID views in some patients with implants. It is also sometimes used for axillary views. **B:** Standard 18 × 24 cm compression paddle. **C:** Larger, standard 18 × 30 cm compression paddle. Although this larger paddle facilitates the imaging of some women with no extra views, some patients may still require more than two images to adequately include all of the tissue in the two standard projections. The red markings centrally on the paddles indicate available photocell positions with the particular unit being used.

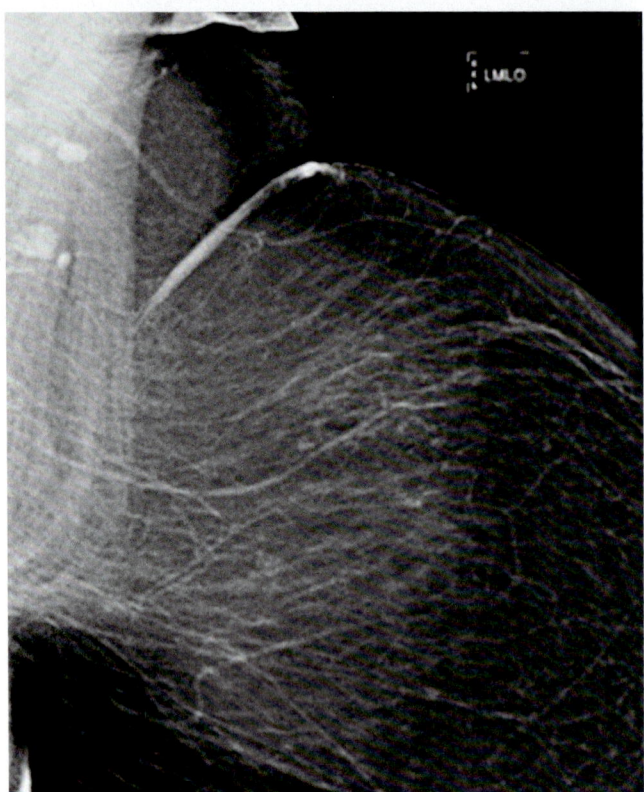

FIG. 2.3 • **Tissue exclusion, need for additional views to include all tissue in standard screening projections.** MLO view, left breast. Although the 18 × 30 cm paddle is used for this image, anterior and inferior tissue is excluded and as such additional views are needed to be able to evaluate all of the breast tissue in two projections.

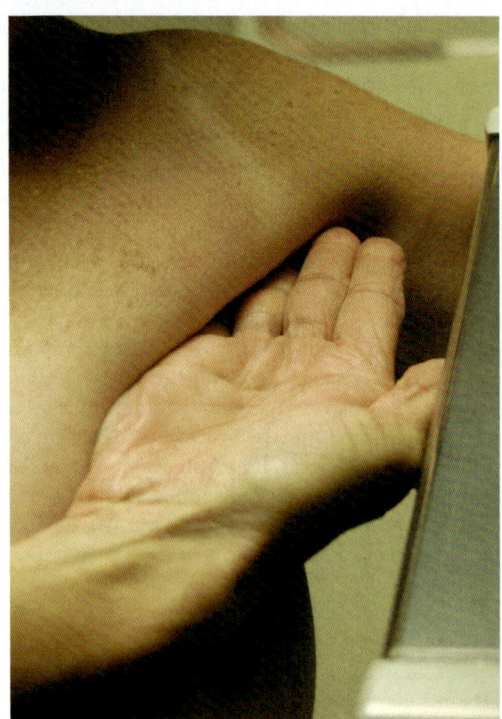

FIG. 2.4 • **Determining angle of obliquity for MLO view.** With the patient's arm relaxed as she stands by the digital detector, the technologist can determine the optimal angle of obliquity and adjust the gantry accordingly for the MLO views. The angle of obliquity used for the MLO views is based on the patient's body habitus and orientation of the underlying pectoral muscle; it is different for different patients.

are followed routinely, a maximal amount of tissue is included on the images while compression-related discomfort is minimized.

In positioning patients for MLO views, four separate concepts need to be considered, understood, and applied consistently: selection of a patient-specific angle of obliquity, relaxation of the pectoral muscle, medial mobilization of the breast and underlying pectoral muscle, and the need for an out and upward pull of the breast tissue and underlying

Table 2.2 FACTORS TO BE CONSIDERED IN POSITIONING FOR MLO VIEWS

Technologist works from behind and the medial side of patient
Angle of obliquity
   Specific for each patient
   Determined by technologist based on the obliquity of the pectoral muscle
Relaxation of the pectoral muscle
   Inward rotation of humeral head
   Ipsilateral arm down
Medial mobilization of breast tissue and pectoral muscle
   Need to maintain medial mobilization
   Minimizes skin stretching in the upper inner quadrant
Patient needs to stay in unit (tendency is to pull back out)
Breast pulled up and out
   Open IMF
   Include a small amount of abdomen

muscle. The breasts are skin appendages. In trying to maximize the outward pull of a skin appendage so it can be imaged, it is best to pull the appendage out parallel to the underlying muscle; the pectoral muscle is the muscle underlying the breast. Consequently, the technologist needs to assess the orientation of the pectoral muscle for the individual patient (Fig. 2.4) and use this to determine the angle of obliquity for the MLO view. By necessity, the angle will be different for different patients. Tall women will have a more vertically oriented pectoral muscle compared to short women. In an effort to include as much tissue as possible on MLO views, the breasts should be pulled away from the body parallel to an underlying relaxed pectoral muscle (7).

In addition to selecting an appropriate angle of obliquity, the technologist needs to make sure that the pectoral muscle is relaxed; otherwise, she may be fighting the resistance added by a tense muscle. The pectoralis major muscle inserts on the upper third of the humerus; so the muscle tenses if the arm is elevated and the humeral head is externally rotated. During positioning, the patient's arm should be kept down (behind or on the bucky) while making sure that she inwardly rotates her humeral head. The amount of tissue and muscle included on the images is increased if the pectoral muscle is relaxed.

With respect to the importance of breast mobility, consider the basics of breast anatomy. The lateral and inferior aspects of the breasts are the most mobile (Fig. 2.5A). Tissue in the upper and particularly inner quadrants has little inherent mobility. Unfortunately, most of our equipment is designed so that, for MLO views, the compression paddle travels from the upper inner quadrant toward the lower outer quadrant (Fig. 2.5B). As the compression paddle is engaged, we are attempting to mobilize tissue with little inherent mobility in the upper inner quadrants into the field of view. Inevitably, as the compression paddle

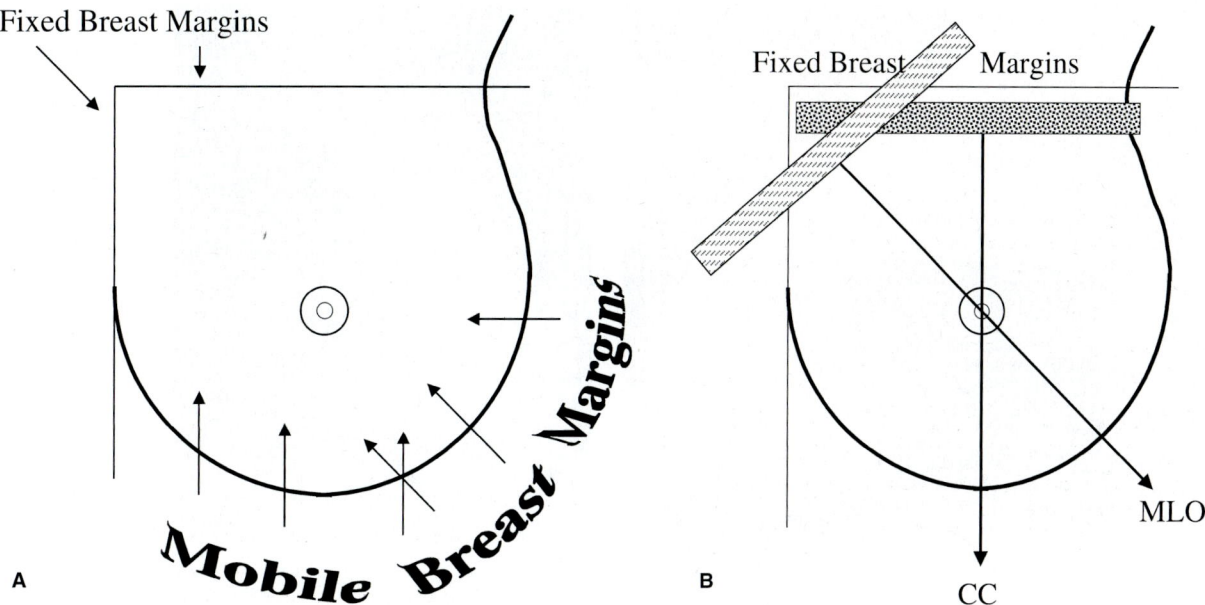

FIG. 2.5 • **Breast mobility. A:** Lateral and inferior breast tissue is mobile. Upper and medial breast tissue has little inherent mobility. During positioning, tissue should be mobilized so as to minimize the amount of fixed tissue passed over by the compression paddle. **B:** For the MLO view, the compression paddle moves from the upper inner quadrant toward the lower outer quadrant. With little inherent mobility, upper inner quadrant tissue is excluded from the field of view as the compression paddle is mobilized for the MLO views. The skin is stretched and sometimes scraped as the paddle moves over this tissue. Similarly, for craniocaudal (CC) views, the compression paddle moves from upper to lower quadrants. As the paddle moves downward, superior tissue, and possibly lesions, can roll out from the under the paddle. Skin stretching, resulting from the compression paddle scraping over this portion of the breast, accounts for some of the discomfort patients associate with breast compression. (From Cardeñosa G. *Breast Imaging* [*The Core Curriculum Series*]. Philadelphia, PA: Lippincott Williams & Wilkins; 2003.)

moves, tissue and potentially lesions roll out from under the paddle and are excluded from the field of view. The movement of the compression paddle over fixed tissue in the upper inner quadrant of the breast also results in skin stretching that almost certainly accounts for much of the discomfort patients associate with mammography and attribute to breast compression. If we use natural breast mobility effectively, we can minimize the amount of tissue that is excluded as well as the amount of skin stretching (7). Every 1 mm that we are able to mobilize tissue and underlying muscle medially represents 1 mm less of the compression paddle travelling over fixed tissue. In addition to mobilizing the breast and muscle medially, the breast tissue needs to be actively pulled out away from the body to include a maximal amount of posterior tissue, and upwardly, so that the inframammary fold (IMF) is opened. Ideally, a small amount of upper abdomen is included on the image.

The tip of the digital detector is positioned at the apex of the axilla so that it is snug against the body along the mid-axillary line. As the patient is rotated toward the digital detector and the breast is mobilized, the technologist needs to smooth the tissue going up against the detector; otherwise, skinfolds can develop (Figs. 2.6 and 2.7A). Also, there should be no air gap (Fig. 2.7A) between the pectoral muscle and upper portion of the breast and the digital detector. If the air gap is not cleared, uneven exposure (overexposure) of the pectoral muscle and axillary tissue will be apparent (Fig. 2.7A, B). Last, there should be no space between the digital detector and the breast posteriorly (Fig. 2.7C); otherwise, posterior tissue is excluded. The technologist should not be able to advance her index finger into the apex of the axilla.

If the correct angle of obliquity for the individual patient is selected, the pectoral muscle is relaxed, the breast is medially mobilized and maintained there as the breast is pulled up and out, the amount

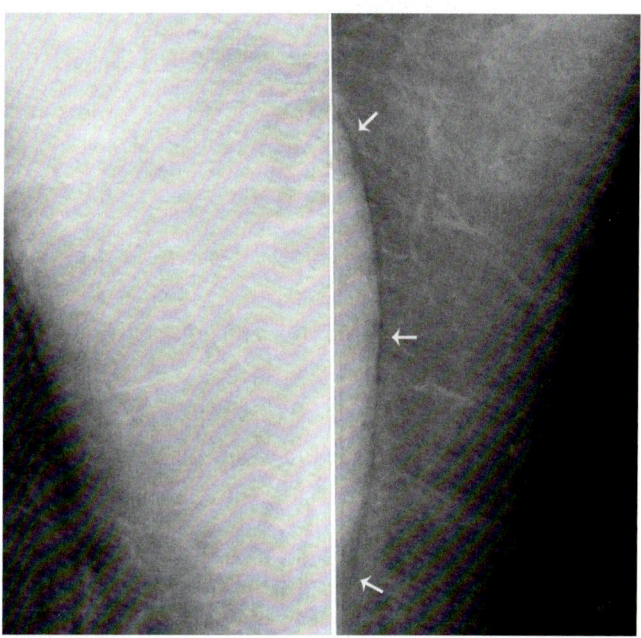

FIG. 2.6 • **Skinfold.** MLO views photographically coned to superior tissue. Skinfold develops laterally as the breast is being mobilized medially. Since the skinfold develops on the portion of breast up against the digital detector, it is not readily apparent to the technologist during positioning. Air (lucency) outlines the edge of the skinfold (*arrows*). When skinfolds are present, compression may be compromised; consequently, the tissue surrounding a skinfold needs to be evaluated carefully for motion (blur). If the skinfold is adequately penetrated, and there is no associated blur, it is not absolutely necessary to repeat the image. (From Cardeñosa G. *Breast Imaging* [*The Core Curriculum Series*]. Philadelphia, PA: Lippincott Williams & Wilkins; 2003.)

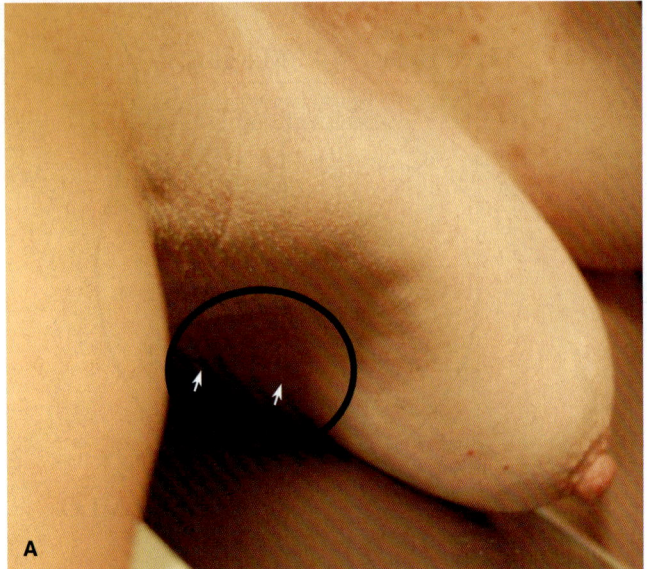
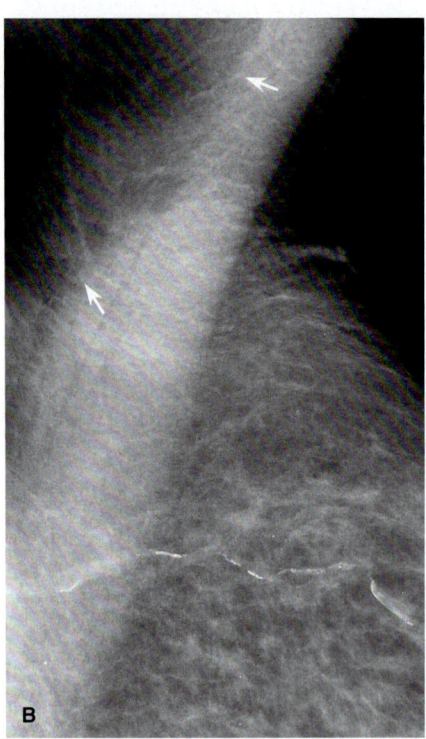
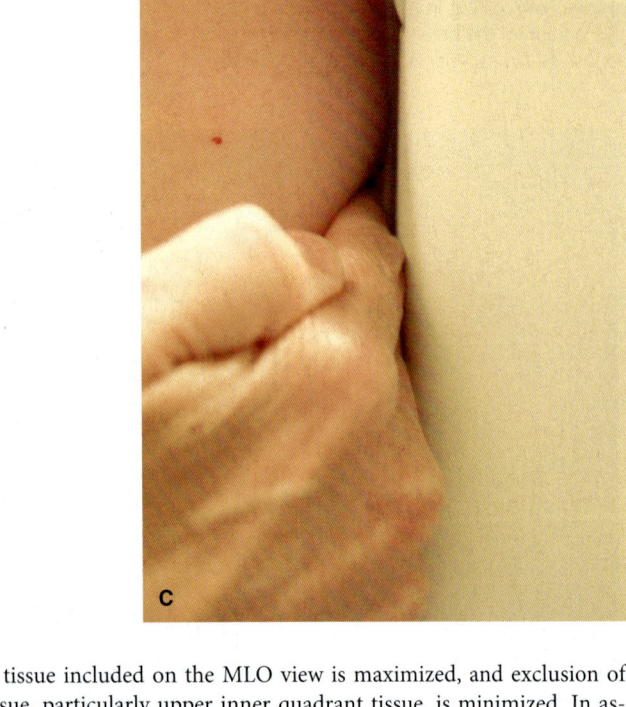

FIG. 2.7 • Positioning, MLO views. A: In positioning the patient's breast for the MLO view, breast, pectoral muscle, and axillary tissue need to be directly in contact with the digital detector. If the tissue is not flush on the detector, the resulting air gap (*black oval*) leads to suboptimal breast compression and apparent overexposure of axillary tissue and pectoral muscle. Also, the technologist needs to be sure no skinfolds develop in the tissue (*arrows*) going up against the detector. **B:** Uneven exposure (*arrows*) resulting from the presence of an air gap between axillary tissue and the detector (e.g., the tissue was not directly up against the detector). When areas of uneven exposure are seen related to air gaps, compression of the tissue in the area is not optimal and as such the tissue needs to be evaluated carefully for blur. Arterial calcification is noted incidentally. (From Cardeñosa G. *Breast Imaging* [*The Core Curriculum Series*]. Philadelphia, PA: Lippincott Williams & Wilkins; 2003.) **C:** The corner of the detector is in the apex of the axilla and the edge of the detector is flush with the skin along the mid-axillary line. The technologist should not be able to interpose her fingers between the detector and the patient in the axilla or along the edge of the detector.

of tissue included on the MLO view is maximized, and exclusion of tissue, particularly upper inner quadrant tissue, is minimized. In assessing the adequacy of positioning on MLO views, the interpreting radiologist should consider the factors listed in Table 2.3. Consider the length and shape of the pectoral muscle on the MLO views (8). The pectoral muscle should be thick (wide) at the axilla, have an anterior convex margin, and extend to the level of the nipple (Fig. 2.8). Selection of an inappropriate angle of obliquity, inadequate relaxation of the muscle, failure to medially mobilize or maintain medial mobilization of breast tissue, or allowing the patient to lean back slightly can result in a concave pectoral muscle edge, a triangular pectoral muscle, or a muscle that is parallel to the edge of the film (Fig. 2.9). The IMF should be open with a small amount of abdomen included on the image. The technologist should exercise care to not include too much

abdomen, or allow a skinfold (Fig. 2.6) to develop up against the bucky laterally, since this may limit compression. A small triangular density superimposed on the pectoralis major muscle in a small number of women is the pectoralis minor muscle (Fig. 2.10).

Table 2.3 ASSESSING POSITIONING ON MLO VIEWS
Wide (thick) pectoral muscle (PM) at the axilla
PM to level of nipple
Convex anterior margin of PM
Breast pulled up and out (no sagging)
Open IMF
Small amount of upper abdomen

Screening Mammography

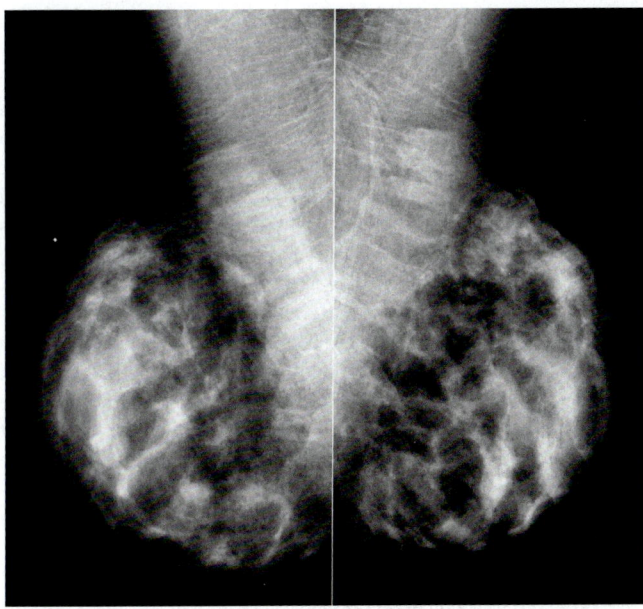

FIG. 2.8 • **MLO views.** The pectoral muscles are thick in the axillae; the anterior borders are convex and extend to the level of the nipples. The tissue is pulled up and out, adequately compressed, and optimally exposed. The IMFs are open. (From Cardeñosa G. *Breast Imaging* [*The Core Curriculum Series*]. Philadelphia, PA: Lippincott Williams & Wilkins; 2003.)

In some women, positioning may be limited secondary to a physical disability such as kyphosis, paraplegia, a frozen shoulder, Parkinson disease, or absence of the pectoral muscle (Poland syndrome) (9) (Fig. 2.11A, B). In these situations, we work closely with the patient to obtain the best images possible and document the limitations and our efforts to obtain adequate images on the patient's history form. If the limitations are significant, we describe this in our breast imaging consultation report. In contrast to patients with Poland syndrome in whom there is absence of a pectoral muscle, rarely, in patients with a history of prolonged steroid (Fig. 2.11C) exposure, or those with disuse (e.g., paralysis of the ipsilateral arm, polio) of the chest wall musculature (Fig. 2.11D), it may appear as though there is no pectoral muscle, yet on close review of the images, the "ghost" of a pectoral muscle is apparent as the striations of the pectoral muscle are seen in an otherwise fatty replaced muscle.

CRANIOCAUDAL VIEWS

Factors to be considered in obtaining optimal positioning of the breasts on CC views are listed in Table 2.4. If these concepts are followed routinely, a maximal amount of tissue is included on the images and compression-related discomfort is minimized.

In positioning patients for CC views, several concepts need to be considered, understood, and applied consistently: upward mobilization of the breast to the extent permitted by the natural mobility of the IMF, placement of the imaging receptor up against the chest wall, positioning of the contralateral breast on the image receptor, outward pull of the breast, and the lateral tug. In considering the CC view, keep in mind that the breast is mobile inferiorly while upper tissue, particularly close to the chest wall, is relatively fixed in position. Yet, when the compression paddle is engaged, it moves over upper inherently fixed tissue posteriorly in an attempt to mobilize it inferiorly. The technologist should identify the natural position of the IMF as she holds and lifts the breast as far as the natural mobility of the IMF allows. If the technologist is able to mobilize the breast upward to meet the paddle, exclusion of upper posterior tissue can be minimized. Every millimeter the breast is moved upward to meet the paddle is 1 mm less that the paddle will need to move down over fixed tissue (7); this results in inclusion of a maximal amount of tissue and minimizes skin stretching

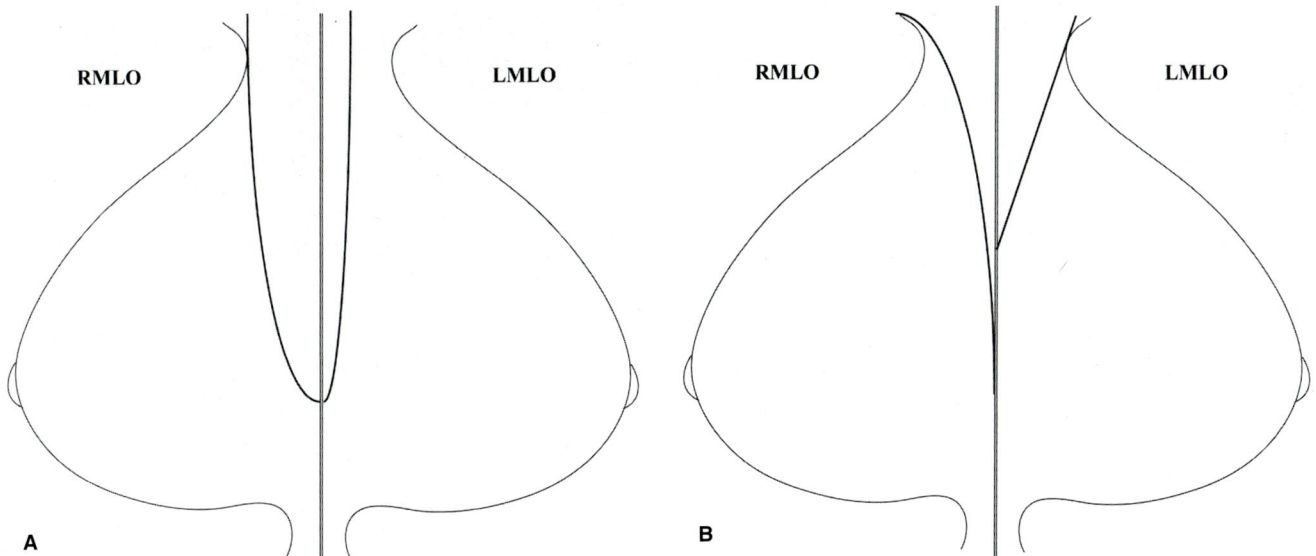

FIG. 2.9 • **The pectoral muscle shape and MLO views. A:** Evaluation of the pectoral muscle is helpful in assessing positioning on MLO views. Ideally, as illustrated on the right MLO (RMLO), the pectoral muscle is thick in the axilla, with a convex anterior border that extends to the level of the nipple. To accomplish this with a cooperative patient, the technologist determines the angle of obliquity based on the orientation of the pectoral muscle for the individual patient. The technologist needs to make sure that the pectoral muscle is relaxed, mobilized medially, and maintained there as compression is applied. If the patient moves back slightly out of the machine, the pectoral muscle is thin and parallel to the edge of the image as illustrated on the left MLO (LMLO). **B:** If an incorrect angle of obliquity is selected or the muscle is not relaxed, the muscle may have a concave contour as illustrated on the right MLO or be triangular in shape as shown on the left MLO. For each of these, inferior and posterior tissue may have been excluded from the image. (From Cardeñosa G. *Breast Imaging* [*The Core Curriculum Series*]. Philadelphia, PA: Lippincott Williams & Wilkins; 2003.)

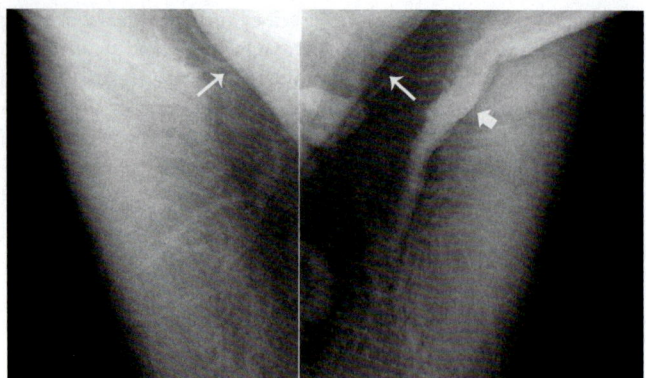

FIG. 2.10 • **Pectoralis minor muscle.** A triangular density superimposed on the pectoral major muscle is the pectoralis minor muscle (*thin arrows*). In this woman, the pectoralis minor muscle is seen bilaterally. The pectoralis minor muscle is imaged in a small percentage of women and is sometimes only imaged on one side. A skinfold is noted on the left (*thick arrow*). Also note air gap with uneven exposure particularly prominent on the left. (From Cardeñosa G. *Breast Imaging* [*The Core Curriculum Series*]. Philadelphia, PA: Lippincott Williams & Wilkins; 2003.)

and the associated discomfort. The image receptor should not be placed higher than the elevated IMF position; otherwise, posterior tissue is excluded. As the breast is lifted, the technologist needs to be careful so that a skinfold doesn't develop between the inferior aspect of the breast and the IMF or that a portion of abdomen is not included on the image. When present, this skinfold (or abdomen) can simulate the pectoral muscle. A sharp lucency (air) outlines the edge of a skinfold but is not seen associated with the pectoral muscle (Fig. 2.12). Also, as the breast is lifted upward it also needs to be actively pulled out away from the body.

The position of the contralateral breast needs to be considered. If the contralateral breast is left pendulous, it can become an impediment to the digital detector being placed against the chest wall. The technologist needs to place the contralateral breast on the edge of the imaging receptor so that the detector can go up against the chest wall (Fig. 2.13A). The technologist should check to make sure there is no space (air gap) between the chest wall and digital detector; she should not be able to put her index finger through the cleavage (Fig. 2.13B).

The inclusion of medial tissue on CC views needs to be emphasized; however, as much as 2 cm of lateral tissue can be pulled into the

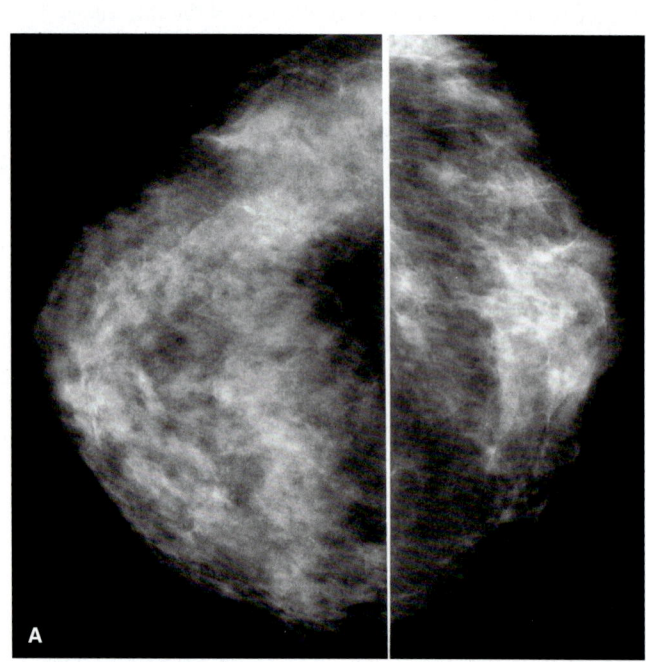

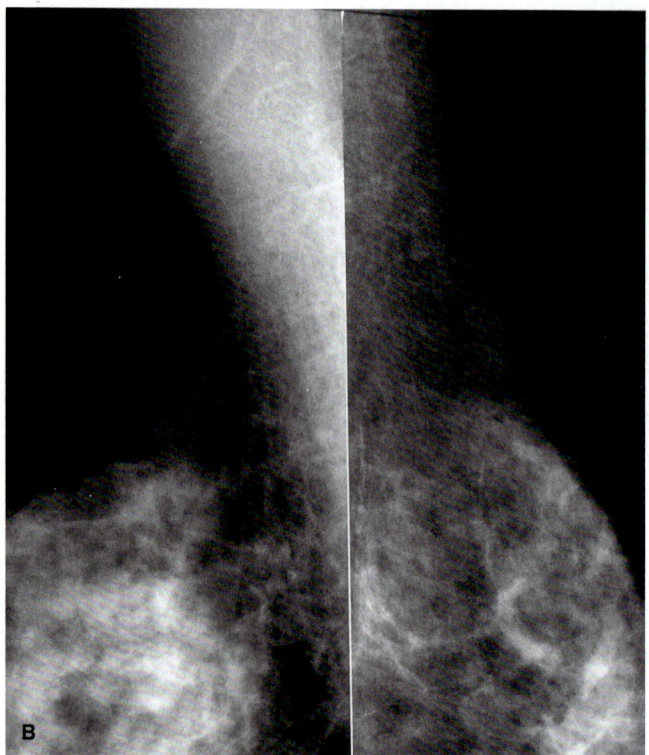

FIG. 2.11 • **Poland syndrome and fatty replaced pectoral muscles.** CC **(A)** and MLO **(B)** views from a screening study. The left breast is smaller than the right. No pectoral muscle is imaged on the left MLO view. As in this patient with Poland syndrome, the breast on the affected side is usually smaller than the contralateral breast. Other ipsilateral chest wall abnormalities, including absence of the clavicle, may be seen in patients with Poland syndrome. (From Cardeñosa G. *Breast Imaging* [*The Core Curriculum Series*]. Philadelphia, PA: Lippincott Williams & Wilkins; 2003.) **C:** MLO views in a different patient. On initial review, you might think the patient is missing the pectoral muscles bilaterally or that positioning is suboptimal with triangularly shaped muscles high up on the image; however, on close review, striations are noted on the MLO views (*arrows*) in largely fatty replaced pectoral muscles. Less fat replacement is seen superiorly in the muscle particularly on the right. This patient has a long history of steroid use. The round radiopaque marker seen on the right MLO is marking a skin lesion. **D:** MLO views in a different patient. You might initially think this is a patient with Poland syndrome with no pectoral muscle on the left, however, if you look carefully you can see the "ghost" of the pectoral muscle with internal striations. This patient has a history of polio with limited mobility on the left side of her body resulting in disuse atrophy. Morphologically normal-appearing lymph nodes are seen in the left axilla.

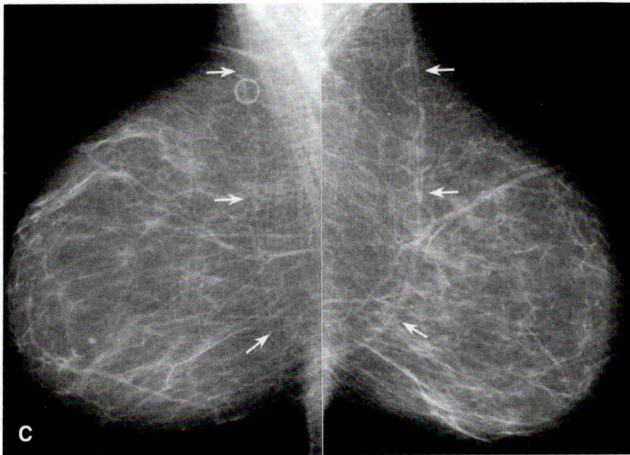

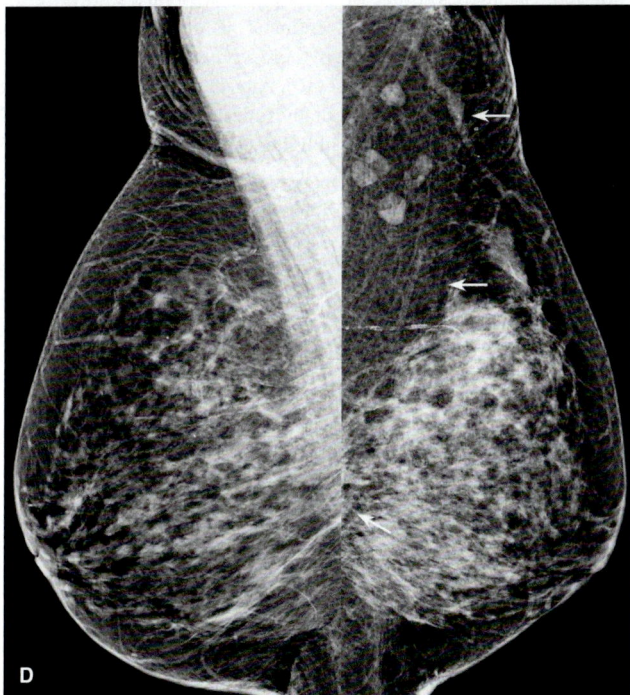

FIG. 2.11 • (Continued)

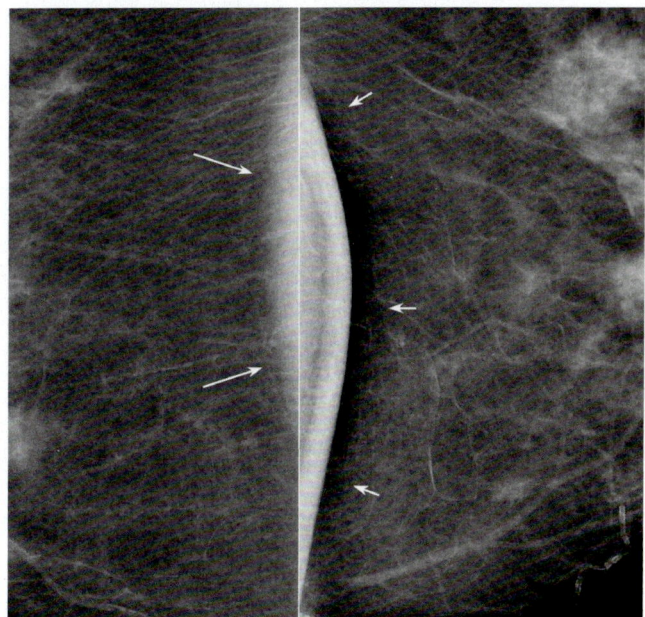

FIG. 2.12 • **Skinfold.** As the breast is mobilized upward for positioning on CC views, a skinfold can develop inferiorly or a portion of the abdominal wall is included on the image. This skinfold simulates the pectoral muscle, however, if evaluated carefully, air (lucency) outlines the skinfold (*short arrows*) on the left CC view; this lucency is not seen outlining the anterior contour of the pectoral muscle (*long arrows*) on the right. Since the skinfold develops up against the digital detector inferiorly, the technologist does not see it during positioning. (From Cardeñosa G. *Breast Imaging* [*The Core Curriculum Series*]. Philadelphia, PA: Lippincott Williams & Wilkins; 2003.)

Table 2.4 **FACTORS TO BE CONSIDERED IN POSITIONING FOR CC VIEWS**
Technologist works from medial side of patient
Neutral position of IMF is identified
Breast tissue is lifted to the extent of natural mobility of IMF
Pull breast tissue out
Lateral tug: active pull of lateral tissue into field of view
Contralateral breast up on digital detector (not left pendulous)
Detector to chest wall
In women with no history of breast surgery the nipple should point straight out
Suspect medial exaggeration if nipple is pointing laterally
Suspect lateral exaggeration if nipple points medially

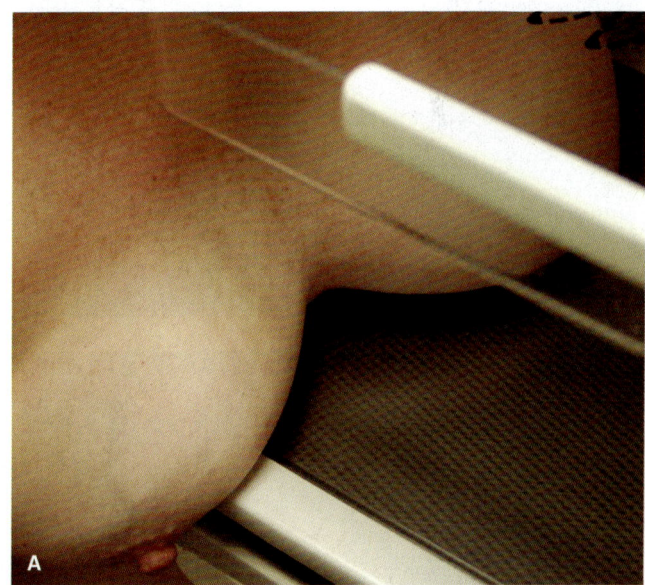

FIG. 2.13 • **Positioning, CC views. A:** In positioning the breast for a CC view, the contralateral breast should be draped over the edge of the digital detector. If the breast is left pendulous, it becomes an impediment to the imaging receptor being placed as far posteriorly as possible. **B:** If the technologist is able to advance her fingers through the cleavage as is demonstrated on this image, posteromedial tissue is being excluded from the field of view. Note that on this image the contralateral breast is not on the imaging receptor but rather has been left pendulous.

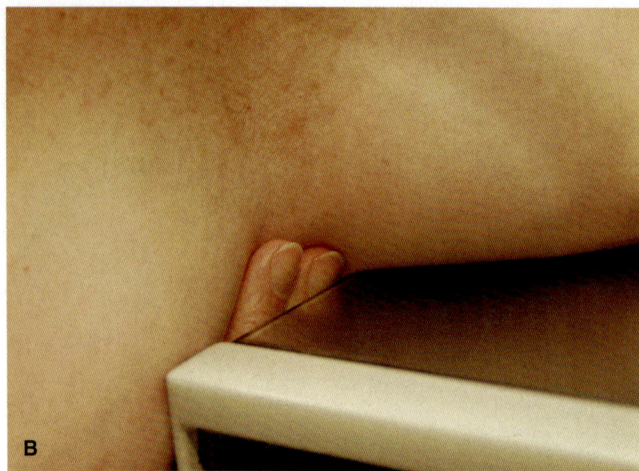

FIG. 2.13 • (continued)

image without giving up medial tissue (Fig. 2.14). The lateral aspect of the breast is mobile and has to be pulled actively into the image by the technologist as compression is applied. As the lateral aspect of the breast is tugged, a skinfold often develops laterally. This skinfold can sometimes be rolled out if the technologist puts her finger under the paddle and rolls it out with the skinfold.

In women who have had no breast surgery, the nipple can be used as an indicator of unwanted exaggeration on CC views. In an optimally positioned CC view, the nipple should point straight out. If the nipple points medially, there may be lateral exaggeration and similarly, if the nipple points laterally, medial exaggeration may be present. Caution should be exercised, however, because in women with significant tissue mobility laterally, a routine CC may seem exaggerated laterally when it is not; the apparent exaggeration laterally is a reflection of an optimal lateral tug.

In assessing the adequacy of positioning on CC views (Table 2.5), pectoral muscle should be seen in 30% to 40% of patients (7,8) (Fig. 2.15A); in younger women, the pectoral muscle may be imaged more commonly than in older patients. If the pectoral muscle is not seen, look for cleavage (Fig. 2.15B). If pectoral muscle or cleavage is seen, you are assured that medial tissue has not been excluded from the image; if neither is seen, consider measuring the posterior nipple line (PNL) (see below). Laterally, retroglandular fat should be seen; if tissue is seen to the edge of the film, an XCCL view may be indicated.

In some women, the pectoral muscle is atrophied and only the sternal insertion is seen medially on the CC view. The rounded or triangular appearance of the muscle in these women can simulate the anterior portion of a mass (Fig 2.16) (10). Alternatively, a round density partially seen on the CC view medially superimposed on the pectoral muscle (with no correlate on the oblique view) can represent the sternalis muscle (Fig. 2.17; also see Fig. 10.1). Even with spot compression views, it is usually only partially seen. The sternalis muscle is an uncommon normal variant in chest wall musculature; it is the remnant of a muscle that would extend from the infraclavicular region to the caudal aspect of the sternum (11). It is commonly a unilateral finding. When the MLO view is reviewed in these patients, no abnormality is seen.

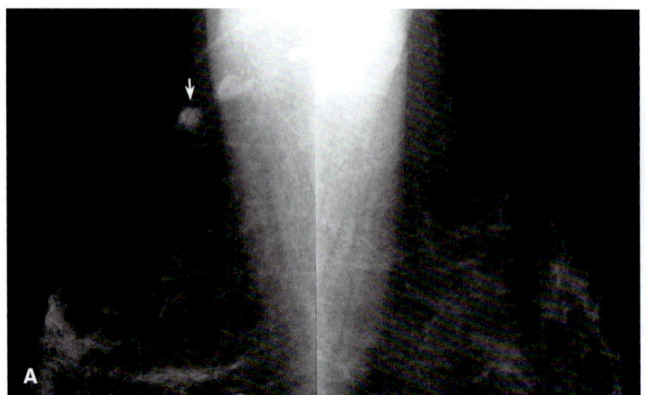

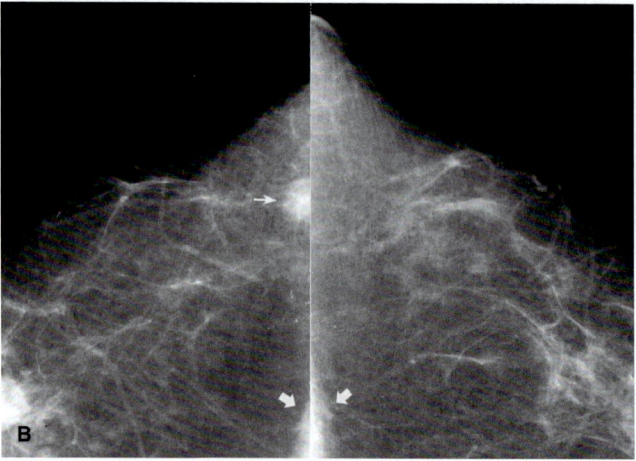

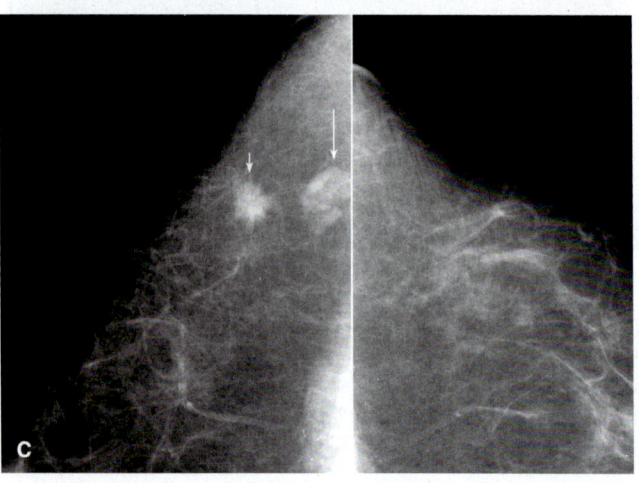

FIG. 2.14 • **Lateral tug for CC view. Invasive ductal carcinoma.** MLO **(A)** and CC **(B)** views photographically coned to the upper and lateral portions of the images, respectively. A mass is seen on the right MLO view (*arrow*). It is partially imaged on the CC view (*thin arrow*). Pectoral muscle is seen (*thick arrow*) centrally on the CC views. **C:** Repeat right CC view with attention to the lateral tug. The mass (*short arrow*) and additional posterior tissue, including a lymph node (*long arrow*), are now included on the image. During positioning for CC views, the technologist needs to actively pull on the lateral aspect of the breast to include as much tissue as possible into the image. This will increase the amount of lateral tissue that is imaged without sacrificing the inclusion of medial tissue. (From Cardeñosa G. *Breast Imaging* [*The Core Curriculum Series*]. Philadelphia, PA: Lippincott Williams & Wilkins; 2003.)

Table 2.5 ASSESSING POSITIONING ON CC VIEWS
Is pectoral muscle imaged? If not
Is there cleavage? If not
Measure PNL—(PNL between MLO and CC views to be within 1 cm of each other)
Retroglandular fat laterally

POSTERIOR NIPPLE LINE

The PNL can be used to determine if a significant amount of posterior tissue is excluded when no pectoral muscle or cleavage is seen on the CC view. This is most accurate when measured on a well-positioned MLO (Fig. 2.18A, D). If positioning on the MLO view

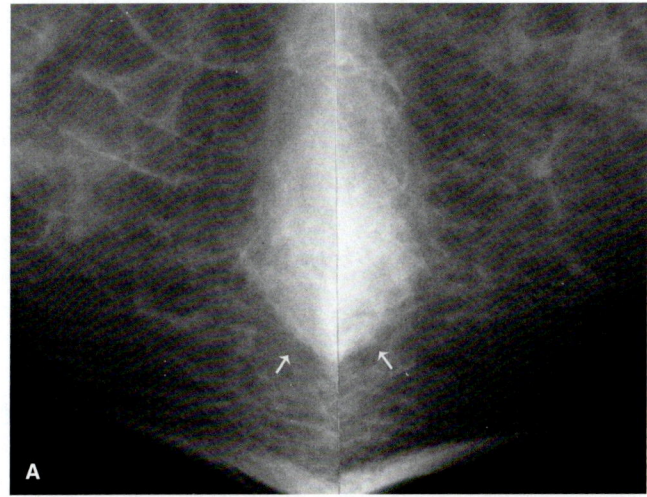

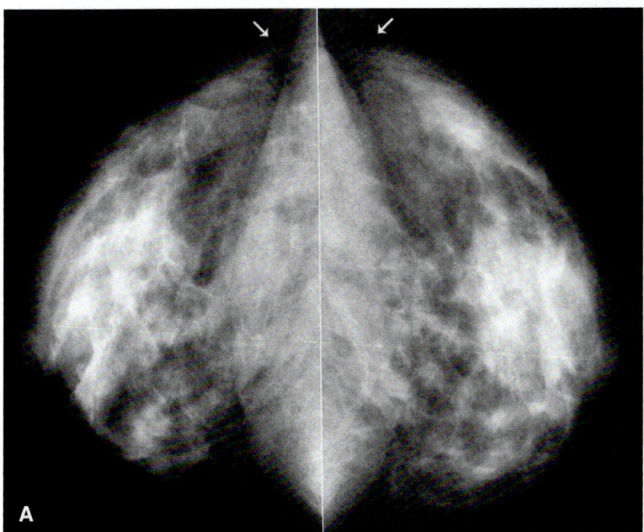

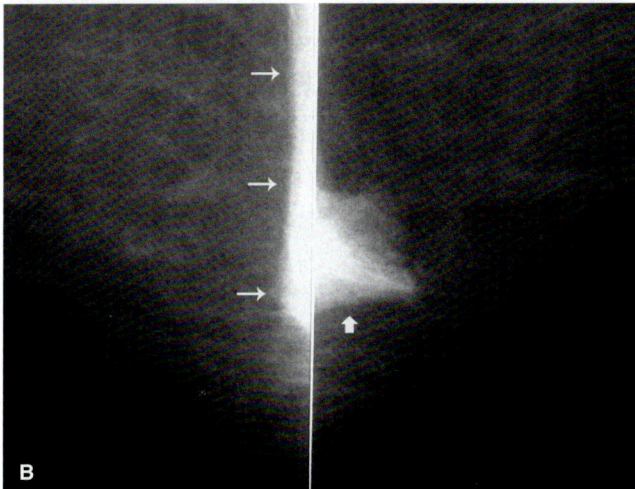

FIG. 2.16 • **Pectoral muscle insertion, medially. A:** Round, mass-like appearance of the pectoral muscle (*arrows*). **B:** In some patients, the pectoral insertion may have a triangular-like shape (*thick arrow*). A more characteristic appearance of the pectoral muscle is noted on the right (*thin arrows*). (From Cardeñosa G. *Breast Imaging* [*The Core Curriculum Series*]. Philadelphia, PA: Lippincott Williams & Wilkins; 2003.)

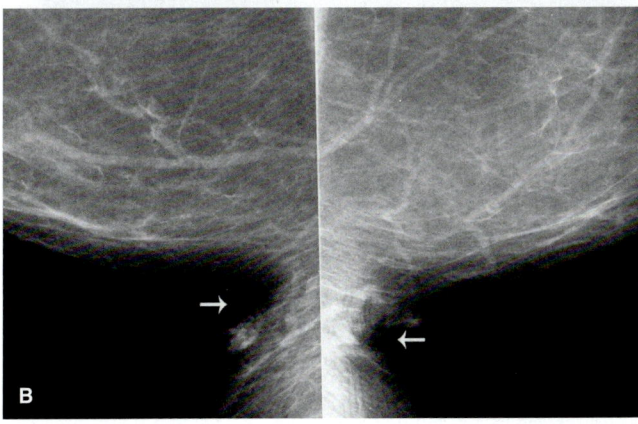

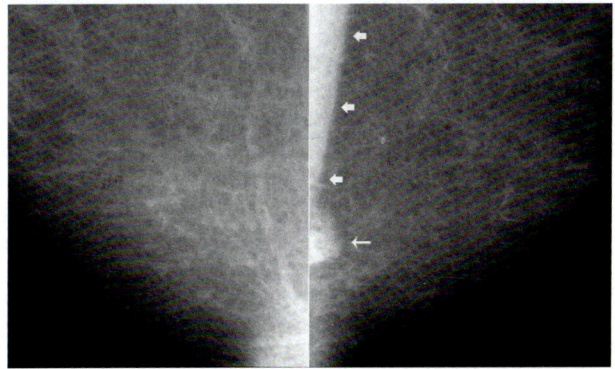

FIG. 2.15 • **CC views. A:** Pectoral muscle is seen in 30% to 40% of CC views. When pectoral muscle is seen, we are assured that posterior tissue has been maximally included in the image. Retroglandular fat should be seen laterally (*arrows*). **B:** If pectoral muscle is not seen, look for cleavage. When cleavage is seen on CC views, we are assured that medial tissue has not been excluded. It also indicates that the contralateral breast is placed appropriately on the edge of the detector (not pendulous) and the digital detector is back to the chest wall. If neither pectoral muscle nor cleavage is seen, measure the PNL to assure that as much posterior tissue as possible is included on the CC views. (From Cardeñosa G. *Breast Imaging* [*The Core Curriculum Series*]. Philadelphia, PA: Lippincott Williams & Wilkins; 2003.)

FIG. 2.17 • **Sternalis muscle.** Rarely, a round mass-like density (*thin arrow*) is partially imaged posteromedially at the edge of the image on the CC view either in isolation or overlying the pectoral muscle (*thick arrows*). No abnormality is seen on the MLO view (not shown). Also see Figure 10.1 for another example of the sternalis muscle, including ultrasound and CT scan images. (From Cardeñosa G. *Breast Imaging* [*The Core Curriculum Series*]. Philadelphia, PA: Lippincott Williams & Wilkins; 2003.)

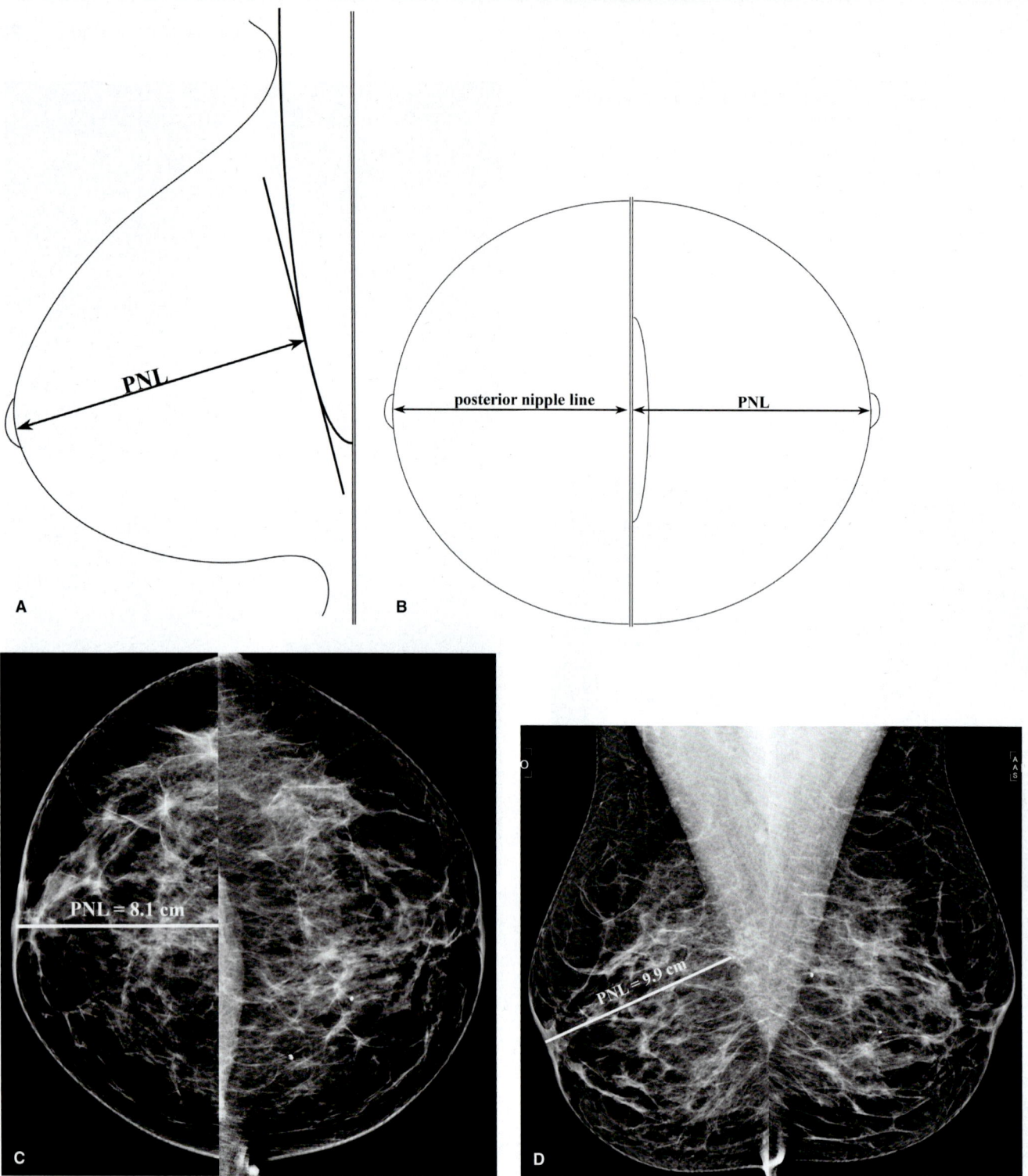

FIG. 2.18 • PNL measurement. A: The PNL is used to assess inclusion of posterior tissue on CC views when pectoral muscle or cleavage is not seen. It is most useful when measured on an optimally positioned MLO view. The distance from the nipple to the anterior edge of the pectoral muscle is measured on the MLO view. The line that is dropped from the nipple to the muscle should be perpendicular to the edge of the muscle. This is the PNL. **B:** On the CC view, the distance from the nipple to the edge of the film is measured (even if pectoral muscle is seen on the CC view, the PNL measurement on the CC needs to be extended to the edge of the image, not the pectoral muscle). These two measurements should be within 1 cm of each other. CC **(C)** and MLO **(D)** views from a screening study. The MLO views are optimally positioned: the pectoral muscles are thick in the axilla, the anterior border of the muscles is convex, and they extend to the level of the nipples. For the CC views, pectoral muscle and cleavage are noted on the left, however, neither is seen on the right; also note that the size of the breasts is symmetric on the MLO views but appears asymmetric in the CC views. Comparison with prior films for the amount of tissue included on the CC views can also be helpful. A PNL measurement is done to confirm the suspicion that posterior tissue is excluded. The PNL on the optimally positioned right MLO view measures 9.9 cm. The PNL measures 8.1 cm on the right CC view. The discrepancy of more than 1 cm between these measurements confirms that posterior tissue is excluded on the right CC. A repeat CC view of the right breast is indicated. **E:** Repeat right CC view includes more posterior tissue such that retroglandular fat, pectoral muscle, and cleavage are now seen on the image.

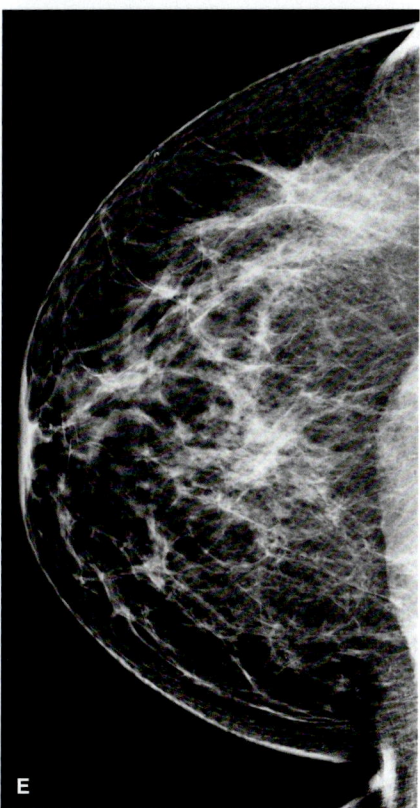

FIG. 2.18 • *(Continued)*

to be considered in assessing adequacy of positioning on XCCL views include seeing retroglandular fat laterally and a small (sliver) amount of pectoral muscle laterally (Figs. 2.19C and 2.20B).

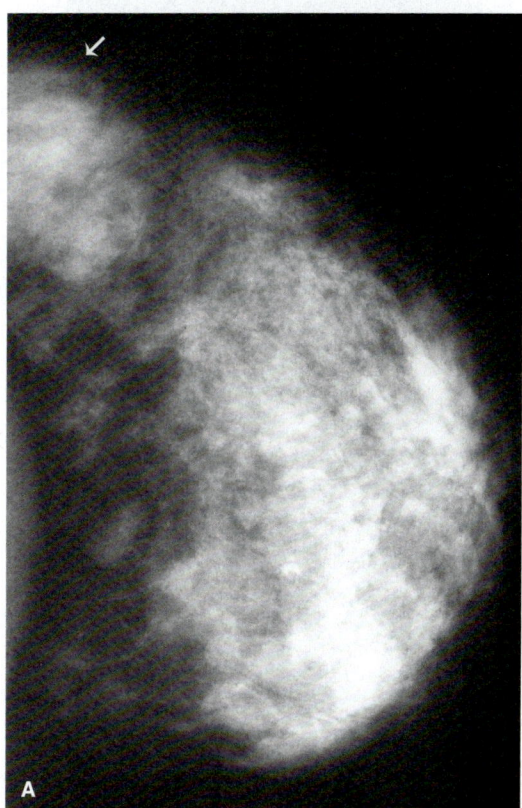

is suboptimal, the usefulness of the PNL measurement is limited. The distance from the nipple to the anterior edge of the muscle is measured on the MLO view. The distance from the nipple to the edge of the film is then measured on the CC view (Fig. 2.18B, C). These two measurements should be within 1 cm of each other. If the PNL measures 10 and 8 cm on MLO and CC views, respectively, posterior tissue is excluded on the CC view and it should be repeated (Fig. 2.18E) (7,8).

EXAGGERATED CRANIOCAUDAL VIEWS

There are two indications for XCCL views. In the screening setting, when tissue extends to the edge of the film on the CC view after the lateral tug is done, and tissue is seen projecting over the upper aspect of the pectoral muscle on the MLO view, an XCCL view is done to image lateral breast tissue in the craniocaudal projection (Fig. 2.19). In the problem-solving setting, the XCCL projection can be combined with spot compression to evaluate potential lesions in the lateral aspect of the breast (Fig. 2.20).

Factors to consider in positioning women for an XCCL view are listed in Table 2.6.

In positioning for an XCCL view, the woman is asked to rotate slightly so that the digital detector is placed at the mid-axillary line. The tube may need to be angled slightly so that the compression paddle clears the humeral head (7). The tube should not, however, be angled more than 5 degrees and the patient should not be leaning back; otherwise, a shallow oblique rather than a CC view is obtained. If the pectoral muscle seen on the XCCL is prominent, convex, and bulging (like what is seen on MLO views), it is likely that the tube was angled more than 5 degrees or the patient had leaned back during positioning, and the image represents a shallow oblique and not an XCCL view. Factors

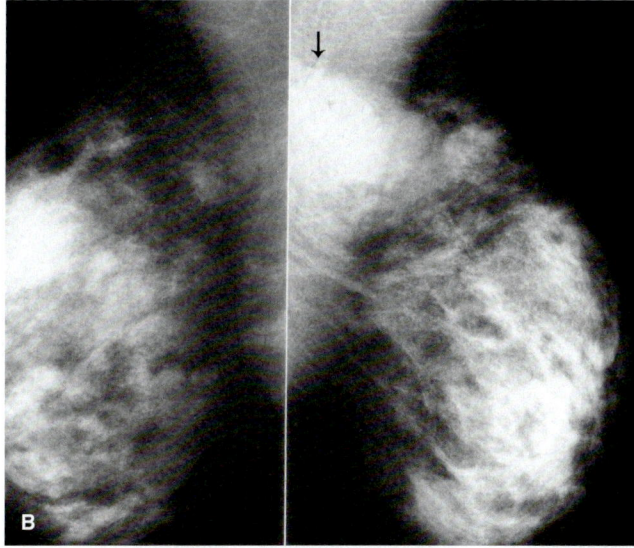

FIG. 2.19 • **XCCL view.** Left CC **(A)** and MLO **(B)** views. Glandular tissue is seen to the edge of the film on the CC view (*arrow*). On the MLO view dense tissue is noted superimposed on the left pectoral muscle. Although the lateral tug may add some additional lateral tissue on the CC view, it is unlikely to include this relatively sizeable island of accessory tissue. An XCCL is indicated in this patient on the left. **C:** Left XCCL view. On this image the accessory tissue can be evaluated in the CC projection. Retroglandular fat is now seen (*thick arrow*). A small amount of pectoral muscle (*thin arrows*) is included on all well-positioned XCCL views. (From Cardeñosa G. *Breast Imaging* [*The Core Curriculum Series*]. Philadelphia, PA: Lippincott Williams & Wilkins; 2003.)

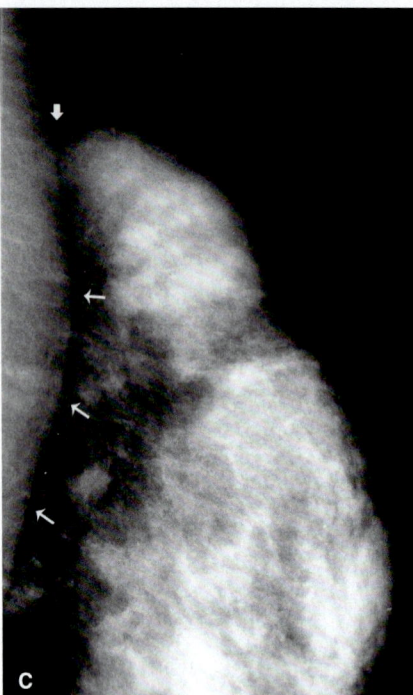

FIG. 2.19 • (continued)

Table 2.6	**FACTORS TO BE CONSIDERED IN POSITIONING FOR XCCL VIEWS**

Rotate patient slightly
   Digital receptor is placed at mid-axillary line
Angle x-ray tube but not more than 5 degrees
   (to clear humeral head)
Do not lean patient back

COMPRESSION AND THE USE OF ANTERIOR COMPRESSION VIEWS

Maximal tissue compression is ideal for optimal image quality (7,8). As breast tissue is thinned, optimal exposure with lower radiation doses is facilitated and scatter radiation, a deterrent to optimal contrast, is reduced. Immobilization of the breast minimizes geometric unsharpness and, as tissue is thinned, superimposition is decreased so that lesions become more apparent. Detrimental effects on image quality related to inadequate compression are listed in Table 2.7. These effects can be localized or involve the entire image (Figs. 2.21 through 2.28).

In evaluating images for blurring, it is important to prepare your brain to see it; otherwise it may go undetected. In other words, when reviewing images, specifically ask yourself: is the trabecular pattern sharp (Fig. 2.21)? Is the pectoral muscle edge sharp (Fig. 2.21)? If there are vessels or calcifications, are they sharp (Fig. 2.24)? Also evaluate those areas in which compression may be compromised, specifically, the subareolar areas and the tissue just above the IMF on MLO views, particularly if the breast is sagging. If you see areas of uneven exposure or skinfolds, consider the possibility of suboptimal exposure and review the underlying tissue specifically looking for blurring.

Recognizing potential factors that can limit compression is important in preventing suboptimal studies and troubleshooting blurry images. Potential limiting factors to adequate compression include patient issues (e.g., pain, body habitus), breast thickness, prominent pectoral muscles, inclusion of other body parts (upper arm, chin, abdomen) on the image, skinfolds, technique used for exposure, and aging compression paddles.

The technologist needs to work closely with the patient. The importance of compression is explained to the patient and the amount of time compression lasts is approximated. The patient is made to feel in charge of how much compression is applied and is asked to let the technologist know when she finds compression uncomfortable so it can be stopped (7). If the patient's breast discomfort is cyclical, scheduling the exam when her breast tissue is less sensitive may be helpful. Alternatively, the patient can try taking an analgesic half-an-hour to an hour prior to the mammogram so as to decrease any associated discomfort.

The breast is a conical structure with the base being the thickest part. Consequently, as compression is applied, the base of the breast is what limits compression such that tissue in the anterior aspect of the breast may be inadequately compressed (Figs. 2.23 and 2.26). Likewise,

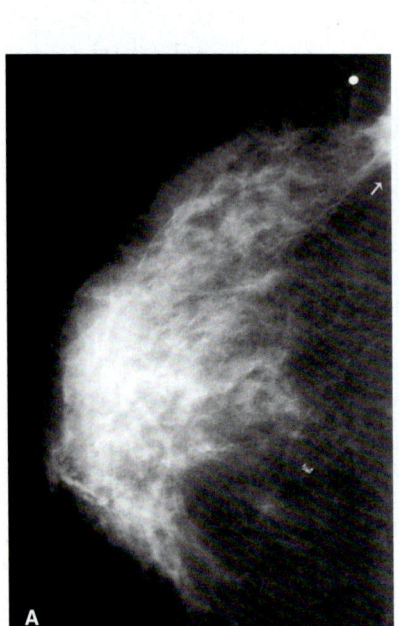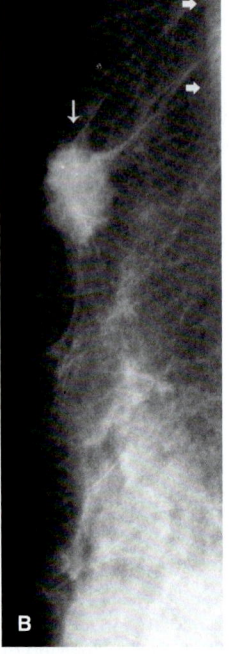

FIG. 2.20 • **XCCL view. Invasive ductal carcinoma.** Left CC **(A)** and XCCL **(B)** views. A mass (*arrow*) is partially seen laterally on the CC view (*arrow*). The mass (*thin arrow*) is imaged in its entirety on the XCCL view. Retroglandular fat is now seen. On a well-positioned XCCL view, a small amount of pectoral muscle is seen (*thick arrows*). (From Cardeñosa G. *Breast Imaging* [*The Core Curriculum Series*]. Philadelphia, PA: Lippincott Williams & Wilkins; 2003.)

Table 2.7	**ASSESSING ADEQUACY OF COMPRESSION**

Blurring (motion) (Fig. 2.21)
Uneven exposure (Figs. 2.7B and 2.22)
Inadequate exposure
Poor separation of parenchymal densities (Fig. 2.23)
Interposition of other body parts in the image (Fig. 2.26)

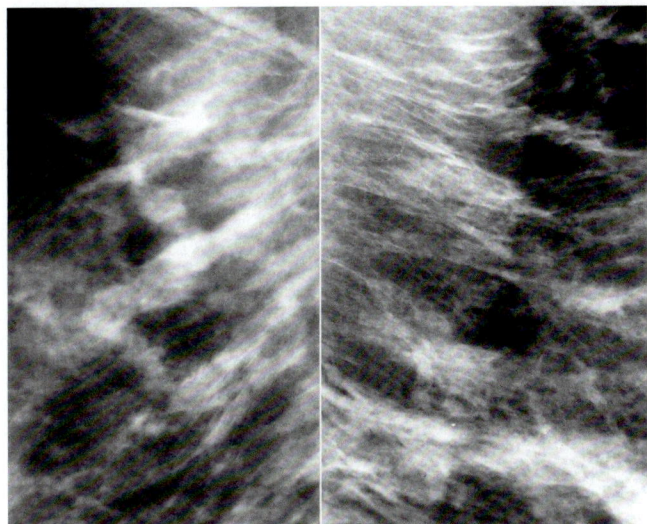

FIG. 2.21 • **Geometric unsharpness (blur, motion).** MLO views photographically coned to the upper portion of the images. Compare the trabecular pattern and pectoral muscle edges on these two images. The trabeculae and pectoral muscle edge are blurred on the right. Note the apparent loss of contrast on the right. Our brains perceive blur as an apparent loss of contrast (also see Figs. 2.24 and 2.37). Adequate compression and working with the patient are critical in minimizing the likelihood of motion. (From Cardeñosa G. *Breast Imaging* [*The Core Curriculum Series*]. Philadelphia, PA: Lippincott Williams & Wilkins; 2003.)

in women with prominent pectoral muscles, a thick muscle may limit compression of anterior tissue. In these women, obtaining an anterior compression view may be indicated so that evaluation of anterior tissue is optimized. Since the technologist is in the room with the patient, she can evaluate to see if anterior tissue is doughy (as opposed to taut) in which case she will obtain one or as many anterior compression views needed for the individual patient. For anterior compression views, the compression paddle is moved forward off the base of the breast, or the pectoral muscle, so that maximal compression of anterior tissue is

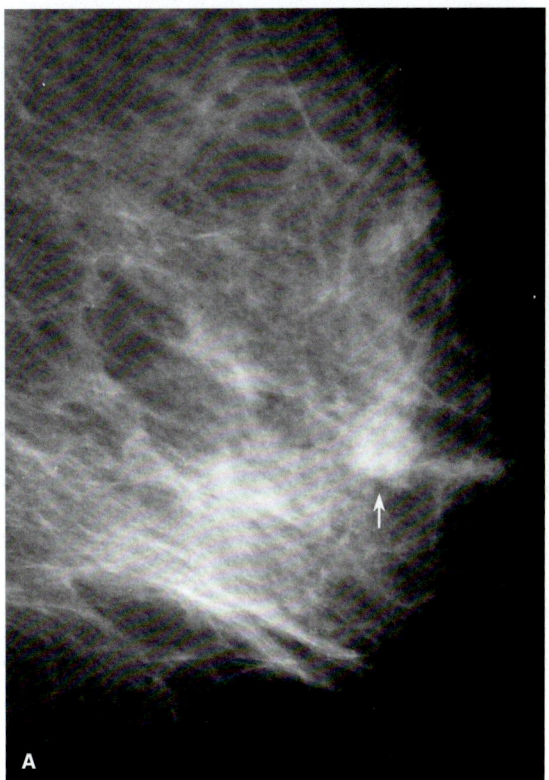

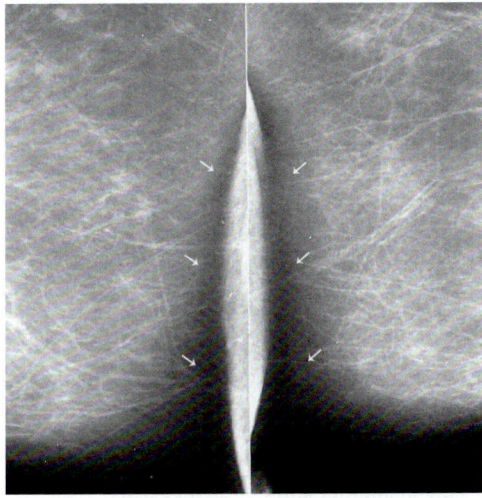

FIG. 2.22 • **Uneven exposure.** CC views photographically coned to the posteromedial aspect of the breasts. Areas of uneven exposure (*arrows*) are seen bilaterally secondary to skinfolds. When areas of uneven exposure are detected, compression is likely compromised and as such, the tissue in these areas needs to be evaluated specifically looking for motion (blur). (From Cardeñosa G. *Breast Imaging* [*The Core Curriculum Series*]. Philadelphia, PA: Lippincott Williams & Wilkins; 2003.)

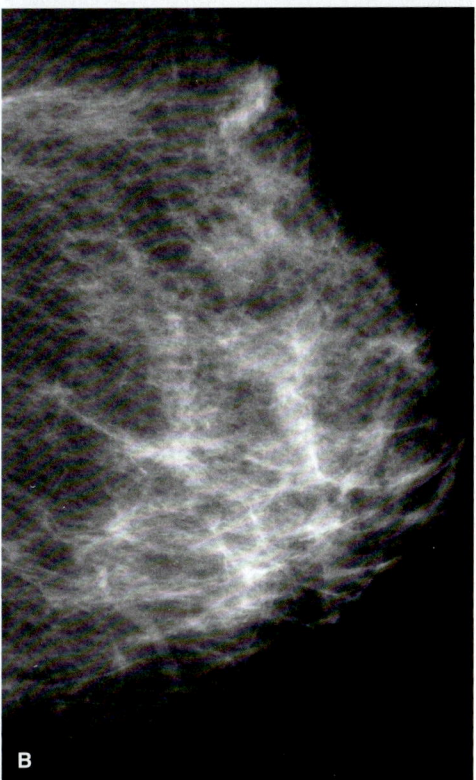

FIG. 2.23 • **Poor separation of parenchyma. A:** MLO view, left breast photographically coned to the anterior aspect of the breast. Poor separation of anterior tissue and a possible mass are noted (*arrow*). The tissue is also relatively underexposed. **B:** Anterior compression view obtained by the technologist at the time of the screening study. Parenchyma is now adequately compressed, exposure is improved, and no mass is present. A patient recall is averted. (From Cardeñosa G. *Breast Imaging* [*The Core Curriculum Series*]. Philadelphia, PA: Lippincott Williams & Wilkins; 2003.

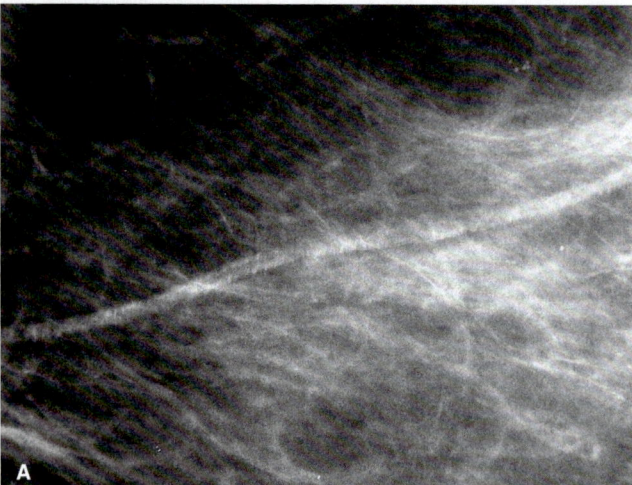 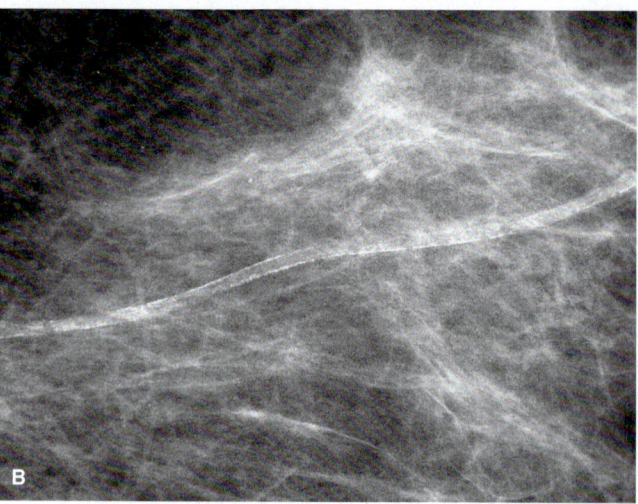

FIG. 2.24 • **Motion, effect on vascular calcification. A:** In evaluating this image consider contrast, the trabeculae, and the sharpness of the vessel included on the image. Can you state with confidence if there is calcification of the vessel wall? **B:** Repeat image with no motion demonstrates sharp vessel with associated mural calcification. Note the difference in contrast and the sharpness of the trabeculae in this image compared to that shown in part **A**. Do not settle for images with blur since calcifications and small masses can be "tomogramed" off the image as illustrated in this patient with vascular calcification. (From Cardeñosa G. *Breast Imaging* [*The Core Curriculum Series*]. Philadelphia, PA: Lippincott Williams & Wilkins; 2003.)

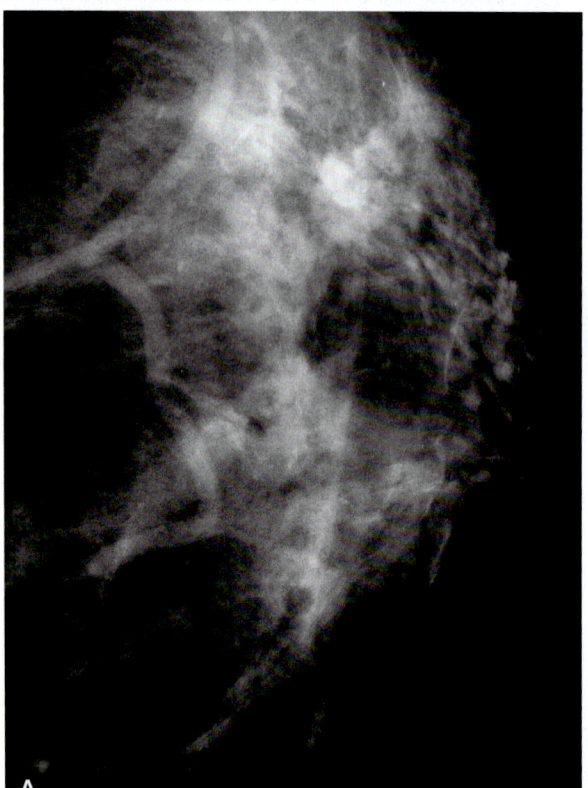 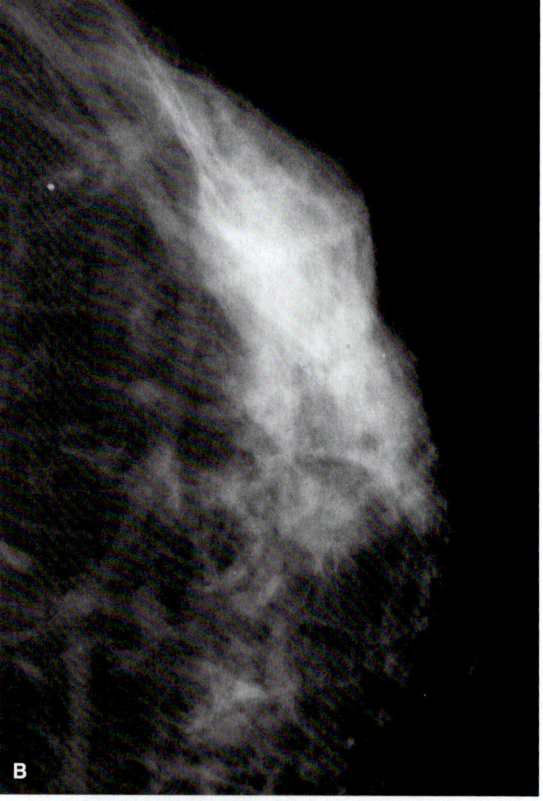

FIG. 2.25 • **Suboptimal compression and use of anterior compression view in identification of an invasive ductal carcinoma.** CC **(A)** and MLO **(B)** views (5.6 cm of compression) photographically coned to the anterior aspect of the left breast. The base of the breast is thick resulting in poor separation of the parenchyma anteriorly. **C:** Anterior compression (4.4 cm of compression) view in the CC projection obtained by the technologist as part of the screening study. A high-density mass (*arrow*) with indistinct margins is detected on this image and confirmed on spot compression views (not shown). Ultrasound-guided biopsy done to establish diagnosis. Optimal compression is critical to our ability to detect early potential curable breast cancer mammographically. (From Cardeñosa G. *Breast Imaging* [*The Core Curriculum Series*]. Philadelphia, PA: Lippincott Williams & Wilkins; 2003.)

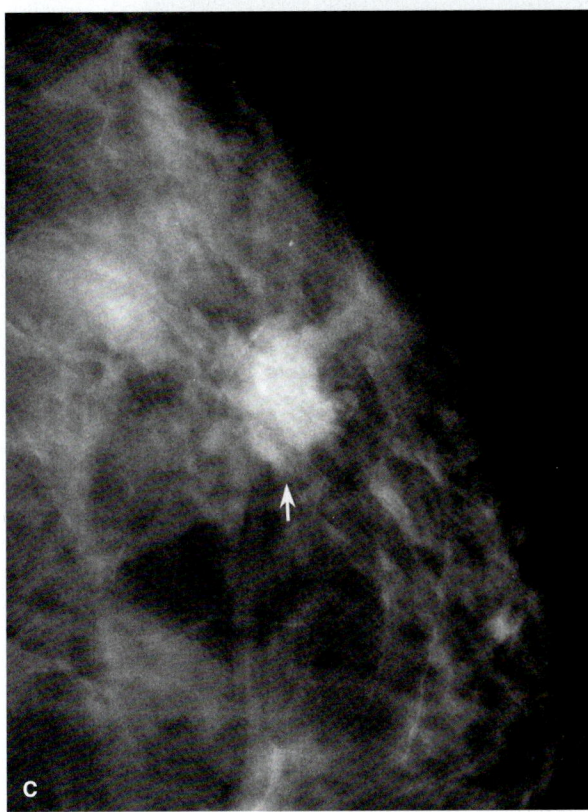

FIG. 2.25 • *(continued)*

obtained. In some patients, anterior compression views can be done using a spot compression paddle.

Interposition of other body parts (e.g., chin, arm on MLO views) between the compression paddle and the digital receptor can compromise compression and adequate positioning (Fig. 2.26A, B). Uneven exposures or blurring can be seen in these images limited to the upper portion of the breast on the MLO views. If the chin (Fig. 2.26) or arm is visible on the image, focus your attention on the adjacent breast tissue to ensure that image quality has not been compromised. If the breast is sagging (Figs. 2.27 and 2.28), too much abdomen (Fig. 2.28) is included on the image or a skinfold is seen posterolaterally on the MLO view, compression may be compromised particularly in the area of the IMF. Uneven exposure (Fig. 2.28) and blurring limited to tissue just above the IMF can sometimes be seen in these patients. Large skinfolds can also lead to inadequate compression and often result in uneven exposures.

IMAGING WOMEN WITH IMPLANTS

Women with implants have been included in the screening chapter because, unless these women have a specific sign or symptom that may indicate the presence of breast cancer (e.g., palpable finding, skin or nipple changes), we schedule them as screening studies. At some facilities, women with implants are done as diagnostics since a double set of images is required to adequately evaluate these patients. On the basis of the ACR practice guidelines on screening and diagnostic mammography (4), either one of these approaches is acceptable; the decision on how to schedule asymptomatic women with implants is left to the discretion of the imaging facility.

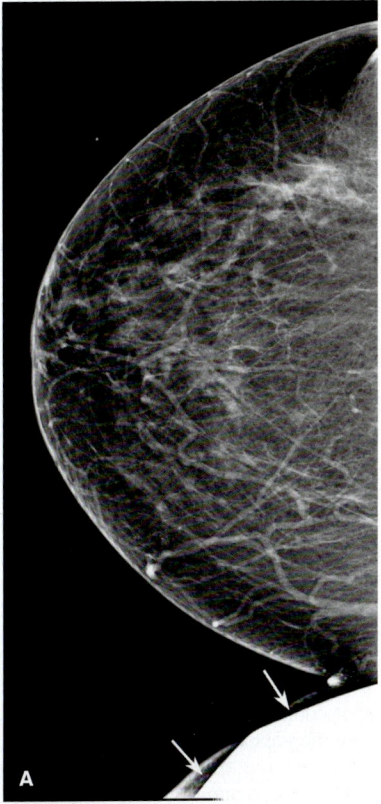
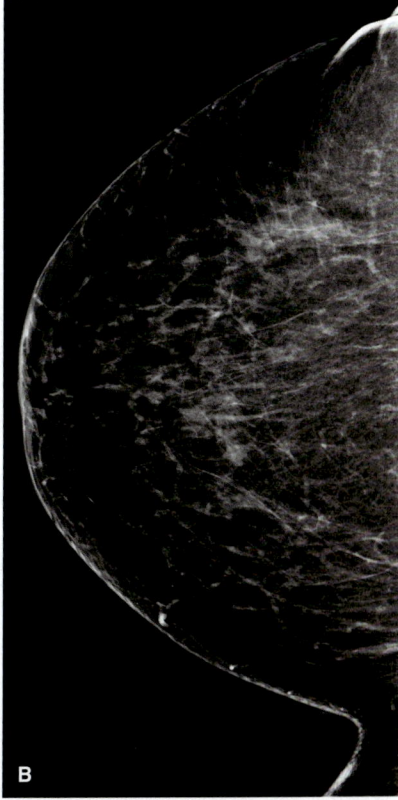

FIG. 2.26 • **Chin, limiting compression. A:** Right CC view with the patient's chin (*arrows*) projecting in the image medially. The inclusion of other body parts (abdomen, chin, upper aspect of the arm) in the image may preclude optimal compression. **B:** Repeat right CC view. Compression of the glandular tissue is improved and more posterior tissue is included in the image.

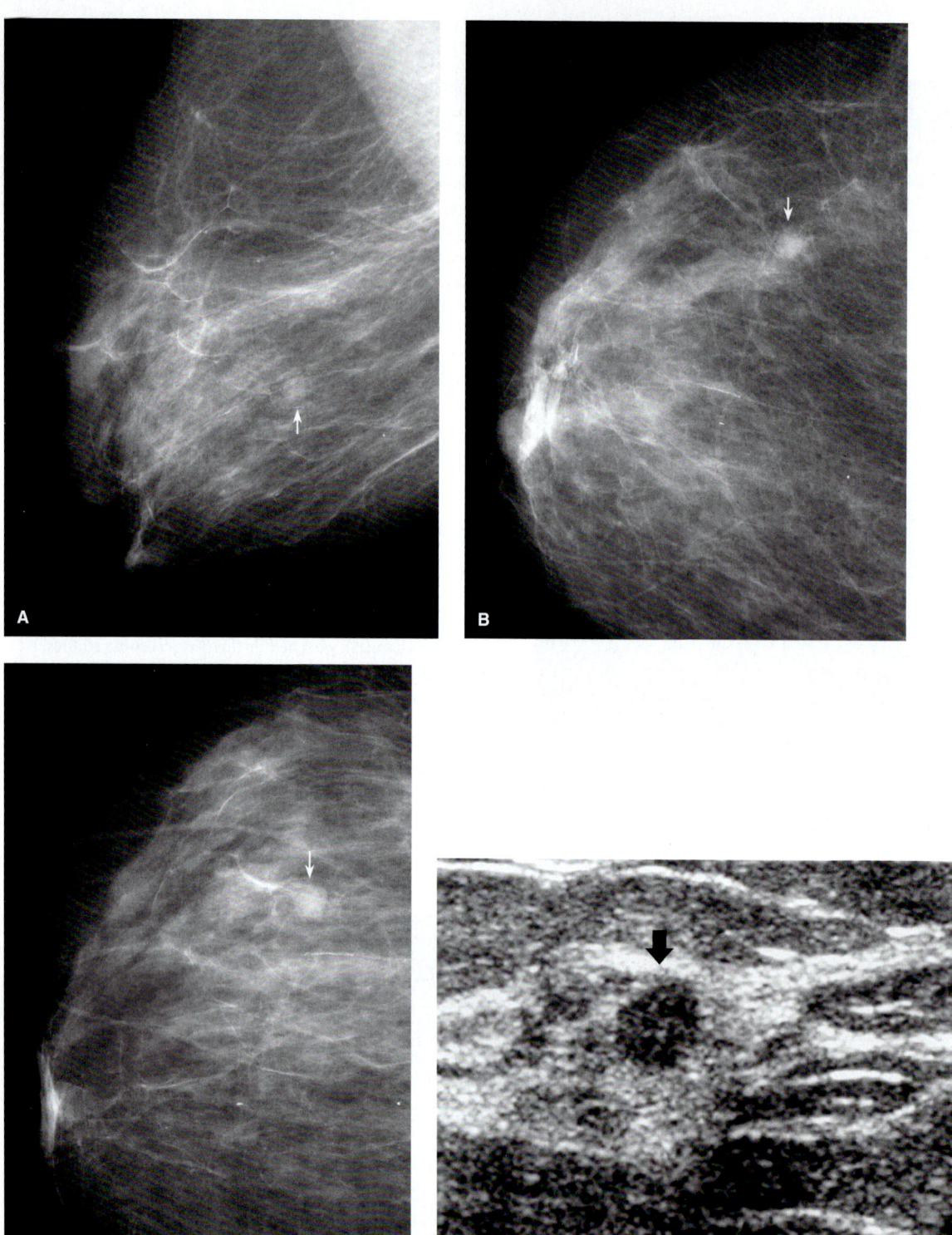

FIG. 2.27 • Sagging breast, suboptimal compression limiting ability to detect an invasive ductal carcinoma with ductal carcinoma in situ of the micropapillary and cribriform type, low nuclear grade. **A:** MLO view (compression = 7.5 cm, kV = 32, mAs = 122) in a 72-year-old patient photographically coned to the anterior aspect of the left breast. The breast is large, with a thick prominent pectoral muscle. The anterior aspect of the breast is sagging such that compression is likely suboptimal resulting in poor separation of the tissue anteriorly. A possible mass (*arrow*) may be present. **B:** CC view. Mass (*arrow*) is seen. This mass is new compared with prior studies (not shown). **C:** Anterior compression in the MLO projection (compression = 5 cm, kV = 27, mAs = 75) obtained by the technologist as part of the screening study (photographically coned to anterior portion of the breast). Anterior tissue is now optimally compressed. Mass (*arrow*) is apparent at the approximate location expected for what is seen on the CC view. Isodense mass with indistinct margins is confirmed on spot compression views (not shown). **D:** Round mass with indistinct margins (*arrow*) corresponding to the mass seen mammographically. A new solid mass in a 72-year-old patient warrants biopsy. Ultrasound-guided biopsy is done to establish the diagnosis of invasive ductal carcinoma with ductal carcinoma in situ of the micropapillary and cribriform type, low nuclear grade. (From Cardeñosa G. *Breast Imaging* [*The Core Curriculum Series*]. Philadelphia, PA: Lippincott Williams & Wilkins; 2003.)

Screening Mammography

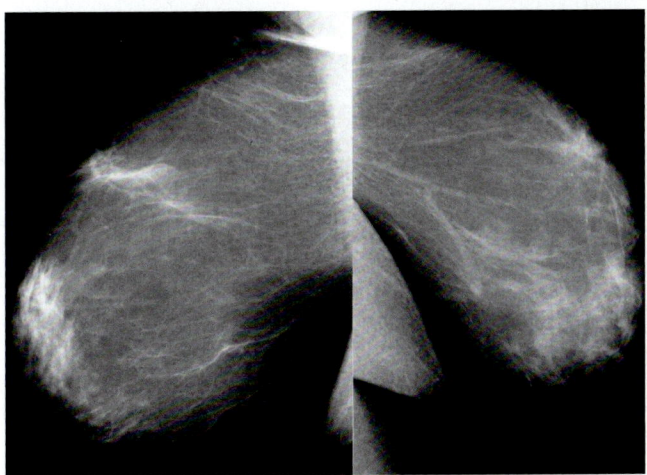

FIG. 2.28 • **Sagging of the breasts, inclusion of too much abdomen, and suboptimal compression.** MLO views demonstrate sagging of the breasts anteriorly, too much abdomen, and not enough pectoral muscle included on the images. Notice uneven exposure in the area of IMF consistent with suboptimal compression. Additional images needed for this patient in the MLO projection include anterior compression views and MLO views done to image superior tissue and axilla (e.g., include more muscle on the images). (From Cardeñosa G. *Breast Imaging* [*The Core Curriculum Series*]. Philadelphia, PA: Lippincott Williams & Wilkins; 2003.)

In women with implants, four views of each breast are done: CC and MLO views with the implants in the field of view and CC and MLO views with the implants displaced (ID) out of the field of view (Figs. 2.29 and 2.30). On the images done with the implant in the field of view, compression is limited by the implants, and so compression is applied mostly to immobilize the breast (6). Attempts to increase compression only serve to increase tissue superimposition and underexposure anteriorly as the implant impinges and pushes tissue out against the skin. On the implant in the field of view images, carefully evaluate the tissue surrounding the posterior aspect of the implants, particularly in women with subglandular implants, since this tissue may not be included on the ID views.

For ID views, the technologist pulls tissues out away from the implant as she pushes the implant back toward the chest wall. Compression is applied on the tissue with the implants out of the field of view (6). Depending on the location of the implants (e.g., subglandular or subpectoral), and the amount of encapsulation, variable amounts of tissue are imaged on implant displaced views (Figs. 2.29 and 2.30). As a general rule, more tissue is imaged when the implants are subpectoral in location. Tissue visualization may be limited significantly in women with subglandular implants, particularly those with encapsulated implants (see Fig. 11.49).

ARTIFACTS

Artifacts are defined as density variations in an image that do not reflect true attenuation differences in the patient. Artifacts with digital systems can originate from the equipment (Table 2.8), they can be related to software processing (Table 2.9), or to the patient (Table 2.10) (12). Except for patient-related artifacts, some of the others may vary depending on detector technology and manufacturer.

The detectors are intended to operate within the temperature range specified by the equipment manufacturer. Field inhomogeneity can result if imaging is attempted before the detector reaches the temperature specified by the manufacturer. Detector-related artifacts include ghosting, gouging, and horizontal line artifacts. Ghosting results when the latent image from the last exposure is superimposed on a newly acquired image; recalibration is needed to resolve this artifact. With some units, if the detector array is inadvertently damaged, the

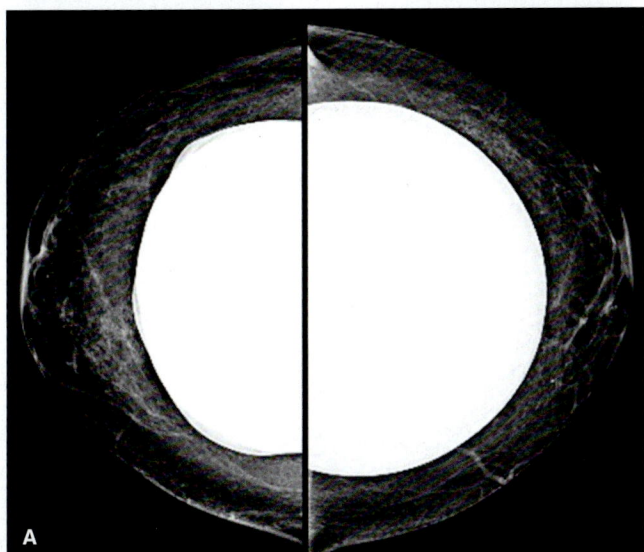

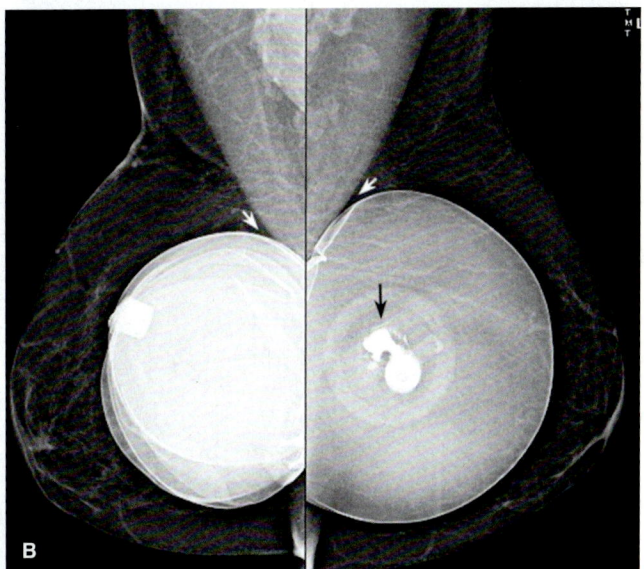

FIG. 2.29 • **Screening study in a woman with implants in a subglandular location.** CC **(A)** and MLO **(B)** views with saline implants in the field of view. The right implant is smaller than the left with minor contour changes and more wrinkles (partially collapsed). On the oblique views, the pectoral muscles (*white arrows*) are noted deep to the implants superiorly. Also note dense calcification (*black arrow*) associated with the valve on the left implant. CC **(C)** and MLO **(D)** ID views. On the oblique views, part of the implants and the implant valves are seen. When the implants are subglandular in location, only a small amount of the pectoral muscles is included on the ID images and the muscles often take on a triangular shape superiorly. Since in many of these women only a small amount of muscle is included on the MLO ID views, the shape of the breasts may simulate the shape of the breasts on CC views.

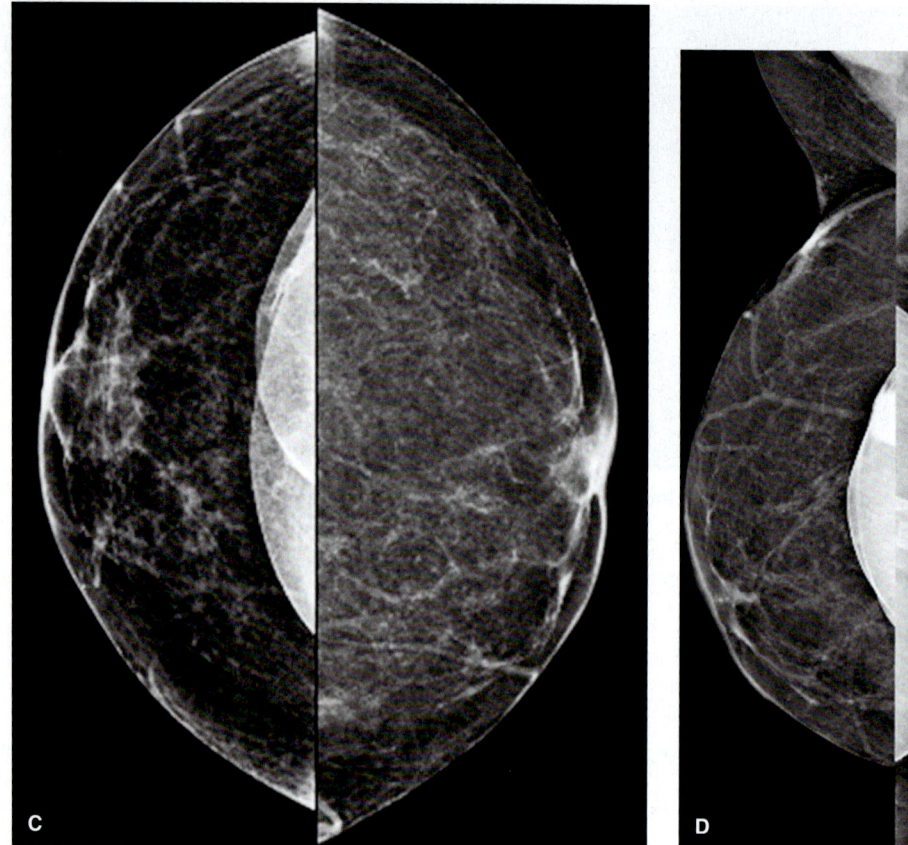
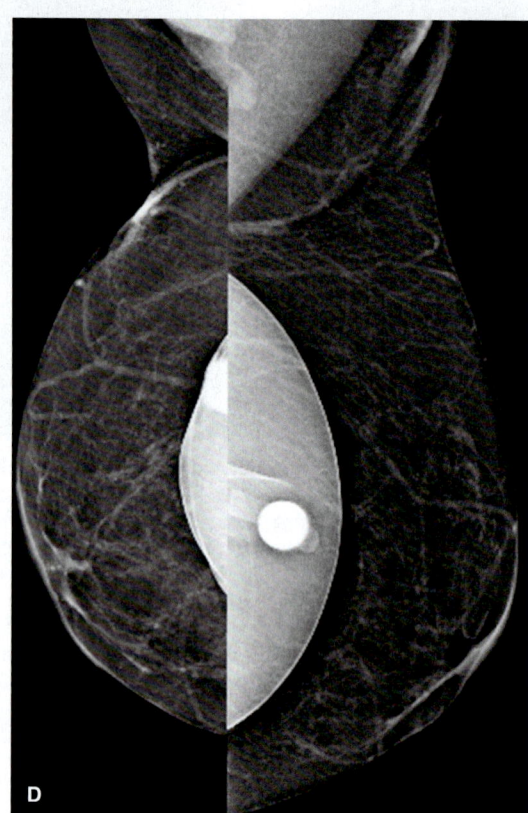

FIG. 2.29 • *(continued)*

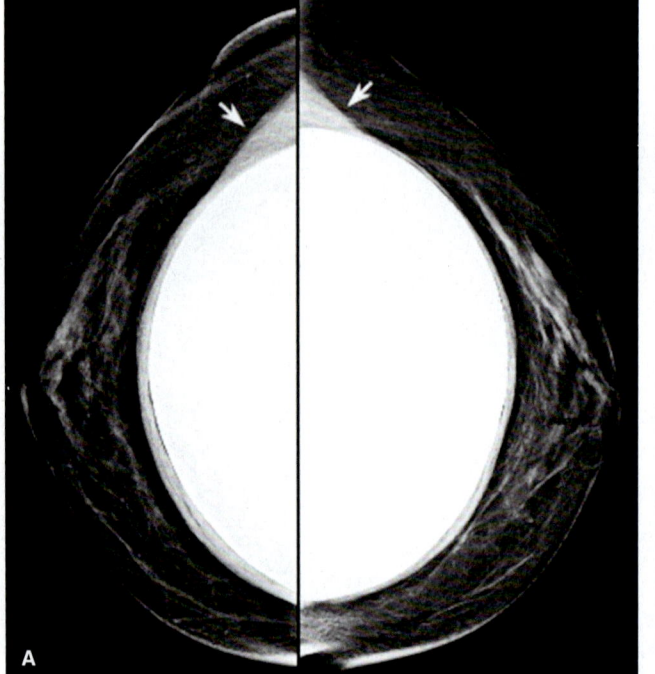
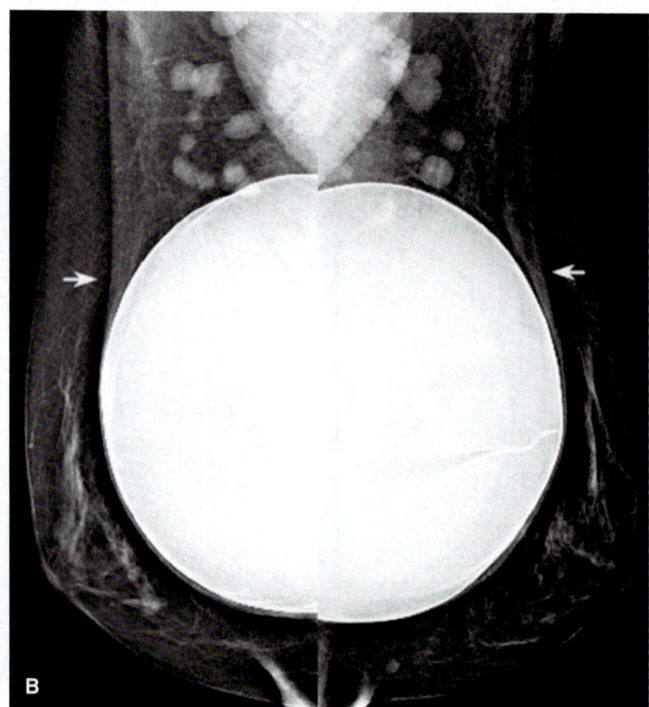

FIG. 2.30 • **Screening study in a woman with implants in a subpectoral location.** CC **(A)** and MLO **(B)** views with saline implants in the field of view. A slip of the pectoral muscle (*arrows*) is seen draped over the superior aspect of the saline implants and can be seen surrounding the implants on the craniocaudal views. Do not mistake the pectoral muscle for a capsule. Unless calcified, the capsule is not apparent mammographically. Also, note multiple lymph nodes in the axillae. CC **(C)** and MLO **(D)** ID views. When the implants are in a subpectoral location, glandular tissue can usually be evaluated optimally. Notice that the contour of the breasts particularly on the oblique views is similar to that seen in women who do not have implants. In some patients, the implants may not be seen on the displaced views at all. Note the implant valve (*arrow*) seen on the left oblique ID view.

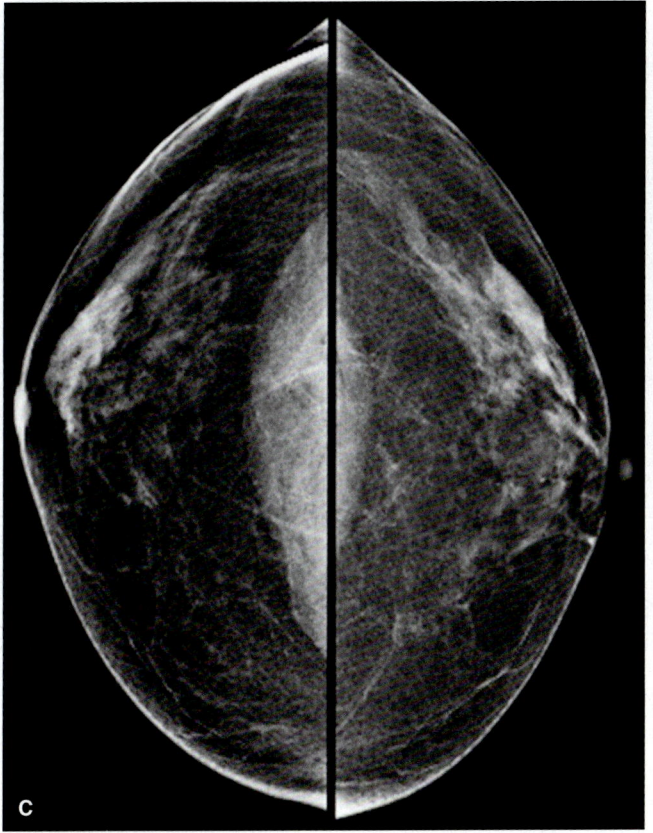
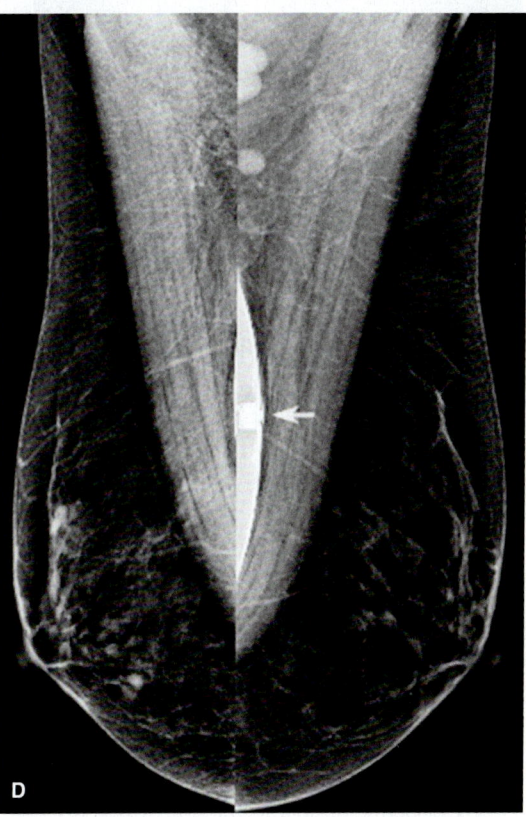

FIG. 2.30 • *(continued)*

Table 2.8 **EQUIPMENT-RELATED ARTIFACTS**
Field inhomogeneity
Detector-related
Ghosting
Gouging
Horizontal line artifacts
Collimator misalignment
Underexposure
Grid (lines, malpositioning, not used)
Vibration artifact
High-density materials on paddle or surface of detector

Table 2.10 **PATIENT-RELATED ARTIFACTS**
Motion (blur)
Deodorant
Talc on skin
Hair, hair products
Jewelry (nipple rings, ear rings)
Tattoos
Other body parts projecting on image
Pacemaker
Central venous catheters

Table 2.9 **SOFTWARE PROCESSING–RELATED ARTIFACTS**
High density
Breast within a breast
Loss of edge
Vertical processing bars

indentations (gouges) on the array result in an inhomogeneous field with circular artifacts noted corresponding to the sites of gouging on the array (12). If this occurs, the detector needs to be replaced. A horizontal line artifact will be apparent on the images if there is a defective line of pixels or incorrect readout of the data. Since this results in the elimination of potentially diagnostic information, this artifact needs to be recognized and addressed effectively. Calibration of the unit may be sufficient; however, if it persists, servicing is indicated, since the detector may need to be replaced.

Additional equipment-related artifacts include collimator misalignments, grid-related issues (lines, malpositioned or inadvertently not used), vibration, underexposure, and high-density objects on the surface of the detector or compression paddle (12). Misalignment of the collimator with respect to the detector results in a vertical white line of variable thickness depending on the degree of misalignment. It is most commonly noted affecting images along the chest wall edge (Fig. 2.31) where it potentially impacts diagnostic information; however, it can involve any edge of the image. As with film-screen mammography, if the grid slows down, grid lines (Fig. 2.32) may be seen on digital images and the pattern of the lines depends on the configuration of the grid. If the grid is not used, scatter radiation can result in suboptimal images with field inhomogeneity. Alternating black and white thick horizontal lines may be seen secondary to electrical interference on the data

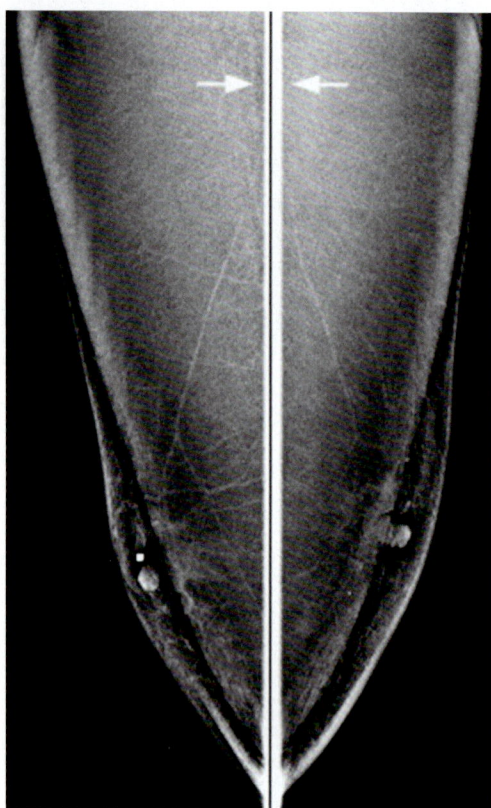

FIG. 2.31 • **Collimator misalignment.** MLO views in a man. Thin solid white line (*arrows*) along the chest wall side of the detector on both images, more prominent on the left MLO, reflects a misalignment of the collimator with respect to the detector.

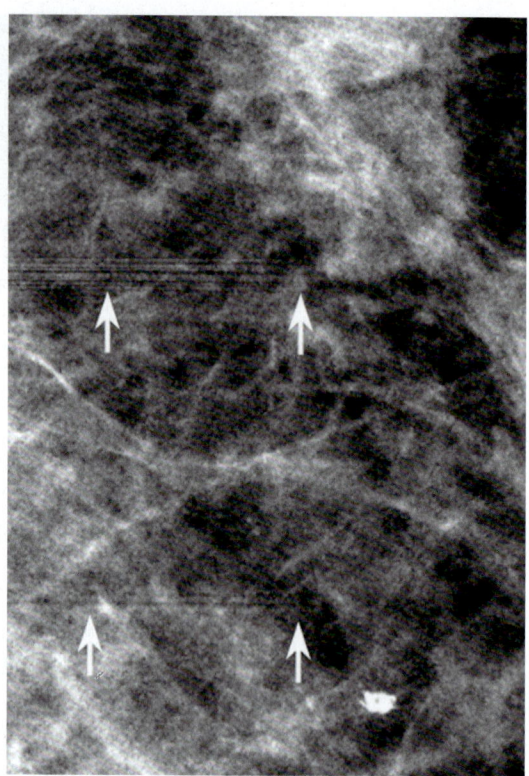

FIG. 2.33 • **Vibration and electrical interference–related artifacts.** CC view photographically coned to the posterolateral aspect of the left breast. Clusters of a random number of black lines (*arrows*) randomly spaced along the chest wall portion of the image reflecting vibration artifact. If this artifact is intermittently seen affecting images done on a single unit, the array may need to be changed.

readout resulting from the vibration of the cooling fans in the detector (Fig. 2.33). When the SNR is low, as a result of underexposure, the image has a distinctive "salt and pepper"–like appearance (Fig. 2.34). Dark speckled areas are seen scattered throughout the image. Photocell cell placement and the technical factors used for exposure need to

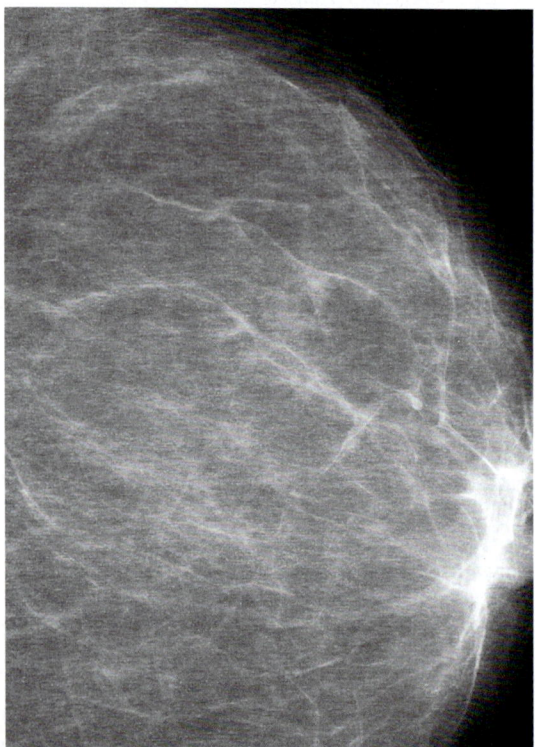

FIG. 2.32 • **Artifact.** Grid lines related to a malfunction of the grid. (From Cardeñosa G. *Breast Imaging* [*The Core Curriculum Series*]. Philadelphia, PA: Lippincott Williams & Wilkins; 2003.)

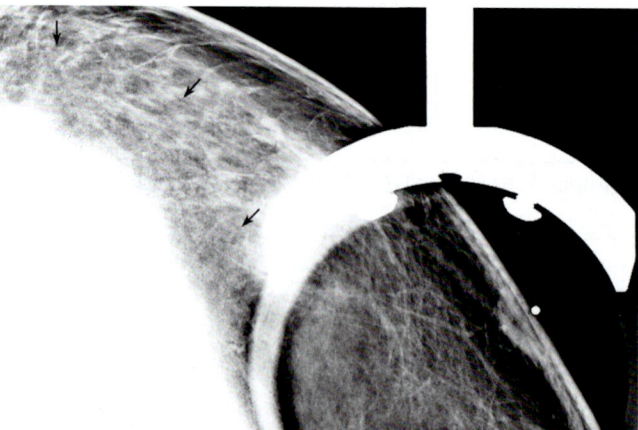

FIG. 2.34 • **Underexposure effect.** Spot tangential view of a palpable finding. The metallic BB denotes the palpable finding. On physical examination this correlates to a sebaceous cyst. Note the underexposed tissue adjacent to the edge of the spot compression paddle. A "salt and pepper" appearance (*arrows*) is seen resulting from the underexposure of the tissue at the edge of the paddle.

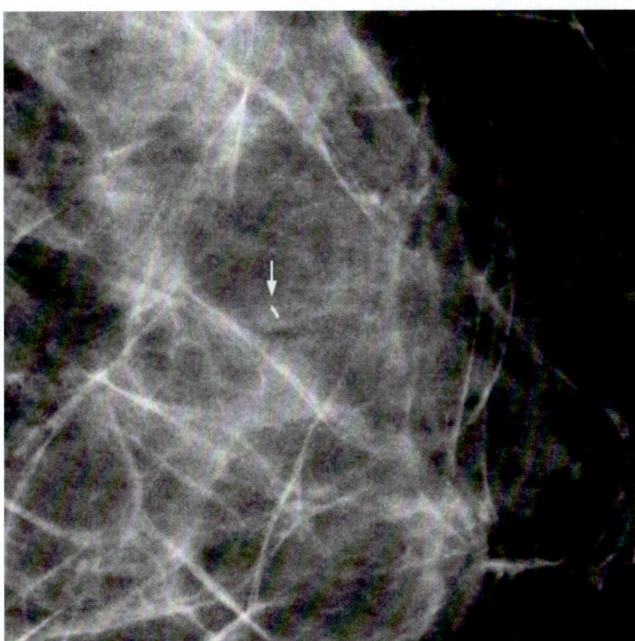

FIG. 2.35 • **High-density object on compression paddle.** CC view photographically coned to highlight artifact. As you are reviewing images, be vigilant for the presence of subtle artifacts like this one that repeat among patients. This linear, high-density artifact (*arrow*) was noted on the images for several different patients. It was identical in appearance and location on the images. All of the patients who had images with the artifact were done in the same mammography room. After meticulous inspection of the surface of the detector and the compression paddle, a metal shaving was identified on the compression paddle.

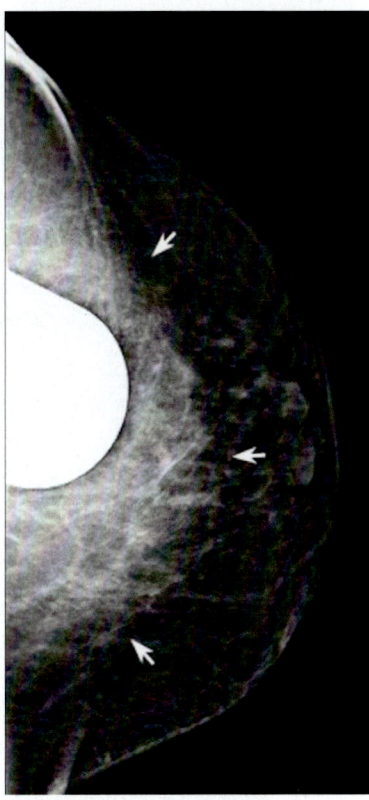

FIG. 2.36 • **"Breast within a breast" artifact.** From-below (FB) view of the left breast in a patient with a pacemaker. An abrupt change in the thickness of the breast can create an exaggerated and misleading boundary between the central and peripheral aspects (*arrows*) of the breast. This artifact can also be seen with abrupt changes in the density of the tissue.

be considered in troubleshooting and resolving this artifact. Any high-density object that is small and not easily noticed on the surface of the detector or compression paddle may be seen repeatedly on images done with the affected mammography unit or compression paddle (12). The artifact can be traced to the specific mammographic room (Fig. 2.35).

High density, breast within a breast, loss of edge, and vertical processing bars are some of the artifacts that can be seen attributable to software processing (12). High-density related artifacts do not impact interpretation, but they may be apparent when, for example, a spot compression view is done and the surrounding uncompressed tissue is thick and not penetrated or if there is a high-density object in the field. A "salt and pepper" appearance may be assigned to the high-density tissue or object (Fig. 2.34). The "breast within a breast" (not to be confused with the use of this term when referring to fibroadenolipomas) artifact is the result of an abrupt change in the thickness of the breast or in tissue composition such that the processing software creates an exaggerated and false boundary between the central and peripheral aspects of the breast (Fig. 2.36). This is more likely to be seen in women with large breasts or those with implants and easier to perceive in predominantly fatty breasts. If the imaging algorithm cannot properly detect the edge of the breast, loss of an edge may be noted affecting a part of the breast. Images need to be repeated only if the artifact potentially affects interpretation.

Patient-related artifacts are many and varied. As already discussed, motion is a significant problem because calcifications and small masses can be made imperceptible. Unless there are patient-related issues (e.g., stretcher-bound patient, Parkinson disease) precluding motion-free images, stop and have the images repeated rather than interpreting them (Fig. 2.37A, B). Deodorant is typically seen in the axillary regions (see Fig. 6.48A) and can simulate malignant-type calcifications. Women can be asked not to wear deodorant to their mammogram appointment, in which case, we give small stick deodorants to patients so they can use it after the mammogram is done. Alternatively, the woman can be asked to wipe the deodorant off at the time of the study. Other patient-related artifacts include hair (Fig. 2.37C), portions of the ear lobes, earrings, nipple rings (Fig. 2.37D), tattoos, talc or other products applied to the skin (see Fig. 6.48B), pacemakers (Fig. 2.37A), implanted defibrillators, and central venous catheter ports (see Fig. 11.19D). During positioning, other body parts (chin, portion of the upper arm on the MLO view) may be inadvertently included on the image (Fig. 2.26); these can sometimes limit compression so when seen, they should prompt careful evaluation for motion/blur.

SCREENING

Basically, screening is the search for unsuspected disease, and most screening mammograms are normal. When you consider all comers to a screening program, four to eight cancers can be expected per 1,000 screening mammograms. In contrast, the likelihood of malignancy among diagnostic patients is much higher. Screening and diagnostic studies should be approached differently. The purpose of screening is the detection of potential abnormalities, not characterization. So streamlining the screening process—batch interpretation of studies so that the radiologist is focused on the images with no interruptions—is important. There are different ways to increase the efficiency of the interpreting radiologist, maximize lesion detection, and minimize the

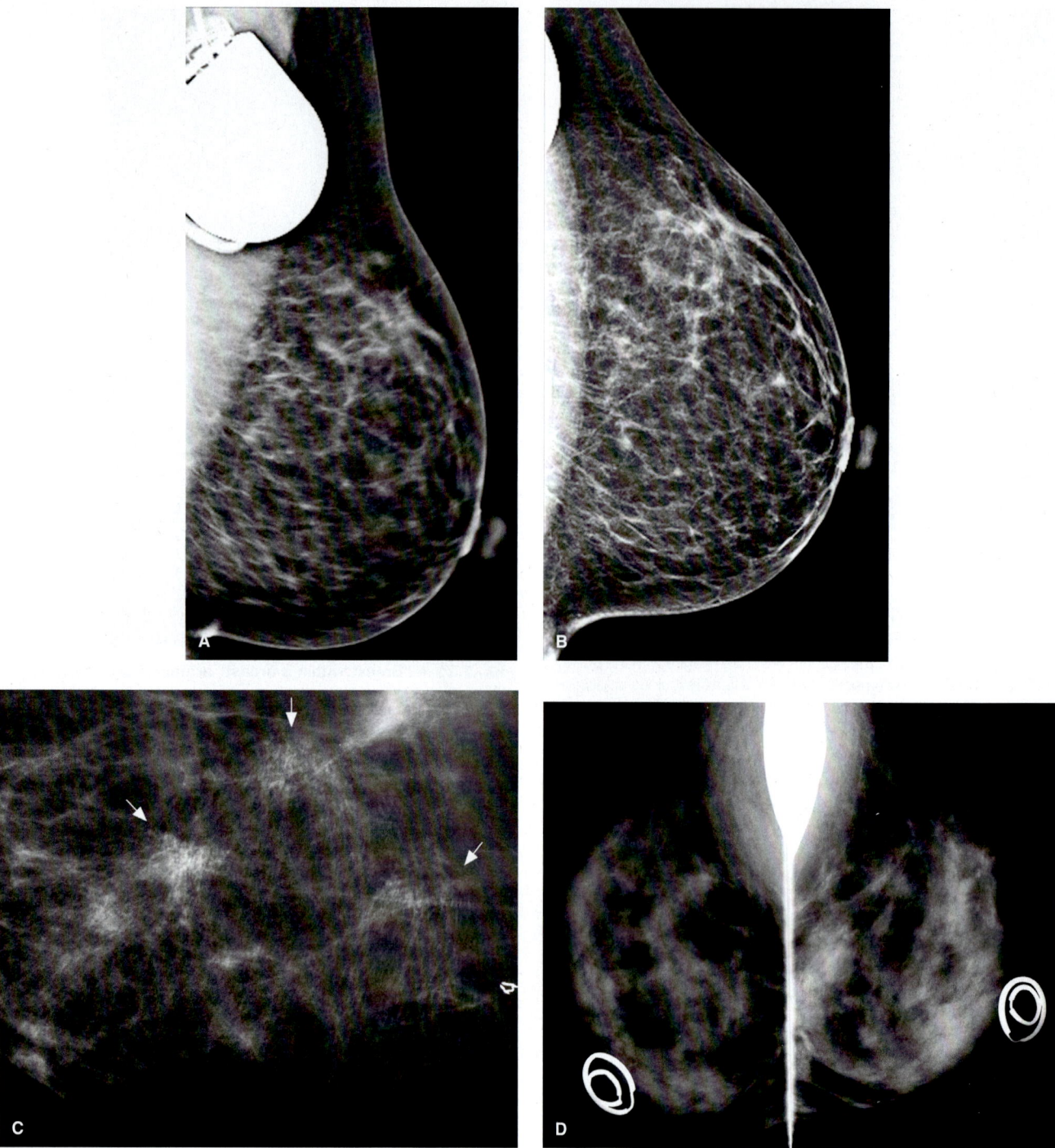

FIG. 2.37 • **Gross motion, likely pacemaker-related. A:** Left MLO view in a patient with a pacemaker. The pacemaker is partially imaged superimposed on the pectoral muscle, possibly limiting compression of the tissue anteriorly. The trabecular markings, edge of the pectoral muscle, and the nipple are blurry as a result of gross motion. Note image contrast. **B:** Repeat MLO view focusing on the anterior aspect of the breast (e.g., coming off of the pacemaker). The trabecular markings and edge of the pectoral muscle are now sharp; also note the difference in contrast between the images. Our brains perceive blurriness, as a loss of contrast. **C:** CC view photographically coned to the medial aspect of the left breast. An irregular swirling pattern of thin white lines (*arrows*) is detected medially in the left breast. When seen, hair is almost always noted posteromedially on the CC views. As the patient is positioning for the CC views she is asked to turn her head away from the face shield, as she turns her head, hair can fall into the field of view. If the technologist is not vigilant in repositioning the hair, it may be seen as an artifact. Also noted at the edge of this image is a micromark biopsy clip. (From Cardeñosa G. *Breast Imaging* [*The Core Curriculum Series*]. Philadelphia, PA: Lippincott Williams & Wilkins; 2003.) **D:** MLO ID views. Nipple rings are noted. We do not ask women with nipple rings to remove them at the time of the mammogram. A portion of the implants is noted in a subpectoral location. (From Cardeñosa G. *Breast Imaging* [*The Core Curriculum Series*]. Philadelphia, PA: Lippincott Williams & Wilkins; 2003.)

number of women called back for additional studies. While a discussion of all the viable strategies is beyond the scope of this text, we will discuss some of the issues to consider.

Spatial, and if this is not possible, temporal separation of screening and diagnostic studies is encouraged; different tactics are used for each. One of the most critical ongoing tasks is the education of referring physicians and patients regarding the differences between screening and diagnostic studies. Screening is done in asymptomatic women. A radiologist does not need to monitor these studies or be on site when screening studies are done; in fact, if the process is to be efficient, it is best that a radiologist not be involved at the time the study is done. A set schedule with rapid throughput and minimal overhead costs is important for a screening program, particularly given the low reimbursement rates for this study type. The configuration of the mammography and dressing rooms is important in obtaining these goals. Ideally, the mammography room is not used as the dressing room. From the interpretation standpoint, it is more efficient to batch interpret the studies while providing a rapid turnaround time.

The online reading of screening studies while the patient is still in the breast center is not optimal. On a busy, hectic day with interruptions, a screening mammogram is not likely to get the time and attention it requires from the interpreting radiologist. A quick answer is not always the right answer. Additionally, since the patient is still in the environment, the tendency to do extra images is likely to be exercised by the interpreting radiologist. This calls into question the statistics and medical audit information on the screening program (e.g., are patients in whom "just one" extra image is done tracked as screening callbacks? And if so, how?). It is a mistake to set up the expectation that women having a screening mammogram will get their results at the time of the study. In contrast, diagnostic studies are done in patients who have a potentially abnormal screening mammogram or signs and symptoms possibly indicating the presence of a cancer. A radiologist should be available to monitor all diagnostic studies. Although discussed at greater length in Chapter 3, flexibility and the ability to see patients expeditiously is critical for the diagnostic program.

With respect to interpretation, we batch interpret all of our screening studies. The current study is reviewed with images from 2 and, if available, 4 years, previously. If the woman has multiple prior studies, these are all available to us so that, if needed, we can assess the evolution of potential findings easily. Current and past history forms are electronically available to us as are pathology reports on those patients who have had a previous breast biopsy. The viewing protocol is individualized but standardized for the radiologist. Ambient light and other distractions are eliminated. Paperwork is minimized and we use standardized ("canned") reports for our patients, including those with implants and for women in whom a potential abnormality is seen and additional evaluation or outside prior films are indicated.

We recommend annual screening mammography starting at age 40. For women with a high risk of breast cancer, we may start annual screening at age 30. Most of our patients are scheduled following referral from one of our clinical colleagues. However, we have chosen to see self-referred and self-requesting women. Self-referred women are those who have no identified primary health care provider. Although we do not encourage self-referral, we do see these patients and have a robust mechanism in place for referral if any abnormality is identified on the mammogram. The self-requesting woman provides the name of a primary health care provider, but the woman herself schedules the mammogram. We treat this group of patients as the self-referred women, if for some reason, the health care provider they list declines to accept the mammography report (e.g., we make referrals as needed based on any significant findings) (4).

VIEWING CONDITIONS

Viewing conditions must be considered and optimized prior to the evaluation of clinical images for potential abnormalities. A qualified medical physicist should test soft copy display devices used for interpretation regularly to ensure compliance with MQSA. The luminance of the monitor should be at least 400 cd/m^2 with greater than 450 cd/m^2 recommended for optimized contrast; at least an 8-bit luminance resolution is required (2). Depending on the luminance, consistency in the grayscale presentation of the images needs to be maintained. We have 5 megapixel monitors at all of the interpretation workstations and provide our technologists with 3 megapixel monitors in the mammography rooms. All images need to be viewed at 1:1 or 100% size as well as routinely zooming the image 200% to 2:1. Image displays systems must also be able to display: (a) computed aided detection (CAD) markings, (b) images in "true" size, and at the "same" physical size even though they may come from different acquisition stations, (c) annotated image information, image identification, and technical factor information, (d) a scale, (e) current and prior four-view screening studies, and (f) a black background outside of the breast even after contrast adjustments are made to the image (2). Current and prior studies should be easily and rapidly accessible with flexible hanging protocols as specified by the user. For mammography, no specifications are in place regarding the use of monochrome versus color displays. Efforts should be made to minimize glare and reflection; ambient light should be consistent and low, however, total darkness is not recommended. Room temperature should be adjustable to accommodate personal preferences and distractions should be minimized. Although expensive, adjustable, ergonomically focused desks and chairs are a worthwhile investment minimizing radiologist strain while increasing efficiency (2).

EVALUATION OF IMAGES

After ensuring optimal viewing conditions and as the starting point, evaluate images for overall quality (Fig. 2.38). As the radiologist, you set the height of the quality bar at your center: the higher you set it, the better the quality of the images generated at your facility. Set it high and watch your technologist rise to the occasion time and time again. Unless there is a specific patient-related reason for suboptimal images (e.g., patient is imaged on a stretcher, Parkinson disease, stroke, shoulder surgery limiting range of motion), do not interpret inadequate images and hide behind disclaimers. If tissue is excluded, or if there are other technical limitations (Fig. 2.39), the images need to be repeated, and it is your responsibility to have it done.

In evaluating screening images for potential abnormalities, consider adopting three basic principles: develop a standardized way of reviewing mammograms, prepare your brain to find abnormalities ("chance favors a prepared mind") in specific locations (13), and make no assumptions. I encourage you to evaluate the current study completely before looking at prior films. Although prior studies are useful (Fig. 2.40), they can sometimes create a false sense of security relative to findings that should be pursued, and would be pursued, if you didn't have prior studies (e.g., stability does not assure benignity). If you detect an area of distortion, or a mass with potentially spiculated margins, and the patient has *no* history of surgery or trauma specifically localized to the site of the distortion or mass, do not let stability talk you out of further evaluation. This is particularly true if only last year's study is used for the comparison.

After you determine that the films are of interpretable quality methodically, and in a standardized approach, review the images for

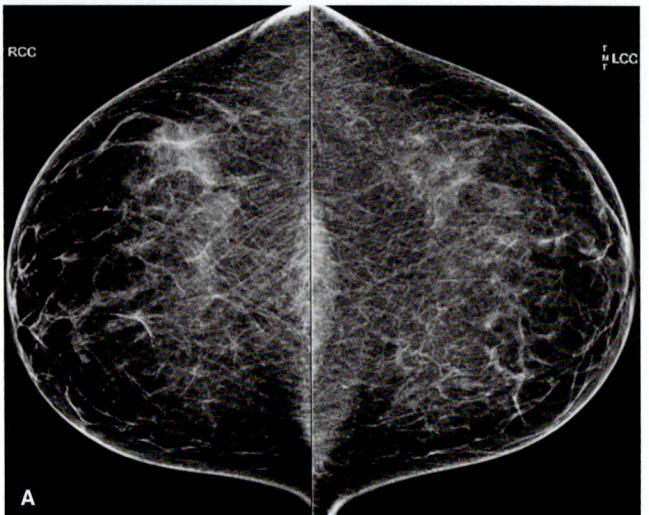
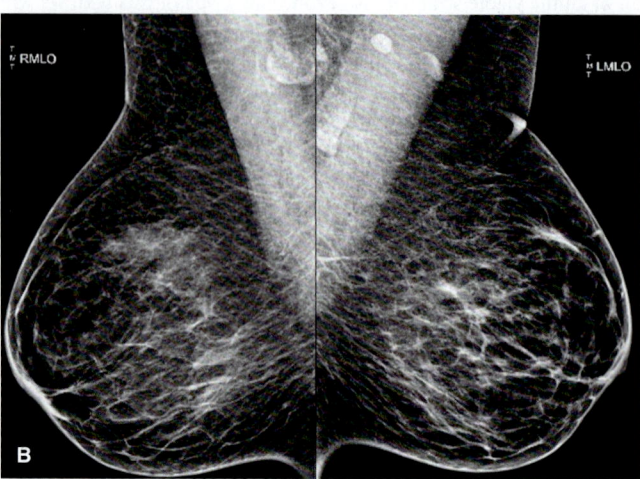

FIG. 2.38 • **Image quality, optimal.** CC **(A)** and MLO **(B)** views from a screening study. Assess image quality before focusing on finding potential abnormalities. In this patient, positioning is optimal in both projections. Labeling of the images is correct (not all included on what is shown). There is no motion. The tissue is adequately penetrated and contrast is high. A small skinfold is noted superiorly on the left MLO (this results from the technologist lifting the breast up as much as possible). Although not optimal, this does affect our ability to detect a potential abnormality. At this point, we start evaluating the images for possible abnormalities. Benign-appearing lymph nodes are noted in the axillae. BI-RADS 1: negative.

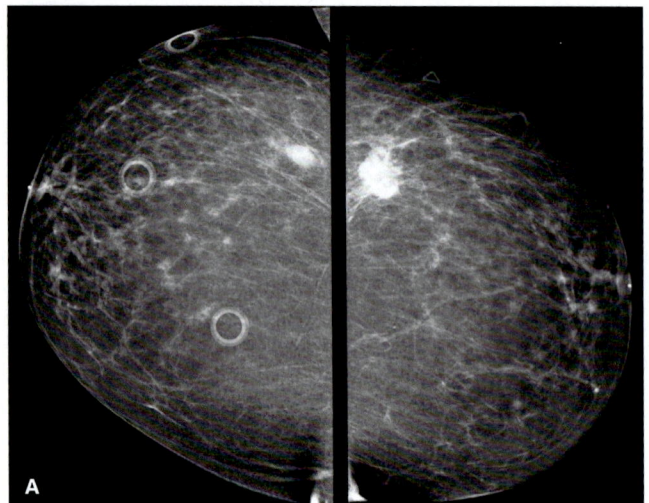
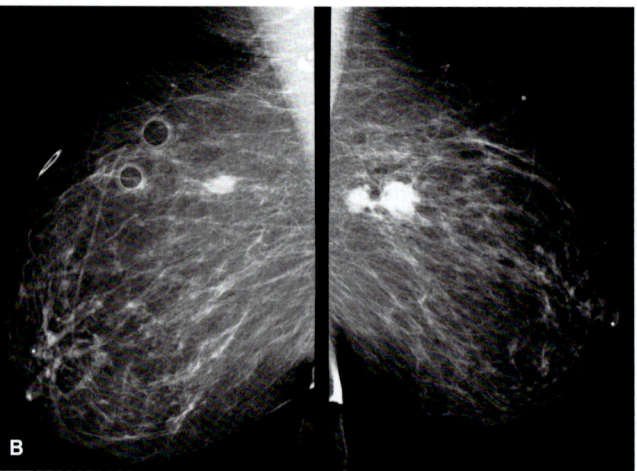

FIG. 2.39 • **Image quality, suboptimal.** CC **(A)** and MLO **(B)** views from a screening study. Radiopaque round markers used to denote skin lesions; also metallic BBs have been used to mark the nipples. Are these optimal images? Are you willing to put your name on these images? Can we do better? The technologist has not indicated any patient-related issues that might result in suboptimal positioning. As a starting point, review the MLO views. An insufficient amount of pectoral muscle is included on the images, particularly on the left. The breasts are sagging and there is uneven exposure just above the IMF bilaterally. In considering the CC views, no pectoral muscle is seen on either side and cleavage is not included even on the right CC, which is exaggerated medially (notice that right nipple is pointing laterally). Given the suboptimal positioning on the MLO views, posterior nipple line measurements are not necessarily accurate and yet there is almost 2 cm of posterior tissue excluded on the CC views. So much so that the second, slightly more posterior high-density mass imaged in the left MLO view is not included on the left CC view. When image quality is grossly suboptimal with no apparent explanation: STOP. Do not interpret images that can be improved and hide behind disclaimers. At the end of the day, you are responsible for the quality of the images you interpret. Repeat CC **(C)** and MLO **(D)** views of the left breast. Pectoral muscle is thicker in the axilla, extends to the level of the nipple, and has a convex contour anteriorly. The breast is lifted such that the IMF is included and open. Lymph nodes can now be seen in the left axilla. On the CC view, not only is the second lesion included on the image but almost a centimeter more tissue is included posterior to the lesion and although pectoral muscle is noted included, cleavage is seen. If screening mammography is going to be used effectively to diagnose early breast cancer, it is incumbent upon us, the radiologists, to demand the highest quality possible for our patients.

Screening Mammography

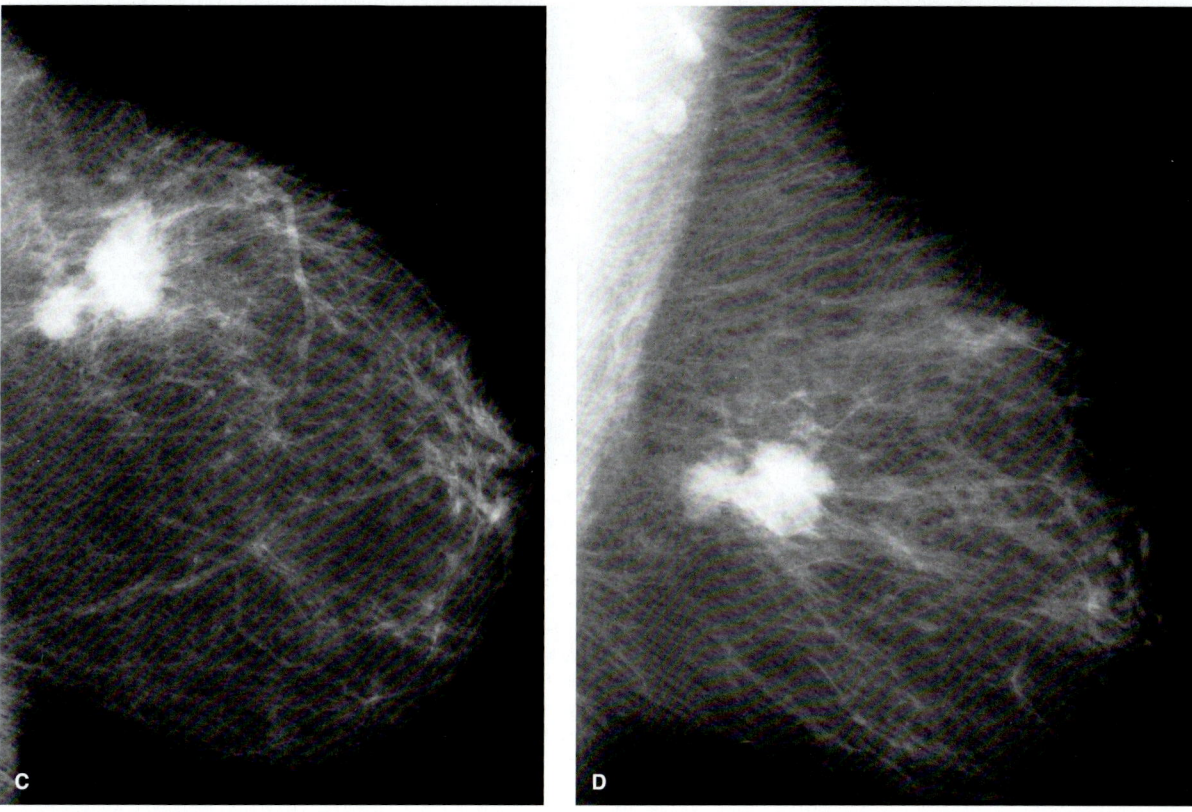

FIG. 2.39 • (continued)

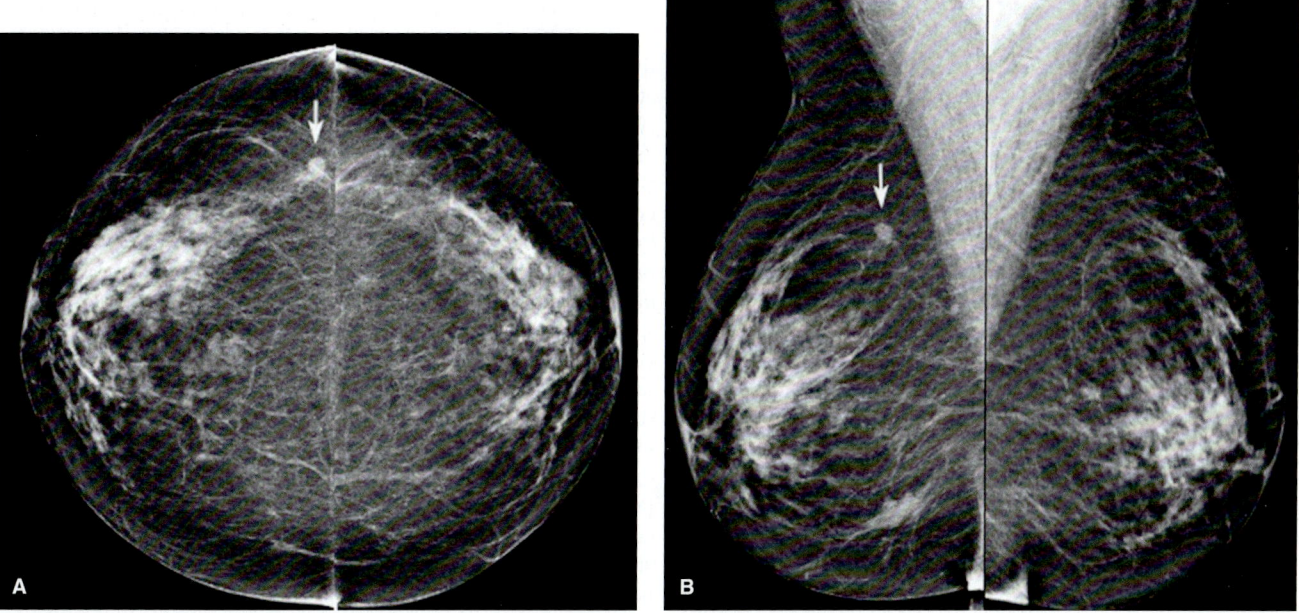

FIG. 2.40 • **Use of comparison study.** CC **(A)** and MLO **(B)** views from a screening study in a 62-year-old woman. **C:** MLO view, right breast 1 year previously. On the current study a mass (arrows) is identified in the CC view posterolaterally with a correlate identified superiorly in the MLO view. Given the location of this mass, a lymph node is a consideration; however, on close inspection no fatty notch is identified on either view, the margins do not appear circumscribed, and this is not seen previously. In a 62-year-old woman, a new mass with possibly spiculated and indistinct margins requires additional evaluation that will likely include biopsy. BI-RADS 0: need additional imaging evaluation. Please see Figures 3.11 and 4.39B for the additional studies done to evaluate this patient.

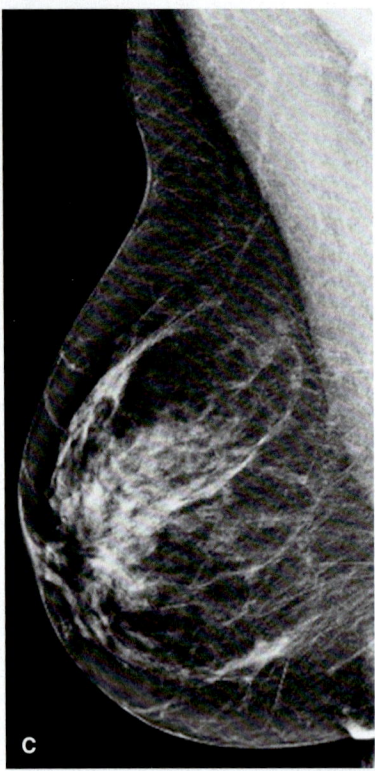

FIG. 2.40 • *(continued)*

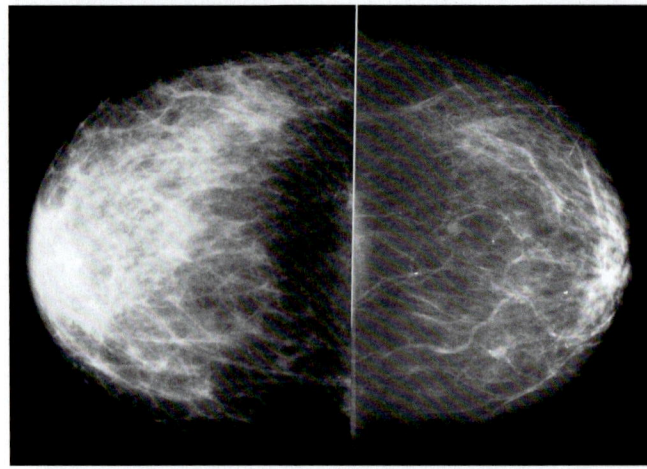

FIG. 2.41 • **Diffuse changes, right breast.** CC views. The right breast is larger and less compressible than the left. The overall density of the parenchyma is increased, as is the prominence of the trabecular markings. Diffuse changes may be readily apparent when unilateral but are more difficult to establish when bilateral. If you immediately focus your attention on finding a small mass or cluster of calcifications, diffuse changes may go undetected particularly if the findings are bilateral. Make a habit of reviewing the technical factors (centimeters of compression, kVp, mAs, angle of obliquity for the MLO) used for exposure particularly when you suspect a diffuse abnormality (in this patient for the right CC: compression = 47 mm, kVp = 28, mAs = 84.9; for the left CC: compression = 32 mm, kVp = 25, mAs = 45.2). The findings in this patient are related to fluid overload.

possible abnormalities. Start by looking at the images from a distance for gross findings (e.g., breast size, parenchymal asymmetry, diffuse change). As mentioned previously, prepare your brain for the detection of potential abnormalities. In evaluating the images from a distance, specifically ask yourself: are the breasts symmetric in size? Are there areas of parenchymal asymmetry? Is there skin thickening (focal, diffuse)? Are there diffuse changes (unilateral, bilateral)? If you are not actively looking for these things, or if you immediately focus your attention on finding a small cluster of calcifications, you are likely to overlook gross findings (Fig. 2.41). If you perceive asymmetry or possible diffuse changes, look at the technical factors used for exposure. How many centimeters of compression were used for each breast in each view? What kVp was used for the different images and what was the resulting mA for each? Compare the technical factors for the breast you think may be abnormal with those used on the other breast as well as the technical factors used on prior studies. Needless to say if the changes are bilateral, your ability to perceive diffuse changes is decreased unless you are specifically assessing the images for diffuse changes and comparing with prior studies (see Chapter 11 for additional discussion).

After evaluating the images from a distance, move in for a closer inspection. Using a magnifying lens (yes, even for digital images), scrutinize the images specifically looking for calcifications (Fig. 2.42), masses (Fig. 2.43), or distortion (Fig. 2.44; also see Figs. 8.22 and 8.45); don't sit passively waiting for the abnormalities to jump out at you or rely on CAD markings. Also, rather than viewing the entire image, systematically evaluate the upper, mid, and inferior portions of the breast on the MLO views and lateral, mid, and medial portions on the CC views (13). Go back and forth from one side to the other. If there are obvious findings, do not focus on them to the exclusion of the remaining tissue and contralateral breast. Obvious findings serve as distractors that keep us from identifying the small potentially curable cancers (Fig. 2.45; also see Figs. 8.37 and 8.45).

In addition to looking for specific findings, focus your attention on areas that may be troublesome (e.g., subareolar, where compression may be suboptimal) or the areas in which breast cancers are commonly identified (e.g., medial quadrants). On CC views specifically, evaluate medial (Fig. 2.46) and retroglandular tissue, particularly the tissue-fat interface (see Fig. 8.17). In most women, the medial portion of the breast is relatively fatty. Any developing density medially warrants additional evaluation (Fig. 2.47). On the MLO views, evaluate the upper cone of tissue (Fig. 2.48), the lower fatty regions just above the IMF (Fig. 2.49), and the usually fatty strip of tissue between pectoral muscle and glandular tissue (Figs. 2.14A and 2.38B; also see Figs. 3.33, 3.20, and 8.48). If the upper cone of tissue starts to round off (Fig. 2.48), or densities begin to develop in this area, additional views are warranted (13). Developing distortion or alteration in the contour of the fat-glandular interface posteriorly likewise warrants evaluation. Scrutinize and focus your attention on the subareolar area (Fig. 2.50). Remember that compression in the subareolar areas may be inadequate when the base of the breast or the pectoral muscle is thick (7,8). Also, when you identify a possible malignancy on a screening study, keep looking. Additional sites of disease may be present in either breast (Figs. 2.50 and 2.51; also see Figs. 8.37 and 8.45).

Last, make no assumptions. This is applicable to every step of the process in taking care of patients. The minute you make an assumption, critical thinking stops. Keep your mind open. If you detect a potential abnormality, describe it and provide a differential. Every finding has benign and malignant correlates; so don't assume that something is benign or malignant until you have proved it by the clinical and imaging features of a finding or a biopsy.

In determining the appropriateness of calling a patient with vague densities (greater than 1 cm in size) back for additional evaluation, consider the position of the potential lesion and its apparent size. The location of a potential lesion on the CC view should be compatible with the location noted on the MLO view. If you see a potential

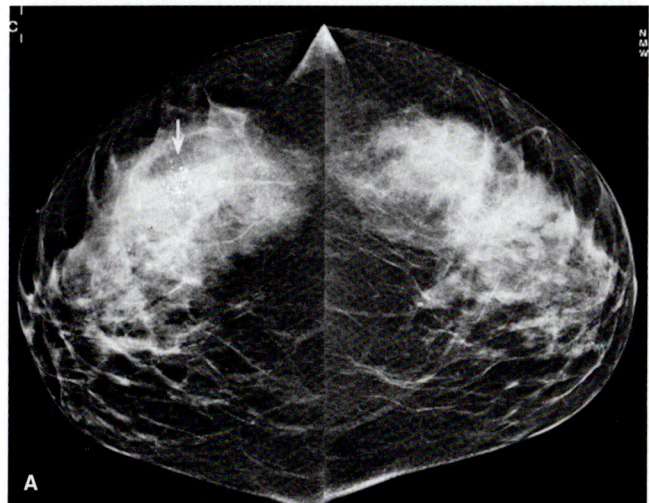

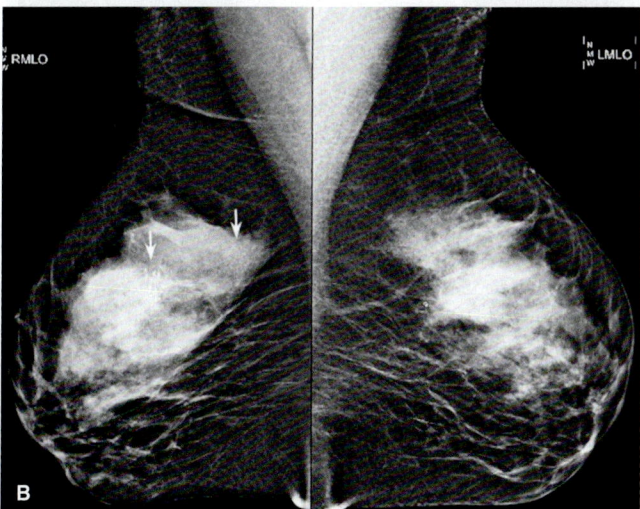

FIG. 2.42 • **Calcifications.** CC **(A)** and MLO **(B)** views from a screening study in a 47-year-old woman. After establishing optimal image quality and evaluating the images for gross findings, focus in and send your brain looking for distortion, small masses, calcifications, and evaluate specific locations (medial quadrants, fat-glandular interfaces, subareolar areas, tissue between pectoral muscle, and glandular tissue on MLO views). A cluster of calcifications (*arrows*) is detected in the upper outer quadrant of the right breast in zone **B** with apparent extension posteriorly noted on the MLO view. Spot compression magnification views are indicated for further evaluation and characterization of the calcifications. BI-RADS 0: need additional imaging evaluation. Please see Figure 3.15 for the additional images done to evaluate this patient.

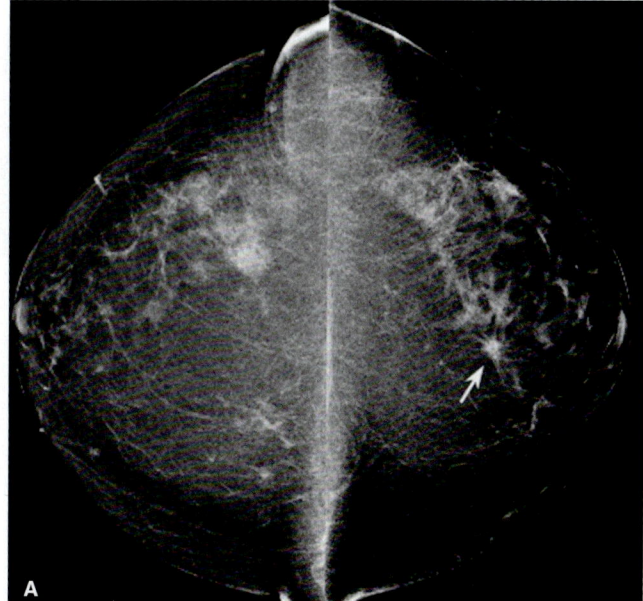

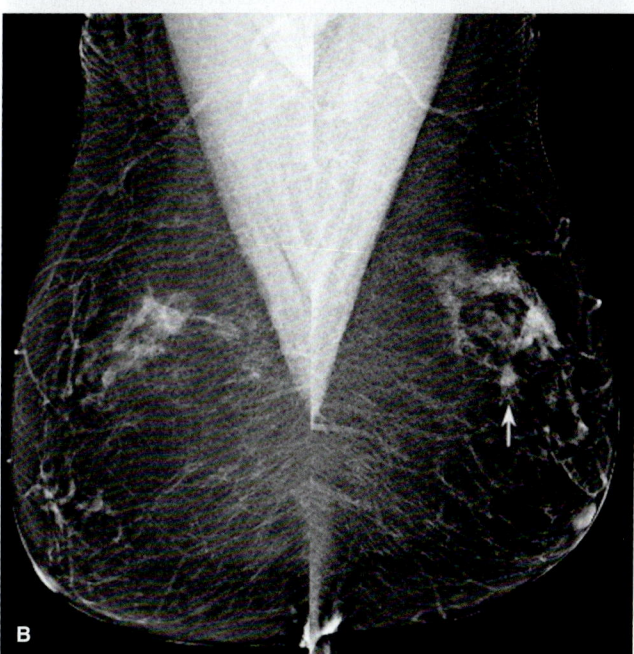

FIG. 2.43 • **Possible mass, left breast.** CC **(A)** and MLO **(B)** views from a screening study in a 67-year-old woman. A possible mass (*arrow*) is initially detected in the left CC view. Given the location of this finding in the CC view, a possible correlate of approximately the same size and density (*arrow*) is seen in the MLO view. Additional evaluation with spot compression views is indicated. BI-RADS 0: need additional imaging evaluation. Please see Figure 3.6 for the additional studies done to evaluate this patient.

abnormality within a centimeter of the nipple and what concerns you on the MLO is far posteriorly, it is unlikely that these two findings represent the same thing. Also, although there are exceptions (e.g., some invasive lobular carcinomas, complex sclerosing lesions), most cancers are three-dimensional. If a 1.5-cm area of concern is noted on one of the screening views, and no comparably sized abnormality is identified on the other view (at the approximate distance from the nipple), it is unlikely to represent a significant finding.

CALLBACKS

As mentioned previously, screening studies are for detection, not characterization. Consequently, we make no efforts to describe or be definitive about a potential abnormality on the screening mammogram report and the only BI-RADS assessment categories (14) we use on screening studies are: "1" = negative; "2" = benign finding, negative, and "0" = incomplete, additional imaging evaluation is needed. We assign category "0" to women in whom we request prior films for comparison or women for whom we recommend additional studies. At the time of a screening study, the patient is informed by the technologist of the possibility of a callback for additional evaluation.

Our protocol relative to women in whom prior films are needed requires that these studies be dictated. We do not hold them aside

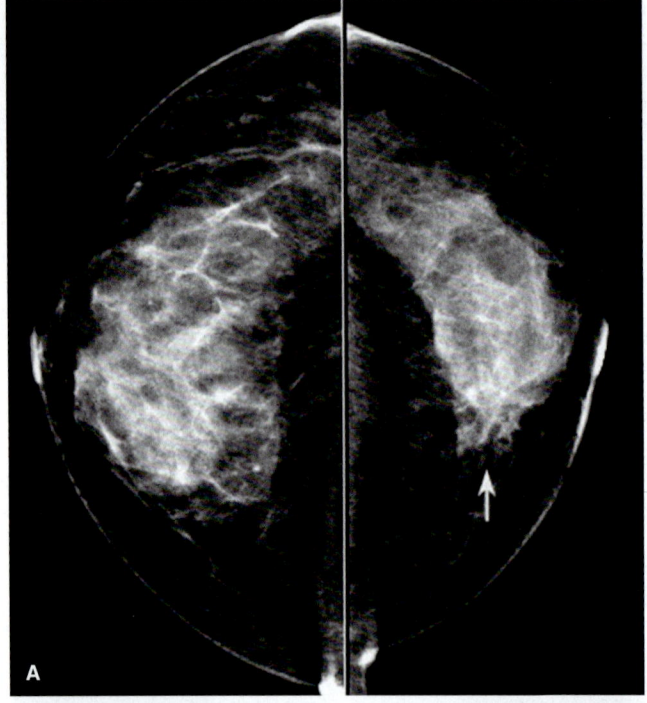

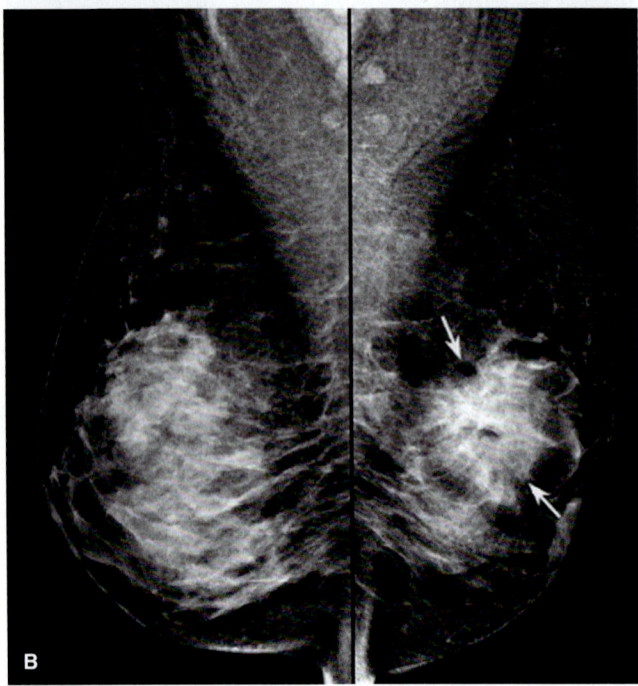

FIG. 2.44 • **Possible distortion, left breast.** CC **(A)** and MLO **(B)** views from a screening study in a 51-year-old woman. The left breast is smaller than the right. Possible distortion (*arrows*), with apparent spicules, particularly noticeably along the posterior edge of this area, is detected in the left breast in the MLO projection. In reviewing the CC view, no definite correlate is identified; however, consider the appearance of the tissue in the medial aspect of the breast (*arrow*). Also note the appearance of the left nipple: it appears retracted on the oblique view and flattened on the CC view. Additional evaluation with spot compression views and correlative physical examination is indicated. BI-RADS 0: need additional imaging evaluation. Please see Figures 3.13 and 5.22A for the additional studies and MRI done to evaluate this patient.

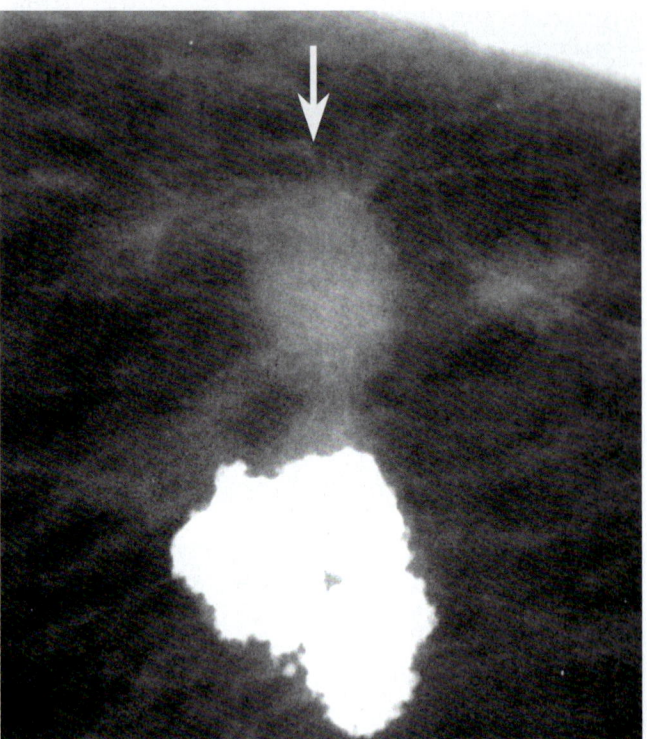

FIG. 2.45 • **Hyalinized fibroadenoma and invasive ductal carcinoma.** Your eye is likely to be drawn to the coarse, popcorn calcification present in this image. However, on closer inspection, an isodense mass with indistinct and spiculated margins (*arrow*) is present in the tissue adjacent to the benign calcification. When there are obvious findings, or the patient presents describing a focal finding, make sure you evaluate the mammogram in its entirety before focusing in on clinical or obvious findings. (From Cardeñosa G. *Breast Imaging* [*The Core Curriculum Series*]. Philadelphia, PA: Lippincott Williams & Wilkins; 2003.)

without a dictation waiting for the old films to come in. In a busy practice, putting undictated films aside is fraught with potential problems. We dictate the study and classify it as a category "0" study. This sets in motion attempts to procure prior studies and helps keep the referring physician informed. The steps we follow are listed in Table 2.11. Every step taken is documented so as to show that there is a "reasonable" effort made to locate prior studies. If prior films have not been received 2 weeks after the date of the screening study, we dictate an addendum and proceed with our recommendations as though the patient has no prior films.

For those women in whom a potential abnormality is identified, the interpreting radiologist qualifies the callback. This is used exclusively as an internal means to communicate with our schedulers relative to the time slot that should be assigned to that given patient. Category I callbacks are assigned a 15-minute time slot. For these patients, the radiologist has a low level of concern and thinks that with one or two additional views the issue will be resolved. Category II callbacks are assigned a 30-minute time slot. For these patients, the interpreting radiologist believes that additional views and an ultrasound, or additional views and a ductogram, may be needed. Category III callbacks are patients in whom the radiologist considers an imaging-guided biopsy a likely possibility. An hour time slot is provided for these patients. This system is not intended to be an exact science but an internal effort to

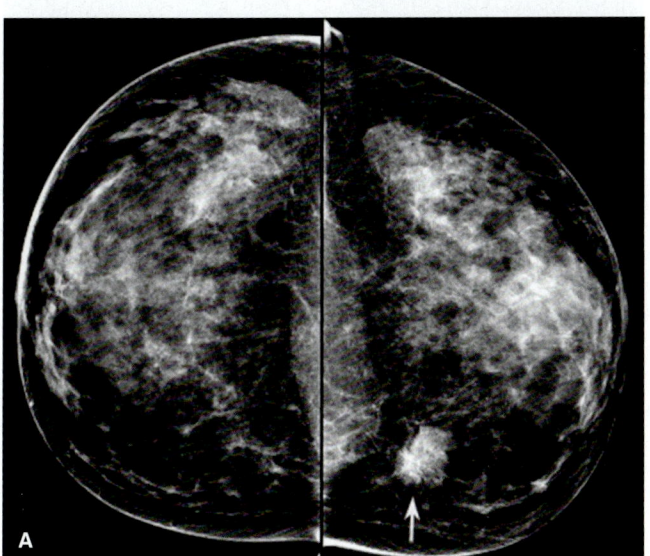
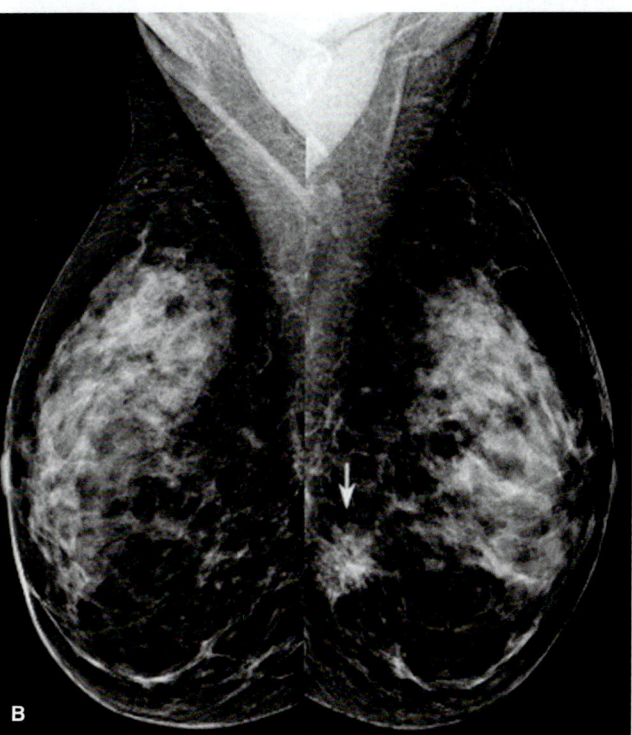

FIG. 2.46 • **Mass, lower inner aspect left breast.** CC **(A)** and MLO **(B)** views from a screening study is a 36-year-old woman. A mass with indistinct margins is imaged in the lower inner aspect of the left breast. Since the patient has no history of trauma or surgery at this site, spot compression views, physical examination, and ultrasound are indicated. BI-RADS 0: need additional imaging evaluation. Please see Figures 3.7, 4.39D and 5.21 for the additional studies and MRI done to evaluate this patient.

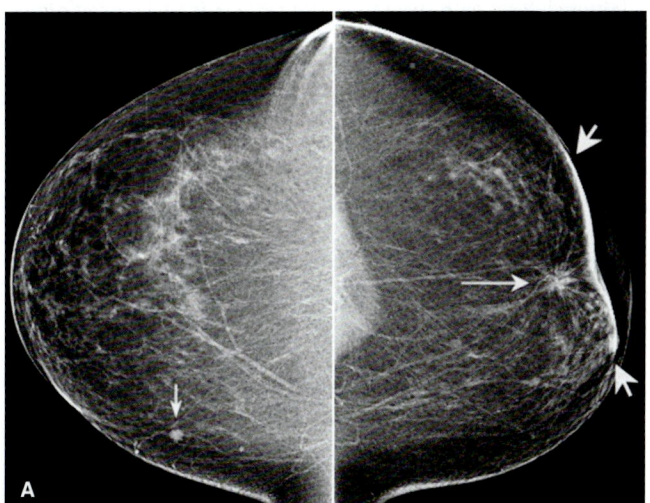
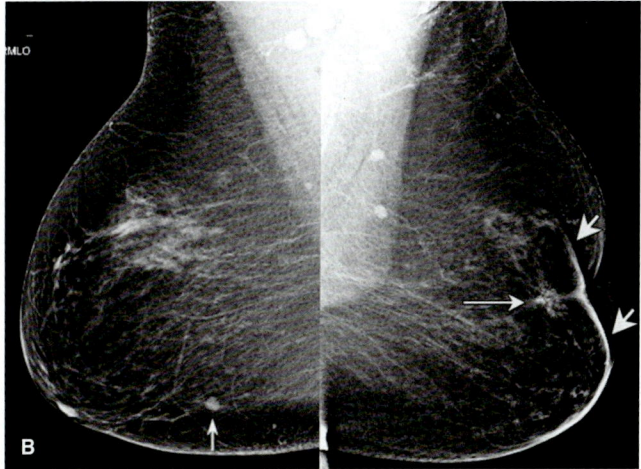

FIG. 2.47 • **Mass, medial location.** CC **(A)** and MLO **(B)** views from a screening study in a 62-year-old woman with a previous lumpectomy and radiation therapy for cancer in the left breast 9 years ago. A high-density mass (*arrow*) with possibly lobulated but circumscribed margins is detected in the upper inner quadrant of the right breast in zone **B**. This is new compared with the patient's earlier study 1 year ago. Developing masses medially in postmenopausal women require additional evaluation. Given the density of this mass and the patient's history of breast cancer in the left breast, the likelihood of malignancy is high. In the left breast a low-density mass, with spiculated margins (*long arrow*) somewhat more prominent on the CC view, is noted corresponding to the lumpectomy site. Associated skin thickening and retraction (*thick arrows*) are also noted related to the prior surgery. The findings in the left breast can be seen on prior studies. BI-RADS 0: need additional imaging evaluation. Please see Figure 3.8 for the additional studies done to evaluate this patient.

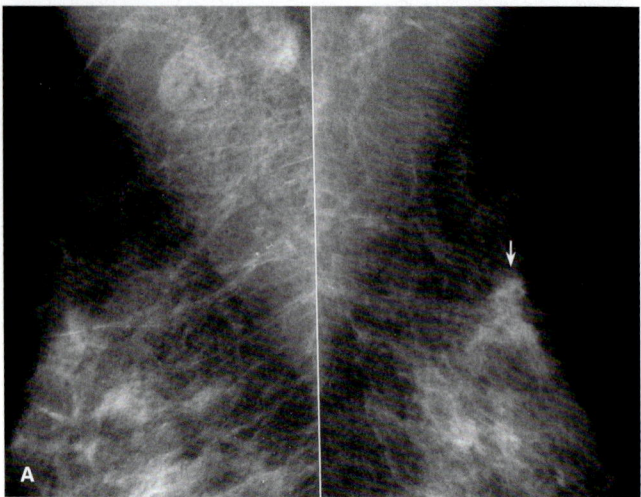 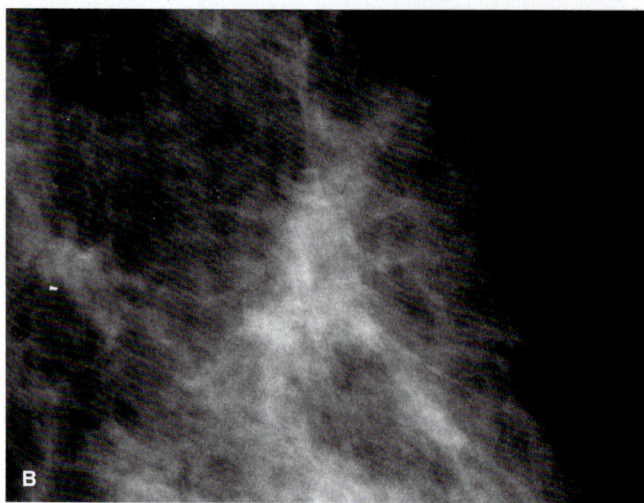

FIG. 2.48 • **Upper cone of tissue, invasive ductal carcinoma, not otherwise specified. A:** MLO views photographically coned to the upper aspect of the images. Notice the asymmetry and rounded appearance of the upper cone of tissue on the left (*arrow*) compared to the right. Additional evaluation with spot compression views is indicated. BI-RADS 0: need additional imaging evaluation. **B:** Spot compression view, MLO projection confirms the presence of an irregular, isodense mass with spiculated margins. Biopsy is indicated. BI-RADS 4C: suspicious abnormality, biopsy is indicated. (From Cardeñosa G. *Breast Imaging* [*The Core Curriculum Series*]. Philadelphia, PA: Lippincott Williams & Wilkins; 2003.)

control the diagnostic schedule and run it efficiently. The system actually works well and has eliminated bottlenecks or slow periods when radiologists and technologists are sitting around waiting for the next patient. Most importantly, it has given us the capability of doing biopsies at the time the patient returns for her evaluation. This helps expedite patient care since it has virtually eliminated the need for rescheduling patients for biopsy or an ultrasound and yet we do not generate significant delays for other patients. The capability of completing workups, including needed biopsies, is appreciated greatly since most patients, when told of a possible abnormality, want a definitive answer as soon as possible.

As is done by many facilities now, we do our own callbacks. The benefits of the imaging facility scheduling callbacks are immeasurable (15,16). The reason for the callback is communicated appropriately to the patient; if this responsibility is relegated to individuals who don't understand the process, the patient is often misinformed about why more images are needed (e.g., "they didn't get it right and need to repeat your films"). These are not repeat images, but rather additional views with special techniques to evaluate a specific area of concern. When we control the callbacks, patients are scheduled in a manner that is convenient for the patient and provides us the ability to assign appropriate time slots for the individual patient's potential

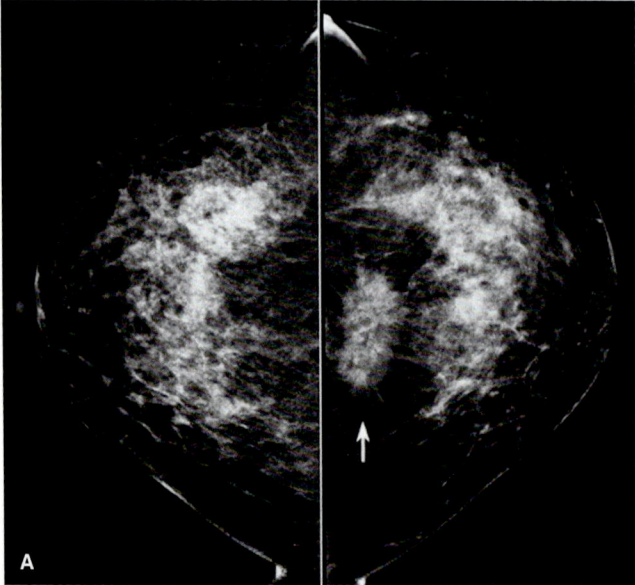 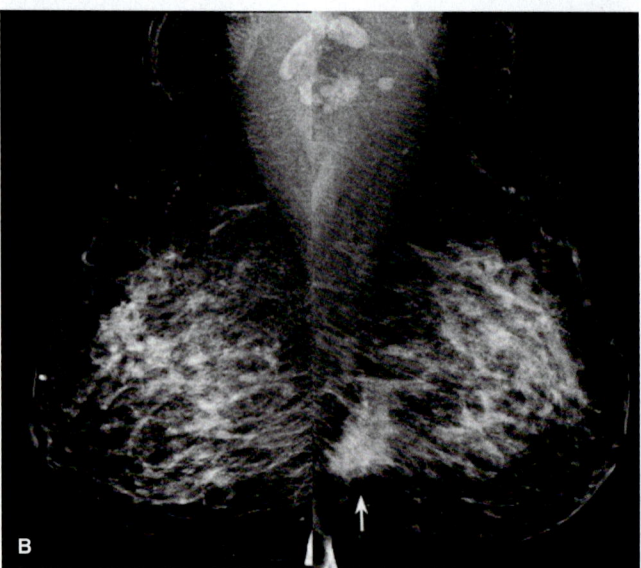

FIG. 2.49 • **Mass.** CC **(A)** and MLO **(B)** views from a screening study in a 43-year-old woman. A mass with spiculated margins (*arrows*) is present in the retroglandular fat in the lower (just above the IMF) central aspect of the left breast posteriorly. Benign-appearing lymph nodes are incidentally noted in the axillae. Additional evaluation is indicated. BI-RADS 0: need additional imaging evaluation. Please see Figures 3.9 and 4.39C for the spot and ultrasound done to evaluate this patient, respectively.

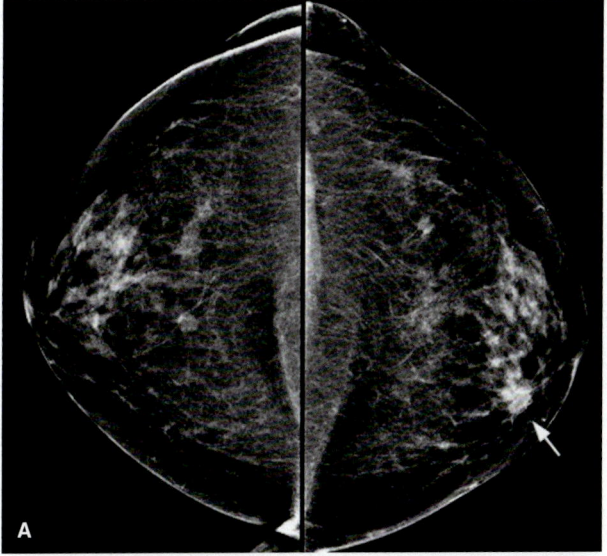
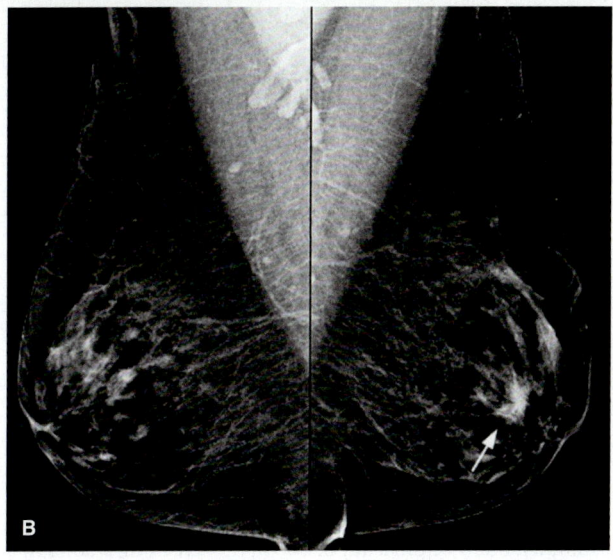
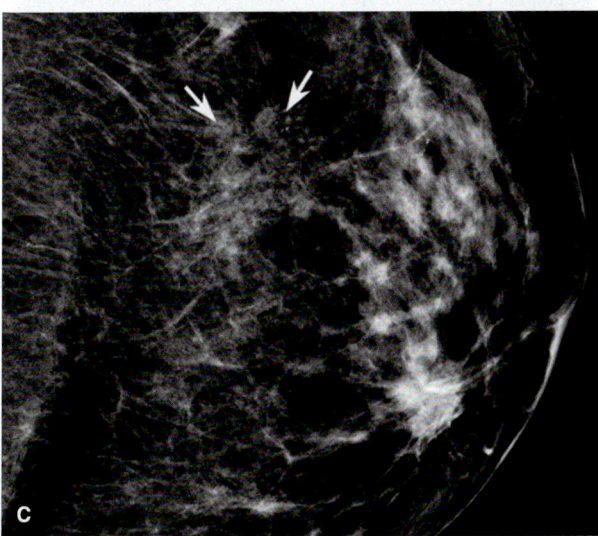

FIG. 2.50 • **Mass and cluster of calcifications.** CC **(A)** and MLO **(B)** views from a screening study in a 62-year-old woman. A high-density mass (*arrow*) is detected on the left CC view anteriorly. When the distance from the nipple and size of the potential lesion is placed in the context of the MLO view, a likely correlative finding (*arrow*) is identified. Benign-appearing lymph nodes are incidentally noted in the axillae. After you identify one potential lesion, keep looking. **C:** Photographically coned image of the anterior aspect of the left breast in the craniocaudal projection. In addition to the possible mass already discussed, a cluster of calcifications is noted in the upper outer aspect of the breast (*arrows*). Additional imaging evaluation is indicated: spot compression for the mass and spot compression magnification for the cluster of calcifications. BI-RADS 0: need additional imaging evaluation. Please see Figures 3.10 and 4.39E for the spots and ultrasound done to evaluate this patient, respectively. Remember: once you find a possible cancer, keep looking.

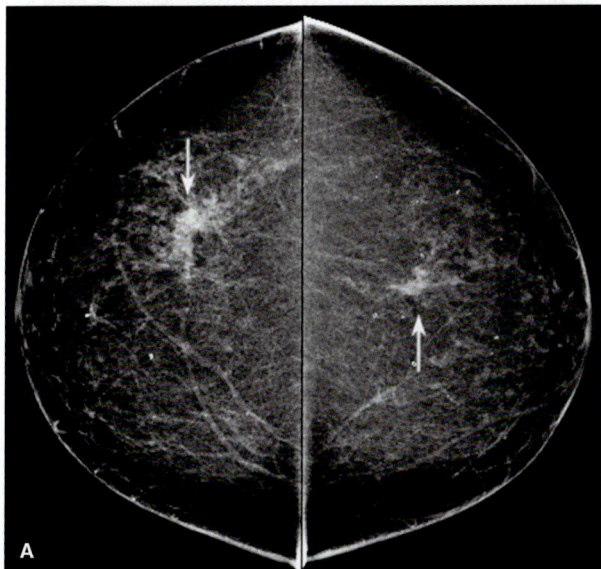
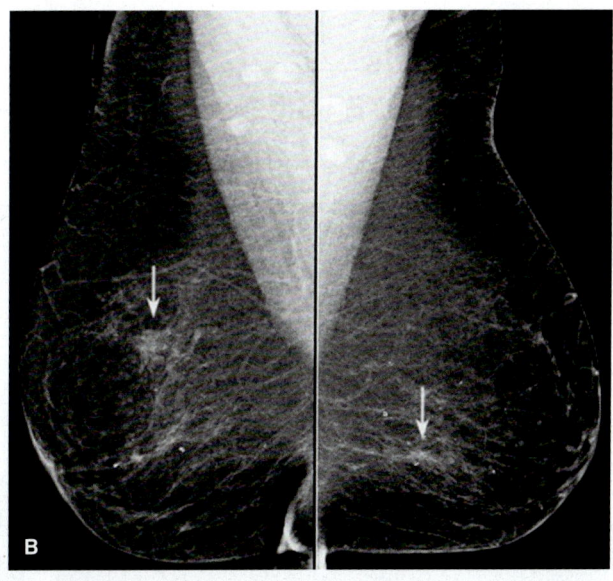

FIG. 2.51 • **Masses, synchronous breast cancers.** CC **(A)** and MLO **(B)** views from a screening study in a 62-year-old woman. In this patient a mass is apparent in the right breast. When you identify one significant finding, don't stop reviewing the images. Keep looking for additional findings in the ipsilateral breast as well as the contralateral side. A second possible mass is imaged in the left CC view; this is harder to identify on the oblique view. Additional evaluation is indicated bilaterally. BI-RADS 0: need additional imaging evaluation. Spot compression views bilaterally (not shown) confirm the suspected masses, one in each breast. An invasive ductal carcinoma is diagnosed following an ultrasound-guided biopsy on the right and an invasive ductal carcinoma with lobular features is diagnosed following an ultrasound-guided biopsy of the mass in the left breast.

Table 2.11 STEPS FOLLOWED IN PROCURING PRIOR STUDIES

Patient signs a release form for outside film/report requests

Contact the facility listed by the patient on the release form

If the facility listed has no studies, we contact the referring physician for a prior report (the report provides the date and name of facility where prior study was done)

If needed as last resort, the patient is contacted to verify site of prior study

problem. Handling the callbacks assures you that patients are scheduled promptly, often within a day or two of the screening studies. If a patient cannot be reached, steps are put in motion to attempt to communicate with her. If after three attempts within a 48-hour period we are unable to reach the patient by phone, we send a certified letter to the patient. Every effort made is documented. It is important to be able to show that a "reasonable" effort was made to communicate with the patient directly. The individuals doing the "callbacks" for your facility need to be empathetic, compassionate, and considerate. The patient needs to be informed that most of the time nothing significant is found on the additional views. She is also assured that she will be given her results at the time of the study by a radiologist.

In addition to the above, we print a monthly report of all unsettled category "0" patients from our data tracking system. Each outstanding case is investigated and a last effort is made to communicate with the patient.

References

1. Department of Health and Human Services. FDA Mammography Quality Standards, Final Rule. *Fed Regist*. 1997;62(208):21 CFR parts 16 and 900.
2. American College of Radiology. *ACR-AAPM-SIIM Practice Guideline for Determinants of Image Quality in Digital Mammography*. Reston, VA: American College of Radiology; 2012:Resolution 36.
3. American College of Radiology. *Mammography Quality Control Manual*. Reston, VA: American College of Radiology; 1999.
4. American College of Radiology. *ACR Practice Guideline for the Performance of Screening and Diagnostic Mammography*. Reston, VA: American College of Radiology; 2008:Resolution 24.
5. Saslow D, Boetes C, Burke W, et al. American Cancer Society guidelines for breast screening with MRI as an adjunct to mammography. *CA Cancer J Clin*. 2007;57:75–89.
6. Eklund GW, Busby RC, Miller SH, et al. Improved imaging of the augmented breast. *AJR Am J Roentgenol*. 1988;151:469–473.
7. Eklund GW, Cardenosa G. The art of mammographic positioning. *Radiol Clin North Am*. 1992;30:21–53.
8. Eklund GW, Cardenosa G, Parsons W. Assessing adequacy of mammographic image quality. *Radiology*. 1994;190:297–307.
9. Samuels TH, Haider MA, Kirkbride P. Poland's syndrome: a mammographic presentation. *AJR Am J Roentgenol*. 1996;166:347–348.
10. Meyer JE, Stomper PC, Lee RR. Pectoralis muscles simulating a breast mass. *AJR Am J Roentgenol*. 1989;152:481–482.
11. Bradley FM, Hoover HC, Hulka CA, et al. The sternalis muscle: an unusual normal finding seen on mammography. *AJR Am J Roentgenol*. 1996;166:33–36.
12. Ayyala RS, Chorlton MA, Behrman RH, et al. Digital mammographic artifacts on full-field systems: what are they and how do I fix them? *Radiographics*. 2008;28:1999–2008.
13. Tabar L, Dean PB. *Teaching Atlas of Mammography*. 4th ed. New York, NY: Thieme; 2011.
14. D'Orsi CJ, Sickles EA, Mendelson EB Morris EA et al. ACR BI-RADS® Atlas, Breast Imaging Reporting and Data System. Reston, VA, American College of Radiology; 2013.
15. Cardenosa G, Eklund GW. Rate of compliance with recommendations for additional mammographic views and biopsies. *Radiology*. 1991;181:359–361.
16. Robertson CL, Kopans DB. Communication problems after mammographic screening. *Radiology*. 1989;172(2):443–444.

CHAPTER SELF-ASSESSMENT QUESTIONS

1. Screening mammogram in a 45-year-old woman. No prior studies.

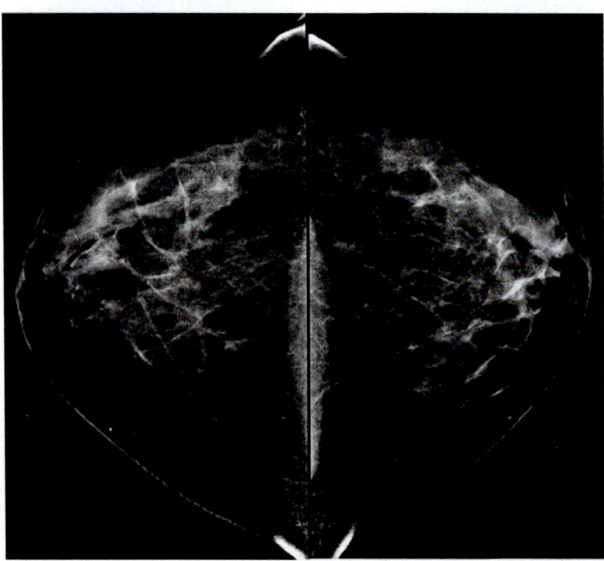
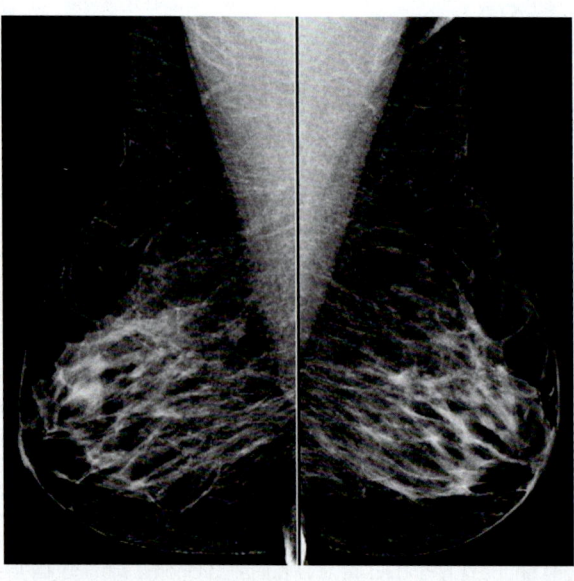

- A BI-RADS 1—screening mammogram in 1 year
- B BI-RADS 0—need additional imaging evaluation bilaterally
- C BI-RADS 0—need additional imaging evaluation of the left breast
- D BI-RADS 0—need additional imaging evaluation of the right breast

2. For this screening mammogram, what additional view of the left breast would be helpful?

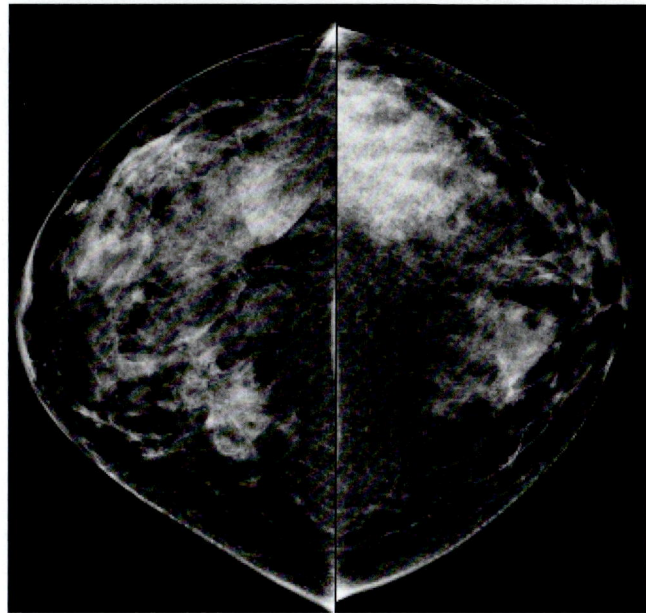

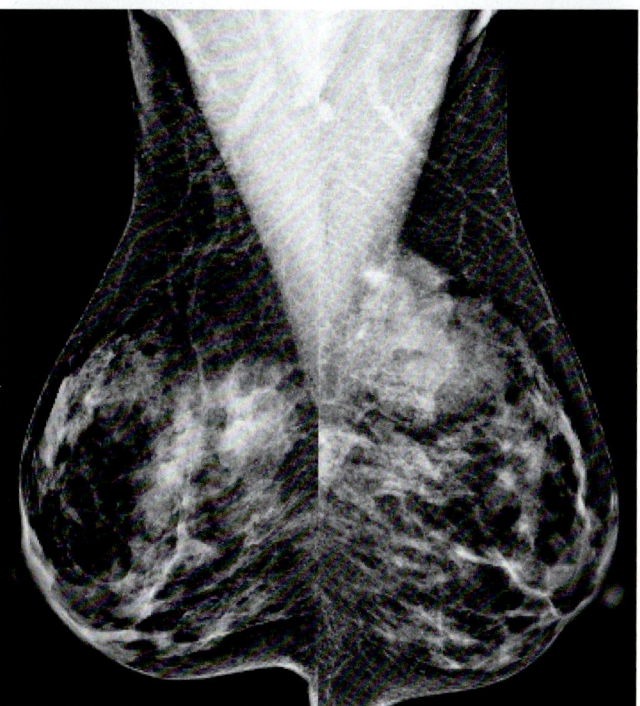

- A XCCL
- B Ninety-degree lateral (ML)
- C Ninety-degree lateral (LM)
- D Cleavage

Answers to Chapter Self-Assessment Questions

1. D A possible mass is apparent on the right mediolateral oblique (MLO) anterior to the pectoral muscle and posteromedially on the right craniocaudal (CC) view. The location, size, and density of this possible finding correlate on the CC and MLO views. See Chapter 3 Question 1.

2. A On the left craniocaudal view, tissue is seen extending to the edge of the film laterally. This observation should prompt the technologist to consider the need for an exaggerated craniocaudal view laterally (XCCL). The need for an XCCL is confirmed by reviewing the mediolateral oblique view: if tissue is present superimposed on the pectoral muscle, then an XCCL should be done. In this patient, the island of asymmetric tissue seen superimposed on the left pectoral muscle is incompletely imaged in the craniocaudal projection. In comparison, retroglandular fat is seen laterally on the right and no tissue is apparent superimposed on the right pectoral muscle. In this patient, an XCCL is needed on the left only.

Diagnostic Breast Imaging 3

LEARNING OBJECTIVES

1. What is diagnostic mammography, and how is it defined?
   - Studies directed by radiologists
   - At least a few images are done with spot compression paddle
   - Patient groups commonly undergoing diagnostic mammography
     Symptomatic (women and men)
     Callback from screening for evaluation of a potential abnormality
     Post lumpectomy and radiation for the first 7 years
     Patient with a probably benign lesion undergoing follow-up
   - Standardization of imaging algorithms
2. What are the common indications for various additional views, and how is each done?
   - Spot compression—how we define "spot" compression and why
     Spot compression paddle
     Frameless spot compression paddle
   - Spot compression magnification
   - Spot compression tangential
   - Spot compression rolled
   - 90-Degree lateral (lateromedial [LM] and mediolateral [ML])
   - Cleavage
   - Lateromedial oblique (LMO)
   - Superolateral to inferomedial oblique (SIO)
   - From below (FB)
3. For lesions initially seen in one view and in establishing mammographic–ultrasound concordance, how do you apply triangulation concepts?
   - Use of rolled views
   - Use of 90-degree lateral views
     In conjunction with the mediolateral oblique (MLO) view
     In conjunction with MLO and craniocaudal (CC) views
   - Stepwise approach

APPROACH TO DIAGNOSTIC BREAST IMAGING

In our practice, the diagnostic patient population is composed primarily of three groups of patients. Those who require additional evaluation of potential abnormalities detected on their screening mammograms, patients presenting with signs and symptoms possibly reflecting the presence of breast cancer, and women who have a history of lumpectomy and radiation therapy (we consider this last group of women as diagnostics for the first 7 years following their treatment, after which they are returned to the screening population—see Chapter 11). Additional but relatively small groups of diagnostic patients are women with probably benign lesions undergoing short interval follow-up and men with breast-related symptoms (1). Many different approaches to diagnostic mammography are available. In general, diagnostic studies usually include at least one or more images done using the spot compression paddle.

Our approach has been to develop a consultative breast service such that we run the Center more like a clinical practice than like a radiology service. We believe that as breast imagers we are in a unique position to provide a desperately needed comprehensive breast health service. In many communities, breast care is disjointed with no standardization and provided haphazardly by general surgeons, gynecologists, family practitioners, and internists. Having someone who can put things together for patients is quite helpful. As radiologists, we have at our disposal all of the imaging modalities that are critical in the diagnosis and subsequent management of patients. If we complement this with clinical acumen, we can provide a much-needed service. Functioning as a team member, we can serve a pivotal role in patient care. We have elected to develop our service with these concepts in mind: the radiologist as a clinical breast imager. Our approach to patients with possible breast cancer is to evaluate them as needed to reassure them of benign findings, low likelihood of malignancy, or undertake the necessary procedures to establish a definitive diagnosis.

As discussed in Chapter 2, women with potentially abnormal mammograms are scheduled for diagnostic studies in 15-, 30-, and 60-minute time slots, depending on the abnormality detected at screening. Our approach to these patients is to do whatever it takes, on their return trip, to arrive at a definitive, justifiable recommendation. In some patients, this may take one or two additional mammographic images, while in others, additional mammographic images, correlative physical examination, ultrasound, and an interventional procedure (cyst aspiration, ductogram, FNA, and biopsy) may be indicated. For those patients in whom a biopsy is indicated, we offer the patient the option of having it done immediately. Unless requested by the patient, we do not reschedule them for ultrasounds, aspirations, ductograms, or biopsies. Approximately 99% of patients opt for having the biopsy the same day. Most patients are appreciative of being offered this option. Additionally, we have a commitment from our Pathology Department for a 24-hour turnaround time on core biopsies. Consequently, we see our biopsy patients the day following their procedure, at which time findings are discussed directly with the patient and referrals are made as needed on the basis of the results: (i) Screening mammogram in one year for patients with benign congruent results; (ii) Surgical consultation for patients with high-risk lesions (e.g., atypical ductal hyperplasia); and (iii) MRI and surgical consultation for patients with a malignant lesion.

Although there are many projections available to us during diagnostic mammography, I have purposely limited the discussion to those used most often. Having a handle on the material discussed in this chapter will enable you to evaluate the vast majority of patients presenting to your diagnostic center in a logical and efficient manner. I encourage the standardization of diagnostic imaging evaluations. Appropriate and justifiable recommendations become self-evident, and confidence in your work is increased greatly.

SYMPTOMATIC PATIENTS: IMAGING ALGORITHMS

Our basic imaging algorithms for symptomatic patients are listed in Table 3.1. In symptomatic women who are 30 years or older presenting with a "lump," focal tenderness, skin dimpling, nipple retraction, or other focal symptoms, a metallic BB is placed at the site of concern and CC and mediolateral oblique (MLO) views are obtained

Table 3.1 **IMAGING ALGORITHMS FOR SYMPTOMATIC PATIENTS**

Symptomatic Patient (30 y of age or older)
("Lump," focal tenderness, dimpling, nipple retraction)
Metallic BB placed at the site of concern
Bilateral CC and MLO views
Spot tangential view at the site of concern
Physical examination and ultrasound (unless area of concern is totally fatty and there is no chance, the finding is excluded from the field of view)
Symptomatic Patient (under age 30; pregnant or lactating regardless of age)
("lump," focal tenderness, dimpling, nipple retraction)
Physical examination
Ultrasound
Mammogram (bilateral) if cancer is suspected on physical examination and ultrasound

bilaterally. In addition to the standard images, the technologist obtains a spot tangential view of the site of concern as pinpointed by the patient. Correlative physical examination and an ultrasound are done unless completely fatty tissue is imaged at the site of concern on the routine and spot tangential views, and there is no possibility that the area of concern is excluded from the image. If the metallic BB is at the edge of the film (Fig. 3.1), not seen on CC and MLO images, or marks an area from which tissue may be excluded (e.g., axilla, upper inner quadrant posteriorly, areas of inframammary fold [IMF]) (Fig. 3.2), correlative physical examination and ultrasound are indicated. In women with nipple discharge, a ductogram may be done if it is determined that the discharge is spontaneous and arising from one duct on physical examination (see Chapter 12). We do not consider diffuse, cyclical tenderness as an indication for a diagnostic study; these women are scheduled for screening mammography.

In symptomatic women under the age of 30, or those who are pregnant or lactating (regardless of age), physical examination and ultrasound (see Figs. 4.45 and 4.47) are our starting point (2,3). If cancer is suspected on the basis of this initial evaluation, a full mammogram is obtained to more completely evaluate the lesion, as well as the rest of the tissue in that breast, the contralateral breast, and the axillae.

SPOT COMPRESSION VIEWS

Spot compression views are the most common additional views obtained in our practice. The area of concern is immobilized and maximally compressed in two projections unless it is seen only in one view initially. Spot compression views minimize superimposition and geometric unsharpness, and resolution is improved as the object to film distance is decreased. When evaluating spot compression views, it is important to ensure that the area of concern is included in the field of view (Fig. 3.3). As focal compression is applied, lesions can "roll," or "squeeze," out of the field of view. For purposes of orienting ourselves on the spot compression views, we like to include surrounding tissue on the image. Consequently, we do not cone down on spot compression views, and, although not compressed, surrounding tissue is evaluated and used to assure inclusion of the area of concern. While at the point of reviewing a spot, you are clearly evaluating a specific potential finding, keep an open mind (eye), and be sure to evaluate all of the tissue on the image and that surrounding the paddle. The original focus of attention may turn out to be benign, and an unsuspected malignant process may become apparent (Fig. 3.3).

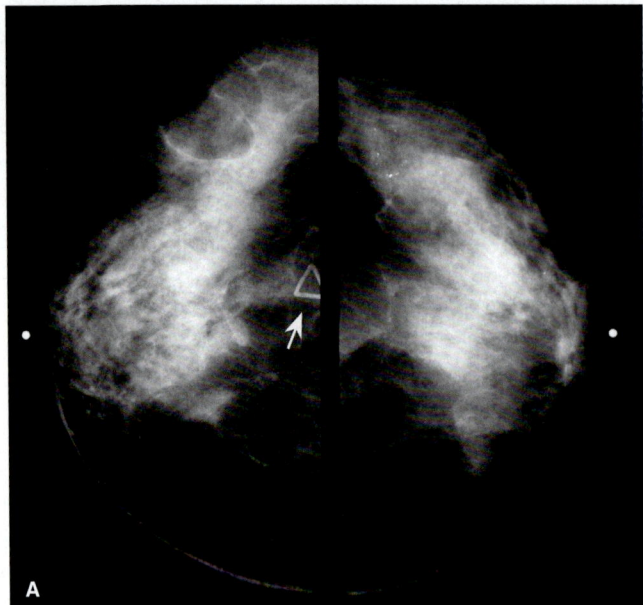
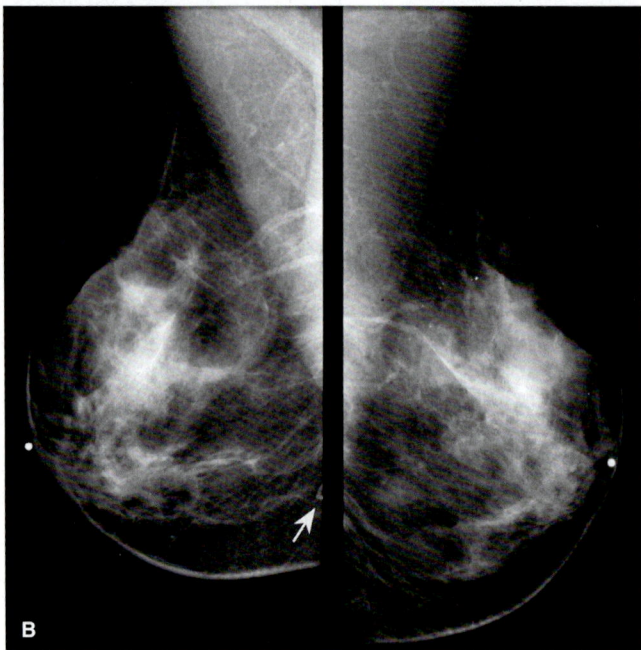
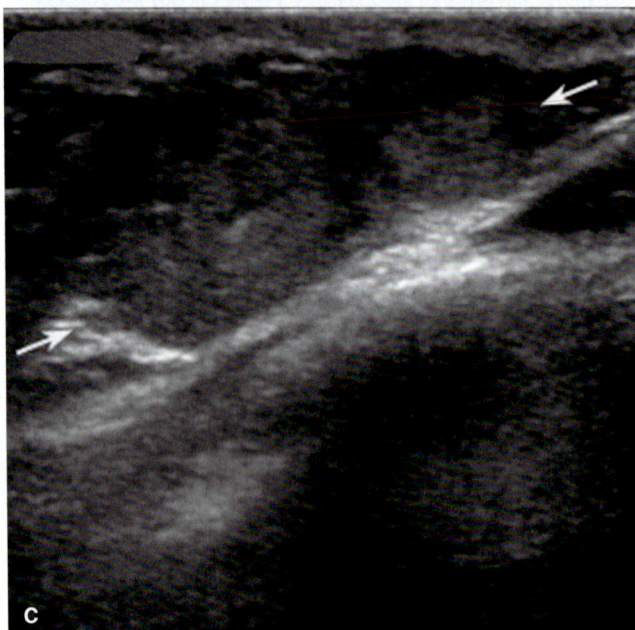

FIG. 3.1 • **Lesion exclusion, invasive ductal carcinoma not otherwise specified.** CC **(A)** and MLO **(B)** views done in a 53-year-old patient presenting with a "lump" in the right breast. A radiopaque triangular marker is used to denote the location of the palpable finding, and metallic BBs mark the nipples. Loosely clustered round calcifications are noted in the upper outer quadrant of the left posteriorly; these are stable. The radiopaque marker *(arrow)* is at the edge of the film on the CC view and is barely seen on the MLO view such that the lesion may have been excluded from the field of view. When the metallic marker used to denote a site of clinical concern is at the edge of the images, or not included on the images at all, correlative physical examination and ultrasound are indicated even if fatty tissue is imaged. **C:** Ultrasound. On physical examination, a hard mass is readily apparent just above the IMF on the right. An oval iso-to-slightly hyperechoic mass *(arrows)* with posterior acoustic enhancement is imaged interposed between the skin and one of the lower ribs. BI-RADS 4B: Suspicious abnormality, biopsy is indicated.

To obtain the maximum benefit of spot compression views, we use a small round paddle (Fig. 3.4A) or a frameless spot paddle (Fig. 3.4B). The frameless spot paddle centers a 7.5-cm spot compression cup into an 18 × 24 cm paddle and eliminates the metal frame around the spot device; this permits visualization of the surrounding tissue with some compression and eliminates the artifact (distraction) generated by the metal frame of the paddle. All of the diagnostic images done at our facilities are done with the paddles shown in Figure 3.4A, B; we have removed the larger rectangular and square paddles from our mammography rooms (Fig. 3.4B, C). Although in women with larger breasts using the round spot presents a challenge in getting the area in the field of view, it is a challenge we welcome and overcome routinely. Using larger "spot" paddles to make it easier for the technologist to include the area in the field of view in many ways defeats the purpose of *focal* compression. If your "spot" compression views include more than half of the breast (Fig. 3.4E), what are you really accomplishing?

Indications for spot compression views are listed in Table 3.2. As a general rule, if we are not sure a lesion is present, our starting point is spot compression. Spot compression views are used to evaluate densities seen in only one view (Fig. 3.5), masses with possibly obscured margins (Figs. 3.6 through 3.11), asymmetric tissue (Fig. 3.12), and possible areas of distortion (Fig. 3.13). Additionally, spot compression can be used to reach and image lesions that are excluded from routine screening views (Fig. 3.14): lesions close to the chest wall, in the axillary tail, or high in the upper inner quadrants (4–6). If there is blurring

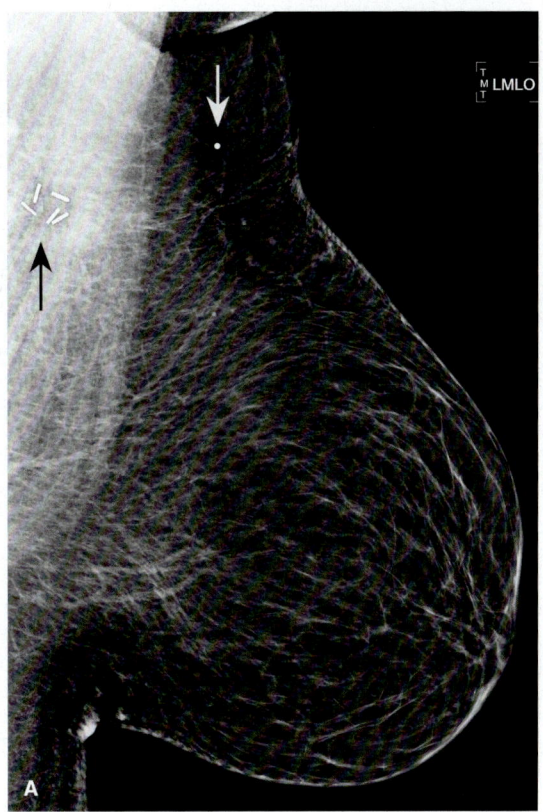
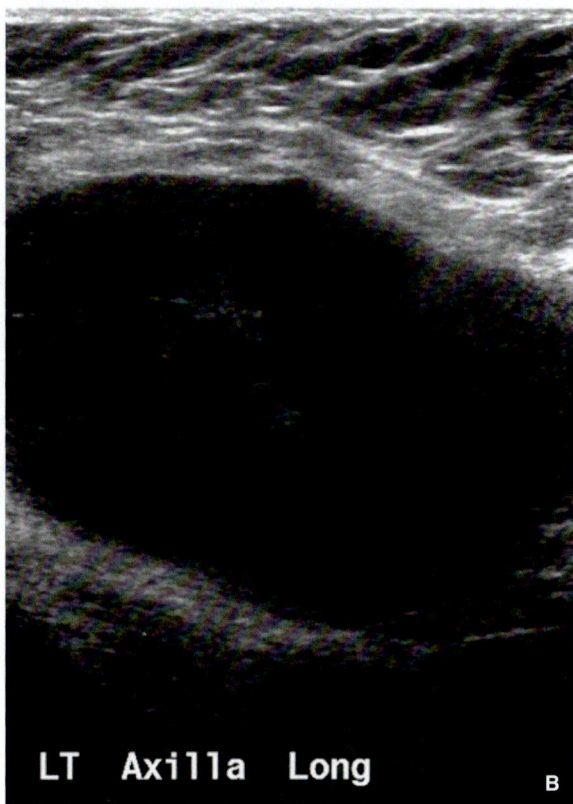
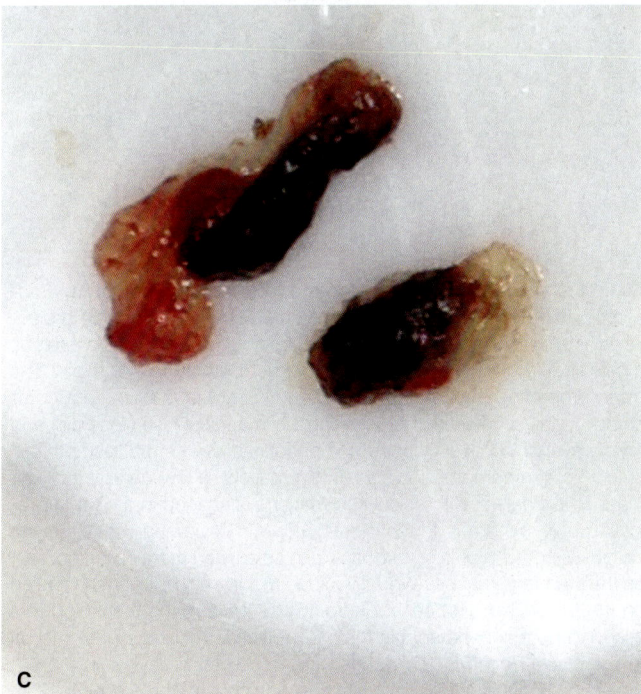

FIG. 3.2 • **Lesion exclusion, metastatic melanoma. A:** MLO view of the left breast in a 41-year-old woman presenting with a painful "lump" underneath her left arm. The metallic BB *(white arrow)* used to mark the site of the "lump" is apparent on the MLO, but it is not seen on the CC view (not shown). Fatty tissue is imaged in the area of concern to the patient on the MLO and the spot tangential view (not shown). Surgical clips *(black arrow)* are imaged in the left axilla related to a sentinel lymph node biopsy done at the time of surgery for a melanoma on her back 2 years ago. Even though these images are normal, a described clinical finding in the axilla requires additional evaluation because as compression is applied, masses can roll out from under the paddle and may not be included on the images. Correlative physical examination and an ultrasound are indicated. **B:** Ultrasound. A hard mobile mass is palpated in the left axilla; tenderness is elicited on palpation. A lobulated, markedly hypoechoic mass with circumscribed margins is correlated with the palpable finding. Biopsy is indicated. BI-RADS 4C: Suspicious abnormality, biopsy is indicated. **C:** Cores. Portions of the cores are dark brown, highly suggestive of metastatic melanoma. This diagnosis is confirmed histologically.

related to inadequate compression (e.g., subareolar or IMF areas), or focal areas of underexposed tissue, spot compression can help overcome these technical limitations.

It is important to emphasize that for most patients spot compression views are done in two projections. It is only when a potential lesion is seen in only one view (Fig. 3.5) that we limit the spots to the projection in which the potential abnormality is seen. If no abnormality is confirmed on the spot compression view, we do no additional images. If the spot compression view confirms a mass or distortion, we need to determine its location in the orthogonal plane by using

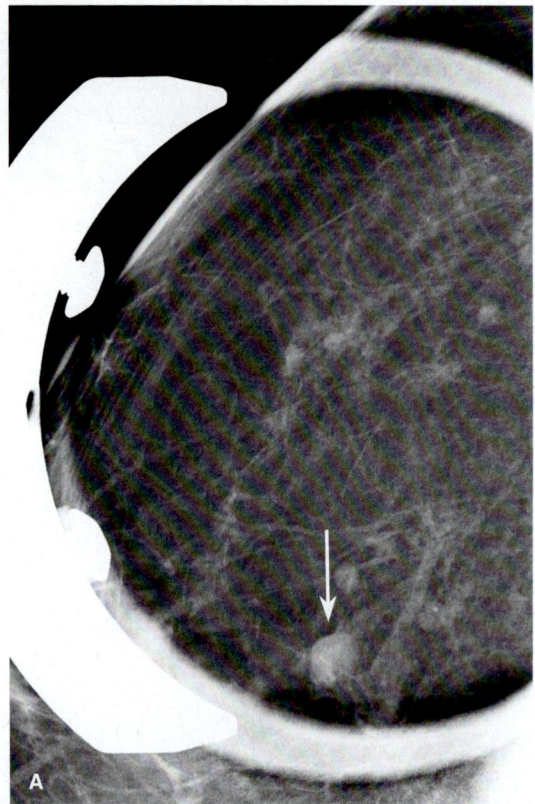
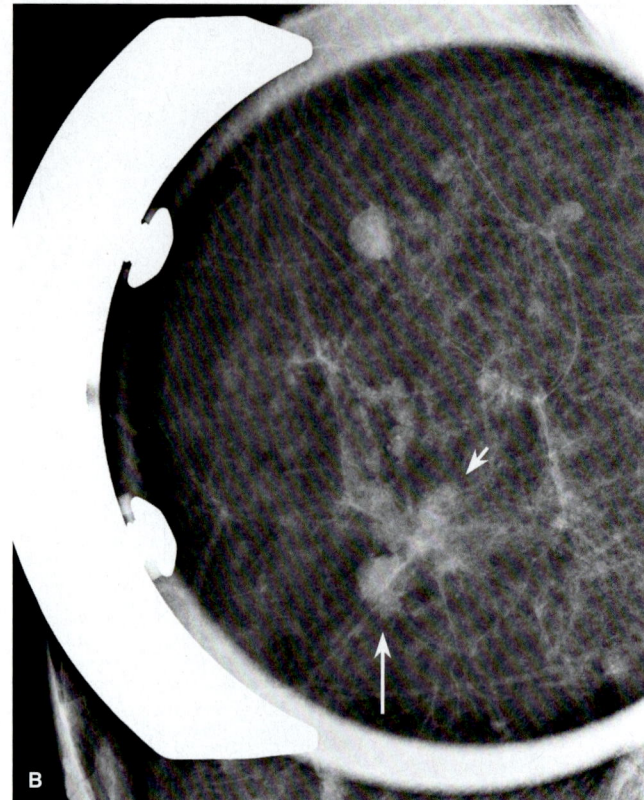
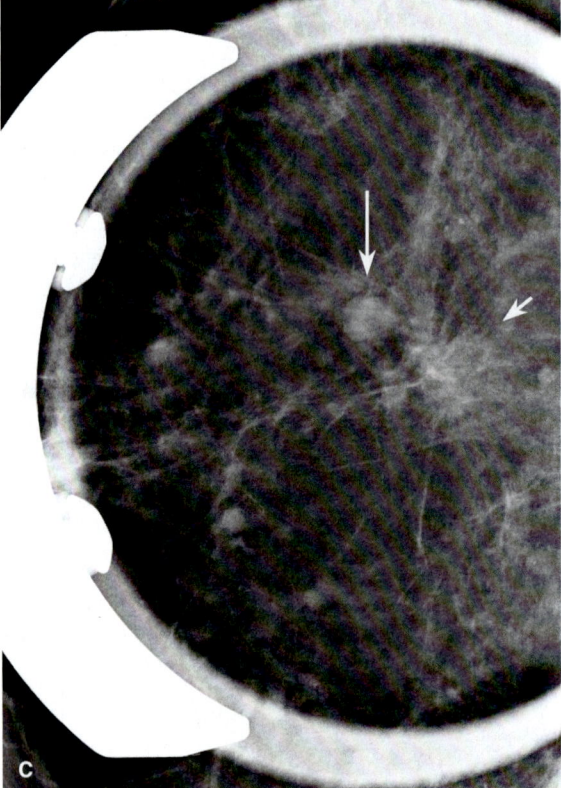

FIG. 3.3 • **Spot compression paddle, lesion inclusion.** Spot compression views of the right breast in CC **(A)** and MLO **(B)** projections. The patient is called back for evaluation of a round mass noted as a new finding on the screening mammogram. What do you think? The mass prompting the callback *(long arrow)* is noted in both spot compression views; however, in evaluating the images please step back and review everything directly under the paddle as well as the tissue that is outside of the compression field. In this patient, a low-density irregular mass *(short arrow)* with spiculated margins is imaged in the MLO projection only. Where is this on the CC spot? Reviewing the screening images is not helpful (e.g., no mass with spiculated margins is apparent on the standard images). Would you do anything else? Given the finding on the MLO view, you cannot stop. In this patient, the technologist is asked to do a second spot in the CC projection moving slightly medial to the current position. **C:** Second spot compression view in the CC projection. On this additional projection, you confirm the presence of an irregular mass *(short arrow)* with spiculated margins in the CC projection and again image the round mass with circumscribed margins prompting the callback *(long arrow)*. The round mass is a cyst; the mass with spiculated margins is an invasive ductal carcinoma.

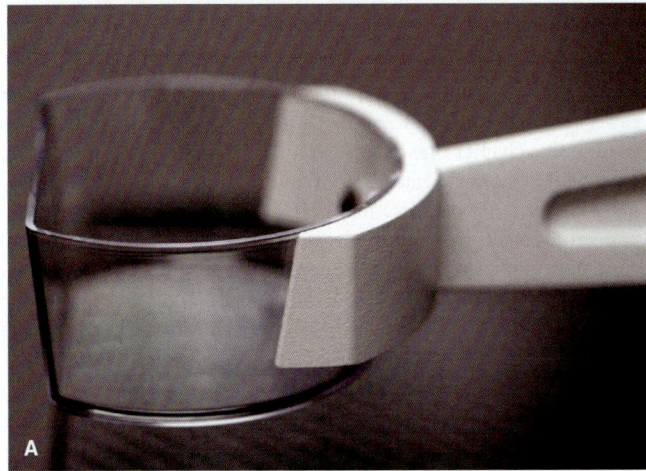
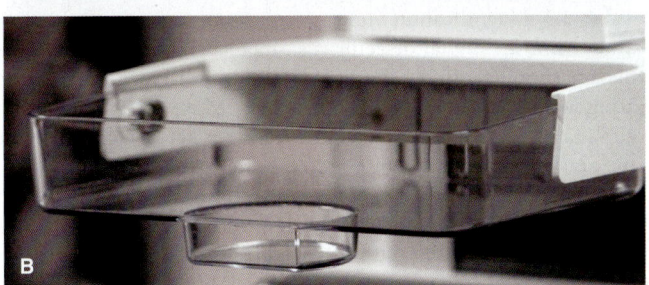
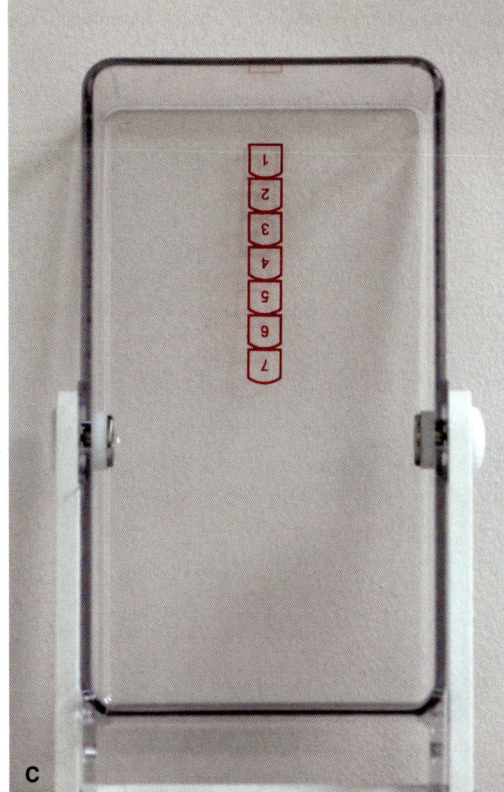
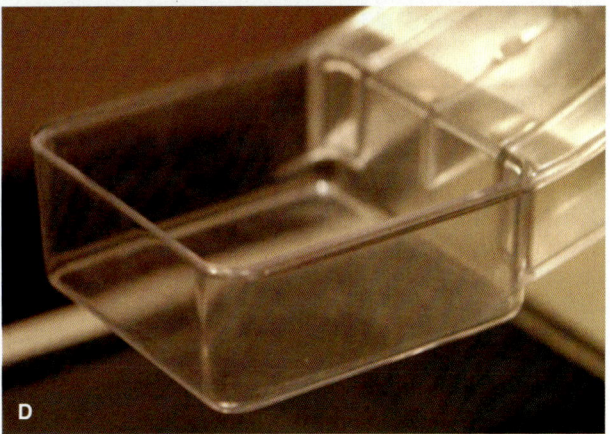
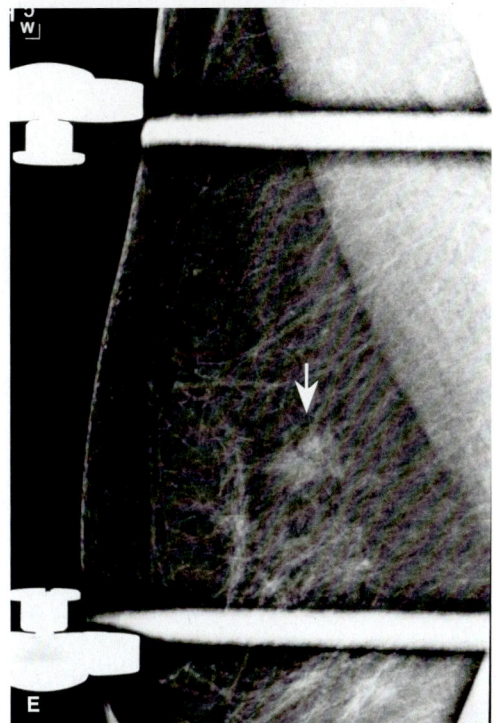

FIG. 3.4 • **Spot compression paddles. A:** This is one of the paddles that we use for our spot compression images (spot compression, spot compression magnification, spot tangential, and spot rolled views). This paddle is particularly helpful in evaluating potential lesions that are posterior or axillary in location. **B:** Frameless spot paddle. A 7.5-cm compression cup is centered on an 18 × 24 cm paddle. This, in combination with the paddle shown in part **A**, is the paddle we use for *all* of our spot compression views. The absence of a metal frame permits evaluation of all of the tissue surrounding the spot and eliminates the metallic arm artifact that is seen on images when the paddle in part **A** is used. The diagnostic images shown throughout this chapter and the book were done with the spot paddle shown in part **A** or this frameless paddle. Rectangular **(C)** and square **(D)** compression paddles. We do not use these two types of paddles (we do not even have them in our facility). Their geometry and size are such that they preclude obtaining maximal compression to a small area of the breast. In many patients, paddles of this size include more than half or the entire breast, negating the benefit of "focal" compression. **E:** Spot compression image done with rectangular paddle. Irregular mass with indistinct margins *(arrow)* is present. Note the amount of breast tissue and pectoral muscle included in the image. When this amount of pectoral muscle is included on the image, compression of the tissue anteriorly (where the mass is located) is likely to be limited, negating the benefits of doing "spot" compression views. We define spot as that obtained with the compression paddles shown in part **A** or **B**; we do not use the paddles shown in parts **C** and **D** in our diagnostic evaluations.

Table 3.2	INDICATIONS FOR SPOT COMPRESSION VIEWS

Evaluation of questionable areas
   Density
   Asymmetry
   Distortion
Evaluation of masses
   Characterization of margins
   Effect on surrounding tissue
Inclusion of tissue
   Posterior
   Axillary
   Upper inner quadrant
Technical issues
   Blurring
   Underexposure (focal)
Localizations (preoperative)
   See Chapter 12

views, mammographic–ultrasound concordance can be established easily (see discussion in Chapter 4). Although for many of the figures used in this chapter one mammographic and ultrasound projection is provided, orthogonal images are done routinely in the evaluation of patients (e.g., spot compression views are obtained in two projections, and orthogonal images of the lesion are taken on ultrasound); space constraints limit the number of images I can present. Also as described in subsequent sections, we do not do 90-degree lateral views routinely in our diagnostic evaluations. We relegate the use of these projections to specific situations and to answer specific questions.

MAGNIFICATION VIEWS

Factors to consider when doing magnification views are listed in Table 3.3. Magnification views are obtained by moving the breast away from the digital detector (i.e., increasing the object to image distance and decreasing the source to object distance), thereby creating an air gap. A grid is not needed because scatter radiation is eliminated in the air gap. As the object to image distance increases, the amount of magnification increases (e.g., 1.5×, 1.8×); however, this is associated with a loss of resolution from an increasing penumbra effect. The use of a small focal spot (0.1 mm) helps overcome the loss of resolution. With the small focal spot, however, exposure time is increased, leading potentially to motion. In an effort to obtain acceptable exposure times, the kilovolt used to obtain magnification views can be increased by at least 2 compared with that used for screening views.

rolled views or a 90-degree lateral view (see triangulation). We make *no* assumptions about the possible location of the lesion in the orthogonal plane. If on the screening images a potential lesion is seen in both projections, spot compression views are done in both before any effort is made to take the patient to ultrasound. Once the lesion is identified and fully evaluated with CC and MLO spot compression

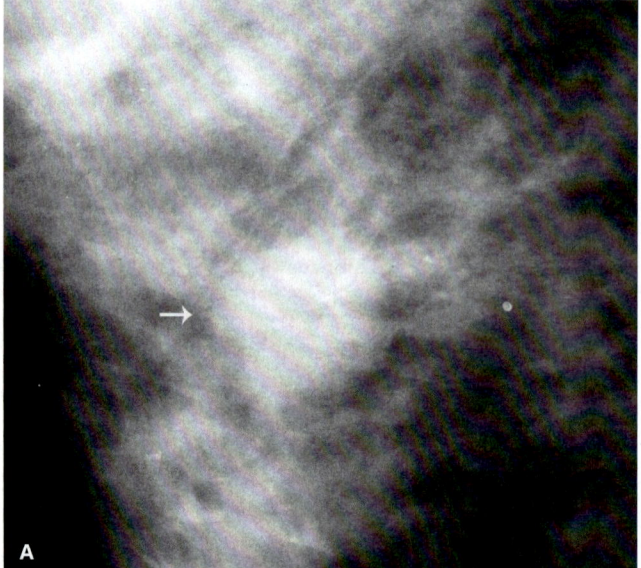 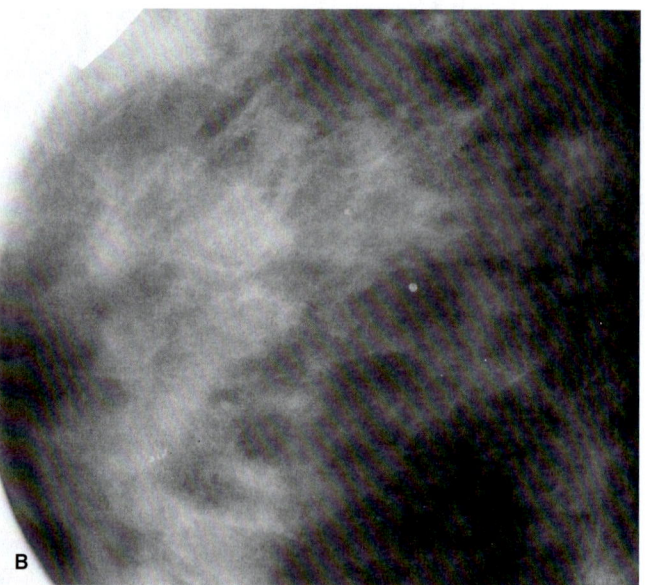

FIG. 3.5 • **Pseudolesion, superimposed glandular tissue. A:** CC view, right breast photographically coned. A round density *(arrow)* possibly representing a mass is noted on the screening study. Time and time again, you will find that what you perceive on screening studies may be misleading. "Lesions" of concern on the screening study turn out to be "imaginomas," and true lesions look innocuous. Screening is for detection, not characterization. We make no attempt to describe features or arrive at any conclusion of possible lesions detected on a screening mammogram. Even in women who have an obvious cancer, additional views are helpful in characterizing the imaging features of the lesion, extent of the lesion, detecting additional unsuspected lesions, allowing us to establish rapport with the patient and expedite her care by undertaking imaging-guided biopsy when she returns for additional views. **B:** Spot compression view. No abnormality is identified. Surrounding benign calcifications confirm that the right area of tissue has been evaluated on the compression view. The original density represents superimposition of normal glandular tissue (presumably tissue that is inadequately compressed). Since the "potential mass" is not confirmed on the view in which it is seen, no additional views need to be done in the CC or oblique projections. (From Cardeñosa G. *Breast Imaging [The Core Curriculum Series]*. Philadelphia, PA: Lippincott Williams & Wilkins; 2003.)

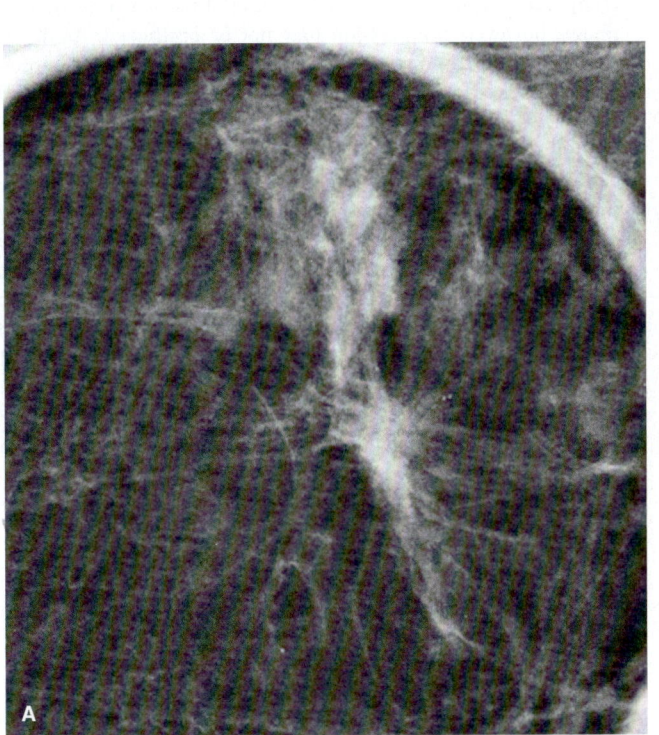
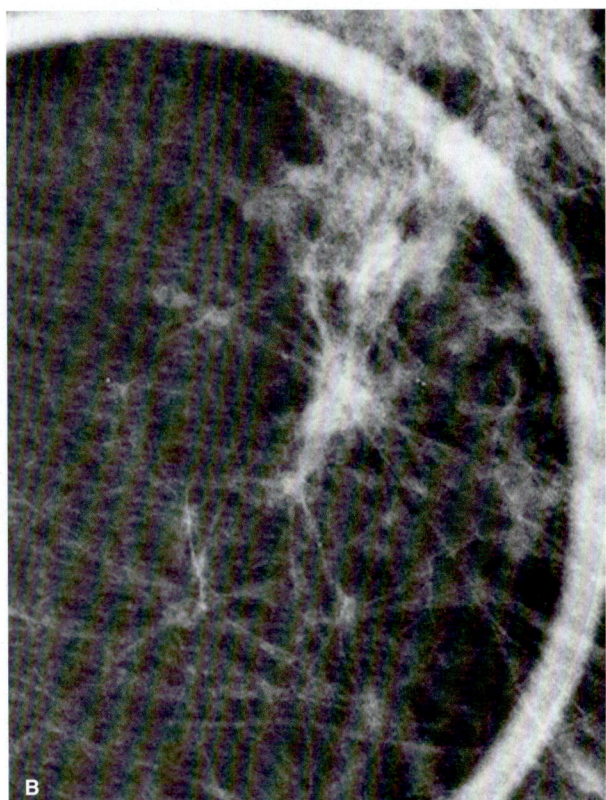
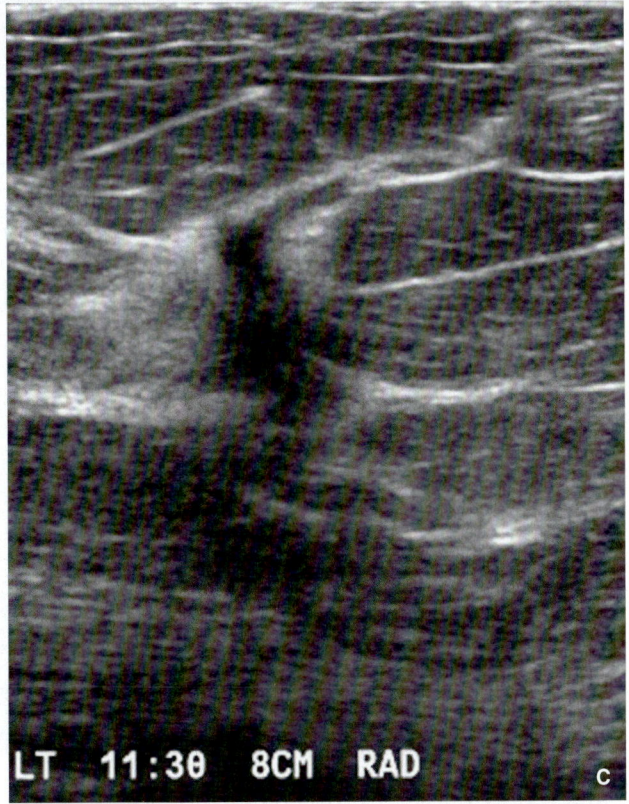

FIG. 3.6 • **Invasive ductal carcinoma with lobular features.** CC **(A)** and MLO **(B)** spot compression views (done using the frameless paddle). An irregular isodense mass with spiculated margins and two associated round calcifications is confirmed in the left breast (see Fig. 2.43 for the screening views on this patient). **C:** Ultrasound. On the basis of the location of the lesion on the mammographic images, we walk into the ultrasound with a specific anticipated location for the mass. An irregular, vertically oriented mass with spiculated and angular margins, an echogenic rim, and shadowing is identified at the 11:30 o'clock position, 8 cm from the left nipple as expected on the basis of the mammogram. As with the spots, orthogonal images of the mass are done as part of our ultrasound evaluation, only the radial *(RAD)* projection is shown here. At the time of the ultrasound, ultrasound-guided palpation is done to determine whether the finding is palpable; the mass is not palpable in this patient. BI-RADS 4C: Suspicious abnormality, biopsy is indicated. Ultrasound-guided biopsy is done to establish the diagnosis.

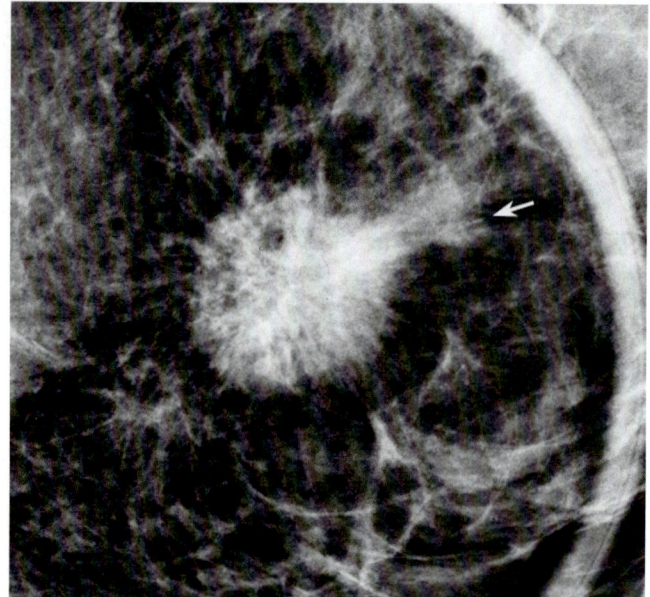

FIG. 3.7 • **Invasive ductal carcinoma, intermediate to high grade.** Spot compression view (done using the frameless paddle), CC projection. A dense round mass with indistinct and spiculated margins as well as associated calcifications *(arrow)* is present in the lower inner aspect of the left breast. See Figures 2.46, 4.39D, and 5.21 for screening, ultrasound, and MRI images on this patient, respectively. Spot compression view in the oblique projection is not shown. BI-RADS 4C: Suspicious abnormality, biopsy is indicated. Ultrasound-guided core biopsy is done.

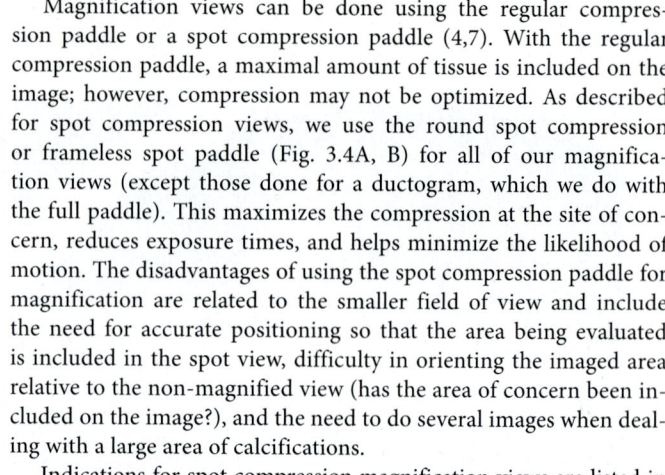

Magnification views can be done using the regular compression paddle or a spot compression paddle (4,7). With the regular compression paddle, a maximal amount of tissue is included on the image; however, compression may not be optimized. As described for spot compression views, we use the round spot compression or frameless spot paddle (Fig. 3.4A, B) for all of our magnification views (except those done for a ductogram, which we do with the full paddle). This maximizes the compression at the site of concern, reduces exposure times, and helps minimize the likelihood of motion. The disadvantages of using the spot compression paddle for magnification are related to the smaller field of view and include the need for accurate positioning so that the area being evaluated is included in the spot view, difficulty in orienting the imaged area relative to the non-magnified view (has the area of concern been included on the image?), and the need to do several images when dealing with a large area of calcifications.

Indications for spot compression magnification views are listed in Table 3.4. Although many use magnification views to evaluate masses and possible areas of distortion regardless of the presence of calcifications, we use spot compression magnification views almost exclusively to evaluate and characterize calcifications (Figs. 3.10B, 3.15, and 3.16) and masses (Fig. 3.17) or areas of distortion having associated calcifications.

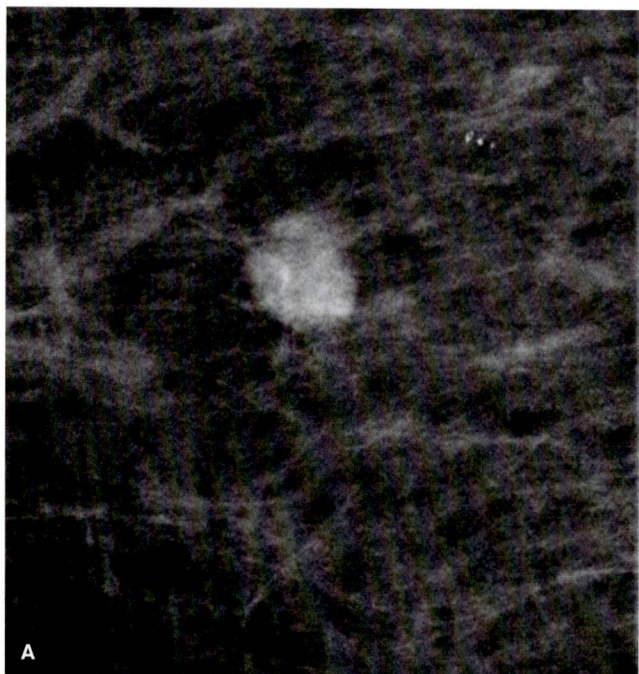
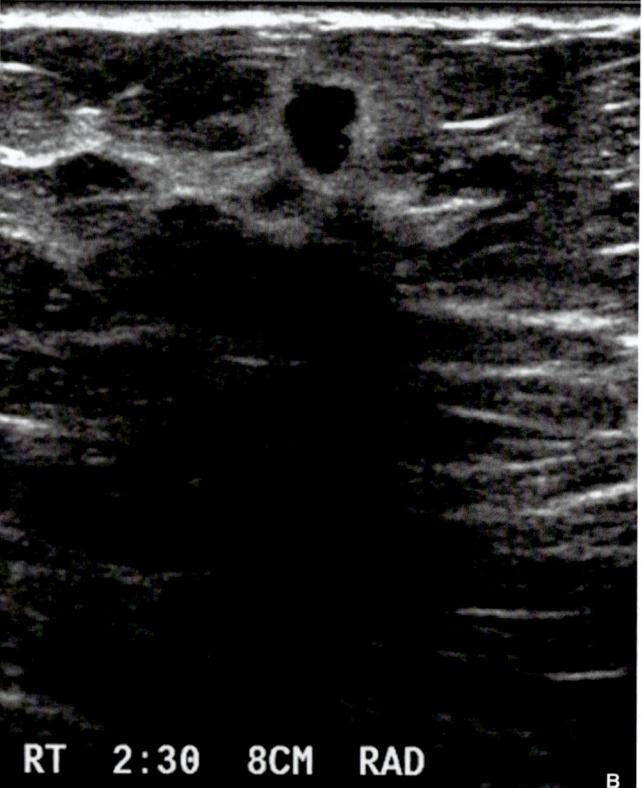

FIG. 3.8 • **Invasive ductal carcinoma, low to intermediate grade. A:** Spot compression view, mediolateral oblique projection. A dense round mass with indistinct margins is confirmed on the spot compression views (only MLO projection is shown). See Figure 2.47 for the screening views on this patient. At what location (be specific) would you expect to find this lesion on ultrasound? **B:** Ultrasound. Even though this lesion projects below the level of the nipple on the MLO view, it is actually above the level of the nipple and is identified at the 2:30 o'clock position, 8 cm from the nipple (see triangulation discussion). The mass is vertically oriented with angular margins and an echogenic rim and correlates with the mammographic findings. Only the radial *(RAD)* projection is shown. In a patient with a personal history of breast cancer and the development of a new dense mass with these mammographic and ultrasound features, a malignancy is expected. BI-RADS 4C: Suspicious abnormality, biopsy is indicated. Ultrasound-guided core biopsy is done.

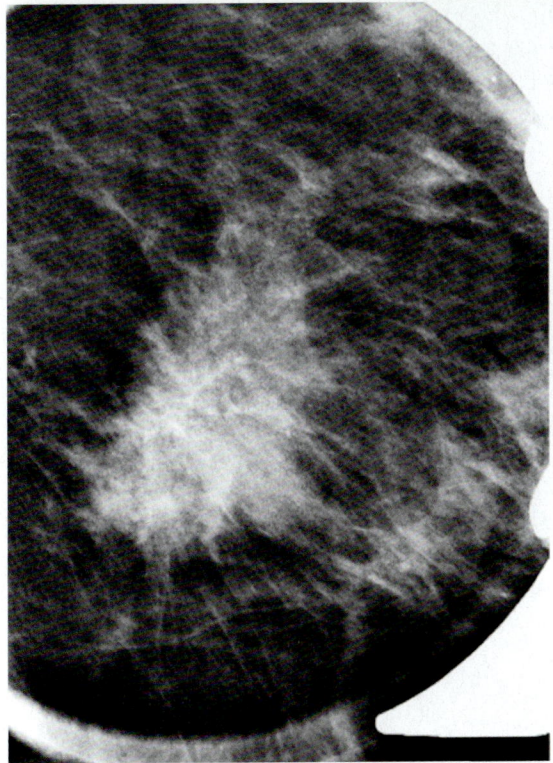

FIG. 3.9 • **Invasive ductal carcinoma, low nuclear grade.** Spot compression view, MLO projection. An irregular isodense mass with spiculated margins is confirmed on the spot compression views (only MLO projection shown). See Figure 2.49 for the screening views on this patient. At what specific location do you expect to find this lesion on ultrasound? See Figure 4.39C for the ultrasound on this patient. BI-RADS 4C: Suspicious abnormality, biopsy is indicated and done. The spot compression paddle was used for this image; a portion of the metal frame is seen surrounding the paddle.

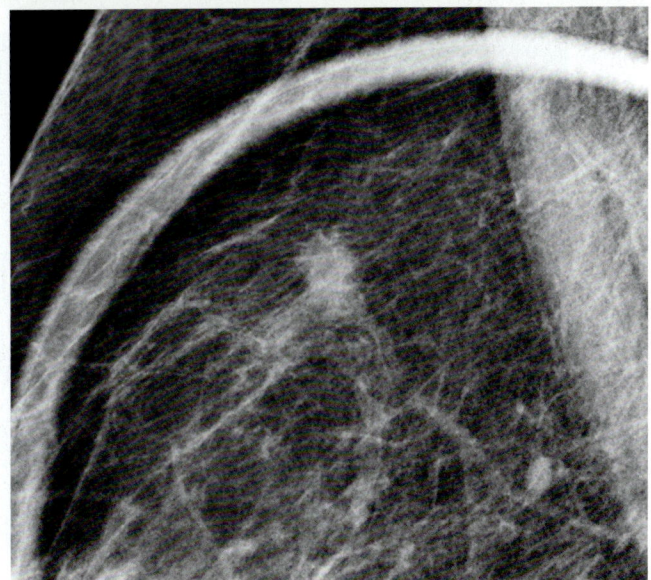

FIG. 3.11 • **Invasive ductal carcinoma, intermediate nuclear grade.** Spot compression view (done using the frameless paddle) in the MLO projection. An oval isodense mass with partially obscured and indistinct margins is confirmed on the spot compression views (CC projection not shown). BI-RADS 4C: Suspicious abnormality biopsy is indicated. Ultrasound-guided core biopsy is done. See Figures 2.40 and 4.39B for the screening and an ultrasound image on this patient, respectively.

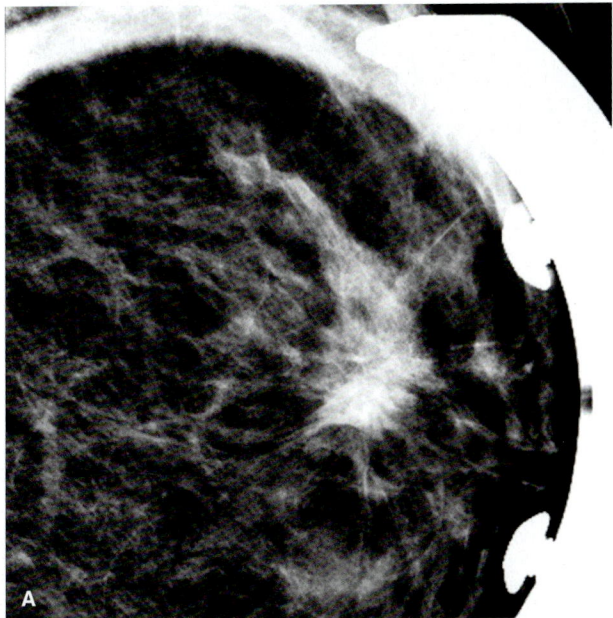
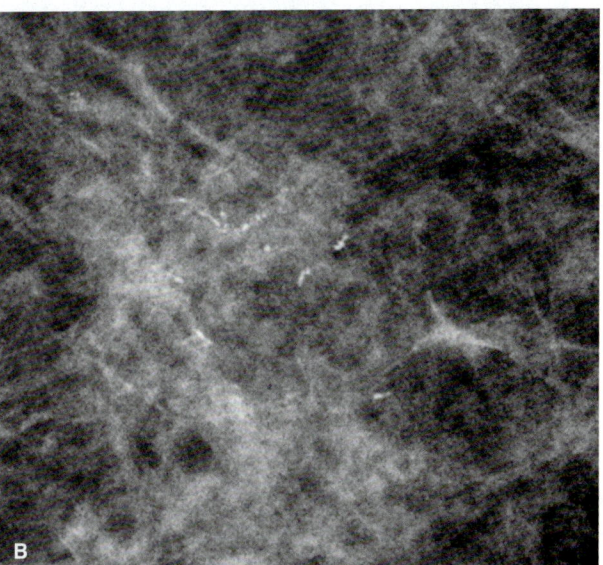

FIG. 3.10 • **Multicentric disease: invasive carcinoma with lobular features and ductal carcinoma in situ. A:** Spot compression view in the MLO projection. An irregular high-density mass with spiculated margins is confirmed on the spot compression views (CC projection not shown). The spot compression paddle was used for this image; a portion of the metal frame is seen surrounding the paddle. See Fig. 2.50 for screening views on this patient. BI-RADS 4C: Suspicious abnormality biopsy is indicated. At what location (be specific) would you expect to find this lesion on ultrasound? See Figure 4.39E for the ultrasound on this patient. Ultrasound-guided core biopsy is done to establish the diagnosis of invasive carcinoma with lobular features. You will recall that in addition to the mass, a cluster of calcifications was also detected in the lateral aspect of the breast of this patient. **B:** Spot compression magnification view in the CC projection confirms a cluster of pleomorphic calcifications that includes linear forms, and some of the calcifications demonstrate a linear orientation. BI-RADS 4C: Suspicious abnormality biopsy is indicated. Stereotactically guided core biopsy is done to establish the diagnosis of DCIS.

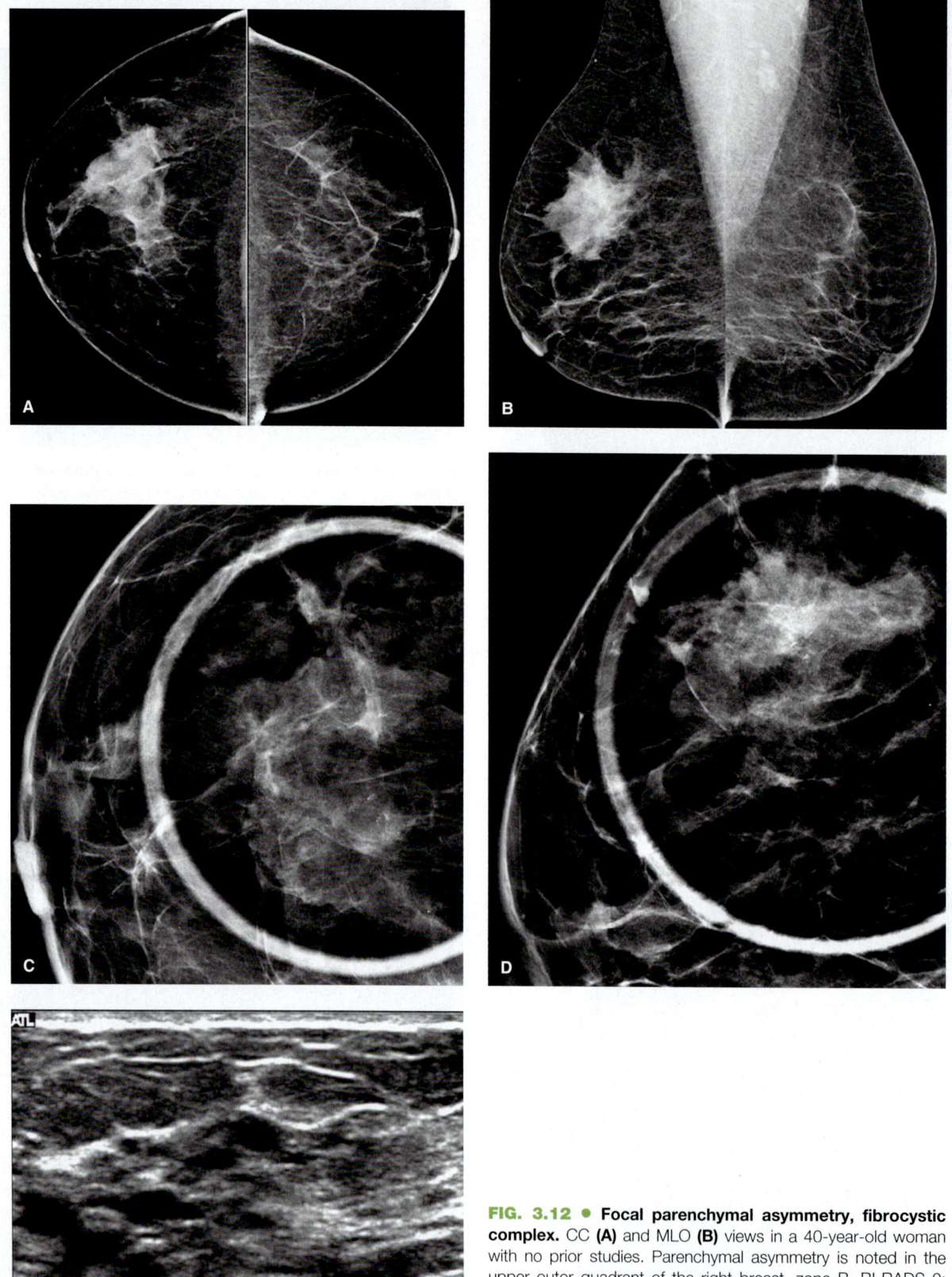

FIG. 3.12 • **Focal parenchymal asymmetry, fibrocystic complex.** CC **(A)** and MLO **(B)** views in a 40-year-old woman with no prior studies. Parenchymal asymmetry is noted in the upper outer quadrant of the right breast, zone B. BI-RADS 0: Need additional imaging evaluation. CC **(C)** and MLO **(D)** spot compression views (done with the frameless paddle) demonstrate glandular tissue with intermingled fat, areas of scalloping, and no bulging contours. Since this is the patient's first mammogram, correlative physical examination and ultrasound are done. On physical examination, globular, mobile tissue is palpated corresponding to the parenchymal asymmetry seen mammographically. **E:** On ultrasound (orthogonal images not shown), dense fibrous tissue with multiple cysts of varying sizes is imaged corresponding to the asymmetric tissue. BI-RADS 2: Benign finding.

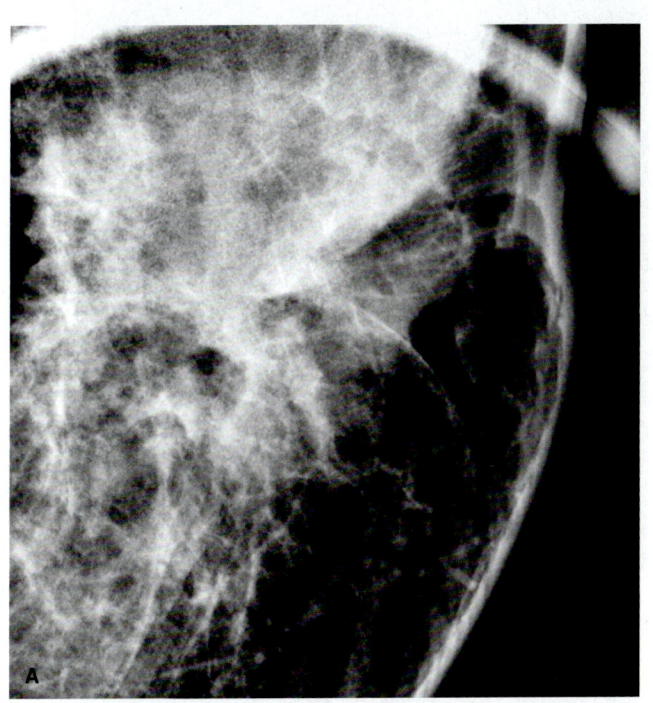
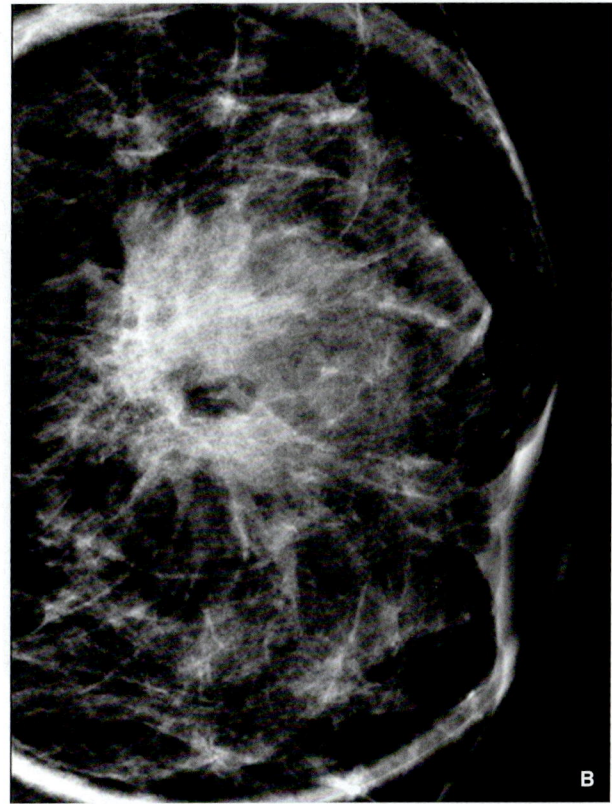
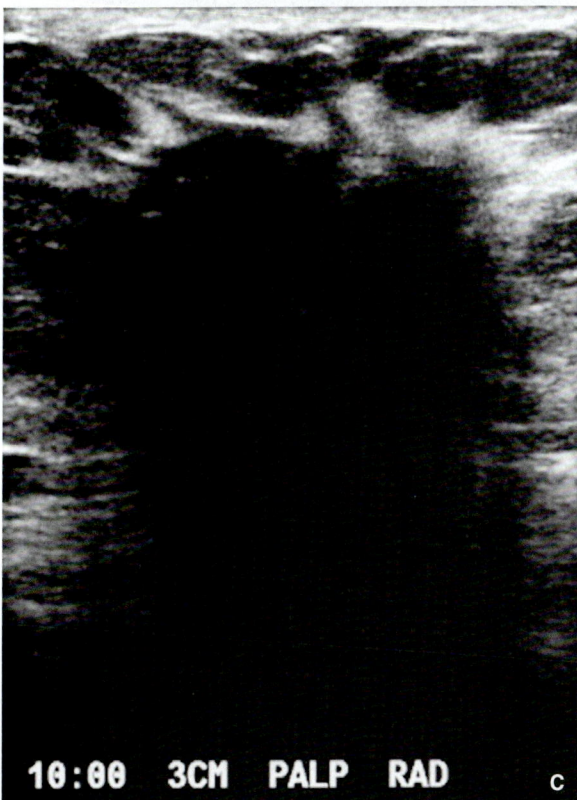

FIG. 3.13 • **Invasive lobular carcinoma.** CC **(A)** and MLO **(B)** spot compression views of the left breast. Distortion without a definable mass is the predominant finding on the CC spot compression view. This is more mass-like on the oblique spot. See Figure 2.44 for the screening views on this patient. **C:** Ultrasound. On physical examination, a hard mass is readily palpable *(PALP)*. A mass with intense shadowing and spiculated margins is imaged in the upper inner quadrant of the left breast; only radial *(RAD)* plane is shown. BI-RADS 4C: Suspicious abnormality, biopsy is indicated. Ultrasound-guided core biopsy is done. See Figure 5.22A for an MRI image on this patient.

ROLLED OR CHANGE OF ANGLE VIEWS

Rolled or change of angle views are commonly used in conjunction with spot compression views in establishing the presence of a lesion (8). For rolled views, we also use the round spot compression paddle. Breast tissue is often planar and changes in appearance as tissue is rolled or the angle of the incident beam is changed (Fig. 3.18). In contrast, most breast cancers (except some invasive lobular carcinoma and, small, <5-mm, invasive ductal carcinomas) are three dimensional. As tissue

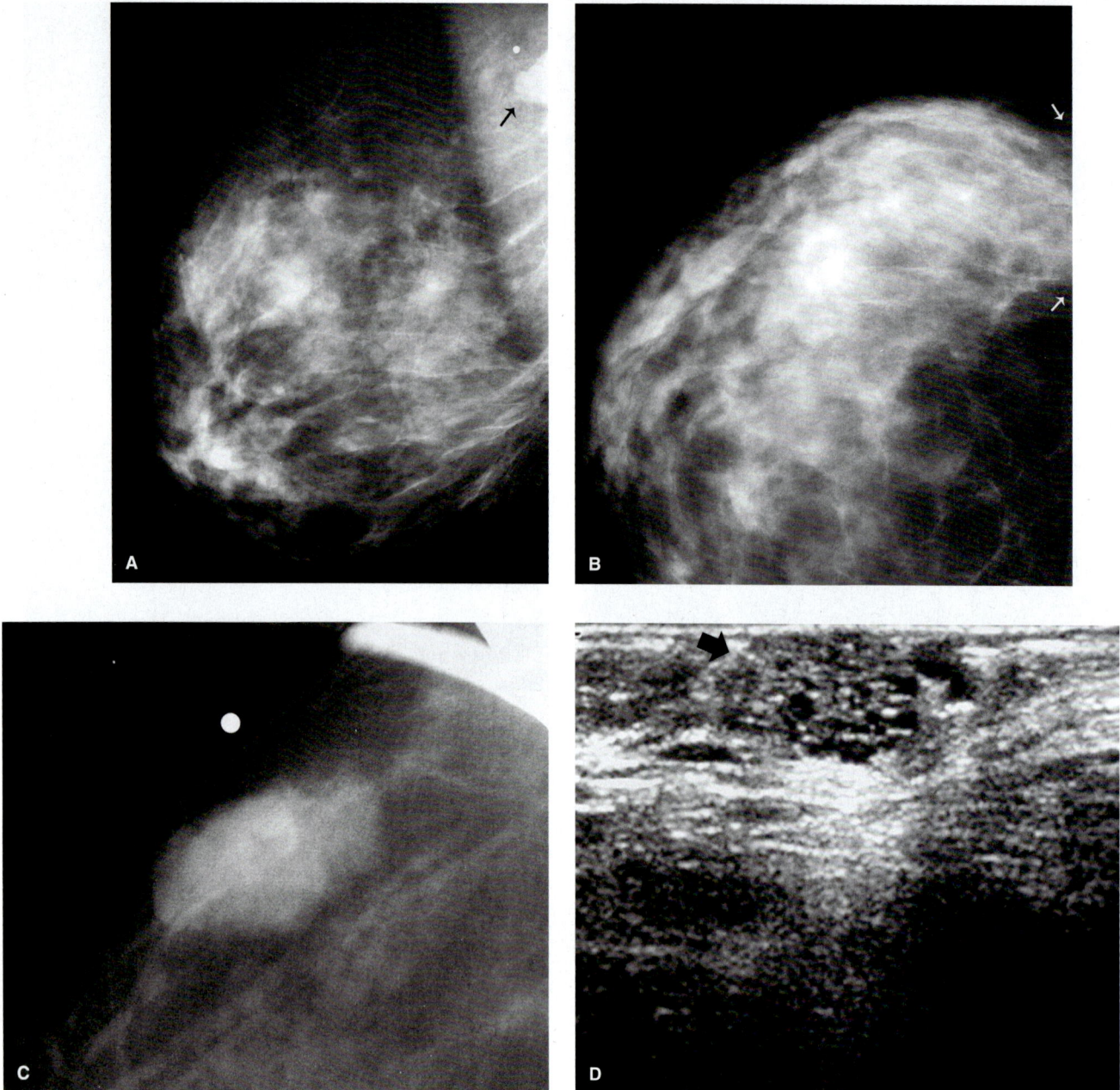

FIG. 3.14 • **Use of spot compression to include more tissue in the field of view.** MLO **(A)** and CC **(B)** views of the right breast in a 40-year-old patient who presents with a "lump" in the right breast. A mass is partially seen on the MLO view superimposed on the pectoral muscle *(arrow)*. Metallic BB is noted above the partially imaged mass close to the edge of the image. Neither the lesion nor the metallic BB is included on the CC view; however, tissue is seen extending to the edge of the film *(arrows)*. **C:** Spot compression view in an exaggerated craniocaudal lateral (XCCL) projection. Isodense oval mass with circumscribed margins is now seen in its entirety surrounded by subcutaneous fat. Spot compression views can be helpful in evaluating areas that may be excluded from the field of view (e.g., axillary tail, axilla, upper inner quadrants posteriorly, etc.). **D:** Ultrasound demonstrates a hypoechoic mass with small anechoic round areas and posterior acoustic enhancement *(arrow)*. BI-RADS 4A: Suspicious abnormality, biopsy is indicated. Ultrasound-guided core biopsy is done. The lesion decreased significantly in size following the first core sample and completely resolved following the second core sample, consistent with the findings described histologically of fibrocystic change with apocrine and epithelial lined cysts. (From Cardeñosa G. *Breast Imaging [The Core Curriculum Series]*. Philadelphia, PA: Lippincott Williams & Wilkins; 2003.)

is rolled, the contour and appearance of most cancers do not change significantly. Rolled or change of angle views can also be used to triangulate the location of a lesion (Fig. 3.19), or to move a lesion away from glandular tissue so that it is surrounded by fat and evaluated more completely.

For triangulation purposes, rolled or change of angle views can give the approximate location of a lesion seen in only one view on the screening study. You can expect lesions to move with their surrounding tissue. If there is a lesion on the CC view that cannot be identified

Table 3.3 MAGNIFICATION VIEWS

Air gap
No grid used (scatter radiation eliminated in air gap)
Small focal spot (0.1 mm) to overcome loss or resolution resulting from the penumbra effect
Small focal spot increases exposure times
    Increase kilovolt used for screening images by at least 2
Spot compression paddle

Table 3.4 INDICATION FOR SPOT COMPRESSION MAGNIFICATION VIEWS

Evaluation of masses
    Margins
    Shape
    Associated calcifications
    Effect on surrounding tissue
    Presence of satellite lesion(s)
Evaluation of calcifications
    Morphology
    Extent
    Associated mass or distortion
Evaluation of architectural distortion
    Isolated
    Associated with mass
    Associated with calcifications
Ductography (Chapter 12)

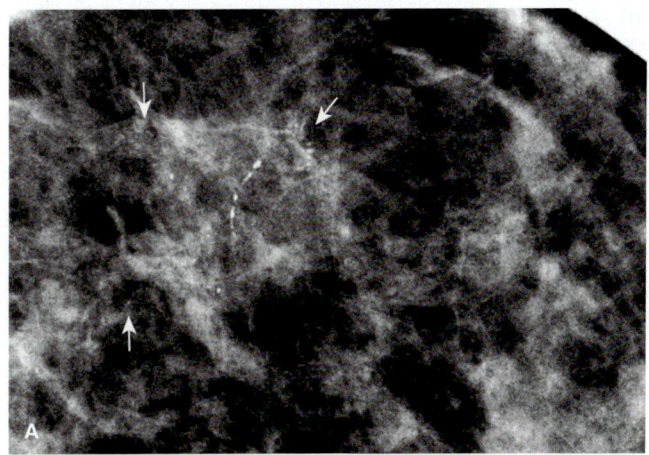

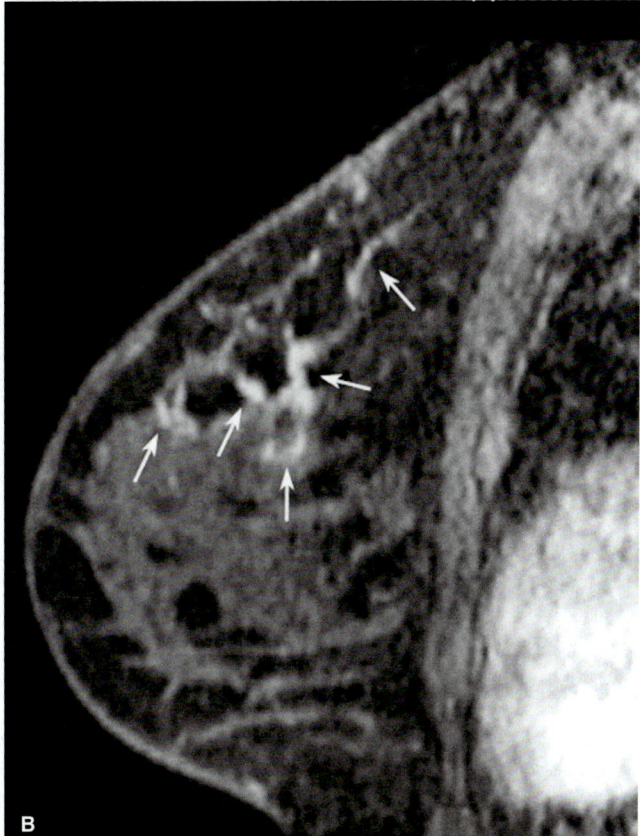

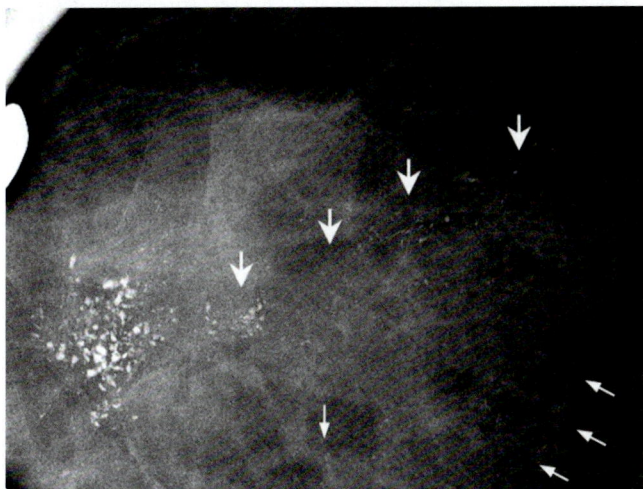

FIG. 3.15 • Ductal carcinoma in situ. Spot compression magnification view in the CC projection. A dominant cluster of pleomorphic, high-density calcifications *(thick arrows)* is identified. Segmentally distributed coarse heterogeneous (round, punctate, and linear) calcifications are noted extending posteriorly from the dominant cluster for approximately 3 cm. Additionally, amorphous calcifications *(thin arrows)* are noted scattered and encompassing even more tissue. Spot compression magnification view in the oblique projection is not shown. See Figure 2.42 for the screening views on this patient. BI-RADS 4C: Suspicious abnormality, biopsy is indicated.

FIG. 3.16 • Ductal carcinoma in situ (DCIS). A: Spot compression magnification view in the MLO projection in a 48-year-old patient called back from screening for evaluation of a cluster of calcifications in the left breast (spot compression magnification view in the CC projection not shown). A cluster of calcifications *(arrows)* that includes linear calcifications in a linear distribution as well as round and punctate calcifications is confirmed in the upper outer aspect of the left breast posteriorly. BI-RADS 4C: Suspicious abnormality, biopsy is indicated. Stereotactically guided biopsy is done to establish the diagnosis. **B:** Magnetic resonance imaging, sagittal T1 reconstruction image of the left breast postcontrast demonstrates approximately 6 cm of linear enhancement *(arrows)*. An MRI-guided biopsy of the anterior most extent of the enhancement is done to confirm the suspected extent of the disease. DCIS is confirmed anteriorly. Although conservative therapy was initially planned, given the extent of the disease demonstrated on the MRI and confirmed histologically, a mastectomy is done. Sentinel lymph node is negative.

FIG. 3.17 • Invasive ductal carcinoma with associated DCIS. Spot compression magnification view in the CC projection (spot compression magnification in oblique projection is not shown). A dense round mass *(thick arrow)* with spiculated margins and associated linear and punctate calcifications in a linear orientation *(thin arrows)* are imaged in the subareolar area of the right breast. BI-RADS 5: Highly suspicious abnormality biopsy is indicated.

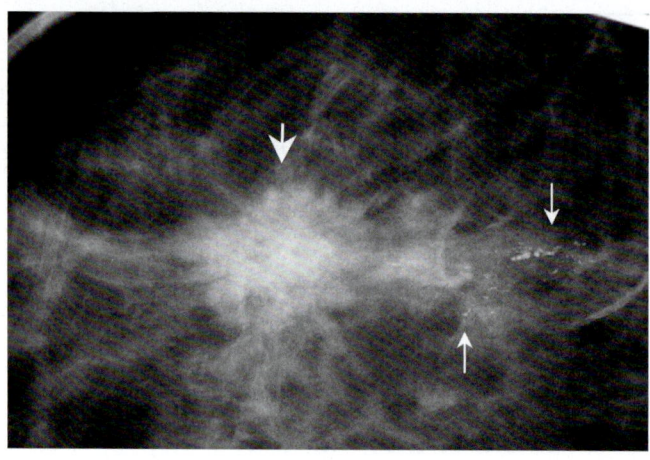

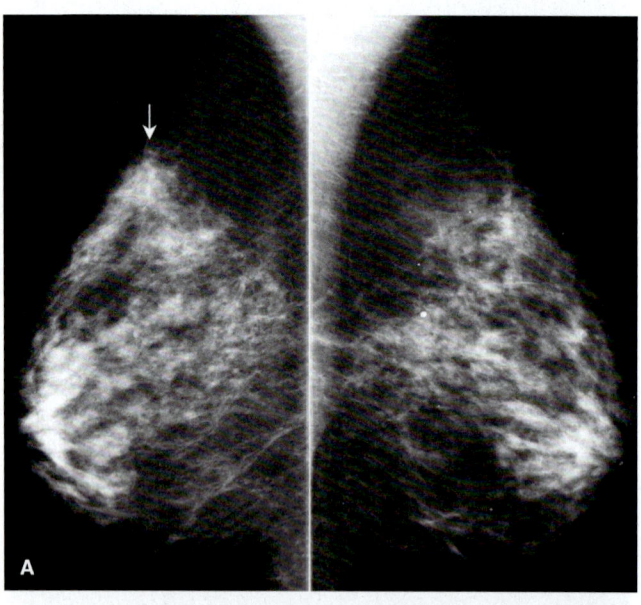

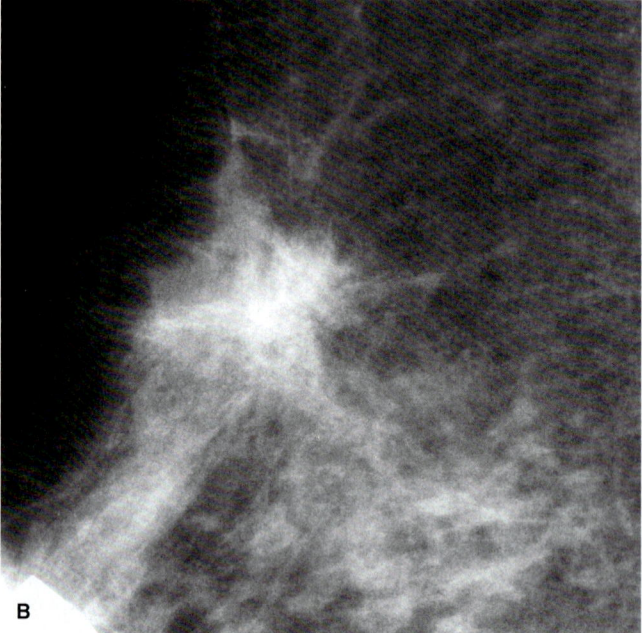

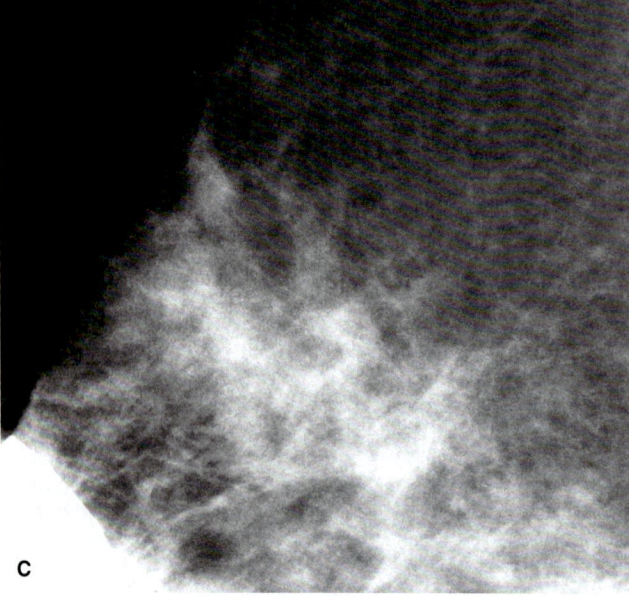

FIG. 3.18 • **Use of spot rolled views in the evaluation of a possible mass seen in only one view. A:** MLO views, screening study. Asymmetric rounded tissue *(arrow)* is noted superiorly on the right MLO. No correlate is identified in the CC projection. Rather than making assumptions of where this could be on the CC view, we need to establish whether it is real or possibly superimposed tissue. We stay in the projection in which we see it and obtain a spot compression view. **B:** Spot compression view in the oblique projection suggests that this may persist. Spot rolled views are done to further evaluate this area as well as possibly determine the expected location on the CC view. **C** and **D:** Spot rolled views in the oblique projection demonstrate a significant change in the appearance of this tissue with no underlying mass identified. **E:** Ninety-degree lateral (LM) view of the right breast is done as an additional change of angle view. No mass is identified superiorly in the right breast. BI-RADS 1: Negative.

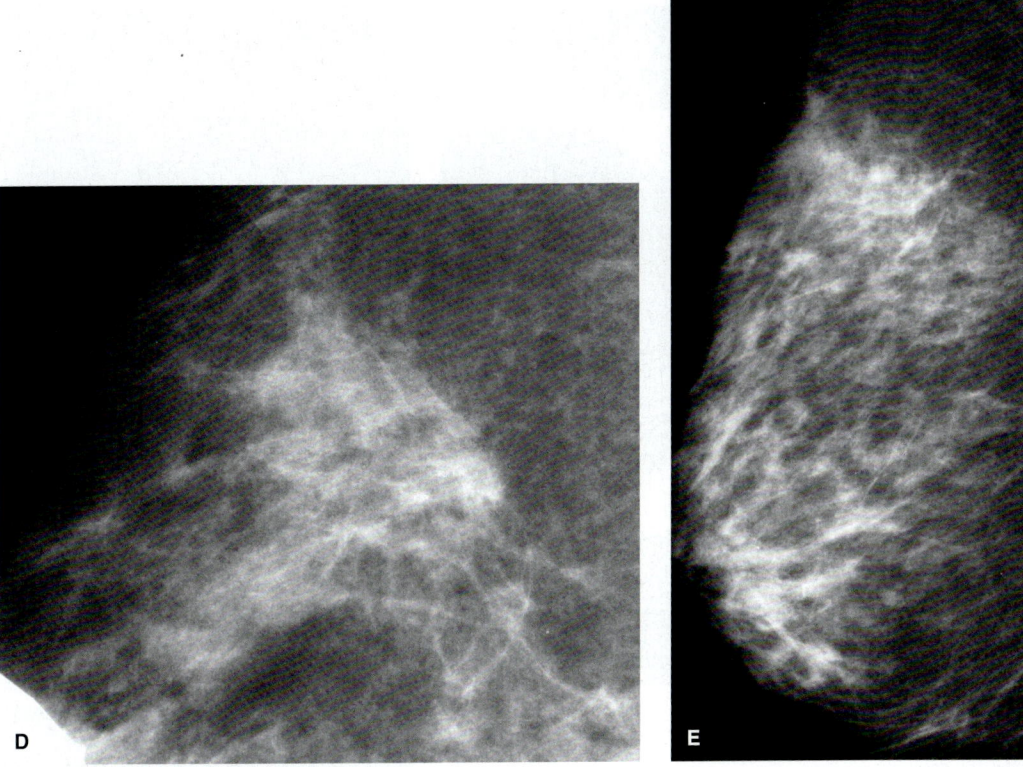

FIG. 3.18 • (continued)

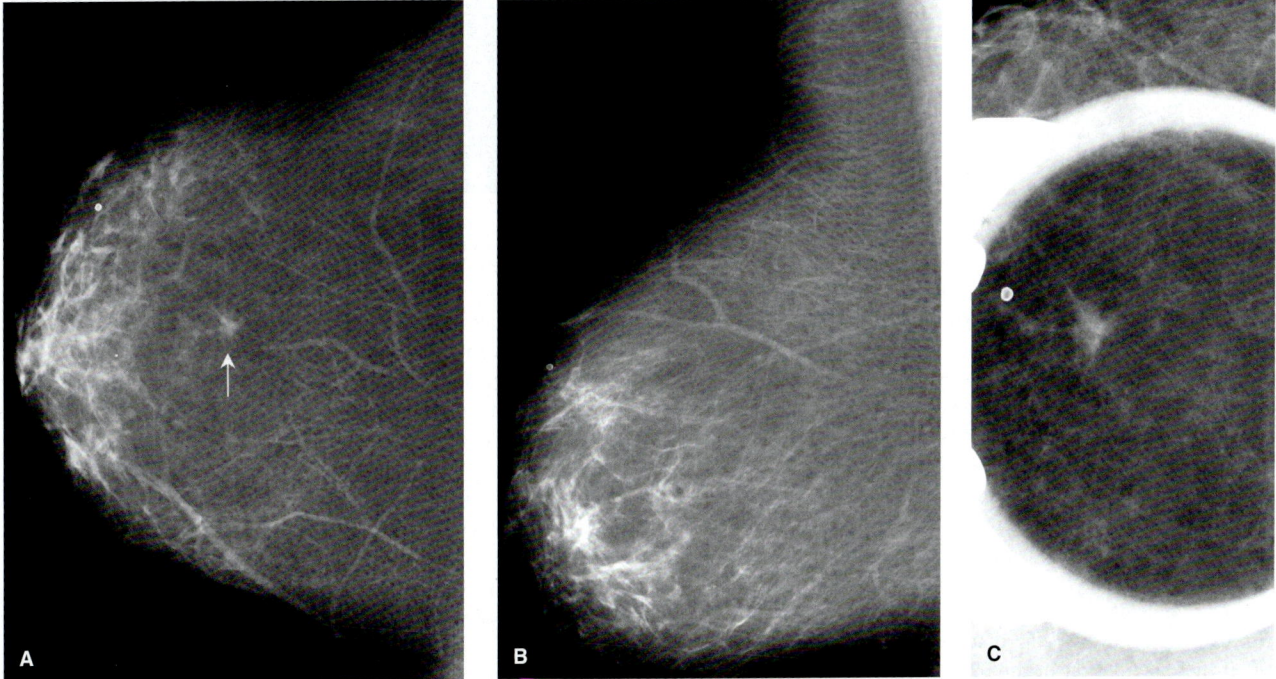

FIG. 3.19 • **Use of rolled views, triangulation.** CC **(A)** and MLO **(B)** views of the right breast in a 63-year-old woman who has had a left mastectomy for breast cancer. A new mass (arrow) is noted in the CC view, but no abnormality is apparent in the MLO view. Even though no finding is readily identified in the oblique projection, the appearance of the finding on the CC view in a patient with a previous left mastectomy for breast cancer warrants additional evaluation. BI-RADS 0: Need additional imaging evaluation. When the patient returns, we stay in the projection in which the finding is noted and determine if it is a real finding. **C:** Spot compression view, right CC projection. Is it real? Yes, it is real and the margins are spiculated. Rather than make any assumptions (which may be wrong) of where this is on the oblique projection, spot rolled view is done.

FIG. 3.19 • (continued) **D:** Spot rolled view with inferior tissue rolled medially. First, the lesion persists, further supporting that it is a true lesion and second, it moves with inferior tissue. This is consistent with the lesion being in the inferior aspect of the breast; the amount of movement suggests that it is far inferiorly (the more the lesion moves, the farther away it is from the central aspect of the breast). **E:** Spot compression view oblique view, inferiorly. This confirms the presence of the mass that is now localized precisely. When you ultrasound this patient, you know exactly where to look for the lesion, facilitating correlation between mammographic and ultrasound findings. We are no longer making any assumptions about this lesion and where it might be in the breast. **F:** Ultrasound. An irregular, vertically oriented mass with angular margins, disrupting soft tissue planes is readily identified at 6 o'clock, 4 cm from the right nipple. As expected, this mass is superficial in location. BI-RADS 4C: Suspicious abnormality, biopsy is indicated. An invasive ductal carcinoma low nuclear grade is diagnosed on the ultrasound-guided core biopsy.

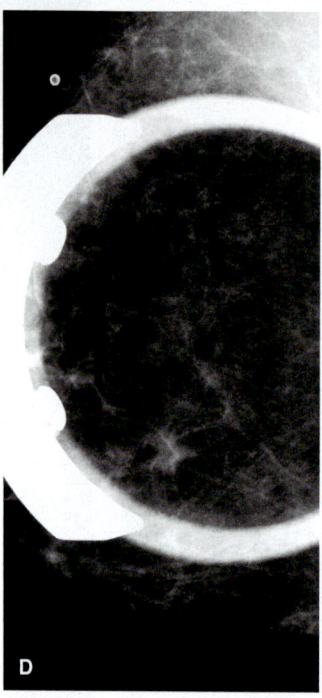
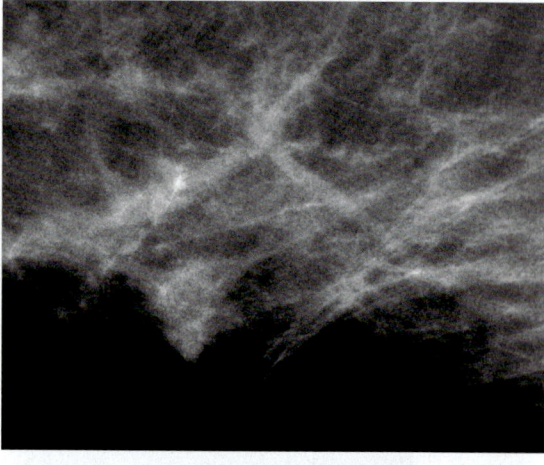
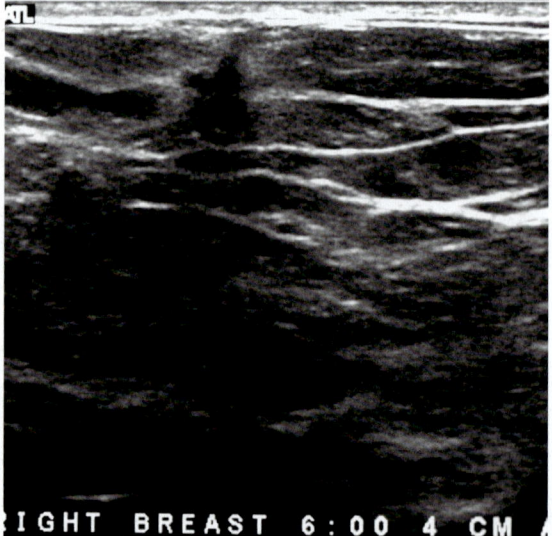

with certainty on the MLO view, rolled views can be done. If the top of the breast is rolled medially while the lower part is rolled laterally and the lesion moves medially, this suggests the lesion is in the superior portion of the breast. If the lesion does not shift in position significantly, the lesion is in the central portion of the breast, and if the lesion moves laterally (Figs. 3.19 and 3.20), it is in the inferior aspect of the breast. This can be confirmed by repeating the image and rolling the upper portion of the breast laterally and the lower portion medially. Given an approximate location for the lesion, the MLO, or a 90-degree lateral view, can now be reviewed, and additional workup of the upper, central, or lower portions of the breast is undertaken.

Rolled or change of angle views can also be used to move a lesion away from surrounding tissue so that it can be better evaluated. For example, if there is a lesion in the inferior and medial aspect of the breast that is partially visualized on the CC view medially, the lower portion of the breast can be rolled medially so that the lesion is moved away from surrounding glandular tissue into a fatty area (Fig. 3.21).

TANGENTIAL VIEWS

Tangential views are used in evaluating women with palpable masses (9), focal tenderness, a history of lumpectomy and radiation therapy for breast cancer, and in localizing lesions to the skin. We do all of our tangential views using the spot compression paddle (Fig. 3.4A, B).

For women presenting with a palpable abnormality or focal tenderness, a metallic BB is used to mark the location of the mass or focal findings on routine CC and MLO views. Additionally, a tangential view of the area of concern is obtained (Fig. 3.22) (4). This is particularly helpful in women with dense tissue (Fig. 3.23). The purpose of the tangential view is to try to at least partially surround the area of concern with subcutaneous fat (Fig. 3.24; also see Fig. 7.58B).

On any two views of the breast, only a small amount of skin is in tangent to the incident x-rays; most of the skin is superimposed on the breast parenchyma (in fact, most of the radiation used in exposing the breast on any given image is expended in penetrating the two layers of skin). Consequently, skin calcifications and masses are commonly superimposed on the breast parenchyma on screening views and mischaracterized as potential breast lesions. By placing a marker on the skin lesion, a tangential view is obtained to document that the lesion is in the skin (see Figs. 7.9 and 7.11) rather than in the breast. To localize calcifications to the skin, you can follow some of the principles described for preoperative wire localizations (see Chapter 12) so as to demonstrate on a spot tangential view that the calcifications are in the skin. Orthogonal views (CC and 90-degree lateral) of the breast are reviewed, and the shortest distance from the skin to the calcification is determined. A fenestrated alphanumeric compression paddle is used to compress the skin surface thought to contain the calcifications, and an image is obtained (e.g., a CC view using the alphanumeric compression paddle is done if the calcifications are closest to the superior skin

FIG. 3.20 • Diagram, use of rolled views for triangulation purposes. A: Lesion seen on the CC view, not identified with certainty on MLO. M, medial; L, lateral; S, superior or cranial, I, inferior or caudal. In *scenario 1*, the lesion is in the superior aspect of the breast. The lesion will move with superior tissue. If superior tissue is moved laterally and inferior tissue is moved medially, the lesion moves laterally. If superior tissue is moved medially and inferior tissue is moved laterally, the lesion moves medially. In *scenario 2*, the lesion is central in the breast. No significant shifts in position are noted when tissue is rolled. In *scenario 3*, the lesion is in the inferior aspect of the breast. If superior tissue is moved laterally and inferior tissue is moved medially, the lesion will move medially. If superior tissue is moved medially and inferior tissue laterally, the lesion will move laterally. **B:** Lesion seen on the lateral view, not identified with certainty on the CC view. In *scenario 1*, the lesion is lateral in the breast. If lateral tissue is rolled superiorly and medial tissue inferiorly, the lesion moves up on the rolled view. If lateral tissue is rolled inferiorly and medial tissue superiorly, the lesion moves inferiorly. When the lesion is central in the breast *(scenario 2)*, no significant movement of the lesion is seen when tissue is rolled. In *scenario 3*, the lesion is in medial tissue. As lateral tissue is rolled superiorly and medial tissue inferiorly, the lesion moves down. As lateral tissue is rolled inferiorly and medial tissue superiorly, the lesion moves superiorly. (From Cardeñosa G. *Breast Imaging [The Core Curriculum Series]*. Philadelphia, PA: Lippincott Williams & Wilkins; 2003.)

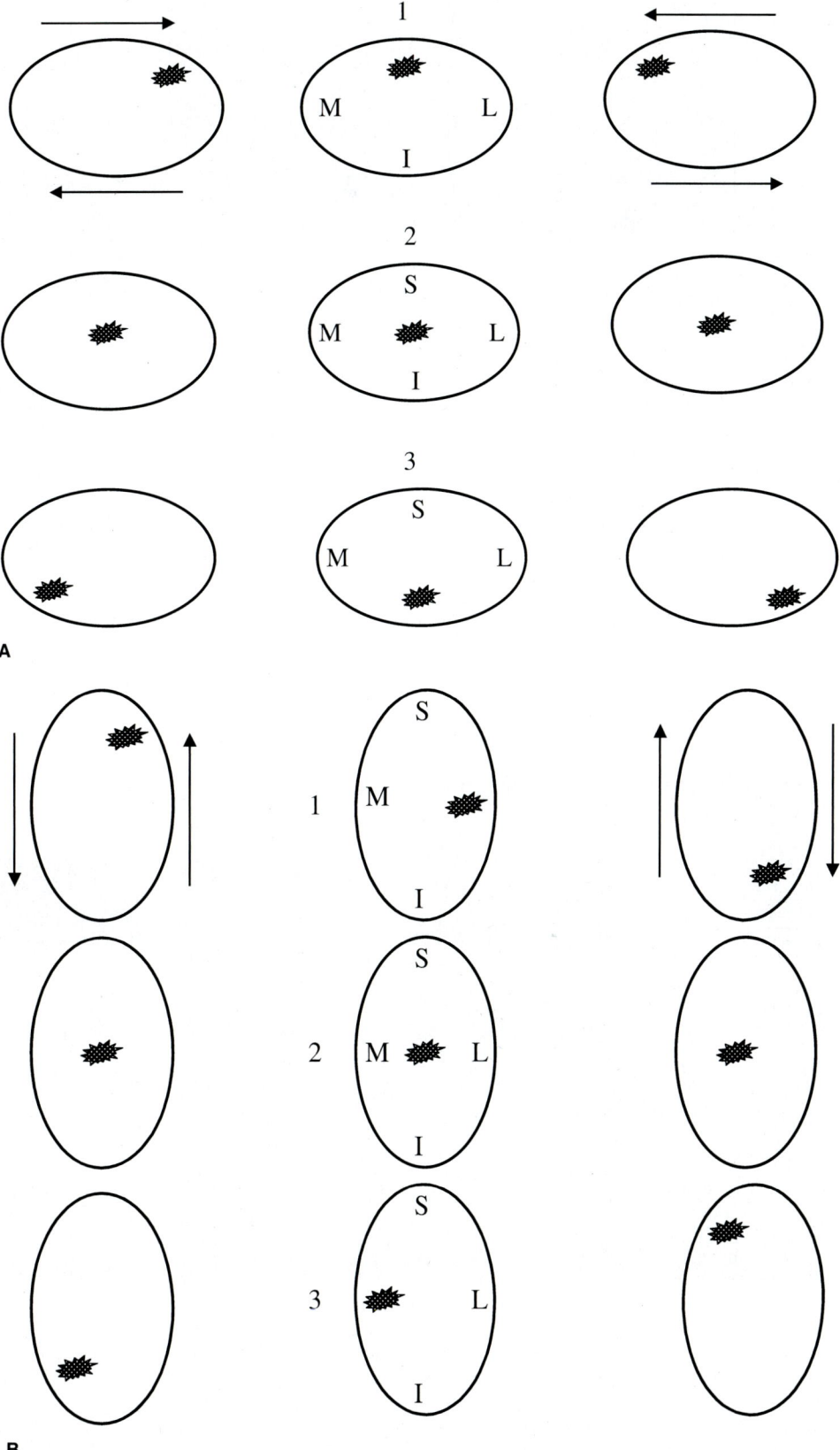

surface on the 90-degree lateral). A BB is then placed at the coordinates for the calcifications, and a tangential view of the BB is obtained to show that the calcifications are in the skin (Fig. 3.25).

Skin thickening and distortion are seen in women following lumpectomy and radiation therapy. These skin changes can project on the lumpectomy site, thereby limiting the evaluation for recurrent disease. If the lumpectomy site is imaged in tangent to the x-ray beam, skin changes can be separated from the underlying parenchymal changes (10). In these patients, the tangential views can be done using the magnification technique (Fig. 3.26).

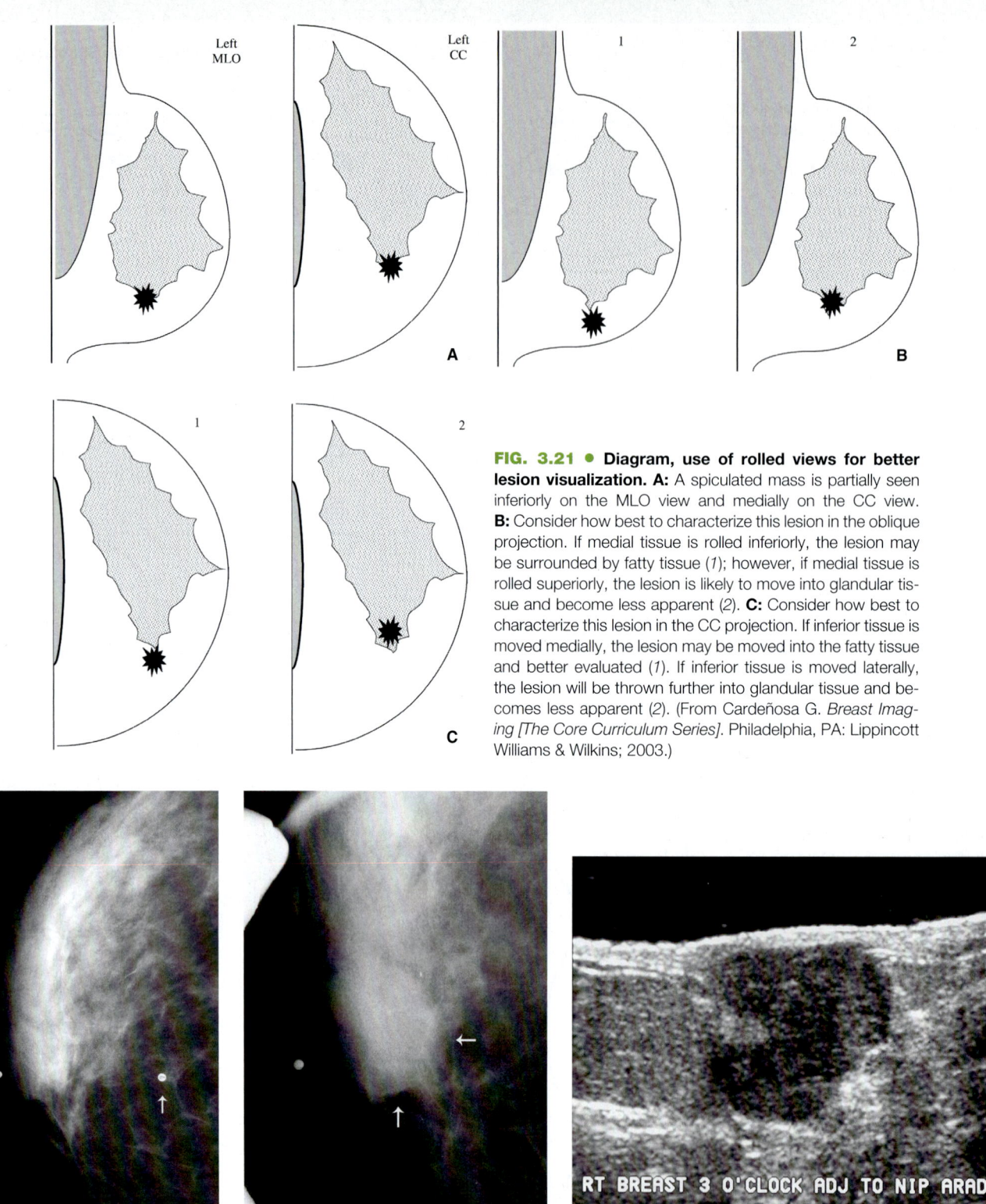

FIG. 3.21 • **Diagram, use of rolled views for better lesion visualization. A:** A spiculated mass is partially seen inferiorly on the MLO view and medially on the CC view. **B:** Consider how best to characterize this lesion in the oblique projection. If medial tissue is rolled inferiorly, the lesion may be surrounded by fatty tissue (*1*); however, if medial tissue is rolled superiorly, the lesion is likely to move into glandular tissue and become less apparent (*2*). **C:** Consider how best to characterize this lesion in the CC projection. If inferior tissue is moved medially, the lesion may be moved into the fatty tissue and better evaluated (*1*). If inferior tissue is moved laterally, the lesion will be thrown further into glandular tissue and becomes less apparent (*2*). (From Cardeñosa G. *Breast Imaging [The Core Curriculum Series]*. Philadelphia, PA: Lippincott Williams & Wilkins; 2003.)

FIG. 3.22 • **Use of spot tangential view, palpable finding. A:** MLO view photographically coned to anterior aspect of the breast. Patient presents describing a "lump" adjacent to her right nipple. A metallic BB is used to mark the location of the "lump." Dense tissue is present in the subareolar area with no abnormality identified on the routine views. A lucent centered calcification is noted incidentally *(arrow)*. **B:** Spot tangential view of the area of clinical concern. A round dense mass with partially circumscribed margins is imaged *(arrows)*. If appropriate positioning technique is used for the spot tangential view in women with dense tissue, these can be helpful by partially or completely surrounding the lesion with subcutaneous fat. **C:** Ultrasound demonstrates a superficial, solid mass with circumscribed margins, heterogeneous echotexture, and posterior acoustic enhancement. What is your differential? What additional piece of information would you like on this patient? In formulating a differential for this lesion, the age of the patient is most helpful. In a young woman, a fibroadenoma would be a primary consideration. In an 88-year-old patient, however, a fibroadenoma is unlikely. A new palpable mass in a patient this age is likely to represent breast cancer. BI-RADS 4C: Suspicious abnormality, biopsy is indicated. An invasive ductal carcinoma, not otherwise specified, is diagnosed on the ultrasound-guided biopsy. (From Cardeñosa G. *Breast Imaging [The Core Curriculum Series]*. Philadelphia, PA: Lippincott Williams & Wilkins; 2003.)

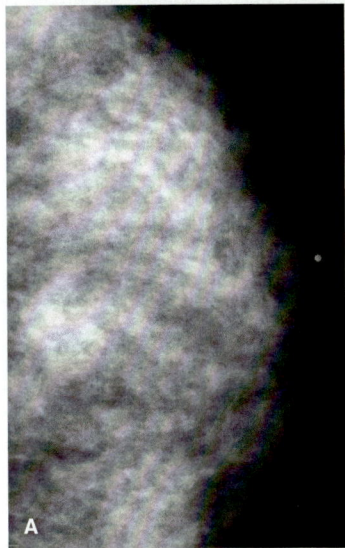 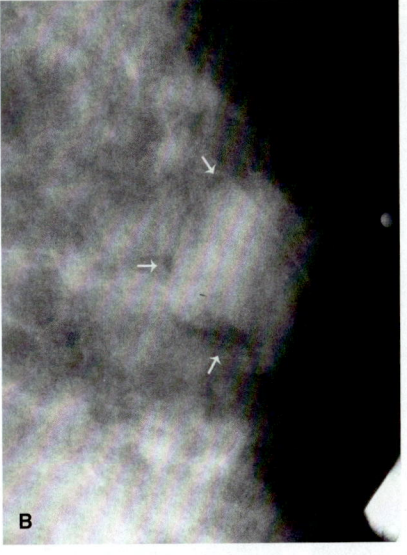 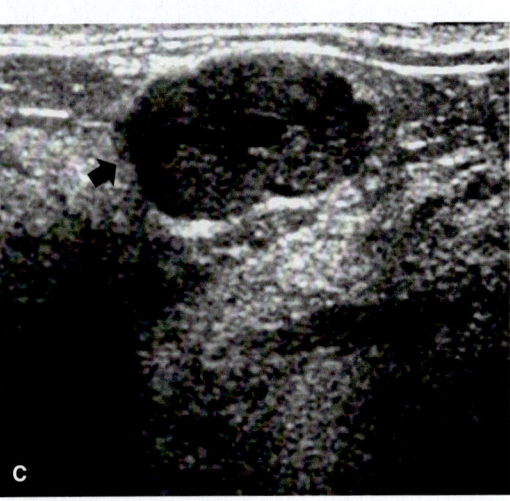

FIG. 3.23 • **Use of spot tangential view, palpable finding. A:** MLO view, left breast photographically coned anteriorly in a 36-year-old patient who presents describing a "lump" in her left breast. A metallic BB is used to mark the site of the "lump." Dense glandular tissue is present. No abnormality is apparent at the site of clinical concern. **B:** Spot tangential view demonstrates a macrolobulated isodense mass with circumscribed margins *(arrows)*. Although dense tissue is present, the mass is now seen, and the margins can be characterized. **C:** Ultrasound demonstrates an oval mass with circumscribed margins, two small central cystic areas, gentle macrolobulations, and posterior acoustic enhancement. A fibroadenoma is the primary consideration in a 36-year-old woman with a mass with these imaging features. BI-RADS 4A: Suspicious abnormality, biopsy is indicated. A fibroadenoma is diagnosed following ultrasound-guided biopsy. (From Cardeñosa G. *Breast Imaging [The Core Curriculum Series]*. Philadelphia, PA: Lippincott Williams & Wilkins; 2003.)

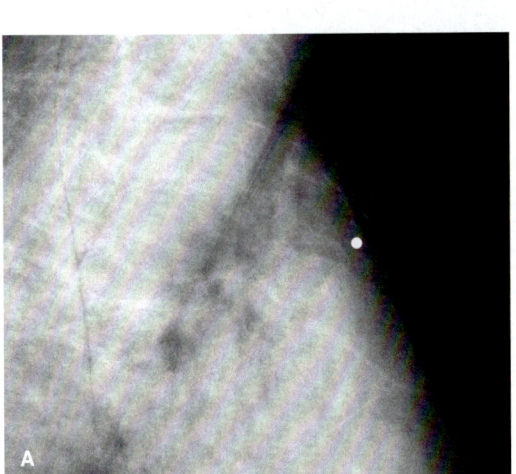 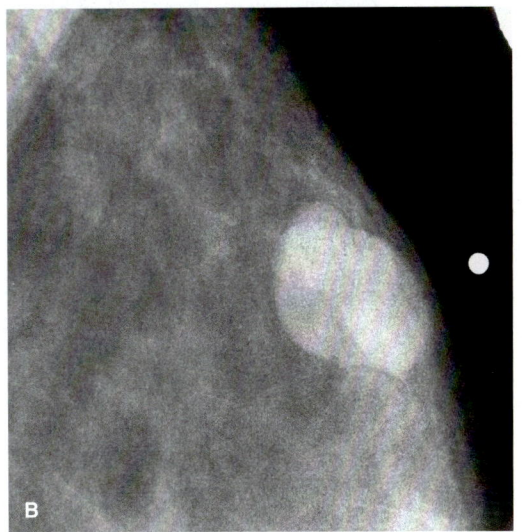

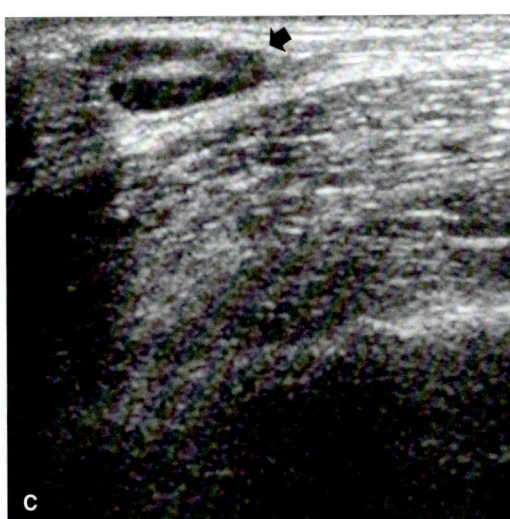

FIG. 3.24 • **Use of spot tangential view, palpable finding. A:** MLO view photographically coned superiorly in a 41-year-old patient who presents describing a "lump" in her left breast. The metallic BB denotes the site of the "lump." What are you going to say? With what degree of certainty can you say it? Dense tissue. No abnormality is apparent on the routine views. **B:** Spot tangential view. A macrolobulated oval mass with circumscribed margins is present corresponding to the palpable finding. **C:** Ultrasound demonstrates an oval mass with circumscribed margins and a central hyperechoic area. These findings are consistent with an intramammary lymph node *(arrow)*. No "atypical" features are noted. BI-RADS 2: Benign finding; negative. The patient is reassured of the benign etiology of the palpable finding. No further intervention or short interval follow-up is warranted. (From Cardeñosa G. *Breast Imaging [The Core Curriculum Series]*. Philadelphia, PA: Lippincott Williams & Wilkins; 2003.)

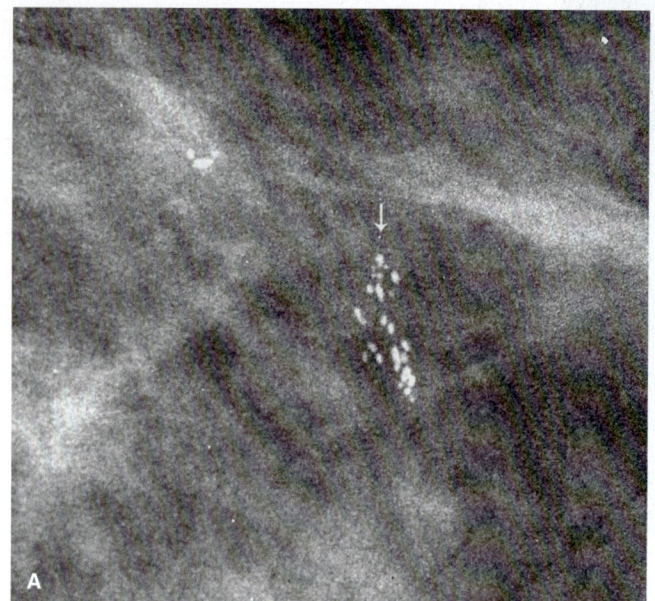
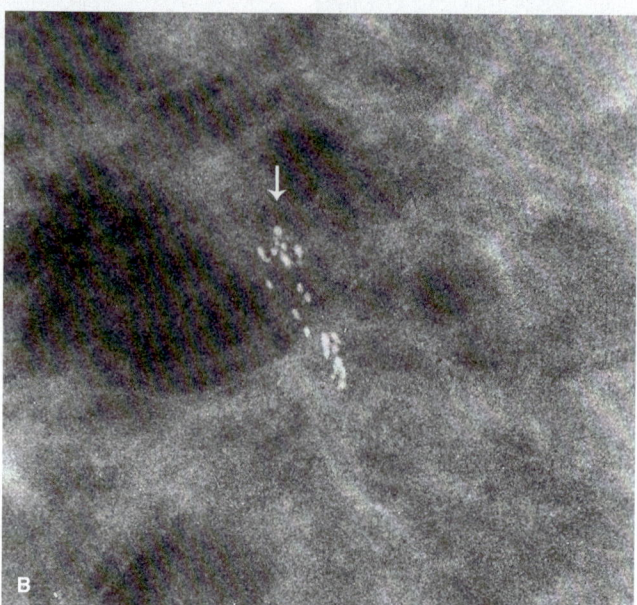
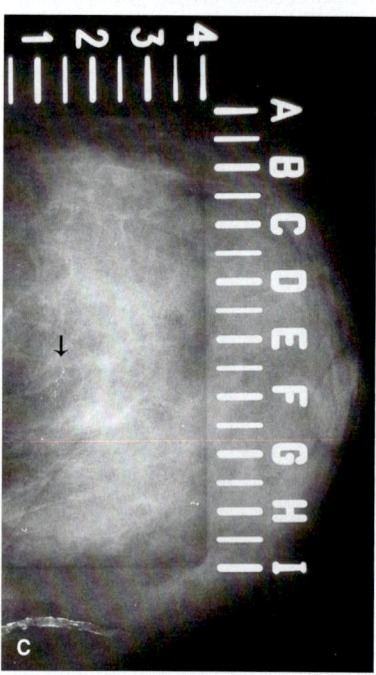
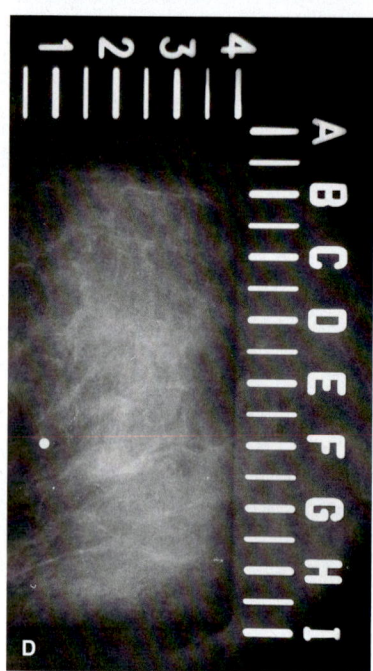
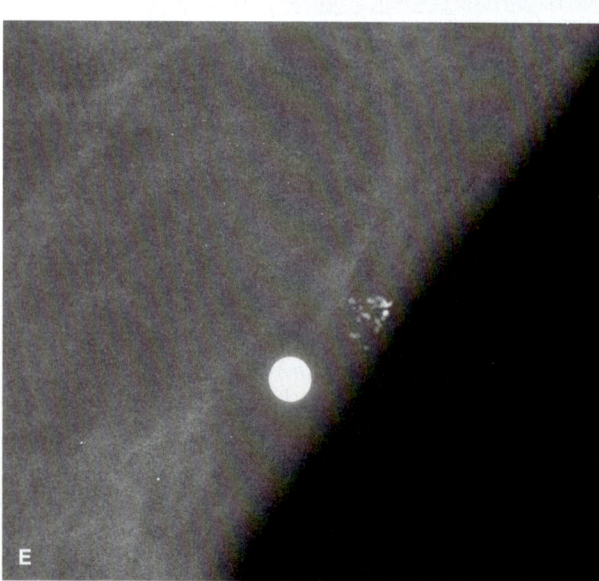

FIG. 3.25 • **Use of spot tangential view, localization of calcifications to the skin.** MLO **(A)** and CC **(B)** views photographically coned demonstrate a cluster of calcifications *(arrows)*. These appear to be closest to the inferior aspect of the breast. **C:** A FB view (CC) is done using the alphanumeric fenestrated paddle. The coordinates for the calcifications are determined *(arrow)* on this image, and a metallic BB is placed on the skin surface at the intersection of the coordinates. **D:** Follow-up image demonstrates the BB in close proximity to the calcifications. **E:** Spot tangential view is taken at the location of the BB. This confirms the dermal location for these calcifications. BI-RADS 2: Benign finding, negative. The patient is reassured of a benign finding. No further intervention is warranted. Screening mammogram is recommended in one year. (From Cardeñosa G. *Breast Imaging [The Core Curriculum Series]*. Philadelphia, PA: Lippincott Williams & Wilkins; 2003.)

Diagnostic Breast Imaging 69

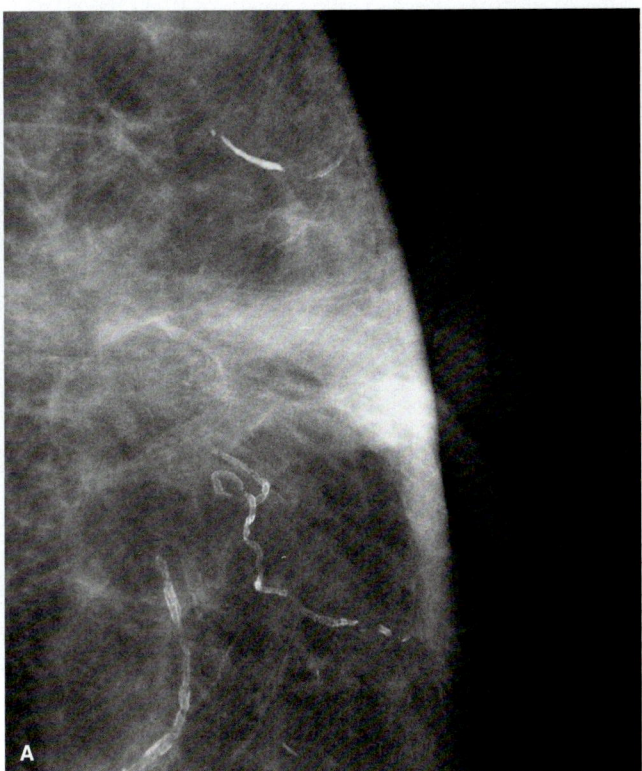 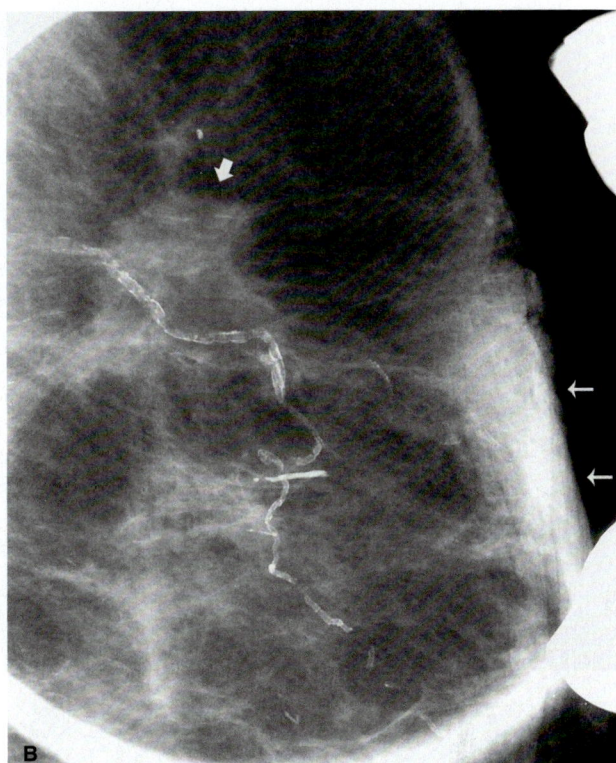

FIG. 3.26 • **Use of tangential view, lumpectomy site. A:** CC view photographically coned to the anterior aspect of the breast in a patient following lumpectomy and radiation therapy. Thickened skin is superimposed on the lumpectomy site and may preclude good evaluation of the lumpectomy site. **B:** Spot tangential view done at the lumpectomy site using magnification technique. Skin thickening *(thin arrows)* is now in tangent to the x-ray beam and no longer superimposed on the lumpectomy site *(thick arrow)*. Early changes of a local recurrence are easier to appreciate on spot tangential views such as these. Incidentally noted is extensive vascular calcification. (From Cardeñosa G. *Breast Imaging [The Core Curriculum Series]*. Philadelphia, PA: Lippincott Williams & Wilkins; 2003.)

CLEAVAGE VIEWS

Cleavage views are used to evaluate medial and posterior tissue in the CC projection. The film holder is placed up against the chest wall while medial and posterior tissue is imaged. Manual timing is needed, or, if phototiming is used, the technologist needs to offset the breasts so that the breast being evaluated is placed over the photocell (4). If the breasts are centered on the bucky and phototiming is used, the exposure may not be optimal since the phototimer sees air (Fig. 3.27).

90-DEGREE LATERAL VIEWS

Lateral views can be done in two different ways: LM and ML. For the 90-degree LM view, the digital detector is placed up against the sternum so that medial tissue is closest to the film and compression is applied from the lateral aspect of the breast. For 90-degree ML views, lateral tissue is closest to the digital detector, and compression is applied from the medial aspect of the breast. Since medial tissue has less mobility, tissue may be excluded as the compression moves over the medial quadrants.

90-Degree LM view

Maximal inclusion of medial tissue and the evaluation of medial lesions are the major advantages of 90-degree LM views. This view is also used in the localization of lesions closest to the lateral aspect of the breast and in triangulating the location of lesions. Unless we are evaluating a lateral lesion, we prefer and default to LM views. The

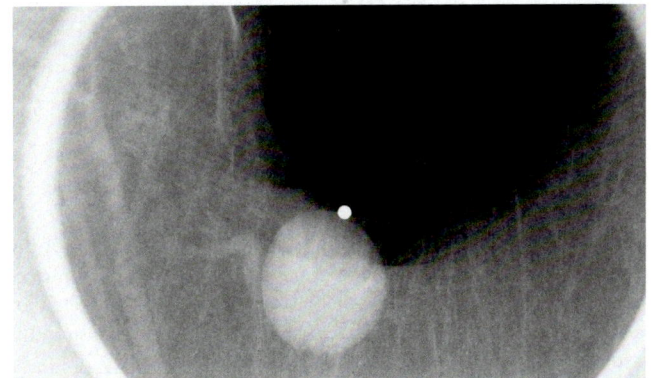

FIG. 3.27 • **Cleavage view. Sebaceous cyst.** Patient presents describing a "lump" medially on the right. A cleavage view is needed to image the lesion. This is a round isodense mass with circumscribed margins (metallic BB). On physical examination, a readily mobile mass that moves with the skin is palpated. On careful inspection, a "black head" is noted in the skin overlying the lesion. With gentle pressure, a small amount of white, thick material can be expressed. BI-RADS 2: Benign finding. (From Cardeñosa G. *Breast Imaging [The Core Curriculum Series]*. Philadelphia, PA: Lippincott Williams & Wilkins; 2003.)

digital detector is placed against the sternum, and the patient is asked to lower her chin onto the upper surface of the detector, while compression is applied from the lateral aspect of the breast. By placing the film holder up against the sternum, it is unlikely that a medial lesion

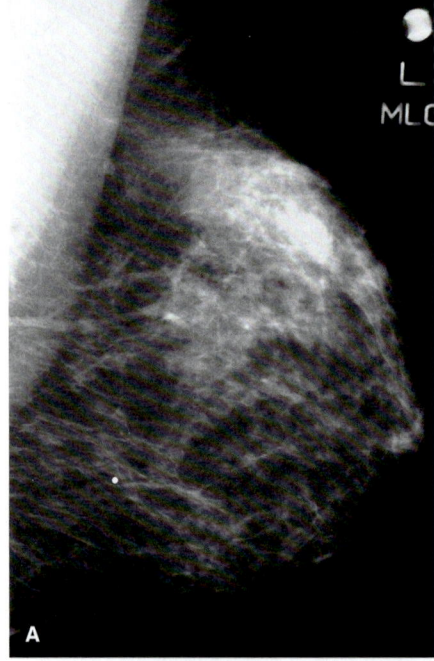
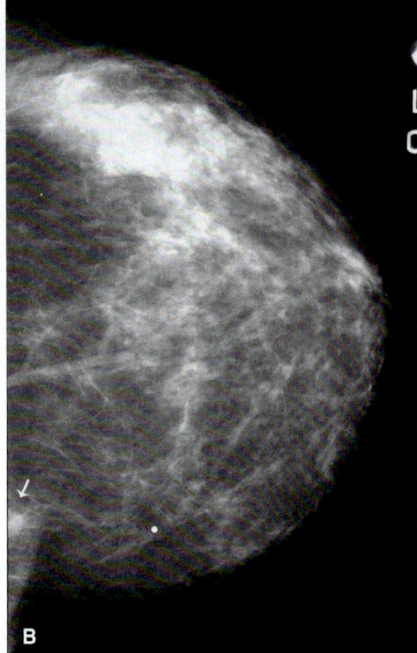
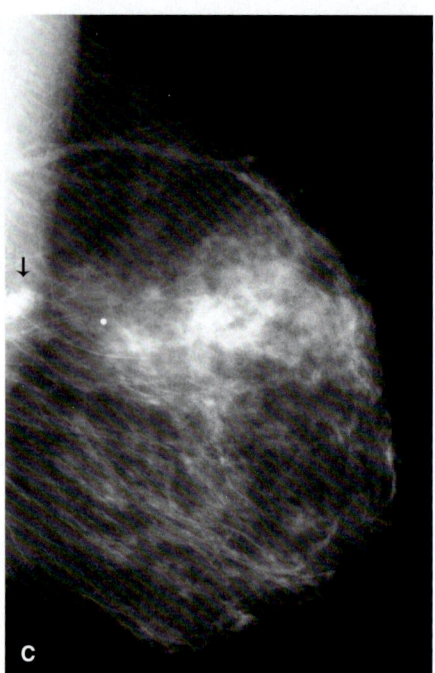
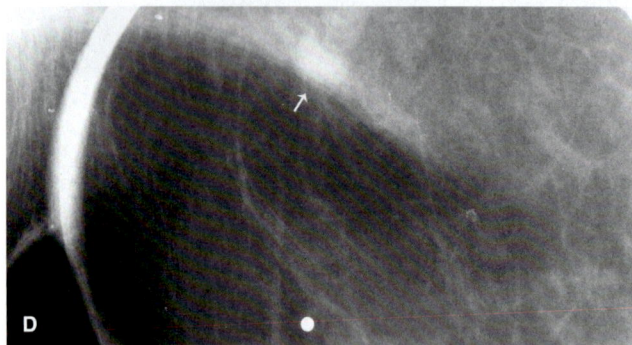

FIG. 3.28 • **Use of 90-degree lateral (LM) and cleavage views.** MLO **(A)** and CC **(B)** views of the left breast in a 44-year-old patient presenting with a "lump." The metallic BB purportedly marks area. The MLO view is normal. On the CC view, a round density is partially seen posteromedially *(arrow)*. Note that the BB is 2 to 3 cm anterior to the potential lesion. Since the lesion is on the medial aspect of the breast, 90-degree lateral and cleavage views may be helpful. In selecting between LM and ML 90-degree lateral views, the LM is selected since, on this view, medial tissue is up against the detector. **C:** Ninety-degree LM view. A high-density oval mass is now partially imaged in this view *(arrow)*. Note the upward movement of the metallic BB as one goes from the MLO view to the LM view: medial lesions (BB in example) move up as you go from MLO to LM views. **D:** Cleavage view. A round mass is seen *(arrow)* corresponding to the area of concern to the patient. On ultrasound (not shown), an irregular mass is imaged in the upper inner quadrant of the left breast corresponding to the palpable finding. Ultrasound is helpful in reaching areas that are difficult to image mammographically. This includes upper inner quadrants and axillary tissue. BI-RADS 4C: Suspicious abnormality, biopsy is indicated. Ultrasound-guided biopsy is done to establish the diagnosis of an invasive ductal carcinoma, not otherwise specified. (From Cardeñosa G. *Breast Imaging [The Core Curriculum Series]*. Philadelphia, PA: Lippincott Williams & Wilkins; 2003.)

will be excluded from the image and, since the medial aspect of the breast is close to the detector, resolution of medial tissue is optimized. In a small number of patients, medial lesions may be completely or partially excluded even on 90-degree LM views. Breast ultrasound is particularly helpful in evaluating these patients (Fig. 3.28).

90-Degree ML view

The evaluation of lateral lesions, localization of medial lesions, and lesion triangulation are done with the 90-degree ML view. The digital detector is placed on the lateral aspect of the breast, and compression is applied from the medial side. Resolution of lateral tissue is maximized since lateral tissue is placed closest to the detector (Fig. 3.29).

FROM BELOW

Analogous to what is described for 90-degree lateral views, tissue can be evaluated in the CC projection or from below (FB—caudocranial). The FB projection is not used commonly; however, it can be helpful in specific circumstances. CC views may be difficult to do on patients who are on a stretcher and unable to sit or stand; an FB may be easier to do (Fig. 3.30). FB views can also be done in an attempt to include superior tissue or image a lesion in the superior aspect of the breast posteriorly. Alternatively, in combination with the spot compression paddle, a lesion in the inferior and posterior aspect of the breast just above the IMF may be included (Fig. 3.31) more easily on the image, particularly if the breast is imaged at the neutral IMF position (e.g., the tissue is not lifted as is usually done for positioning on CC views). This projection is also used during preoperative wire localizations or in localizing calcifications to the skin (Fig. 3.25C) if the lesion being localized is closest to the inferior aspect of the breast.

LMO AND SIO VIEWS

These are two additional projections available to the mammographer. For the LMO, the x-ray beam travels from the lower outer aspect of the breast toward the upper inner quadrant of the breast. The digital detector is placed just below the clavicle against upper inner quadrant tissue,

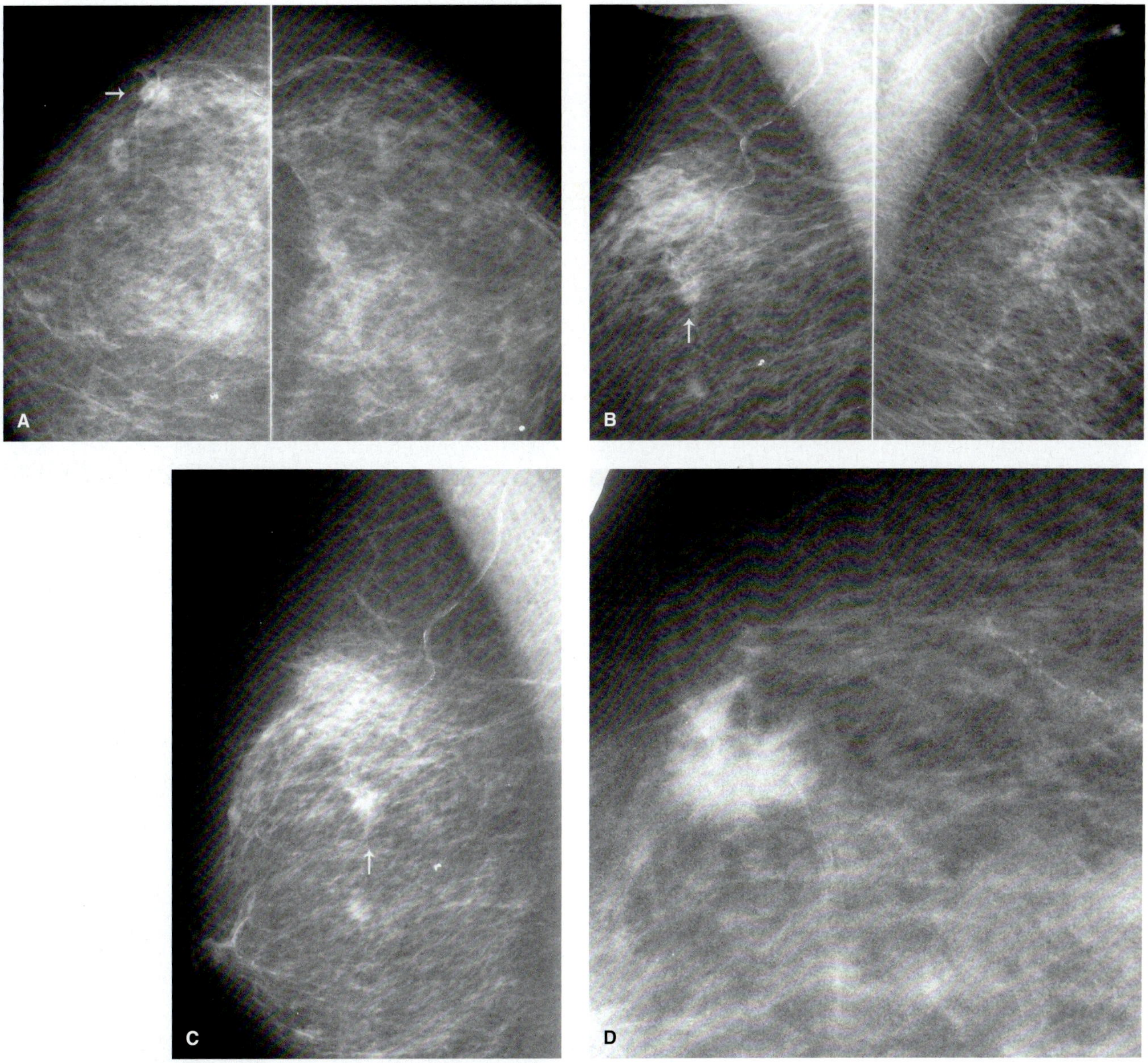

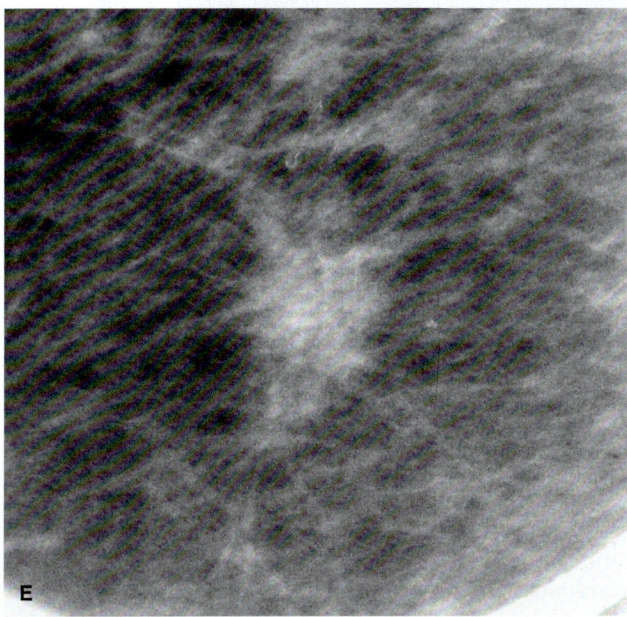

FIG. 3.29 • **Use of 90-degree ML.** CC **(A)** and MLO **(B)** views photographically coned from a screening study in a 74-year-old patient. A mass (*arrow*) is readily apparent on the right CC view. It is not as easily identified on the MLO view; however, if one measures back from the nipple and scans the MLO along this expected location, a potential corresponding abnormality is seen (*arrow*). BI-RADS 0: Need additional imaging evaluation. **C:** Ninety-degree lateral (ML) view. On this projection, lateral tissue is up against the film or detector for maximal resolution. As expected, the potential lesion noted on the MLO moves inferiorly ("down and out") on the ML view (*arrow*). CC **(D)** and ML **(E)** spot compression views demonstrate an irregular mass with spiculated margins. A new mass with this appearance in a 74-year-old woman is likely to be malignant, particularly if there is no history of surgery or trauma to this site. BI-RADS 4C: Suspicious abnormality, biopsy is indicated. Ultrasound (not shown) guided biopsy is done to establish diagnosis of invasive lobular carcinoma. (From Cardeñosa G. *Breast Imaging [The Core Curriculum Series]*. Philadelphia, PA: Lippincott Williams & Wilkins; 2003.)

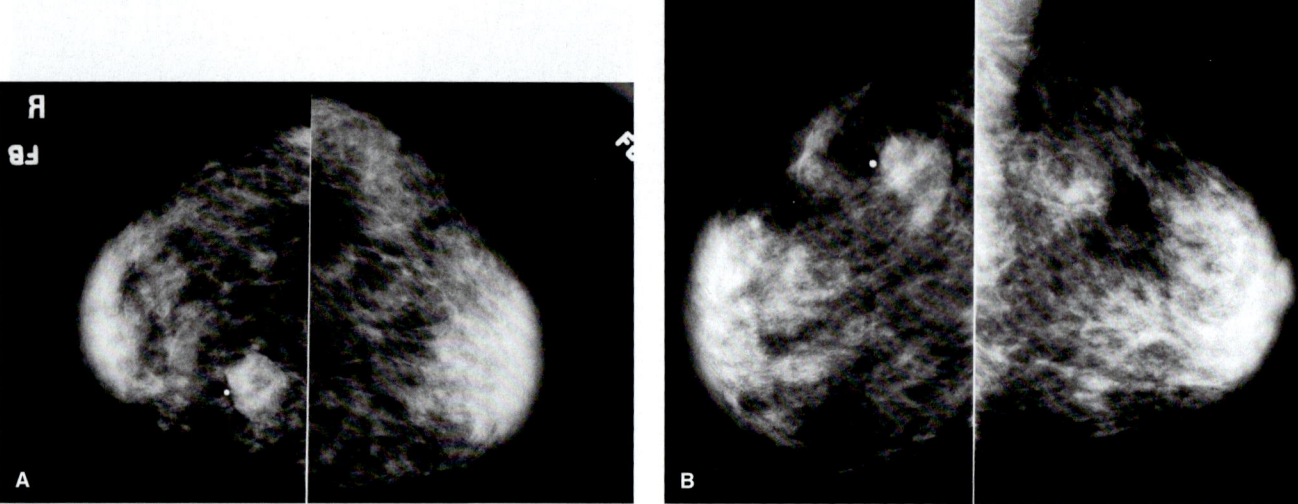

FIG. 3.30 • **Use of FB view, patient on stretcher.** FB **(A)** and MLO **(B)** views (anterior compression on the right) in a patient with a "lump" in the right breast. Metallic BB is used to denote the palpable finding. She is on a stretcher and unable to sit or stand. FB views are done because CC views are not possible. Under the circumstances, these are good images and include the palpable finding.

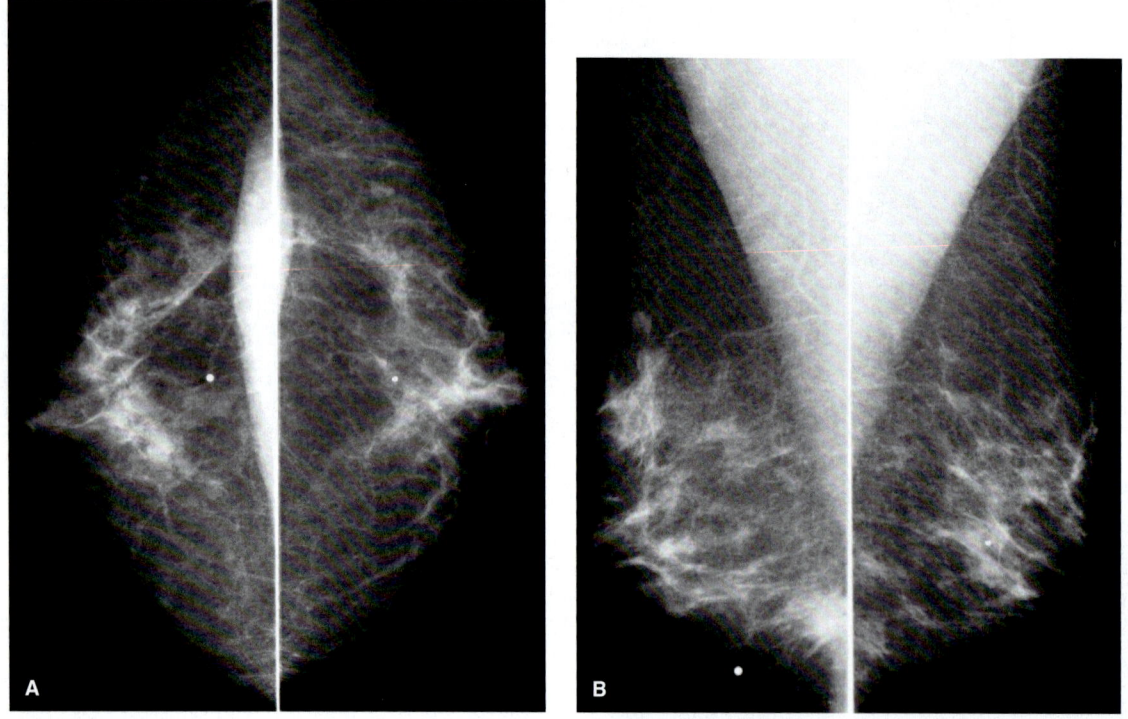

FIG. 3.31 • **Use of FB view to image a lesion.** CC **(A)** and MLO **(B)** views in a 65-year-old patient with a "lump" in the right breast. A metallic BB is used to mark the location of the "lump." A mass corresponding to the site of the palpable finding (metallic BB) is apparent on the right MLO just above the IMF. No abnormality is identified on the right CC view. Keep in mind that in positioning the breast for a CC view, the technologist identifies the neutral position of the IMF and lifts the breast up. In this patient, as the breast is lifted, the lesion likely rolls out and is excluded from the image. To overcome this, the technologist is asked to do an FB view using the spot paddle to reach back as far as possible and to place the detector at the neutral IMF position. **C:** FB spot compression view confirms the presence of a low-density mass with ill-defined margins and associated calcifications that include linear and round forms (MLO spot not shown). **D:** Ultrasound. An irregular predominantly hyperechoic mass is imaged at the 7 o'clock position, 5 cm from the right nipple corresponding to the clinical (*PALP*) and mammographic finding. Although hyperechoic masses are often benign, this is not always the case. Given the mammographic features of this mass, an invasive ductal carcinoma (mass) with associated DCIS (calcifications) is the expected diagnosis. BI-RADS 5: Highly suspicious abnormality, biopsy is indicated. An invasive ductal carcinoma with DCIS is confirmed on an ultrasound-guided core biopsy.

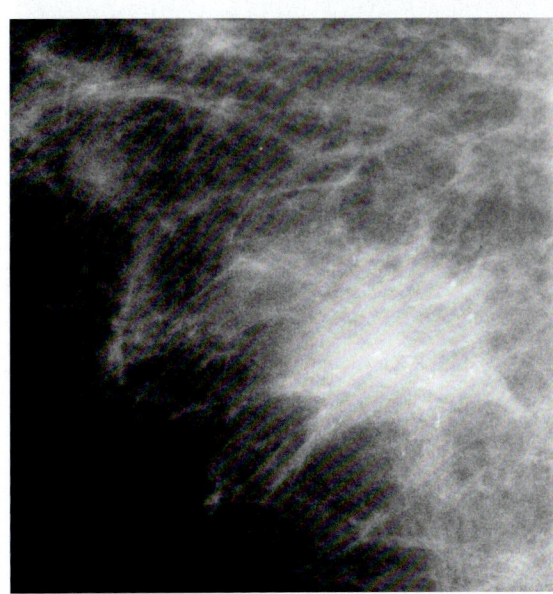
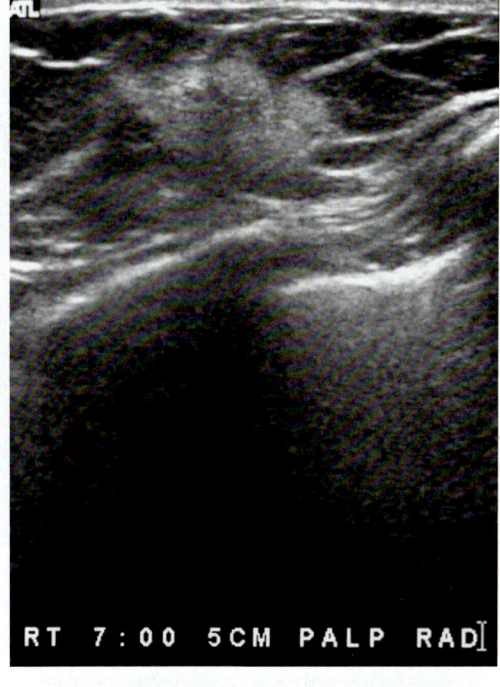

C   D

FIG. 3.31 • (continued)

and compression is applied from the lower outer aspect of the breast (in essence, the opposite of what is done for an MLO view). This projection can be helpful in evaluating upper inner quadrant tissue since this is now up against the receptor for maximal resolution. It is also sometimes used to image patients with severe kyphosis, pectus excavatum, pectus carinatum, or those with pacemakers (Fig. 3.32). The angle of obliquity is established as described for MLO views.

The SIO view is of limited usefulness. For the SIO view, the x-ray beam travels from the upper outer quadrant of the breast toward the lower inner quadrant. The digital detector is placed in the lower inner aspect of the breast, and compression is applied from the upper outer quadrant of the breast toward the lower inner quadrant. Rarely, this projection is used for stereotactically guided biopsies of lesions in the axillary tail (upper outer quadrant posteriorly) of the breast.

TRIANGULATION

The ability to accurately locate lesions on ultrasound and establish mammographic and ultrasound concordance is critical (also see discussion in Chapter 4). Before doing an ultrasound to evaluate a mammographic finding, the location of the lesion needs to be established accurately on the mammogram. Incomplete workups account for many of the described "seen in only one view lesions." If a logical approach is taken in the evaluation of potential lesions seen in only one view initially, the location of the lesion in the orthogonal image can be established reliably in most patients.

Our approach to an area of concern seen in only one view is to first establish whether it represents superimposition of normal tissue on the view in which the abnormality is seen initially (Figs. 3.5, 3.18, and 3.19). For example, if a potential lesion is seen on an MLO view and not identified with certainty on the CC view, we first obtain a spot compression view (and sometimes rolled views) in the MLO projection to determine whether the lesion persists or whether it represents the superimposition of normal parenchymal structures (Figs. 3.18, 3.33, and 3.34). If the abnormality is real, we need to establish its location on the CC view. It is important to emphasize that we make

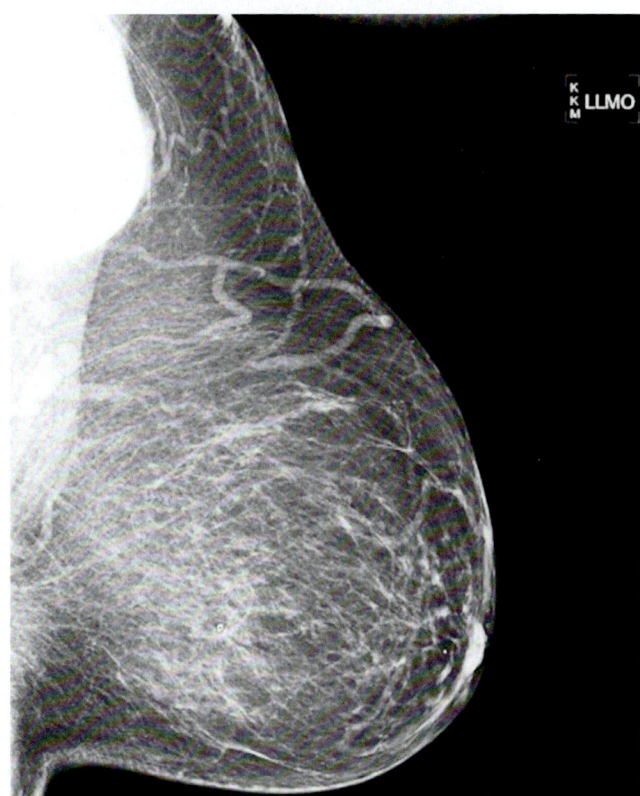

FIG. 3.32 • **Lateromedial oblique (LMO) view.** This is an LMO view done on a patient who has a pacemaker. Without the LMO label, it is hard to distinguish this from an MLO view. For an LMO view, the digital detector is placed on the upper inner quadrant of the breast, and compression is applied from the lower outer quadrant toward the upper inner quadrant. The x-ray beam travels from the lower outer aspect toward the upper inner quadrant of the breast. This projection is sometimes used to image patients with severe kyphosis, pectus excavatum, pectus carinatum, or, as in this woman, those with pacemakers.

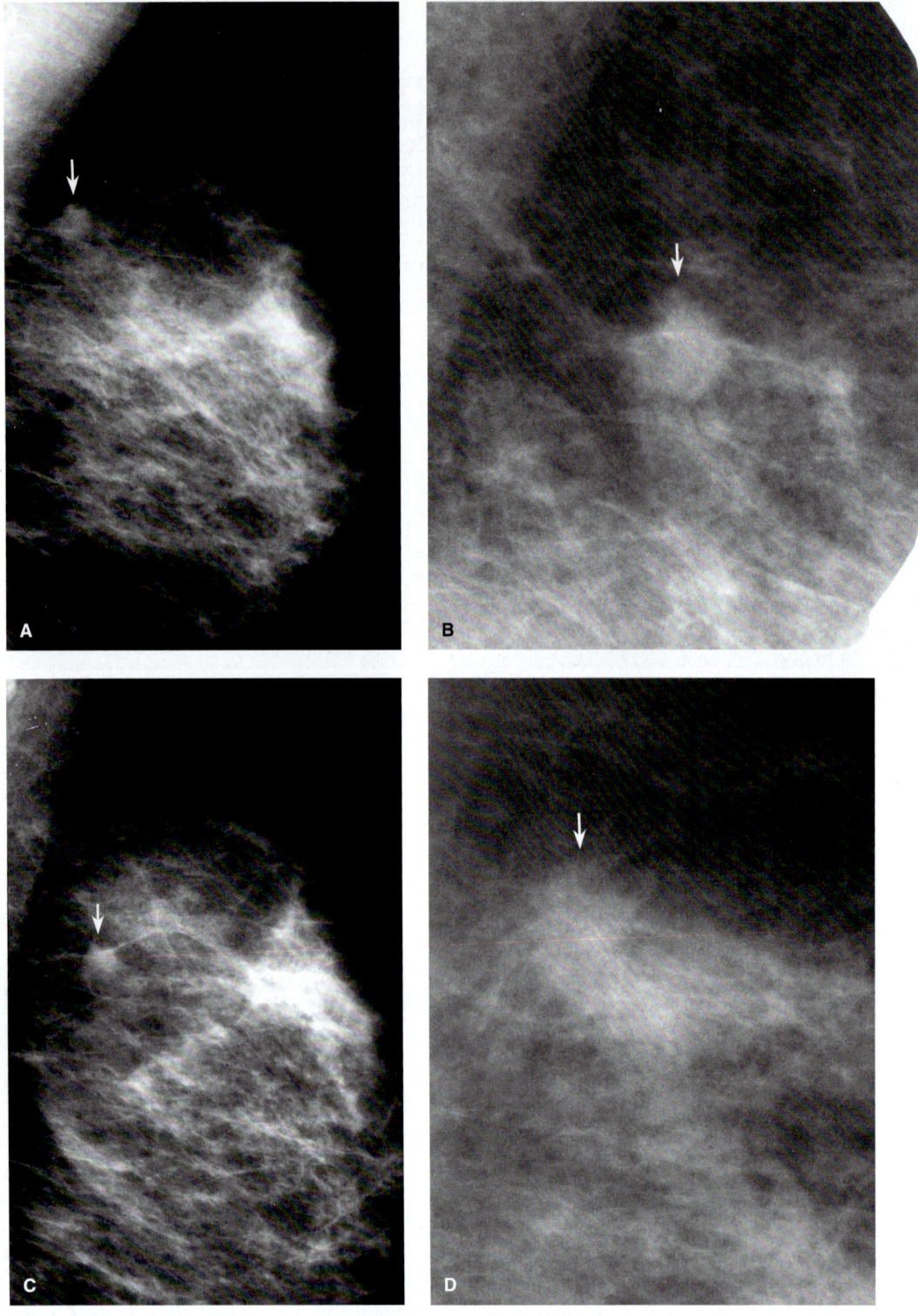

FIG. 3.33 • **Lesion localization, triangulation concepts. A:** MLO views of the left breast from a screening study in a 45-year-old woman. The CC view (not shown) is normal. When the strip of fatty tissue anterior to pectoral muscle is evaluated, a possible mass *(arrow)* is detected. At this point, it is unclear if this is a significant finding. BI-RADS 0: Need additional imaging evaluation. When the patient returns for her diagnostic study, our approach is to first establish whether what we are seeing on the MLO view is real. **B:** Spot compression view, MLO projection. An isodense round mass with spiculated margins *(arrow)* is confirmed on the spot compression view. The location of this mass now needs to be determined on the CC projection. Is this a lateral, medial, or central lesion? Instead of making any assumptions and blindly evaluating potential areas for the location of the lesion, a 90-degree lateral view is obtained. If the lesion moves down in going from the MLO to the lateral view, the lesion is in lateral tissue, and an XCCL view would be appropriate. If the lesion moves up in going from the MLO to the lateral view, the lesion is in medial tissue, and a cleavage view would be appropriate. If the lesion does not shift significantly, it is retroareolar in location. **C:** Ninety-degree lateral (LM) view. Lesion moves down on the lateral view. **D:** Spot compression view, in an exaggerated craniocaudal projection laterally (XCCL). The mass *(arrow)* is identified, and the location of the lesion is now known precisely. BI-RADS 4C: Suspicious abnormality, biopsy is indicated. Ultrasound (not shown) guided biopsy is done to establish the diagnosis of an invasive ductal carcinoma, not otherwise specified. (From Cardeñosa G. *Breast Imaging [The Core Curriculum Series]*. Philadelphia, PA: Lippincott Williams & Wilkins; 2003.)

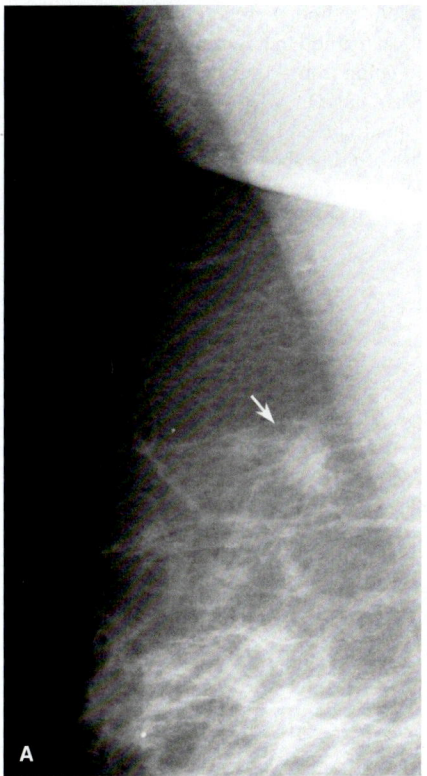
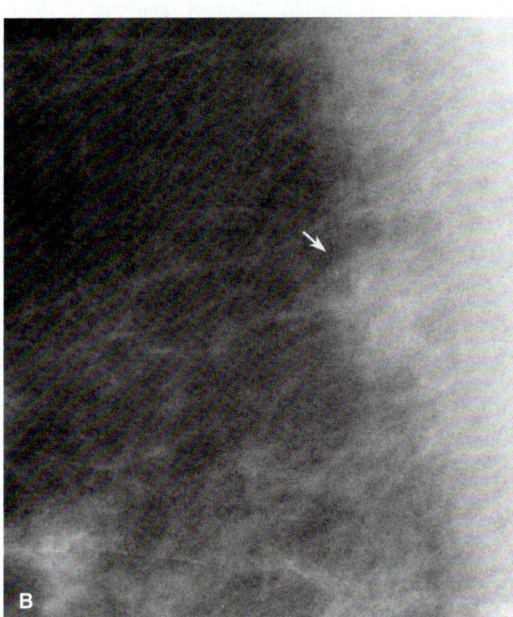
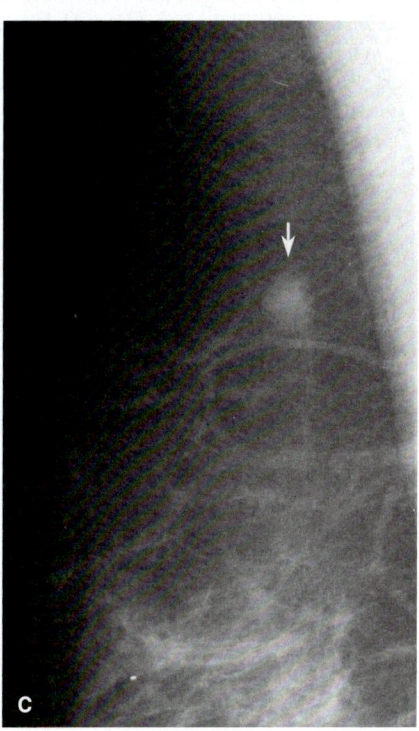
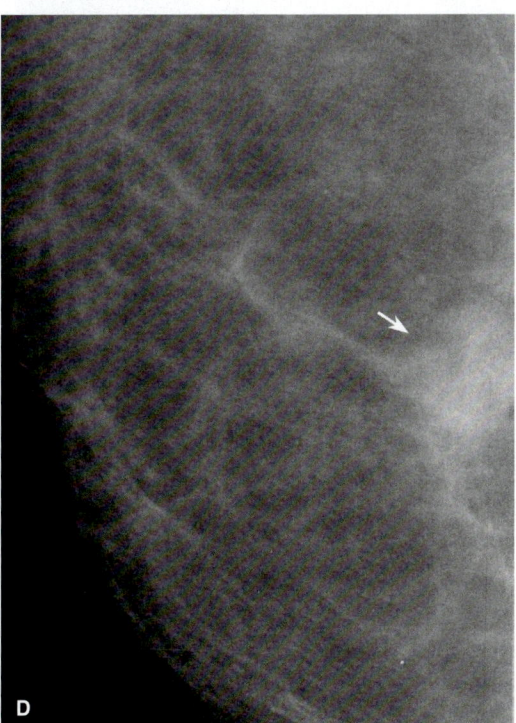

FIG. 3.34 • **Lesion localization, triangulation concepts. A:** Right MLO, screening study in a 61-year-old woman. A possible mass *(arrow)* is perceived anterior to the pectoral muscle on the oblique view. The CC view is normal (not shown). This patient had been evaluated at two other facilities, and both groups had obtained multiple views. The assumption was made that the lesion was lateral in location, yet no mass could be seen in the XCCL images. She presents to us with a purportedly "seen-in-only-one-view lesion." As discussed, we first establish whether the lesion is real in the projection in which it is seen. **B:** Spot compression view, MLO projection. A low-density mass with ill-defined margins persists *(arrow)* on the spot compression view. Instead of making any assumptions and blindly evaluating areas in the CC projection, a 90-degree lateral (LM) view is done. If the mass moves down in going from the MLO to the lateral view, the lesion is in lateral tissue, and an XCCL view would be appropriate. If the lesion moves up in going from the MLO to the lateral view, the lesion is in medial tissue, and a cleavage view would be appropriate. If it does not move very much, a spot of retroareolar tissue would be appropriate. **C:** Ninety-degree lateral (LM) view, right breast. The mass *(arrow)* moves up as you go from the MLO view to the 90-degree lateral view. The lesion is in medial tissue. **D:** Spot compression view, of medial tissue in the CC projection. A mass with indistinct margins is imaged *(arrow)*. Using the spot compression paddle enables us to include more tissue in the field of view compared with the regular CC view. With two additional views, the possible mass detected on the screening study is confirmed to be real, and its exact location is established on orthogonal projections; this enables us to establish mammographic–ultrasound concordance. BI-RADS 4C: Suspicious abnormality, biopsy is indicated. Ultrasound (not shown) can now be done knowing exactly where to scan. Ultrasound-guided biopsy is done to establish diagnosis of invasive ductal carcinoma, not otherwise as specified. Make no assumptions about the nature or location of a lesion during diagnostic studies; otherwise, you will overlook the obvious. If patients and workups are approached logically and one step at a time, most things are resolved easily, appropriate recommendations become self-evident, and your confidence in them is increased greatly. (From Cardeñosa G. *Breast Imaging [The Core Curriculum Series]*. Philadelphia, PA: Lippincott Williams & Wilkins; 2003.)

no assumptions regarding the location of the lesion on the orthogonal view (e.g., we don't just start spotting in the orthogonal projection). Rolled views can be obtained to see if the lesion moves with lateral or medial tissue. Another crude way of establishing the approximate location of a lesion on the CC view is to make use of the movement of the lesion between MLO and 90-degree lateral views. If the lesion moves up from the MLO to the 90-degree lateral view, the lesion is in the medial aspect of the breast (Fig. 3.34). If the lesion moves down ("down and out") between the MLO and 90-degree lateral views, the lesion is in the lateral aspect of the breast (Fig. 3.33). If the location of the lesion does not change significantly between the MLO and 90-degree lateral views, it is in the central area (e.g., retroareolar—deep to the nipple). In general, the more the lesion moves, the more peripheral the location of the lesion.

A useful approach described by Sickles (11) involves lining up the CC, MLO, and 90-degree lateral views with the nipple on the same horizontal plane for all three images, and drawing a line connecting the lesion in the two views in which the lesion is seen. If this line is extended onto the third image, the lesion will be found along the course of that line (Fig. 3.35). The distance from the nipple to the lesion can be used to approximate the location of the lesion along the line on the third view.

G.W. Eklund (Triangulation method, *personal communication*, August 1998) described a practical method that is useful in approximating the location of lesions when going from MLO and CC views to ultrasound (Fig. 3.36; also see Fig. 4.52). On MLO views, x-rays pass from upper inner to lower outer quadrants so that some tissue in the lower outer quadrant of the breast projects above the nipple on the MLO view; the PNL approximates the course of the x-ray beam. Likewise,

FIG. 3.35 • **Triangulation of lesions.** If, for example, a lesion is seen on the MLO view and not on the CC view, a lateral view can be done. The lateral, oblique, and CC views are lined up with the nipple on the same horizontal plane. A line is drawn connecting the lesion on the lateral and MLO views and extended into the CC view. The lesion will be along the course of this line. If you then measure the distance from the nipple to the lesion on the lateral view (*x* cm), this measurement can be used to determine where along the course of the line the lesion is located on the CC view. Note that this is a medial lesion. As you go from MLO to 90-degree lateral view, the lesion moves up, as discussed above. (From Cardeñosa G. *Breast Imaging [The Core Curriculum Series]*. Philadelphia, PA: Lippincott Williams & Wilkins; 2003.)

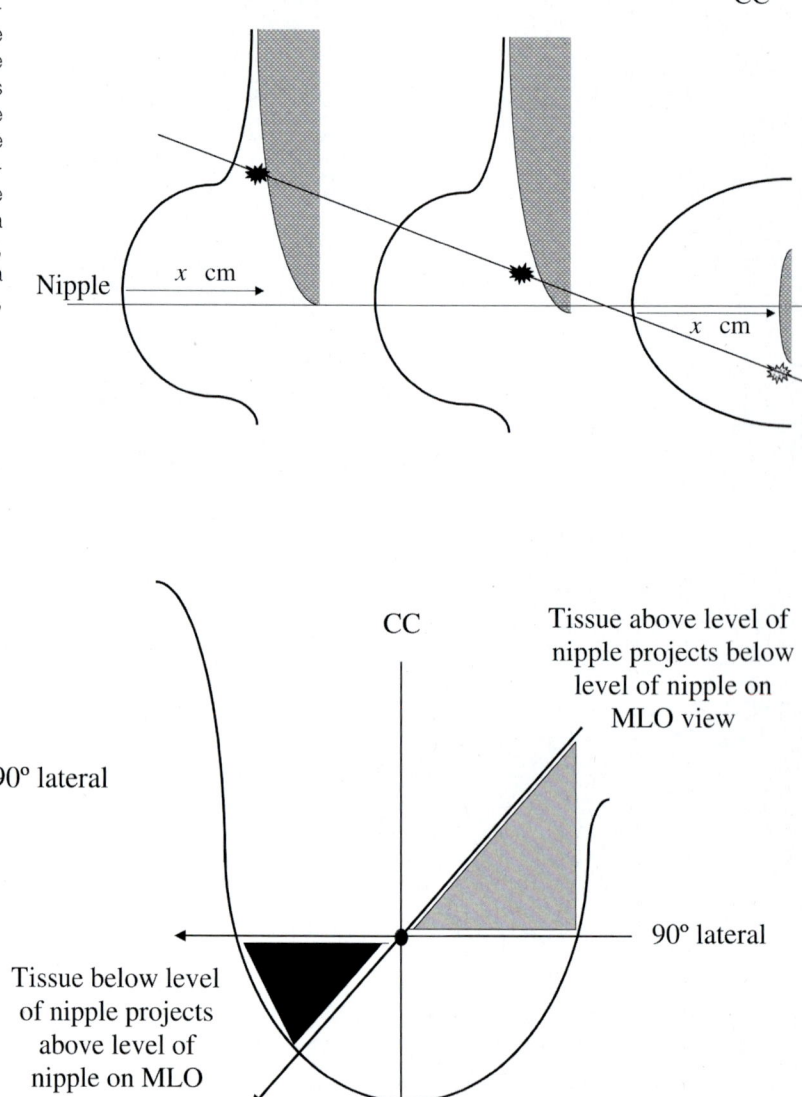

FIG. 3.36 • "Eklund" method of determining the location of lesion based on ML and CC views. **A:** On CC views, lateral tissue is lateral to the nipple, and medial tissue is medial to the nipple. On 90-degree lateral views, tissue projecting above the nipple is above the nipple, and tissue projecting below the nipple is below the nipple. For the MLO view, the x-rays pass from the upper inner quadrant through the breast and out at the lower outer quadrant. All of the tissue below the MLO line (actually the posterior nipple line, PNL) projects below the level of the nipple, and tissue above this line projects above the nipple on MLO views. **B:** Diagrammatically, on an MLO view, a small amount of tissue projecting above the nipple is really below the nipple *(black triangle)*, and some tissue projecting below the nipple is really above the nipple *(gray triangle)*. **C:** The PNL can be used on the frontal view of the breast to establish the approximate o'clock position of a lesion for correlating and targeting ultrasound studies appropriately. **D:** A lesion is seen approximately 1 cm below the PNL on the MLO view. This lesion is medial in location on the CC view. On a frontal view of the right breast, a line is drawn 1 cm below the PNL. The lesion is medial on the CC view such that the lesion is in the upper inner quadrant of the breast (2 o'clock). **E:** A lesion is seen on the MLO approximately 2 cm above the PNL. A line is drawn on the frontal view 2 cm above the PNL. Using the CC view, we determine that the lesion is lateral in location. We now have a fairly accurate idea of the o'clock location of the lesion for the purposes of doing targeted breast ultrasound. (From Cardeñosa G. *Breast Imaging [The Core Curriculum Series]*. Philadelphia, PA: Lippincott Williams & Wilkins; 2003.)

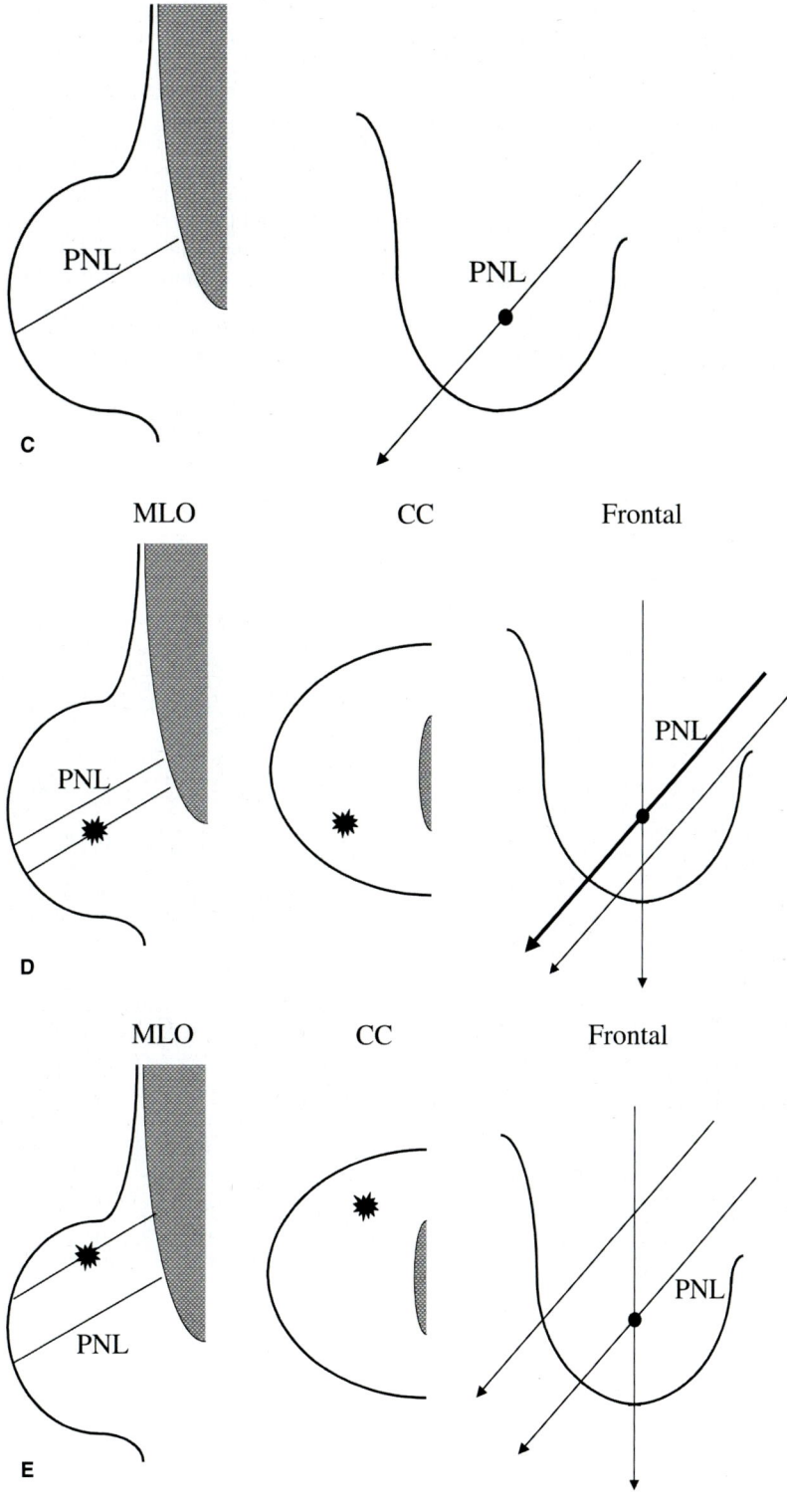

FIG. 3.36 • *(continued)*

some tissue in the upper inner quadrant of the breast projects below the nipple (Fig. 3.8). If one assumes that the MLO view has been taken at a 45-degree angle, lesions along the course of the x-ray beam will project behind the nipple on the MLO view along the course of the PNL. If a lesion is 1 cm above the PNL on the MLO view, a line drawn 1 cm above and parallel to the PNL of the incident x-ray beam on a frontal diagram of the breast will describe the possible locations of the lesion. In combination with the CC view, one can establish whether the lesion is in the upper inner quadrant at the 11 o'clock position (e.g., medial on the CC view), at the 12 o'clock position (e.g., retroareolar on the CC view), or at the 3:30 o'clock position (e.g., lateral on the CC view).

Lastly, a stepwise approach can be taken to finding the lesion on an orthogonal view (12). If a lesion is confirmed to be real on the CC view, and not identified with certainty on the MLO view, small amounts of angulation are incrementally added and the lesion is followed (e.g., 0, 15, 30, 45, 60, 75, and 90 degrees).

References

1. American College of Radiology. *ACR Practice Guideline for the Performance of Screening and Diagnostic Mammography*. Reston, VA: American College of Radiology; 2008 (Resolution 24).
2. Vade A, Lafita VS, Ward KA, et al. Role of breast sonography in imaging adolescents with palpable solid breast masses. *AJR Am J Roentgenol*. 2008;191:659–663.
3. Robbins J, Jeffries D, Roubidoux M, et al. Accuracy of diagnostic mammography and breast ultrasound during pregnancy and lactation. *AJR Am J Roentgenol*. 2011;196:716–722.
4. Eklund GW, Cardenosa G. The art of mammographic positioning. *Radiol Clin North Am*. 1992;30:21–53.
5. Berkowitz JE, Gatewood OMB, Gayler BW. Equivocal mammographic findings: evaluation with spot compression. *Radiology*. 1989; 171:369–371.
6. Logan WW, Janus J. Use of special mammographic views to maximize radiographic information. *Radiol Clin North Am*. 1987;25:953–959.
7. Sickles EA. Combining spot compression and other special views to maximize mammographic information. *Radiology*. 1989;173:571.
8. Alimoglu E, Ceken K, Kabaalioglu A, et al. An effective way to solve equivocal mammography findings: the rolled views. *Breast Care*. 2010;5:241–245.
9. Faulk RM, Sickles EA. Efficacy of spot compression-magnification and tangential views in mammographic evaluation of palpable breast masses. *Radiology*. 1992;185:87–90.
10. Karstaedt PJ, Jeske JM, Mendelson EB. Tangential magnification view of lumpectomy site: should it be standard in mammographic follow up after breast conservation? [abstract]. In: *Society of Breast Imaging Meeting*; 1997.
11. Sickles EA. Practical solutions to common mammographic problems: tailoring the examination. *AJR Am J Roentgenol*. 1988;151:31–39.
12. Pearson KL, Sickles EA, Frankel SD, et al. Efficacy of step-oblique mammography for confirmation and localization of densities seen on only one standard mammographic view. *AJR Am J Roentgenol*. 2000;174:745–752.

CHAPTER SELF-ASSESSMENT QUESTIONS

1. One of two spot compression views (left) and representative ultrasound (US) image (right) in a 45-year-old patient called back from screening (see screening mammogram Chapter 2 Question 1).

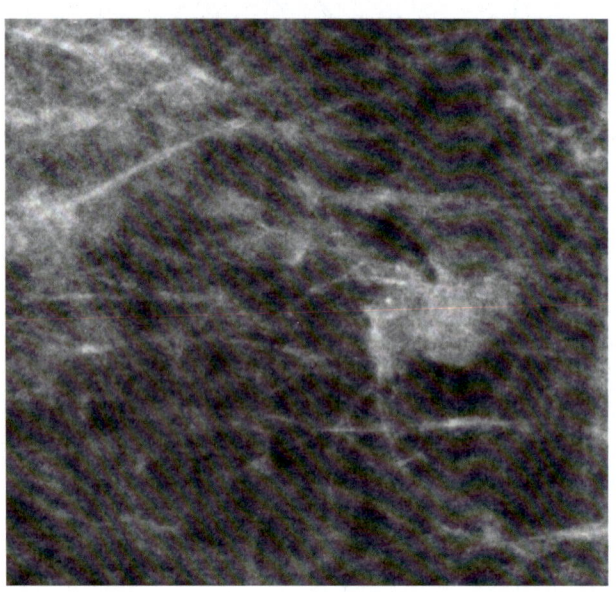
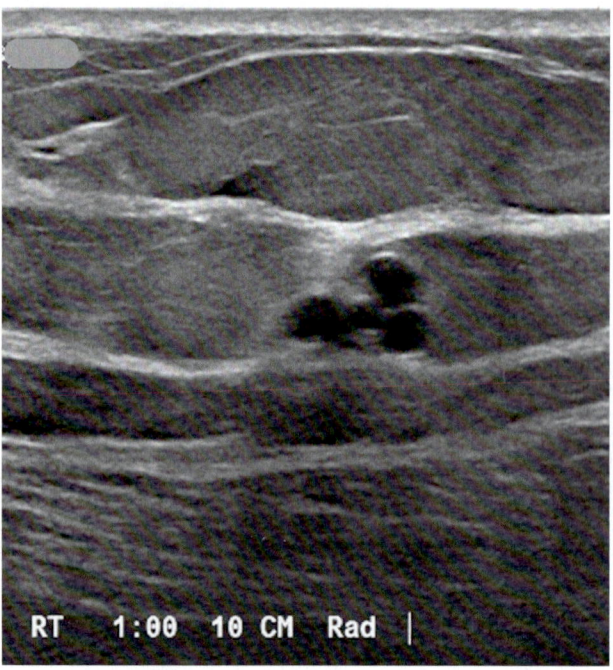

   A. Lesion imaged on US does not correlate with the mammographic finding
   B. BI-RADS 2: benign finding—screening mammogram in 1 year
   C. BI-RADS 3: probably benign finding, follow-up US in 6 months
   D. BI-RADS 4A: Suspicious finding, biopsy is indicated

2. Screening mammogram images (top and bottom) and one of two spot compression views (right, mediolateral oblique spot not shown) of the right breast posteromedially. Physical examination and ultrasound of the right breast are normal. What is indicated?

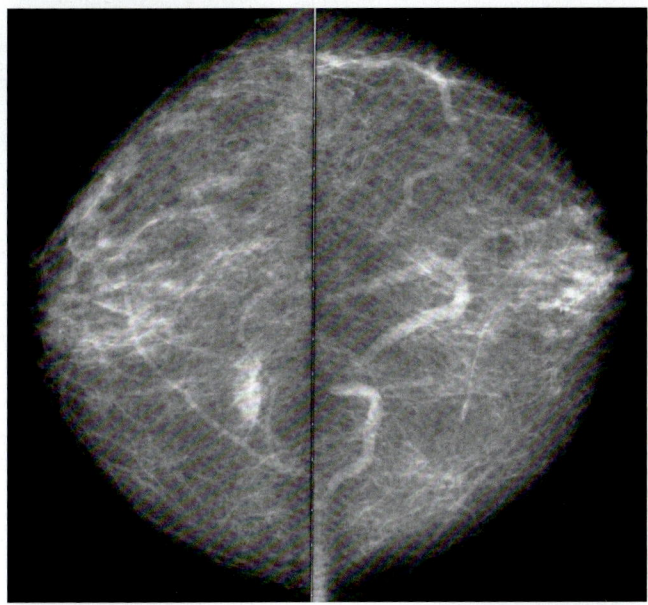

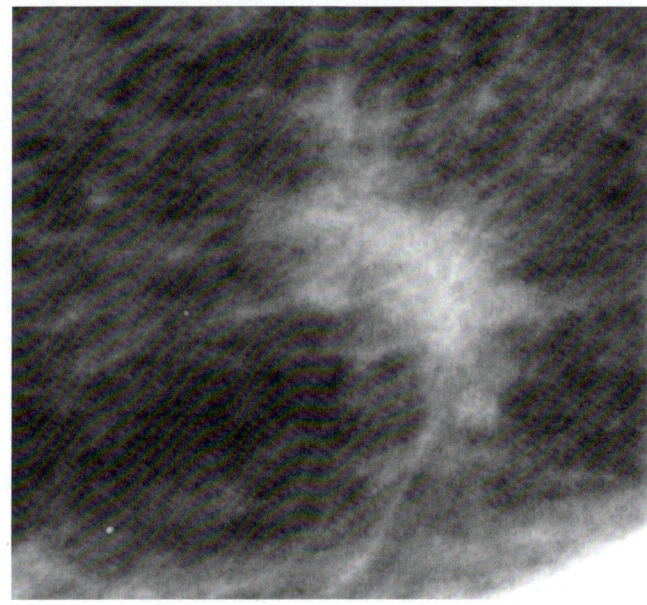

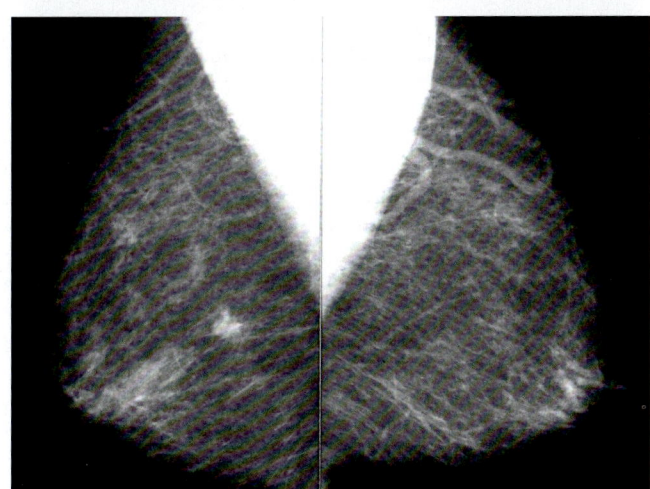

A. Six-month mammographic follow-up
B. Magnetic resonance imaging
C. Stereotactically guided breast biopsy
D. Reassure patient of benign parenchymal asymmetry, screening in 1 year

Answers to Chapter Self-Assessment Questions

1. B The spot compression views confirm the presence of a low-density mass with indistinct margins in the upper inner quadrant of the right breast posteriorly. A cluster of developing cysts is identified on ultrasound at the expected location of the mammographic finding. This is a benign finding requiring no additional intervention or short-term follow-up. A screening mammogram is indicated in 1 year.

2. C The images demonstrate an irregular mass with indistinct margins in the upper inner quadrant of the right breast posteriorly. On the basis of the location and mammographic features, this mass requires biopsy, not a 6-month follow-up; also, this is not benign parenchymal asymmetry. Although an MRI will be done after the suspected diagnosis of invasive disease is established, it would not be done prior to the biopsy (also, even if no MRI correlate is identified, the mammographic finding requires biopsy). One can argue that in this patient, the ultrasound is done for the purpose of determining the biopsy method to be used—if the mass is identified with ultrasound, it can be biopsied using ultrasound guidance. The lack of an identifiable ultrasound correlate speaks to the solid nature of the mammographic finding and does not eliminate the need for a biopsy. Biopsy to establish diagnosis of invasive ductal carcinoma done stereotactically.

Breast Ultrasound

LEARNING OBJECTIVES

1. Equipment and scanning techniques used in breast ultrasound
2. Image labeling of breast ultrasound images
3. Technical considerations in breast ultrasound
4. Normal breast anatomy on ultrasound
5. Breast ultrasound terminology
6. Indications for breast ultrasound
7. Ultrasound features of benign lesions
8. Ultrasound features of malignant lesions
   - Establishing clinical, mammographic, and ultrasound concordance

EQUIPMENT AND TECHNICAL ISSUES

Our dedicated ultrasound equipment is in immediate proximity to the mammography, stereotactic and magnetic resonance (MR) equipment. The ultrasound units are equipped with 12.5- and 17.5-MHz transducers. Optimization of the scanning parameters is critical. As discussed with mammographic image quality, it is important that you maximize ultrasound image quality. Set your quality standards high, and monitor image quality on a patient-by-patient basis. Do not settle for suboptimal equipment or images (1,2). Review and become familiar with the guidelines from the American College of Radiology regarding breast ultrasound (3). Unfortunately, and somewhat reminiscent of the experience with mammography image quality in the 1980s and early 1990s, breast ultrasound image quality at many facilities may not be what is required for good diagnostic work. On a review of 152 breast ultrasound examinations from 86 different institutions, Baker and Soo reported noncompliance with at least one of the ACR guidelines for breast ultrasound in 60.5% of studies (4). It is only when optimized equipment, image quality, and meticulous scanning technique are used that ultrasound becomes an invaluable tool in the evaluation and management of women with breast-related diseases. Anything else is often misleading and may be worse than nothing.

The number and positioning of the focal zones need to be set appropriately. The focal zone(s) should be at the level of the lesion or, at most, 1 cm superficial or deep to the anterior and posterior margins of the mass, respectively. Gain settings should enable the distinction between a simple cyst and solid mass. In the absence of a cyst, fat lobules should have varying shades of gray and not be so light as to be white or so dark as to be black. The field of view is adjusted so that an adequate amount of tissue is seen surrounding the lesion being evaluated; ideally, the images include the pectoral muscle (chest wall); however, depending on the location of the lesion and the size of the breast, this may not be achievable. It should be possible to establish the distance from the skin to the mass, and there should be enough posterior tissue to assess any changes in the transmission of the ultrasound beam beyond or deep to the lesion (2,3). Lesions can be excluded from the image if the field of view is inappropriately "zoomed" (Fig. 4.1A, B). In patients with large masses, it may be difficult to image the entire lesion and surrounding tissue using a rectangular image; a trapezoidal acquisition of the image may be used to include more of the lesion. Depending on the unit and transducer used, a standoff pad may be needed to evaluate superficial lesions. The standoff pad increases the distance from the transducer to the lesion, helping position the lesion at an appropriate depth of focus for the transducer. If the standoff pad is not used for superficial lesions, near-field artifacts may be created, leading to an inaccurate characterization of lesions. Some of the main technical considerations when doing breast ultrasounds are shown in Table 4.1.

SCANNING TECHNIQUE

Currently, breast ultrasound is an adjunctive tool used to evaluate areas of mammographic, MR, or clinical concern. Although the entire breast can be scanned, studies limited to the area of mammographic or clinical concern are common. Whole breast ultrasound units are now available on the market to facilitate automated scanning of the entire breast. For targeted ultrasound, the patient is positioned so that the tissue in the area of interest is thinned as much as possible. Supine positioning is used when evaluating the inner quadrants, and oblique positioning for tissue in the lateral quadrants and axilla; depending on breast size, the patient may be in a decubitus position to evaluate potential findings laterally. In evaluating the outer quadrants and axillae,

Breast Ultrasound

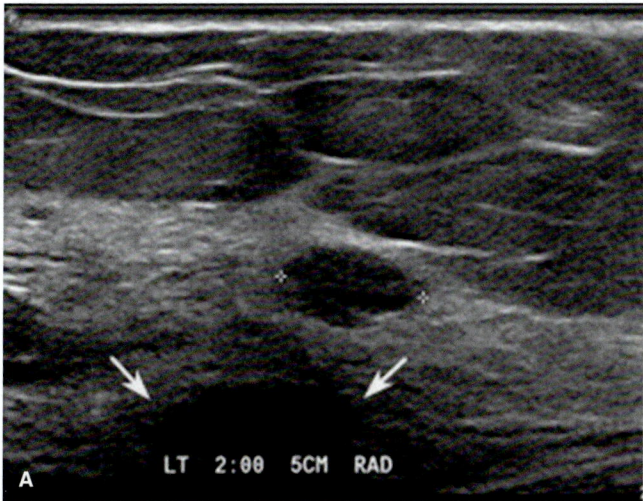

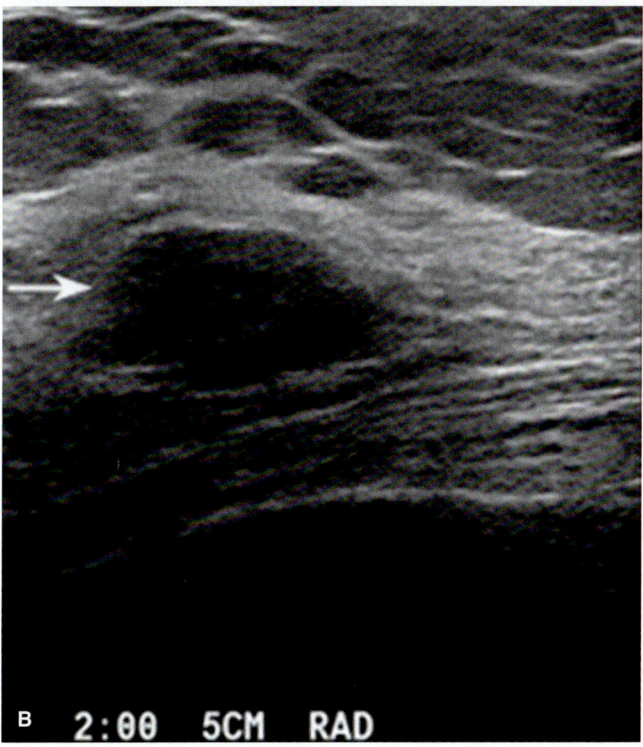

FIG. 4.1 • **Field of view. A:** Inappropriate field of view (FOV). The mass being followed is only partially included on the image *(arrows)*, and image annotation has been placed over the lesion. The calipers were placed on a fatty lobule assumed to be the lesion not included with FOV. **B:** An appropriate FOV includes the mass *(arrow)* as well as the surrounding tissue preferably to include pectoral muscle. Although "zooming" on a lesion is sometimes done, in establishing the presence of a lesion, it is important to have a field of view that includes enough of the tissue to be sure that a lesion is not excluded. In most patients, if the tissue in the area of lesion has been thinned out as much as possible, the relationship to the pectoral muscle, ribs, and chest wall is demonstrated.

Table 4.1	**BREAST ULTRASOUND: TECHNICAL CONSIDERATIONS**

High transducer frequency (12.5 MHz, 17.5 MHz), linear array transducer
Focal zone(s) positioning
Gain setting
Field of view
Lesion in perpendicular (orthogonal) projections
Maximal dimensions for the lesion in orthogonal projections
Image annotations: laterality, lesion location (o'clock position, quadrant, or shown on diagram of breast), probe orientation
Film labeling: patient's first and last names, unique identification number, facility name, location of facility date of study, and operator's identification

position, she is scanned initially in an upright position. When there are significant physical limitations, patients can be scanned in a wheelchair or stretcher.

The reason for the study and how the study is done are explained to the patient. The coupling gel is pre-warmed in commercially available warmers. If the gel is used at room temperature, it can be uncomfortably cold, particularly in the winter months. As with positioning for the mammographic study, it is important to consider the patient's modesty. Only the breast to be examined and scanned is exposed. The contralateral breast is kept covered unless comparison needs to be made. At the completion of the study, the patient is provided a towel to wipe the coupling gel off her breast. A second person is always in the room when we scan patients.

Scanning by the radiologist is encouraged strongly. The breast imaging radiologists do all of the breast ultrasounds at our facility. We do not have an ultrasound technologist. A mammography technologist, or an assistant, helps us during diagnostic and interventional ultrasounds, but they do not scan. We have several reasons for taking this approach. First, by having the radiologist do the ultrasound studies, we are able to examine the patient and correlate what is described, or seen on the mammogram, with our own physical exam and what is imaged on the ultrasound. Real-time scanning and palpation are critical to our final impression. The information obtained during the physical examination is as important as the imaging information. Second, ultrasound is an operator-dependent study. Normal tissue can be made to simulate a lesion, and "true" lesions can be overlooked easily. To establish the presence of a lesion, the transducer needs to be rotated over the potential finding as variable amounts of pressure are applied to eliminate artifactual shadowing generated by ligaments. Third, as physical examination is done, and an impression is generated during the real-time scan portion of the study, selective images are taken to document the features of the lesion, leading us to make a specific recommendation (Table 4.2). We do not take images of normal tissue. Lastly, by doing the ultrasound ourselves, we can establish rapport with patients. We can elicit a pertinent history, reassure the patient we are doing everything possible to take care of her, and discuss findings and recommendations. The patient's input is sought, and she is involved in the decision-making process. After discussing all reasonable alternatives, and taking clinical and imaging data into consideration, we provide patients with a specific recommendation.

Visual inspection of the breast is done with the lights up in the room prior to scanning. We specifically evaluate the breasts for changes in size

the patient is asked to raise the ipsilateral arm and place it comfortably under her head. This helps to further thin the area being scanned. One of the major advantages of ultrasound is the real-time capability. Patients are positioned as needed to evaluate the area of concern, and physical examination is done as the transducer is rotated and varying amounts of pressure are applied over a potential or real lesion. If the patient describes an abnormality as more apparent in the upright

Table 4.2	FEATURES OF LESIONS TO CONSIDER ON ULTRASOUND		
Malignant	Benign	Indeterminate	
Spiculation	Intensely hyperechoic, homogeneous	Isoechoic	
Angular margins	Oval, ellipsoid shape	Mildly hypoechoic	
Marked hypoechogenicity	Gentle bi- or trilobulation	Heterogeneous echotexture	
Shadowing	Thin echogenic pseudocapsule	Homogeneous echotexture	
Calcifications	Anechoic	Normal sound transmission	
Duct extension	No malignant features	Posterior enhancement	
Branch pattern			
Microlobulation			
Echogenic rim			
Vertical orientation (taller than wide)			

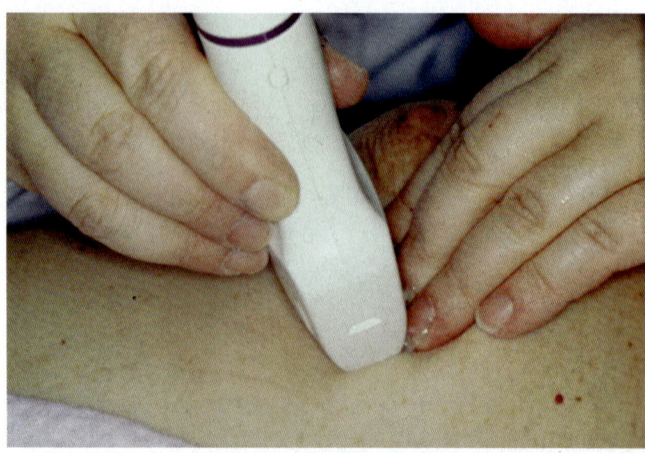

FIG. 4.2 • **Breast ultrasound scanning.** One hand holds the transducer, while the index, middle, and ring fingers of the contralateral hand are placed at the leading edge of the transducer palpating the area being scanned (e.g., putting an eyeball at the tip of our fingers). The transducer is rotated over the area as varying amounts of pressure are applied. The ultrasound coupling gel is helpful in that it appears to facility and possibly improves palpation.

and contour. We evaluate the nipple areolar complex for any erosion and nipple discharge. We establish the presence of skin findings, including skin dimpling, retraction, erythema, ecchymosis, localized thickening or thinning, peau d'orange changes (localized or generalized), eczematous changes, bullae, discoloration, or hyperpigmentation (see Figs. 8.1 through 8.7 and 9.30 for examples of findings on physical examination). In examining the breast, is the temperature of one increased compared with the contralateral side? If the patient presents with a localized finding, she is asked to pinpoint its location. If you palpate a mass, is it tender? Is it mobile or fixed? Are there any findings in the axilla? After the visual inspection and initial palpation, the lights in the room are dimmed. In further establishing the presence and physical characteristics of a mass, the transducer coupling gel is helpful in that it appears to facility and improves palpation. By combining palpation of the tissue with transducer movements, you are in essence placing an eyeball at the tips of your fingers (Fig. 4.2).

The transducer is moved in small increments over the area of concern to the patient or the specific area (e.g., o'clock position and expected distance from the nipple) in which you are expecting to locate a mammographically or MRI-detected abnormality. One hand holds the transducer while the index, middle, and ring fingers of the contralateral hand are placed at the leading edge of the transducer palpating the area being scanned (Fig. 4.2). If a possible abnormality is detected, the transducer is rotated 360 degrees over the area to help distinguish a mass from a fat lobule in cross section. A mass maintains a round, oval, or irregular shape as the transducer is rotated, whereas fatty tissue elongates and fuses with surrounding structures (Fig. 4.3). Varying amounts of pressure can be applied over the area being scanned and any possible abnormality detected. Traditionally, transverse and sagittal orientations are used for imaging, but because ductal structures radiate out from the nipple toward the chest wall, radial and antiradial scan orientations are recommended by some for breast ultrasound (2).

Images are not taken until a decision is made about the presence of a mass or an ongoing process (e.g., inflammatory) in the breast. Making this determination involves correlation with mammographic and clinical findings, slow movements and rotations of the transducer over the area of concern, gradations in compression, time gain compensation (TGC) curve and power setting manipulations, positioning of the focal zone(s), correct field of view, and, if indicated, use of a standoff pad. In some patients, particularly those with an inflammatory or possibly diffuse change related to trauma, scanning the contralateral breast may be helpful for comparison and assessing the patient's

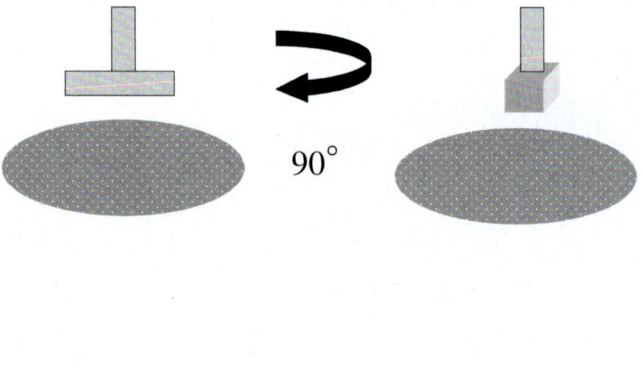

FIG. 4.3 • **Importance of transducer rotation in distinguishing pseudolesions from masses. A:** Cooper ligaments create a honeycomb-like "skeletal" framework for breast tissue. Oblong bundles of glandular and fatty tissues are found within the honeycombs created by the ligaments. When the tissue is imaged longitudinally, the oblong tissue bundles are easily detected as normal tissue. When viewed in cross section, however, they can sometimes closely mimic a mass. Rotation (90 degrees) and sometimes minor rocking of the transducer over a suspected mass is critical in determining the significance of any potential finding. **B:** If a mass is present in the tissue bundles, it is seen three-dimensionally as the transducer is manipulated and rotated over the suspected mass. Palpation is undertaken as the tissue is scanned. (From Cardeñosa G. *Breast Imaging [The Core Curriculum Series]*. Philadelphia, PA: Lippincott Williams & Wilkins; 2003.)

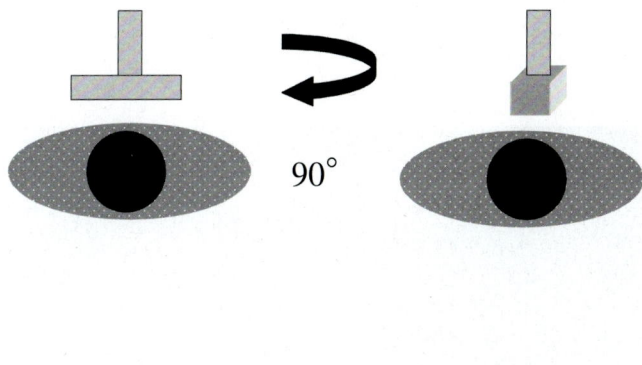

FIG. 4.3 • (Continued)

normal tissue echogenicity and soft tissue planes. If during real-time scanning it is determined that a lesion is present, images are then taken to document the presence and features of the lesion. Using whatever orientations demonstrate the features of the mass best, orthogonal images are taken with and without measurements for a total of four images per lesion.

The study (2–4) should include the name of the patient, unique patient identifying number, date of study, name and location of facility, as well as the initials of the individual doing the ultrasound. The images need to be further annotated with respect to the breast being imaged, clock location of the lesion (Fig. 4.4A), distance of the lesion from the nipple, transducer orientation (radial/antiradial, transverse/sagittal, or longitudinal) (Fig. 4.4B), and depth in the breast (retroareolar, anterior third, middle portion, posterior third, axillary tail, axilla).

Some ultrasound units provide diagrams that adequately annotate the location and scan plane used for a given image. As the transducer is manipulated, the size of the lesion varies. In providing a measurement, an attempt is made to use the largest dimensions of the lesion (2–4). If the mass demonstrates a thick echogenic rim, that rim should be included in the measurements. It is also useful to indicate on the image if the lesion is palpable. As mentioned in Chapter 3, many screen-detected abnormalities are palpable when, based on the mammographic findings, one knows exactly where to palpate.

TERMINOLOGY

Several terms are used to characterize the appearance of tissue and lesions on ultrasound. In the breast, the echogenicity of an area of interest is compared with the appearance of subcutaneous fat (2). If the area contains fewer echoes (i.e., appears darker) compared with subcutaneous fat, it is hypoechoic; if it contains more echoes (i.e., appears whiter), it is hyperechoic; if it contains no echoes (i.e., it is black), it is anechoic, and if it is of the same echogenicity as subcutaneous fat, it is isoechoic. At the junction of tissues with significant acoustic impedance differences, variable amounts of the sound beam are reflected back, and a shadow is seen. The size of the shadow depends on the size of the interface. Shadowing is a feature of some lesions, and although more common with malignant lesions, it is also seen with benign masses (Fig. 4.5A). In masses with associated calcifications, shadowing can sometimes be seen distal to the calcifications (Fig. 4.5B, C).

Simple cysts do not attenuate sound energy. Consequently, a proportionately greater amount of sound energy reaches the tissues deep to a cyst. The TGC curve, however, compensates for presumed decreases in echo strength as the distance from the transducer is increased. The resulting effect is that tissue deep to cysts appears more echogenic than adjacent tissue. This increased echogenicity deep to fluid-filled structures is called posterior acoustic enhancement or increased sound (through) transmission. Enhancement is common with cysts; however, it can be seen with benign (Fig. 4.5) and malignant masses.

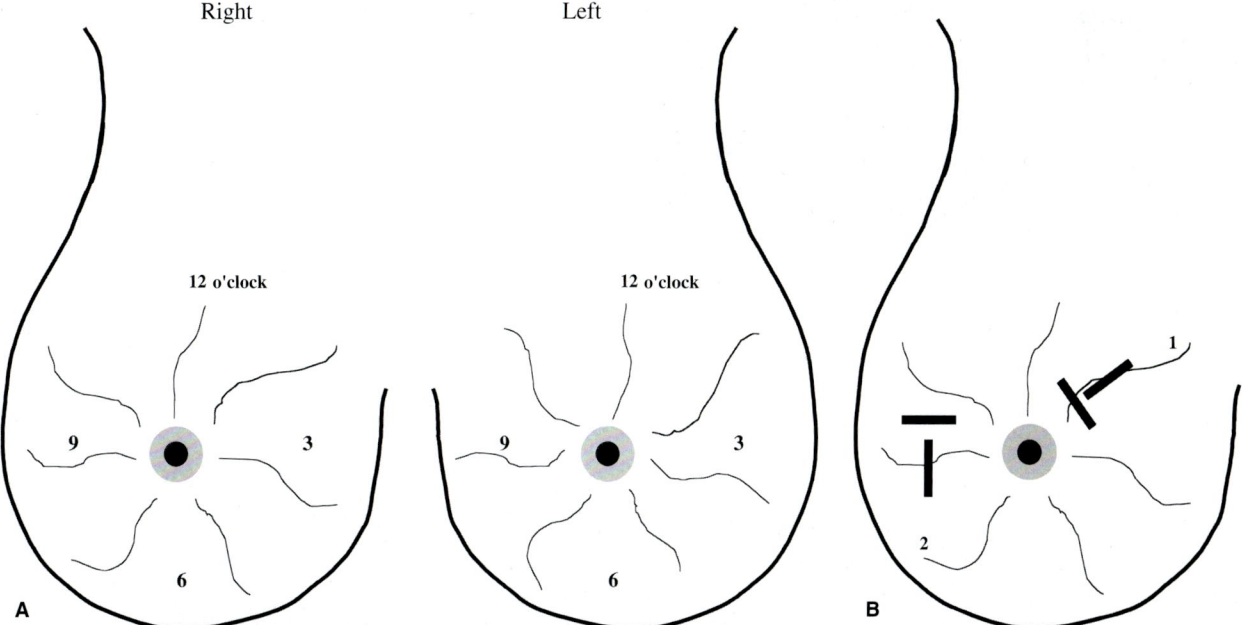

FIG. 4.4 • **Image labeling, ultrasound. A:** Lesion location is indicated by using the o'clock position of the lesion in the breast and the distance of the lesion from the nipple. **B:** Images are obtained in orthogonal projections. This includes (1) radial *(rad)* and antiradial *(arad)* or (2) transverse *(trv)* and sagittal or longitudinal *(sag, long)*. (From Cardeñosa G. *Breast Imaging [The Core Curriculum Series]*. Philadelphia, PA: Lippincott Williams & Wilkins; 2003.)

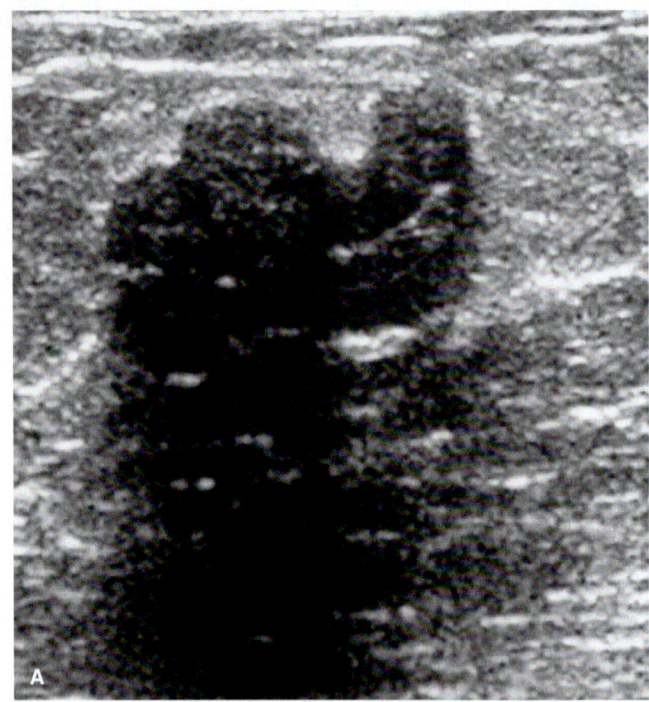

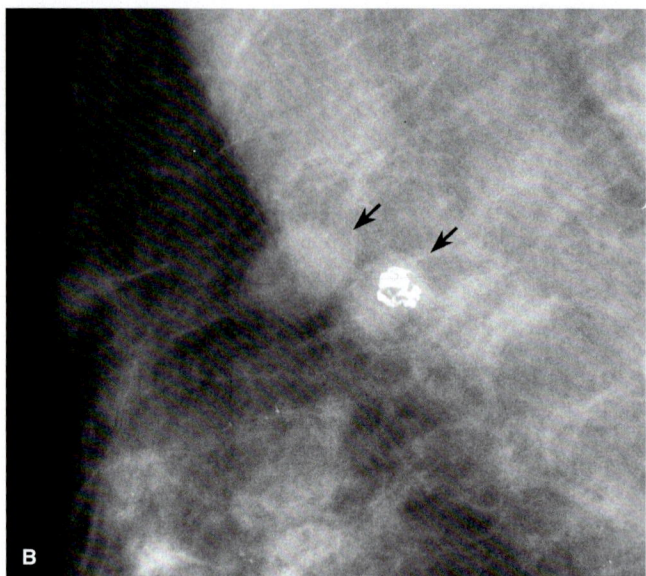

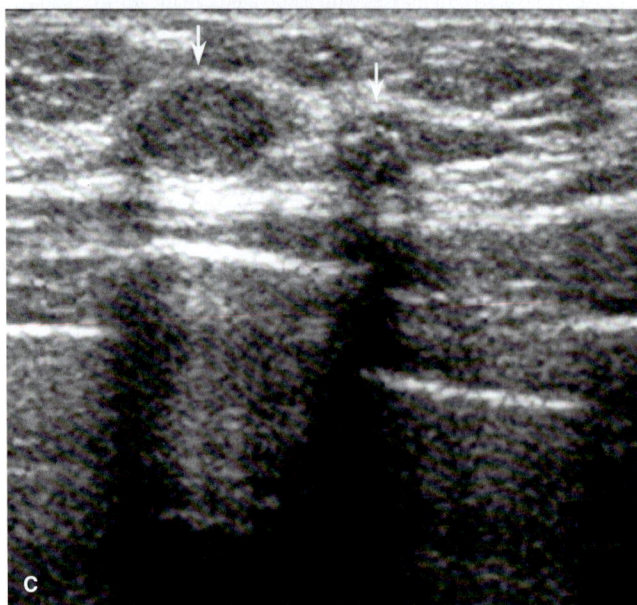

FIG. 4.5 • **Hyalinized fibroadenomas; multiple peripheral papillomas. A:** An irregular, lobulated hypoechoic mass with shadowing is imaged. No calcifications are seen mammographically. Shadowing is more commonly associated with malignant masses; however, it can be seen with benign lesions, including hyalinized fibroadenomas, focal fibrosis, and masses with associated calcifications. BI-RADS 2: Benign finding. **B:** Mediolateral oblique (MLO) view photographically coned to the upper portion of the image in a different patient. Two low-density oval masses *(arrows)* are new compared with the study done a year ago. A coarse calcification is noted associated with the smaller of the two masses. **C:** Two adjacent masses *(arrows)* are seen on ultrasound corresponding to the masses seen on the mammogram. The larger of the two is oval with circumscribed margins and posterior acoustic enhancement. The smaller mass contains internal specular echoes and associated shadowing reflecting the presence of the calcifications seen on the mammogram. BI-RADS 4A: Suspicious abnormality, biopsy is indicated. Papillomas are diagnosed on core biopsy and confirmed on excisional biopsy. (From Cardeñosa G. Breast Imaging [The Core Curriculum Series]. Philadelphia, PA: Lippincott Williams & Wilkins; 2003.)

Please see Appendix A (Table A.2) for the ACR BI-RADS® ultrasound lexicon. This provides the terminology to be used, and what needs to be described in reports, with respect to ultrasound findings. You should familiarize yourself with this and apply it consistently when describing breast ultrasound findings.

BREAST ANATOMY ON ULTRASOUND

Understanding the anatomy of the breast and its surroundings on ultrasound is helpful in evaluating potential lesions and their sites of origin (see Figs. 8.57 and 11.22). The pleural reflection, ribs, and pectoral muscles are deep to breast tissue and usually imaged during scanning. The pleural reflection is a hyperechoic band deep to the ribs. The tissue air interface usually leads to shadowing deep to the pleural reflection. Simulating lesions, ribs in cross section are circumscribed oval hypoechoic structures (Fig. 4.6A). Recognizing the relationship of the ribs to the pleural reflection and overlying pectoral muscles is important in distinguishing a rib in cross section from a lesion. Longitudinally, ribs are echogenic bands of variable thickness with shadowing (Fig. 4.6B). The pectoral muscles are hypoechoic with associated specular echoes that may be seen as bright spots in the muscle when in cross-section or echogenic, parallel hyperechoic bands when imaged longitudinally (Fig. 4.6C). The deep pectoral fascia is an echogenic line on the surface of the pectoral muscle that separates the muscle from overlying breast tissue.

Cooper ligaments connect deep and superficial pectoral fascial layers, thereby providing a honeycomb-like structure or a "skeleton" for breast tissue. The ligaments are hyperechoic bands that crisscross the breast, isolating oval and oblong-shaped areas of glandular and fatty tissues. Superficially, Cooper ligaments extend to the superficial

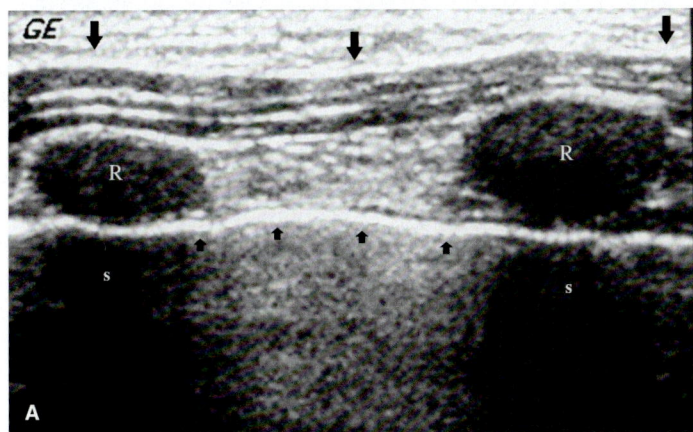
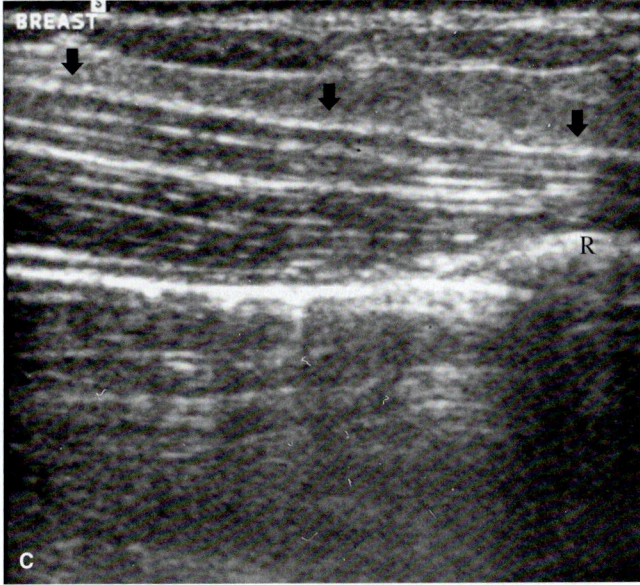
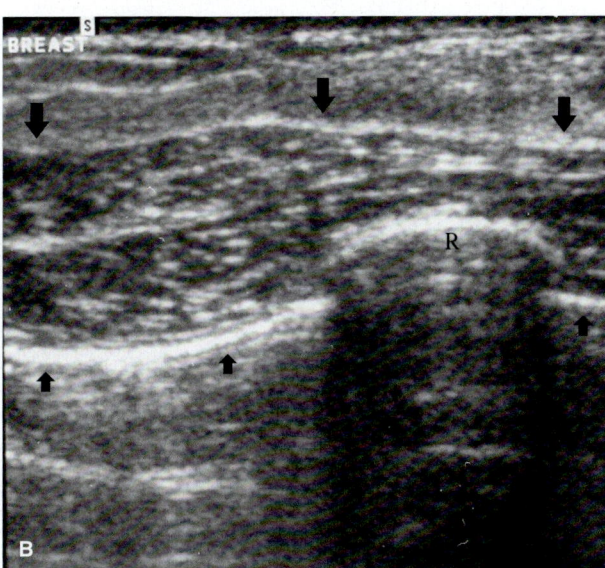

FIG. 4.6 • **Normal breast anatomy on ultrasound. A:** Ribs *(R)* in cross section simulate oval hypoechoic masses; these are often associated with shadowing *(s)*. The echogenic line deep to the ribs *(short arrows)* is the pleural reflection. Two parallel echogenic lines are present in the body of the pectoral muscle, directly over the ribs. The echogenic line on the superficial surface of the muscle is the deep pectoral fascia *(long arrow)* and serves as the demarcation between breast tissue and chest wall structures. In this area, the pectoral muscle is thin, and there is not much overlying breast tissue. **B:** Different patient. Longitudinally oriented rib *(R)* with associated shadowing. The pleural reflection is imaged as an echogenic line *(short arrow)* deep to the pectoral muscle. In this orientation, round and oval specular echoes are imaged in the pectoral muscle. The echogenic line *(long arrows)* on the surface of the muscle is the deep pectoral fascia. A small amount of overlying breast tissue is seen on this image. **C:** The specular echoes noted in the muscle on the image in part *B* elongate and become parallel echogenic lines in the substance of the muscle as the transducer is rotated 90 degrees. The pleural reflection is again seen as an echogenic line deep to the muscle; a portion of rib *(R)* with associated shadowing is also noted. The echogenic line associated with the surface of the muscle is the deep pectoral fascia *(arrows)* and separates the muscle from overlying breast tissue. (From Cardeñosa G. *Breast Imaging [The Core Curriculum Series]*. Philadelphia, PA: Lippincott Williams & Wilkins; 2003.)

pectoral fascia in the deep dermis. Given the oval and oblong shape of breast tissue bundles, transducer movements and rotation over an area of concern are important. When breast tissue bundles are imaged in cross section as round or oval structures, they can sometimes simulate a lesion. As the transducer is rotated 90 degrees, breast tissue bundles elongate and fuse with surrounding tissue; a mass maintains its round or oval shape (Fig. 4.2). Fatty breast tissue bundles also commonly have small hyperechoic bands within them not typically seen in solid masses (Fig. 4.7).

Dense glandular tissue is relatively hyperechoic (Fig. 4.8). Since most breast lesions are hypoechoic relative to subcutaneous fat, lesions are identified more readily in women with dense tissue mammographically. Cooper ligaments are not as apparent in hyperechoic fibrous tissue because they are isoechoic with the fibrous tissue. In women with predominantly fatty tissue, however, lesions may be isoechoic with surrounding tissue and not identifiable. In fatty tissue, Cooper ligaments are identified more easily because they are hyperechoic relative to the surrounding tissue (Fig. 4.7). In this patient population, however, mammography is reliable in depicting small water-density lesions. During pregnancy, breast tissue usually becomes more homogeneous with small round and oval anechoic spaces, some of which are vessels (determined with Doppler). Cooper ligaments, fibrous ridges, and tissue bundles are not as readily apparent (Fig. 4.9). Prominent ductal structures may be seen particularly in the subareolar area.

Use of the standoff pad may be required for evaluation of the skin. Normally, skin measures 1 to 2 mm and is made up of a hypoechoic band sandwiched between two hyperechoic lines (Fig. 4.10). Benign masses involving the skin (e.g., sebaceous cysts) can be localized (Fig. 4.10), and their track to the skin surface can sometimes be identified (Fig. 4.11). Edema resulting from radiation therapy acutely, congestive heart failure, benign inflammatory processes, or inflammatory carcinoma can present with skin thickening. The deep hyperechoic line may be disrupted, and there is thickening of the hypoechoic band. Small, anastomosing, serpiginous tubular structures, representing dilated lymphatics or vascular structures, are sometimes seen deep to the thickened skin (Fig. 4.12; also see Fig. 9.5B, C). Malignant and inflammatory processes arising in breast tissue can extend to involve the skin with disruption of the deep hyperechoic stripe and expansion of

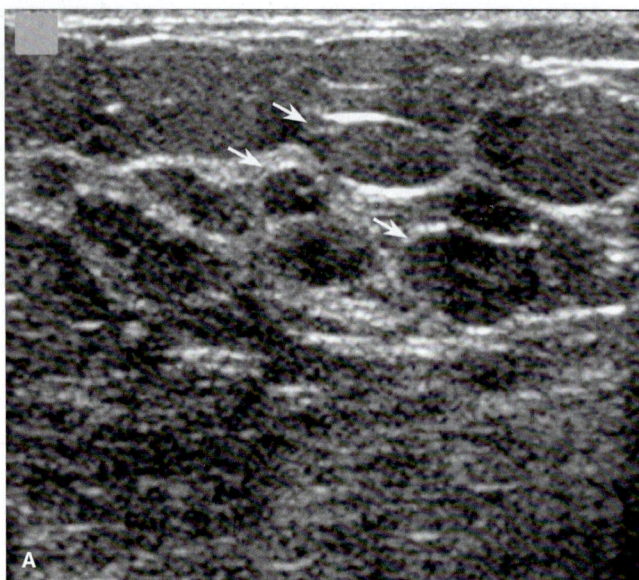 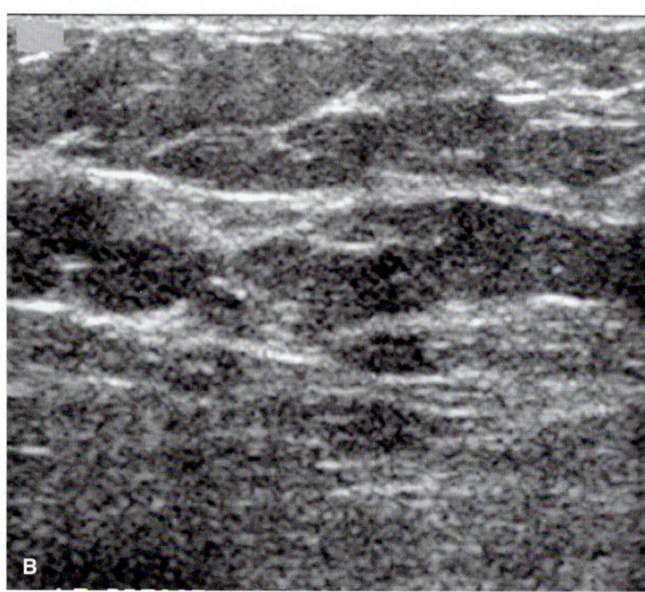

FIG. 4.7 • **Fatty tissue and lobulation. A:** Round and oval mass-like areas *(arrows)* of fatty lobulation can be mistaken for lesions on a single static image. **B:** As the transducer is rotated 90 degrees, these areas fuse and elongate with surrounding tissue consistent with normal fatty lobulation. A true mass will maintain its three-dimensional shape as the transducer is rotated. (From Cardeñosa G. Breast Imaging [The Core Curriculum Series]. Philadelphia, PA: Lippincott Williams & Wilkins; 2003.)

the hypoechoic band (Fig. 4.13; also see Fig. 9.14B). Rarely, metastatic disease to the skin can be imaged as thickening of the hypoechoic band with disruption of the superficial echogenic line when there is associated skin ulceration (Fig. 4.14).

The nipple contains connective tissue and smooth muscle. In some women, it can produce intense shadowing, and in others it can be made to simulate a solid mass (Fig. 4.15A, B). In many patients, the transducer needs to be angled around the nipple to evaluate the subareolar area adequately. Ductal structures can be seen in the subareolar area coursing toward the nipple (Fig. 4.16). These are most commonly tubular in appearance and anechoic. In cross section, they may look more like an anechoic mass (e.g., a cyst). Rarely, they can be homogeneously hyperechoic in appearance (see Fig. 9.32B). Intraductal lesions such as papillomas can sometimes be identified, particularly if

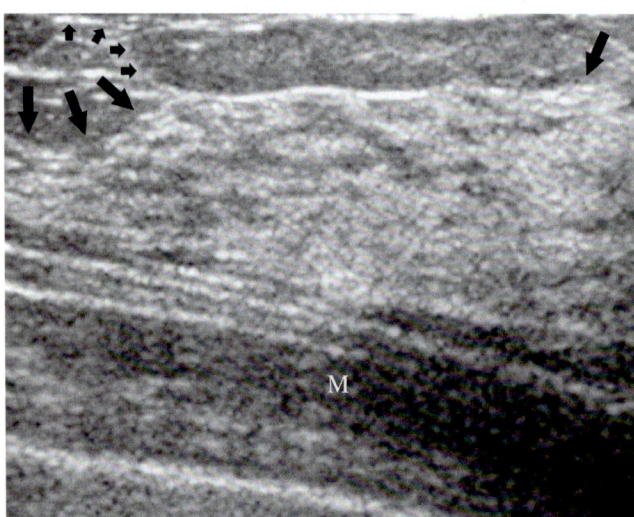 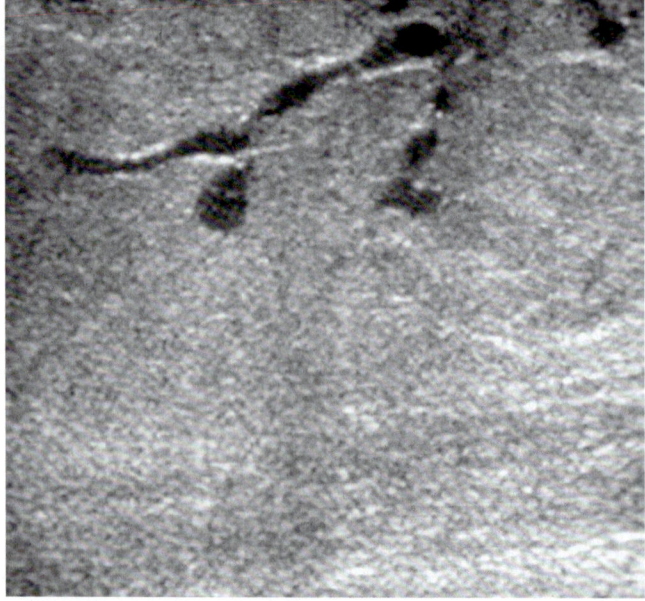

FIG. 4.8 • **Dense tissue.** Dense tissue is relatively hyperechoic on ultrasound *(large arrows)*. Visualization of Cooper ligaments is limited in this type of tissue. Small hypoechoic round and oval areas are seen in the echogenic fibrous tissue, likely reflecting ducts and lobular units. Relatively hypoechoic fatty tissue is seen superficially *(small arrows)*. Ligaments are more easily seen in fatty tissue as echogenic lines. Muscle *(M)* is seen deep to the glandular tissue. (From Cardeñosa G. *Breast Imaging [The Core Curriculum Series]*. Philadelphia, PA: Lippincott Williams & Wilkins; 2003.)

FIG. 4.9 • **Lactational changes.** During late pregnancy and lactation, breast tissue is more homogeneously hyperechoic, and demarcation of tissue bundles is less apparent. Mild-to-moderately dilated ducts with a somewhat beaded appearance can be seen coursing through the tissue for variable distances from the nipple. These can be more or less distended depending on when the last breast feeding or pumping occurred. (From Cardeñosa G. *Breast Imaging [The Core Curriculum Series]*. Philadelphia, PA: Lippincott Williams & Wilkins; 2003.)

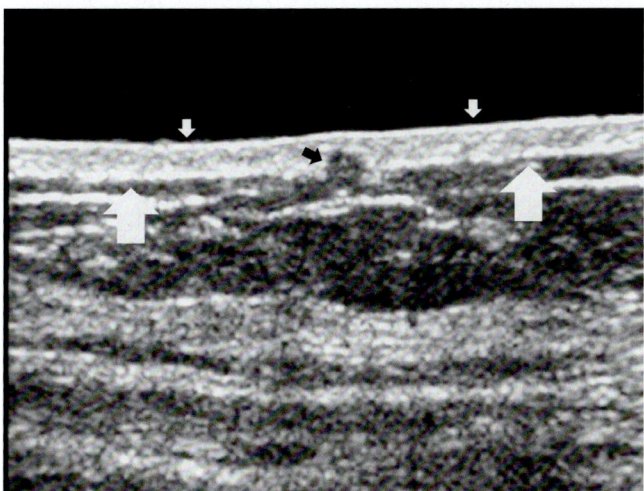

FIG. 4.10 • **Skin and developing skin lesion.** Spacer used to evaluate a superficial palpable mass (*black arrow*). Normal skin is 1 to 2 mm thick and is characterized by a hypoechoic band sandwiched between two echogenic lines. The superficial (*small white arrows*) and deep echogenic lines (*big white arrows*) are well seen in this patient. The palpable mass arises in the hypoechoic band, disrupts the deep echogenic line, and extends minimally into the subcutaneous fat of the breast. (From Cardeñosa G. *Breast Imaging [The Core Curriculum Series]*. Philadelphia, PA: Lippincott Williams & Wilkins; 2003.)

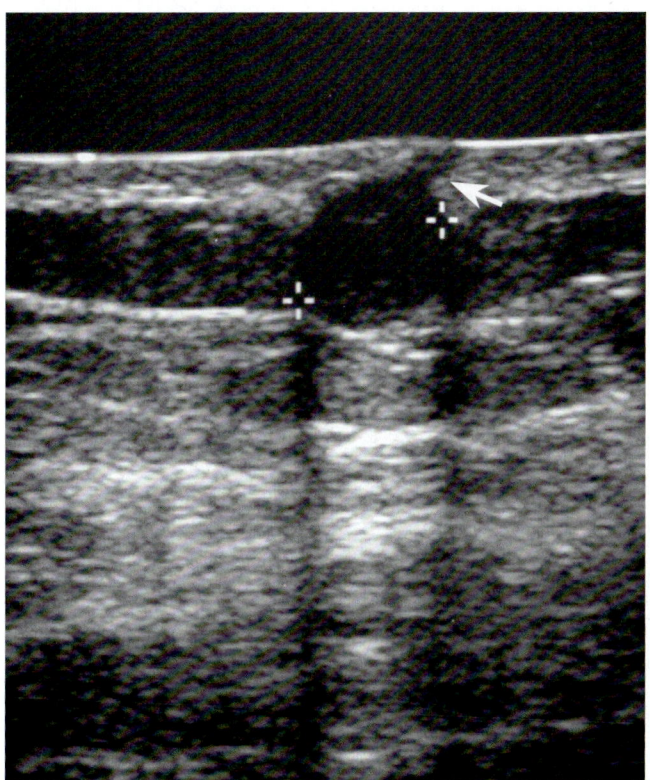

FIG. 4.11 • **Sebaceous cyst.** On physical examination, a punctum is seen on the skin, and a mass that moves with the skin is palpated. Using the standoff pad, a vertically oriented hypoechoic mass (*calipers*) with circumscribed margins, posterior acoustic enhancement, and a track (*arrow*) to the skin is imaged on ultrasound corresponding to the palpable finding and a round isodense mass with circumscribed margins seen on the mammogram (not shown). The patient is reassured of the benign nature of the finding. This requires no additional intervention or short-term follow-up unless it becomes infected or painful, in which case surgical excision may be needed. BI-RADS 2: Benign finding.

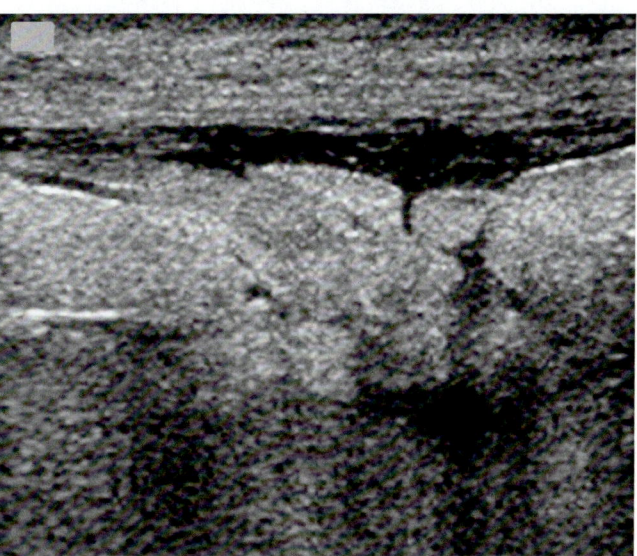

FIG. 4.12 • **Skin thickening and dilated subcutaneous lymphatics in a patient with congestive heart failure.** Skin thickening is noted in this patient with congestive heart failure. The superficial and deep echogenic lines are not apparent, and the hypoechoic band is thickened. Tubular, anastomosing, serpiginous structures deep to the skin are dilated lymphatics; rarely, some of these represent vascular structures and can be characterized as such with Doppler (see Fig. 9.5B). The tissue is echogenic, and normal tissue planes are disrupted related to edematous changes. (From Cardeñosa G. *Breast Imaging [The Core Curriculum Series]*. Philadelphia, PA: Lippincott Williams & Wilkins; 2003.)

the lesion is in the subareolar portion of the duct and the duct is dilated (Fig. 4.17). However, keep in mind that ductal structures often come into and out of the scan plane, potentially causing misleading interpretations regarding the presence or absence of an intraductal mass. Radial scanning may be helpful in demonstrating the ducts coursing for variable distances away from the nipple. As the distance from the nipple increases, the likelihood of identifying intraductal lesions decreases unless the duct remains dilated.

Vascular structures can sometimes be imaged in cross section, less commonly longitudinally (Fig. 4.18), and are more likely to be identified in patients with ongoing inflammatory or edematous changes in the breasts (see Fig. 9.5B). Vessels are often anechoic

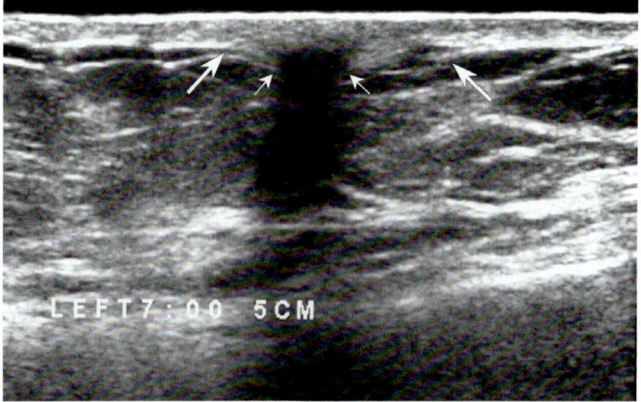

FIG. 4.13 • **Invasive ductal carcinoma, not otherwise specified secondarily involving the skin.** A mass with shadowing is imaged disrupting the echogenic deep dermal line (*large arrows*). It focally thickens and extends into the hypoechoic layer (*thin arrows*) of the skin (also see Fig. 9.14B).

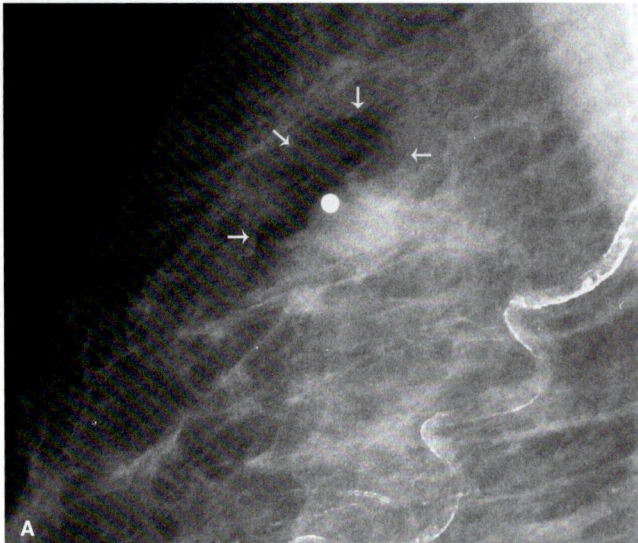 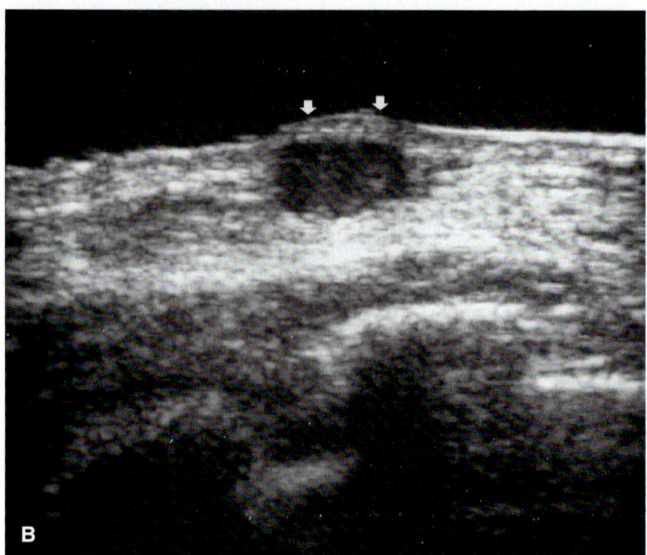

FIG. 4.14 • **Leiomyosarcoma, metastatic to skin. A:** MLO view photographically coned to the superior aspect of the right breast in a patient presenting with an ulcerating mass. The patient's history is notable for previous treatment of a leiomyosarcoma. The metallic BB denotes the site of the palpable finding. Air (lucency) pocket *(arrows)* outlines the ulcerative portion of the mass. Vascular calcification is present. **B:** Ultrasound with standoff pad. A mass involves the hypoechoic band of the skin extending and disrupting the superficial *(arrows)* and deep echogenic lines of the skin. (From Cardeñosa G. *Breast Imaging [The Core Curriculum Series]*. Philadelphia, PA: Lippincott Williams & Wilkins; 2003.)

simulating small cysts; however, pulsations are apparent if the transducer is held steady over the anechoic structure. Doppler is helpful in establishing the nature of the finding. In women with extensive, dense vascular calcification, the calcified vessels can sometimes be seen on ultrasound (Fig. 4.19). In patients presenting with Mondor disease (see Chapter 9), the dilated thrombosed vein is often imaged subcutaneously (Fig. 4.20; also see Figs. 9.39 and 9.40); no flow is seen in the vein.

On ultrasound, intramammary and axillary lymph nodes are characterized by the presence of a hypoechoic cortical region that partially

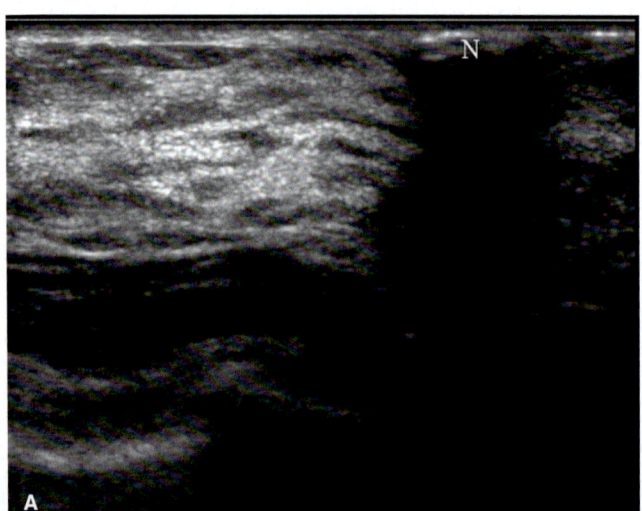 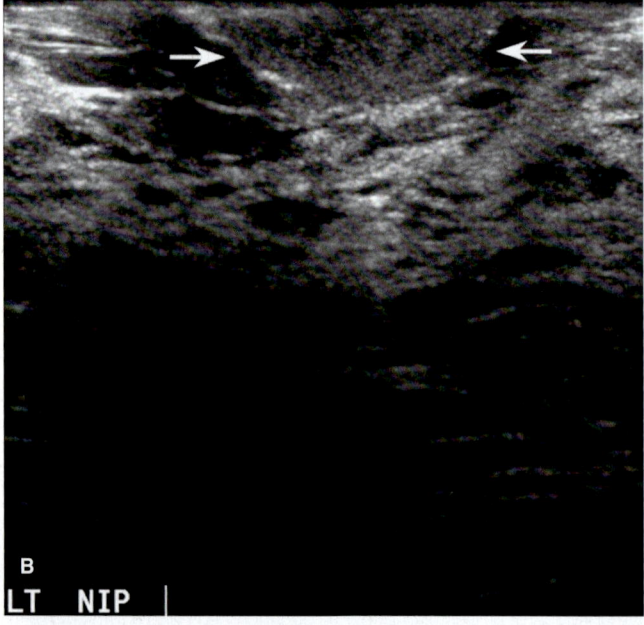

FIG. 4.15 • **Nipple. A:** In many women, the nipple *(N)* produces an intense shadow that limits evaluation of the subareolar area and may be mistaken for a malignant lesion on a static image. **B:** In others, if generous amounts of coupling gel are put over the nipple and some pressure is applied, the nipple simulates an oval hypoechoic mass *(arrows)* that may be mistaken for a lesion on a static image. During real-time scanning, this can easily be identified as the nipple and not a mass in the subareolar area. To evaluate the subareolar area adequately, the transducer needs to be placed at the base of the nipple and angled toward the subareolar area.

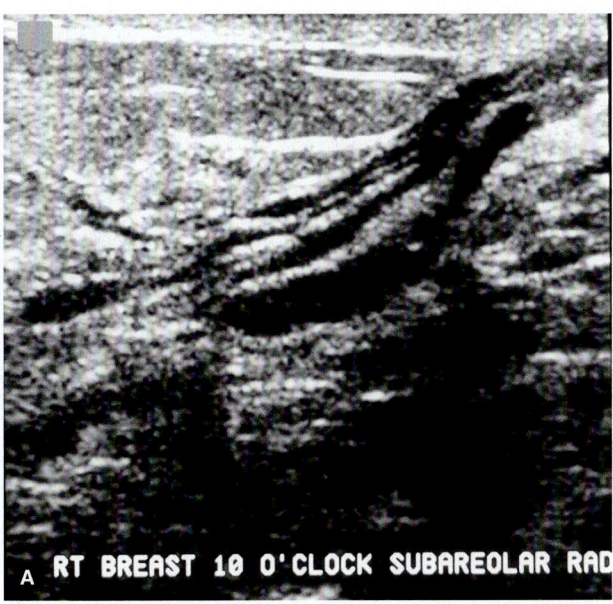
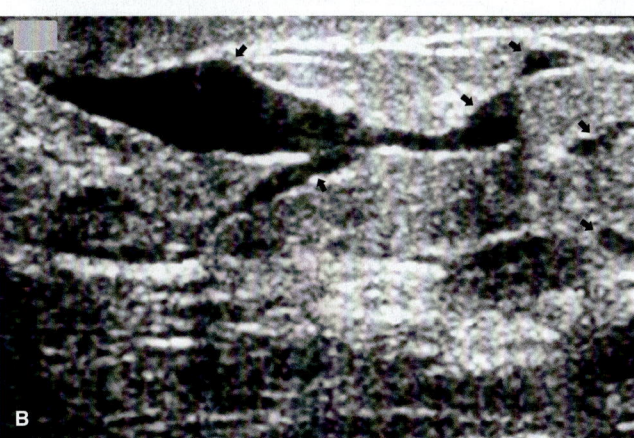

FIG. 4.16 • **Ductal structures in the subareolar area. A:** Several ducts are imaged coursing proximally from the nipple. Since ducts and their branches course in and out of the plane of the transducer, it can be difficult to follow and image them. **B:** Different patient. A duct *(arrows)* with focal areas of dilatation can be followed from the nipple proximally. During real time it could be connected to some of the tubular structures in this image that appear separate from the main duct. This is common since ducts course in and out of the scan plane. (From Cardeñosa G. *Breast Imaging [The Core Curriculum Series]*. Philadelphia, PA: Lippincott Williams & Wilkins; 2003.)

or completely surrounds an eccentrically or centrally located hyperechoic hilar region (Fig. 4.21). Bulging and thickening of a markedly hypoechoic cortical region, and attenuation (mass effect) or complete loss of the hyperechoic fatty hilar region are nonspecific findings that may be related to metastatic disease, lymphoma, or, less commonly, benign reactive changes (Fig. 4.22). In general, the echogenicity of the cortex, even when prominent and bulging, is helpful in assessing benign from malignant lymph nodes. Benign processes involving the lymph nodes may thicken the cortex; however, the echogenicity of the cortex is often characterized as iso- to slightly hyperechoic (Fig. 4.22A). In contrast, marked hypoechogenicity of the cortex (close

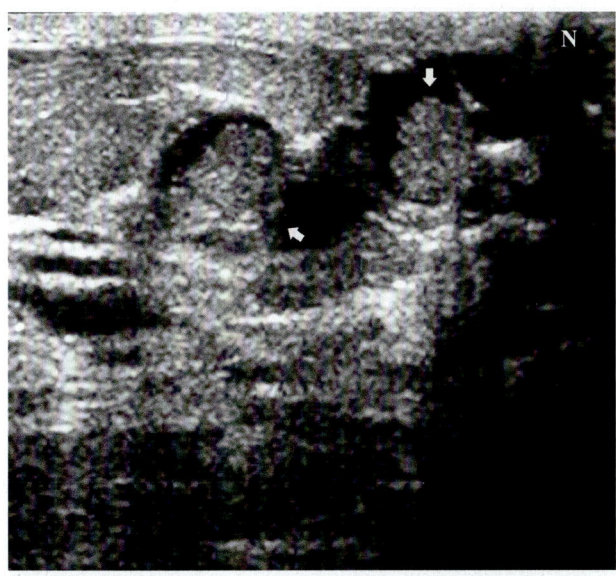
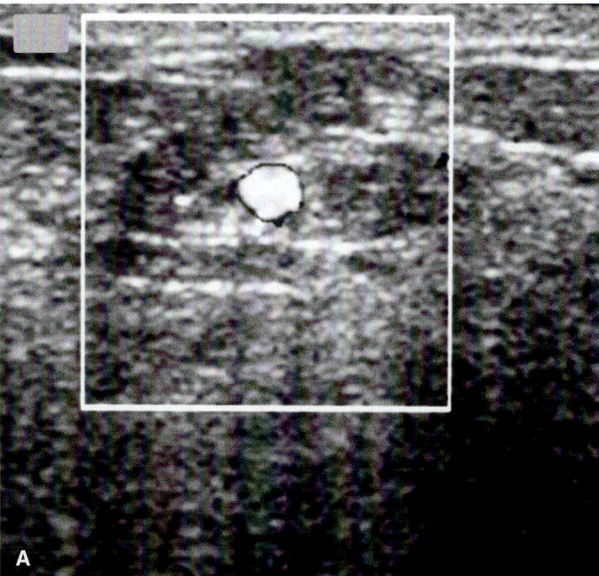

FIG. 4.17 • **Papilloma in the subareolar portions of duct.** Two intraductal lobulated masses *(arrows)* with circumscribed margins and posterior acoustic enhancement are imaged in a dilated duct in the subareolar area. Shadowing is noted associated with the nipple *(N)*. To evaluate the subareolar area adequately, the transducer needs to be placed at the base of the nipple and angled toward the subareolar area. (From Cardeñosa G. *Breast Imaging [The Core Curriculum Series]*. Philadelphia, PA: Lippincott Williams & Wilkins; 2003.)

FIG. 4.18 • **Vascular structures. A:** Artery in cross-section with Doppler on. These are imaged as anechoic round structures that can simulate a cyst when imaged in cross section. As the transducer is manipulated, they can sometimes be seen longitudinally. While holding the transducer over the anechoic structures, pulsations are evident during real-time scanning. Doppler is helpful in confirming these as vascular structures. **B:** As the transducer is rotated over the round mass, the tubular nature of the structure, and with Doppler, the vascular etiology is established. (From Cardeñosa G. *Breast Imaging [The Core Curriculum Series]*. Philadelphia, PA: Lippincott Williams & Wilkins; 2003.)

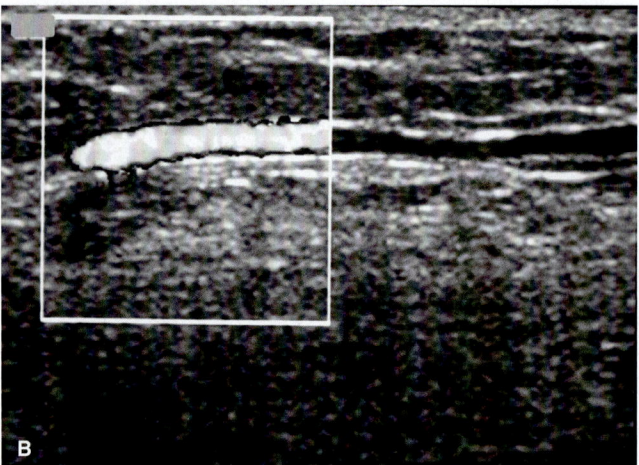

FIG. 4.18 • *(continued)*

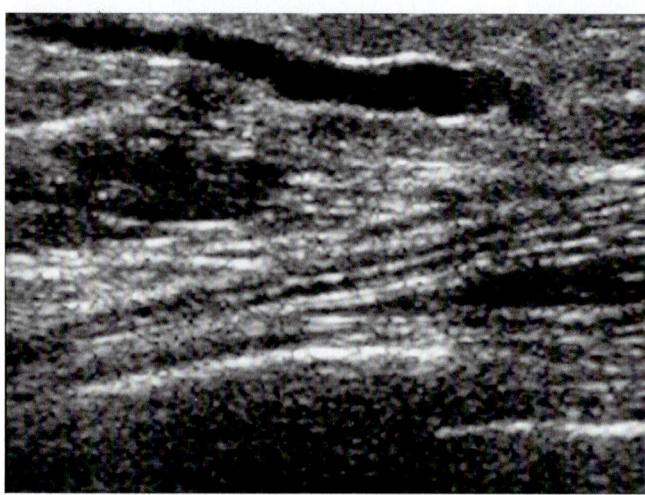

FIG. 4.20 • **Mondor disease.** A 32-year-old patient presents describing a linear area of dimpling in the right breast associated with tenderness. A tubular structure is imaged subcutaneously along the linear dimpling. No flow is seen in the acute phase of Mondor disease. With spontaneous resolution of the thrombophlebitis and recannulation of the vessel, this structure is no longer apparent 8 weeks later. (From Cardeñosa G. *Breast Imaging [The Core Curriculum Series]*. Philadelphia, PA: Lippincott Williams & Wilkins; 2003.)

to anechoic) is more suggestive of metastatic disease (Fig. 4.22B). Please see Chapters 7 and 8 for more on lymph nodes.

INDICATIONS FOR ULTRASOUND

For many years, ultrasound was used sparingly and almost exclusively to characterize breast masses as cystic or solid. While this remains an important use, improvements in equipment have led to increases in the indications for breast ultrasound. It is now an indispensable tool in evaluating women with imaging (mammography, magnetic resonance imaging [MRI]) or clinically detected abnormalities (2). The indications include (i) Matrix characterization of palpable or mammographically detected masses; (ii) Characterization of solid masses as indeterminate or likely benign or malignant; (iii) Evaluation of nonspecific mammographic findings (e.g., developing parenchymal asymmetry, possible area of distortion); (iv) Evaluation of tissue or lesions potentially excluded on routine mammographic views (e.g., upper inner quadrants, axillary tissue, etc.); (v) Evaluation of

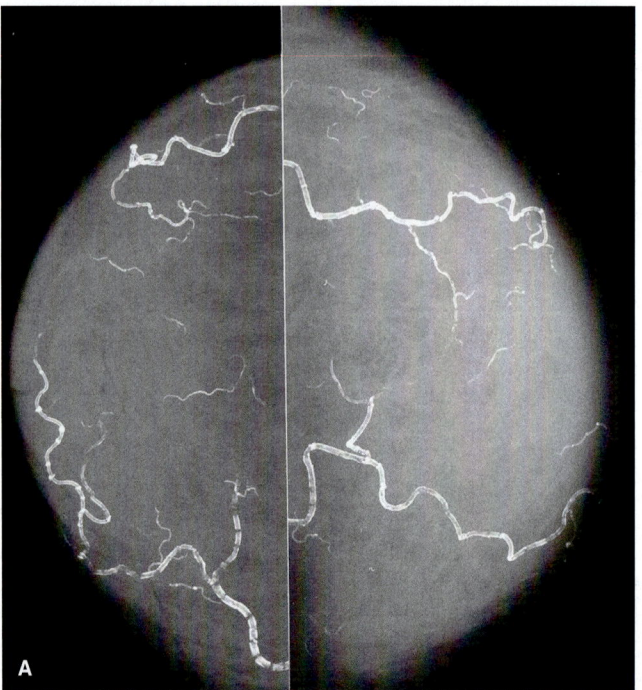

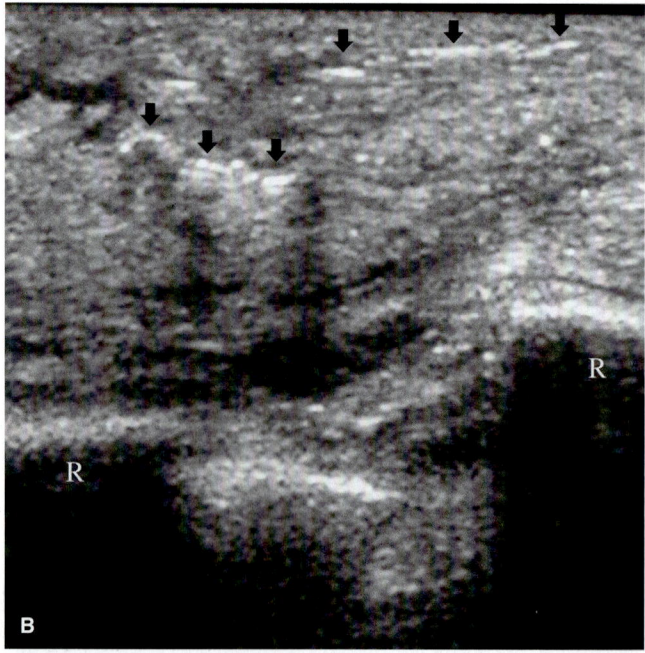

FIG. 4.19 • **Vascular calcification. A:** Craniocaudal (CC) views in a 77-year-old patient. Dense tissue. Extensive vascular calcification is present bilaterally. **B:** Ultrasound. Irregular, linear areas of echogenicity *(arrows)* can be seen rarely when the vascular calcification is dense and extensive as in this patient. Shadowing is seen associated with some of the calcifications. Longitudinally oriented ribs *(R)* are seen. (From Cardeñosa G. *Breast Imaging [The Core Curriculum Series]*. Philadelphia, PA: Lippincott Williams & Wilkins; 2003.)

MRI-detected abnormalities; (vi) Evaluation of women with inflammatory symptoms to distinguish mastitis from an abscess or a locally advanced breast cancer from inflammatory carcinoma; (vii) In conjunction with ductography in the evaluation of women presenting with spontaneous nipple discharge (see Chapter 12); (viii) To guide interventional procedures (Chapter 12); and (ix) For specimen evaluation (specimen sonography, see Chapter 12).

The use of ultrasound for screening purposes is controversial but increasing in use. As ultrasound units, in particular whole breast ultrasound units, improve and we continue to learn, a role for screening women with dense tissue, particularly those who are at high risk for cancer development, is likely to become more common (5–11). Kolb and colleagues (6) reported a 42% increase in the detection of breast cancer with screening ultrasound in women with dense tissue mammographically. In this study, the cancers detected with screening ultrasound were similar in size and stage to those detected with screening mammography. False-positive screening ultrasound studies were reported as 2.4% by these investigators (6).

Screening ultrasound in women with predominantly fatty tissue adds little and may be misleading. In these patients, however, mammography is an excellent screening tool with a sensitivity of 98% (6). The most likely and appropriate role for screening ultrasound would be to evaluate women, particularly those with increased breast cancer risk, who have dense tissue mammographically in whom we know that breast cancers are missed on mammography; the sensitivity of mammography in women with dense tissue may be as low as 48% (6–10). Limitations of ultrasound, and arguments against its routine use for

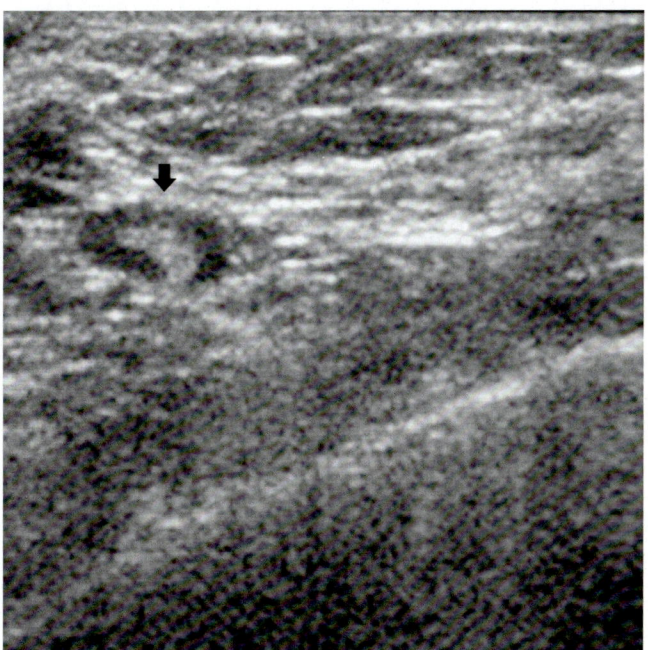

FIG. 4.21 • **Intramammary lymph node.** Oval mass *(arrow)* with a hypoechoic cortex almost completely surrounding ("hugging") the hyperechoic fatty hilar region is imaged in the parenchyma. (From Cardeñosa G. *Breast Imaging [The Core Curriculum Series]*. Philadelphia, PA: Lippincott Williams & Wilkins; 2003.)

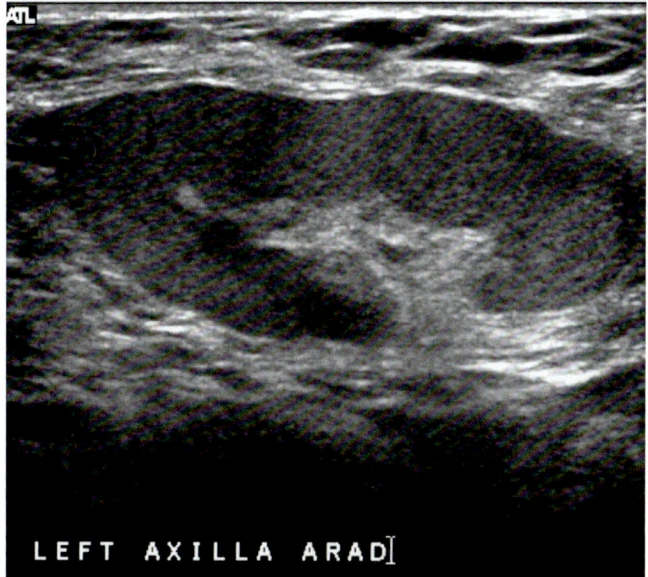
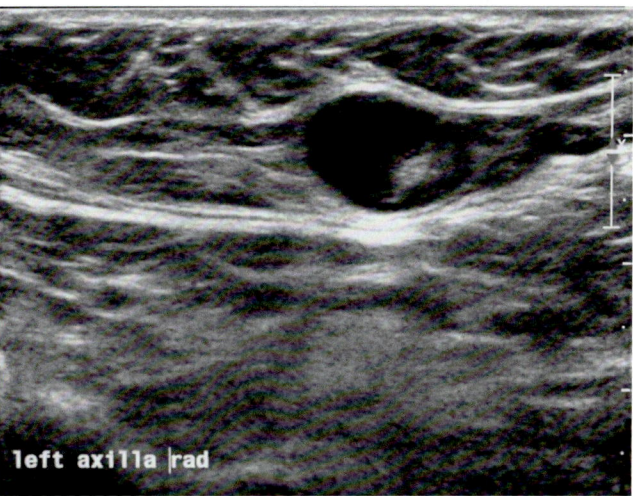

FIG. 4.22 • **Abnormal, lymph nodes. A:** Ultrasound done to evaluate a new dense round mass with circumscribed margins noted in the left axilla on a screening mammogram (not shown) in a 53-year-old woman with a history of sarcoid; she has been symptom-free for several years. A lymph node with circumscribed margins and a prominent, gently lobulated, slightly hyperechoic cortical region is imaged in the axilla corresponding to the dominant mass seen mammographically. Although no fatty hilum is identified mammographically, a fatty hilum is readily apparent on ultrasound, confirming the mass as a lymph node. There is no apparent mass effect on the hilum. Other smaller lymph nodes (not shown) with similar ultrasound features are imaged bilaterally. The echogenicity of the cortex and the presence of a prominent fatty suggest a benign process, particularly in a patient with a history of sarcoid; however, given the change noted mammographically, a biopsy is done. BI-RADS 4A: Suspicious abnormality, biopsy is indicated. A portion of a lymph node with numerous non-necrotizing granulomas and fibrosis without evidence of infection is reported histologically; the findings are consistent with sarcoid. **B:** Ultrasound in a different patient. A lymph node with a markedly hypoechoic thickened and bulging cortex and posterior acoustic enhancement is imaged in the left axilla. The fatty hilum is attenuated and eccentric in position. Compare the echogenicity of the cortex in this patient with that of the lymph node in the patient shown in part **A**. BI-RADS 4C: Suspicious abnormality, biopsy is indicated. Metastatic disease is diagnosed on a core biopsy.

screening, relate to the inability to reliably detect calcifications, false-positive studies (6,10), and the operator dependence of the study (something that may be overcome with the use of automated whole breast units). As with mammography, quality issues and standardization of techniques and equipment would seem to be appropriate before widespread use. Also, it should be made clear to patients, referring physicians, and third-party payors that screening ultrasound would be used in conjunction with mammography and not as a replacement.

MATRIX DETERMINATION

One of the most important roles of breast ultrasound is to help establish whether a clinical apparent mass is real or dense fibrous tissue. If the clinical or mammographically apparent mass is real, is it cystic or solid? Breast ultrasound is 96% to 100% accurate in the diagnosis of cysts when appropriate criteria are used (2,12). Simple cysts are anechoic masses, with circumscribed margins, sharp anterior and posterior walls, thin-edge shadows, posterior acoustic enhancement (Fig. 4.23; also see Fig. 7.44), and compressibility (13). Slight movements or changes in the orientation of the transducer may be needed to demonstrate posterior acoustic enhancement. Also, with small (approximately <5 mm) or deep cysts, posterior acoustic enhancement may not be demonstrable. Unless the cyst is under tension, pressure applied with the transducer leads to compression and elongation of the cyst. Reverberation artifacts can involve the anterior wall of some cysts (Fig. 4.24). If the criteria for a simple cyst are fulfilled, and the patient is asymptomatic, we do not recommend aspiration. We try to educate and reassure the patient that cysts are common, benign masses that fluctuate in size and tenderness with the menstrual cycle, may regress spontaneously, and often recur if aspirated. If the patient is symptomatic, aspiration is undertaken. Likewise, if we are not sure whether the finding is a cyst because it is complicated in appearance on the ultrasound, aspiration and sometimes pneumocystography are done (see Chapter 12).

In the early phases of cyst formation, as acini begin to distend with fluid, tightly clustered, round, 1- to 2-mm sized anechoic areas are seen on ultrasound. The clustered microcysts are separated by thin echogenic septations (Fig. 4.25; also see Fig. 7.47). Posterior

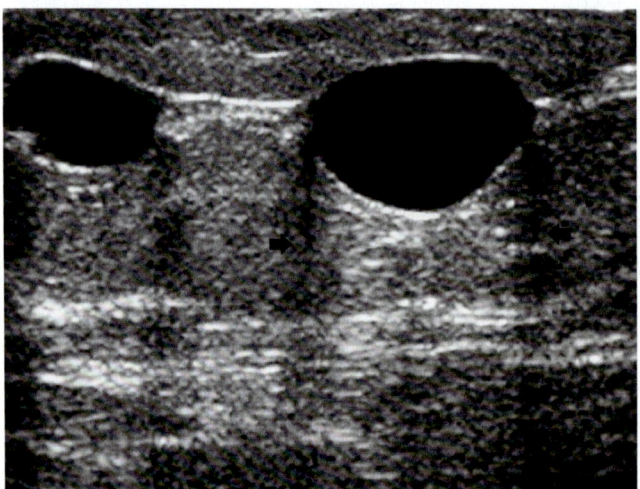

FIG. 4.23 • **Simple cysts.** Two adjacent simple cysts. Anechoic masses with circumscribed margins, thin edge shadows *(arrows)*, sharp anterior and posterior walls, and posterior acoustic enhancement. The enhancement is seen best in the larger of the two cysts. (From Cardeñosa G. *Breast Imaging [The Core Curriculum Series]*. Philadelphia, PA: Lippincott Williams & Wilkins; 2003.)

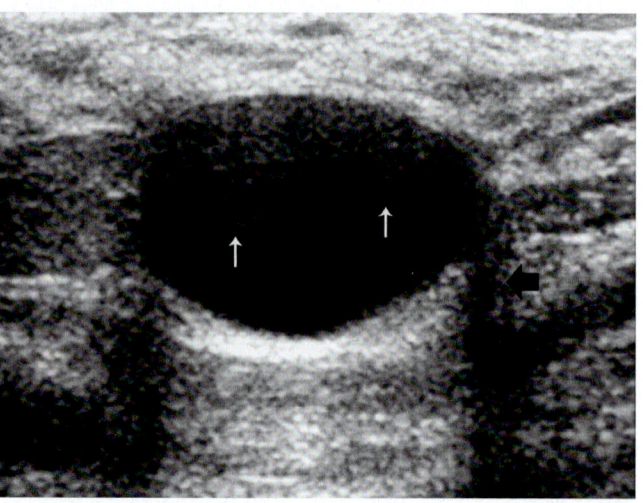

FIG. 4.24 • **Simple cyst, reverberation artifact.** Oval, anechoic mass with circumscribed margins, thin-edge shadows *(black arrow)*, and enhancement. Echoes in the superficial aspect of the cyst *(white arrows)* reflect reverberation artifact. (From Cardeñosa G. *Breast Imaging [The Core Curriculum Series]*. Philadelphia, PA: Lippincott Williams & Wilkins; 2003.)

acoustic enhancement may be present. Although initially described as apocrine-lined cysts (13,14), histologically these areas are commonly a combination of small cystic spaces lined with either epithelial cells or cells characterized by apocrine metaplasia (see Fig. 7.48). As the acini continue to distend with fluid, clusters of small cysts may be seen. As these small cysts coalesce, the more characteristic appearance of the "single" cyst is seen.

The presence of internal echoes that move in the fluid (Fig. 4.26; see also Fig. 7.46) during real-time scanning ("gurgling," swirling) and septations are relatively common variants (2,13). Nondependent, nongurgling internal echoes that partially or completely fill the cyst (Fig. 4.27) and irregular or thickened walls when inflamed may represent "complicated" cysts. If not all of the criteria for the diagnosis of a cyst are present, or the diagnosis of a cyst is otherwise in question, aspiration is undertaken. Cysts should collapse completely, and no residual abnormality should be seen post aspiration. If an intracystic or mural lesion is suspected, pneumocystography or a biopsy of the residual solid component can be done (see Chapter 12). Cyst fluid is not routinely submitted for cytologic evaluation unless the fluid is bloody.

Galactoceles are cysts that contain milky fluid (13). They present in women during lactation, but may be diagnosed several years following the cessation of breast-feeding. Ultrasound findings in women with galactoceles are variable. They are often indistinguishable from simple cysts, but they can be associated with atypical features, including solid appearance, complex cystic mass, or a mass with significant shadowing (Fig. 4.28; also see Fig. 7.56).

Complex cystic and solid masses can be seen in a variety of circumstances (see Chapter 7 and 8 for more complete discussions) (13). Although there can be significant overlap in the diagnostic considerations, we characterize these masses as predominantly cystic with solid components or predominantly solid with cystic components (Table 4.3). Included in the first group are postoperative or traumatic fluid collections. Following surgery, particularly in women undergoing a lumpectomy and radiation therapy or trauma, fluid collections may develop. In some patients these may appear indistinguishable from a cyst. In other patients, these fluid collections have a variable ultrasound appearance, including mural nodules, intracystic septations,

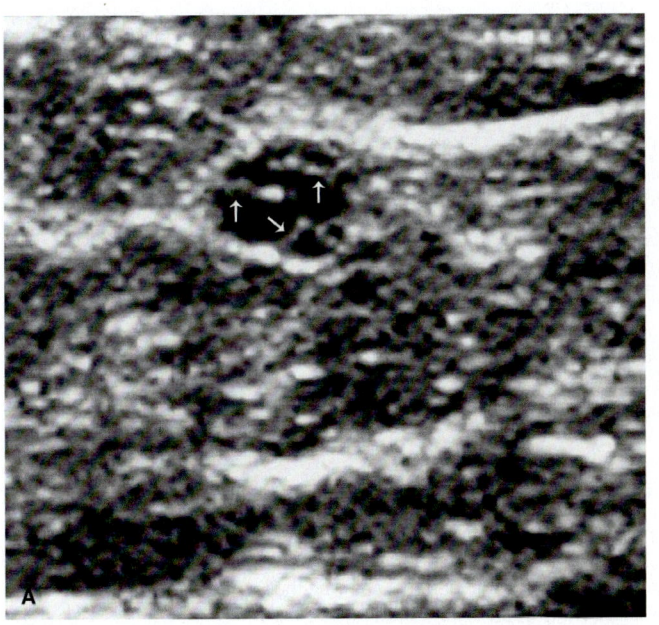
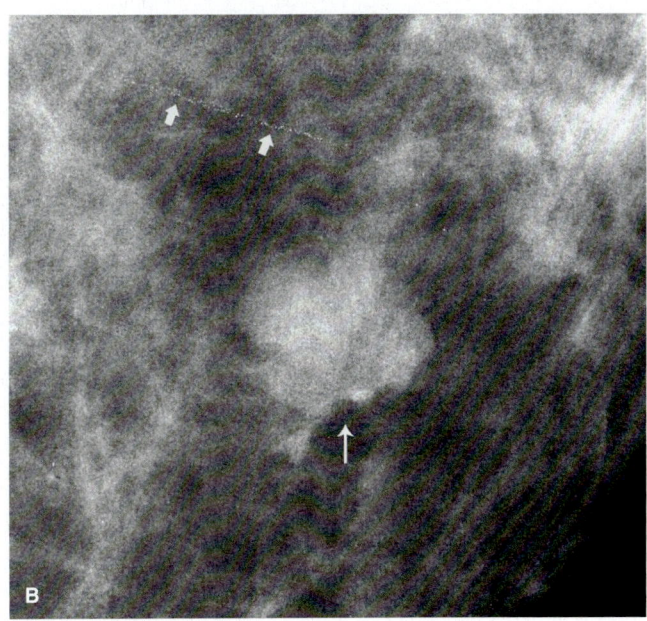
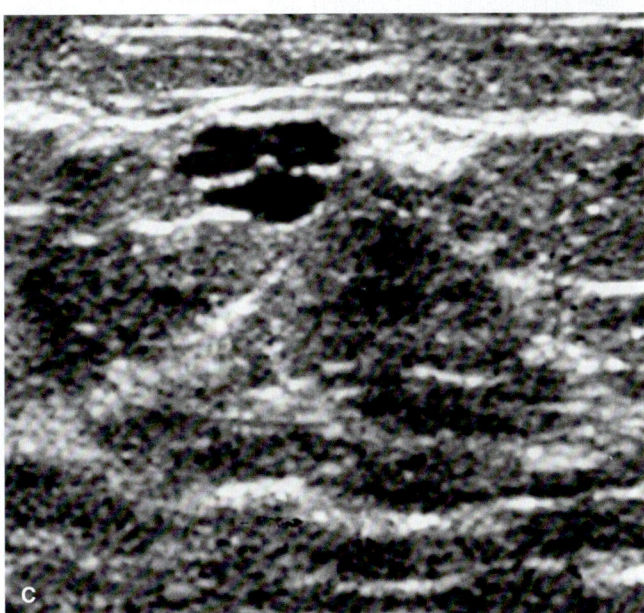

FIG. 4.25 • **Clustered microcysts. A:** A cluster of small, round and oval anechoic masses. The thin walls of the distending acini are evident *(arrows)*. BI-RADS 2: Benign finding. Although not usually indicated, if a core biopsy is done, these lesions tend to disappear after the first or second pass of the needle. Epithelial- and apocrine-lined cysts are reported histologically. **B:** Different patient. Spot compression view of a new finding on screening mammography demonstrates a lobulated mass with partially circumscribed and indistinct margins *(thin arrow)*. Incidentally noted is nail polish artifact *(thick arrows)*. **C:** Ultrasound image corresponding to the area of mammographic concern demonstrating a cluster of oval anechoic masses. The thin walls of the distending acini are evident as thin echogenic lines separating the anechoic components. Epithelial and apocrine-lined cysts are reported histologically. As we have acquired experience, and with our medical audit data to support our approach, we no longer routinely biopsy patients with lesions having these mammographic and ultrasound features. (From Cardeñosa G. *Breast Imaging [The Core Curriculum Series]*. Philadelphia, PA: Lippincott Williams & Wilkins; 2003.)

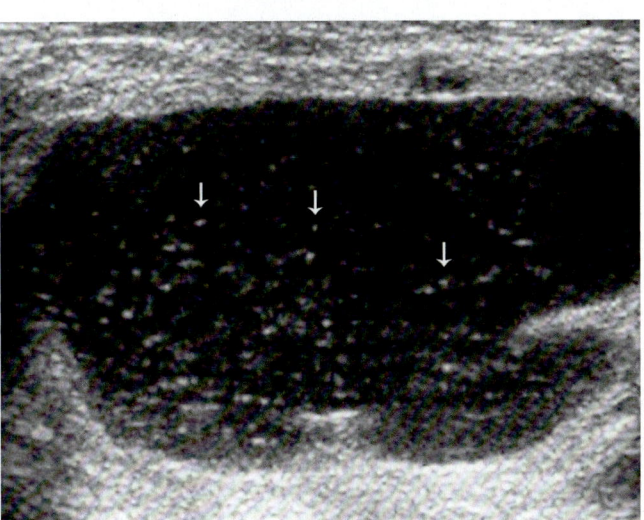

FIG. 4.26 • **Gurgling cyst ("complicated").** Specular echoes (few marked with *arrows*) in otherwise anechoic mass with circumscribed margins and posterior acoustic enhancement. During real-time scanning, the echoes can be seen moving and sometimes swirling in the fluid. Unless the patient is symptomatic, or requests an aspiration, we do not routinely intervene when this feature is seen during real-time scanning. BI-RADS 2: Benign finding. (From Cardeñosa G. *Breast Imaging [The Core Curriculum Series]*. Philadelphia, PA: Lippincott Williams & Wilkins; 2003.)

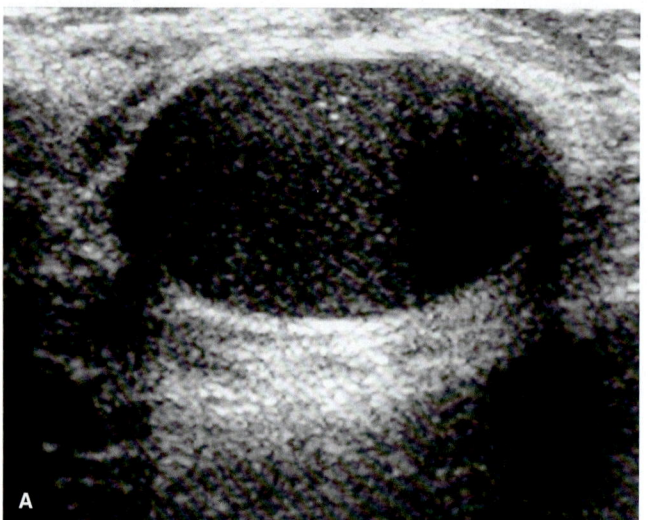 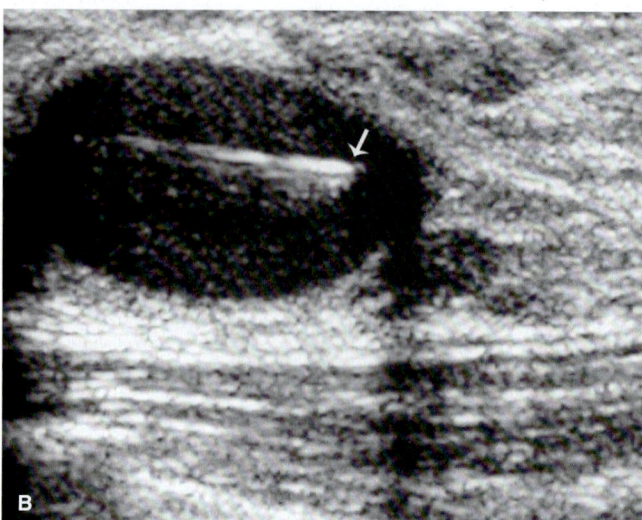

FIG. 4.27 • **Cyst ("complicated"). A:** Oval mass with circumscribed margins, thin-edge shadows, and posterior acoustic enhancement. Internal echoes make distinction from a solid mass difficult. However, when masses with these types of internal echoes (you can almost identify the individual echoes) are seen in the subareolar area, they are commonly cysts. **B:** Needle *(arrow)* in cyst. During the aspiration, the echoes are seen being sucked into the needle along with the fluid. No residual abnormality is seen post aspiration, and thin walls are seen in these patients if a pneumocystography is done following the aspiration. On visual inspection of the fluid, the fluid in these types of cysts appears no different from that in cysts with no internal echoes. Unless we can unequivocally call a mass a cyst, however, we do an aspiration to establish the diagnosis. (From Cardeñosa G. *Breast Imaging [The Core Curriculum Series]*. Philadelphia, PA: Lippincott Williams & Wilkins; 2003.)

or a combination of these. The walls may be irregular, lobulated, and thickened (Fig. 4.29; also see Fig. 11.26). It is important to recognize the benign nature of these collections. Unless an infection is suspected, these should be left alone. Aspiration often leads to re-accumulation of fluid, and rarely, aspiration may lead to the development of draining sinuses that can be difficult to manage (Fig. 4.30; also see Fig. 11.27). Papillomas are commonly imaged as intraductal lesions (Fig. 4.18), particularly if solitary, or as intracystic mass(es) of variable sizes (Figs. 4.31 and 4.32). In some women, they may be solid or predominantly solid with cystic components (Fig. 4.33). Oil cysts and evolving areas of fat necrosis may have stages characterized on ultrasound as a cystic lesion with mural and solid-appearing intracystic nodules (Fig. 4.34; also see Fig. 7.24). Papillary carcinomas presenting centrally as solitary lesions are often characterized as a complex cystic and solid mass (see Chapter 8).

Benign complex cystic masses that are often predominantly solid with cystic components include complex fibroadenomas (Fig. 4.35; also see Fig. 7.62), pseudoangiomatous stromal hyperplasia, and phyllodes tumors. Fat necrosis and posttraumatic changes in the acute setting are often imaged as a hyperechoic mass with cystic components (Fig. 4.36; also see Fig. 7.41C). Malignant lesions presenting as complex cystic and solid masses include invasive ductal carcinomas associated with necrosis (Fig. 4.37), malignant phyllodes, metastatic lesions, and rarely mucinous carcinomas (see Figs. 8.30, 8.33, 8.37, and 8.49) (13).

CHARACTERIZATION OF SOLID MASSES

With a solid mass, features that suggest a benign lesion include oval or ellipsoid shape, gentle bi- or trilobulation, homogeneous hyperechogenicity, and a thin, echogenic pseudocapsule (2,15) (Fig. 4.38). In classifying a mass as likely benign, a combination of features is sought, and, more importantly, no malignant features should be identified. Indeterminate features include isoechogenicity, mild hypoechogenicity, normal or enhancement of sound transmission, and homogeneous or heterogeneous echotexture. In the absence of a malignant feature or a combination of benign features, the mass is considered indeterminate, and biopsy is recommended (15).

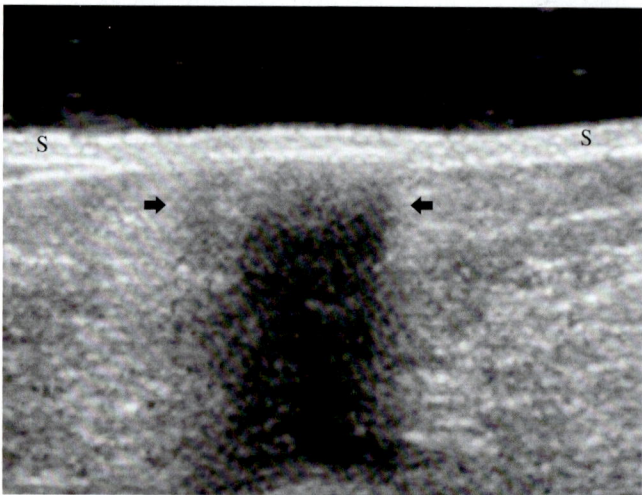

FIG. 4.28 • **Galactocele.** This 28-year-old patient is breast-feeding and presents with a "lump." She thinks it might fluctuate in size. An oval mass with indistinct margins and a heterogeneous echotexture is imaged at the site of concern to the patient. A portion of the mass is nearly isoechoic with surrounding tissue. Another portion of the mass is hypoechoic and associated with an intense shadow. Thick milky fluid is obtained on aspiration. Galactoceles are variable in their presentation. Normal skin *(S)* is seen well since the standoff pad was used to evaluate the patient. Also note the appearance of the tissue: homogeneous and relatively hyperechoic, a common appearance of breast tissue during lactation. (From Cardeñosa G. *Breast Imaging [The Core Curriculum Series]*. Philadelphia, PA: Lippincott Williams & Wilkins; 2003.)

Table 4.3 **COMPLEX CYSTIC AND SOLID MASSES**

Cystic with Solid Elements	Solid with Cystic Features
Postoperative fluid collections	Complex fibroadenomas
Posttraumatic fluid collections (hematoma)	Pseudoangiomatous stromal hyperplasia
Abscess	Fat necrosis
Papilloma (solitary, multiple)	Phyllodes
Oil cyst (fat necrosis)	Invasive ductal carcinoma (necrosis)
Galactoceles	Mucinous carcinoma
Papillary carcinoma (central, solitary)	Metastatic disease

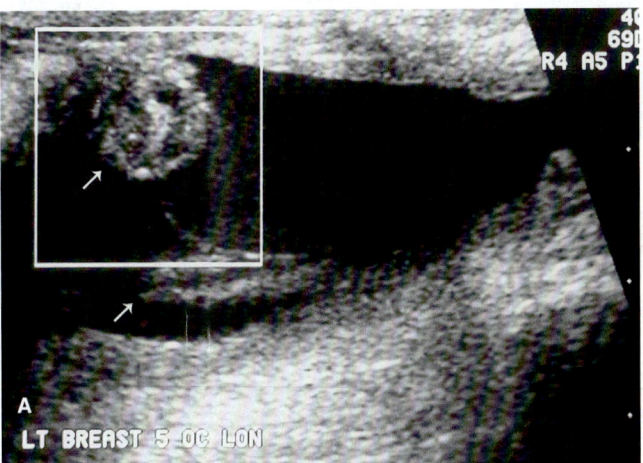

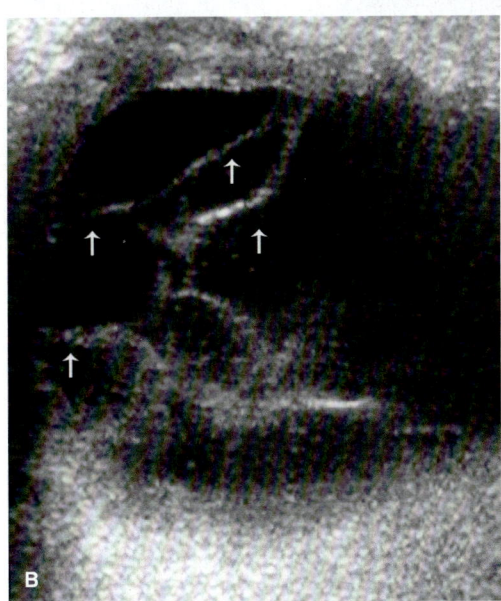

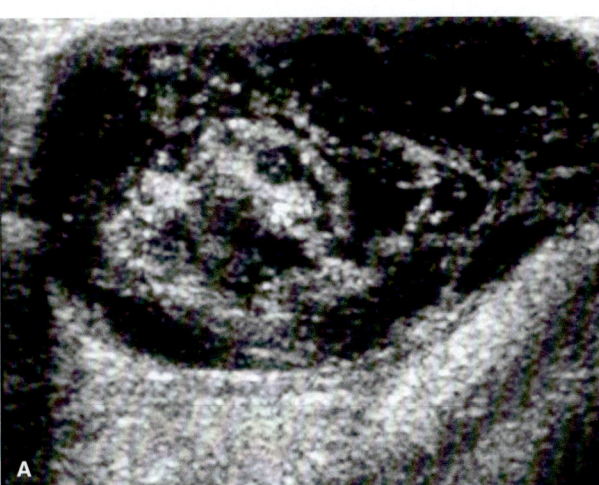

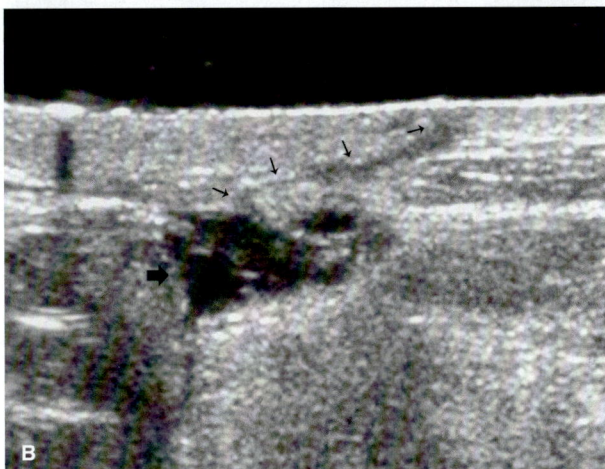

FIG. 4.29 • **Postoperative fluid collections. A:** Cystic mass with mural nodules (arrows) corresponding to lumpectomy site. These nodules simulate intracystic masses; however, if these correlate with the lumpectomy site, and superimposed infection is not suspected, no intervention is warranted. **B:** Complex cystic and solid mass with irregular, thick walls, septations (arrows), and posterior acoustic enhancement at the lumpectomy site. During real-time scanning, the septations are seen shifting in position and "flapping" in the fluid. Unless an infection is suspected clinically, no intervention is warranted in these patients. Aspirations often lead to rapid reaccumulation of fluid, and in some patients, the development of a draining sinus. If left alone, they often slowly resolve spontaneously. (From Cardeñosa G. *Breast Imaging [The Core Curriculum Series]*. Philadelphia, PA: Lippincott Williams & Wilkins; 2003.)

FIG. 4.30 • **Development of a draining sinus in a patient with a postoperative fluid collection. A:** Complex cystic and solid mass at a lumpectomy site. For unclear reasons (superimposed infection was not suspected clinically), the patient was aspirated and the fluid re-accumulated rapidly, prompting a second aspiration, after which the patient describes the development of a slow continuous drainage of fluid. **B:** A complex cystic and solid mass (thick arrow) persists at the lumpectomy site. When pressure is applied to this area, fluid drains just inferior to the nipple. Tract to the skin is evident (thin arrows) on ultrasound. When these develop, they can be difficult to eradicate, often requiring surgical intervention. Unless an infection is suspected clinically, no intervention is warranted in patients with postoperative fluid collections. As in this patient, repeated aspirations often lead to rapid reaccumulation of fluid, and in some patients, the development of a draining sinus. If left alone, postoperative fluid collections often resolve spontaneously. (From Cardeñosa G. *Breast Imaging [The Core Curriculum Series]*. Philadelphia, PA: Lippincott Williams & Wilkins; 2003.)

FIG. 4.31 • **Intracystic papilloma.** Mass detected on screening mammogram (not shown). A complex cystic and solid mass *(arrow)* with circumscribed margins and posterior acoustic enhancement is seen on ultrasound corresponding to the mammographic abnormality. This mass is predominantly cystic with a solid component. A papilloma is diagnosed on excisional biopsy. (From Cardeñosa G. *Breast Imaging [The Core Curriculum Series]*. Philadelphia, PA: Lippincott Williams & Wilkins; 2003.)

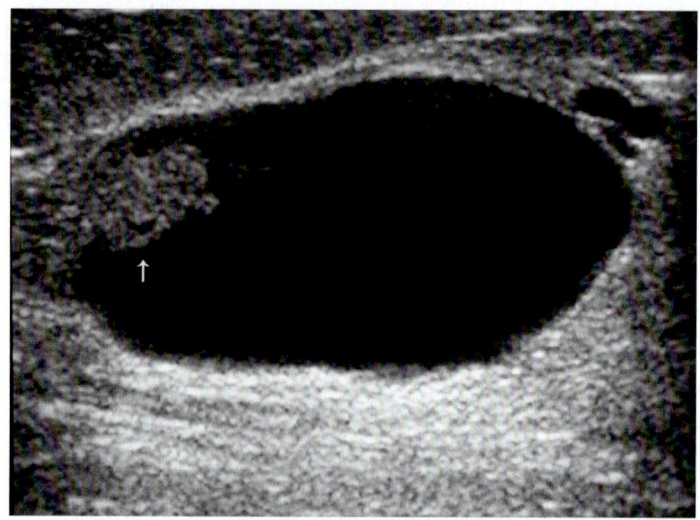

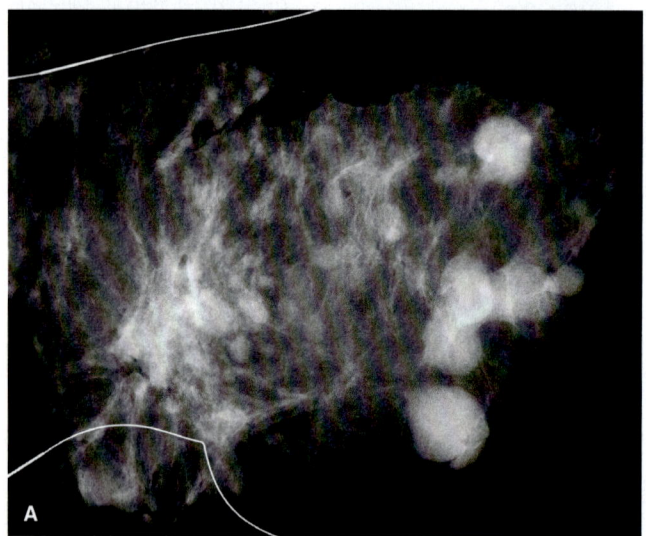

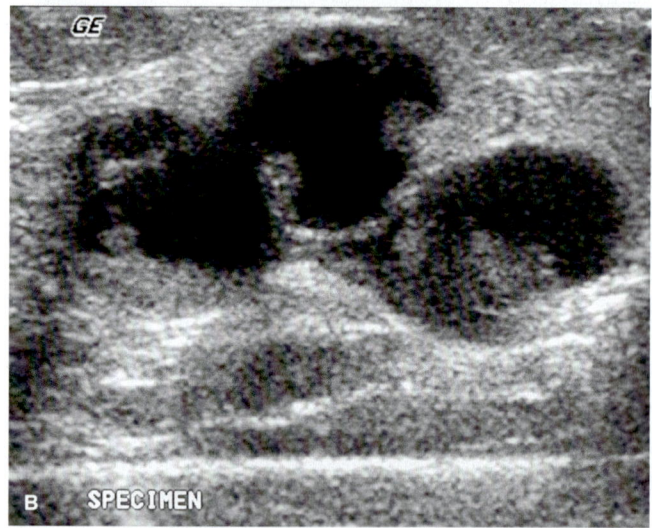

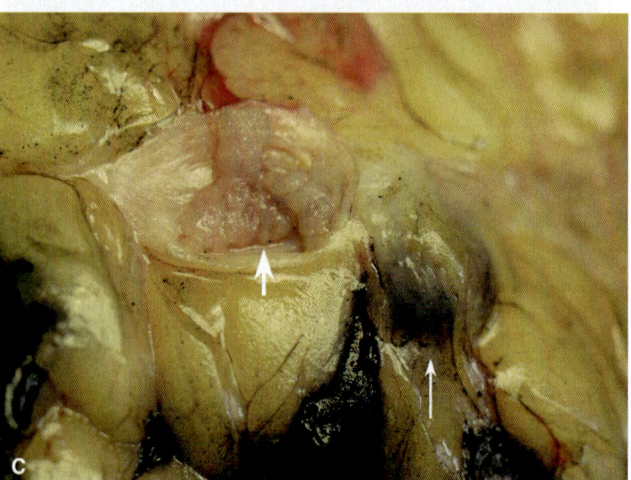

FIG. 4.32 • **Multiple peripheral papillomas, recurrent. A:** Specimen radiograph in a 32-year-old patient with multiple masses of varying sizes and densities; bracketing wires are noted at the ends of the specimen. These masses developed at a prior excisional biopsy site done for peripheral papillomas. **B:** Ultrasound evaluation of the specimen demonstrates multiple complex cystic masses. In this area, three predominantly cystic masses with solid components are imaged. **C:** Correlation between gross pathology and ultrasound images is undertaken. As many of these masses are dissected, fluid is released. In some of these lesions, the fluid is bloody. With sectioning, a complex cystic and solid mass is seen with a partially smooth wall and an irregular solid component *(thick arrow)* adjacent to a "blue domed" cyst *(thin arrow)*. When this second lesion is sectioned, fluid is obtained and an intracystic mural lesion is identified. Multiple peripheral papillomas, some with associated low-grade DCIS, are diagnosed histologically. In our experience, approximately 43% of patients with multiple peripheral papillomas have associated high-risk lesions, including atypical ductal hyperplasia and lobular carcinoma in situ. Synchronous or metachronous low-grade DCIS or low-grade invasive ductal carcinoma is also sometimes diagnosed in patients with multiple peripheral papillomas. (From Cardeñosa G. *Breast Imaging [The Core Curriculum Series]*. Philadelphia, PA: Lippincott Williams & Wilkins; 2003.)

Breast Ultrasound   97

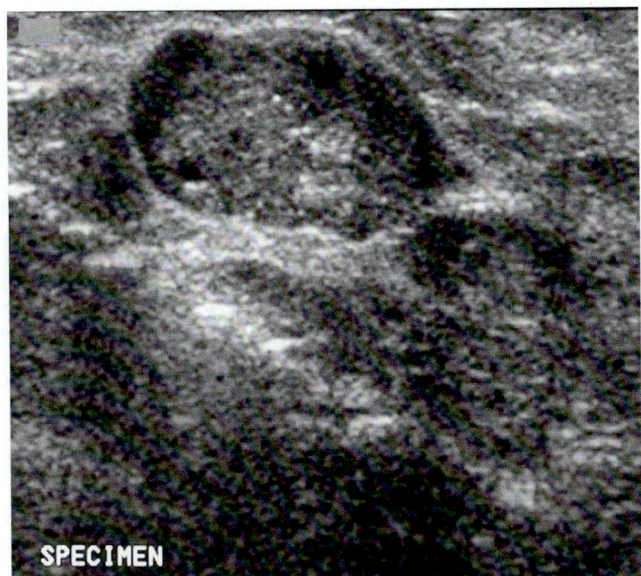

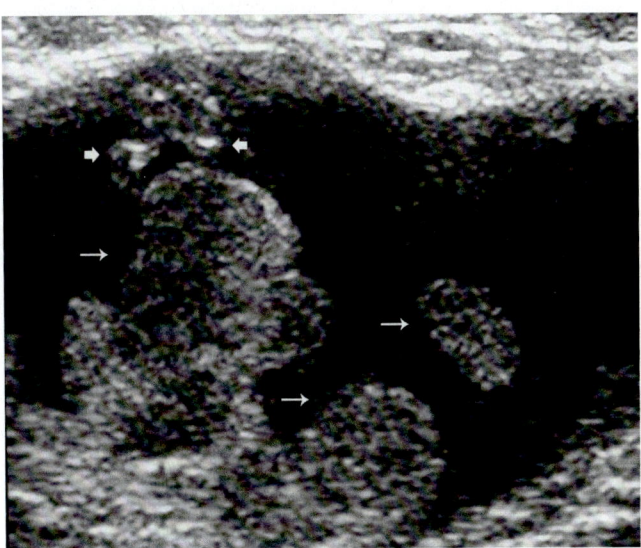

FIG. 4.34 • **Oil cyst.** Same patient as shown in Figure 7.24. Patient presents describing a "lump" in the left breast. A complex cystic and solid mass with multiple solid-appearing intracystic nodules *(arrows)* is imaged corresponding to the palpable finding. The diagnosis in this patient is made mammographically. An oil cyst is imaged at the site of concern to the patient. Although the ultrasound appearance is concerning, the diagnosis is made based on the presence of a lucent mass on the mammogram. No intervention is indicated. The patient needs to be reassured of the benign etiology of the "lump," and the mammography report needs to be definitive. BI-RADS 2: Benign finding, negative. (From Cardeñosa G. *Breast Imaging [The Core Curriculum Series]*. Philadelphia, PA: Lippincott Williams & Wilkins; 2003.)

not included in this list). Rarely, invasive ductal carcinoma, invasive lobular carcinoma, ductal carcinoma in situ (DCIS), lymphoma (see Fig. 9.29D), metastatic lesions, angiosarcoma and liposarcomas present as hyperechoic or predominantly hyperechoic masses (16–18). Hyperechogenicity may be more common among patients with invasive lobular and mucinous carcinomas. Linda et al. (17) reported that

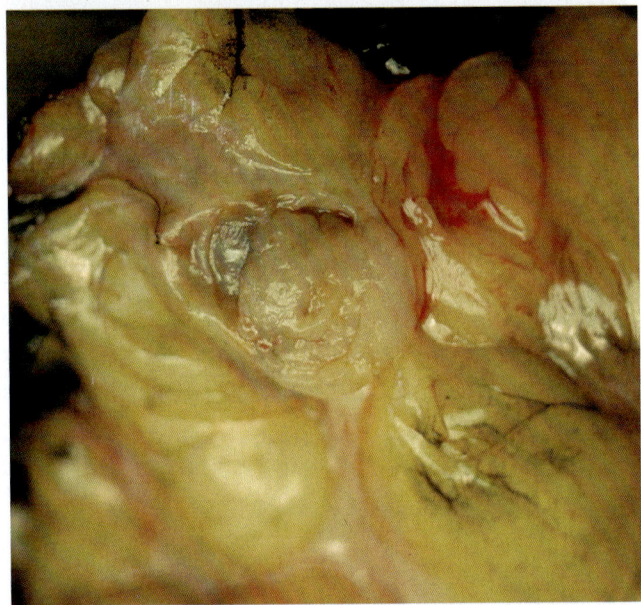

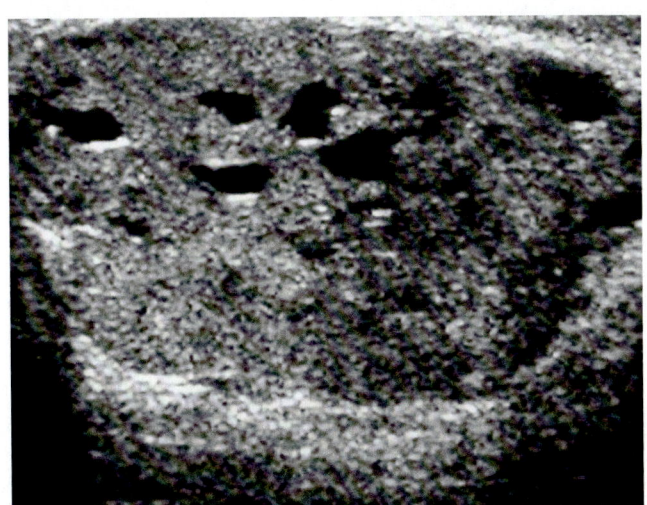

FIG. 4.33 • **Multiple peripheral papillomas.** Same picture as shown in Fig. 4.32. **A:** A complex cystic and solid mass is seen in another portion of the specimen. This is a predominantly solid mass with small cystic spaces and posterior acoustic enhancement. **B:** Specimen with lesion sectioned. Although the papilloma almost completely fills the cyst, only a small portion of it is actually attached to the wall of the cyst. Multiple peripheral papillomas, some with associated low-grade DCIS, are diagnosed histologically. In our experience, approximately 43% of patients with multiple peripheral papillomas have associated high-risk lesions, including atypical ductal hyperplasia and lobular carcinoma in situ. Synchronous or metachronous low-grade DCIS or low-grade invasive ductal carcinoma is also sometimes diagnosed in patients with multiple peripheral papillomas. (From Cardeñosa G. *Breast Imaging [The Core Curriculum Series]*. Philadelphia, PA: Lippincott Williams & Wilkins; 2003.)

FIG. 4.35 • **Complex fibroadenoma.** A complex cystic mass that is predominantly solid with associated cystic spaces and posterior acoustic enhancement is imaged. Complex fibroadenomas are fibroadenomas with superimposed fibrocystic changes, including cysts measuring at least 3 mm in size (see Chapter 7). (From Cardeñosa G. *Breast Imaging [The Core Curriculum Series]*. Philadelphia, PA: Lippincott Williams & Wilkins; 2003.)

In classifying a lesion as hyperechoic and likely benign, the lesion should be homogeneously hyperechoic relative to subcutaneous fat. Lipomas, angiolipomas, hemangiomas, focal fibrosis, hematomas, abscess, galactoceles, and fat necrosis are the more common benign lesions that can present with masses that are hyperechoic (fibroadenolipomas are not usually homogeneously hyperechoic and therefore

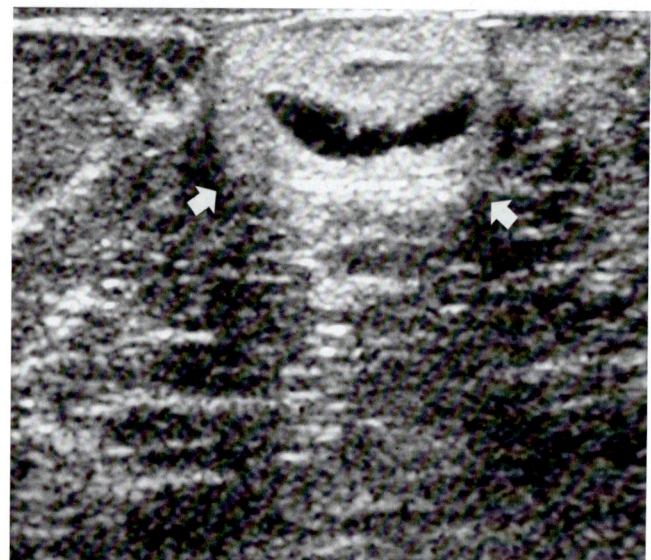

FIG. 4.36 • **Posttraumatic changes.** Oval, hyperechoic mass *(arrows)* with an internal oval cystic space and focal posterior acoustic enhancement is imaged at a prior site of trauma. In our experience, this is a common appearance for acute fat necrosis (posttraumatic). (From Cardeñosa G. *Breast Imaging [The Core Curriculum Series]*. Philadelphia, PA: Lippincott Williams & Wilkins; 2003.)

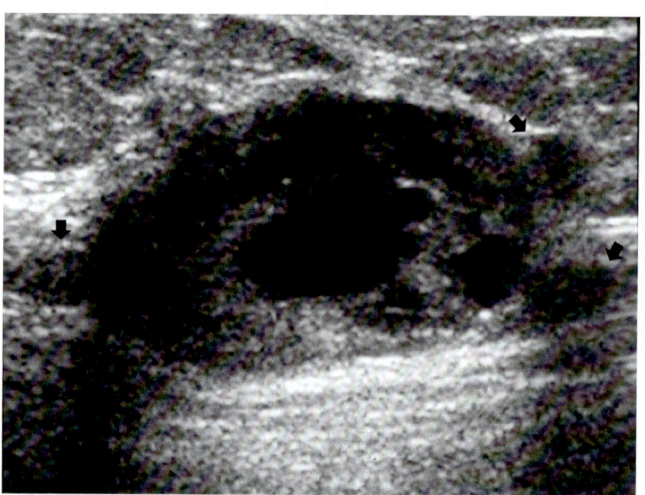

FIG. 4.37 • **Invasive ductal carcinoma, not otherwise specified, with areas of necrosis.** Solid oval mass with macrolobulated margins, cystic spaces, nodular projections *(arrows)*, and posterior acoustic enhancement is imaged corresponding to a clinical and mammographically apparent mass in a 49-year-old patient. Ultrasound-guided biopsy is done to establish the diagnosis. (From Cardeñosa G. *Breast Imaging [The Core Curriculum Series]*. Philadelphia, PA: Lippincott Williams & Wilkins; 2003.)

among 4,511 consecutive ultrasound-guided core needle biopsies, 25 (0.6%) were for hyperechoic masses, with 9 (0.4%) of these being diagnosed as malignant. It is important to emphasize the need for careful evaluation of these lesions and the strict application of diagnostic criteria before presuming a benign etiology: the mass needs to be homogeneously hyperechoic relative to subcutaneous fat, with circumscribed margins and parallel orientation.

Malignant masses may demonstrate one or more of the following features, including spiculation, angular margins, microlobulation,

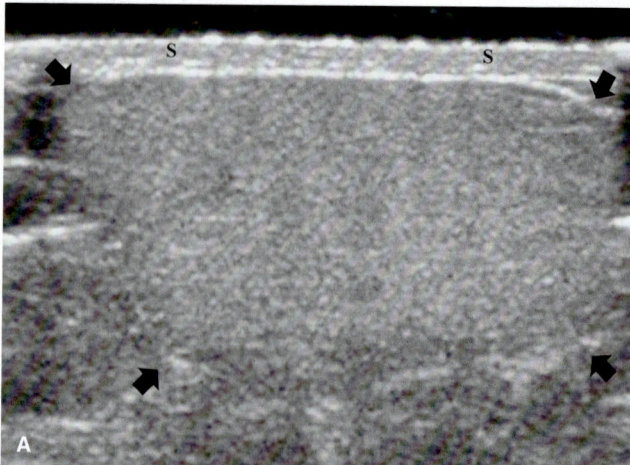

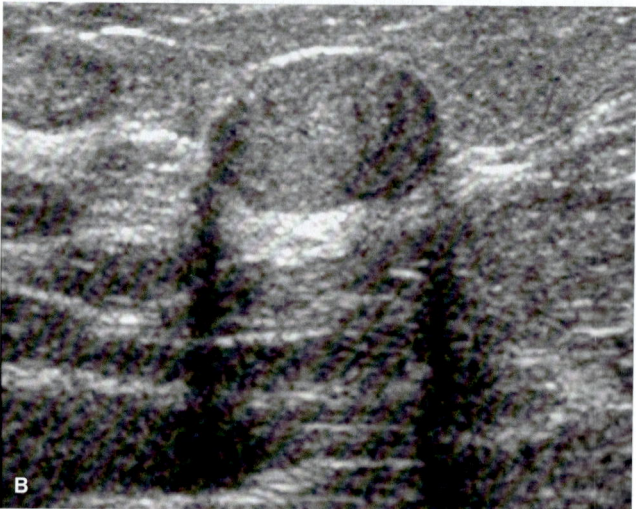

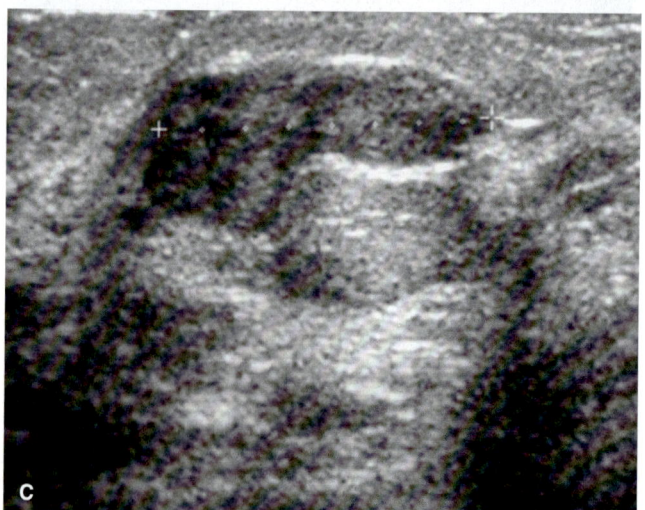

FIG. 4.38 • **Masses with benign features on ultrasound. A:** Homogeneously hyperechoic mass *(arrows)* in a patient with a lipoma mammographically. Homogeneously hyperechoic masses with no malignant features are usually benign. Normal skin *(s)* is noted. **B:** Oval mass with circumscribed margins, thin-edge shadows, and posterior acoustic enhancement. Fibroadenoma. **C:** Oval mass with gentle macrolobulation. Fibroadenoma. (From Cardeñosa G. *Breast Imaging [The Core Curriculum Series]*. Philadelphia, PA: Lippincott Williams & Wilkins; 2003.)

shadowing, marked hypoechogenicity (Fig. 4.39), calcifications (Fig. 4.40), duct extension, and branch pattern (2,15). Malignant masses usually demonstrate several of these features in addition to commonly having an echogenic rim and being taller than they are wide (vertically oriented). Duct extension and branch pattern are determined during real-time scanning (15). Duct extension refers to tubular extension of the lesion toward the nipple, presumably within a duct (Figs. 4.40E and 4.41). A branch pattern refers to a duct-like structure extending from the mass away from the nipple (Fig. 4.42). Posterior acoustic enhancement may be seen with malignant masses. These masses are typically round (e.g., expansile, "blow up") and, in our experience, are often poorly differentiated, rapidly growing invasive ductal carcinomas not otherwise specified; some of these are triple-negative tumors (estrogen and progesterone receptor-negative and HER-2-neu negative). Mucinous and papillary carcinomas are other malignant lesions associated with posterior acoustic

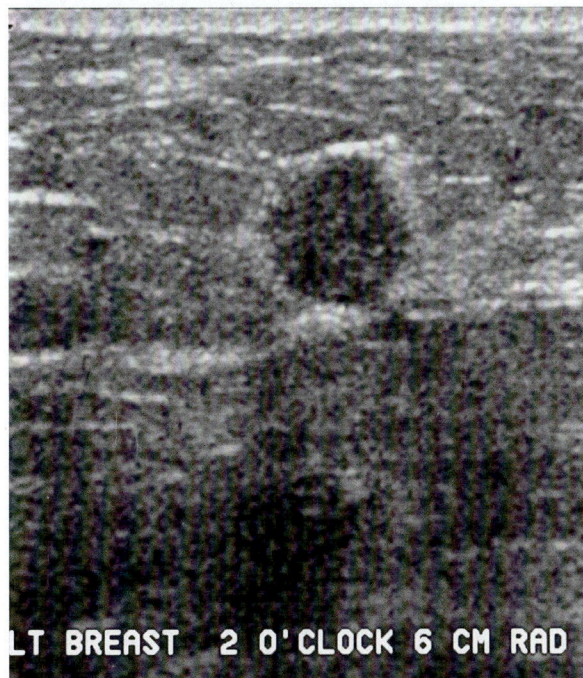

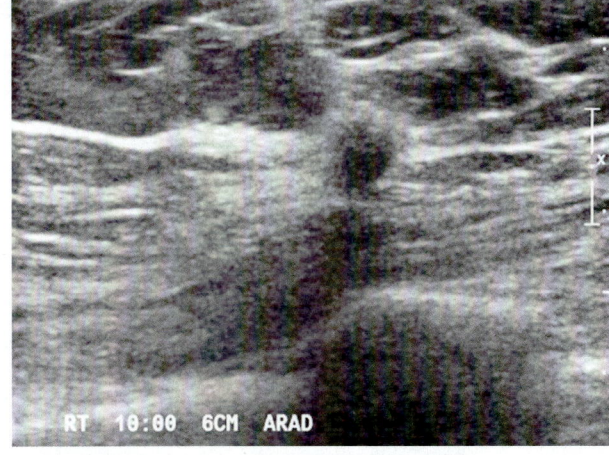

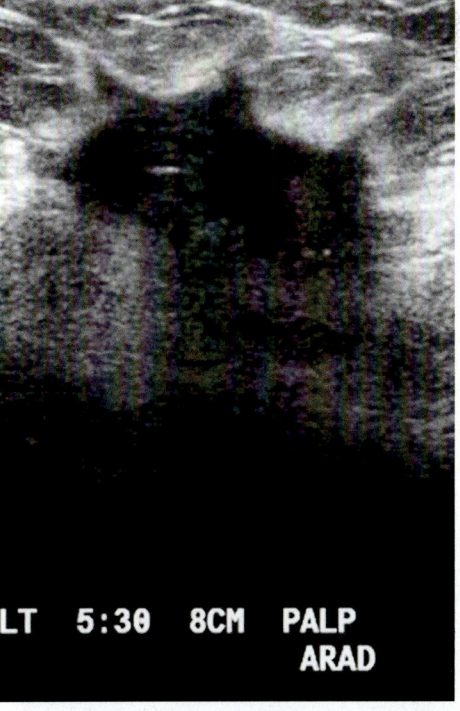

FIG. 4.39 • **Masses with malignant features on ultrasound.** **A:** Round mass with indistinct and spiculated margins and a thickened echogenic rim. Thin spicules can be seen extending from the mass into the echogenic rim. **B:** Round mass with indistinct margins disrupting tissue planes is imaged at the 10 o'clock, 6 cm from the right nipple corresponding to the mammographic abnormality (see Figs. 2.40 and 3.11 for screening and spot compression views on this patient, respectively). Only the anti-radial *(ARAD)* projection is shown. **C:** An irregular mass with spiculated and angular margins and shadowing is imaged at 5:30 o'clock, 8 cm from the left nipple. Only the anti-radial *(ARAD)* projection is shown here (see Figs. 2.49 and 3.9 for screening and spot compression views on this patient, respectively). **D:** An irregular, vertically oriented mass with angular and spiculated margins as well as a thick echogenic rim and some shadowing is imaged at 7:30 o'clock, 7 cm from the left nipple. Only the sagittal ("long") scan plane is shown here. Also, although this is a screen-detected abnormality, as the ultrasound is done, it is determined that the mass is palpable *(PALP)*; the images are annotated accordingly, and the physical findings are described in our consultation report. Many screen-detected abnormalities are palpable, particularly when you have the information from the mammogram and know exactly where to examine (you have placed eyeballs at the tips of your fingers). See Figures 2.46, 3.7, and 5.21 screening, spot compression, and MRI images on this patient, respectively. **E:** Irregular mass with spiculated and angular margins, an echogenic rim, and shadowing is imaged at 10 o'clock, 1 cm from the nipple (only sagittal *LONG* plane shown). Although this is a screen-detected abnormality, at the time of the ultrasound this mass is palpable *(PALP)*. See Figures 2.50 and 3.10A for screening and spot compression views on this patient, respectively.

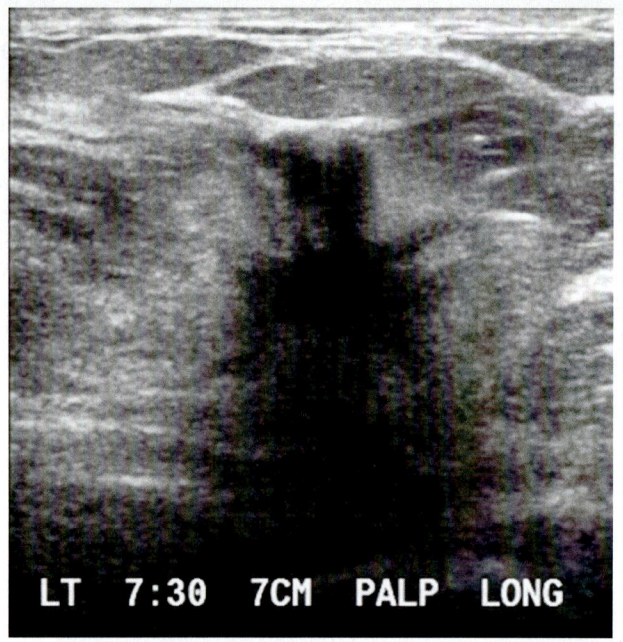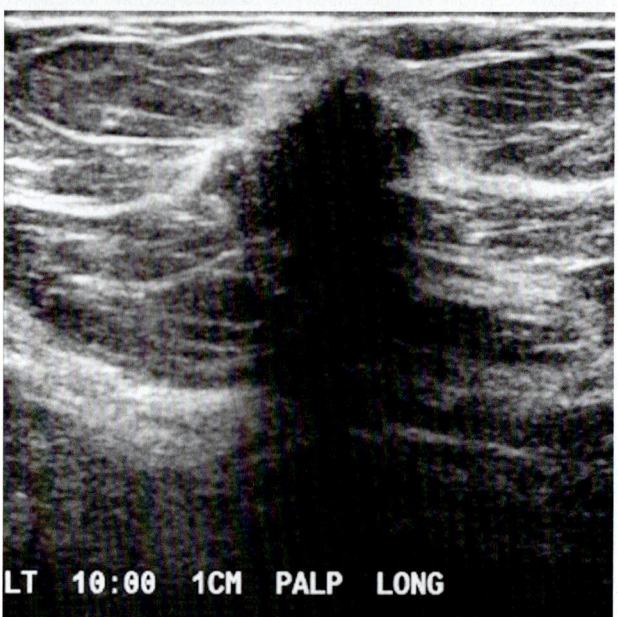

FIG. 4.39 • (continued)

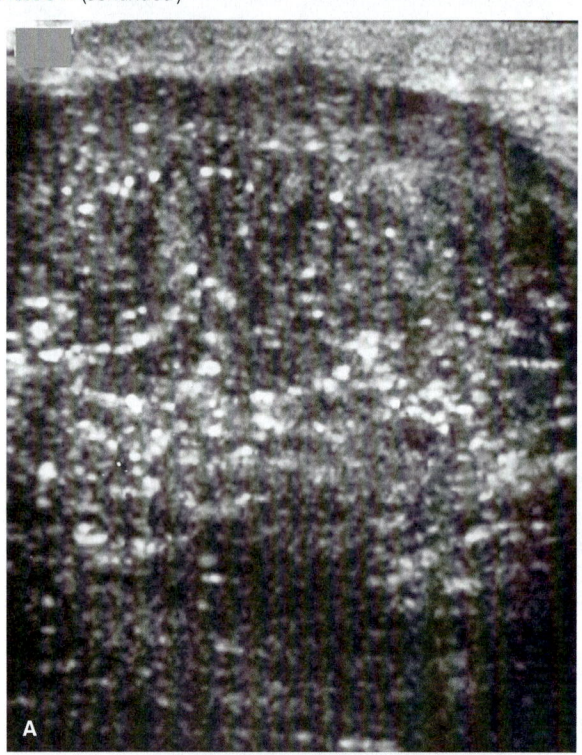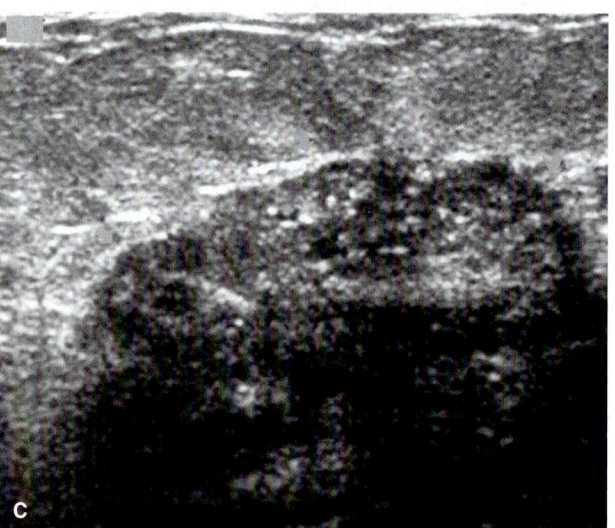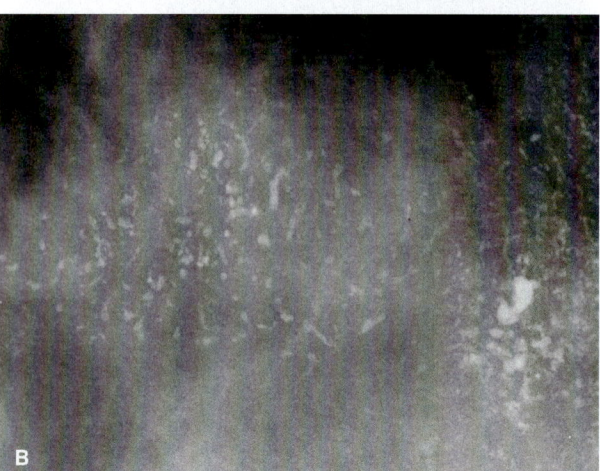

FIG. 4.40 • **Malignant masses with calcifications, invasive ductal carcinomas with extensive DCIS. A:** Round mass studded with high specular echoes corresponding to calcifications seen mammographically (mammogram not shown). These are not associated with shadowing. **B:** Different patient. Area of pleomorphic calcifications, including linear forms, is consistent with a DCIS characterized by central necrosis with associated calcifications. **C:** Mass with high specular echoes related to the calcifications seen mammographically. Although shadowing is noted, this is likely unrelated to the calcifications. **D:** Scan through a different plane demonstrates a dilated ductal structure *(arrows)* with associated luminal calcifications. **E:** Different patient. A round mass with posterior acoustic enhancement is imaged *(long, thick arrow)*. Extension of tumor into a dilated ductal structure *(thin arrows)* is noted associated with luminal calcifications *(short, thick arrows)*. The duct tapers distal to the mass. (From Cardeñosa G. Breast Imaging [The Core Curriculum Series]. Philadelphia, PA: Lippincott Williams & Wilkins; 2003.)

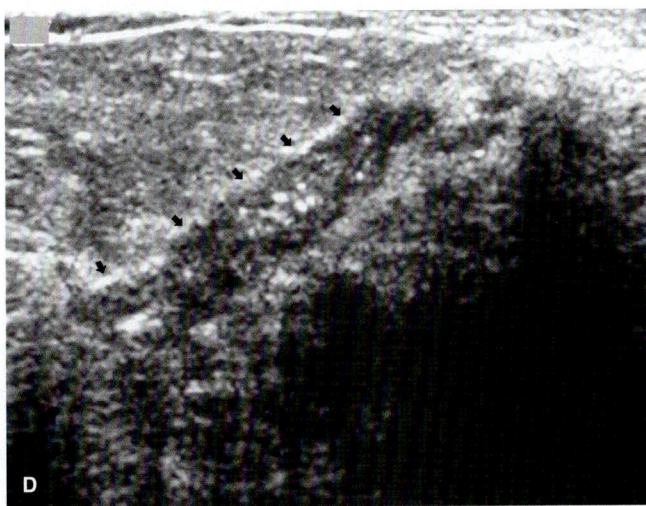
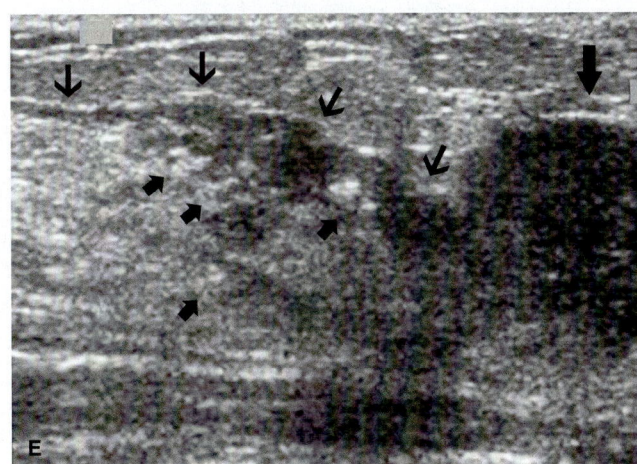

FIG. 4.40 • (Continued)

enhancement (see Figs. 8.26 through 8.31 and 8.33 through 8.38). As mentioned previously, most malignant masses demonstrate more than one feature suggestive of a malignant process; however, if only one is seen, a biopsy is usually done. Additionally, as discussed in Chapter 8, when a malignancy is suspected on the basis of clinical, mammographic, and ultrasound findings, we scan the ipsilateral axilla. In patients with potentially abnormal lymph nodes, imaging-guided sampling of the lymph node is done at the time the mass in the breast is sampled.

If on the basis of mammographic and ultrasound findings a mass is thought to be likely benign, options discussed with the patient include ultrasound and clinical follow-up in 6 months, imaging-guided biopsy, or excisional biopsy. Depending on the physical attributes of the mass, imaging features, patient history, and input, we will make a specific recommendation from among these three choices. It is critical, however, that before a 6-month follow-up recommendation is made, the lesion be scrutinized carefully for any malignant features (Fig. 4.43). If at least one malignant feature is present, a biopsy needs to be done.

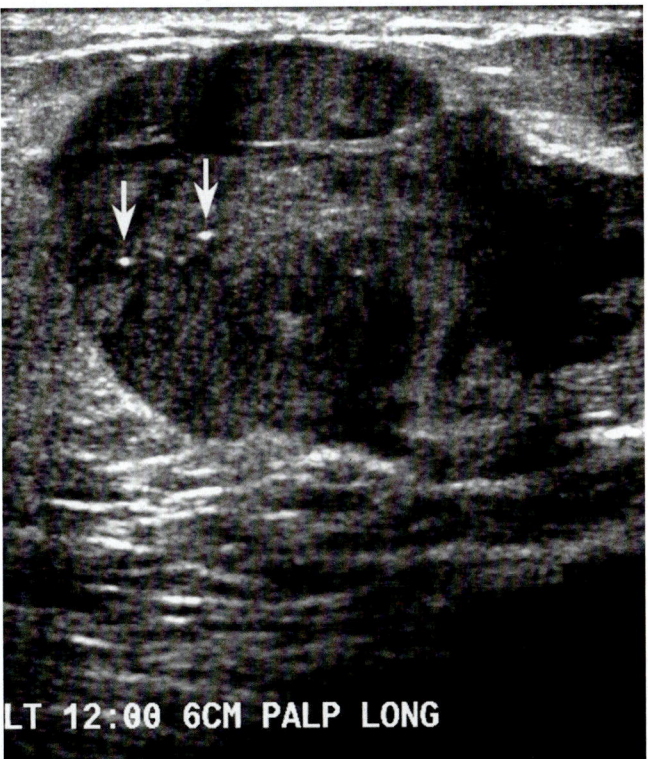
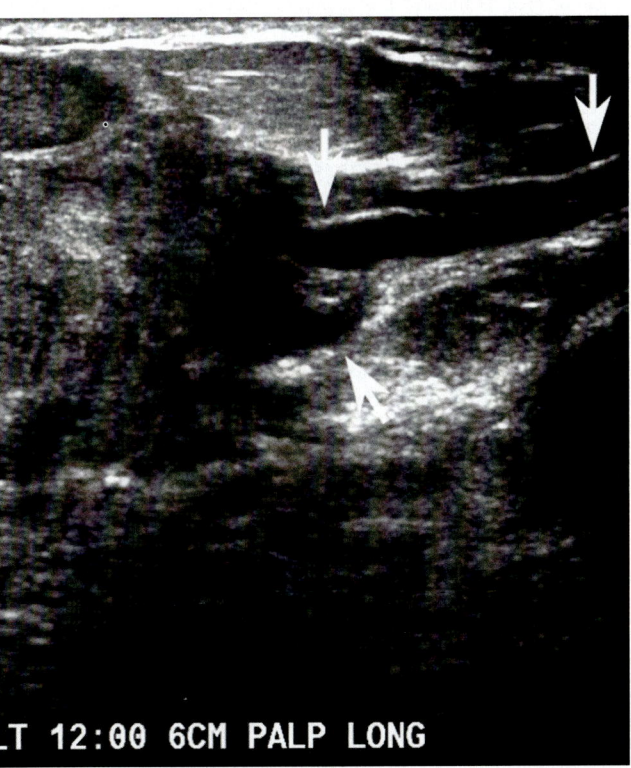

FIG. 4.41 • **Duct extension and posterior acoustic enhancement. A:** Round mass with circumscribed and indistinct margins, calcifications (arrows), and posterior acoustic enhancement. Enhancement is associated with benign masses; however, it can be seen with a variety of malignant lesions. In our experience, it is common with poorly differentiated, rapidly growing invasive ductal carcinomas not otherwise specified, particularly those with necrosis as well as mucinous and papillary carcinomas. **B:** Ductal structures (arrows) are imaged extending from the mass toward the nipple. Invasive ductal carcinoma, not otherwise specified, high nuclear grade is diagnosed on an ultrasound-guided biopsy.

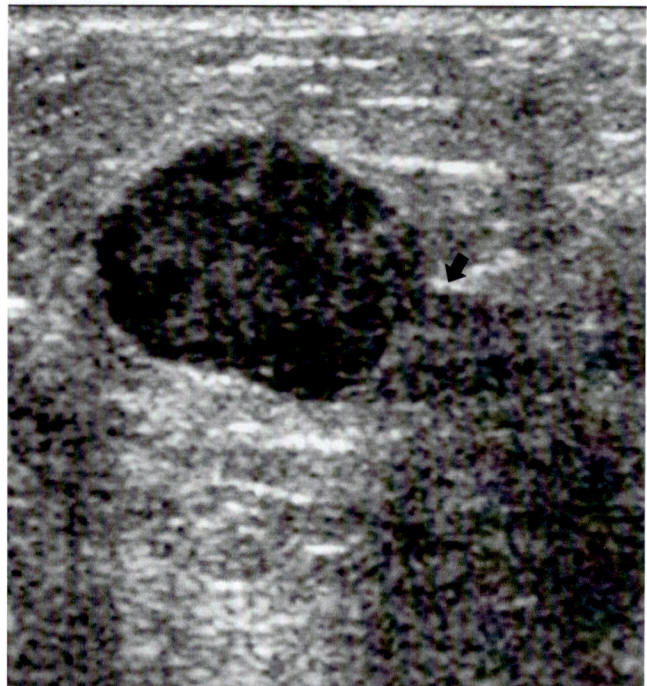

FIG. 4.42 • **Duct branching and posterior acoustic enhancement.** Mass with circumscribed margins, posterior acoustic enhancement, and extension of tumor *(arrow)* into a dilated ductal structure coursing away from the nipple. Posterior acoustic enhancement is commonly associated with benign lesions; however, it is also seen with malignant lesions, including poorly differentiated invasive ductal carcinomas, particularly those with necrosis as well as mucinous and papillary carcinomas. Invasive ductal carcinoma is diagnosed on the ultrasound-guided biopsy. (From Cardeñosa G. *Breast Imaging [The Core Curriculum Series]*. Philadelphia, PA: Lippincott Williams & Wilkins; 2003.)

EVALUATION OF NONSPECIFIC MAMMOGRAPHIC FINDINGS AND POTENTIAL AREAS OF TISSUE EXCLUSION

Breast ultrasound is well suited for the evaluation of mammographically detected masses, developing densities (Fig. 4.44A), and asymmetric tissue (Fig. 4.44B; also see Fig. 3.12). With ultrasound, cysts can be diagnosed with a high degree of accuracy. Solid masses can be separated into those likely to be benign or malignant, and developing densities or asymmetric tissue can be characterized as fibrous breast tissue, a fibrous ridge, or likely to be malignant in etiology.

Breast ultrasound is also useful in imaging areas that may be difficult to evaluate on mammography (see Figs. 3.1 and 3.2). Even when using the spot compression paddle, the margins of masses deep in the breast, close to the chest wall, or in the axilla may be difficult to image mammographically; the mass may roll out of the field of view as compression is applied. Superior, medial, axillary, and far lateral tissue may be excluded from mammographic images. With ultrasound, these areas are readily amenable to evaluation and imaging-guided biopsy procedures.

EVALUATION OF CLINICAL FINDINGS

As described in Chapter 3, ultrasound is our starting point in patients under the age of 30, and those who are pregnant, or lactating, regardless of age, presenting with a focal sign or symptom that may be related to an underlying breast cancer (Fig. 4.45). In all other patients with a focal finding, bilateral mammography and a spot tangential view of the site of concern are done before taking the patient to ultrasound. Ultrasound is not done if the area of concern is an obviously benign finding (e.g., mixed density mass, coarse dystrophic calcification, etc.) or completely fatty tissue mammographically. If tissue is imaged at the site of clinical concern (Fig. 4.46; also see Fig. 8.15) or the lesion is possibly excluded from the view (e.g., metallic BB used to mark site of lesion is at the edge of the mammographic images or not seen in one or both routine views), an ultrasound is always done. During the ultrasound,

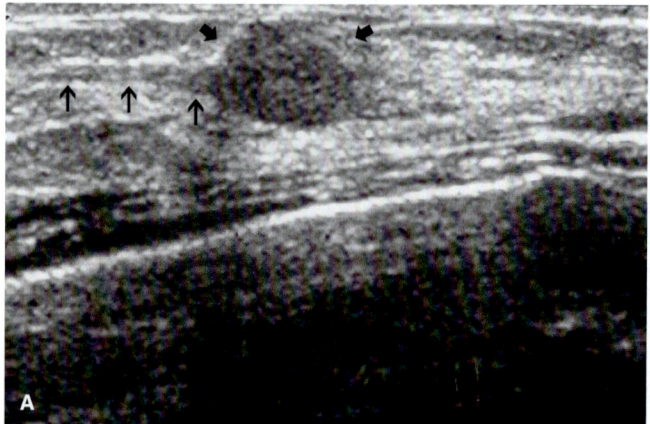

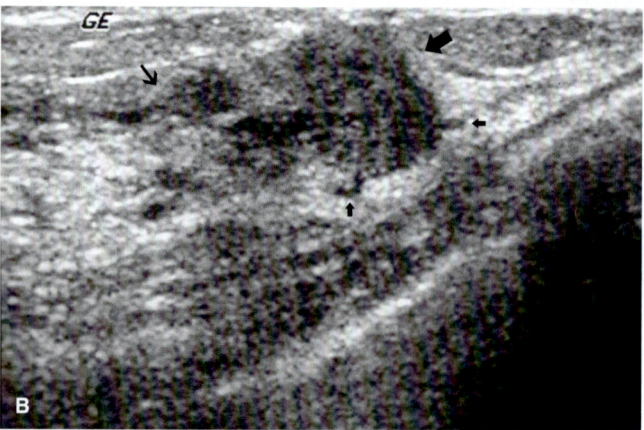

FIG. 4.43 • **Invasive ductal carcinomas, initially classified as probably benign with short interval follow-up recommended.** **A:** Oval isoechoic mass *(thick arrows)* in a 44-year-old patient. This mass is described as a probable fibroadenoma, and a 6-month follow-up ultrasound is recommended. Retrospectively, duct branching *(thin arrows)*, a malignant feature, is seen on the ultrasound images. Please see Chapter 13 for a discussion on probably benign lesions. This is a concept described for mammographic findings. Studies defining probable benign features on ultrasound or MRI and providing the longitudinal data in support of short interval follow-ups have not been done for these modalities. **B:** Six months later. Mass *(thick arrow)* is now larger, irregular with indistinct and spiculated margins. *(thin arrows)* **C:** Different patient. Oval mass with posterior acoustic enhancement is imaged in a 36-year-old patient. This is described as a probable fibroadenoma, and a 6-month follow-up ultrasound is recommended. Retrospectively, duct branching *(arrow)* and indistinct margins, malignant features, are seen on the ultrasound images. **D:** Six months later. The mass is larger and the echotexture is now heterogeneous with ductal branching, angular margins, and posterior acoustic enhancement. It is important to evaluate masses carefully for any malignant feature. Even if one malignant feature is seen, a biopsy should be done. (From Cardeñosa G. *Breast Imaging [The Core Curriculum Series]*. Philadelphia, PA: Lippincott Williams & Wilkins; 2003.)

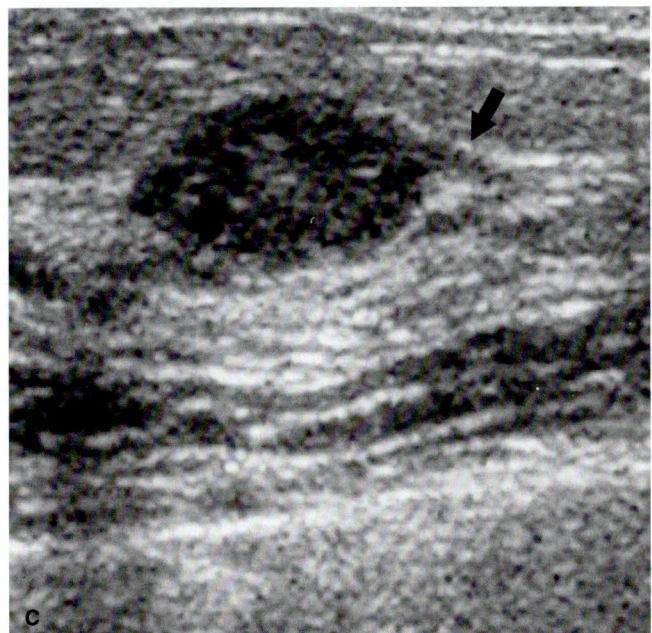
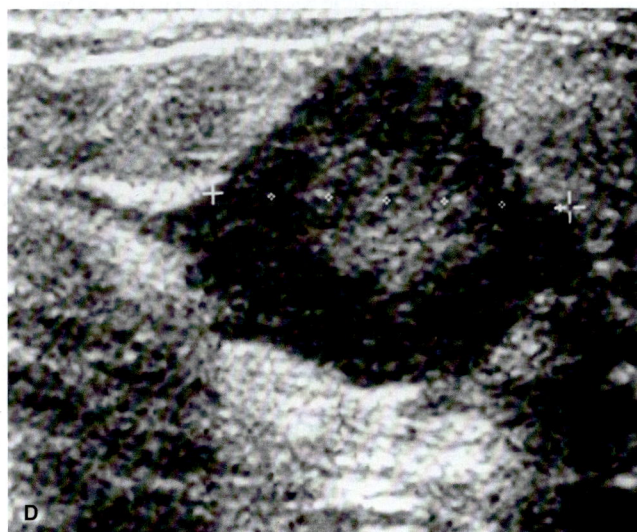

FIG. 4.43 • *(Continued)*

the patient is asked to pinpoint the area of concern, the area and quadrant are palpated, and correlation is made with any imaging findings. If on palpation the finding is not impressive, and the imaging studies are negative, the patient is reassured that what she is feeling is benign breast tissue. Sometimes, showing the patient the appearance of the area of concern and comparing it to a rib in cross section as a reference for what a mass would look like is helpful and reassures the patient. If a cyst is imaged corresponding to the "lump," the patient is reassured that cysts are benign, fluctuate in size relative to the menstrual cycle, are associated with cyclical tenderness, are common, and will not turn into cancer. If the mass demonstrates malignant features, a biopsy is indicated and done.

Cooper ligaments and associated fibrous tissue can be palpated as a discrete mass, particularly if outlined by fat lobules. If on imaging the palpable mass is correlated directly with a fibrous ridge (Fig. 4.47) or fibrocystic area, biopsy is averted. Given the current state of technology, women should not undergo "blind" aspirations or excisional biopsies without an imaging evaluation. Ultrasound provides useful

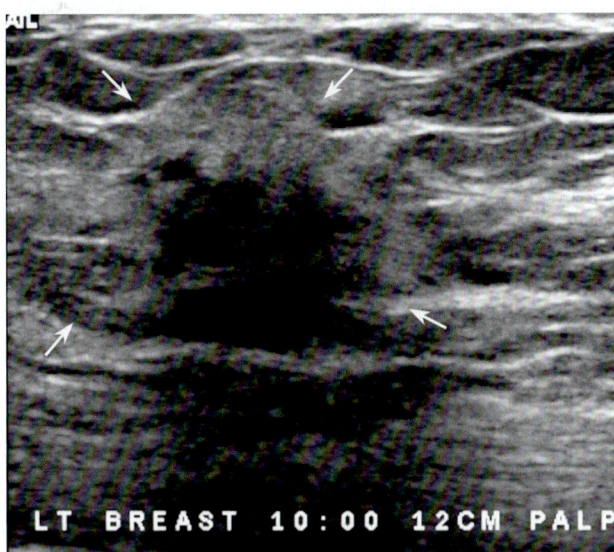
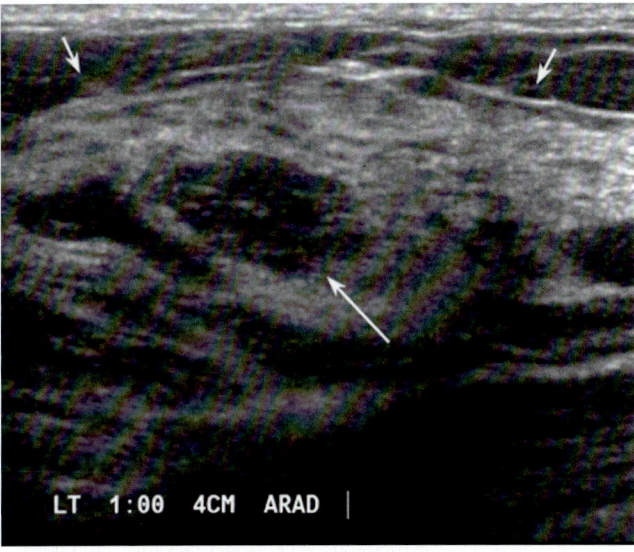

FIG. 4.44 • Evaluation of nonspecific mammographic findings. **A:** Ultrasound. An irregular area of hypoechogenicity is imaged surrounded by a markedly thickened and irregular echogenic rim that crosses and disrupts tissue planes. Shadowing is also apparent *(arrows)*. A hard mass is palpated as this area is scanned. The ultrasound is done to evaluate an area of developing parenchymal asymmetry in the upper inner quadrant of the left breast; tissue persists on spot compression views (not shown), but no mass is identified mammographically. Invasive lobular carcinoma is diagnosed on an ultrasound-guided biopsy. **B:** Ultrasound. A dense fibrous ridge *(small arrows)* within which fatty lobulation *(long arrow)* that elongates as the transducer is rotated is identified corresponding to an area of parenchymal asymmetry noted mammographically. Note thin echogenic lines in the fatty lobule; these are not usually seen in masses. At the time of the ultrasound, no correlate is identified on palpation. This is normal tissue and requires no additional evaluation or short interval follow-up.

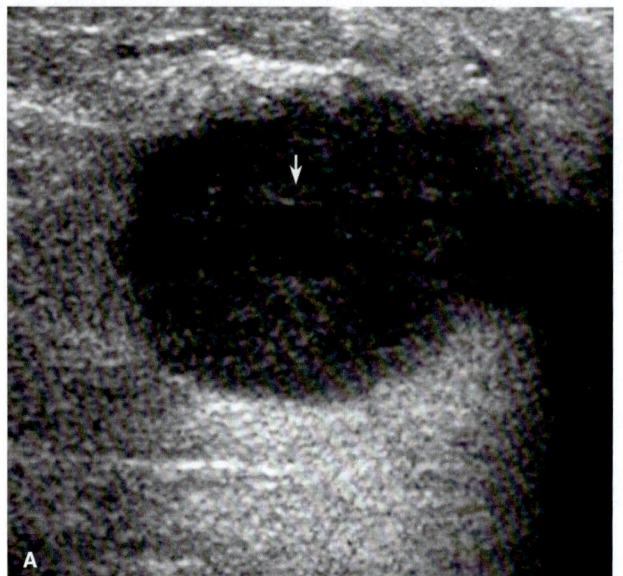

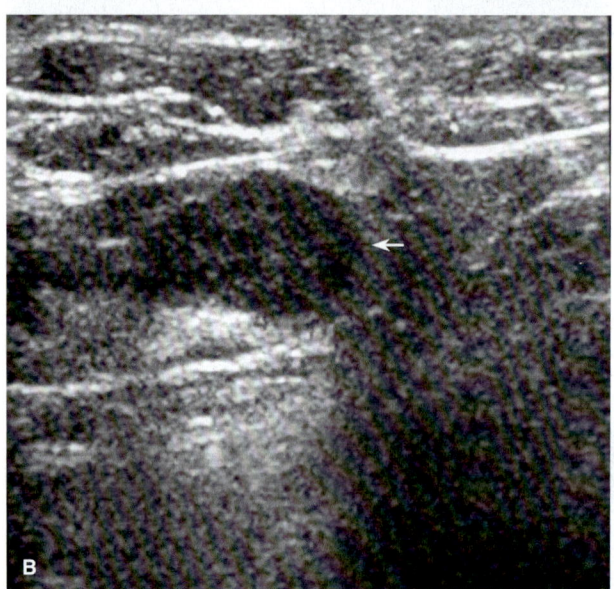

FIG. 4.45 • **Evaluation of patients under the age of 30 or those who are pregnant or lactating. A:** This 29-year-old patient presents describing a "lump" in the upper outer quadrant of her right breast. On physical examination, the upper outer quadrant of the right breast is hard and fixed (particularly when compared with upper outer quadrant tissue on the left). Ultrasound is our starting point. An irregular, lobulated mass with a nearly anechoic central area *(arrow)* and posterior acoustic enhancement is imaged corresponding to the area of clinical concern. The consistency of this mass and surrounding tissue on palpation, coupled with the ultrasound features, suggests a rapidly growing, poorly differentiated invasive ductal carcinoma. **B:** Several hypoechoic masses (only one is shown) are also seen in the right axilla associated with posterior acoustic enhancement *(arrow)*. The echogenic hilum one expects to see with lymph nodes is not seen in these masses. Their appearance suggests metastatic disease. Our starting point with symptomatic women under the age of 30 or, if pregnant or lactating regardless of age, is an ultrasound focused to the area of concern. As in this patient, if the clinical and ultrasound findings suggest the presence of breast cancer, a full, bilateral mammogram (not shown here) is obtained. This helps in evaluating remaining tissue and the contralateral breast. In this patient, an ultrasound-guided core biopsy of the breast mass and a fine needle aspiration of one of the axillary lymph nodes confirm the suspected diagnoses of a poorly differentiated invasive ductal carcinoma and metastatic disease to the axilla.

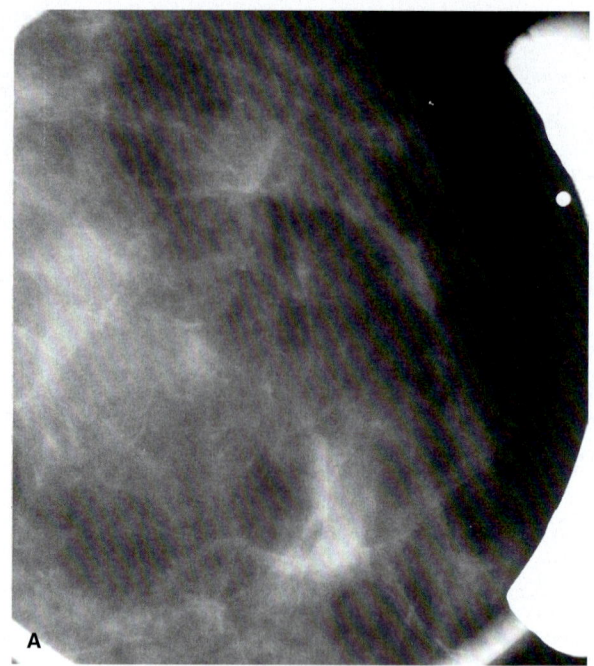

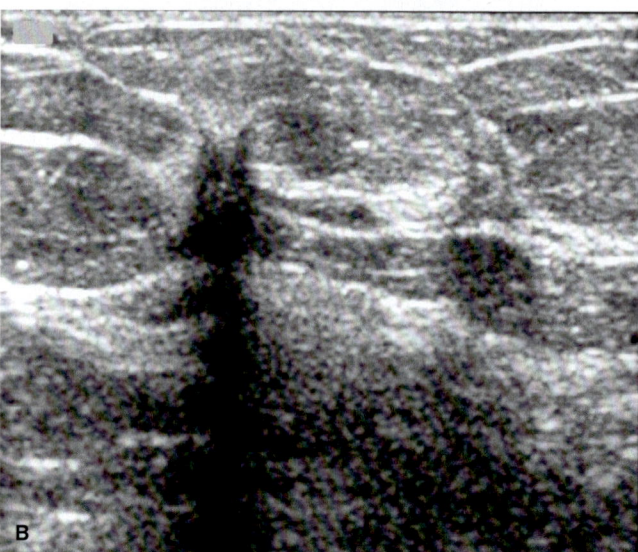

FIG. 4.46 • **Use of ultrasound in evaluating patients with palpable findings and a normal mammogram. A:** Spot tangential view done in a 62-year-old patient who presents describing a "lump" in the left breast. Metallic BB denotes the site of the palpable finding. Normal glandular tissue is imaged on this view as well as on the standard projections (CC and MLO views not shown). The area of concern is anterior such that it is unlikely to have been excluded from the field of view. **B:** On physical examination, a hard mass with little mobility is palpated at the site of concern to the patient. An irregular, vertically oriented mass with indistinct and spiculated margins, an echogenic rim, and shadowing is imaged corresponding to the palpable finding. Clinical, mammographic, and ultrasound findings are factored in making recommendations to patients. In this patient, the mammogram is normal; however, the clinical and correlative ultrasound findings are highly suggestive of a malignancy, and biopsy is indicated. Ultrasound is indicated in patients who present with focal signs and symptoms that may reflect a malignancy, and glandular tissue is imaged at the site of the clinical concern on the mammogram.

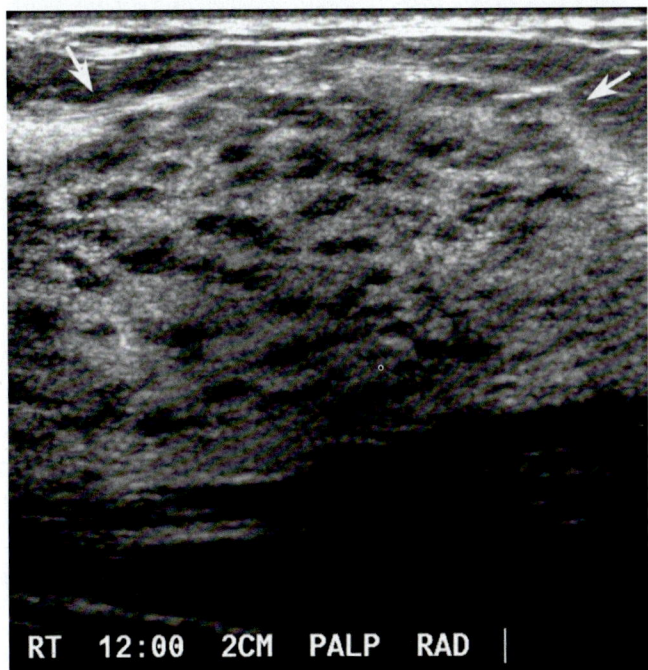 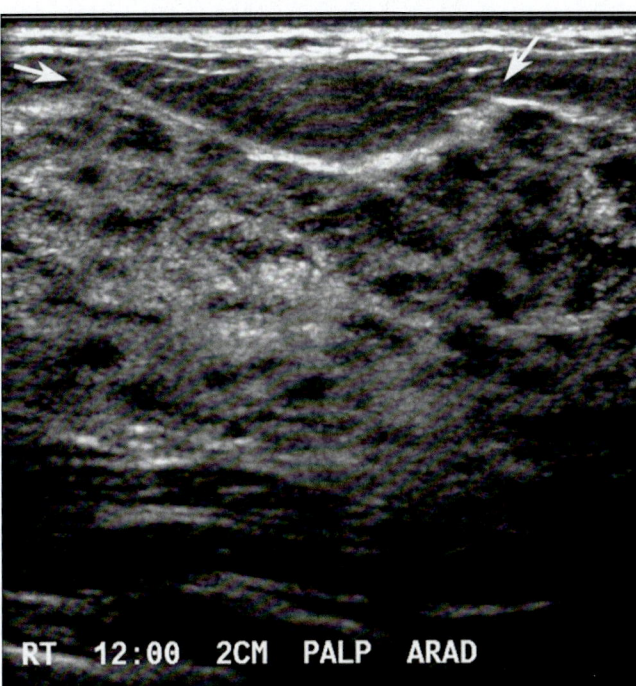

FIG. 4.47 • **Use of ultrasound in evaluating palpable findings. A:** Ultrasound in a 25-year-old woman presenting with a "lump" in her right breast. On physical examination, a discrete mobile mass is palpated at 12 o'clock, 2 cm from the right nipple. When the transducer is placed at the site of the palpable finding, a fibrous ridge of tissue (arrows) is imaged rising to approximate the dermis. This is characterized by the dense fibrous tissue, with a myriad of 2- to 4-mm sized oval and round areas of hypoechogenicity likely representing normal glandular elements (e.g., terminal duct lobular units). Fatty lobulation is noted subcutaneously on either side of the ridge. **B:** As the transducer is moved slightly away from the palpable finding, a second ridge of fibrous tissue is partially imaged with a fat lobule (arrows) separating the two ridges of tissue. When these structures are imaged corresponding to discrete palpable findings, the patient can be reassured that what she feels is normal fibrous tissue made discretely palpable by surrounding fatty tissue.

information, including the identification of unsuspected lesions within or adjacent to the palpable abnormality or mural abnormalities in an otherwise seemingly normal cyst. In many patients with palpable findings, ultrasound reliably identifies a benign etiology, including fibrous ridges, fatty lobulation, and cystic changes. When benign changes are correlated directly with the clinical finding, attempts at blind aspiration and excisional biopsies can be averted (19–21).

It is important to emphasize that clinical and imaging findings need to be considered as equally important pieces of information. Overreliance (or exclusion) of one or the other modality is no longer appropriate. In some patients, the physical examination may be unimpressive or normal in the presence of suspicious imaging findings (e.g., screen-detected malignancies). Conversely, in other patients, the physical examination is highly suggestive of a malignancy, and yet the mammogram is normal (Fig. 4.46). All information available needs to be factored into the decision-making process.

EVALUATION OF MRI-DETECTED FINDINGS

MRI improves sensitivity in the evaluation and diagnosis of breast cancer; however, the specificity for MRI-detected abnormalities ranges from 40% to 80% (22,23). Consequently, tissue diagnosis is indicated in many patients with MRI-detected abnormalities. Ultrasound is done in an effort to identify, further characterize, and, if possible, biopsy the MRI-detected abnormality; some refer to this as a "second-look" ultrasound (even though a first look ultrasound may not have been done). If the lesion is identified with confidence on ultrasound, an ultrasound-guided biopsy can be done to establish a diagnosis. In some patients, the ultrasound features may suggest a benign process, such that a short interval follow-up with ultrasound can be done. Although the lack of a correlate may suggest a benign process for mass lesions, an MRI-guided biopsy should be done in these patients, particularly if the MRI finding is indeterminate or suspicious.

The overall reported frequency with which MRI-detected lesions are seen on ultrasound ranges from 23% to 89% (22–27). Lesion type is the single most important predictor for finding an ultrasound correlate for MRI-detected lesions: the likelihood is higher for masses compared with non–mass-like enhancement (Fig. 4.48; also see Fig. 8.25). Additional predictors for identifying an ultrasound correlate include the size of the lesion, likelihood of malignancy, and type of malignancy (22). Meissnitzer et al. (24) reported 50%, 56%, 72.5%, and 86% detectability for masses less than 5 mm, 6 to 10 mm, 11 to 15 mm, and greater than 15 mm in size, respectively. Detectability rates of 13%, 25%, and 42% were reported by these authors for non–mass-like enhancement measuring 6 to 10 mm, 11 to 15 mm, and more than 15 mm, respectively (24). Malignant lesions are more likely to be identified on ultrasound, and invasive ductal carcinoma is more likely to be identified than invasive lobular carcinoma or DCIS. It is important to emphasize, however, that a suspicious finding on MRI should be biopsied regardless of the ability to detect an ultrasound correlate.

Establishing concordance between MRI and ultrasound findings may be a challenge. Optimal ultrasound equipment and meticulous technique are essential. Differences in the positioning of patients (prone for MRI vs. supine, oblique, or lateral decubitus for US) between these modalities can make exact correlation a significant problem, particularly in patients with larger, more mobile breasts. Lesion type, size, shape, approximate location, and, if present, relationship to

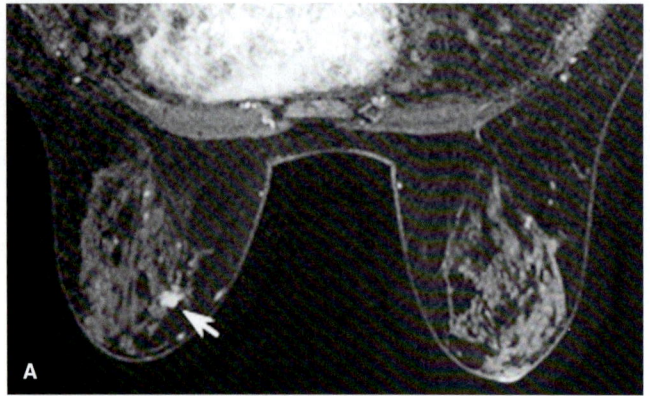
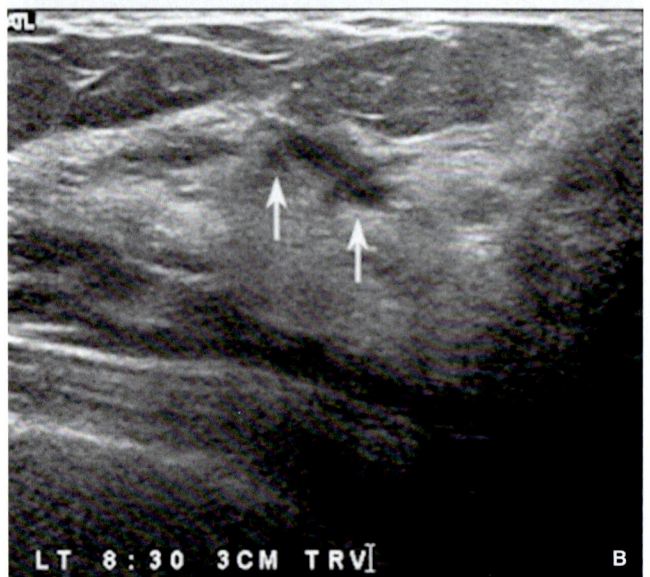
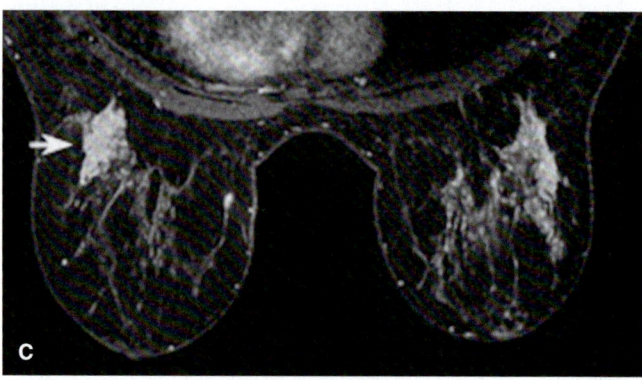

FIG. 4.48 • **Ultrasound evaluation of lesions detected on MRI. A:** MRI T1-weighted axial image post contrast. A homogeneously enhancing mass *(arrow)* with irregular margins and medium-to-rapid wash-in and plateau-type delayed kinetic curve is detected on this screening MRI in a high-risk 44-year-old patient. **B:** Ultrasound. On the basis of location, size, and shape of the enhancing mass on MRI, a targeted ultrasound is done. An irregular mass *(arrow)* with angular and spiculated margins is imaged in the lower inner quadrant of the left breast corresponding to the expected location of the mass seen with MRI. An invasive ductal carcinoma, high nuclear grade, is described on the core following ultrasound-guided biopsy. **C:** MRI, axial T1-weighted image post contrast demonstrates an area of non–mass-like enhancement *(arrow)* posterolaterally in the left breast. Normal tissue is imaged on ultrasound at the expected location of the MRI finding. An ultrasound correlate may not be readily apparent, particularly in patients with non–mass-like enhancement on MRI. In this patient, DCIS is diagnosed on an MRI-guided needle biopsy of this area. If no US correlate is for a suspicious finding on MRI, a biopsy using MRI guidance is indicated. Likewise, if there is any question with respect to the correlation between MRI and ultrasound findings, the biopsy should be done using MRI guidance.

potential landmarks (e.g., cysts) may be helpful. If concerns remain regarding the correlation of US and MRI findings, biopsy should be done using MRI guidance. Imaging–pathology concordance for a biopsy done using ultrasound guidance, for a presumed ultrasound correlate of an MRI-detected lesion, needs to be established on the basis of the ultrasound and MRI findings (not the ultrasound finding alone). Meissnitzer et al. (24) reported that for 80 benign concordant results on presumed US correlates for MRI-detected lesions, the US finding did not correlate with the MRI lesion in 10 patients, 5 of which had a malignancy when the biopsy was repeated with MRI guidance. In an effort to overcome some of the challenges posed by establishing US/MRI and the correlation/reliability of pathology results, some authors have suggested obtaining a limited MRI study following ultrasound-guided biopsy and clip placement (26,28). A single unenhanced T1-weighted nonfat-suppressed pulse sequence can be done following clip placement to verify the correlation between the ultrasound-detected/biopsied lesion and the original MRI-detected abnormality (echo time can be decreased to magnify the resulting metallic artifact from the clip. This sequence takes <5 minutes to complete) (26,28).

INFLAMMATORY PROCESSES: MASTITIS VERSUS ABSCESS

In women with an inflammatory process, ultrasound is useful in distinguishing those with mastitis from those with an abscess that may require drainage. Clinically, these patients present describing pain, redness, increased temperature to the breast (sometimes described as "fever" in the breast), enlargement of the involved breast, and sometimes a "lump." On visual inspection, the involved breast may be larger than the contralateral breast, localized or diffuse erythema, and peau d'orange changes may be apparent as well as skin changes that include oozing, peeling, thinning (or less commonly thickening) or hyperpigmentation in some patients. On physical examination, tenderness is elicited even with gentle compression, a temperature difference is usually appreciated (place one hand on each breast to assess the difference), a mass that is tender may be palpated in the breast, and enlarged tender axillary lymph nodes may also be noted. In some patients, particularly those with a subareolar abscess, fistulas with purulent drainage may be apparent. Rarely, patients with inflammatory process are relatively symptom-free.

Mastitis produces diffuse changes in the appearance of breast tissue on mammography and ultrasound (Fig. 4.49; also see Figs. 9.8 and 9.9). The echogenicity of the tissue is increased, resulting in disruption of normal soft tissue planes. Increased visualization of vascular structures as round or tubular structures (can be confirmed as vessels with Doppler) in the echogenic tissue reflects the hyperemia associated with the ongoing inflammatory process. Skin thickening with dilated subcutaneous lymphatics may be apparent (Fig. 4.49; also see Figs. 9.8 and 9.9). In patients with granulomatous mastitis, tubular areas of hyperechogenicity are intermingled with hypoechoic areas and shadowing (Fig. 4.50; also see Fig. 9.10). If you have any questions regarding the "normal" echogenicity of the individual patient's

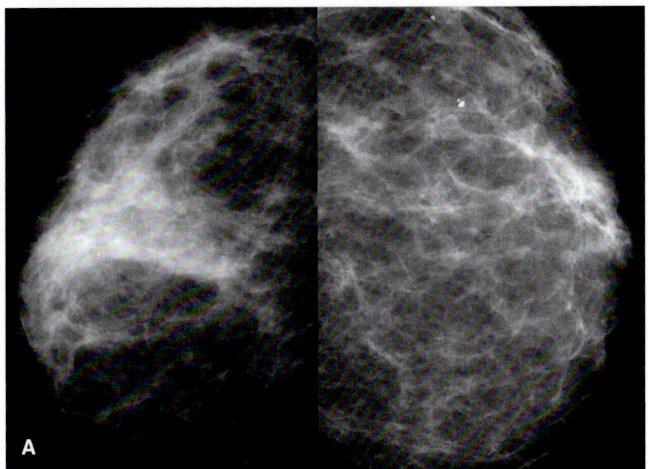

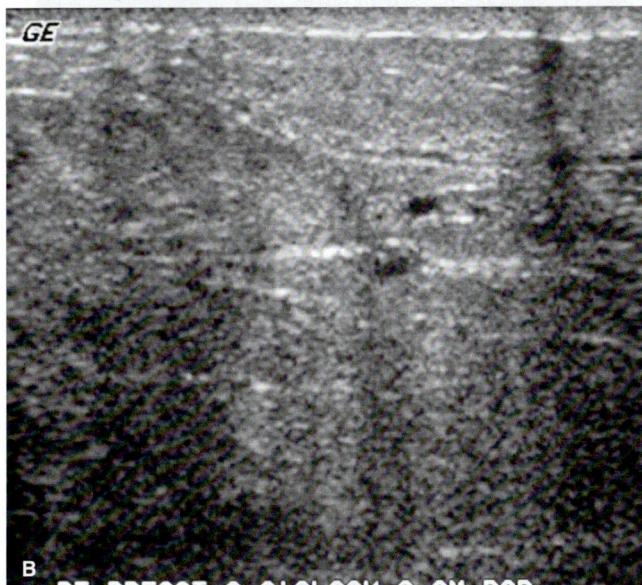

FIG. 4.49 • **Mastitis. A:** Right and left CC views in a patient presenting with the rapid onset of tenderness diffusely involving the right breast associated with redness and swelling. The density of the breast parenchyma is increased on the right. This may be partially related to suboptimal compression because of the discomfort experienced by the patient as compression is applied on the right. **B:** Ultrasound. The echogenicity of the tissue is increased with disruption of normal soft tissue planes. Thin tubular and round anechoic structures reflect hyperemic changes. No skin thickening or dilated subdermal lymphatics are noted. Symptoms and findings resolve completely after a 10-day course of antibiotics.

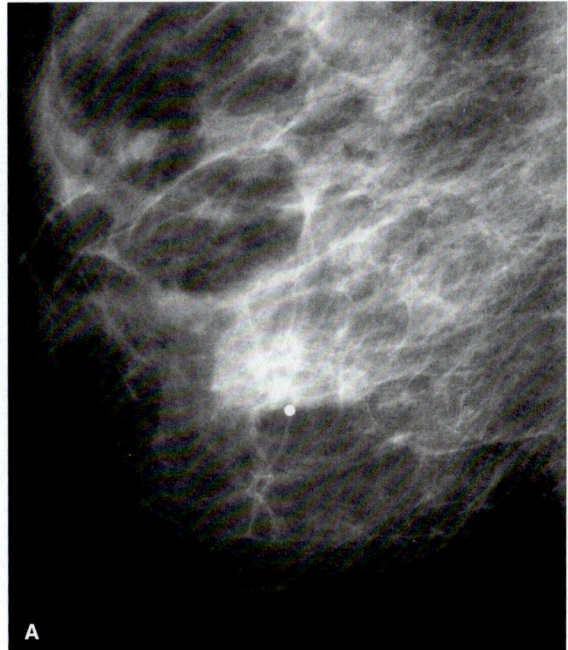

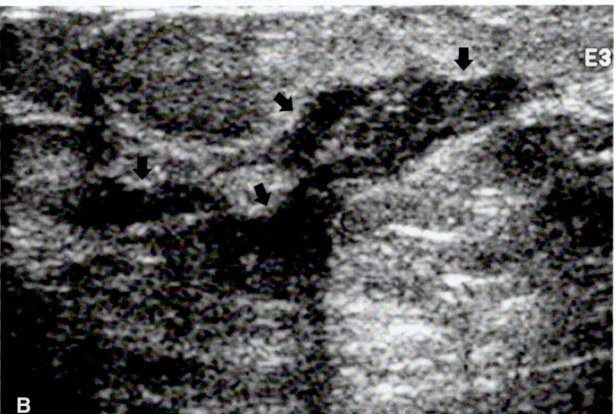

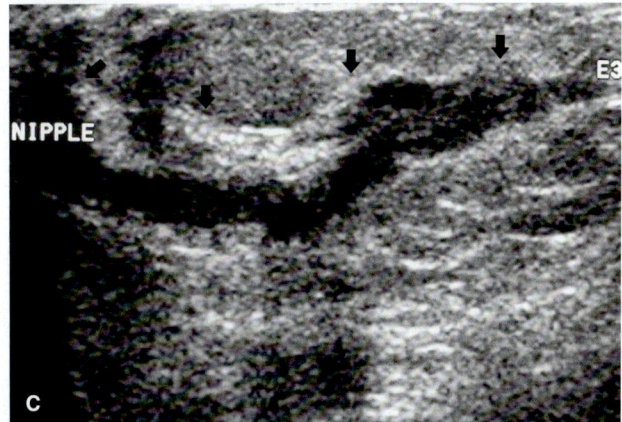

FIG. 4.50 • **Granulomatous mastitis. A:** Right MLO view photographically coned to the lower portion of the image in a patient who presents describing a tender "lump" in the! right breast. Parenchymal asymmetry and increased density is noted at this site of the metallic BB used to denote the location of the "lump" described by the patient. **B:** Ultrasound. An irregular tubular structure *(arrows)* is imaged at the site of the palpable finding; this extends into the subareolar area. **C:** Ultrasound. Portions of the tubular structure closest to the nipple are surrounded by echogenic tissue (see Chapter 9). (From Cardeñosa G. *Breast Imaging [The Core Curriculum Series]*. Philadelphia, PA: Lippincott Williams & Wilkins; 2003.)

tissue, scan in an area not involved by the inflammatory process or the contralateral breast for comparison. In patients with more localized findings, you can see a fairly abrupt change between normal and inflamed tissue.

A complex cystic and solid mass (Fig. 4.51A), tubular-like areas that are hypo to anechoic, or less commonly diffusely increased echogenicity with echoes that move if the transducer is held fixed in place (Fig. 4.51B) are the findings seen in patients with an abscess. Focal areas of marked hyperechogenicity may be noted in the abscess, possibly representing air (Fig. 4.51A). In patients with subareolar abscess, the complex fluid collection almost always extends to involve the skin of the areola (see Figs. 7.51 and 7.52). Drainage under ultrasound

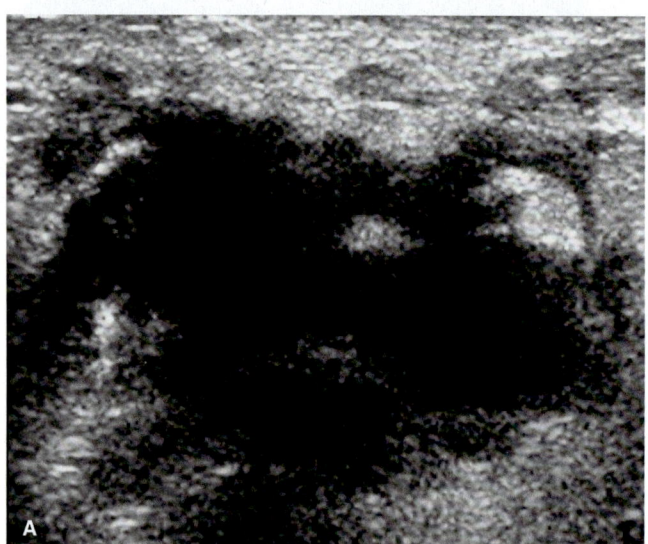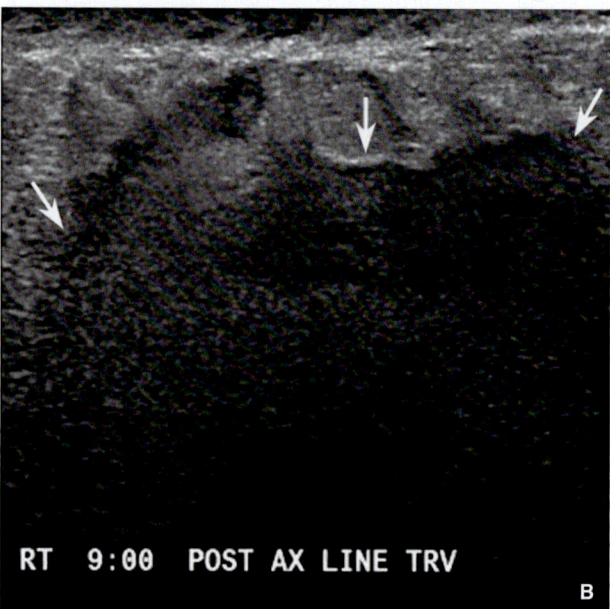

FIG. 4.51 • **Abscesses. A:** Ultrasound. An irregular mass with ill-defined margins and heterogeneous echotexture is imaged corresponding to the site of a painful "lump" described by the patient. Localized areas of marked hyperechogenicity may represent air in the abscess. Pus is aspirated from this mass. No residual abnormality is imaged 2 months after completion of one 10-day antibiotic course. (From Cardeñosa G. *Breast Imaging [The Core Curriculum Series]*. Philadelphia, PA: Lippincott Williams & Wilkins; 2003.) **B:** Ultrasound; different patient who presents described pain, redness, and swelling posterolaterally in the right breast. Tissue echogenicity is increased, and normal soft tissue planes are disrupted in the lateral quadrants of the left breast posteriorly extending to the midaxillary line. Although no apparent discrete fluid collection is initially identified, note a line of demarcation between superficial echogenic tissue and an area of slight hypoechogenicity *(arrows)*. As the transducer was held over this area, the echoes were clearly moving. Using ultrasound guidance, an 18G needle is advanced into this area and purulent material is aspirated. Patient is surgically drained and treated with antibiotics.

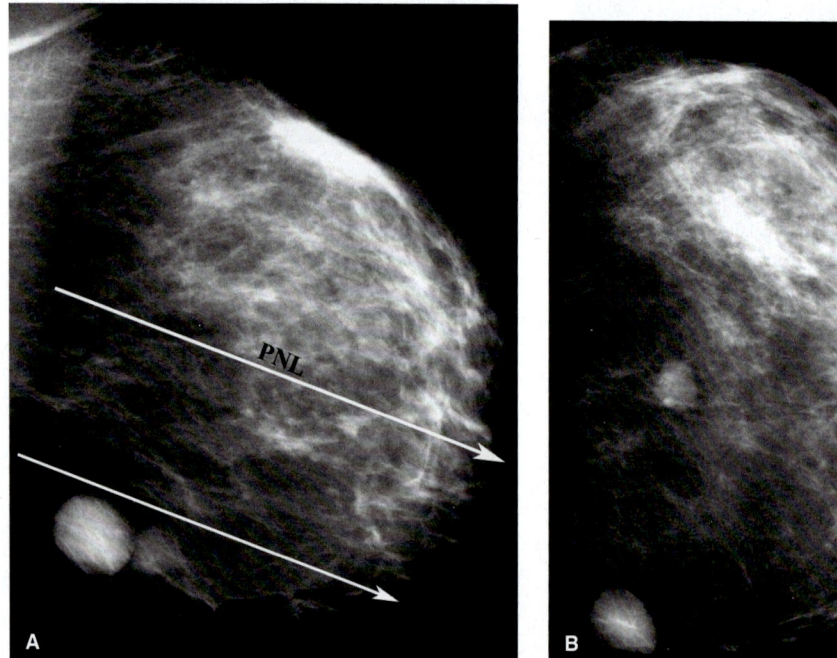

FIG. 4.52 • **Establishing mammographic and ultrasound concordance.** MLO **(A)** and CC **(B)** views demonstrating two round masses in the left breast.

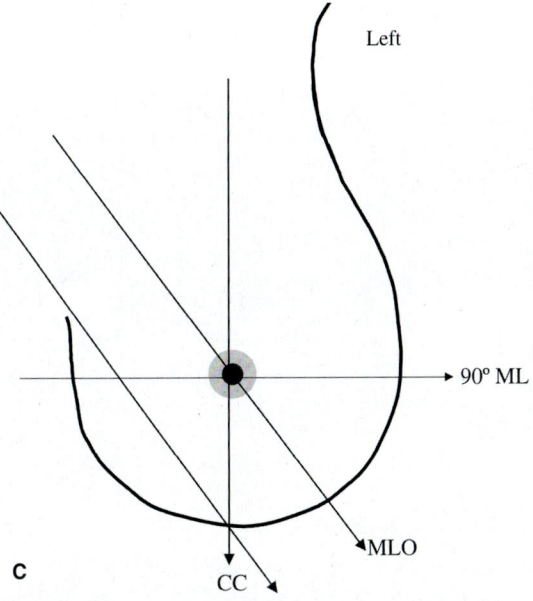

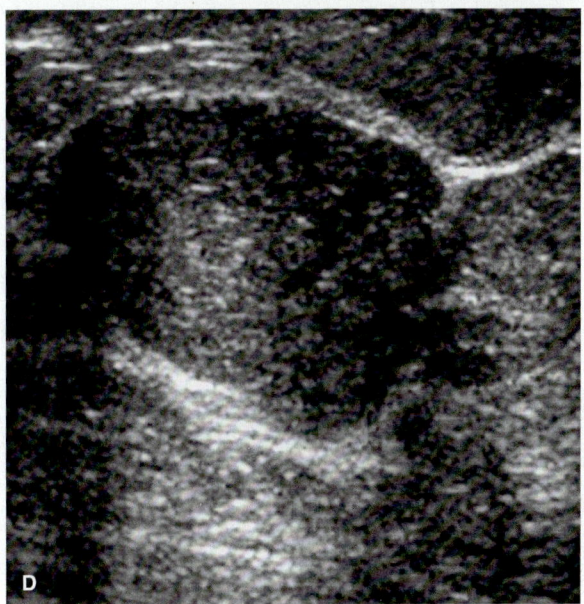

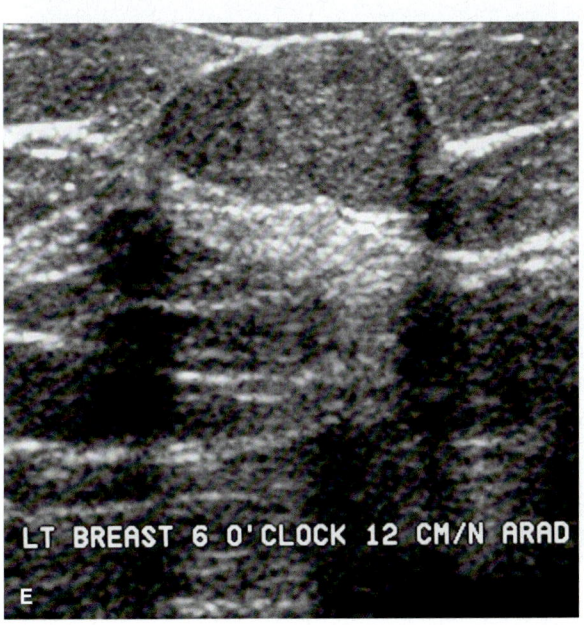

FIG. 4.52 • *(continued)* **C:** Use of the Eklund method (see triangulation section Chapter 3) for determining the approximate o'clock position of lesions seen on CC and MLO views. Keep in mind that on the MLO view, not all tissue projecting below the level of the nipple is anatomically in the lower quadrants. In this patient, on the MLO view both masses project below the level of the nipple and the posterior nipple line (PNL). On the CC view, the largest of the two masses is medial, and the other is directly behind the nipple (retroareolar). On the basis of the frontal diagram, the lesion will be found along the line drawn below the PNL (MLO line). The largest mass should be found at the 10 o'clock position and the second at the 6 o'clock position; you can then measure the distance from the nipple back to the masses on the CC view to approximate the distance (cm) of the masses from the nipple. In doing the ultrasound, the transducer is positioned at these o'clock positions as the starting points. **D:** The largest of the two masses is found at the 10 o'clock position, 12 cm from the nipple. It is an oval mass with circumscribed margins and posterior acoustic enhancement. **E:** A second oval mass with circumscribed margins, thin-edge shadows, and posterior acoustic enhancement is imaged at the 6 o'clock position, 12 cm from the nipple. Both of these are fibroadenomas. It is important to correlate mammographic and sonographic findings. Our approach is to walk into the ultrasound room with the expected o'clock position of the mass based on the mammographic findings. (From Cardeñosa G. *Breast Imaging [The Core Curriculum Series]*. Philadelphia, PA: Lippincott Williams & Wilkins; 2003.)

guidance is helpful in targeting pockets of purulent material. See Chapter 7 for additional discussion on breast abscesses.

IMPORTANCE OF MAMMOGAPHIC AND SONOGRAPHIC CORRELATION

Complete mammographic workups are critical before the patient is taken to ultrasound for evaluation of a mammographically detected mass. If you are not sure about the location of a mass on the mammogram, beware of assuming that what you find on ultrasound correlates with what you are seeing on the mammogram. Based on orthogonal views of the abnormality on the mammogram, an approximate location for the lesion is determined so that the expected o'clock position and distance from the nipple are established prior to starting the ultrasound (Figs. 4.52 and 4.53; also see Fig. 3.36). On the basis of some of the mammographic features of the mass (size and margins), you should have an idea of what you will image on ultrasound. If the mass measures 3 cm on the mammogram, a 1-cm cyst cannot be used to explain the mammographic finding. If any uncertainty persists on the ultrasound–mammographic concordance of a mass, the mass seen on the ultrasound can be marked with a metallic BB, and follow-up mammographic images can help establish correlation. Alternatively, if a biopsy is indicated, a needle can be placed through the presumed lesion under ultrasound, and a follow-up mammographic image done to confirm correlation (see Fig. 12.24).

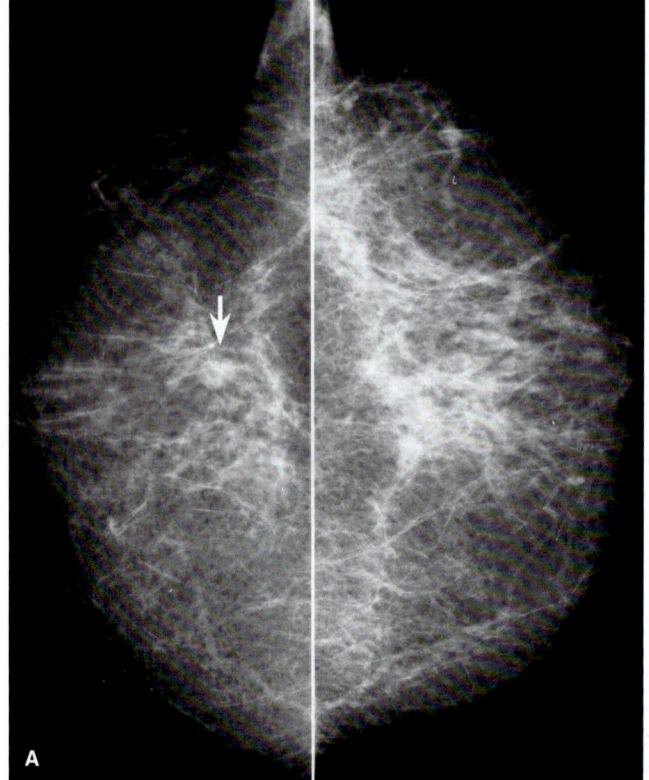
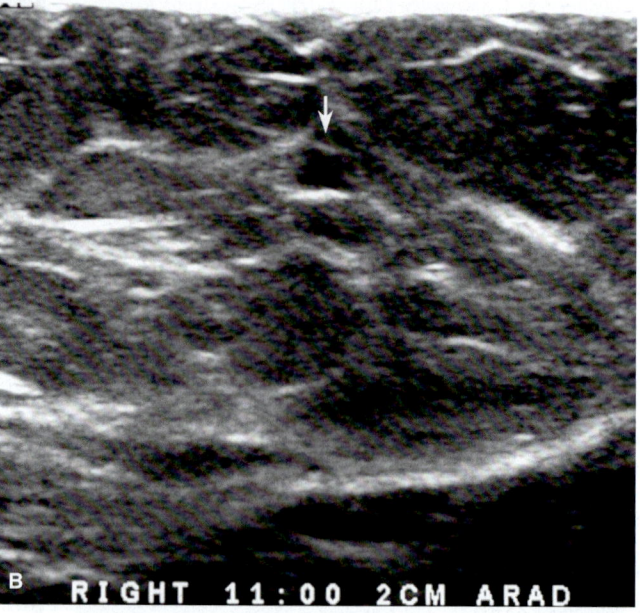
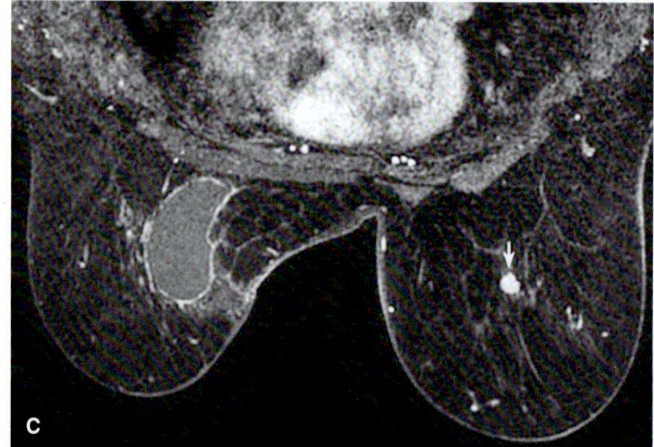

FIG. 4.53 • **Invasive ductal carcinoma, misdiagnosed as a cyst with ultrasound. A:** CC views in a 61-year-old patient. A round mass *(arrow)* is identified in the right breast on CC and MLO (not shown) views. The presence of a mass with indistinct margins is confirmed on spot compression views (not shown). Notice the location of the mass with respect to the nipple; the mass is central and approximately 4 cm from the nipple. **B:** Ultrasound. A "cyst" *(arrow)* is imaged at the 11 o'clock position, 2 cm from the nipple. Neither the size nor the location of the mass correlates with what is seen mammographically. The diagnosis of a cyst should also be questioned given the margins of this lesion seen on the mammogram. **C:** MRI, axial postcontrast image done approximately 3 weeks following the images shown in parts **A** and **B** after an invasive lobular carcinoma is diagnosed and excised in the left breast. Fluid collection with thin enhancing wall is imaged centrally in the left breast. A lobulated mass *(arrow)* with homogeneous enhancement is imaged centrally in the right breast approximately 4 cm from the right nipple. The size, imaging features, and location correlate with the mass seen mammographically. When going from a mammogram to ultrasound make sure you have an o'clock position, expected distance from the nipple, and approximate size for the lesion you are trying to identify on ultrasound. Similarly, on the basis of the morphologic features of the mass on mammography, have an idea of what you will accept as a diagnosis on ultrasound. If you have any questions about the mammographic–ultrasound correlation, put a needle in what you see on ultrasound, and obtain mammographic images to be sure the findings correlate.

References

1. Baker JA, Soo MS, Rosen EL. Artifacts and pitfalls in sonographic imaging of the breast. *AJR Am J Roentgenol.* 2001;176:1261–1266.
2. Stavros AT. *Breast Ultrasound.* Philadelphia, PA: Lippincott Williams & Wilkins; 2004.
3. American College of Radiology. *ACR Practice Guideline for the Performance of a Breast Ultrasound Examination.* Reston, VA: American College of Radiology; 2011 (Resolution 11).
4. Baker JA, Soo MS. Breast US: assessment of technical quality and image interpretation. *Radiology.* 2002;223:229–238.
5. Kolb TM, Lichy J, Newhouse JH. Occult cancer in women with dense breasts: detection with screening US—diagnostic yield and tumor characteristics. *Radiology.* 1998;207:191–199.
6. Kolb TM, Lichy J, Newhouse JH. Comparison of the performance of screening mammography, physical examination, and breast US and evaluation of factors that influence them: an analysis of 27,825 patient evaluations. *Radiology.* 2002;225:165–175.

7. Kelly KM, Richwald GA. Automated whole-breast ultrasound: advancing the performance of breast cancer screening. *Semin Ultrasound CT MR*. 2011;32:273–280.
8. Kelly KM, Dean J, Comulada WS, et al. Breast cancer detection using automated whole breast ultrasound and mammography in radiographically dense breasts. *Eur Radiol*. 2010;20:734–742.
9. Kaplan SS. Clinical utility of bilateral whole-breast US in the evaluation of women with dense breast tissue. *Radiology*. 2001;221:641–649.
10. Berg WA, Zhang, Z, Lehrer D, et al. Detection of breast cancer with addition of annual screening ultrasound or single screening MRI to mammography in women with elevated breast cancer risk. *JAMA*. 2012;307:1394–1404.
11. Moon WK, Noh DY, Im JG. Multifocal, multicentric and contralateral breast cancers: bilateral whole-breast US in the preoperative evaluation of patients. *Radiology*. 2002;224:569–576.
12. Feig S. Breast masses: mammographic and sonographic evaluation. *Radiol Clin North Am*. 1992;30:67–92.
13. Berg WA, Sechtin AG, Marques H, et al. Cystic breast masses and the ACRIN 6666 experience. *Radiol Clin North Am*. 2010;48:931–987.
14. Werner JK, Kumar D, Berg WA. Apocrine metaplasia: mammographic and sonographic appearances. *AJR Am J Roentgenol*. 1998;170:1375–1379.
15. Stavros AT, Thickman D, Rapp CL, et al. Solid breast nodules: use of sonography to distinguish between benign and malignant lesions. *Radiology*. 1995;196:123–134.
16. Adrada B, Wu Y, Yang W. Hyperechoic lesions of the breast: radiologic-histopathologic correlation. *AJR Am J Roentgenol*. 2013;200:W518–W530.
17. Linda A, Zulani C, Lorenzon M, et al. Hyperechoic lesions of the breast: not always benign. *AJR Am J Roentgenol*. 2011;196:1219–1224.
18. Linda A, Zulani C, Lorenzon M, et al. The wide spectrum of hyperechoic lesions of the breast. *Clin Radiol*. 2011;66:559–565.
19. Soo MS, Rosen EL, Baker JA, et al. Negative predictive value of sonography with mammography in patients with palpable breast lesions. *AJR Am J Roentgenol*. 2001;177:1167–1170.
20. Dennis MA, Parker SH, Klaus AJ, et al. Breast biopsy avoidance: the value of normal mammograms and normal sonograms in the setting of a palpable lump. *Radiology*. 2001;219:186–191.
21. Moy L, Slanetz PJ, Moore R, et al. Specificity of mammography and US in the evaluation of a palpable abnormality: retrospective review. *Radiology*. 2002;225:176–181.
22. Leung JWT. Utility of second-look ultrasound in the evaluation of MRI-detected breast lesions. *Semin Roentgenol*. 2011;46:260–274.
23. Abe H, Schmidt RA, Shah RN, et al. MR-directed ("second-look") ultrasound examination for breast lesions detected initially on MRI: MR and sonographic findings. *AJR Am J Roentgenol*. 2010;194:370–377.
24. Meissnitzer M, Dershaw DD, Lee CH, et al. Targeted ultrasound of the breast in women with abnormal MRI findings for whom biopsy has been recommended. *AJR Am J Roentgenol*. 2009;193:1025–1029.
25. Candelaria R, Fornage BD. Second-look US examination of MR-detected breast lesions. *J Clin Ultrasound*. 2010;39:115–121.
26. Trop I, Labelle M, David J, et al. Second-look targeted studies after breast magnetic resonance imaging: practical tips to improve lesion identification. *Curr Probl Diagn Radiol*. 2010;39:200–211.
27. Wiratkapun C, Duke D, Nordmann AS, et al. Indeterminate or suspicious breast lesions detected initially with MR imaging: value of MRI-directed breast ultrasound. *Acad Radiol*. 2008;15:618–625.
28. Monticciolo DL. Postbiopsy confirmation of MR-detected lesions biopsied using ultrasound. *AJR Am J Roentgenol*. 2012;198:W618–W620.

CHAPTER SELF-ASSESSMENT QUESTIONS

1. Representative image from an ultrasound study in a 20-year-old patient presenting with a "lump" in the right breast. What is indicated next?

   A. Follow-up ultrasound in 3 months
   B. Mammogram
   C. Ultrasound-guided biopsy
   D. Annual screening mammography starting at age 40

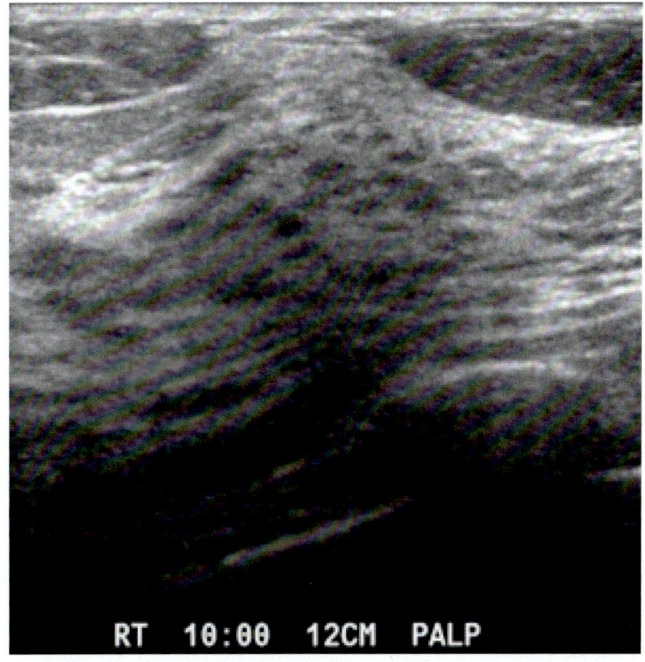

2. Spot tangential view (metallic BB at upper right-hand edge of image) (left) and representative ultrasound image (right) in a patient presenting with a "lump" in the left breast. What would you recommend?

A. Core needle biopsy
B. Aspiration
C. Screening mammogram in 1 year
D. Follow-up ultrasound in 6 months

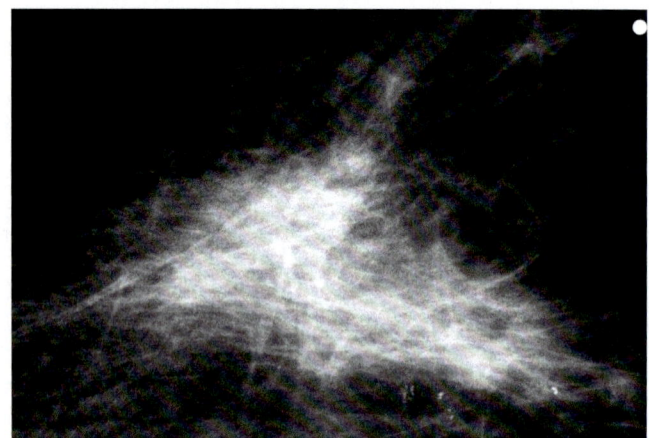

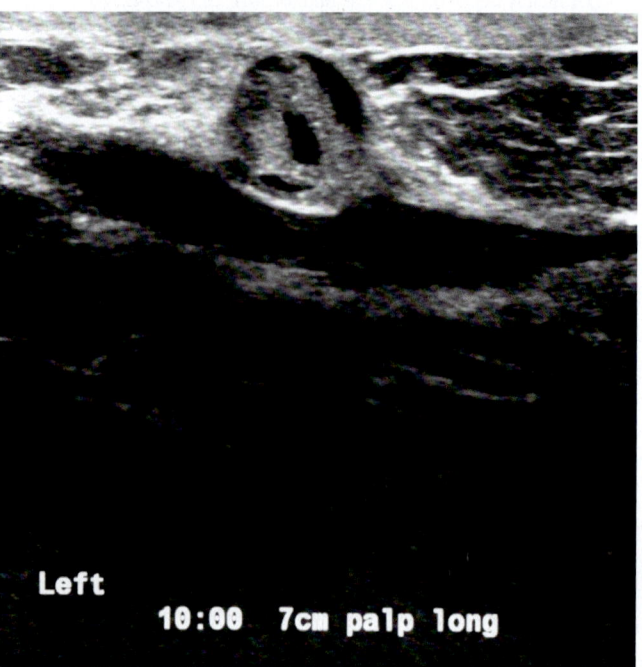

Answers to Chapter Self-Assessment Questions

1. D Correlative physical examination and an ultrasound is our starting point in patients who are below the age of 30 or those who are pregnant or lactating who present with focal breast findings. A mammogram is only done in these groups of patients if cancer is suspected on the basis of the physical examination and ultrasound. In this patient, a fibrous ridge is imaged corresponding to the palpable finding. Provided the fibrous ridge correlates directly to the palpable finding at the time the patient is being scanned, no additional evaluation or short-term follow-up is required. A mammogram is not indicated for this normal finding. Unless there are other intervening clinical concerns, the patient should be reassured that her "lump" is normal tissue and annual screening mammography is recommended starting at age 40.

2. C The ultrasound demonstrates a complex cystic and solid mass. The differential for this lesion includes papillary lesion, surgical or trauma-related change, fat necrosis (oil cyst), galactocele, abscess, and invasive ductal carcinoma with necrosis. Correlation with the patient's history and mammogram is critical before subjecting the patient to unneeded procedures or additional imaging. In this patient, you should be asking "Why was an ultrasound done?" An oil cyst is imaged at the posterior edge of tissue (with benign dystrophic-type calcifications) corresponding to the "lump" described by the patient; this correlates to a site of prior trauma. In this patient, the benign diagnosis is established mammographically and an ultrasound is not indicated (in fact, the complex cystic and solid mass seen with ultrasound might cause some to question the need for intervention).

Breast Magnetic Resonance Imaging

5

LEARNING OBJECTIVES

1. Factors to consider when doing breast magnetic resonance imaging (MRI)
   - Magnet field strength
   - Temporal and spatial resolution
   - Scanning plane (axial, sagittal, coronal)
   - Unilateral versus bilateral studies
   - Contrast administration
   - Fat suppression
   - Kinetic curve analysis
   - Timing of study to the menstrual cycle
     Screening versus diagnostic MRIs
   - Patient issues (breast size, claustrophobia)
2. Common artifacts that may be seen when doing breast MRI
3. Contraindications to breast MRI
4. Indications for breast MRI
5. Lesion evaluation, description, and differentials considerations
6. Masses (location, size, shape, margins, enhancement features, T1- and T2-signal characteristics)
   - Non–mass-like enhancement (distribution modifier, enhancement features)
7. Foci

If one considers the current breast imaging technologies, contrast-enhanced breast MRI has the highest sensitivity rates for the detection of invasive and intraductal cancers. The sensitivity ranges from 89% to 100% (1–3). False-negative MRI studies are not common but have been reported in patients with ductal carcinoma in situ (DCIS), low nuclear grade invasive lesions, or, rarely, in women with early and strong parenchymal enhancement in whom a small enhancing lesion may be masked (4). The reported specificity for breast MRI is variable and ranges from 37% to 97%; this high variation likely relates to differences in imaging protocols and the diagnostic criteria used in the various studies (1–3). The specificity is likely to improve as MR systems improve spatial and temporal resolution, experience with breast MRI increases, and when information other than just the presence of enhancement is factored into the consideration of differentials and management decisions.

In considering a breast MRI program, it is our contention that this is best handled by breast imagers who can provide the needed correlation between physical examination, mammography, ultrasound, MRI, imaging-guided biopsies, and pathology. The integration of breast MRI, and with it MRI-guided breast biopsies, into preexisting breast imaging programs can progress rapidly and seamlessly. The need for concurrently developing MRI-guided biopsy capability is apparent if you consider that breast MRI is done primarily for the early detection of breast cancers not depicted by other modalities. In this situation, patients with enhancing abnormalities not identified mammographically, or on ultrasound, will require biopsies done with MRI guidance (see Chapter 12).

The ability to schedule patients expeditiously is critical, particularly those in whom the MRI is being done for preoperative staging purposes following a breast cancer diagnosis. Likewise, if an MRI-guided biopsy is indicated in any of these patients, scheduling the biopsy needs to be prompt. We schedule all of our patients with a new breast cancer diagnosis for a breast MRI within a day or two of their initial diagnostic biopsy and ahead of the appointment with the surgeon. If, on the basis of the MRI, a biopsy or ultrasound evaluation is indicated, we contact the patient directly to expedite scheduling the needed evaluation. We also contact patients directly when a screening MRI is indicated following a screening mammogram (e.g., known *BRCA* carrier, first-degree relative of a known *BRCA* carrier, multiple first-degree relatives with premenopausal breast cancer, and patients with a history of chest wall radiation during adolescence). Our office personnel obtain insurance authorization for these patients prior to scheduling the MRI. In women with a history of claustrophobia we prescribe medications (Ativan, less commonly valium) so as to relax the patient and minimize the likelihood of motion during the study.

TECHNICAL CONSIDERATIONS

When thinking about the implementation of a breast MRI program, several decisions regarding scanning parameters need to be considered. These include field strength, temporal and spatial resolution, scanning plane (sagittal, coronal, and axial), bilateral or unilateral scanning, contrast administration, fat suppression, kinetic analysis, and timing of the study in premenopausal women (1). Analogous to mammography and ultrasound, MRI provides morphologic information regarding lesions in the breast. Unlike these modalities, MR affords functional information (kinetic curves) as well as the T1- and T2-relaxation times of lesions; this functional information is critical in the diagnostic evaluation of lesions.

A characteristic that is universal to viable malignant lesions is the ability to stimulate the development of their own vascular supply (e.g., angiogenesis) that is not under usual physiologic control mechanisms (1,2). The capillary leakage and arteriovenous shunting characteristic of these abnormal vessels underlie the described kinetic features (kinetics) of invasive lesions seen on breast MRI, and provides the needed differentiation from normal tissue and benign lesions. Although certain enhancement patterns are consistently associated with most malignant lesions, they are not a pathognomonic finding for breast cancer. They can also be seen in normal breast tissue under hormonal stimulation, inflammatory processes, lymph nodes, and benign tumors such as papillomas, fat necrosis, and fibroadenomas. Conversely, by virtue of their growth patterns, some breast cancers (DCIS low nuclear grade and rarely invasive lobular and tubular carcinomas) can demonstrate variable angiogenic activity, making detectability on MRI a challenge.

With this in mind, consider the importance of temporal resolution. To image malignant lesions optimally, the breasts need to be scanned rapidly enough to capture their transient enhancement in a background of progressive parenchymal enhancement. Consequently, the kinetic (dynamic) evaluation of lesions is predicated on the ability to rapidly, repeatedly, and with minimal patient motion, obtain the same stack of images several times after the administration of contrast. Similarly, the ability to characterize morphologic features is maximal in the early postcontrast phase of the study before washout of contrast occurs and surrounding parenchyma enhances. For breast MRI, a temporal resolution of 1 to 2 minutes (ideally closer to 1 minute) is optimal (1).

Spatial resolution is important in the morphologic characterization of lesions; however, spatial resolution comes at the expense of temporal resolution. Within the constraints imposed by an optimal temporal resolution (1 to 2 minutes), maximize the matrix for spatial resolution. An acquisition matrix of 512 × 512 for transverse imaging with a field of view (FOV) ranging from 320 to 350 translates into plane pixel sizes of 0.5 × 0.5 to 0.8 × 0.8 mm and a section thickness (through-plane pixel size) of 1 to 3 mm (1).

A magnet with field strength of 1.5 T is preferred. As field strength decreases, so does the signal-to-noise ratio, potentially leading to a compromise in diagnostic information. Higher field strengths (e.g., 3 T systems) improve spatial and temporal resolution; however, it is not clear how much additional clinical information is provided by higher field strengths (1). A dedicated breast coil and attention to the positioning of the breasts in the coil are imperative in obtaining optimal images of the breasts. Unfortunately, only one coil size is currently available to encompass the significant variation in breast and lesion size encountered in practice. In patients with large breasts or lesions,

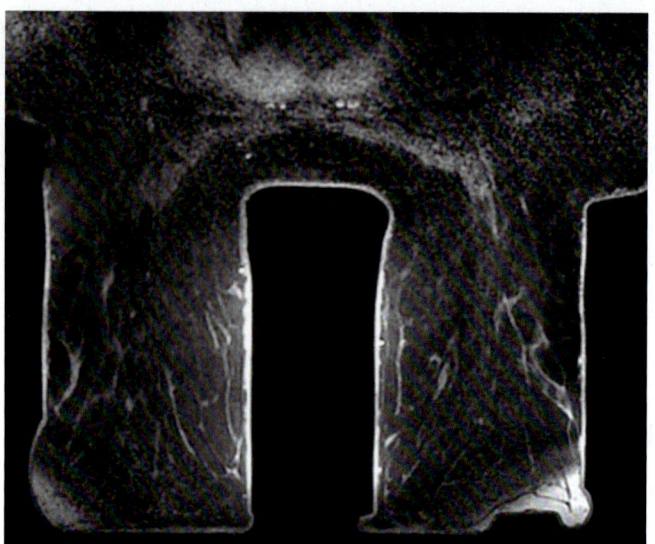

FIG. 5.1 • **Coil size limitations.** MRI, axial T1-weighted image post-contrast. The anterior aspect of the breasts is compressed and flattened against the coil with associated signal flaring. The distortion and compression of tissue anteriorly in these patients could theoretically impact enhancement and our ability to detect lesions. Currently, the dedicated breast coil comes in one size and shape. For women with larger breasts, large lesions, those with variable amounts of axillary tissue or an increased distance between the breasts, limitations in positioning may be apparent and cannot always be addressed optimally. Sometimes, you can use pads to lift the patient up away from the table; however, this can result in exclusion of axillary and posterior tissue. Ideally, different sized breast coils will be developed.

positioning may be compromised and artifacts may be seen (Fig. 5.1). Similarly, with some units, patient size and body weight impose limits on our ability to scan all patients.

The dose of gadolinium (T1-shortening agents) used ranges from 0.1 to 0.2 mmol perkg of body weight. A power injector is used at a rate of 2 to 3 mL per second followed by a 20-mL saline flush. These contrast agents are fairly well tolerated with less than 2% likelihood of adverse reactions. Renal excretion of the gadolinium is dependent on glomerular filtration rates (GFR). Contrast administration is contraindicated in patients with GFRs lower than 30 mL per minute/1.73 m^2. Nephrogenic systemic fibrosis (NSF) is a rare complication related to gadolinium agents in patients with poor renal function (5,6). Patients with NSF develop skin thickening in the extremities, less commonly the torso, and usually there is sparing of the face. With progression, patients develop joint contractures, and in some, systemic involvement may lead to a cardiomyopathy, pulmonary fibrosis, pulmonary hypertension, diaphragmatic paralysis, and death. Point of care testing for eGFR is done on all patients before a breast MRI is done. In patients with eGFRs less than 30 mL per minute/1.73 m^2, MRI is deferred pending discussion with the clinicians and patient. Rarely, if the patient is undergoing dialysis, we do the MRI immediately preceding a scheduled dialysis appointment.

We image the breasts in the axial plane obtaining a precontrast set of axial images (Vibrant) with contiguous 1-mm slice thickness followed by five stacks of images postcontrast for the dynamic T1-weighted fat-suppressed phase of the study. We also obtain axial non–fat-suppressed T2-weighted images as well as sagittal fat-suppressed T2-weighted and non–fat-suppressed T1-weighted images. The axial plane used for the dynamic sequences is analogous to craniocaudal images, and simultaneously scanning the breasts enables us to evaluate for symmetry. We do not do unilateral MRIs. Since contrast is being administered, it makes sense to evaluate both breasts; additionally, the ability to compare one breast with the other is an important reason to do bilateral studies. Scanning in the axial or sagittal planes facilitates characterization of the anterior to posterior extent of disease, a question that is particularly important in patients with DCIS (1,2). In reviewing images, the maximum intensity projection (MIP), subtraction images, multiplanar reconstructions in coronal and sagittal planes, kinetic curves, and color overlays are routinely reviewed for detection and characterization of lesions. Multiplanar reconstructions are particularly helpful in evaluating areas of enhancement to determine whether they represent parenchyma, a mass, or a non–mass-like enhancement. Reconstructions are also helpful in assessing lymph node morphology (e.g., cortical bulging).

Contraindications to breast MRI include the presence of a pacemaker, artificial heart valves, surgical clips in the heart or brain made of MR-incompatible materials, recent heart or brain surgery, cochlear implants, insulin pumps, shrapnel in the orbits, some of the tissue expanders used for breast reconstruction, weight greater than 300 pounds, claustrophobia not controlled with medications, and, as mentioned previously, poor renal function.

When scheduling high-risk premenopausal women for a screening MRI, consider timing it to the menstrual cycle. Breast tissue is most quiescent during the second week of the cycle. Consequently, if a patient's cycle is predictable, screening MRIs should be timed to the second week of the cycle to minimize the enhancement of breast parenchyma sometimes seen when breast tissue is under hormonal stimulation. For patients with breast cancer, in whom the MRI is being done for staging purposes, it is not usually practical to time the MRI evaluation to the patient's cycle.

ARTIFACTS

As with any imaging modality, meticulous attention to detail is imperative in obtaining the highest quality images possible. We should never settle for mediocrity or suboptimal image quality and hide behind disclaimers. The technologists need to work closely with the patient so that during positioning the breasts are centered in the coil. Additionally, making sure the patient is comfortable before starting is important in minimizing the likelihood of motion. If the patient is claustrophobic, consider medicating her so she is more relaxed and less likely to move during the study. Patients are given the option of using earplugs or headphones with music to mitigate the noises from the scanner. To the extent that motion can be minimized, particularly during the dynamic portion of the study, the better the quality of the images and resulting subtraction and kinetic curve evaluation.

The presence of ferromagnetic materials (e.g., surgical clips, sternal cerclage wires, etc.) leads to inhomogeneity in the magnetic field, resulting in susceptibility artifacts. These are noted as signal voids with surrounding high signal intensity and distortion of the image; the amount of distortion depends on the shape and composition of the metallic object (Fig. 5.2). Linearly oriented metallic susceptibility artifacts in lesions are common following core needle biopsies; these are not perceptible mammographically but presumably result from tiny metallic fragments deposited in the lesion during the biopsy (Fig. 5.3). Metallic artifacts are more pronounced in higher magnetic fields (e.g., 3 T magnets) (7).

A dedicated breast coil is essential for breast MRI. The technologist needs to make sure the breast coil is plugged in and selected before scanning the patient. If the body coil is inadvertently used, low signal-to-noise ratio will result in grainy images (7). The anatomical area to be imaged must be included in the FOV, keeping in mind that the selected FOV will affect spatial resolution. Too small an FOV, however, may exclude tissue that needs to be evaluated and may result in wraparound artifacts. With a given matrix, a smaller FOV will improve the in-plane spatial resolution. When using the axial scan plane, the FOV needs to

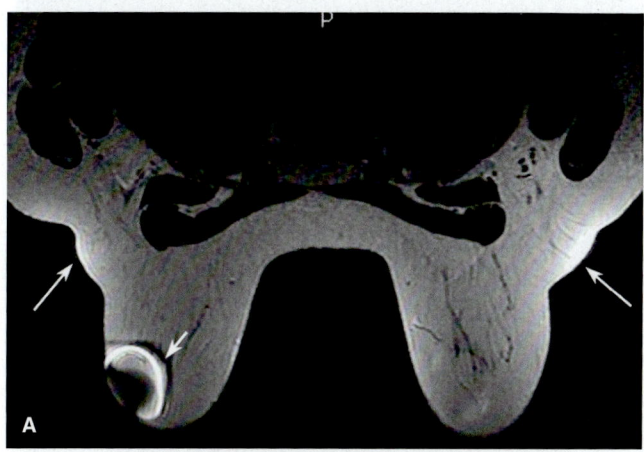
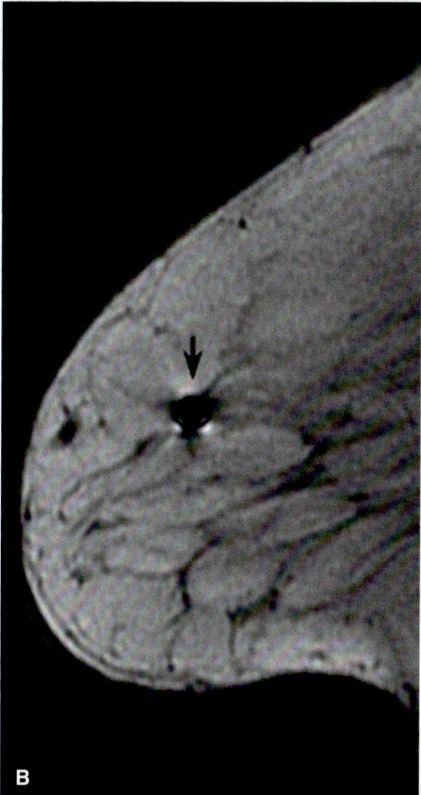

FIG. 5.2 • **Bloom artifact resulting from ferromagnetic objects. A:** MRI, axial T2-weighted image. Bloom artifact (*short arrow*) on the left resulting from a metallic BB on the patient's breast. This limits the evaluation of tissue in this portion of the left breast. The patient's MRI appointment followed evaluation in breast imaging where a metallic BB was used to mark an area of concern; the metallic BB was not removed after the mammogram. Note axillary fat "bulging" (*long arrows*) out from the coil with signal flaring. **B:** MRI, sagittal non–fat-suppressed T1-weighted image in a different patient. Bloom artifact (*arrow*) resulting from a biopsy clip in the breast.

include tissue from the level of the clavicle to just below the inframammary fold, thereby enabling evaluation of the axillae and breasts.

Fat suppression, particularly for the dynamic portion of a study, facilitates the detection of enhancing lesions. If fat suppression is not used, the subtraction images become critical in the assessment of smaller areas of enhancement (Fig. 5.4); for optimal subtraction, patient motion needs to be minimized. After our initial experience with using no fat suppression for the dynamic sequences and a slice thickness of 2 mm, we have switched to the routine use of fat

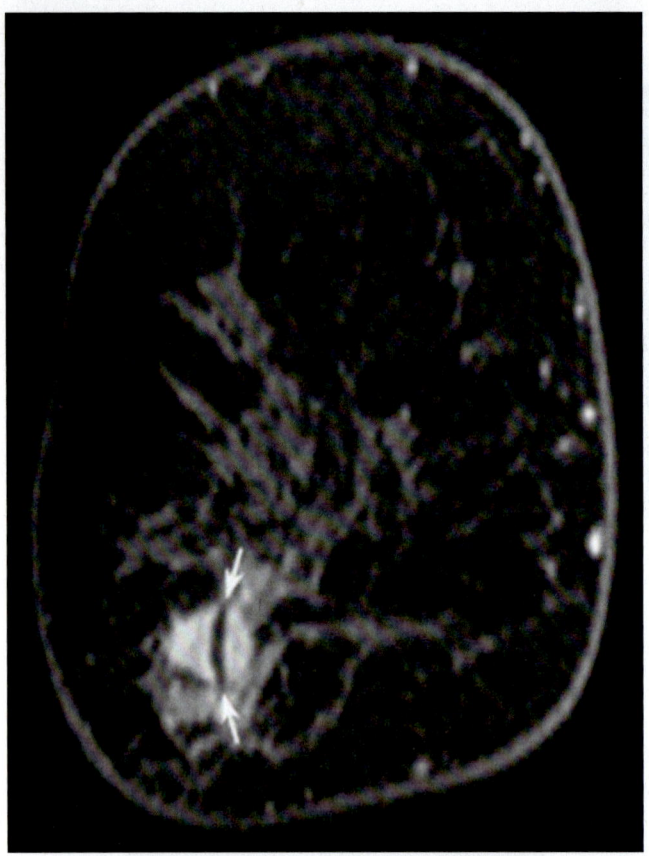

FIG. 5.3 • **Post-biopsy needle artifact, invasive ductal carcinoma high nuclear grade.** MRI, T1-weighted, postcontrast coronal reconstruction of the right breast posteriorly. An irregular mass with heterogeneous enhancement and spiculated margins is imaged in the lower outer aspect of the right breast corresponding to the site of a known invasive ductal carcinoma diagnosed in a 51-year-old patient following an ultrasound-guided biopsy. A linear signal void (*arrows*) through the mass is thought to reflect tiny metallic fragments (shavings) from the needle used for the ultrasound-guided core biopsy. This is a common observation if the MRI study is done immediately following imaging-guided biopsies. The size of the signal void varies depending on the size of the needle used for the biopsy (e.g., 14G vs. 12G).

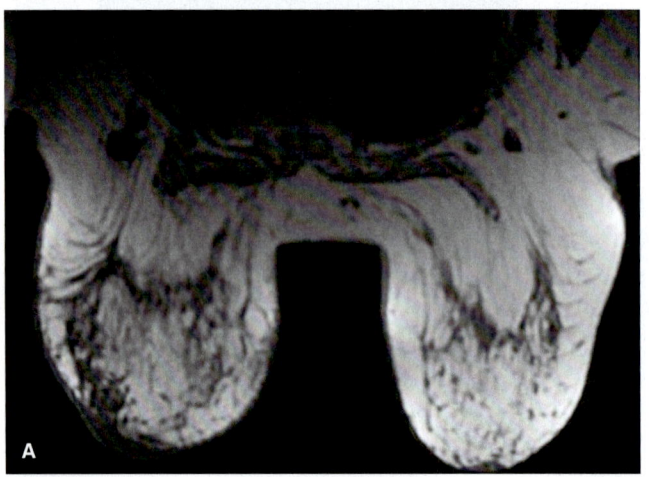

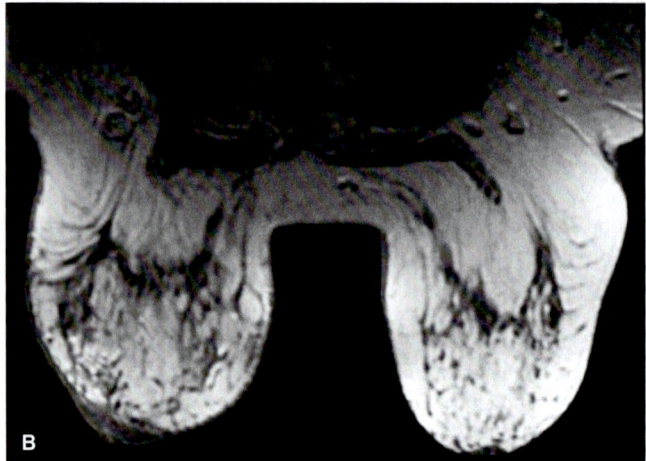

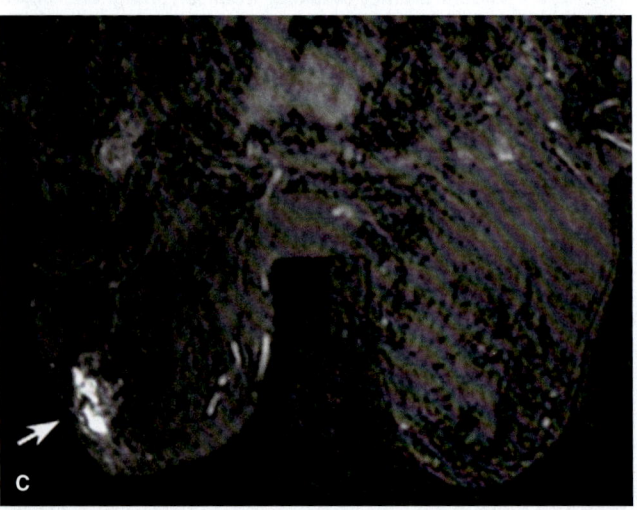

FIG. 5.4 • **Non–fat-suppressed T1-weighted images done using a 2-mm slice thickness. A:** MRI, axial image, precontrast. The left breast is smaller and wider with skin thickening noted anteriorly. Suboptimal positioning of the right breast in the coil is such that tissue in the axillary tail is bulging out of coil; signal flaring is apparent along the edge of this tissue. **B:** MRI, axial image, postcontrast at the same level shown in part **A**. With no fat suppression and 2-mm scan thickness, it can be difficult to establish the presence of enhancement. Similarly, our ability to characterize the morphologic features and distribution of the enhancement is limited. Under these circumstances, subtraction images are critical. **C:** MRI, subtraction image obtained from the images shown in parts **A** and **B**. Non–mass-like enhancement (*arrow*) is present in the left breast anterolaterally. If, as in this patient, the dynamic sequences are done with no fat suppression, you are largely dependent on the subtraction images. Under these circumstances, patient motion can significantly limit the evaluation of the subtractions. Additionally, the 2-mm slice thickness limits morphologic evaluation of lesions. We are now routinely using fat suppression (Vibrant) for the dynamic sequences and scanning at a slice thickness of 1 mm.

suppression for the dynamic sequences and a 1-mm slice thickness. Homogeneous fat suppression may be difficult to obtain, particularly in women with predominantly fatty tissue (Fig. 5.5A) and those with implants (Fig. 5.5B). The software in most MRI units automatically identifies the water peak as the highest signal peak and suppresses the fat by applying saturation pulses at a frequency of 3.5 ppm (224 Hz in a 1.5 T magnet), representing the chemical shift between water and the methyl group of fat. In predominantly fatty breasts, the software may incorrectly identify the fat peak as that of the water peak, resulting in the application of fat suppression pulses at an incorrect frequency (7). Suboptimal fat saturation may also result from inhomogeneities in the magnetic field that may be corrected by shimming of the magnet. Signal flaring (Fig. 5.2B; also see Figs. 7.72C–E, 8.13B, and 8.37E) simulates poor fat saturation but is related to the proximity of the breast to the coil; placing a cushion between the breast and the coil can minimize signal flaring (7).

As mentioned previously, the resonant frequency of the hydrogen in fat differs from that in water by 224 Hz in 1.5 T systems. Chemical shift artifacts reflect spatial misregistrations between fat and glandular tissue (water) in the frequency encoding direction. This artifact can be overcome when fat suppression is used or by increasing the bandwidth used in image acquisition (7).

Ghosting artifacts may be apparent related to blood vessel, cardiac, and pulmonary pulsation. High signal intensity, uniform spacing, and

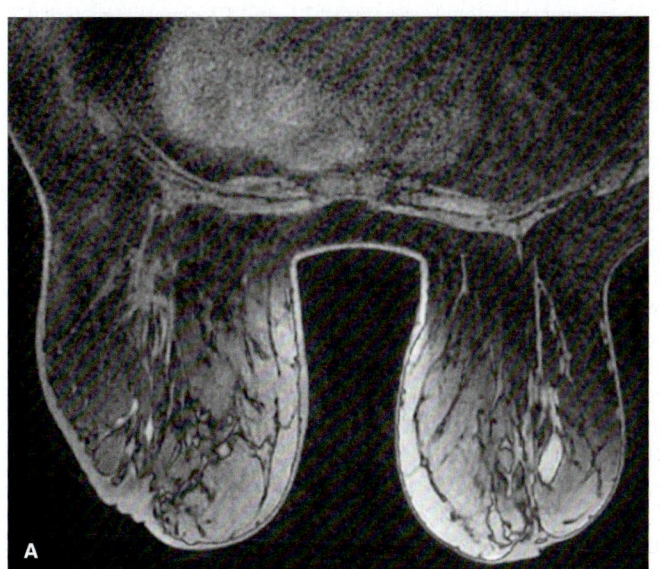

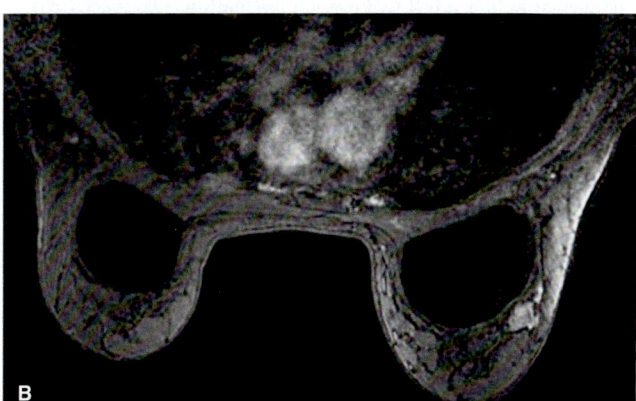

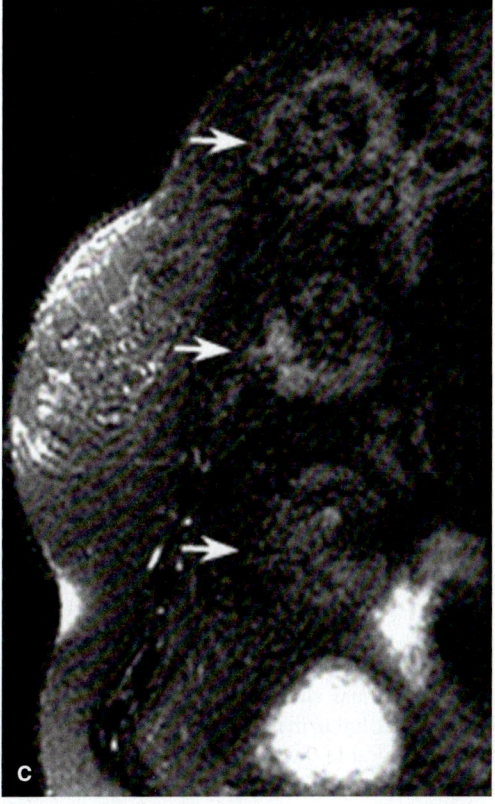

FIG. 5.5 • **Poor fat saturation and ghosting. A:** MRI, precontrast axial T1-weighted image demonstrating poor fat saturation in a patient with predominantly fatty tissue. **B:** MRI, T1-weighted image, postcontrast in a patient with implants. Poor fat saturation is present. A mass with heterogeneous enhancement and lobulated margins is present, abutting the right implant anterolaterally. Although adjustments are made in an effort to improve fat saturation before the contrast is given, poor fat saturation persists on the postcontrast images. In patients with implants, adequate fat saturation can be difficult to obtain. **C:** MRI, sagittal reconstruction. Ghosting resulting from the stomach is seen as a uniformly repeating high signal intensity artifact (*arrows*) simulating the size and shape of the stomach.

sometimes blurring reflecting motion are the characteristics of ghosting artifacts (Fig. 5.5C). These are propagated in the phase-encoding direction so that for breast imaging in the axial and sagittal planes, the left-to-right direction is chosen as opposed to the anterior–posterior direction (e.g., A-P phase encoding results in superimposition of cardiac and vascular pulsations on the breasts). Wraparound artifact is seen when signal-producing tissue is positioned outside the FOV. This type of artifact occurs primarily in the phase-encoding direction and is also known as aliasing or phase wrap (7).

LESION EVALUATION

Analogous to what is discussed with mammography and ultrasound, breast MRIs need to be evaluated for overall quality prior to assessing the images for possible pathology. Are the breasts well positioned in the coil (Fig. 5.6A, B), and has all of the breast tissue been imaged? Is there motion (Fig. 5.6C–E)? Is fat saturation optimal (Fig. 5.5)? Is contrast present (e.g., adequacy of contrast bolus) (Fig. 5.7)? Are there any other artifacts that may affect diagnostic information (Fig. 5.2A)? All MRI studies are reviewed in conjunction with a current mammogram, breast ultrasound, if the patient has had one, and any relevant history (e.g., family history of breast cancer, *BRCA* testing results, prior breast or axillary surgical procedures with pathology and type of implants in women with implants).

In patients with images of diagnostic quality, I usually start by perusing the MIP and subtraction images, as a quick way of establishing the complexity of the study, and the amount of time it will take for me to review the study meticulously. I carefully review all potential lesions in the dynamic portion of the study, toggling between pre- and immediately postcontrast images, followed by sagittal and coronal reconstructions of the area in question, kinetic curve evaluation as well as the precontrast T2- and T1-signal characteristics (Fig. 5.8). In establishing the presence of enhancement, be sure to review the subtraction images and toggle between pre- and postcontrast images. Do not assume that a high T1-signal postcontrast is enhancement without assessing the T1-signal intensity of the area precontrast (Fig. 5.9). In considering kinetic curves, it is important to recognize that these can be variable within a given lesion, depending on where the region of interest (ROI) marker is placed in the lesion. Place the ROI cursor at various locations in the area of enhancement being evaluated and scroll into and out of the plane before formulating an opinion regarding the predominant morphology of the kinetic curve for a given lesion.

If enhancement is present, you need to determine whether it is normal breast parenchyma or a lesion. Background parenchymal enhancement is relatively easy to recognize when diffuse (Fig. 5.10), bilateral, and progressive; however, it may pose more of a challenge when the enhancement is rapid and focal, often localized to the peripheral portions of the parenchyma (what we call parenchymal blushing). Focal parenchymal enhancement is usually planar, follows the shape of the tissue, and does not alter the contour of the parenchyma, particularly when the area is evaluated on reconstructions (e.g., axial, sagittal, and coronal planes). Background parenchymal enhancement is variable. It can be significant in some patients, minimal in others, and may vary with the menstrual cycle. Hormone replacement therapy may cause parenchymal enhancement that may be diffuse or focal, while tamoxifen usually decreases the background enhancement of the parenchyma. When tamoxifen therapy is stopped, background parenchymal enhancement may rebound (Fig. 5.11). Following radiation therapy, the affected breast often appears relatively quiescent when compared with the contralateral breast. If the area of enhancement in question is not parenchyma, what type of lesion is it? Is it a mass? Is it non–mass-like enhancement? Or is it a focus?

Mass

Is the area of abnormal enhancement a mass? Is it space occupying, three-dimensional, and greater than 0.5 cm in size? With a mass, a correlate is usually identified on precontrast T1- and T2-weighted images (Fig. 5.12) (2,3,8). Globally, differential considerations for masses include benign solid masses, invasive breast cancer, or, uncommonly, metastatic disease. For a mass, size, shape (irregular, round, oval), margins (circumscribed, not circumscribed: irregular, spiculated), enhancement features (homogeneous, heterogeneous, rim enhancement, dark internal septations), precontrast T1- and T2-signal characteristics and location should be described (8) and considered in the generation of an appropriate differential. Although not often discussed, we also find the presence of asymmetric edematous changes in tissues surrounding the mass (Fig. 5.12C) and sometimes extending to the pectoral fascia (Fig. 5.13) and the muscle itself as a helpful sign commonly associated with high-grade malignant lesions.

When considering kinetic curves, you need to describe two components: the initial phase, which describes the steepness in the rise of the curve (slow, medium, and fast), and the delayed phase: does the initial uptake decrease rapidly (e.g., washout, type III)? Does it plateau (type II)? Or is there continuous enhancement (e.g., persistent, type I curve) (8); this latter type of curve most commonly reflects benign processes (Fig. 5.10C). Although type I and II curves are associated with malignant lesions (Fig. 5.8F), fibroadenomas in young patients, lymph nodes, fat necrosis, and papillomas may generate rapid washin and washout kinetics. Evaluating all of the features of the lesion (margins, T2 signal, presence of fat, etc.), and correlation with clinical, mammographic, and ultrasound findings is often needed to establish the likely etiology of the finding, and may mitigate the need to biopsy benign lesions with type I and II curves.

In evaluating an enhancing mass, the margin is one of the more reliable indicators of the underlying etiology (2). Benign lesions are more likely to have smooth margins (Fig. 5.14). When considering margins, keep in mind that our ability to characterize them is dependent on spatial resolution. With low-resolution images, irregular margins may appear smooth. Similarly, if there is any patient motion, evaluation of the margins of a mass on subtraction images may be misleading (2,3). The shape and margins of a mass are best evaluated on the first set of images postcontrast. With the progressive enhancement of surrounding tissue on subsequent image sets, evaluation of the shape and margins of a mass may be limited.

For masses that are greater than 1 cm in size, homogeneous enhancement is also a good indicator of a benign process. In masses that are less than 1 cm, this is not a reliable predictor since spatial resolution may affect the evaluation (2). Analogous to mammography, fat-containing masses are usually benign. Fat content can be established on fat-suppressed images in combination with unenhanced, non–fat suppressed T1 and T2 sequences.

Masses with high T2 signal are usually considered benign, provided the entire mass demonstrates a homogeneously high T2 signal. Invasive ductal carcinomas with areas of necrosis (Figs. 5.8 and 5.15), mucinous (Fig. 5.16; also see Figs. 8.26 and 8.27), papillary (see Figs 8.34 and 8.36), and metaplastic carcinomas, as well as phyllodes tumors (see Fig. 7.67) may all demonstrate internal areas of intermediate-to-high T2 signal, but in these lesions, the T2 signal is not homogeneously high and is focal in the mass. Cysts (Fig. 5.17; also see Fig. 7.44C, D) most commonly demonstrate a homogeneously high T2 signal. This

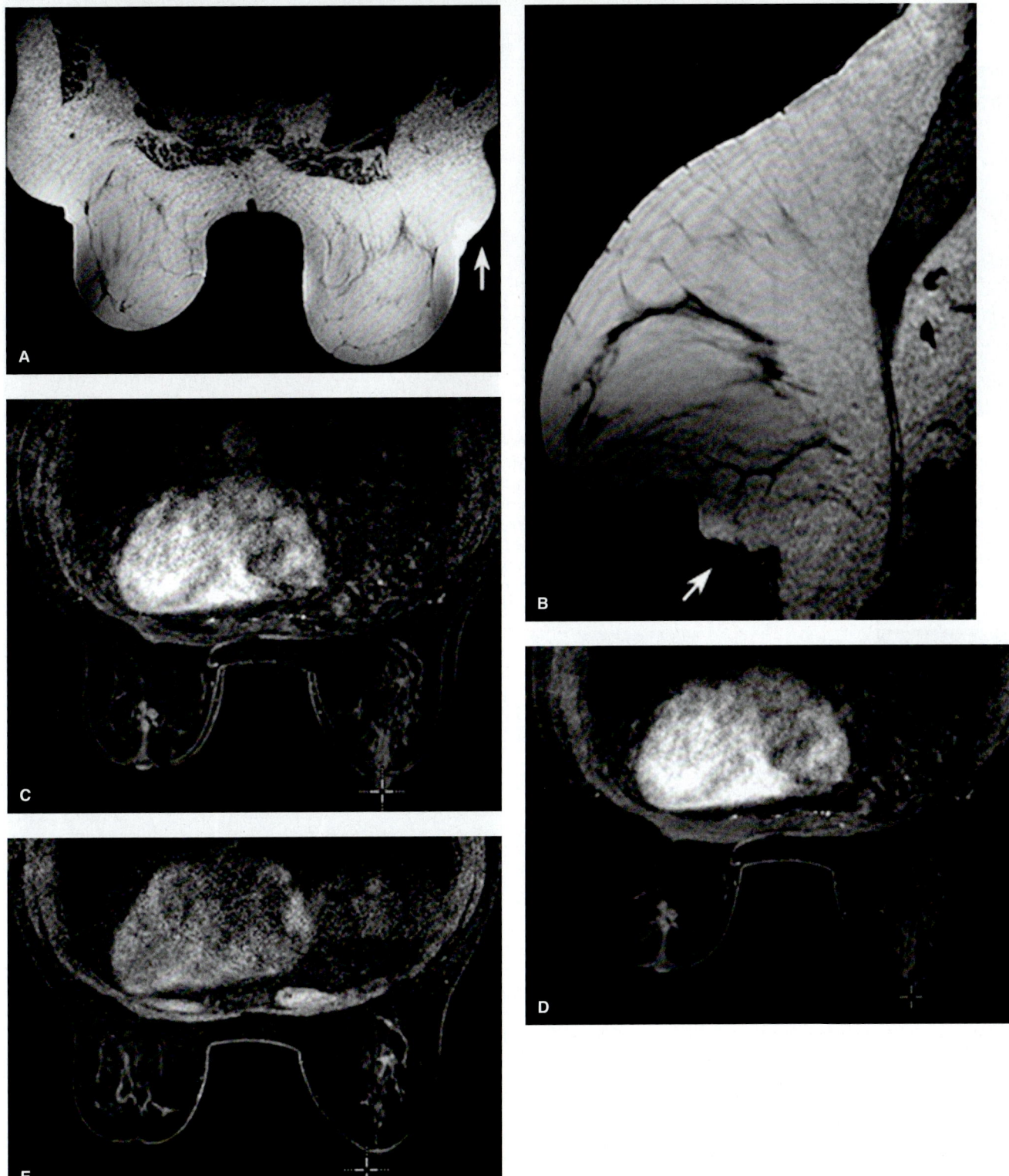

FIG. 5.6 • **Poor positioning and motion. A:** MRI, axial T2-weighted images. The patient is slightly rotated, and the right breast is not completely in the coil. The breasts need to be centered in the coil with every effort made to adequately include the breasts in the coil with no "bulges" (*arrow*) of tissue or skin folds. **B:** MRI, sagittal T1-weighted image with the inferior portion of the right breast (*arrow*) bulging out from the coil. Before scanning, make sure the patient is as comfortable as possible with the breasts centered and all breast tissue in the coil. **C:** MRI, subtraction image on a different patient. Notice doubling of skin line on the image consistent with motion between the pre- and postcontrast set of images. If a region of interest (ROI) is placed in a potential lesion, the kinetic curve will be notable for a steep initial phase (almost vertical). MRI, axial T1-weighted images, postcontrast **(D)** and Precontrast **(E)**. To confirm the observation of motion on the subtraction images, or in trying to determine the presence of subtle motion, the cursor is placed on a clearly identifiable landmark such as the right nipple in this patient and toggled back and forth between pre- and postcontrast images. The position of the nipple relative to the cursor changes between pre- and postcontrast images consistent with patient motion. In evaluating and comparing the pre- and postcontrast images, differences in the appearance of the tissue included on the images can also be appreciated.

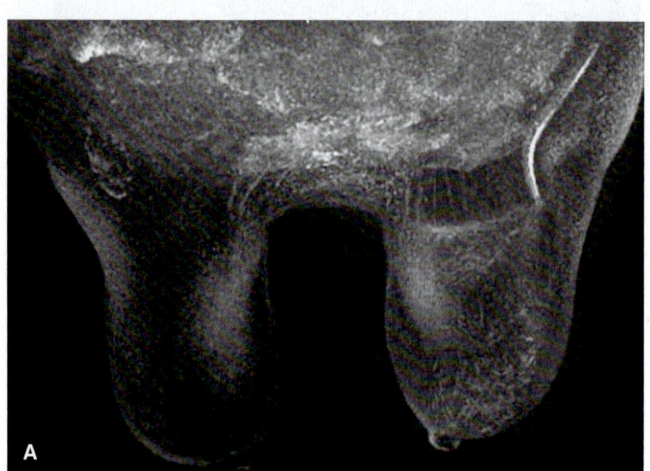
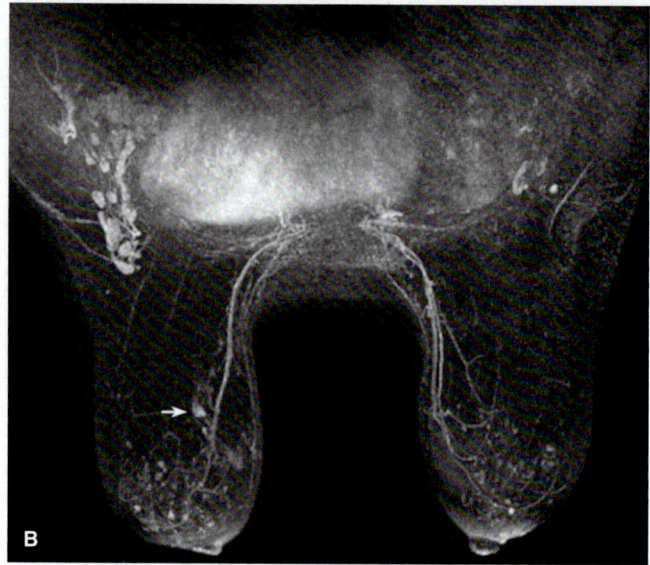

FIG. 5.7 • **Contrast bolus adequacy. A:** MRI, MIP. Initially you might think this is a normal study with quiescent breast tissue. Think again. Where is the heart? Are there no opacified vessels? What about axillary contents? As you review the images, the patient's known cancer is not seen (is this a false-negative breast MRI?). Following questioning, the technologist states that he noted a "puddle of water" on the table when the patient sat up following the study. **B:** MRI, MIP image, repeat study 2 days after image shown in part **A**. The heart is now apparent, as are vessels and axillary contents. Normal enhancement is seen associated with the nipple and, most importantly, the patient's known cancer (*arrow*) is now readily identifiable. As with mammography and breast ultrasound, before immersing yourself in the possible presence and evaluation of lesions, make sure the images are optimal. If they are not optimal, why not, and does the study need to be repeated?

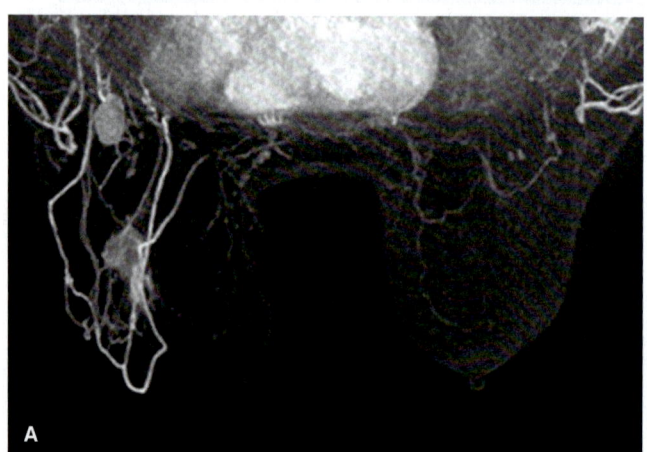
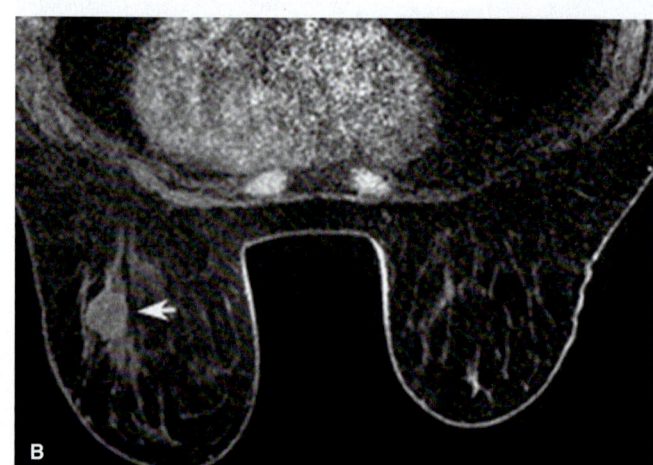

FIG. 5.8 • **Invasive ductal carcinoma, not otherwise specified. A:** MRI, MIP projection. After assessing image quality, I review the MIP, making sure to rotate the image. The relationship and superimposition of lesions can become apparent as the MIP image is rotated. In this patient, masses are apparent in the left breast and axilla; asymmetrically prominent venous structures are also noted in the left breast, a common observation in patients with breast cancer. The right breast appears normal. I follow the overview provided by the MIP image with a careful review of the subtraction images (not shown). MRI, axial T1-weighted precontrast **(B)** and MRI, postcontrast **(C)** images using a 1-mm slice thickness. With the identification of a possible lesion on the MIP and subtraction images, I review the postcontrast images and toggle back and forth between pre- and postcontrast images. In characterizing lesions (mass vs. non–mass-like enhancement), I also routinely do sagittal and coronal reconstructions (not shown). In this patient, a round mass (*short arrow*) with rim enhancement is imaged in the lower outer quadrant of the left breast at the junction of zones B and C. Additionally, heterogeneous non–mass-like clumped and linear enhancement (*long arrow* in **C**) is present, extending anteriorly from the mass for approximately 2 cm. An axillary lymph node (images not shown) demonstrates heterogeneous enhancement and circumscribed margins. **D:** MRI, T2-weighted sagittal fat-suppressed image of the left breast at the level of the mass. After assessing the lesion on the dynamic sequences, I review its T2 signal characteristics. This mass (*short arrow*) demonstrates intermediate T2 signal as well as portions of high T2 signal internally consistent with areas of necrosis. The tissue immediately surrounding the mass is edematous, and the edema is particularly prominent surrounding the non–mass-like enhancement (*long arrow*) extending anteriorly from the mass. Although not shown, the abnormal axillary lymph node is low in T2 signal and contains no internal fat. **E:** Computer-aided detection (CAD), color overlay. Image at scan plane shown in parts **B** and **C**, now with CAD applied. The *red color* overlying the mass usually indicates areas of rapid washin of contrast. The *blue* and *green* areas are more variable in terms of the types of associated kinetic curves. **F:** MRI, representative kinetic curve. This is the predominant type of kinetic curve generated in this patient when selecting ROI in the *red* portions of the CAD markings shown in part **E**. The curve demonstrates rapid initial washin and plateau-type delayed kinetics. CAD can be used to identify potential lesions and the areas within the lesion likely to have rapid washin and washout kinetic curves. I purposely change the location of the ROI within the mass and scroll in and out of the lesion without changing the position of the ROI.

Breast Magnetic Resonance Imaging

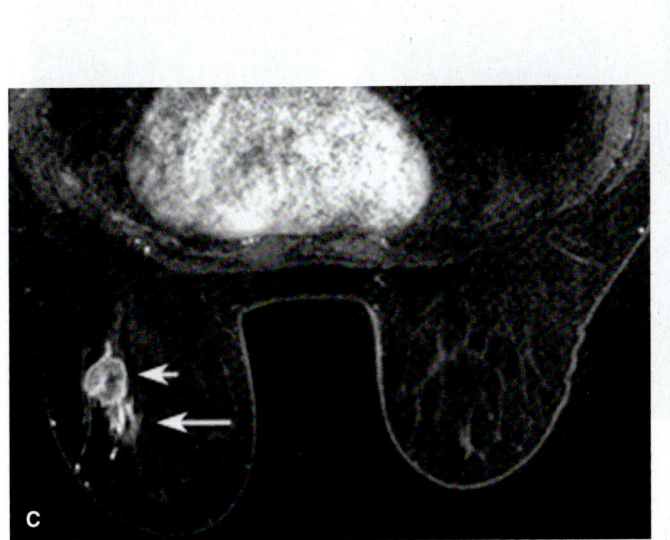

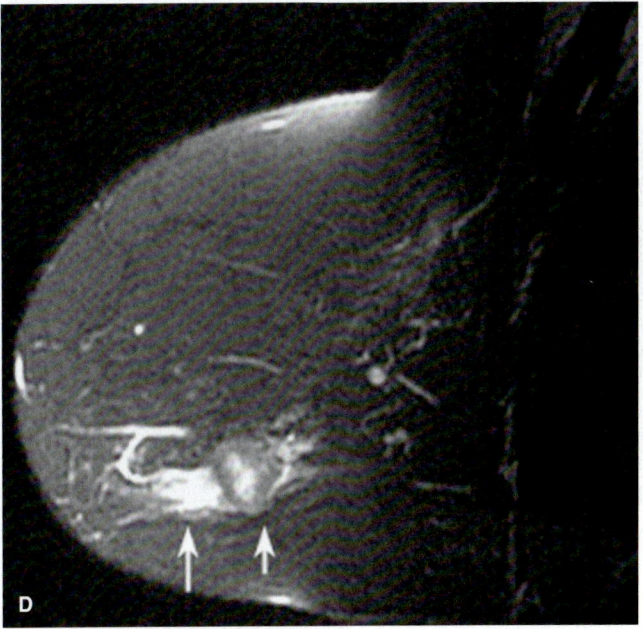

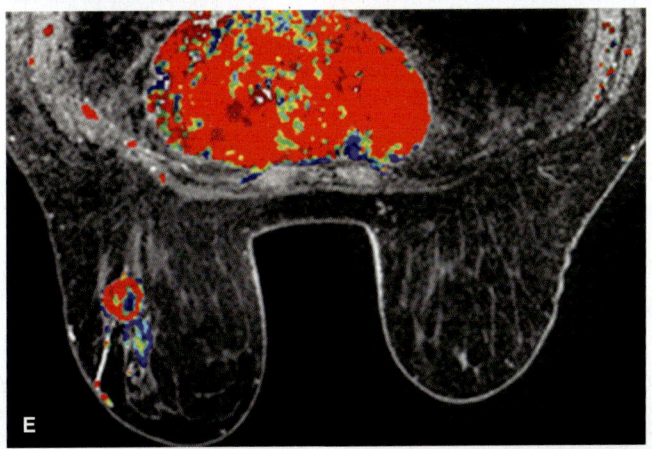

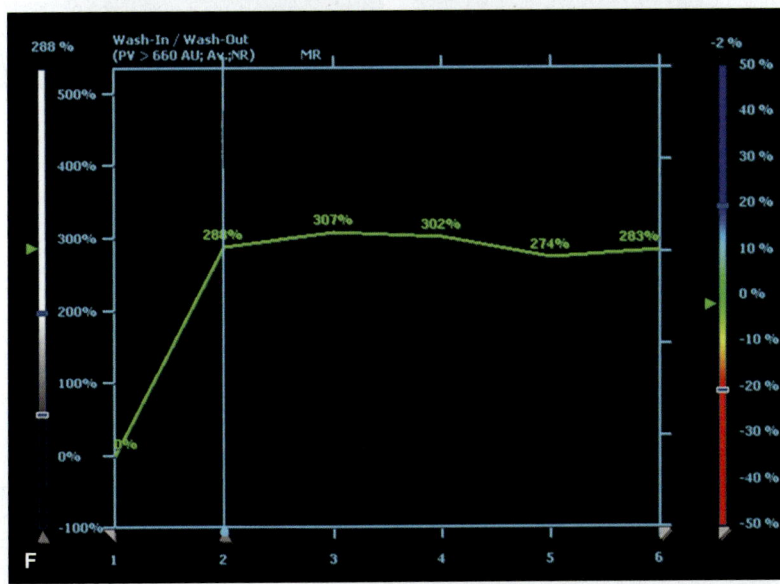

FIG. 5.8 • *(continued)*

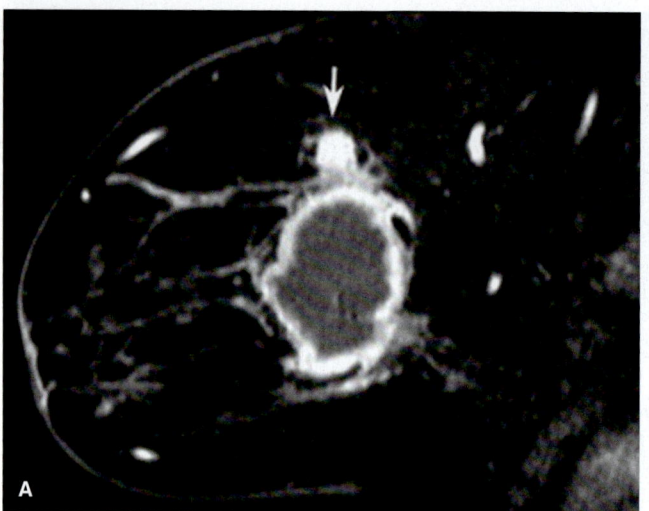 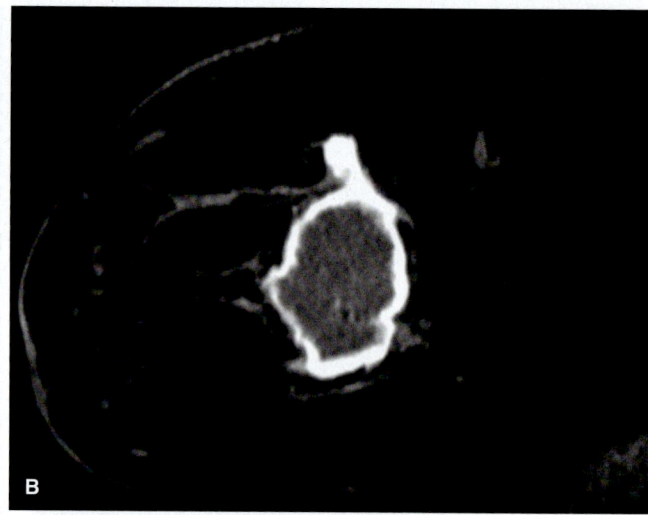

FIG. 5.9 • **Hemorrhage and postoperative fluid collection. A:** MRI, T1-weighted sagittal reconstruction postcontrast. At a quick glance, you might think this is a rim-enhancing mass with an associated enhancing satellite (*arrow*). However, be sure to review the precontrast and subtraction images as well as the kinetic curves in the areas of high T1 signal. **B:** MRI, T1-weighted sagittal reconstruction precontrast. Toggle back and forth between pre- and postcontrast images, review subtraction images, kinetic curves, and T2-weighted images. The T1 signal of the rim of the mass and "satellite" is high precontrast. On the subtraction image (not shown), there is no enhancement. If an ROI is placed on the rim of the mass or the "satellite," the kinetic curve is flat. On sagittal, T2-weighted fat-suppressed images (not shown), a high T2 signal is noted along the rim of this mass as well as the satellite; internally, an intermediate-to-high T2 signal is seen. These findings and imaging characteristics are consistent with hemorrhage at the periphery of a postoperative fluid collection.

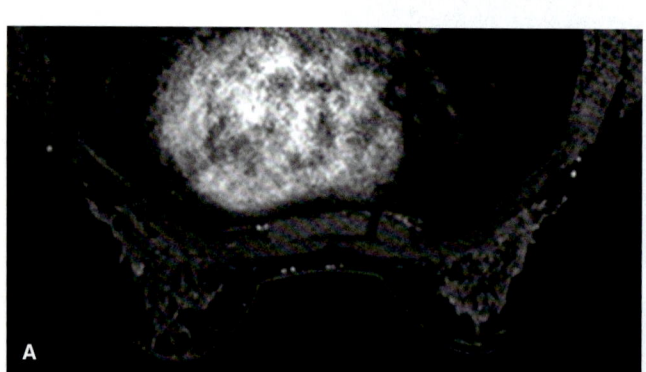 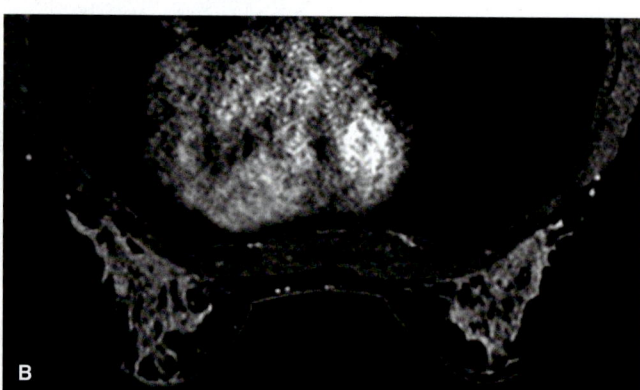

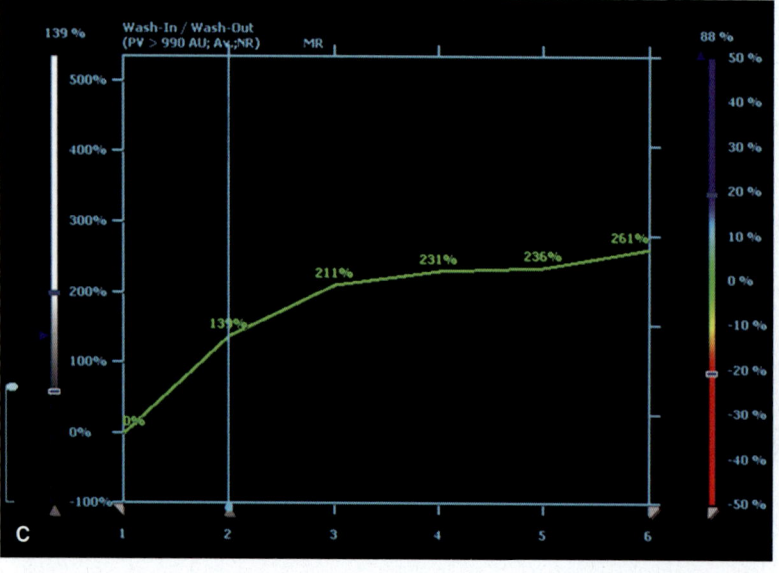

FIG. 5.10 • **Diffuse background parenchymal enhancement. A:** MRI, axial T1-weighted image first time point postcontrast. Minimal enhancement of the parenchyma is apparent at this time. **B:** MRI, axial T1-weighted image, 10 minutes postcontrast administration at the same plane as that shown in part **A**. Diffuse background parenchymal enhancement is present. **C:** MRI, kinetic curve evaluations demonstrate slow initial washin and persistent-type delayed curves bilaterally.

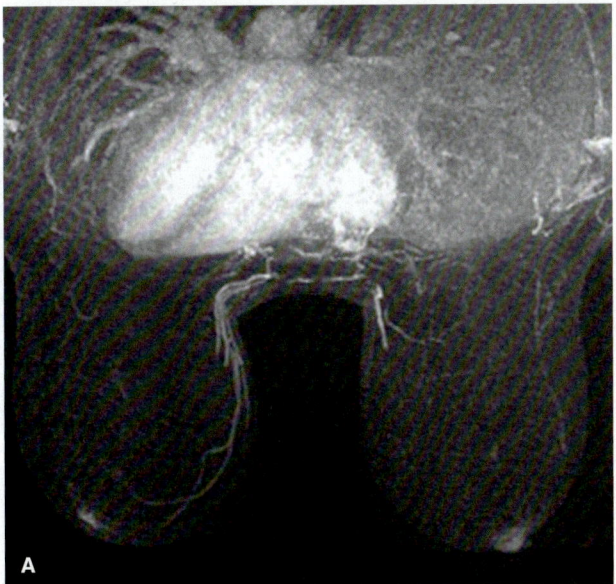
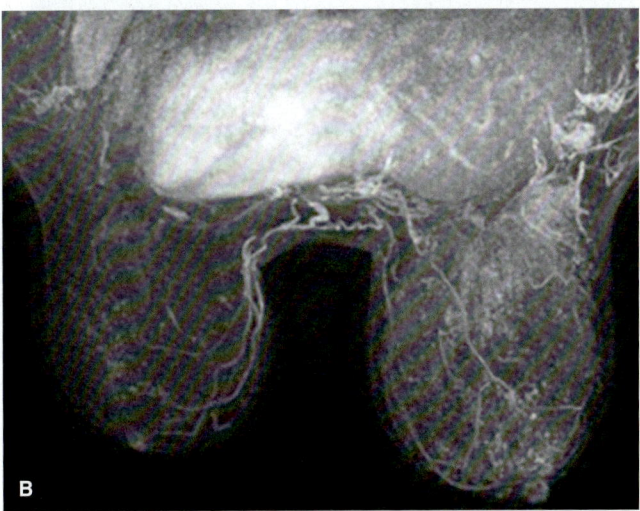

FIG. 5.11 • **Radiation and tamoxifen effect on background parenchymal enhancement. A:** MRI, MIP image in a 30-year-old patient with a history of breast cancer in the left breast treated with lumpectomy and radiation therapy 2 years previously. She was on tamoxifen at the time of this study. The left breast is slightly smaller, consistent with the prior lumpectomy. The breasts are quiescent. **B:** MRI, MIP image 2 years following that shown in part **A**. The patient is no longer on tamoxifen because she is trying to get pregnant. Moderate background parenchymal enhancement is noted diffusely involving the right breast consistent with hormonal effect on the parenchyma following the cessation of tamoxifen. Notice that the left breast remains relatively quiescent, a common observation following radiation therapy.

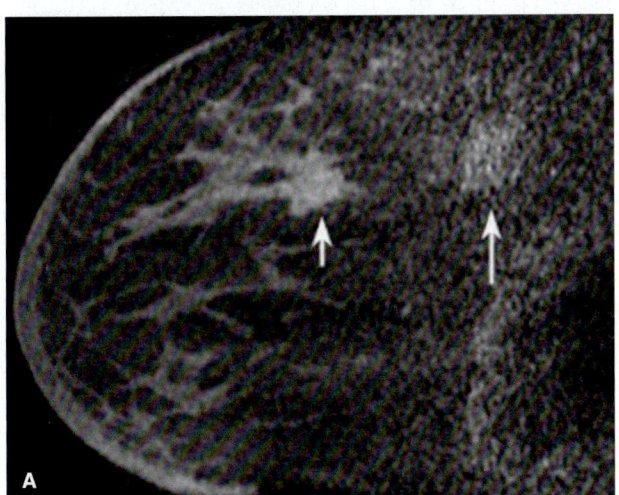
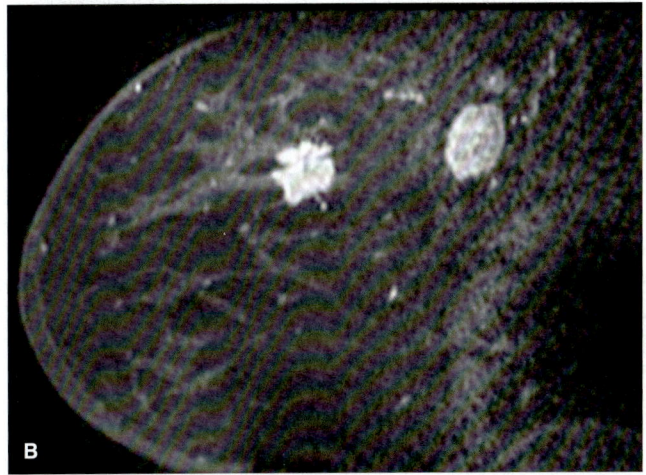

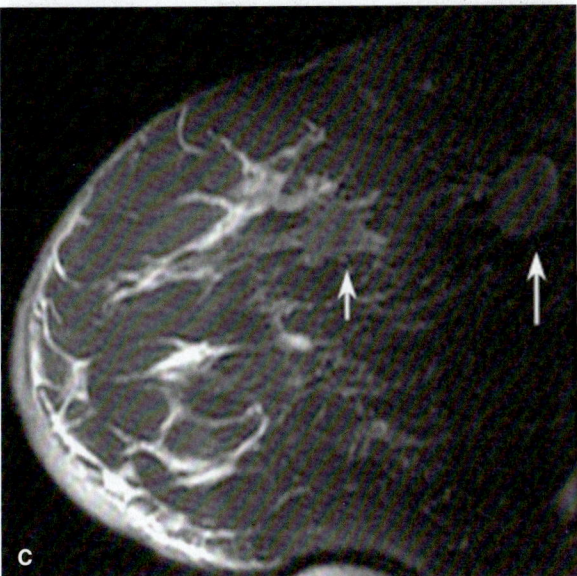

FIG. 5.12 • **Invasive ductal carcinoma, not otherwise specified, with metastatic disease to the axilla. A:** MRI, T1-weighted sagittal reconstruction of the left breast, precontrast in a 50-year-old patient. An irregular mass (*short arrow*) is present in the upper outer quadrant of the left breast posteriorly. A second mass (*long arrow*) is present posteriorly along the chest wall laterally. Note skin thickening anteriorly. **B:** MRI, T1-weighted sagittal reconstruction of the left breast, postcontrast. The irregular mass demonstrates heterogeneous enhancement characterized by rapid washin and washout kinetic curves and spiculated margins. An oval mass with heterogeneous enhancement (stippled) and circumscribed margins is seen posteriorly along the chest wall correlating with known site of metastatic disease to an axillary lymph node. **C:** MRI, T2-weighted sagittal fat-suppressed image of the left breast. The mass (*short arrow*) in the breast demonstrates an intermediate T2 signal. The posterior-most mass (*long arrow*) has no internal fat and is lower in T2 signal than that commonly seen with normal lymph nodes. Skin thickening anteriorly and edematous changes in the subcutaneous tissue and parenchyma are also present.

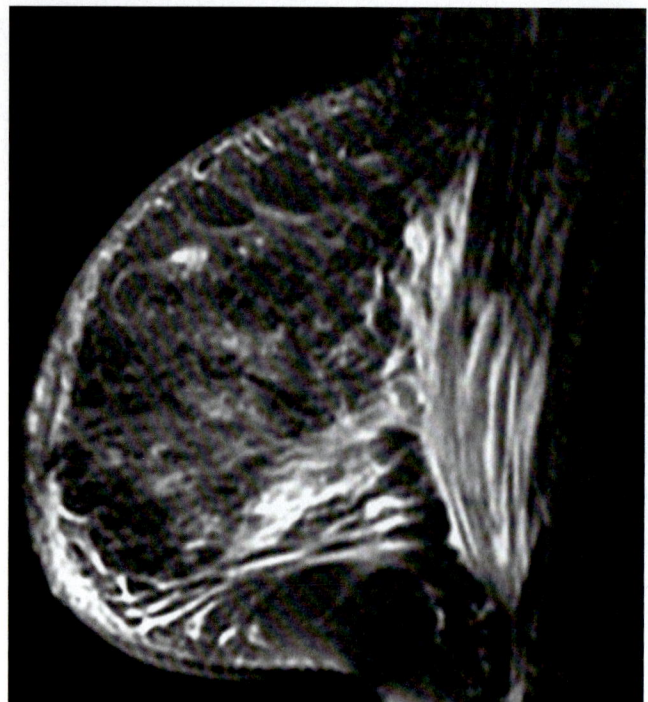

FIG. 5.13 • **Skin thickening and edema extending to the pectoral fascia and pectoral muscle.** MRI, sagittal T2-weighted fat-suppressed image of the left breast demonstrates skin thickening and edematous changes involving the subcutaneous tissue, breast parenchyma, pectoral fascia, and the pectoral muscle. Extensive edematous changes such as these are common associated findings in patients with high-grade invasive lesions. Although it is unknown if there is any significance to this finding, it is likely a poor prognostic indicator.

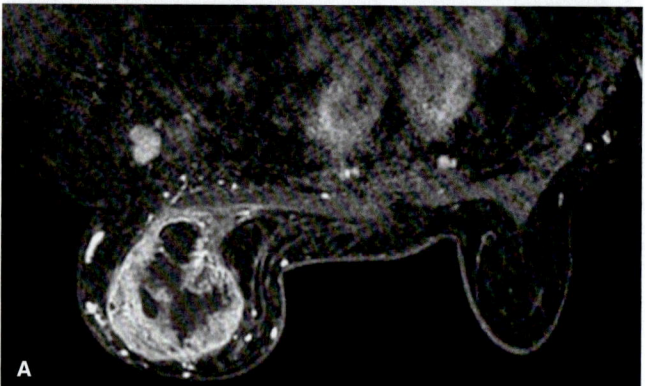

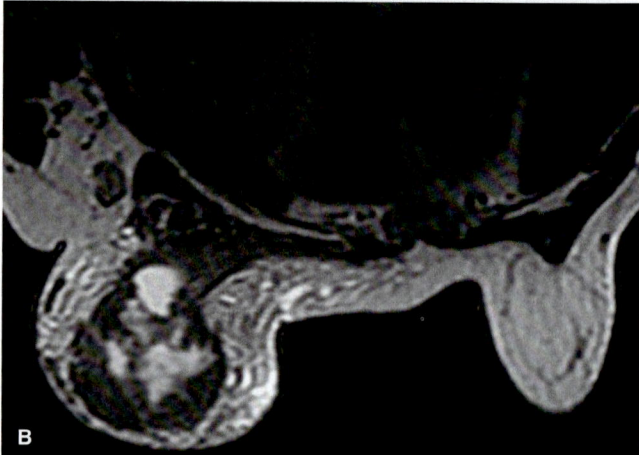

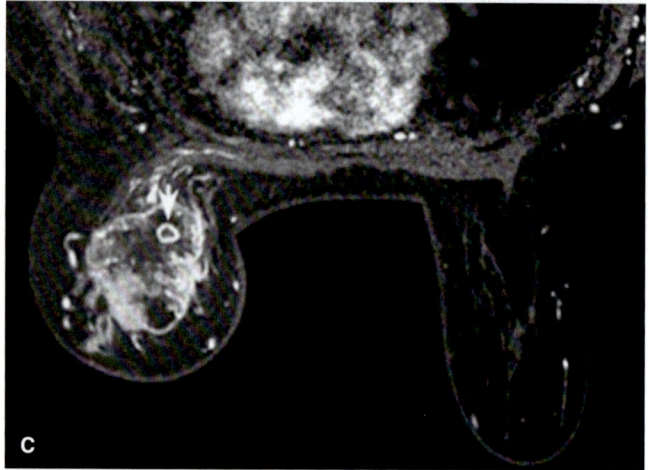

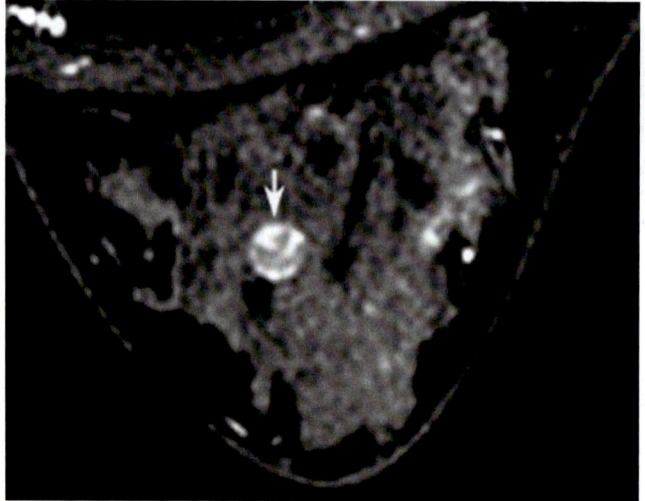

FIG. 5.14 • **Fibroadenoma.** MRI, axial T1-weighted image of the right breast postcontrast. A round mass *(arrow)* with circumscribed margins and nonenhancing internal septations is present centrally in the right breast, consistent with a fibroadenoma. Smooth margins are commonly seen with benign lesions.

FIG. 5.15 • **Invasive ductal carcinomas, high nuclear grade with areas of necrosis.** MRI, axial T1-weighted image postcontrast **(A)** and MRI axial T2-weighted image **(B)**. A mass with heterogeneous enhancement, circumscribed margins, and irregular areas of internal intermediate-to-high T2 signal is present almost completely replacing the left breast at this level. A mass with heterogeneous enhancement, smooth margins, and low T2 signal is also noted in the left axilla consistent with metastatic disease to a lymph node. Edematous changes are also seen in the parenchyma. MRI, axial T1-weighted image postcontrast **(C)** and MRI, sagittal T2-weighted fat-suppressed image of the left breast in a different patient **(D)**. A mass with heterogeneous and central *(arrow* in **C**) enhancement, irregular margins, and areas of intermediate and high T2 signal is present in the upper central aspect of the left breast in zone B and C. Masses that demonstrate homogeneously high T2 signal throughout are often benign. Localized areas of heterogeneous (intermediate to high) T2 signal in masses, however, may indicate necrotic areas in high-grade invasive lesions; they may also be seen in mucinous, metaplastic, and papillary carcinomas or phyllodes tumors.

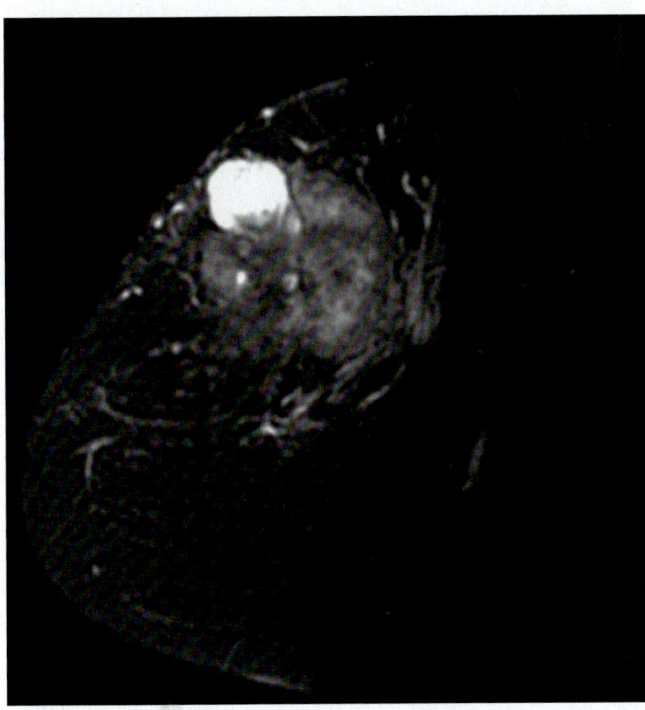

FIG. 5.15 • *(continued)*

may also be seen in myxoid fibroadenomas (see Fig. 7.59) (young fibroadenomas), lymph nodes (Fig. 5.18), and some papillomas (9,10).

Rim enhancement, particularly when the rim is irregularly thickened and spiculated, is usually associated with malignant lesions (Fig. 5.8; also see Figs. 8.17B, 8.27D and 11.33C); however, there are some benign lesions that may demonstrate rim enhancement. Characterization of the internal contents of the mass on additional (T1- and T2-weighted) sequences may be helpful. Smooth and regular rim enhancement may be seen with cysts; this, in conjunction with a homogeneous high T2 signal internally, is diagnostic of cysts (Fig. 5.17A, B; also see Fig. 7.44C, D). Similarly, postoperative fluid collections (see Fig. 11.28C), fat necrosis, and inflammatory (abscess) processes (Fig. 5.17C–E) may demonstrate rim enhancement; however, these also demonstrate high T2 signal, and when correlated with the appropriate history, are not usually a diagnostic dilemma.

Also useful in the assessment of breast masses that are larger than 2 cm in size is the described association of invasive lesions with an enlarged adjacent vessel as well as increased vascularity of the involved breast (Fig 5.8A; also see Figs. 9.15B and 9.21C) (11,12). The adjacent vessel sign is seen in patients with invasive ductal and lobular carcinomas; it is less commonly seen in patients with intraductal lesions. When combined with other lesion features, the adjacent vessel sign and increased ipsilateral vascularity can increase diagnostic accuracy (13) and may be associated with lesions having a poorer prognosis (14). Benign lesions reportedly associated with an adjacent vessel sign include papillomas and phyllodes tumors (15).

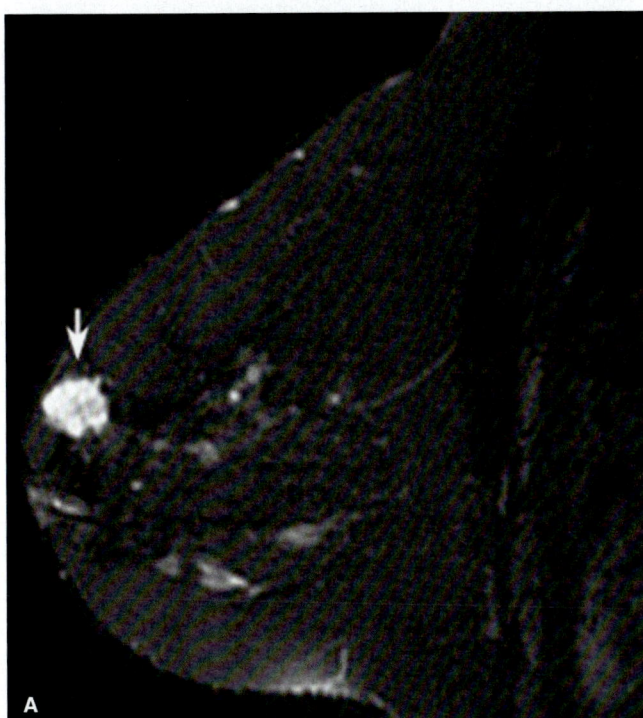

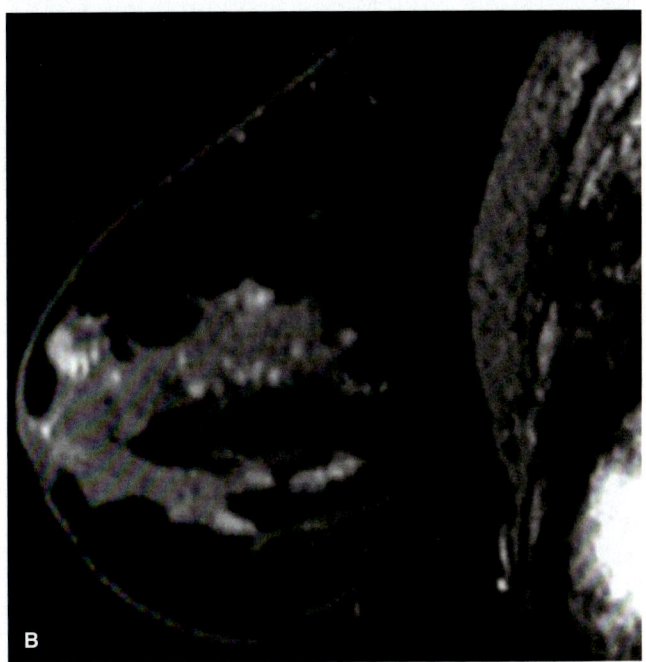

FIG. 5.16 • **Mucinous carcinoma. A:** MRI, sagittal T2-weighted fat-suppressed image of the left breast demonstrates a lobulated mass (*arrow*) with heterogeneously high T2 signal in the superior and anterior aspect of the breast. **B:** MRI, T1-weighted sagittal reconstruction of the left breast, postcontrast. The mass seen in part **A** demonstrates heterogeneous enhancement predominantly inferiorly; type-II (medium washin, plateau delayed) kinetic curves predominate. The superior aspect of the mass does not enhance. Foci of bright signal scattered in the parenchyma are high in signal precontrast (not shown) and do not represent areas of enhancement.

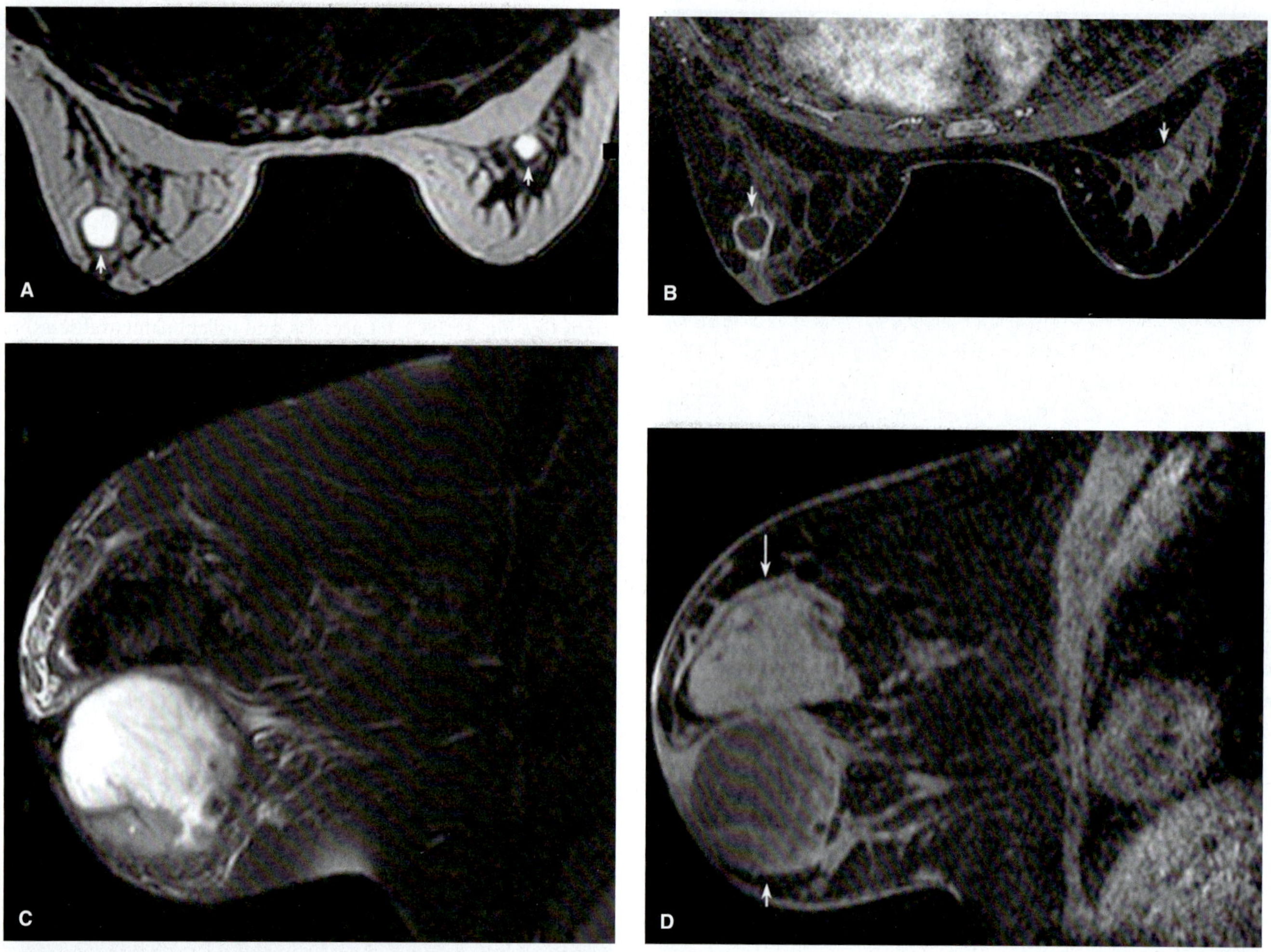

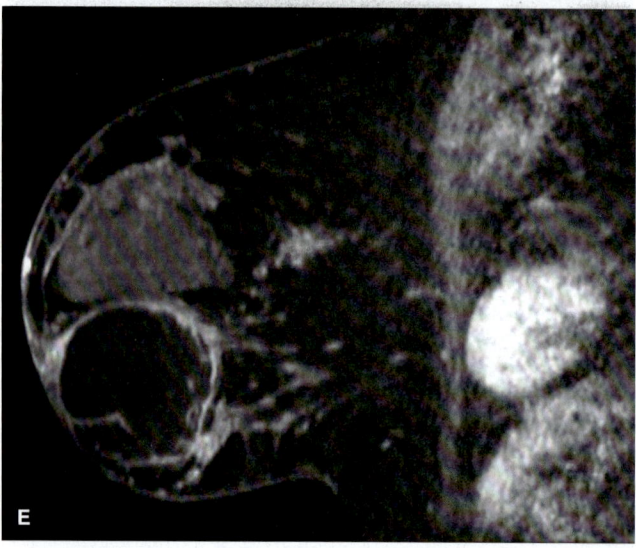

FIG. 5.17 • **Cysts, abscess, and hyalinized fibroadenoma. A:** MRI, axial T2-weighted image. Round masses (*arrows*) with a homogeneously high T2 signal are seen, one in the right breast and another larger one in the left breast. **B:** MRI, axial, T1-weighted image, postcontrast. Rim enhancement is noted involving both masses more prominent on the left than the right. Rim enhancement is sometimes seen with cysts, particularly if inflamed. Signal characteristics, multiplicity of lesions with similar features, and correlation with ultrasound and mammography are all used to confirm the benign etiology of the findings. **C:** MRI, sagittal T2-weighted fat-suppressed image of the left breast on a different patient. Two masses are apparent in the left breast. The superior mass is characterized by a low T2 signal. The inferior mass demonstrates a predominantly heterogeneous high T2 signal with irregular intermediate T2 signal inferiorly and posteriorly. Edema is present subcutaneously and in the parenchyma. MRI, T1-weighted sagittal reconstruction of the left breast, precontrast **(D)** and postcontrast **(E)**. The superior mass (*long arrow*) demonstrates no enhancement and correlates with a biopsy proven hyalinized fibroadenoma. Rim and internal enhancement is seen in the inferior mass (*short arrow*), known to be a subareolar abscess.

Non–mass-like Enhancement

Is the area of enhancement best described as non–mass-like enhancement? This is enhancement that occurs in fibroglandular tissue that appears normal in precontrast images (2,3). No mass effect is identified, and no correlate is usually seen in fat- and non–fat-suppressed T1- and T2-weighted images (Fig. 5.19). This type of enhancement is not a mass or a focus. For this type of enhancement, a distribution modifier (focal, linear, ductal, segmental, regional, multiple regions, or diffuse) should be used, and the features of the enhancement should be characterized (homogeneous, heterogeneous, clumped, or clustered ring) (8). As with masses, the location of the enhancement should be described and, if we think it is related to underlying malignant pathology, we provide a measurement in three planes approximating the amount of tissue encompassed by the enhancement. Kinetic

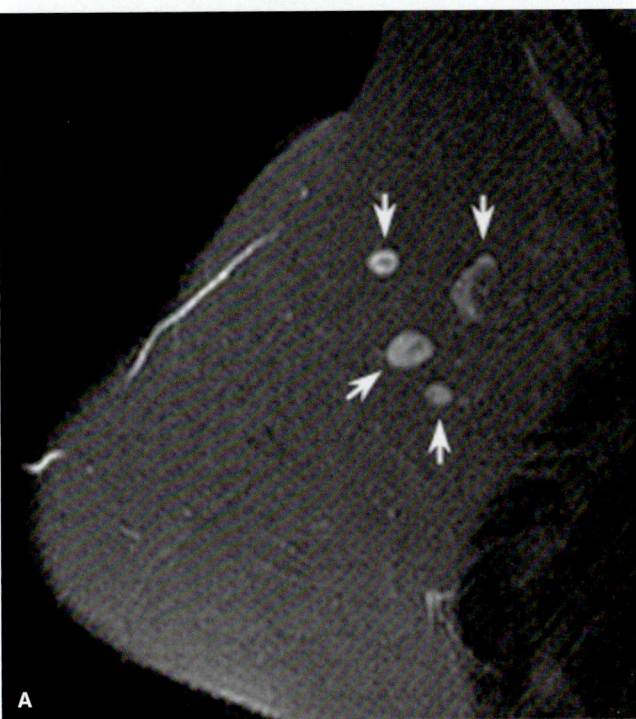

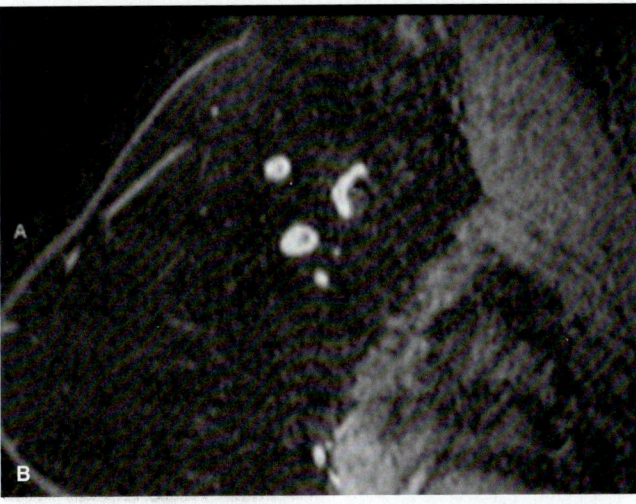

FIG. 5.18 • **Lymph nodes. A:** MRI, sagittal T2-weighted fat-suppressed image. Four masses (*arrows*) demonstrating intermediate-to-high T2 signal, circumscribed margins, and a fatty component are imaged posterolaterally. **B:** MRI, T1-weighted sagittal reconstruction, postcontrast. The masses demonstrate homogeneous enhancement and circumscribed margins. The kinetic curves of most normal lymph nodes simulate that of malignancy with rapid washin and washout of contrast.

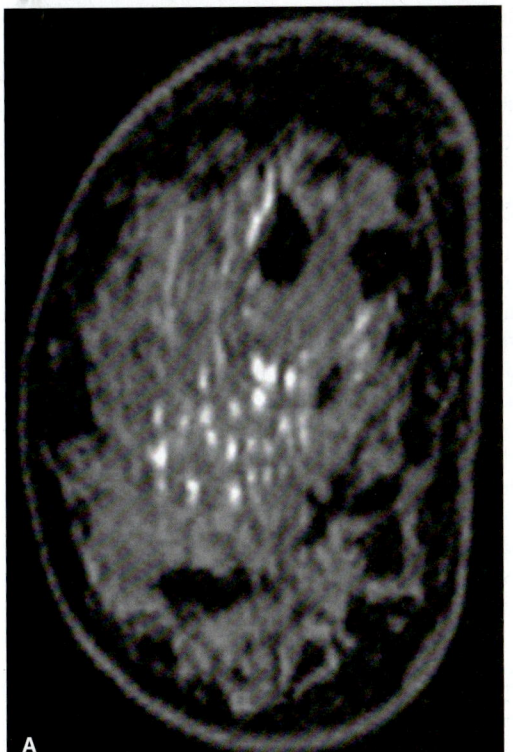

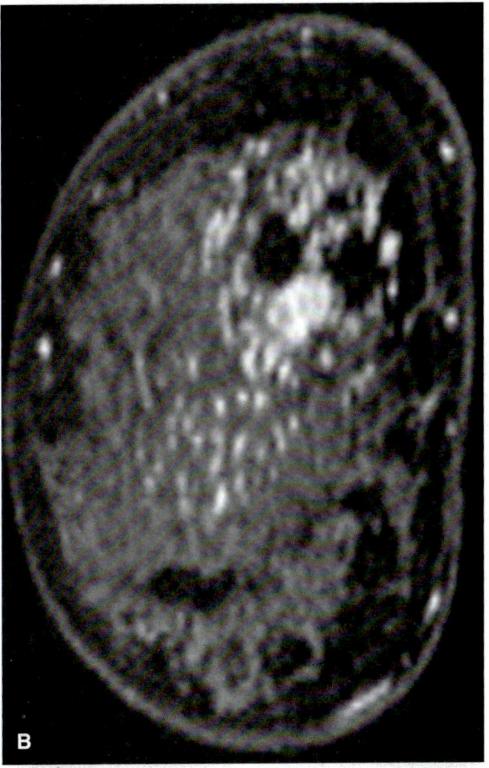

FIG. 5.19 • **Non–mass-like enhancement, invasive ductal carcinoma, and DCIS.** MRI, T1-weighted coronal reconstruction of the right breast precontrast **(A)** and postcontrast **(B)**. On the precontrast image, foci of high T1 signal are noted centrally in the right breast; however, no mass is identified. Non–mass-like enhancement is noted involving the tissue surrounding the foci of high T1 signal precontrast extending segmentally into the upper inner quadrant of the right breast. In establishing enhancement as mass or non–mass-like enhancement, it is critical that the enhancement be evaluated in multiple planes. This patient is diagnosed with invasive ductal carcinoma, high nuclear grade at two separate (distant) sites. Different patient MRI, T1-weighted sagittal reconstruction of the left breast, precontrast **(C)** and postcontrast **(D)**. On the precontrast image, foci of high T1 signal are noted predominantly in the inferior aspect of the left breast. No mass is identified. Non–mass-like heterogeneous, clumped, and linear enhancement is noted diffusely involving the tissue. This patient is diagnosed with invasive ductal carcinoma, high nuclear grade (triple negative) at two separate (distant) sites, and DCIS. No residual tumor is identified histologically following neoadjuvant therapy (e.g., complete pathological response, pCR), and no metastatic disease is reported on sampled axillary lymph nodes (0/24 LNs).

(continued)

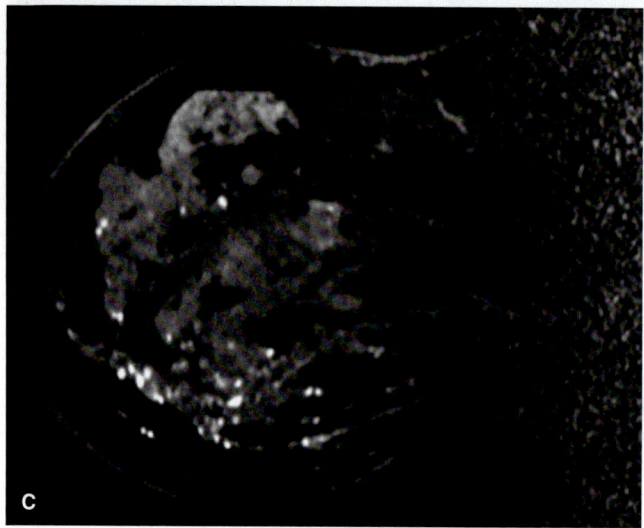
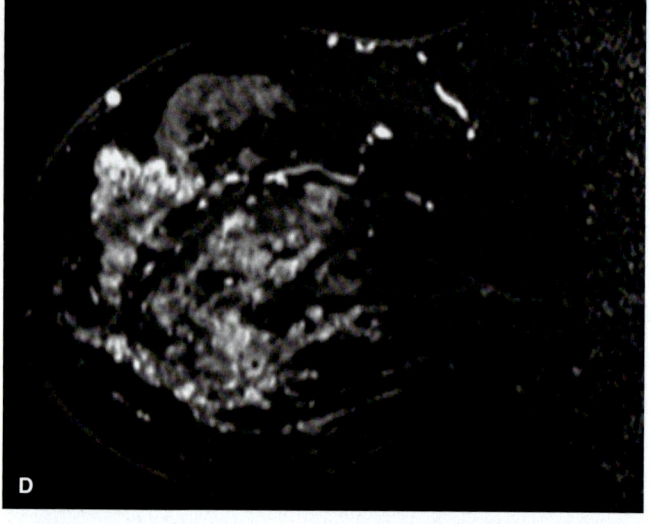

FIG. 5.19 • *(continued)*

curve evaluation in this type of lesion is not usually helpful and may be misleading. The main differential with this type of enhancement is between DCIS (see Fig. 8.22B) or diffuse breast cancer (e.g., invasive lobular) and benign changes, including proliferative fibrocystic changes related to hormonal effect on normal breast parenchyma or an inflammatory process (2,3,9,10). With this type of potentially abnormal enhancement, comparison with the contralateral breast is helpful. If there is non–mass-like enhancement bilaterally, particularly if symmetric, it is more likely to be related to a benign process.

That some DCIS lesions enhance (and the possible biologic significance of this feature of some DCIS lesions) is the subject of much discussion. If DCIS is an intraductal process, why does it enhance, and how can this be explained? Is it likely that enhancing DCIS lesions are prognostically different from those that do not enhance? In considering these observations, Dr. L. Tabar (personal communication) has suggested the possibility that some DCIS lesions are actually invasive lesions that make abnormal ductal structures (e.g., ductogenesis). More recently, on the basis of elegant studies using x-ray fluorescence microscopy and a murine model for DCIS, Jansen and colleagues (16) have shown that the enhancement associated with some DCIS lesions is related to the presence of gadolinium in the DCIS-containing ducts and is not intravascular. They postulate that gadolinium egresses from the intravascular to the extravascular interstitial space and then, as a result of an abnormally permeable basement membrane of some DCIS-containing ducts, gadolinium diffuses into the intraductal space. This theory is consistent with clinical observations regarding the enhancement pattern of DCIS in comparison with that seen with invasive lesions. The enhancement of most DCIS lesions is less than that seen with invasive lesions, and washout is not common. The possibility that the lack of enhancement in some DCIS lesions may be prognostically significant (17) is intriguing and may help advance our understanding of which DCIS lesions require aggressive treatment (e.g., those with enhancement). It may help us identify a subset of patients in whom DCIS can be followed or treated more conservatively.

Focus

Lastly, can the identified enhancement be characterized as a "focus," defined as an area of enhancement measuring less than 0.5 cm (18)? These are often bilateral, multiple, and randomly distributed, likely reflecting sites of focal proliferative fibrocystic changes (Fig. 5.20).

In many patients, these are often associated with small cystic areas on the T2-weighted images. The use of the term focus should not be thought of as implying an underlying benign process but rather recognition that the spatial resolution does not permit further characterization. The management of patients with one or multiple foci should be based on other findings bilaterally, T2 signal characteristics of the tissue surrounding the foci, as well as correlation with history, clinical and mammographic findings.

INDICATIONS FOR BREAST MRI

The indications for breast MRI are evolving, actively being evaluated, and some remain controversial. Indications include preoperative staging evaluation of patients with a new diagnosis of breast cancer, monitoring the effects of neoadjuvant therapy on the tumor, searching for an underlying breast primary in patients with metastatic disease to the axilla and no known primary site, assessment of residual disease in patients with positive margins at the time of the lumpectomy, evaluation of women with implants, screening women with a 20% or higher lifetime risk for breast cancer (using BRCAPRO or Tyrer–Cuzick risk models), problem solving in select patients with equivocal clinical and imaging findings, and assessing the presence of a recurrence in women with equivocal changes (e.g., scar versus recurrence) at a prior lumpectomy site (2,9,10,19).

EVALUATION OF PATIENTS WITH A NEW DIAGNOSIS OF BREAST CANCER

MRI in this group of patients may demonstrate additional sites of disease in the ipsilateral breast (multifocal, multicentric) in as many as 20% to 25% of patients (Figs. 5.21 and 5.22; also see Figs. 8.9C, 8.13B and 8.16C), unsuspected disease in the contralateral breast in 3% to 6% of patients (Fig. 5.23; also see Fig. 8.17B) (2,19–22), metastatic disease to intramammary (see Fig. 8.58E), axillary or internal mammary lymph nodes (Fig. 5.24), and chest wall (Figs. 5.24 and 5.25) or skin involvement (see Fig. 9.14C). If the extent of disease can be accurately established preoperatively, surgical management may be altered. In some patients, a wider excision to encompass all of the disease may reduce the need for re-excisions for positive margins. In others, the extent and distribution of disease, or the presence of histologically proven multicentricity, may indicate the need for mastectomy (Fig. 5.26);

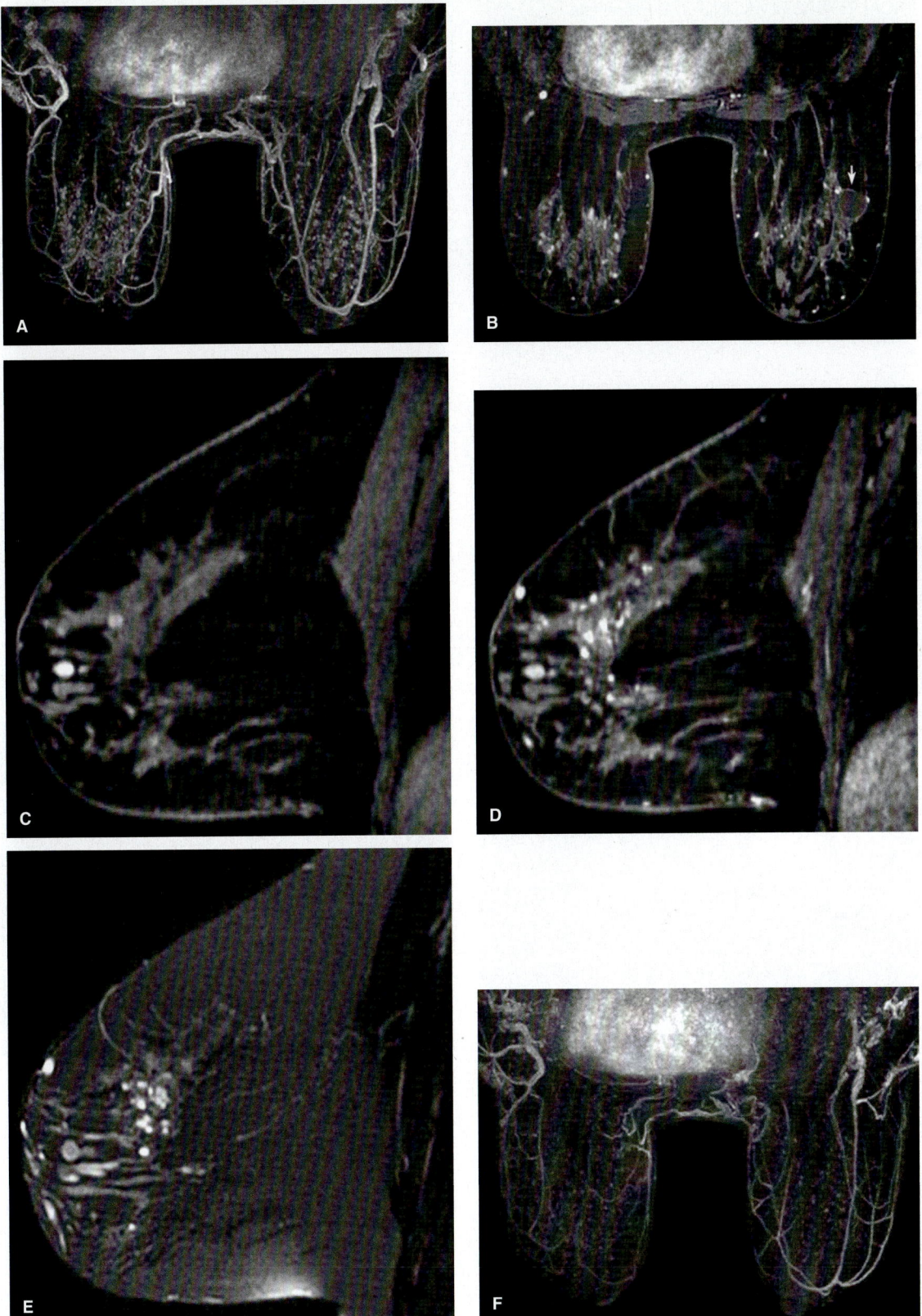

FIG. 5.20 • **Foci, cysts, duct ectasia. A:** MRI, MIP image. Multiple foci of nonspecific enhancement are present bilaterally superimposed on a background of parenchymal enhancement. **B:** MRI axial T1-weighted image, postcontrast image. Multiple foci of enhancement are present randomly distributed in the breast parenchyma. A cyst (*arrow*) is seen in the right breast with some foci of nonspecific enhancement in the surrounding tissue (T2 image not shown here). **C:** MRI, T1-weighted image, sagittal reconstruction, right breast precontrast. Ductal dilation and some cysts are imaged at this scan plane. **D:** MRI, T1-weighted image, sagittal reconstruction, right breast postcontrast at the same plane as that shown in part **B**. Foci of nonspecific enhancement are apparent, randomly distributed in the tissue. **E:** MRI, T2-weighted fat-suppressed images, right breast at the same plane as that shown in parts **B** and **C**. The foci are seen in the tissue surrounding micro and macrocystic changes. **F:** MRI, MIP image one year prior to that shown in part **A**. Based on the time of the study with respect to the menstrual cycle, more or less background enhancement and foci can be seen. Also note changes in the prominence of the vasculature bilaterally.

alternatively, depending on the size and location of the lesions relative to the size of the breast, breast conservation with two separate lumpectomies (Fig. 5.22B, C) may be considered. If a significant amount of tissue is involved and disease is proven histologically, these patients may be better served with mastectomy (Figs. 5.19 and 5.26; also see Fig. 8.46C). Also, the identification of metastatic disease to internal mammary lymph nodes (Fig. 5.24) or chest wall involvement (Figs. 5.24 and 5.25) affects the staging of patients and may lead to a change in management plans; neoadjuvant therapy may be a more appropriate treatment for patients with metastatic disease to internal mammary lymph nodes, and resection of at least a portion of the pectoral muscle may be indicated in those with muscle involvement.

Additionally, knowing the extent of disease, or that there is likely to be multicentric disease, may appropriately alter plans for partial breast irradiation (brachytherapy).

Preoperative breast MRI in women with a new breast cancer is particularly helpful in patients with dense tissue (Fig. 5.26) (however, it is important to note that extensive mammographically occult disease can also be found in patients who do not have dense tissue), those with a diagnosis of invasive lobular carcinoma, or in patients with invasive ductal carcinoma having an extensive intraductal component. In these groups of patients, our ability to delineate the extent of disease on a mammogram or ultrasound may be limited. Clinical, mammographic, and ultrasound evaluation of patients

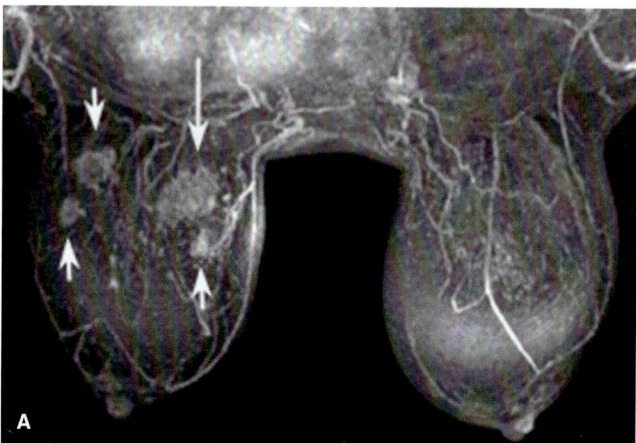

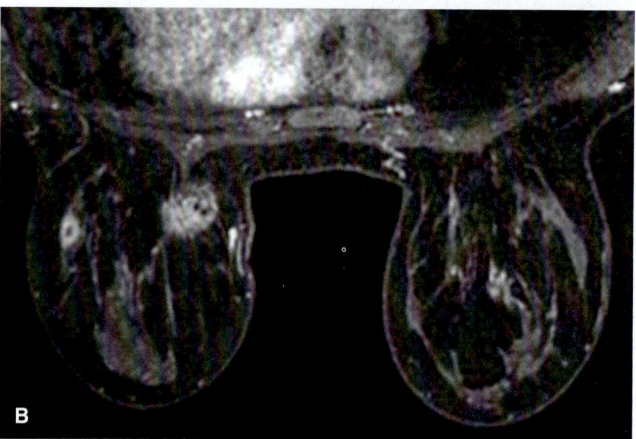

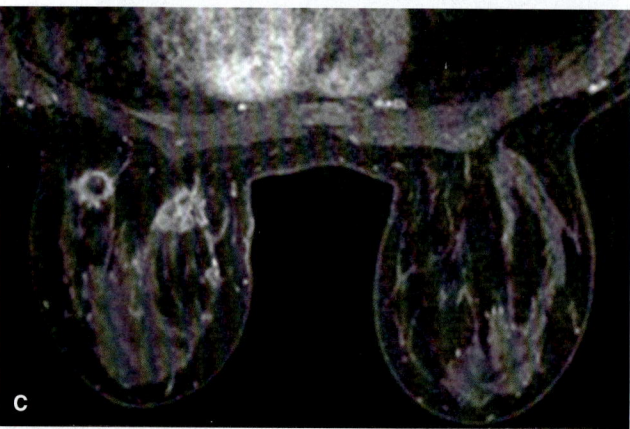

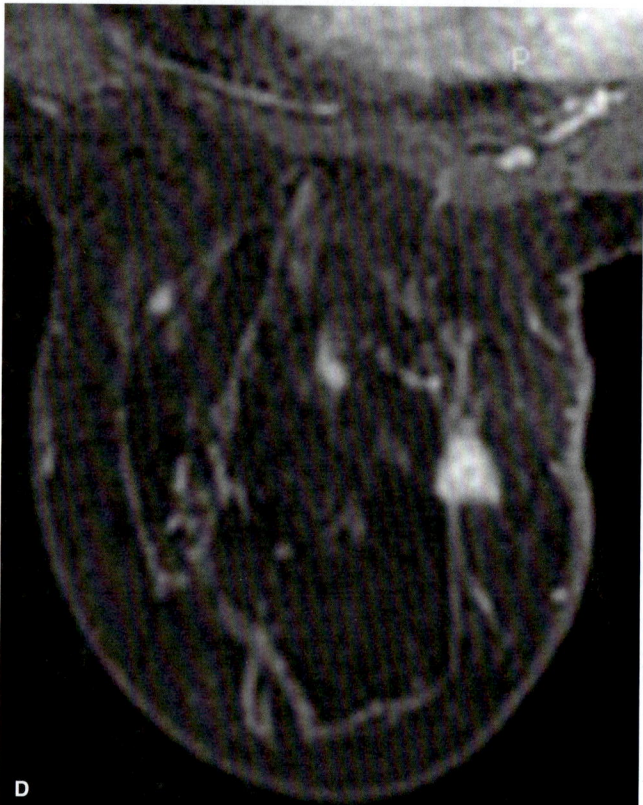

FIG. 5.21 • **Multifocal and multicentric disease. A:** MRI, MIP image. In addition to the patient's known site of invasive ductal carcinoma (*long arrow*), three additional masses (*short arrows*) are identified in the left breast (see Fig. 2.46 for screening images, Fig. 3.7 for spot compression, and Fig. 4.39D for ultrasound image on this patient). **B:** MRI, axial T1-weighted image, postcontrast. Two masses with heterogeneous enhancement are imaged at this level. The medial lesion is further characterized by spiculated margins and correlates with the site of the patient's known, screen-detected invasive ductal carcinoma. The lateral lesion at this level is the more anterior of the two masses seen laterally in the MIP image and demonstrates rim enhancement. **C:** MRI, axial T1-weighted image, postcontrast. The known cancer is still apparent medially on this image. The second of two lateral lesions is seen at this level; it is characterized by rim enhancement and spiculated margins. It is biopsied to confirm suspected multicentric disease. **D:** MRI, axial T1-weighted image, postcontrast. The second of two lesions demonstrated on MRI in the medial aspect of the left breast is imaged demonstrating central enhancement. For those opposed to the routine use of MRI in patients with a new breast cancer diagnosis: Do we really not want to know that this patient has three additional invasive lesions in the left breast? This patient needs a mastectomy, and to suggest that going from the planned lumpectomy to a mastectomy is wrong makes no sense.

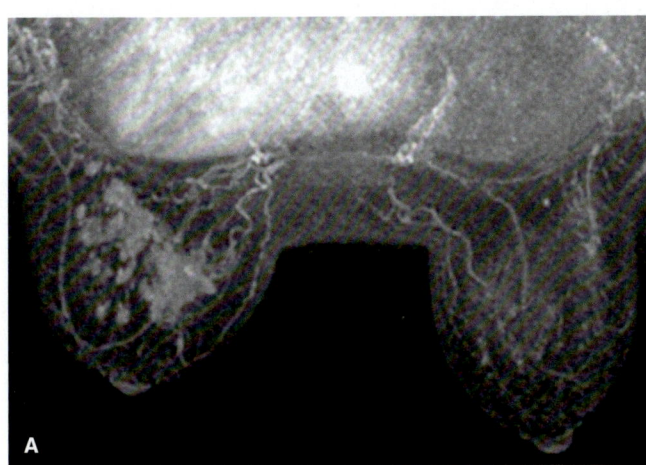
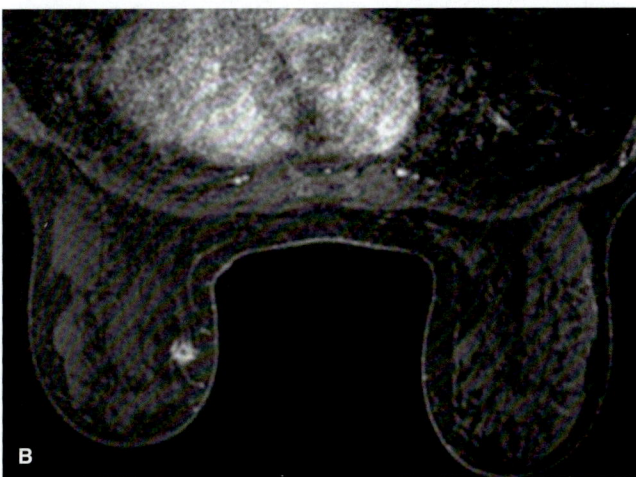
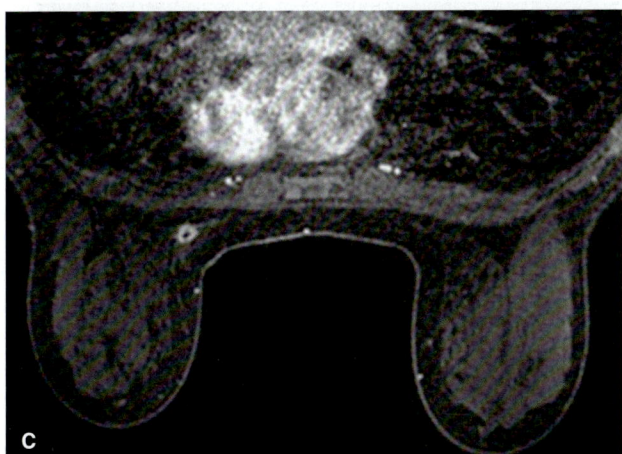

FIG. 5.22 • **Extent of disease and multicentric disease. A:** MRI, MIP in a patient with known invasive lobular carcinoma in the upper inner quadrant of the left breast (see Fig. 2.44 for screening images and Fig. 3.13 for the diagnostic evaluation). In this patient, the mammogram underestimates the extent of disease. Non–mass-like enhancement is apparent extending from the upper inner quadrant of the left breast into the lateral quadrants. The extent of the disease into the lateral quadrants is confirmed on an ultrasound-guided biopsy of a mass identified on second look ultrasound laterally. Given the extent of histologically proven disease, this patient is best served by a mastectomy. **B:** Different patient. MRI, axial T1-weighted image, postcontrast. A round mass with heterogeneous enhancement and spiculated margins is imaged medially in the left breast, zone B corresponding to the site of the patient's known invasive ductal carcinoma with lobular features (ER and PR receptor-positive, HER2/neu positive). **C:** MRI, axial T1-weighted image, postcontrast at a different level than that shown in part **B**. A second mass with rim enhancement and spiculated margins is imaged posteromedially in the left breast. An invasive ductal carcinoma, intermediate-to-high nuclear grade is diagnosed on an ultrasound-guided biopsy. Given normal intervening tissue on MRI, two lumpectomies are done followed by whole breast radiation.

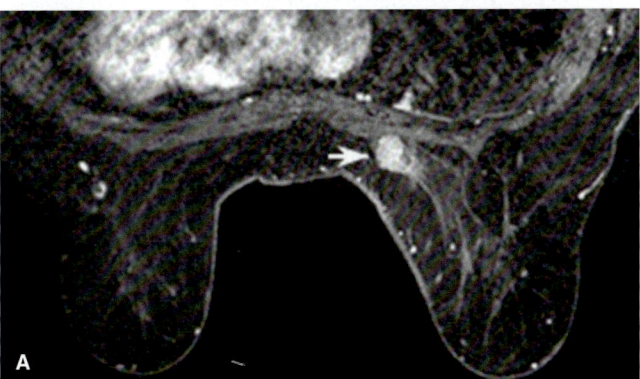
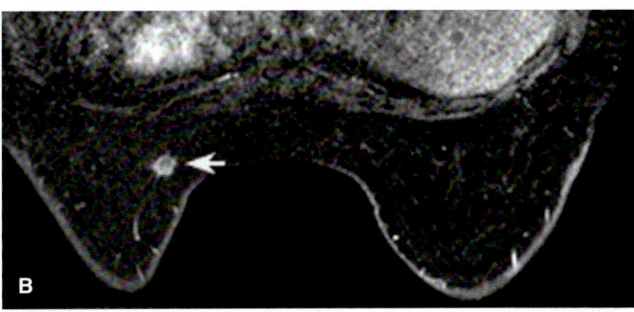

FIG. 5.23 • **Synchronous bilateral disease. A:** MRI, axial T1-weighted image, postcontrast. An oval mass (*arrow*) with heterogeneous enhancement and lobulated margins is imaged in the posteromedial aspect of the right breast abutting the pectoral muscle. This mass is palpable and known to represent a papillary carcinoma with foci of microinvasion. An intramammary lymph node is present in the left breast posterolaterally. **B:** MRI, axial T1-weighted image postcontrast at a different level from that shown in part **A**. A rim-enhancing mass with spiculated margins is detected in the lower inner aspect of the left breast posteriorly. An invasive ductal carcinoma, low nuclear grade is diagnosed on an ultrasound-guided core biopsy.

with invasive lobular carcinoma underestimates the extent of disease in 50%, 70%, and 80% respectively. In patients with invasive lobular carcinoma, additional ipsilateral disease may be identified on MRI in as many as 32% of patients, and contralateral disease in as many as 7% of patients (19).

This use of MRI remains controversial. Multifocality and multicentricity preceded the widespread use of breast MRI. Opponents argue that traditional treatment approaches (e.g., lumpectomy and radiation therapy) have proven successful in patients, some of whom have presumably had multifocal and multicentric disease. They also point to

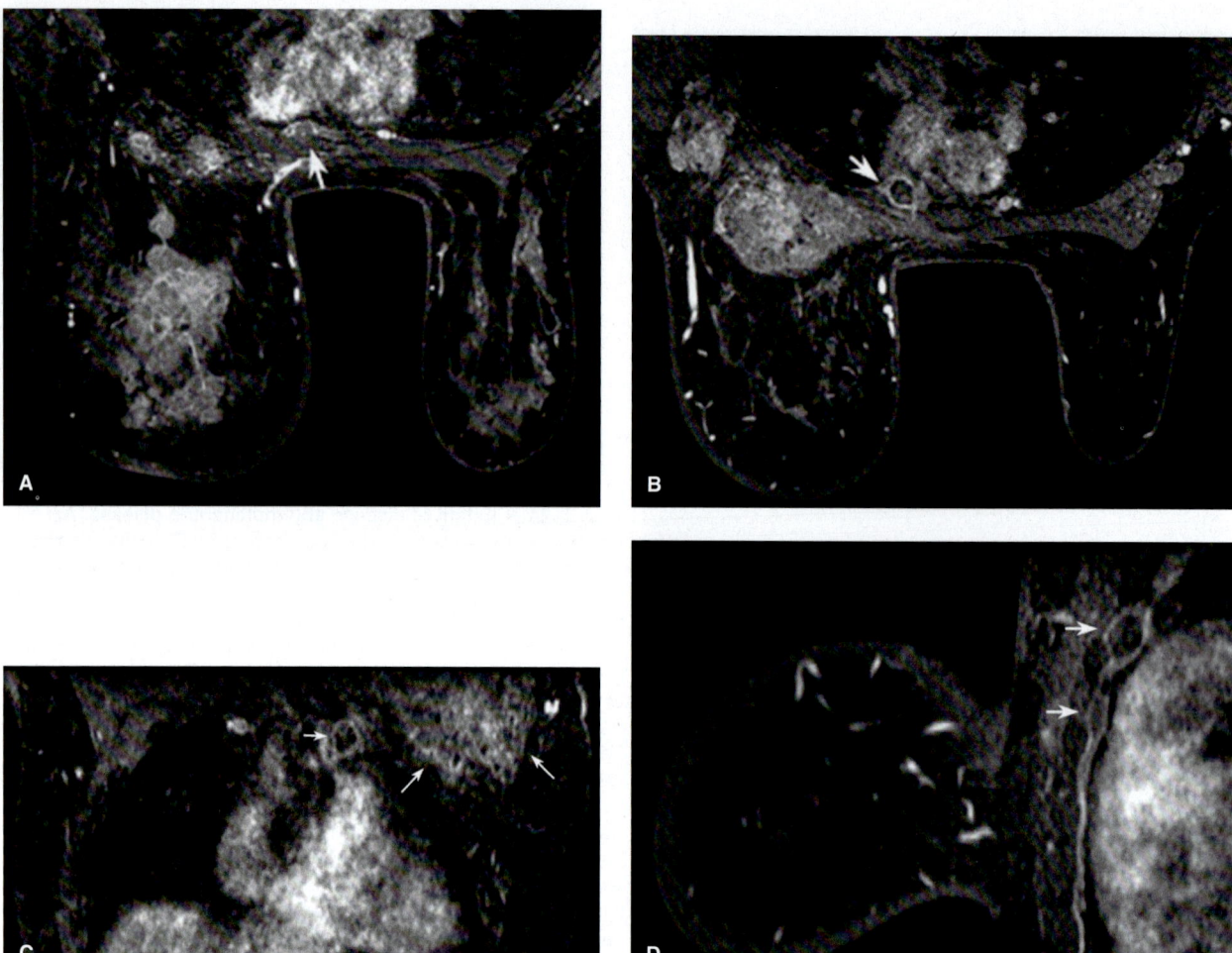

FIG. 5.24 • **Extent of disease, chest wall involvement, internal mammary adenopathy, and matted axillary lymph nodes. A:** MRI, axial T1-weighted image, postcontrast. The left breast is larger and thicker than the right. Multiple lobulated confluent masses with heterogeneous enhancement and irregular margins are imaged centrally in the left breast extending from zone A into zone C. At this level, round areas of enhancement are also noted in the pectoral muscle, and a necrotic internal mammary lymph node (*arrow*) is present. **B:** MRI, axial T1-weighted image, postcontrast superior to the image shown in part A. The pectoral muscle is enlarged, thickened, and enhanced, reflecting replacement with tumor at this level. Matted lymph nodes with heterogeneous enhancement are present in the left axilla, and another necrotic internal mammary lymph node (*arrow*) is noted at this level. **C:** MRI, T1-weighted image, coronal reconstruction postcontrast. A necrotic internal mammary lymph node (*short arrow*) is again noted, as is the replacement of the left pectoral muscle (*long arrows*) with tumor. **D:** MRI, T1-weighted image, sagittal reconstruction along the left internal mammary chain postcontrast. Necrotic internal mammary lymph nodes (*arrows*) are confirmed at two separate levels; note diffuse skin thickening. When evaluating complex disease, multiplanar reconstructions are critical in establishing extent of disease. Histologically, this is an invasive ductal carcinoma, high nuclear grade, ER and PR receptor-negative and HER2/neu negative (e.g., triple negative).

the fact that the likelihood of local recurrence does not approximate the frequency with which MRI detects additional sites of this disease (e.g., multifocal and multicentric disease did not start with the advent of breast MRI). False-positive MRIs resulting in the need for additional biopsies and delays in definitive therapy while the imaging evaluation is completed are additional concerns raised regarding the use of MRI preoperatively for staging patients with a new cancer diagnosis. Lastly, there is concern that a greater number of patients will elect mastectomy over conservative therapy when told of additional disease, and yet we have few data on the impact of this additional disease on overall survival.

As the opposition to evaluating patients with known breast cancer preoperatively with breast MRI continues, it is disconcerting to want to knowingly ignore the potential information that MRI can provide regarding the extent of disease, presence of multicentricity and contralateral disease. By not doing MRIs in these patients, we can certainly avoid the difficult management issues raised by the detection of additional invasive disease, but does this not imply that invasive cancer should be managed differently on the basis of the detection method? If we think surgical excision is required for a clinically or mammographically detected cancer, is it not also the required treatment for MRI-detected invasive disease? Why would we not want to know whether the patient has more than one site of invasive disease? These arguments against MRI also seem particularly perplexing when you consider the attention we have traditionally given to "positive" margins at the time of a lumpectomy. Re-excision is "required" if the margins are focally positive following a lumpectomy, yet we are

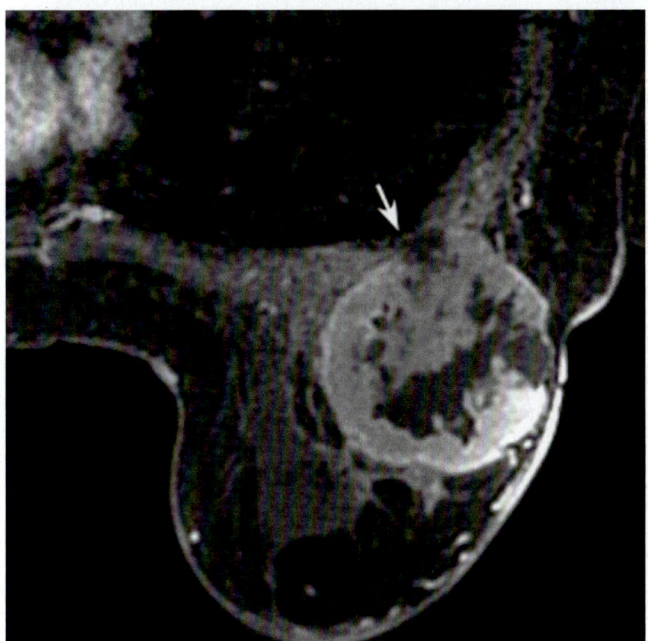

FIG. 5.25 • **Chest wall involvement, invasive ductal carcinoma, high nuclear grade.** MRI, axial T1-weighted image of the right breast postcontrast. A round mass with heterogeneous enhancement and areas of necrosis (T2-weighted images not shown) is present extending into the lateral aspect of the pectoral muscle and chest wall *(arrow)*.

willing to potentially leave invasive disease behind by not looking for it with a study (MRI) we know may identify that disease. How does this make sense? As already stated, we schedule breast MRI on all of our patients with a new breast cancer diagnosis, and we do everything possible to expedite scheduling, so, if additional imaging or a biopsy is required, we minimize the likelihood of a significant delay in definitive treatment.

EVALUATION OF PATIENTS WITH METASTATIC DISEASE TO THE AXILLA BUT NO KNOWN PRIMARY

The evaluation of patients who present with a palpable finding in an axilla, or those with a screen-detected abnormality in the axilla (Fig. 5.27), includes a careful review of their mammogram, particularly the ipsilateral breast, spot tangential or compression views of the finding in the axilla, correlative physical examination, and ultrasound. Depending on the clinical and imaging findings, an ultrasound-guided fine needle aspiration or, more commonly, core biopsy of an abnormal axillary lymph node can be done to establish a diagnosis.

Among the women diagnosed with breast cancer, less than 1% present with metastatic disease to the axilla with an otherwise normal physical examination and mammogram. These patients are generally presumed to have an occult breast primary. Treatment in these patients is variable but has included axillary nodal dissection and radiation therapy to the breast or axillary nodal dissection and mastectomy. Although increased recurrence rates have been reported in patients undergoing axillary dissection and radiation therapy, the overall 5-year survival is comparable in the two groups. In patients

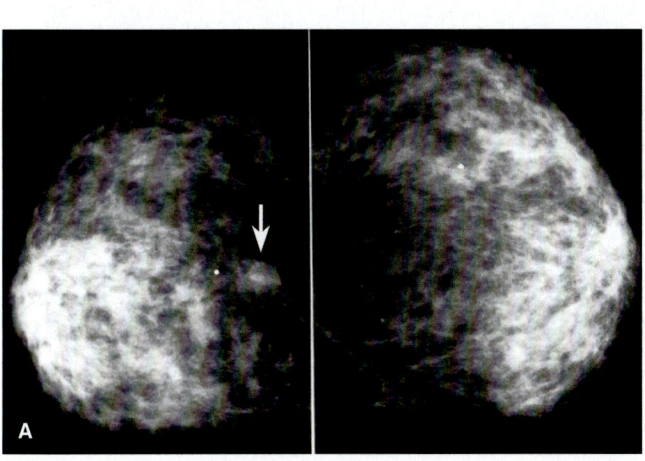

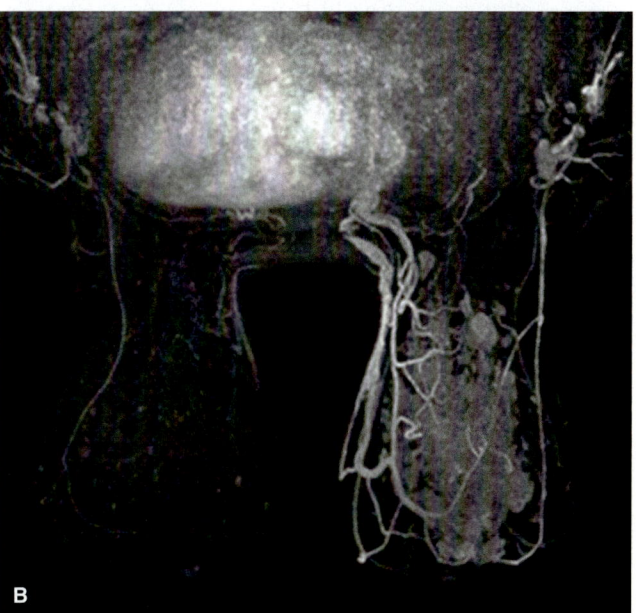

FIG. 5.26 • **Dense tissue and extent of disease. A:** Craniocaudal views in a 49-year-old patient who presents describing a new "lump" in the upper central aspect of the right breast posteriorly. A mass *(arrow)* is seen correlating with the site of the palpable finding. An invasive ductal carcinoma, high nuclear grade, is diagnosed on an ultrasound-guided core biopsy. This patient's previous mammogram, 7 months ago is "normal." **B:** MRI, MIP. Confluent masses with heterogeneous enhancement are identified throughout the upper quadrants of the right breast. In these patients, it is important to obtain histological confirmation of the extent of the disease. The patient is reevaluated with ultrasound, and a mass in the anterior aspect of the breast is biopsied to confirm the diagnosis. Although one might have initially entertained conservative therapy, given the extent of the disease demonstrated on MRI, this patient had neoadjuvant therapy followed by a mastectomy. No metastatic disease is reported in 13 lymph nodes (0/13 LNs). Also note the increased vascularity involving the right breast.

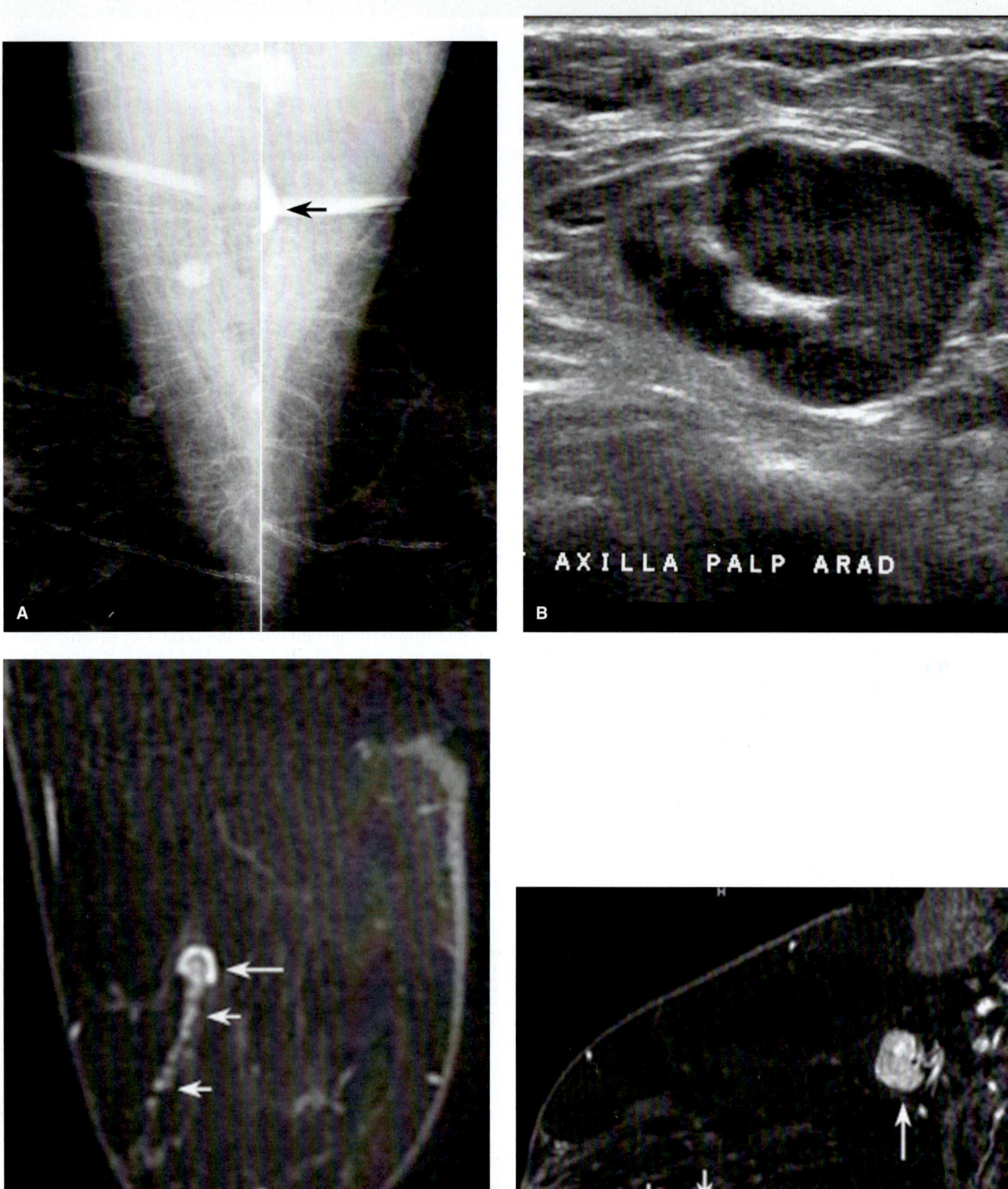

FIG. 5.27 • **Identification of primary lesion in a patient with metastatic disease to the axilla. A:** Mediolateral oblique (MLO) views photographically coned to the upper portion of the image. Screening mammogram in a 68-year-old woman. A dense mass (*arrow*) is partially imaged in the left axilla at the edge of the film. This could not be seen on prior comparably positioned MLOs. BI-RADS 0: need additional imaging evaluation. Spot compression views (not shown) in the oblique projection confirm the presence of a dense mass. **B:** Ultrasound. A hard mobile mass is palpated in the left axilla. A lymph node with cortical bulging and mass effect on an attenuated fatty hilum is imaged corresponding to the palpable finding and mass described on the spot compression view. Metastatic carcinoma consistent with a breast primary is reported on an ultrasound-guided biopsy. Breast MRI is indicated. **C:** MRI, axial T1-weighted image of the left breast, postcontrast. A mass with heterogeneous enhancement and circumscribed margins is imaged in the lower outer aspect of the left breast zone B. Clumped and linear enhancement is present extending anteriorly from the mass for approximately 3 cm. **D:** MRI, T1-weighted sagittal reconstruction of the left breast postcontrast. The mass and associated linear enhancement (*short arrows*) are noted inferiorly in zone B. The abnormal lymph node (*long arrow*) detected mammographically is also apparent, demonstrating heterogeneous internal enhancement and circumscribed margins. Its vascular pedicle is noted on this image. MRI-guided biopsy of the breast findings is done confirming a breast primary in this patient.

undergoing mastectomy, the primary may not be identified in as many as 33% of patients, presumably a function of sampling bias (e.g., tumor is small and not included in the tissue evaluated histologically).

In many patients, special stains to include estrogen (ER) and progesterone (PR) receptors as well as cytokeratins are also done in an effort to elucidate the likely source of the metastatic disease. These stains are most helpful if they are positive. So, for example, if the ER and PR are positive, it is safe to assume that the tumor is likely breast in origin. However, if these are negative, it does not exclude a breast primary. As with any test, it is also important to recognize that there is often overlap in the staining characteristics of some tumors so that ER expression, for example, can also be seen in thyroid, salivary, and sweat gland carcinomas, and in 4% to 15% of lung cancers.

Immunohistochemical stains may suggest a primary source; however, they do not pinpoint the location of the lesion in the breast. So currently, if the mammogram is otherwise normal, and the patient has no known primary (e.g., colon, lung, ovary, etc.), a breast MRI is done. The primary, commonly measuring less than 2 cm in size, is detected in 62% to 86% of patients (19). If the primary is identified with certainty, the patient can be managed appropriately often with neoadjuvant therapy followed by conservative therapy (e.g., lumpectomy and radiation therapy).

EVALUATION OF TUMOR RESPONSE IN PATIENTS ON NEOADJUVANT THERAPY

MRI evaluation of patients undergoing neoadjuvant therapy may be done during therapy to monitor an early response or after therapy to identify residual disease (2,19). Early evaluations in patients undergoing neoadjuvant therapy are intended to identify a metabolic response in the tumor rather than a change in size. If no response is seen after the first course of chemotherapy, patients may benefit from a change in the chemotherapeutic regimen or may be more effectively treated with surgery. Imaging studies providing functional information such as PET, dynamic contrast-enhanced MR imaging, MR spectroscopy, and diffusion-weighted MR imaging are likely to be helpful in assessing early response to therapy (2).

On dynamic contrast-enhanced MRI, changes may be apparent within 6 weeks following the first course of chemotherapy (2,19). Flattening of the kinetic curves with slower washin rates and loss of the washout pattern is one of the earliest changes seen following initial courses of chemotherapy; changes in kinetic curves typically precede any change in the morphology of the lesion. It is reported that with proton MR at higher magnetic field strengths, reductions in the choline peak seen pre-therapy can be identified within 24 hours following treatment and may reliably indicate tumor response. Diffusion imaging may demonstrate changes in interstitial water diffusion rates as an indication of the cytotoxic effect of the chemotherapy (2).

MRI post treatment is used to demonstrate residual disease; however, a negative MRI at the completion of chemotherapy does not indicate absence of viable tumor in as many as 30% of patients (2). This underestimation of residual disease is likely related to the antiangiogenesis effect of some of the chemotherapeutic agents, particularly the taxanes. Compared with other modalities, MRI more accurately predicts final histology in 71% to 90% of patients compared with clinical examination (19% to 60%), mammography (26% to 70%), and ultrasound (35% to 75%) (19). After neoadjuvant therapy, MRI may demonstrate (i) Complete resolution of the findings even when extensive (Fig. 5.28), (ii) Persistence of soft tissue abnormalities with no associated enhancement (Fig. 5.29), (iii) Localized, clustered foci of enhancement at the original tumor site or within areas of persistent, nonenhancing asymmetric tissue (Fig. 5.30), (iv) increased central

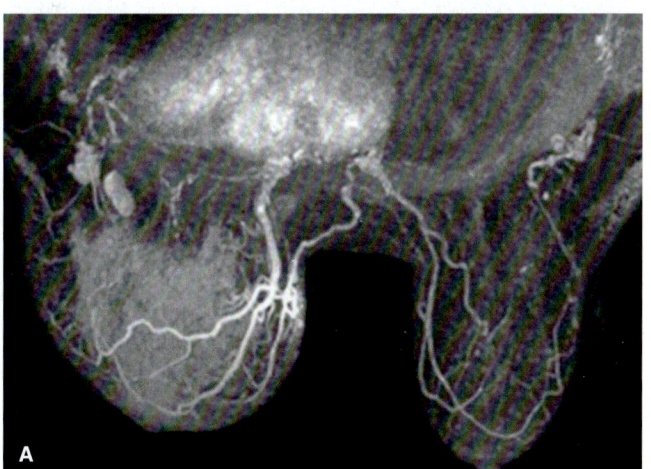 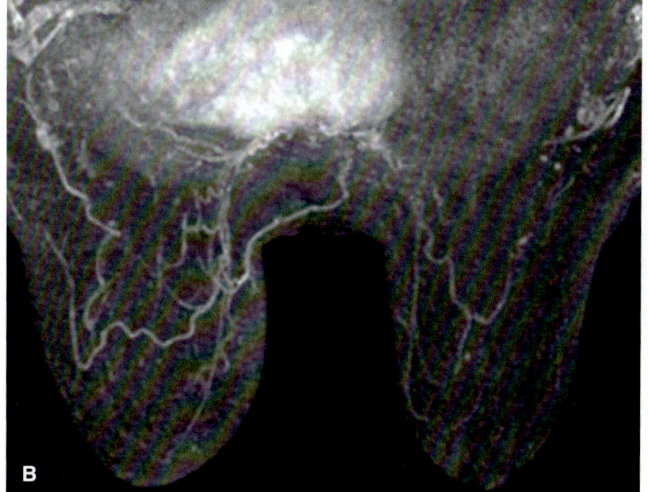

FIG. 5.28 • **Persistent edema but no other soft tissue or enhancing abnormality following neoadjuvant therapy. A:** MRI, MIP in a 72-year-old patient presenting with diffuse changes in the left breast mammographically, including prominence of the trabecular markings and skin thickening and markedly hypoechoic lymph nodes with cortical bulging in the left axilla on ultrasound (not shown). In this image, the left breast is larger and thicker with diffuse non–mass-like enhancement involving the upper and lateral quadrants of the left breast. Diffuse skin thickening and edematous changes (see Fig. 5.13 for a sagittal T2 image of the left breast on this patient) are also present with at least two abnormal lymph nodes in the axillary tail. Also note asymmetric prominence of the venous structures. Histologically, the patient is diagnosed with an invasive ductal carcinoma, high nuclear grade with angiolymphatic invasion apparent on the cores; the tumor is ER and PR receptor-negative, HER2/neu positive. Metastatic disease is diagnosed on cores from one of the lymph nodes in the axillary tail. **B:** MRI, MIP image 4 months following that shown in part **A**. The left breast remains slightly larger; however, no residual soft tissue abnormality or enhancement is apparent, the axillary lymph nodes have decreased significantly in size and are now morphologically normal in appearance. Edematous changes persist (T2 images not shown). Isolated tumor cells are identified in the left breast and in one of 19 lymph nodes sampled at the time of her mastectomy.

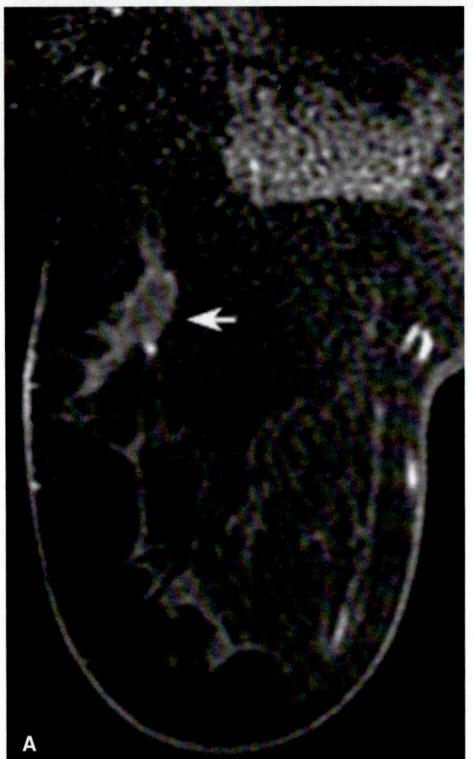
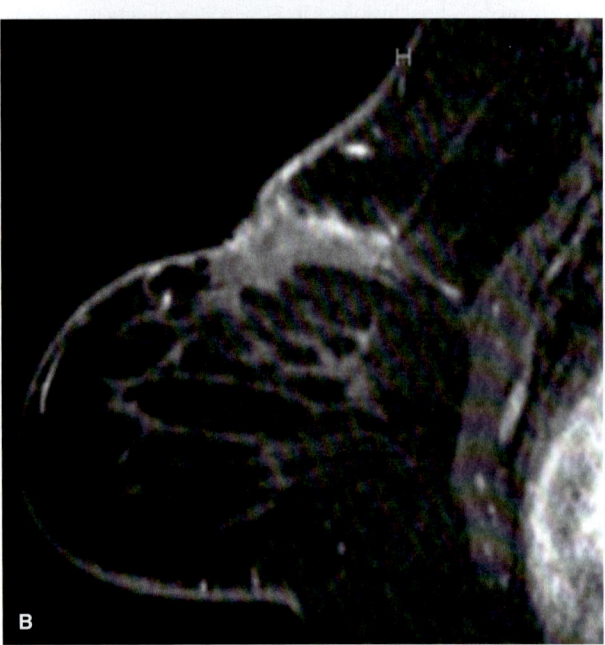
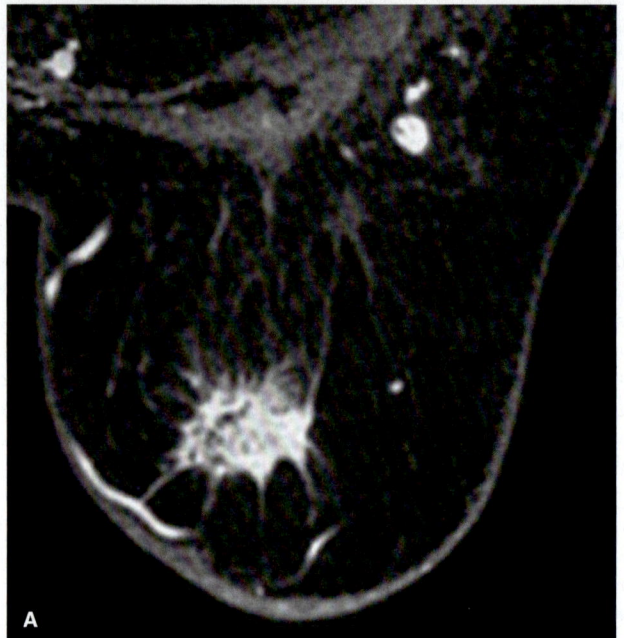
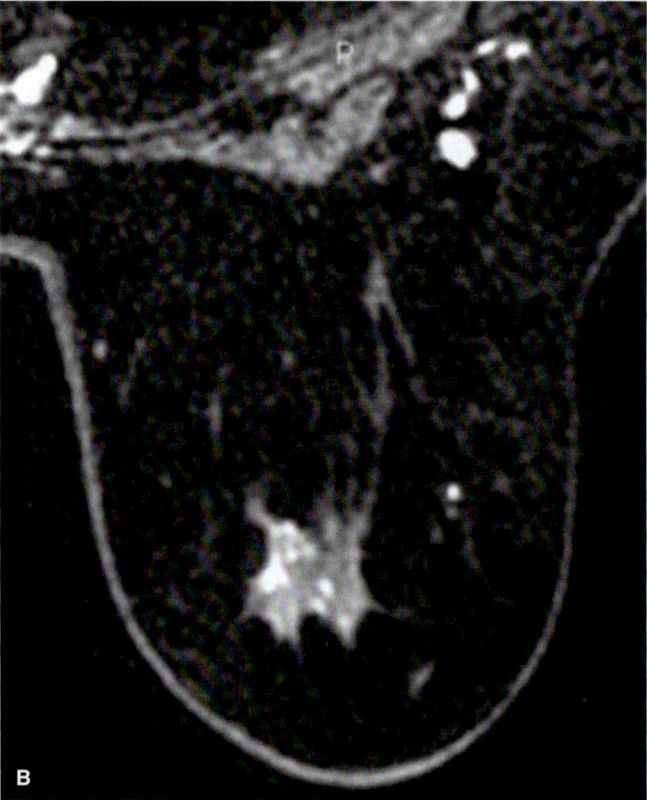

FIG. 5.29 • **Residual nonenhancing soft tissue following neoadjuvant therapy. A:** MRI, axial T1-weighted image of the left breast, postcontrast; study done 7 months after neoadjuvant therapy and the images shown in Figure 5.12. Nonenhancing soft tissue (*arrow*) persists at the site of the patient's original tumor. The axillary lymph node has decreased in size, and is now morphologically normal. Viable tumor measuring 0.6 cm is diagnosed at the time of her lumpectomy, and residual metastatic disease is identified in one of 11 lymph nodes. The tumor (invasive ductal carcinoma, grade 2) is ER and PR receptor-positive, HER2/neu negative. **B:** Different patient. MRI, T1-weighted sagittal reconstruction postcontrast and neoadjuvant therapy. Residual predominantly nonenhancing soft tissue with associated skin retraction is present superiorly at the site of the patient's known invasive ductal carcinoma (see Fig. 8.5C for pre-therapy images). At the time of mastectomy, no residual tumor is identified histologically (complete pathological response, cPR). In patients with persistent nonenhancing soft tissue at the site of the original tumor, you cannot be sure if residual viable tumor is present or if the nonenhancing soft tissue on MRI reflects treatment effect (e.g., chemotherapy-related fibrosis).

FIG. 5.30 • **Residual soft tissue with internal foci of enhancement post neoadjuvant therapy. A:** MRI, axial T1-weighted image of the right breast postcontrast in a 71-year-old patient. An irregular mass with heterogeneous enhancement and spiculated margins is present in the upper central to slightly medial aspect of the right breast anteriorly. This is an invasive ductal carcinoma, intermediate nuclear grade; it is ER and PR receptor-negative, HER2/neu negative (e.g., triple negative). **B:** MRI, axial T1-weighted image of the right breast postcontrast 6 months following that shown in part **A**. The mass is smaller in size with isolated round foci of internal enhancement sprinkled in residual nonenhancing soft tissue. Histologically, extensive fibrosis consistent with chemotherapy effect is reported as is residual invasive ductal carcinoma and DCIS. One of nine lymph nodes is positive for metastatic disease. The presence of enhancing foci in persistent nonenhancing soft tissue suggests residual viable disease; however, caution is again recommended; in some patients, viable tumor is not identified at the time of definitive surgical treatment.

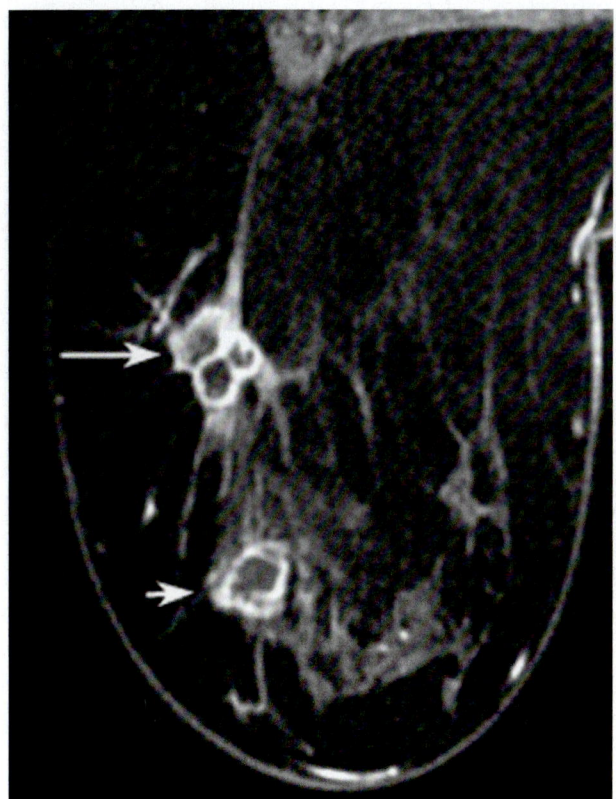

FIG. 5.31 • **Gross residual disease following neoadjuvant therapy.** MRI, axial T1-weighted image of the left breast postcontrast in a 41-year-old patient with a triple negative invasive ductal carcinoma, nuclear grade 3. Two masses (*arrows*) with rim enhancement persist in this patient following neoadjuvant therapy. The posterior mass (*long arrow*) demonstrates internal enhancing septations. In this patient, the enhancement seen on the posttreatment MRI is consistent with residual viable tumor.

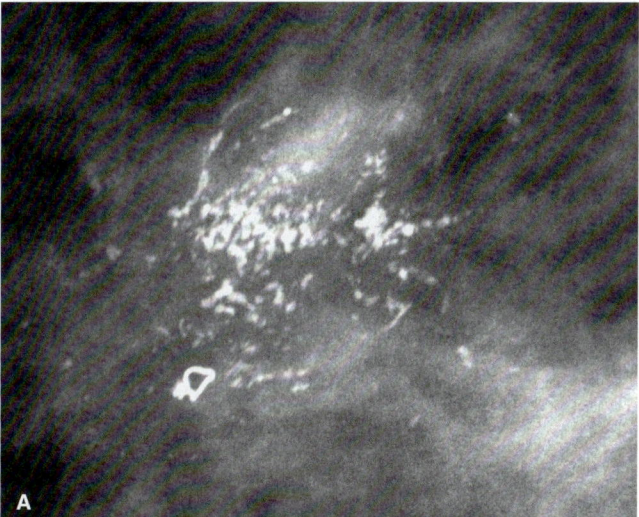
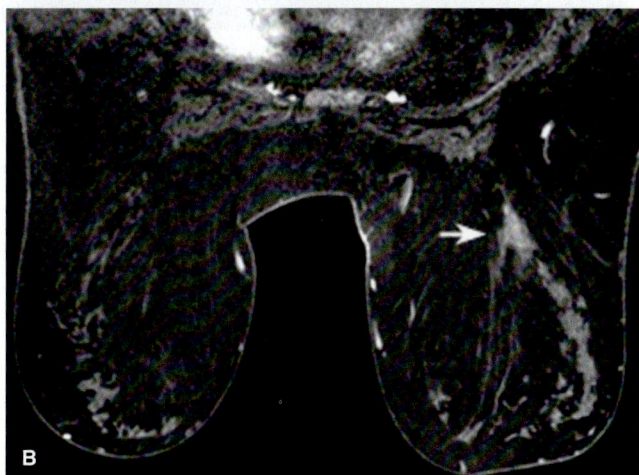

FIG. 5.32 • **Findings post neoadjuvant therapy in patients with an extensive intraductal component. A:** Photographically coned image to a cluster of calcifications in the right breast. Dense pleomorphic calcifications are identified with linear forms and linear orientation (a clip is noted reflecting the diagnostic biopsy site). A previously noted mass is not apparent at this time (see Fig. 7.2A for the mammogram on this patient before neoadjuvant therapy). In most patients with a calcifying extensive intraductal component, calcifications persist and may be more extensive after neoadjuvant therapy. Their significance, however, is not clear. In some patients, DCIS is found histologically; however, not in all. **B:** MRI, axial T1-weighted image of the right breast postcontrast. Residual soft tissue (*arrow*) is noted at the location of the patient's original tumor; however, no associated enhancement is identified following neoadjuvant therapy. At the time of lumpectomy, a 1-cm area of residual invasive ductal carcinoma is described histologically; no DCIS is reported. No metastatic disease is identified in the four excised axillary lymph nodes.

necrosis with persistence of a rim-enhancing mass, or (v) gross residual enhancing tumor (e.g., mass or clumped and linear enhancement) (Fig. 5.31). Unless gross residual disease is apparent, the findings on MRI post neoadjuvant therapy are nonspecific and may reflect complete pathologic response, residual disease, isolated tumor cells, or dense fibrosis (scarring) related to chemotherapy. The effect of neoadjuvant therapy is maximal on invasive lesions; the response of DCIS is variable. In patients with invasive disease and DCIS with calcifications seen mammographically, the calcifications usually do not regress (Fig. 5.32; see Fig. 7.2A for pretreatment image) following neoadjuvant therapy, and in some patients the calcifications may progress; however, progression does not necessarily reflect progression of the DCIS. If lack of response or tumor progression is suspected clinically, an MRI may be done during treatment.

EVALUATION OF PATIENTS WITH POSITIVE MARGINS

If patients with a breast cancer diagnosis are routinely undergoing MRI evaluations preoperatively, the need for re-excisions for positive margins and the use of MRI to postoperatively evaluate patients with positive margins should decrease. Unfortunately, some patients are not being evaluated adequately preoperatively (e.g., some may not have a preoperative tissue diagnosis), and if specimens are not oriented for the pathologist properly, MRI can be helpful in demonstrating the site of marginal disease and delineating the extent of residual malignancy in the breast (19). The role of MRI in this group of patients is to identify those with residual bulky disease (Fig. 5.33) so that the re-excision can be planned appropriately to the area with the disease, and to identify patients with multicentric disease that might benefit from a mastectomy or a second lumpectomy (Fig. 5.34). Although some have suggested that to minimize false-positive MRIs following lumpectomy, it is best to scan patients 35 days after surgery, this is not practical. If the purpose of the MRI study is to identify gross residual disease, we are scanning patients within a week of the surgery without a significant number of false-positive studies (see Fig. 11.28).

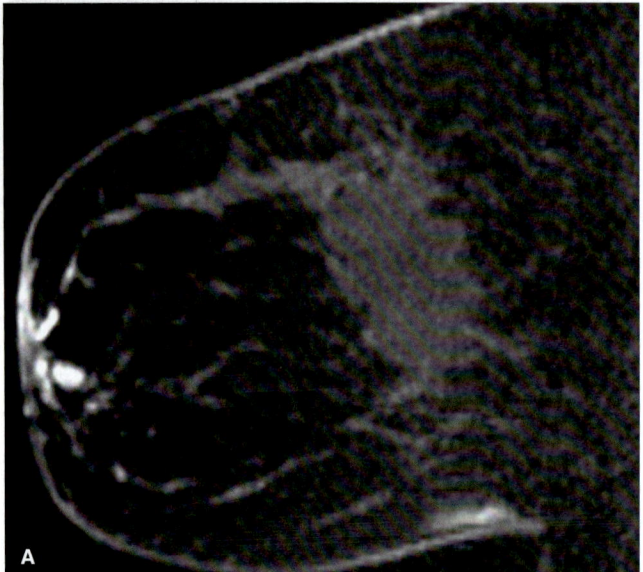 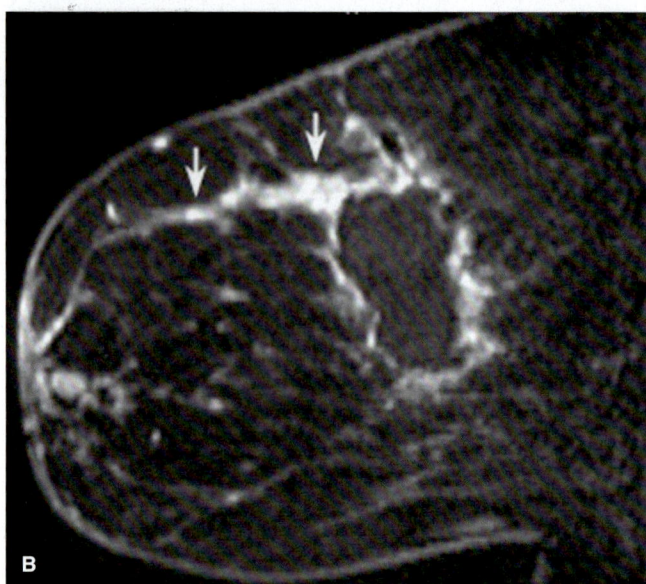

FIG. 5.33 • **Assessment of positive margins. A:** MRI, T1-weighted sagittal reconstruction of the left breast, precontrast. An irregular fluid collection (T2 images not shown) is imaged in the posterior aspect of the left breast following an excisional biopsy. The biopsy was done for diagnosis (e.g., no preoperative needle biopsy was done) and the specimen was not oriented for the pathologist. Positive margins are described. MRI is done in an effort to identify residual or additional disease and to evaluate the contralateral breast. **B:** MRI, T1-weighted sagittal reconstruction of the left breast, postcontrast. Non–mass-like linear and clumped enhancement (*arrows*) is identified arising from the superior aspect of the fluid collection extending anteriorly for approximately 5 cm. An MRI-guided biopsy of the anterior most extent of the enhancement confirms the presence of disease. The patient's re-excision is now appropriately targeted, and negative margins are obtained.

EVALUATION OF WOMEN WITH IMPLANTS

MRI in women with implants may be done for two primary reasons: to assess implant integrity, primarily intracapsular rupture (extracapsular rupture is often evident mammographically) in women with silicone implants (19), and to evaluate patients with implants for the presence of cancer: If the study is being done to evaluate implant integrity, no contrast is needed. Intracapsular rupture (see Fig. 11.54) is characterized by the presence of fragments of the implant shell floating in the free silicone contained by the fibrous capsule formed by the patient (e.g., linguine sign). Wrinkles and radial folds normally occur in implants. When there is silicone signal within a wrinkle (e.g., filling in of keyholes) or external to a radial fold, this may represent the presence of gel-bleed, while others suggest these are signs of intracapsular rupture. On unenhanced silicone hyperintense inversion recovery sequences, extracapsular silicone is readily apparent in the breast or axillae external to the capsule of the implant (see Fig. 11.55D,E).

If the MRI is being done for the detection or evaluation of breast cancer, the same sequences as those used in patients who do not have implants are obtained (Fig. 5.35). As already mentioned, fat suppression in women with implants may be difficult to obtain (Fig. 5.5B).

SCREENING WOMEN WHO ARE AT HIGH RISK FOR DEVELOPING BREAST CANCER

BRCA mutation carriers have a 60% to 80% lifetime risk of developing breast cancer, and *BRCA 1* carriers also have an approximately 40% risk of developing ovarian cancer. In familial breast cancers, *BRCA* mutations account for approximately 40% to 50% of all the breast cancers. Clearly other, as yet unidentified, gene mutations exist, accounting for breast cancer clusters in families who are *BRCA*-negative. Patients who are known carriers of a *BRCA* mutation may elect to have prophylactic mastectomies and oophorectomies. Patients undergoing an oophorectomy to decrease their risk for ovarian cancer also decrease their risk for breast cancer by approximately 30%. Close surveillance is the alternative. If screening is chosen, it should be started by age 30 since more than 50% of familial breast cancers occur in women under the age of 50. Unfortunately, the sensitivity of mammography alone in this group of women is low, and interval cancer rates in the range of 43% to 60% have been reported. The reported sensitivity of breast MRI in this group of women ranges from 80% to 98% with prognostically favorable cancers being identified. Higher rates of false-positives and a low positive predictive value in some of the early trials have been attributed to a relative lack of experience with MRI in the screening setting, since the specificity after several rounds of screening approximates that reported for mammography (2,19,21,22).

Currently, the American Cancer Society (ACS) recommends annual screening MRI for women at high risk, including (23) women with a *BRCA* mutation and their untested first-degree relatives, women who have had chest wall radiation between the ages of 10 and 30, women with syndromes (Li-Fraumeni, Cowden, and Bannayan–Riley–Ruvalcaba syndromes) associated with an increased breast cancer risk, and those women with a lifetime risk of greater than 20% to 25% (Fig. 5.36) as determined by risk models (BRCAPRO, Tyrer–Cuzick) (23).

Insufficient evidence for or against MRI screening is currently available in women with an intermediate (15% to 20% lifetime risk) risk for breast cancer (23). This includes women with prior biopsy-proven atypia or lobular carcinoma in situ, women with dense tissue mammographically, and those patients with a personal history of breast cancer who have no other associated risk factors (e.g., family history). Breast MRI is not recommended for screening women with a less than 15% lifetime risk for breast cancer (23).

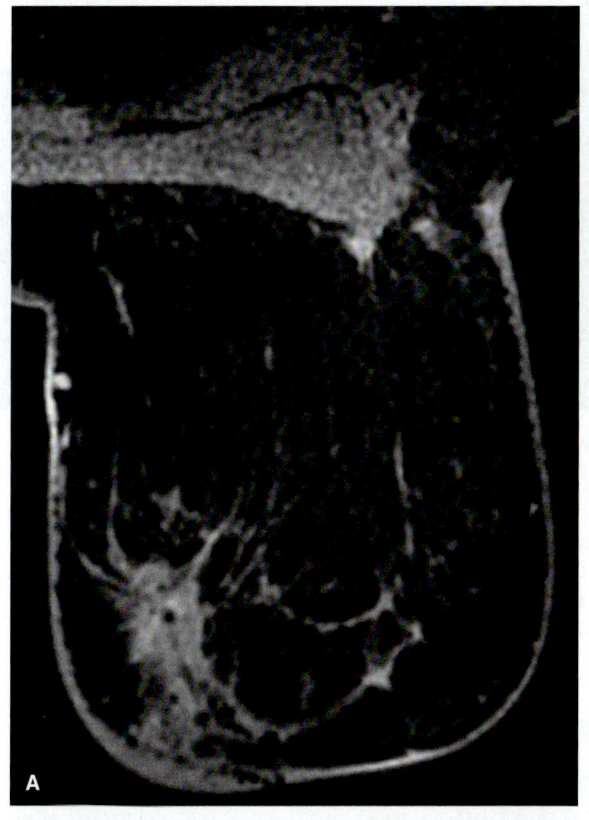
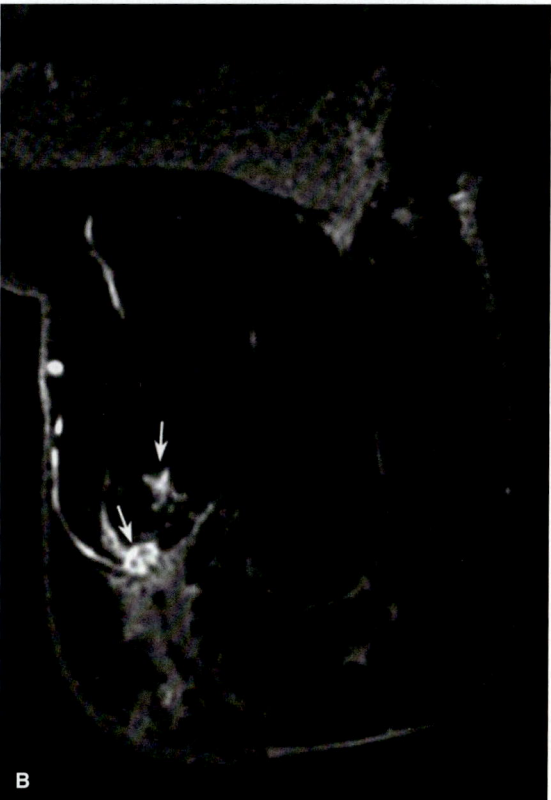
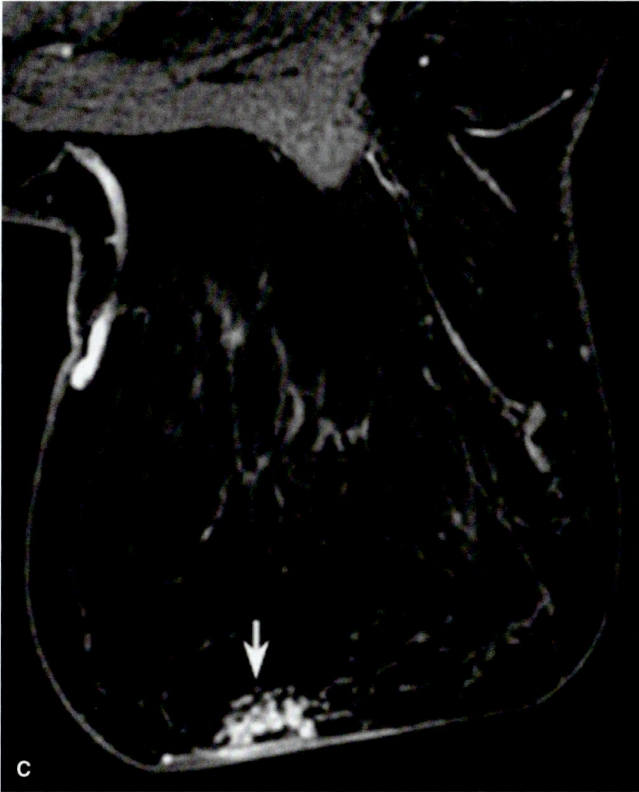

FIG. 5.34 • **Assessment of positive margins. A:** MRI, axial T1-weighted image of the right breast, precontrast. Biopsy changes with distortion are apparent in the anteromedial aspect of the right breast following an excisional biopsy. The biopsy was done for diagnostic purposes (e.g., no preoperative needle biopsy was done), and the specimen was not oriented for the pathologist. Positive margins are described. **B:** MRI, axial T1-weighted image of the right breast, postcontrast. An enhancing mass is imaged at the posterior edge of the biopsy site; however, an additional site of enhancement is present approximately 1 cm posterior to the biopsy site. **C:** MRI, axial T1-weighted image of the right breast, postcontrast. Non–mass-like enhancement (*arrow*) is also identified in the right subareolar area. The likelihood of positive margins is likely to decrease if MRIs to characterize and localize the extent of disease are done before definitive surgery is done. Similarly, additional sites of unsuspected disease that may alter management plans should be identified preoperatively.

PROBLEM SOLVING

This is not yet a commonly used indication for breast MRI, and at the onset it must be made clear that the lack of an MRI correlate for suspicious mammographic (particularly calcifications) or ultrasound findings does not obviate the need for biopsy. Our primary use of MRI in this scenario relates to patients with equivocal clinical or mammographic findings in whom concern remains even after complete mammographic, sonographic, and even in some patients, negative core needle biopsies. Specifically, this is usually in patients with areas of parenchymal asymmetry or distortion (Fig. 5.37). Additionally, in

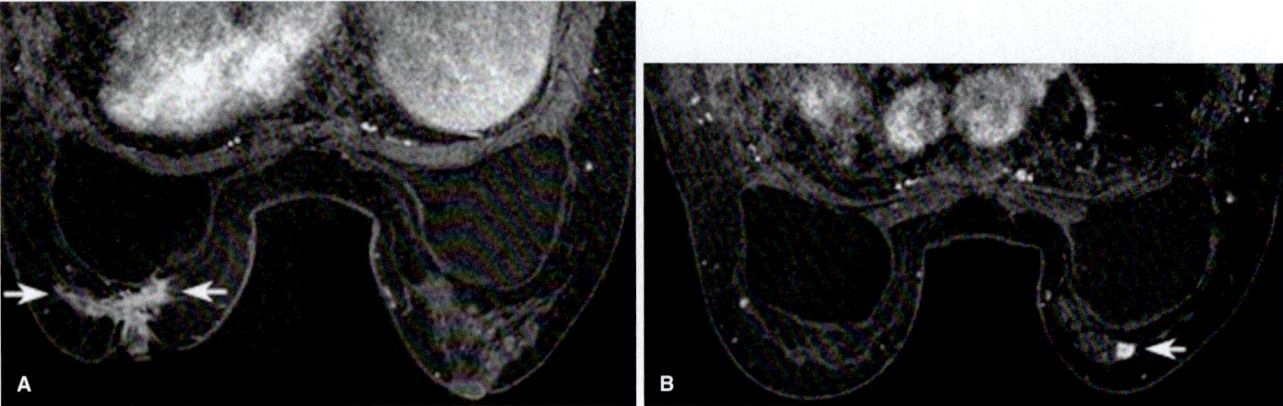

FIG. 5.35 • **Evaluation of patients with implants, synchronous bilateral cancers. A:** MRI, axial T1-weighted image postcontrast in a 53-year-old patient with saline implants in a subglandular location. Heterogeneous non–mass-like reticular enhancement *(arrows)* with distortion and associated nipple retraction is present in the left subareolar area. This corresponds to a site of known invasive ductal carcinoma with lobular features. **B:** MRI, axial T1-weighted image postcontrast at a different level from that shown in part **A**. A mass *(arrow)* with homogeneous enhancement and circumscribed margins is identified in the right breast. The patient is evaluated with ultrasound and a vertically oriented markedly hypoechoic mass with spiculated margins is identified in the right breast corresponding to the MRI finding. An invasive ductal carcinoma, low nuclear grade is diagnosed following ultrasound-guided core biopsy.

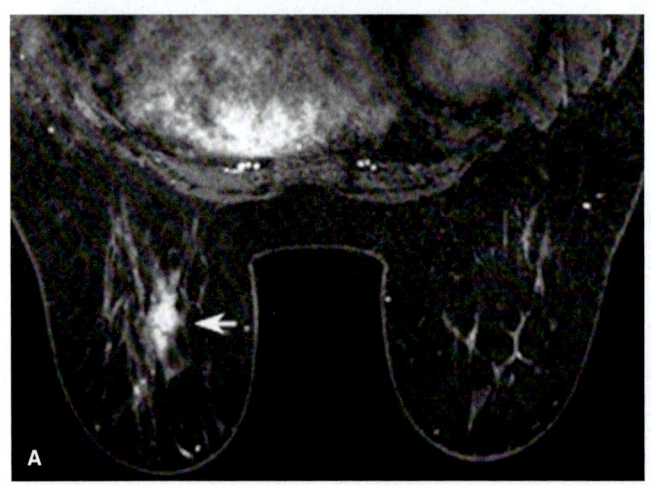

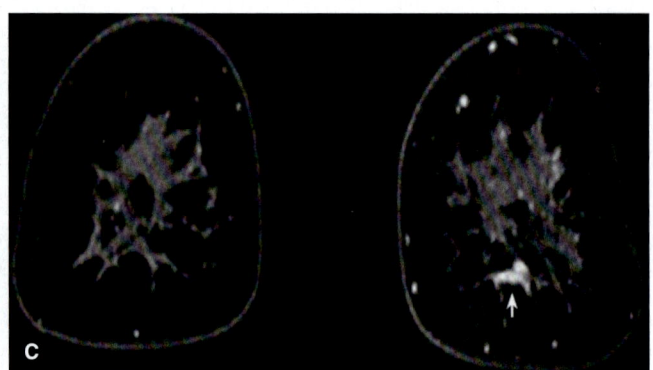

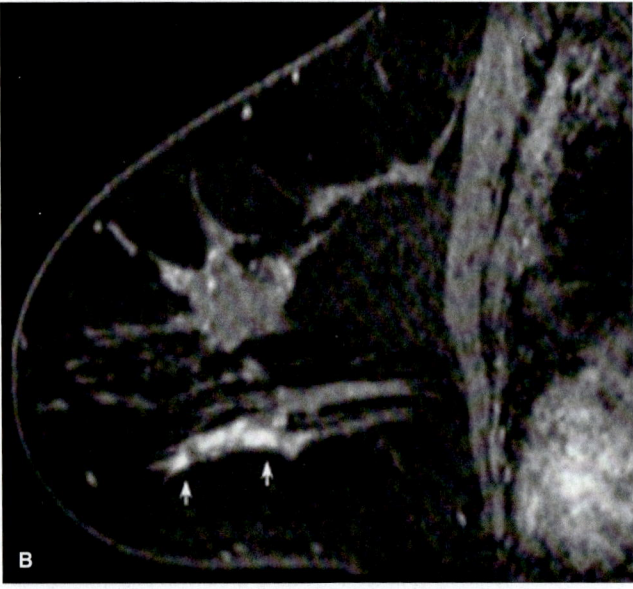

FIG. 5.36 • **Screening high-risk patients. A:** MRI, axial T1-weighted image postcontrast in a patient who, because of family history, is referred for genetic counseling. She is *BRCA* negative; however, her estimated lifetime risk using various models is 25%. Annual screening with mammography and breast MRI is recommended. Non–mass-like enhancement *(arrow)* is identified in the lower central to slightly medial aspect of the left breast, zone B. MRI, T1-weighted sagittal **(B)** and coronal **(C)** reconstructions of the left breast, postcontrast. The features of the enhancement are reviewed in the axial images as well as on the sagittal and coronal reconstruction before characterizing the lesion as focal, heterogeneous, non–mass-like, and linear *(arrows)*. MRI-guided biopsy is done to establish the diagnosis of an invasive ductal carcinoma high nuclear grade with an extensive intraductal component; the tumor is ER and PR receptor-negative, HER2/neu negative (triple negative). One of our genetic counselors comes to our outpatient breast-imaging center 1 day a week to evaluate any self-referred patients or those in whom, by virtue of a known family history, may be at increased risk for breast cancer. Annual screening with mammography and breast MRI is recommended in those women identified with a lifetime risk greater than 20% as determined by various models used by the counselor.

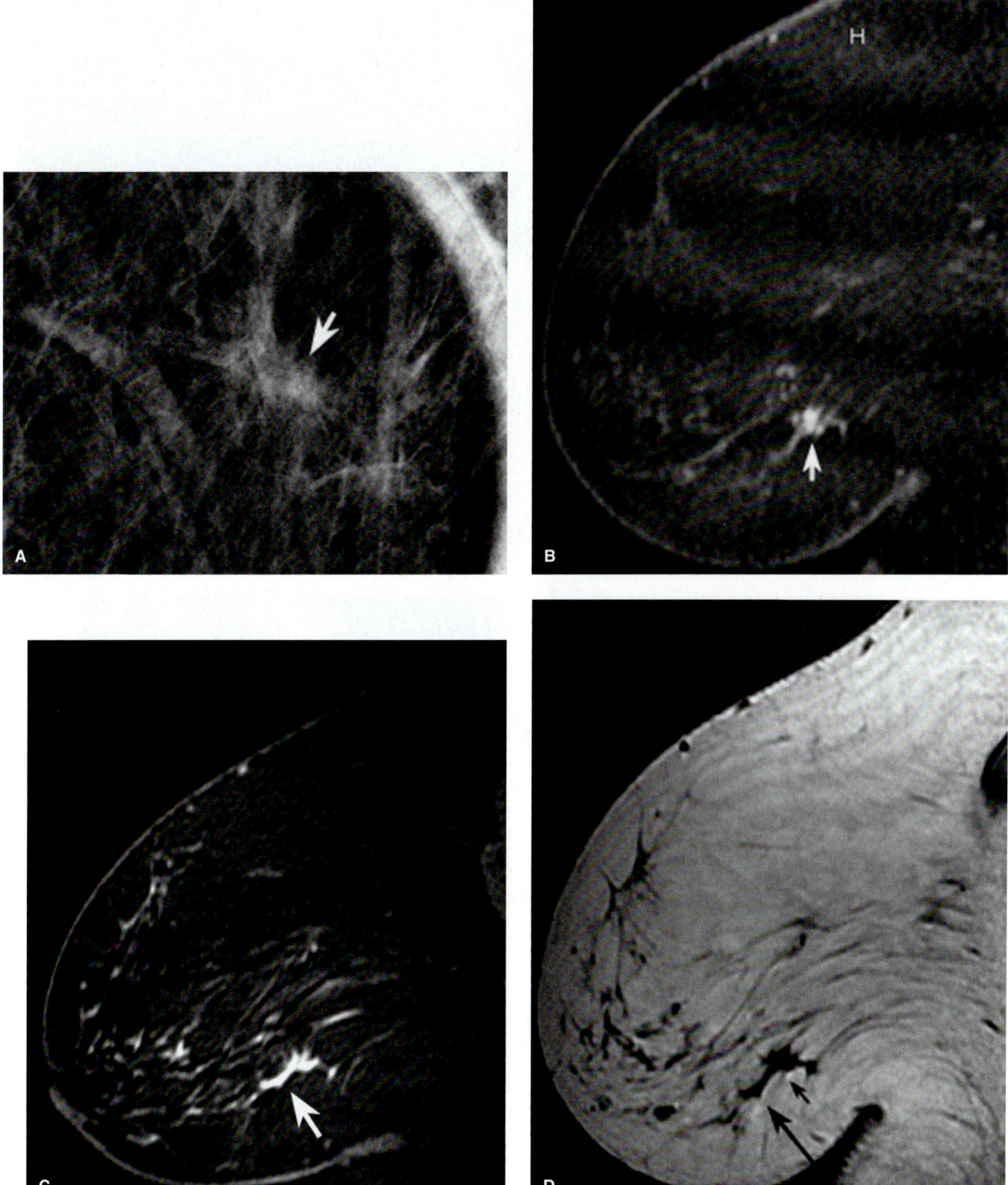

FIG. 5.37 • **Problem solving. A:** Spot compression view of the left breast. One of several spot compression views obtained following a screening mammogram in a 51-year-old woman to evaluate possible distortion in the left breast. Distortion in the lower central aspect of the left breast zone B persists on every spot compression view done, including spot rolled views. No abnormality is identified on ultrasound. Benign breast tissue is described following a stereotactically guided biopsy. This is not congruent with the imaging findings. Options available at this point include re-biopsy or excisional biopsy. Following a lengthy discussion with the patient, we opted for an MRI with the idea that if this lesion enhanced, we could do the biopsy under MRI guidance. However, it is made clear to the patient that if no MRI correlate is seen, an excisional biopsy is needed. MRI, T1-weighted sagittal reconstruction of the left breast at one level **(B)** and the immediately adjacent level **(C)**. A mass (*arrow* in part **B**) with spiculated margins and associated linear enhancement (*arrow* in part **C**) extending anteriorly for approximately 2 cm is imaged correlating with the site of the mammographic finding. **D:** MRI, T1-weighted sagittal non–fat-suppressed image of the left breast. The mass (*short arrow*) with distortion, spiculated margins, and linear extension of disease (*long arrow*) is nicely depicted in this image. Invasive lobular carcinoma is diagnosed on an MRI-guided biopsy.

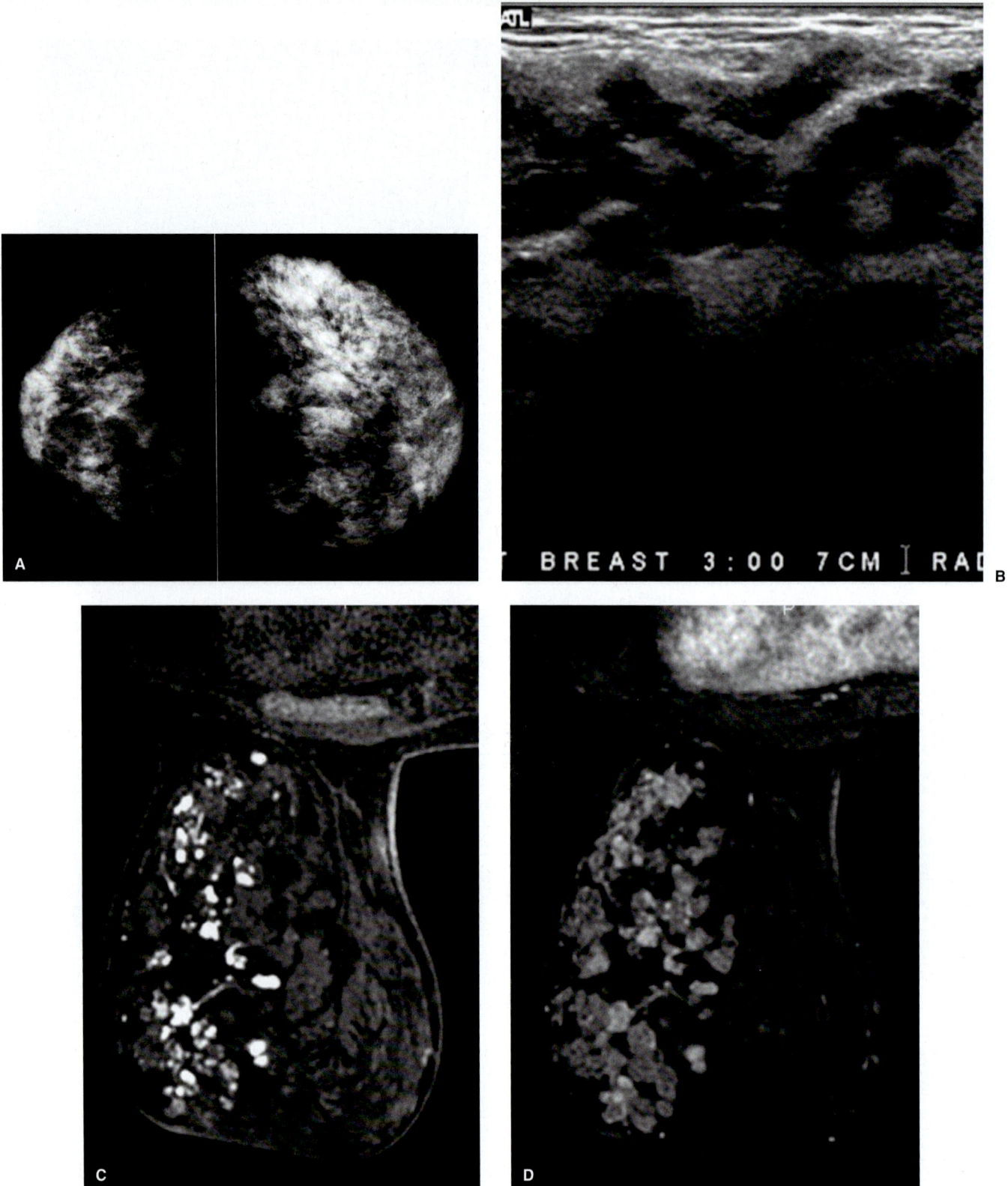

FIG. 5.38 • **Segmentally distributed heterogeneous non–mass-like clumped and linear enhancement; DCIS.**
A: Craniocaudal views in a 46-year-old patient who presents describing progressive heaviness and an increase in the size of her left breast. The left breast is larger and denser; however, no focal abnormality or calcifications are identified on the mammogram. **B:** Ultrasound, representative image. Dilated ducts with scattered echogenic foci likely representing calcifications are imaged in the lateral central to lower aspect of the left breast. No intraductal or focal parenchymal abnormality is identified. No nipple discharge is elicited on physical examination. **C:** MRI, axial T1-weighted image of the left breast precontrast. Segmentally distributed, dilated fluid-filled ducts (bright T1 and T2 signal, proteinaceous fluid) extending posteriorly from the nipple into the lower outer quadrant of the left breast. **D:** MRI, axial T1-weighted image of the left breast postcontrast. Diffuse enhancement surrounding the dilated ductal structures is seen on the postcontrast images. DCIS high nuclear grade (solid, cribriform, and micropapillary types) with comedonecrosis is diagnosed following MRI-guided biopsy of two separate sites (anterior and posterior). DCIS with no invasion is confirmed on the mastectomy specimen. Sentinel lymph node biopsy is negative for metastatic disease.

patients with rapidly developing solitary dilated ducts, MRI may be helpful in identifying the location of the causative intraductal lesion; rarely, some of these patients are diagnosed with DCIS (Fig. 5.38; also see Figs 9.35 and 9.36).

In this indication one can also include the evaluation of patients in whom, following conservative therapy, a question arises regarding changes at the lumpectomy site that may represent progressive fibrosis post radiation therapy or recurrent disease. Scar tissue and fibrosis do not enhance, recurrent disease does.

References

1. Kuhl C. The current status of breast MR imaging, part I: choice of technique, image interpretation, diagnostic accuracy and transfer to clinical practice. *Radiology*. 2007;244:356–378.
2. Kuhl C. The current status of breast MR imaging, part II: clinical applications. *Radiology*. 2007;244:672–691.
3. Millet I, Pages E, Hoa D, et al. Pearls and pitfalls in breast MRI. *Br J Radiol*. 2012;85:197–207.
4. Shimauchi A, Jansen SA, Abe H, et al. Breast cancers not detected at MRI: review of false-negative lesions. *AJR Am J Roentgenol*. 2010;194:1674–1679.
5. Kuo PH, Kanal E, Abu-Alfa AK, et al. Gadolinium-based MR contrast agents and nephrogenic systemic fibrosis. *Radiology*. 2007;242:647–649.
6. Sadowski EA, Bennett LK, Chan MR, et al. Nephrogenic systemic fibrosis: risk factors and incidence estimation. *Radiology*. 2007;243:148–157.
7. Harvey JA, Hendrick RE, Coll JM, et al. Breast MR imaging artifacts: how to recognize and fix them. *Radiographics*. 2007;27:S131–S145.
8. Morris EA, Comstock CE, Lee CH, et al. Magnetic Resonance Imaging. In: ACR BI-RADS® Atlas, Breast Imaging Reporting and Data System. Reston, VA, American College of Radiology; 2013.
9. Morris EA, Liberman L, eds. *Breast MRI: Diagnosis and Intervention*. New York, NY: Springer; 2010.
10. Raza S, Birdwell RL, Ritner JA, et al. *Breast MRI: A Comprehensive Imaging Guide*. Philadelphia, PA: Lippincott Williams & Wilkins; 2009
11. Wright H, Listinsky J, Quinn C, et al. Increased ipsilateral whole breast vascularity as measured by contrast-enhanced magnetic resonance imaging in patients with breast cancer. *Am J Surg*. 2005;190:576–579.
12. Fischer DR, Malich A, Wurdinger S, et al. The adjacent vessel on dynamic contrast-enhanced breast MRI. *AJR Am J Roentgenol*. 2006;187:W147–W151.
13. Schmitz AC, Peters NH, Veldhuis WB, et al. Contrast-enhanced 3.0-T breast MRI for characterization of breast lesions: increased specificity by using vascular maps. *Eur Radiol*. 2008;18:355–364.
14. Han M, Kim TH, Kang DK, et al. Prognostic role of MRI enhancement features in patients with breast cancer: value of adjacent vessel sign and increased ipsilateral whole-breast vascularity. *AJR Am J Roentgenol*. 2012;199:921–928.
15. Dietzel M, Baltzer PAT, Vag T, et al. The adjacent vessel sign on breast MRI: new data and a subgroup analysis for 1084 histologically verified cases. *Korean J Radiol*. 2010;11:178–186.
16. Jansen SA, Paunesku T, Fan X, et al. Ductal carcinoma in situ: x-ray fluoresce microscopy and dynamic contrast-enhanced MR imaging reveals gadolinium uptake within neoplastic mammary ducts in a murine model. *Radiology*. 2009;253:399–406.
17. Kuhl CK. Science to practice: why do purely intraductal cancers enhance on breast MR images? *Radiology*. 2009;253:281–287.
18. Liberman L, Mason G, Morris EA, et al. Does size matter? Positive predictive value of MRI-detected breast lesions as a function of lesion size. *AJR Am J Roentgenol*. 2006;186:426–430.
19. Argus A, Mahoney MC. Indications for breast MRI: case based review. *AJR Am J Roentgenol*. 2011;196:WS1–WS14.
20. Liberman L, Morris EA, Dershaw DD, et al. MR imaging of the ipsilateral breast in women with percutaneously proven breast cancer. *AJR Am J Roentgenol*. 2003;180:901–910.
21. Liberman L, Morris EA, Kim CM, et al. MR imaging findings in the contralateral breast of women with recently diagnosed breast cancer. *AJR Am J Roentgenol*. 2003;180:333–341.
22. Lehman CD, Gatsonis C, Kuhl CK, et al. MRI evaluation of the contralateral breast in women with recently diagnosed breast cancer. *N Engl J Med*. 2007;356:1295–1303.
23. Saslow D, Boetes C, Burke W, et al. American Cancer Society guidelines for breast screening with MRI as an adjunct to mammography. *CA Cancer J Clin*. 2007;57:75–89.

CHAPTER SELF-ASSESSMENT QUESTIONS

1. Representative MRI images of a mass in the left breast: axial T2-weighted (left) and postcontrast T1-weighted (right) images. What is the most likely diagnosis?

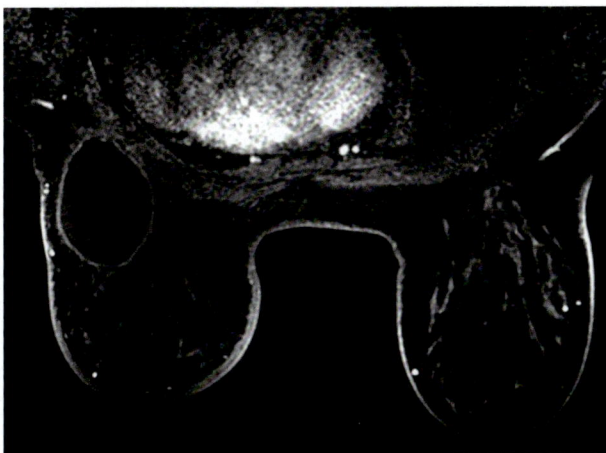
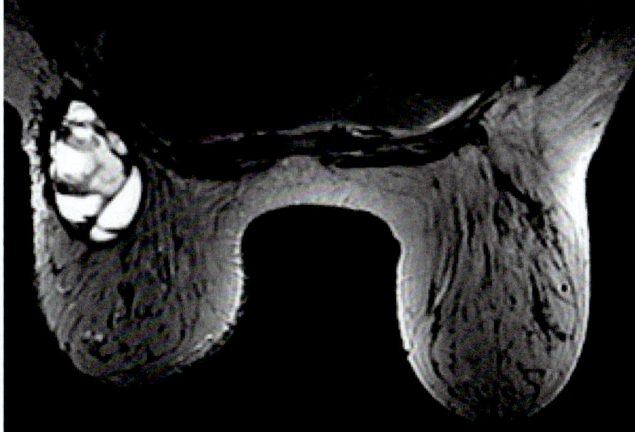

   A. Postoperative fluid collection
   B. Phyllodes tumor
   C. Papillary carcinoma
   D. Abscess

2. Pre- (left) and postcontrast T1-weighted (right) sagittal reconstructions of the left breast in a patient with a normal mammogram. The finding is best described as?

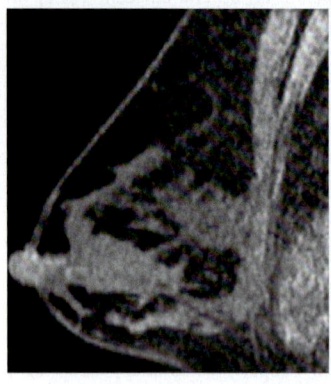 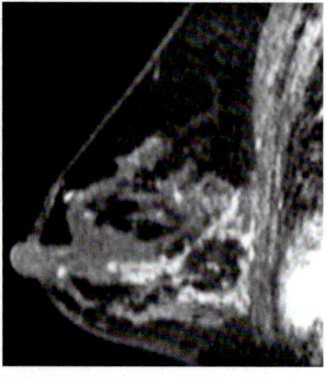

A. Benign parenchymal enhancement
B. Enhancing ductal structures
C. Segmentally distributed non–mass-like enhancement
D. Mass with associated linear enhancement

Answers to Chapter Self-Assessment Questions

1. A   This is a postoperative fluid collection with minimal enhancement of a thin rim. The thin rim with no associated surrounding soft tissue stranding makes an abscess less likely. Also, the lack of any internal enhancement makes any type of a malignancy or phyllodes tumor unlikely.

2. C   This is a nice example of segmentally distributed non–mass-like enhancement. Given the segmental distribution and the lack of ductal structures with high internal signal precontrast makes benign parenchymal enhancement or enhancement of ductal structures unlikely. No mass is identified pre- or postcontrast. If there is no mammographic correlate (e.g., calcifications), MRI-guided biopsies to delineate the anterior and posterior extent of disease would be appropriate. Ductal carcinoma in situ is diagnosed on MRI-guided biopsies.

Breast Calcifications 6

LEARNING OBJECTIVES

1. Describe the appropriate evaluation of breast calcifications that cannot be classified as benign on screening images
2. Features of benign breast calcifications and appropriate descriptors
3. Descriptors used for the distribution of breast calcifications
4. Ductal carcinoma in situ (DCIS)
   - Heterogeneity of the disease
   - Presentations
   - Imaging features
5. Features of calcifications associated with DCIS characterized by central necrosis
6. Features of calcifications that develop in secretions associated with proliferative changes in the ducts (hyperplasia, atypical ductal hyperplasia, low grade DCIS; columnar cell change)

Calcifications developing in the breast and detected on screening mammograms are variable in number and appearance, and most reflect a benign etiology. A small number develop in association with ductal carcinoma in situ (DCIS), less commonly the invasive component of ductal carcinomas or in metastatic disease to the breast or axillary lymph nodes (e.g., psammoma bodies—ovarian or thyroid carcinomas) (see Fig. 8.56). It is incumbent upon the radiologist to detect, evaluate, classify, and make appropriate recommendations for calcifications perceived on mammograms for which, in most patients, there is no clinical correlate.

Complete mammographic workups that include spot compression magnification views in two projections with no motion, coupled with knowledge of breast anatomy and histopathology, are critical in understanding the mammographic appearance of breast calcifications and establishing appropriate and justifiable recommendations. Calcifications developing in a space (i.e., ducts or acini) are molded by that space. Calcifications arising in ducts are tube-like or linear and may demonstrate linear distribution. If they develop in subsegmental ducts, they are large, rod-like, and dense compared with the smaller calcifications of variable density that develop in terminal ducts. When the epithelial lining is attenuated or denuded, the border of the calcifications is smooth (Fig. 6.1) compared with the irregular margins that may be seen when there is active cellular proliferation and necrotic debris in the lumen of the duct (Fig. 6.2). Calcifications forming in acini are round or punctate (Fig. 6.3). If the normally round acini are compressed, elongated, or deformed by proliferation of the surrounding perilobular stroma, the calcifications may demonstrate pleomorphism, including round, punctate, oval, and comma-shaped forms.

As discussed in Chapters 2 and 3, establishing optimal film quality is one of the initial steps in reviewing screening and diagnostic mammograms. Well-exposed, high-contrast images with optimal positioning and no blurring are essential in maximizing our ability to detect microcalcifications, small spiculated masses, and subtle areas of distortion. The acceptance and interpretation of suboptimal films can result in a delay in the diagnosis of breast cancer. With respect to calcifications in particular, generalized or localized blurring on an image can lead to a failure to detect calcifications, or if noted, the morphology of the calcifications may be grossly distorted, potentially resulting in a misdiagnosis (see Fig. 2.24).

When evaluating calcifications, consider the following characteristics: What is the predominate *form* of the individual calcifications? Round or linear, coarse or fine (granular), monomorphic or pleomorphic (heterogeneous), or within a cluster? Monomorphism is not common. Pleomorphism and heterogeneity are seen in most groups of calcifications even when related to a benign etiology. What is the *size* of the calcifications? Large or small and, if in a cluster, are the individual calcifications homogeneous in size? What is the *density* of the calcifications? High or low? In a given cluster is there homogeneity in density among the individual calcifications? What is the *distribution* of the calcifications? Unilateral or bilateral, single cluster or multifocal, diffuse, regional, segmental, or linear? Calcifications that are diffusely

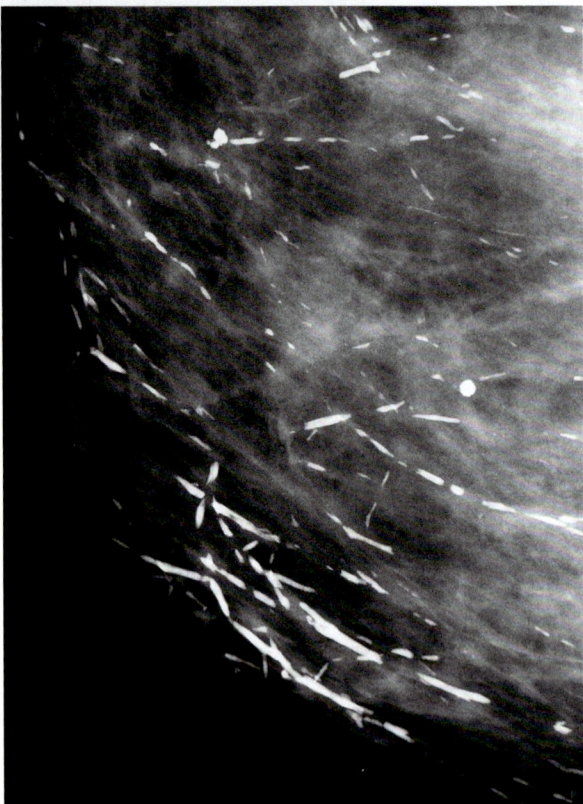

FIG. 6.1 • **Rod-like calcifications.** Forming in subsegmental ducts, these calcifications are dense, rod-like, and linearly oriented toward the nipple. The smooth border of the calcifications reflects a denuded or attenuated epithelial lining in the ducts. They are often identified bilaterally usually with no round, punctate, or amorphous forms in the neighborhood. BI-RADS 2: Benign finding. (From Cardeñosa G. *Breast Imaging [The Core Curriculum Series]*. Philadelphia, PA: Lippincott Williams & Wilkins; 2003.)

scattered in dense tissue bilaterally are typically benign in contrast to linear calcifications in a linear or segmental distribution. Are the calcifications new compared with prior studies, and if so, where in the breast are the calcifications developing?

The emphasis placed previously on the number of calcifications in a given cluster, in our opinion, is not a particularly helpful characteristic. One or two linear calcifications with irregular margins may be related to the presence of DCIS and require a biopsy. Conversely, a tight cluster of many round, pearl-like calcifications of homogeneous density does not usually require a biopsy. There is no question that calcifications related to an underlying DCIS tend to be numerous with variation in form (e.g., linear forms are commonly surrounded by punctate and amorphous forms as well as some larger, dense, coarse calcifications), density and distribution. So it is important to look at not only the individual calcifications, but also the neighborhood in which they reside.

The presence of linear calcifications with irregular borders, variable density, and linear orientation that are grouped, haphazardly or segmentally distributed needs to be considered significant (Figs. 6.2 and 6.4) (1–3). The likelihood of an underlying DCIS (low, intermediate, or high nuclear grade) associated with central necrosis is high; biopsy is indicated in these patients. These types of calcifications are fairly distinctive and uncommonly associated with benign processes, including those listed in Table 6.1. We also consider the linear distribution of round, oval, punctate (fine pleomorphic; coarse heterogeneous),

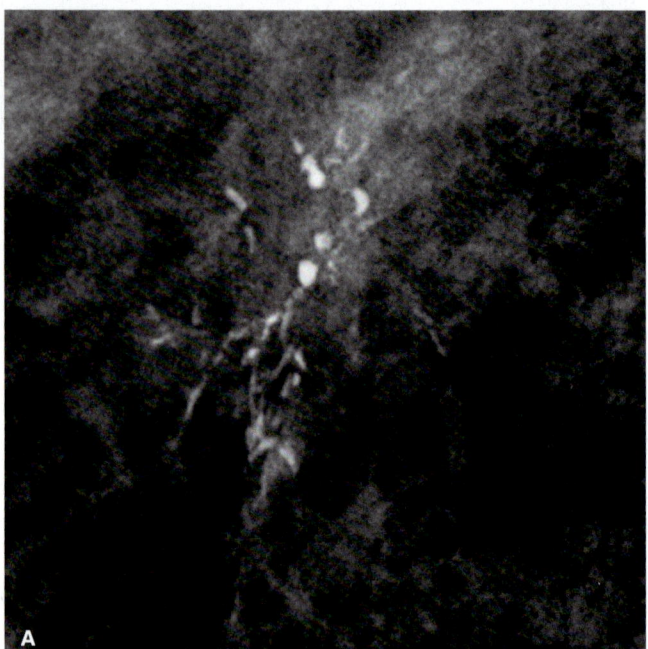

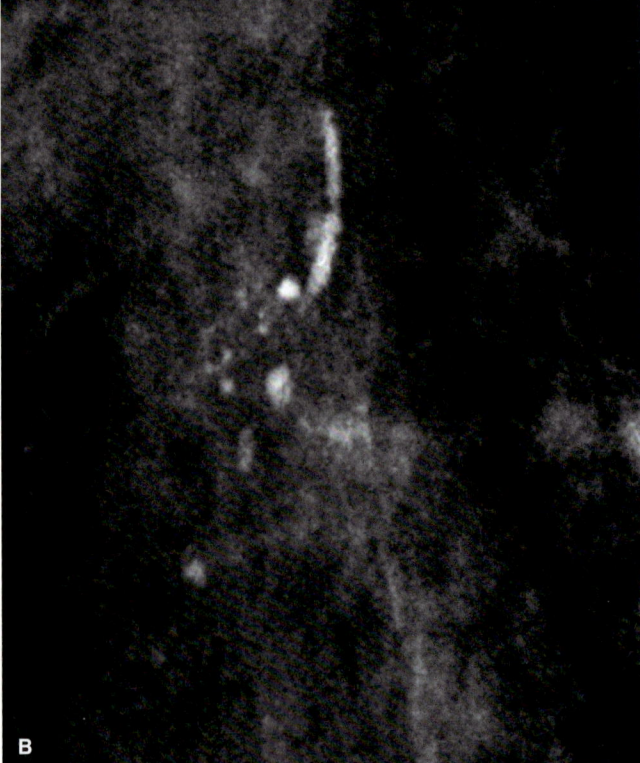

FIG. 6.2 • **Linear calcifications in a linear distribution, DCIS. A:** Spot compression magnification view. Group of calcifications that includes linear calcifications in a linear (ductal) distribution as well as coarse dense heterogeneous calcifications. Note that the density of the calcifications is variable. BI-RADS 4C: Suspicious abnormality, biopsy is indicated. **B:** Spot compression magnification view. Group of calcifications that includes linear calcifications in a linear distribution as well as coarse heterogeneous calcifications. Note the irregular margins of the linear calcifications. These calcifications develop in necrotic cellular debris deposited in the lumen of dilated ducts and are molded by the proliferating epithelial cells. BI-RADS 4C: Suspicious abnormality, biopsy is indicated. Although not pathognomonic of DCIS, be careful before accepting a benign histology for calcifications having these morphologic features.

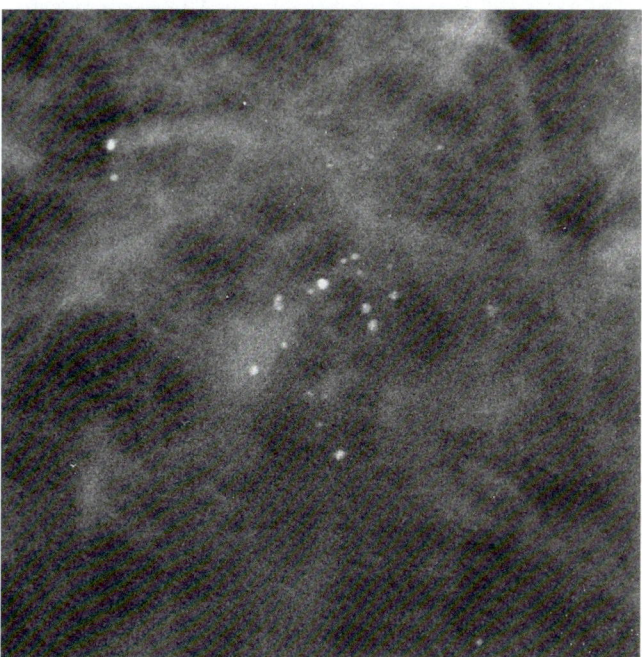

FIG. 6.3 • **Round and punctate calcifications. Lobular.** This group of calcifications is characterized by relatively monomorphic round and punctate calcifications having some variation in density. No linear forms or linear orientation is seen. BI-RADS 2: Benign finding. (From Cardeñosa G. *Breast Imaging [The Core Curriculum Series]*. Philadelphia, PA: Lippincott Williams & Wilkins; 2003.)

Table 6.1 **DIFFERENTIAL: FINE, LINEAR, BRANCHING CALCIFICATIONS IN A GROUP OR LINEAR/SEGMENTAL DISTRIBUTION**

DCIS (w/central necrosis; commonly high nuclear grade DCIS but can also be seen in approximately 15–20% of low- or intermediate-grade DCIS)

Fat necrosis (in the early stages of calcification)
Fibroadenoma
Dystrophic, fibrosis
Autoimmune disorders (dermatomyositis, scleroderma, lupus)
Vascular (early stage)
Secretory (focal)
Suture (cut gut sutures and radiation)
Parasites (serpiginous)

BENIGN BREAST CALCIFICATIONS

For didactic purposes, I take an anatomic approach in describing breast calcifications. The terms provided in the American College of Radiology (ACR) BI-RADS® lexicon (6) for description and distribution modifiers are listed in Tables 6.3 and 6.4, respectively, and used throughout the text. Also please see Appendix A for the ACR BI-RADS® mammography, US and MRI lexicons.

As mentioned previously, when thinking about breast calcifications consider the anatomical structures available for breast calcifications to develop and the potential pathologic processes associated with these structures. This becomes helpful when analyzing calcifications and determining appropriate diagnostic considerations and management. Include the following tissue types: skin, stroma (e.g., fibrous tissue), ducts (large and small), acini grouped into lobules, and arteries. Calcifications developing in masses may be associated with the wall (mural, rim) of the mass, if one is present (e.g., cysts, oil cysts), or the epithelial or stromal elements of the mass. If the mass contains fluid, the calcifications may be in suspension (e.g., milk of calcium). Rarely, calcifications develop in association with foreign bodies such as suture material and parasites.

or amorphous calcifications with variable density as an indication for biopsy (Fig. 6.5). However, in the absence of linear calcifications or a linear distribution, the likelihood of DCIS drops significantly and, when diagnosed, is usually, though not exclusively, low or intermediate grade DCIS with no central necrosis. Diagnostic considerations for groups of round, oval, punctate (Fig. 6.6), and amorphous calcifications (4,5) include those listed in Table 6.2.

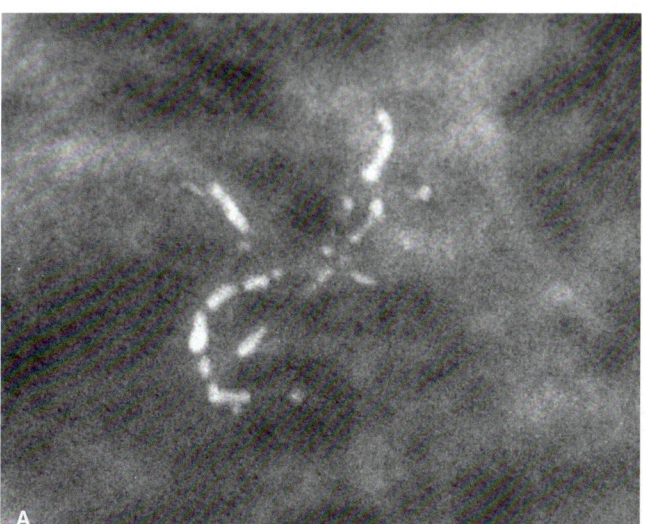
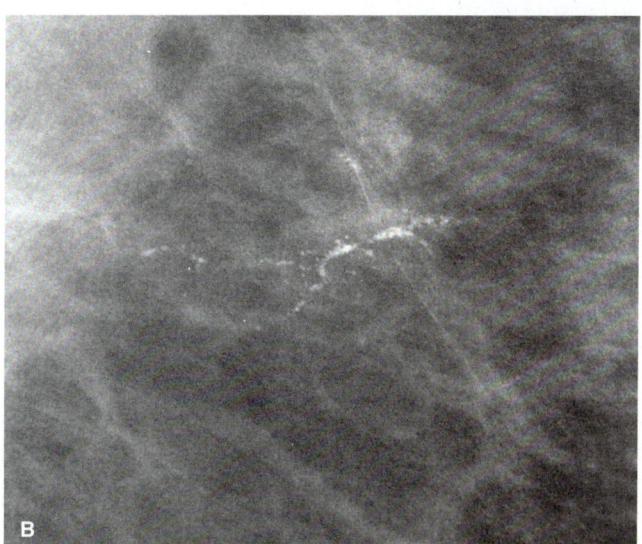

FIG. 6.4 • **Linear calcifications in a linear (ductal) orientation. DCIS. A:** Spot compression magnification view. Dense linear calcifications in a linear (ductal) distribution. BI-RADS 4C: Suspicious abnormality, biopsy is indicated. **B:** Linear calcifications with irregular margins and clefts in a linear, branching distribution. These calcifications develop in intraluminal necrotic debris, reflective of the ongoing proliferative cellular process. Fine pleomorphic calcifications are also present. BI-RADS 4C: Suspicious abnormality, biopsy is indicated.

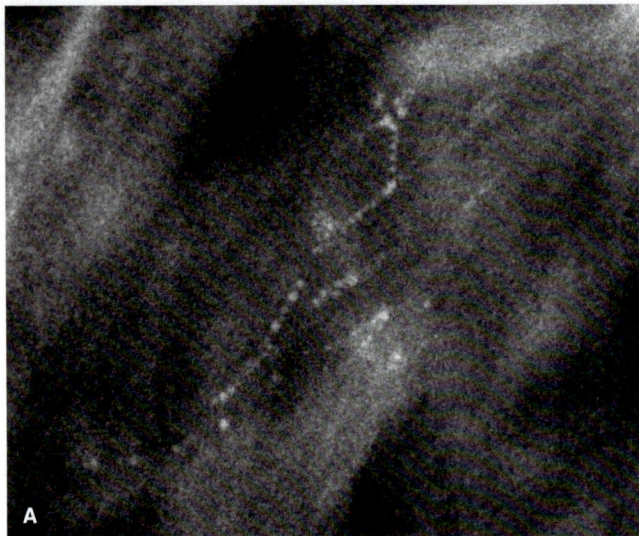
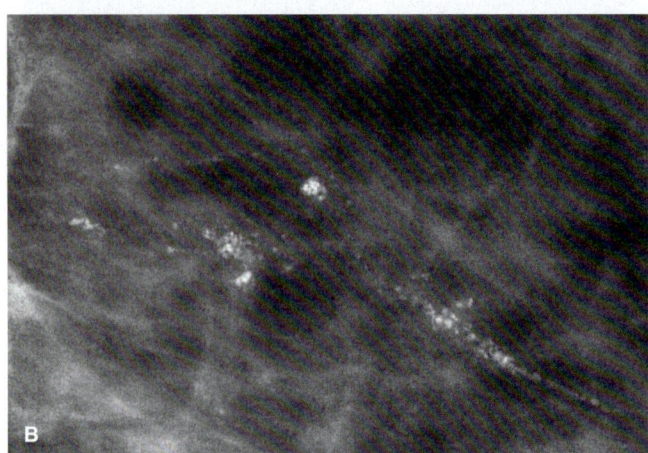

FIG. 6.5 • **Linear (ductal) distribution. DCIS. A:** Coarse heterogeneous and fine pleomorphic calcifications in a linear distribution ("string of pearls"). No linear forms are identified; however, the linear (ductal) distribution of the calcifications warrants biopsy. BI-RADS 4B: Suspicious abnormality, biopsy is indicated. DCIS, low nuclear grade, cribriform is diagnosed on core biopsy and confirmed on the lumpectomy specimen. **B:** Fine pleomorphic calcifications with intermingled coarse heterogeneous calcifications in a linear or segmental distribution. Linearly or segmentally distributed calcifications with the features shown warrant biopsy. BI-RADS 4C: Suspicious abnormality, biopsy is indicated. DCIS, high nuclear grade comedo-type is diagnosed on core biopsy and confirmed on the lumpectomy specimen.

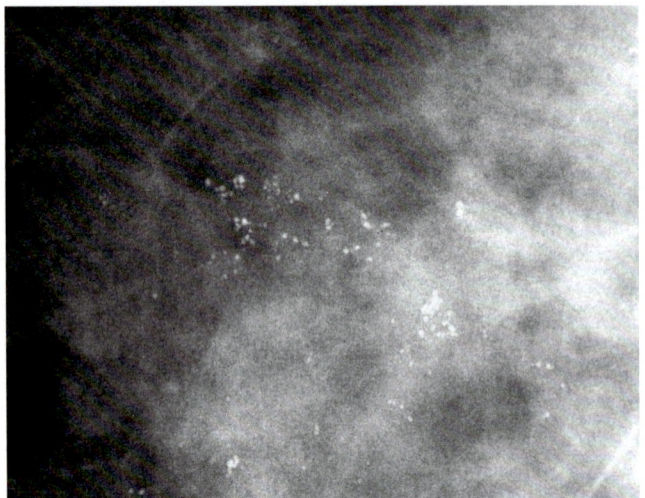

FIG. 6.6 • **Round and punctate calcifications.** Group of predominantly round calcifications with similar density, no linear forms or linear orientation. These may be considered "probably benign" if no prior films are available for comparison. BI-RADS 3: Probably benign finding; however, we recommend follow-up in 1 year for patients with these types of calcifications (e.g., no 6-month follow-up). (From Cardeñosa G. *Breast Imaging [The Core Curriculum Series]*. Philadelphia, PA: Lippincott Williams & Wilkins; 2003.)

SKIN CALCIFICATIONS

Skin calcifications (Fig. 6.7) form in sweat glands following low-grade folliculitis and inspissation of sebaceous material. Consequently, they are round or oval, lucent-centered, isolated, or more commonly, multiple tight clusters bilaterally. A lace-like pattern can be seen when associated with moles (see Fig. 7.8A). In lucent-centered skin calcifications, a punctate calcification may be seen centrally. Commonly, skin calcifications are seen posteromedially projecting on the pectoral muscles on mediolateral oblique (MLO) views, and medially at the cleavage, on craniocaudal (CC) views (Fig. 6.8); they can also involve the skin diffusely. In patients who

Table 6.2 **GROUPS OF FINE PLEOMORPHIC (PUNCTATE, ROUND, OR AMORPHOUS CALCIFICATIONS) AND COARSE HETEROGENEOUS CALCIFICATIONS**

Lobular calcifications
Fibroadenoma
Papilloma
Fibrocystic changes
    Sclerosing adenosis
    Ductal hyperplasia
    Atypical ductal hyperplasia (ADH)
    Flat epithelial atypia
    Columnar cell change (CAPPS with or without atypia)
    Fibrosis
Fat necrosis
Mucocele-like lesions
DCIS (more commonly low or intermediate cribriform, micropapillary DCIS w/no central necrosis)

Table 6.3 **ACR LEXICON, DESCRIPTIVE TERMS FOR CALCIFICATIONS**

Benign	Suspicious
Skin	Amorphous
Vascular	Coarse heterogeneous
Coarse or popcorn-like	Fine pleomorphic
Large rod-like	Fine linear or fine-linear branching
Round	
Rim	
Milk of calcium	
Suture	
Dystrophic	

Table 6.4	ACR LEXICON, DISTRIBUTION MODIFIERS FOR CALCIFICATIONS
Grouped	
Linear	
Segmental	
Regional	
Diffuse	

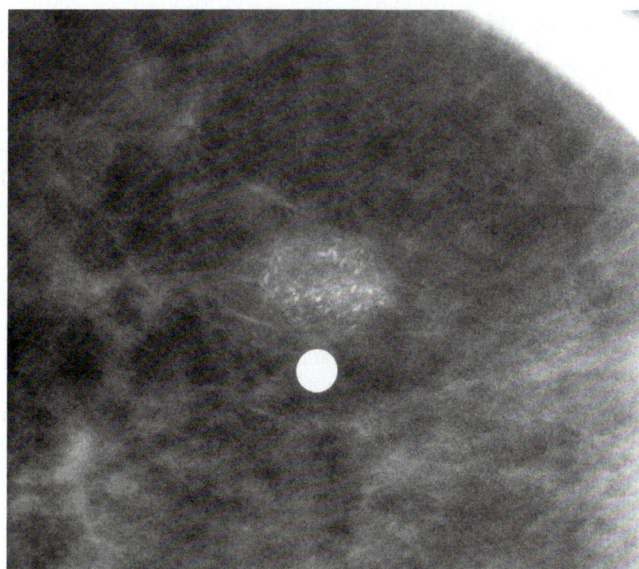

FIG. 6.9 • **Skin mass with associated fine pleomorphic calcifications.** Metallic BB denotes site of skin lesion. A low-density mass with indistinct margins and fine pleomorphic calcifications is imaged correlating with the site of the skin lesion. BI-RADS 2: Benign finding. (From Cardeñosa G. *Breast Imaging [The Core Curriculum Series].* Philadelphia, PA: Lippincott Williams & Wilkins; 2003.)

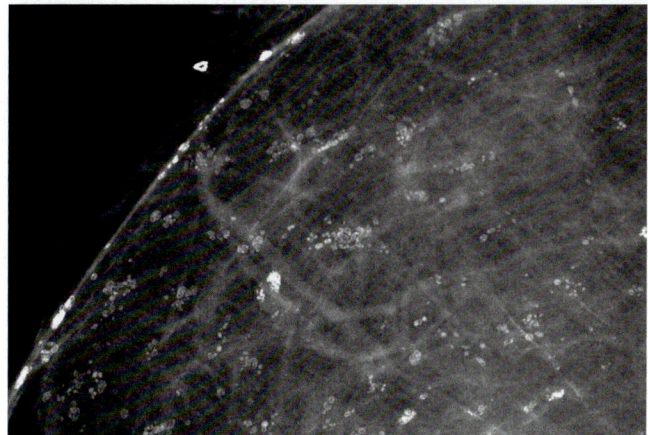

FIG. 6.7 • **Skin calcifications.** Multiple groups of round and oval lucent-centered calcifications. BI-RADS 2: Benign finding. A micromark biopsy clip is noted subcutaneously.

have had a reduction mammoplasty, skin calcifications sometimes develop along the incisions, demonstrating a linear distribution.

On any two views of the breast, much of the skin is superimposed on breast parenchyma; only a small amount of skin is ever in tangent to the x-ray beam, enabling distinction between skin and associated lesions from underlying breast tissue (Fig. 6.8). Although the appearance of most skin calcifications is distinctive, if lucent centers are not readily apparent, definitive diagnosis is made when the skin containing the calcifications is imaged in tangent to the x-ray beam (see Fig. 3.25 and Chapter 3 for a description of skin localization) (7–9).

In some patients, calcifications develop in association with moles or other skin lesions (e.g., sebaceous cysts). These can outline the crevices

of the mole, creating semicircular, lace-like calcifications, or, when developing in the contents of the mass, they may be pleomorphic (Fig. 6.9) or more coarse and dense (see Fig. 7.13). In some women, talc, Desitin, or other high-density products, deposited in the crevices of moles, can simulate calcifications. The overall density of the particles, their morphology and distribution, is usually pathognomonic (Fig. 6.10); alternatively, placing a metallic BB on the skin lesion and demonstrating that the BB moves with the lesion on two views (Fig. 6.9), obtaining a tangential view of the skin lesion (see Figs. 3.25, 7.9B and 7.11B), or wiping the patient's skin and repeating an image can provide a definitive diagnosis.

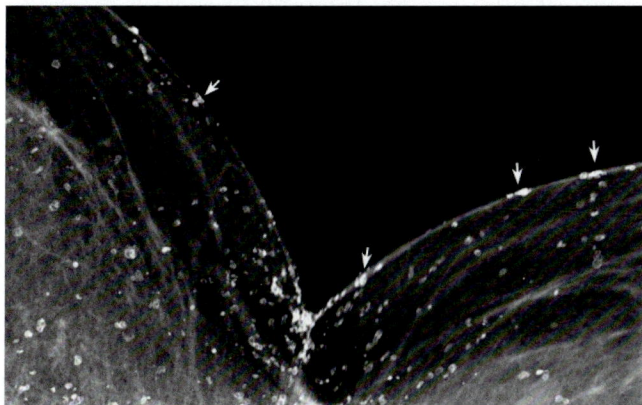

FIG. 6.8 • **Skin calcifications.** Cleavage view. Many round and oval lucent-centered calcifications are noted posteromedially seemingly in the breast. However, keep in mind that only a small amount of skin is captured in tangent to the x-ray beam. On any image of the breast, most of the skin projects on the breast parenchyma. Those calcifications in the skin that are in tangent to the x-ray beam can be localized to the skin *(arrows)*.

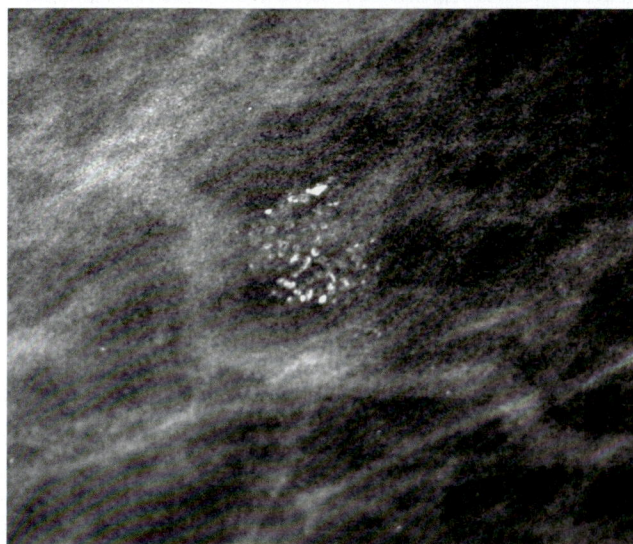

FIG. 6.10 • **High-density particles outlining crevices of skin lesion.** Central lucencies are evident. The density of the particles and their morphology are helpful in establishing the benign etiology. If concerns remain, a metallic BB can be placed on the skin lesion, or the skin can be wiped clean and a follow-up image used to establish correlation. (From Cardeñosa G. *Breast Imaging [The Core Curriculum Series].* Philadelphia, PA: Lippincott Williams & Wilkins; 2003.)

VASCULAR CALCIFICATIONS

Deposition of calcium in the media, at the perimeter of the elastic fibers of arterial walls, results in dense, linear, parallel, or "tram track-like" calcifications most common in postmenopausal women; in some patients, these develop and progress rapidly after menopause (if no hormone replacement therapy is used). When seen in younger premenopausal women, it is often in patients with diabetes (see Fig. 7.80) or in those with underlying renal disease. Interestingly, in some women this is a reversible process with vascular calcifications decreasing or resolving completely on subsequent screening mammograms (Fig. 6.11). When only a portion of the arterial wall is affected, or when small vessels are involved, the calcifications may be linear, irregular, variable in density, and have a linear orientation (Fig. 6.12A), simulating those occurring in DCIS. On careful inspection, early developing arterial calcifications often have a beaded appearance (Fig. 6.12B). Spot compression magnification views in some of these patients demonstrate the contralateral noncalcified vessel wall, noncalcified sections of the vessel coming into and out of the area of the calcifications, or an accompanying vein (Fig. 6.12A and 6.13).

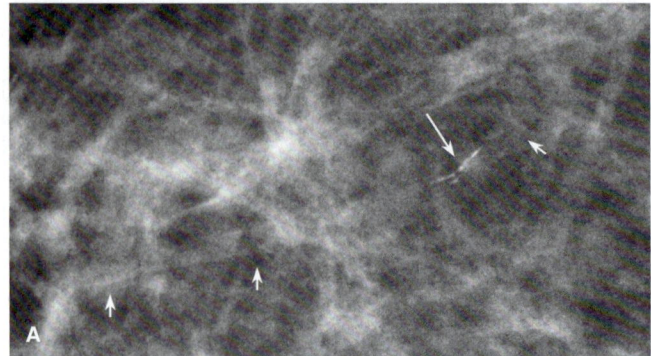

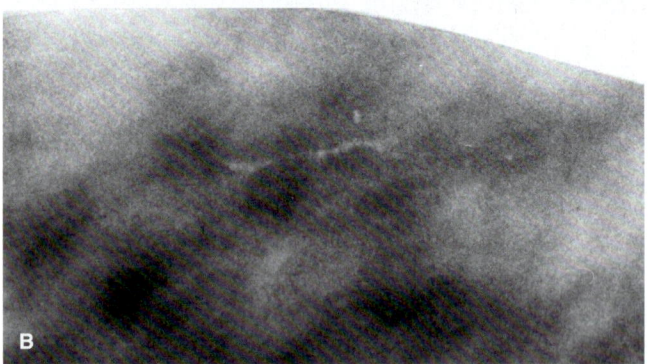

FIG. 6.12 • **Arterial calcifications, early stage. A:** Fine linear calcifications in a linear distribution *(long arrow)* are noted. In this patient, a vessel *(short arrows)* is identified coming into and out of the area of the calcifications. BI-RADS 2: Benign finding. **B:** Linear calcifications with a beaded appearance and linear distribution. In this patient, multiple spot compression magnification views are done, and no association with a vessel is established. Biopsy is done with a sizeable hematoma developing after the first core. Core radiograph (not shown) demonstrates a linear calcification in the one core obtained. Calcification in the media of an artery is diagnosed histologically. It is exceedingly rare not to be able to correlate calcifications to a vessel wall on spot compression magnification views, but it does happen.

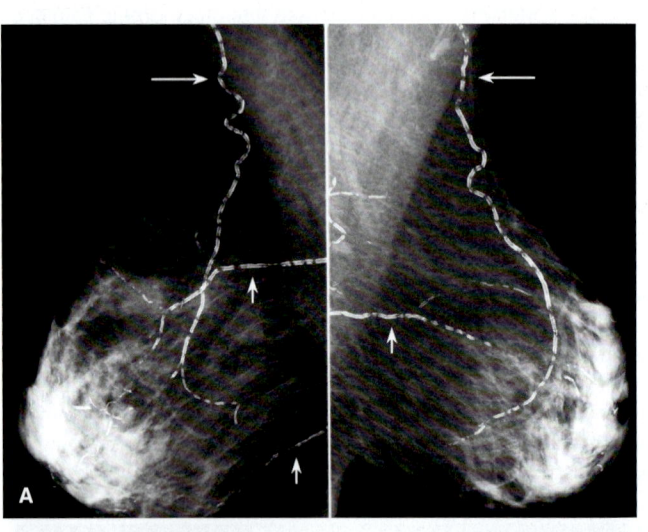

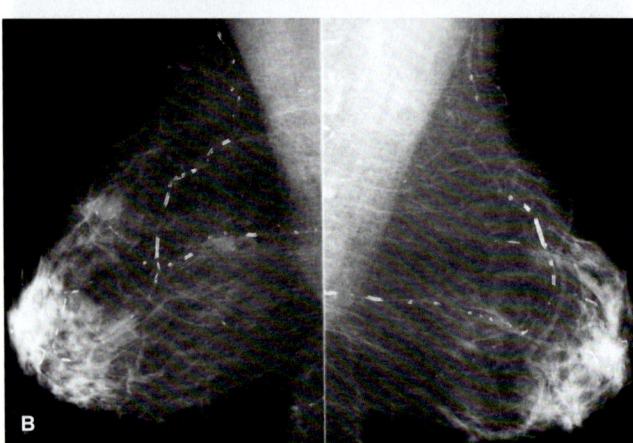

FIG. 6.11 • **Resolving arterial calcifications. A:** MLO views in a 63-year-old woman. The lateral thoracic arteries *(long arrows)* and some branches of the internal mammary arteries *(short arrows)* are densely calcified bilaterally. **B:** MLO views, 2 years after those in part **A**. Arterial calcifications are almost completely resolved. Although in this patient no apparent explanation for the resolution of the calcifications is known, in some patients, with underlying cardiac or renal disease, we have seen vascular calcifications resolve following cardiac or renal transplants; in some postmenopausal women, arterial calcifications may resolve after the patient is started on hormone replacement therapy.

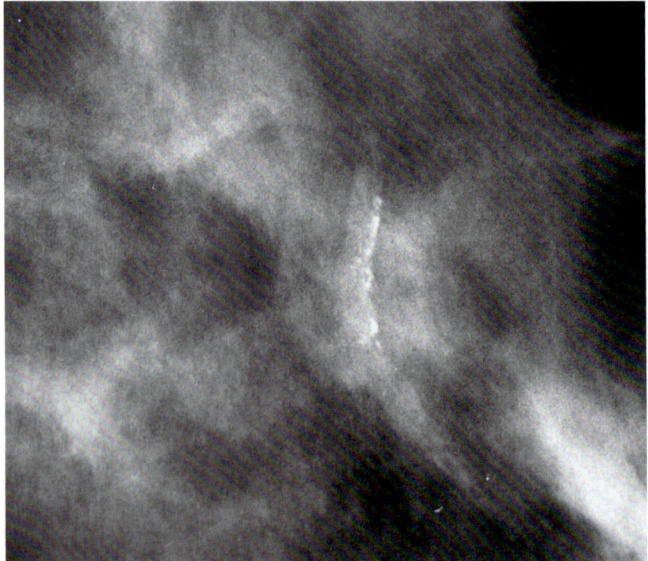

FIG. 6.13 • **Vascular calcifications.** In this patient, the association of linear calcifications with the wall of an artery is established easily on this projection. The contralateral vessel wall and other portions of the vessel are identified readily. BI-RADS 2: Benign finding. (From Cardeñosa G. *Breast Imaging [The Core Curriculum Series]*. Philadelphia, PA: Lippincott Williams & Wilkins; 2003.)

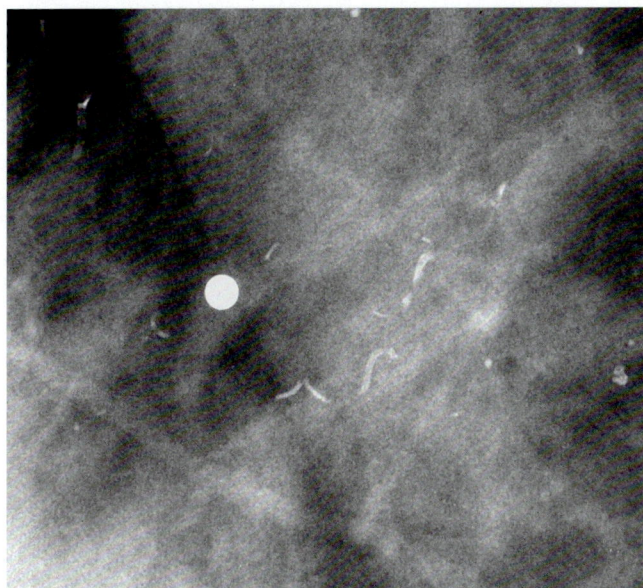

FIG. 6.14 • **Vascular calcifications.** "Quirky" calcifications are identified with smooth margins and central lucencies consistent with arterial calcifications. Similarly, calcifications are noted diffusely scattered bilaterally. BI-RADS 2: Benign finding. (From Cardeñosa G. *Breast Imaging [The Core Curriculum Series]*. Philadelphia, PA: Lippincott Williams & Wilkins; 2003.)

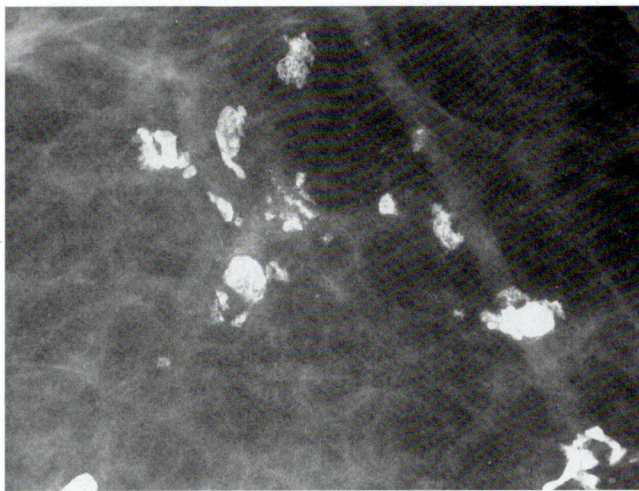

FIG. 6.15 • **Stromal (dystrophic) calcifications.** Dense, coarse calcifications developing in fibrous tissue and not a predefined space are variable in size, density, and shape. They may be focal, limited to areas of prior surgery or trauma or diffuse. (From Cardeñosa G. *Breast Imaging [The Core Curriculum Series]*. Philadelphia, PA: Lippincott Williams & Wilkins; 2003.)

Occasionally, smaller vessels calcify, leading to the appearance of "quirky" types of calcifications. The borders of these calcifications are well defined, and a lucent center is often seen when evaluated closely with a magnifying lens (Fig. 6.14). In our experience, these smaller arterial calcifications tend to be more common in premenopausal women with dense tissue and can fluctuate from year to year; in some patients, they resolve completely. These patients do not usually have a history of diabetes or arteriosclerotic heart disease.

It has been reported by several investigators that there may be a correlation between the extent of arterial calcifications seen on a mammogram and underlying coronary artery disease (10–12). This remains controversial, with some reports refuting the correlation (13,14) particularly since calcifications and plaque in heart disease involve the intima of the vessel wall, not the media as seen in the vessels calcifying in the breast. We describe the presence of arterial calcifications in our consultation reports when they are identified in premenopausal women or when the calcifications develop rapidly from one year to the next (10–12). Rarely, tortuous and serpiginous calcification associated with a venous structure may be seen as long-term sequelae of Mondor disease (15).

STROMAL CALCIFICATIONS

Calcifications developing in the stroma of the breast are dystrophic. Since these develop in fibrous tissue, and not in predefined anatomic spaces, they vary in size, shape, and density; no two of these calcifications are alike. They are coarse, dense, large, irregularly shaped, and may have associated areas of lucency (Fig. 6.15). When diffuse and bilateral (Fig. 6.16), they may reflect the presence of an underlying inflammatory, degenerative, or metabolic process (e.g., renal disease with hyperparathyroidism). Dystrophic calcifications can also be seen in the fibrous capsule that forms around implants (Fig. 6.17; also see Fig. 11.49A, B), remnants of calcified capsule if implants are explanted (see Fig. 11.57C), or in conjunction with the granulomatous response elicited by foreign bodies such as silicone or paraffin injections.

Dystrophic calcifications in areas of dense stromal fibrosis can demonstrate a linear appearance (Fig. 6.18). The margins are sometimes irregular and jagged with some of the calcifications forming acute angles. In a given cluster, some of the linear calcifications are well defined, and on close inspection central lucencies (Fig. 6.19) may be identified. Stromal or dystrophic type calcifications can also develop in the fibrous tissue in masses such as fibroadenomas (see discussion in mass section) and in areas of prior trauma, burns, surgery, or radiation therapy (see Chapter 11) as well as a healed abscess or hematoma.

DUCTAL

The precipitation of calcium salts in entrapped secretions in subsegmental ducts leads to the development of fusiform calcium casts of the dilated ducts (16,17). These calcifications (Figs. 6.1 and 6.20) are "rod-like," cigar shaped, coarse, high in density, smooth bordered, diffuse, bilateral, pointing toward the nipple, and can demonstrate branching. When the calcifications form periductally, a radiolucent center is seen. This type of calcification reflects the presence of duct ectasia with associated inflammatory changes also called periductal mastitis, secretory disease, comedo mastitis, plasma cell mastitis, and mastitis obliterans. Histologically, the dilated ducts contain amorphous debris, foam cells, and, less commonly, a crystalline-like lipid material. The epithelial cells normally lining the ducts are atrophic, appearing attenuated, deformed, and flattened or absent. The elastic tissue layer is disrupted and partially destroyed. In women with mastitis obliterans, fibrous tissue obliterates the epithelial lining and duct lumen. A chronic inflammatory process composed of plasma cells may be seen periductally.

This process is often diffuse and bilateral, less commonly unilateral, and rarely focal (Fig. 6.21). Since the epithelial lining of the ducts is flattened or denuded, the border of these calcifications is smooth (Fig. 6.22). Coarse calcifications, associated with dense fibrotic breast tissue in the subareolar areas, reflect burned out plasma cell mastitis. These patients may describe a tender mass in one or both subareolar areas. A white, thick, cheese-like, and at times foul-smelling discharge may also be present arising from multiple duct openings bilaterally.

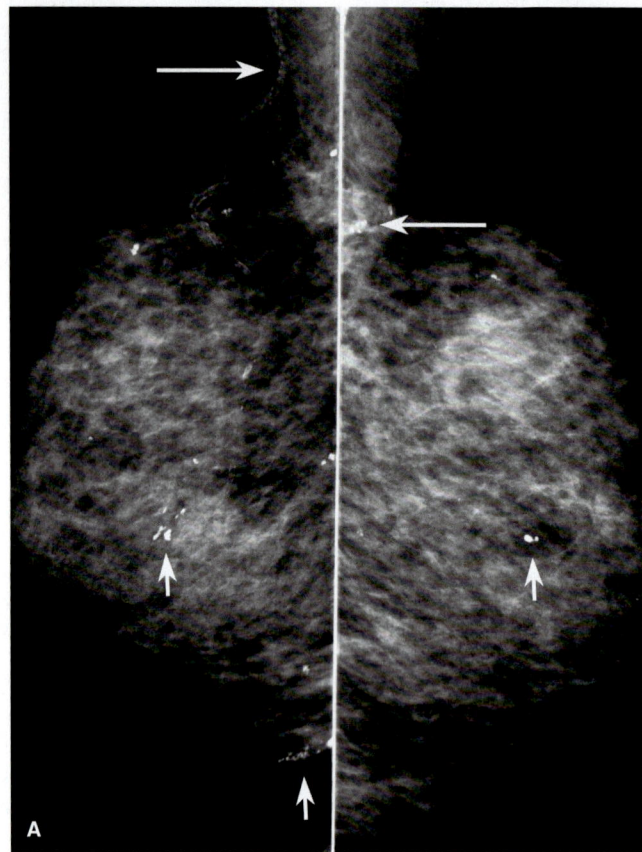

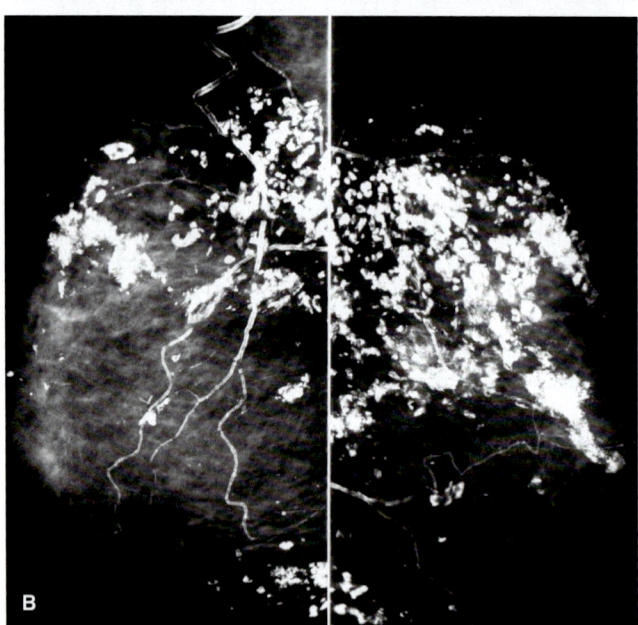

FIG. 6.16 • **Stromal (dystrophic) calcifications developing in a patient with end-stage renal disease and hyperparathyroidism. A:** MLO views. Dense tissue. A few coarse dense calcifications *(short arrows)* are present scattered bilaterally as are arterial calcifications *(long arrows)*. **B:** Follow-up MLO views. The patient has developed many dense, coarse stromal (dystrophic) calcifications reflective of her end-stage renal disease and hyperparathyroidism. Dense arterial calcifications are now also apparent. In these patients, the dystrophic (stromal) and arterial calcifications can resolve completely if the renal disease (and hyperparathyroidism) are well controlled with dialysis or renal transplantation.

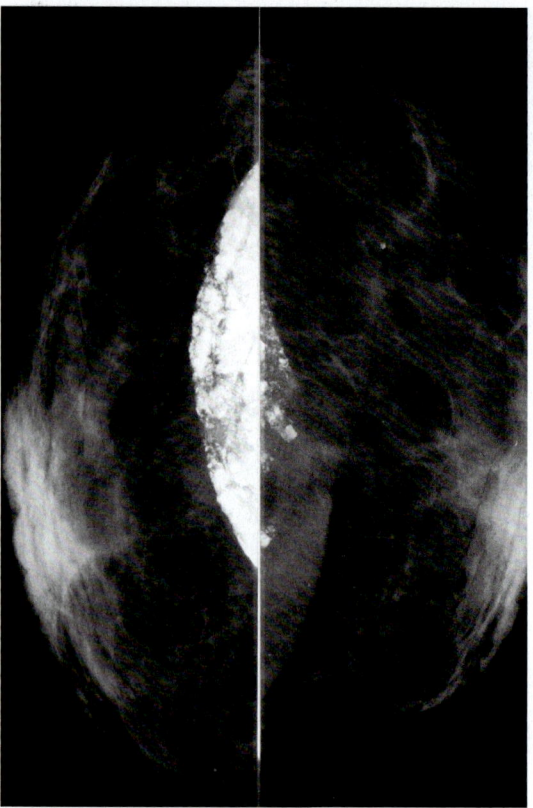

FIG. 6.17 • **Calcification in fibrous capsule around implant.** Implant displaced views. In some patients, dense dystrophic calcifications can be seen in the fibrous capsule that forms around implants and may remain after explantation (see Fig. 11.57C).

LOBULAR

Lobules represent groupings of round glands called acini. It is in the acinar structures that milk is produced during late pregnancy and lactation. If the acini are not altered by proliferations of the surrounding fibrous perilobular tissue, as is seen in fibroadenomas and sclerosing adenosis, calcifications developing in acini are round, relatively high density, well defined, or pearl-like and smooth bordered. If the lumen of the glands is small, the calcifications may be punctate. These can occur as clusters (Fig. 6.23A, B) of predominantly round calcifications or diffusely scattered round calcifications often bilaterally (Fig. 6.23C, D). When there is associated proliferation of perilobular stroma, as is seen with sclerosing adenosis and fibroadenomas, the acinar spaces may be deformed, compressed, and elongated, resulting in grouped pleomorphic calcifications that are indistinguishable from those seen in some forms of DCIS (18).

If the acinar spaces are tiny and tightly apposed, we may not be able to resolve the individual calcification particles but rather see smudgy, ill-defined, or amorphous calcifications. When specimen radiography is done using higher magnification factors than achievable in patients, these amorphous calcification clusters can sometimes be resolved into individual punctate calcifications reflecting tightly packed, adjacent acinar structures. Amorphous calcifications (5) usually reflect the presence of sclerosing adenosis; they can be associated with DCIS, commonly low nuclear grade without central necrosis (Table 6.5). When the amorphous calcifications are diffuse and bilateral in patients with dense tissue (Fig. 6.24), our approach is careful follow-up. When amorphous calcifications are identified grouped (Fig. 6.25),

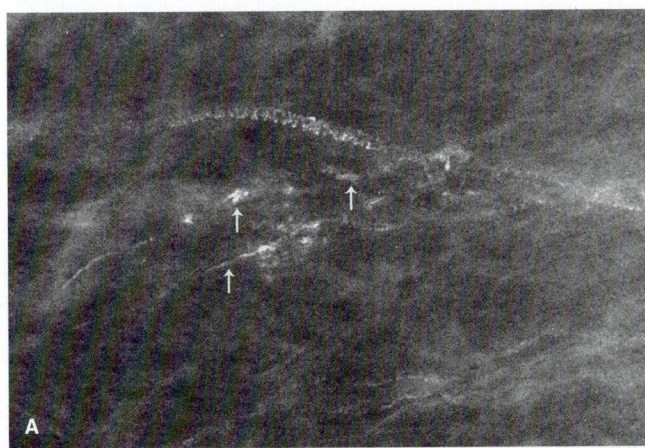

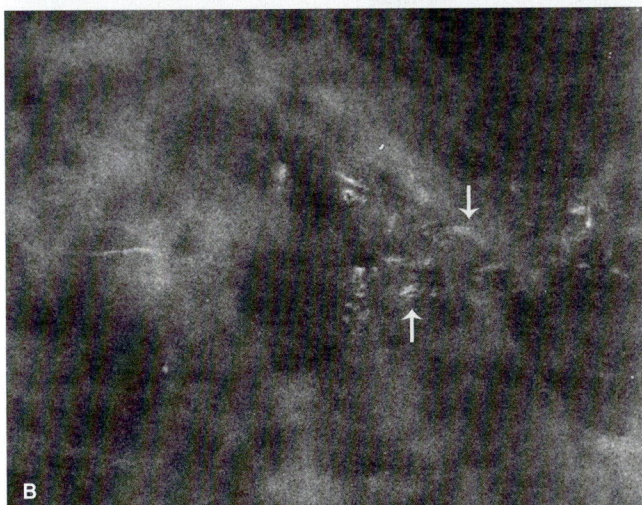

FIG. 6.18 ● **Stromal (dystrophic) calcifications in hyalinized breast tissue.** Spot compression magnification views in the MLO **(A)** and CC **(B)** projections. Linear calcifications in a linear orientation are identified. On careful review with a magnification lens, some have a central lucency (arrows). Although the diagnosis of stromal fibrosis is suspected on the basis of the mammographic appearance of the calcifications, a biopsy is done confirming the diagnosis of dense stromal fibrosis with calcifications. BI-RADS 4A: Suspicious abnormality, biopsy is indicated. On the MLO view, arterial calcifications are also present. (From Cardeñosa G. Breast Imaging [The Core Curriculum Series]. Philadelphia, PA: Lippincott Williams & Wilkins; 2003.)

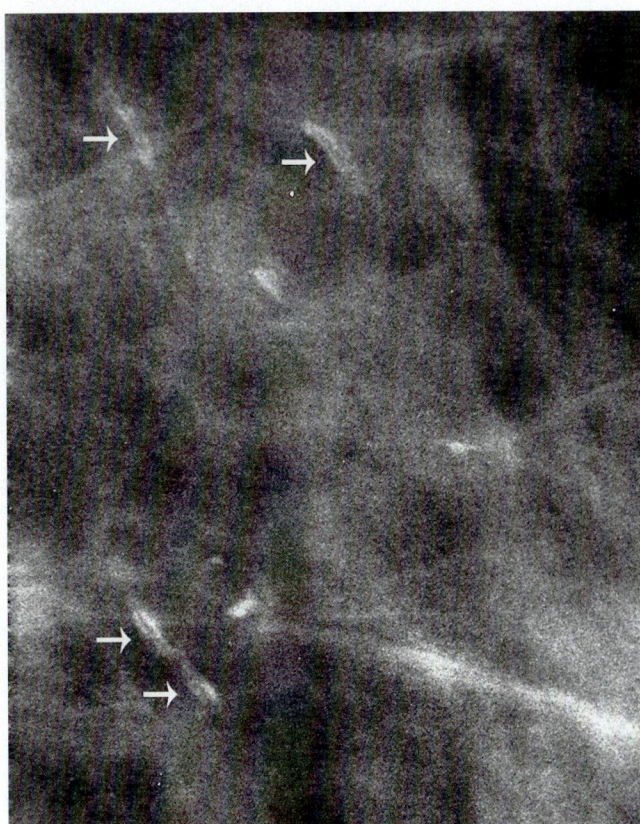

FIG. 6.19 ● **Stromal calcifications.** Spot compression magnification view demonstrating linear calcifications with a central lucency (arrows). BI-RADS 2: Benign finding. Calcifications are stable on subsequent annual screening mammograms. (From Cardeñosa G. Breast Imaging [The Core Curriculum Series]. Philadelphia, PA: Lippincott Williams & Wilkins; 2003.)

particularly if developing compared with prior studies, or if in an unusual location (e.g., upper inner quadrant), we recommend biopsy.

BENIGN-TYPE CALCIFICATIONS DEVELOPING IN MASSES

Curvilinear calcifications can be seen when they form in the wall of a mass, possibly a cyst (Fig. 6.26A), oil cyst (Fig. 6.26B), or in silicone granulomas (Fig. 6.27). Some of these are lucent-centered calcifications (Fig. 6.28) or, rim-type calcifications (Fig. 6.29) (e.g., when developing in the wall of an oil cyst).

Calcium can be present in suspension (Fig. 6.30) or as discrete calcifications in micro- or macrocysts (Fig. 6.31). The hallmark of intracystic calcifications is their variation in appearance on orthogonal views (19–21). When viewed on the CC view, the calcium may appear as an amorphous, ill-defined, round smudge, or a cluster of high-density tightly packed round (polyhedral) calcifications. When viewed in the horizontal plane on a 90-degree lateral view (and often even on the MLO view), the calcium layers in the dependent portion of the cyst and is seen as sharp, high-density curvilinear calcification or individual calcifications assuming a "teacup" or a meniscus-like configuration, enabling definitive diagnosis (Fig. 6.32). Microcysts and milk of calcium can be multifocal and bilateral in women with dense tissue (Fig. 6.30), or focal and unilateral (Fig. 6.32). In some patients, milk of calcium involves macrocysts (Fig. 6.31). Although ultrasound evaluation is not indicated in these patients, micro and macrocysts with associated milk of calcium can be identified on ultrasound (Fig. 6.30C).

In solid masses, calcifications can develop in epithelial elements, stromal components, or peripherally. Popcorn-type calcifications (Fig. 6.33A) are dystrophic, developing in the hyalinized fibrous stroma of fibroadenomas; in some patients with a papilloma, a "hollow" popcorn is seen as the periphery of the lesion calcifies (Fig. 6.33B; also see Fig. 9.34C). Popcorn calcifications are dense and coarse and can occur in one or both breasts and be uni- or multifocal. In the initial stages of hyalinization with calcification, grouped pleomorphic calcifications may be seen with or without an associated mass (Fig. 6.34). Sequential mammograms demonstrate progressive deposition of calcium with coalescence and formation of larger calcifications (Fig. 6.35). Some women with calcified fibroadenomas present describing a hard "lump." In these patients, it is imperative that the interpreting radiologist be unequivocal in their description of the benign finding and its correlation

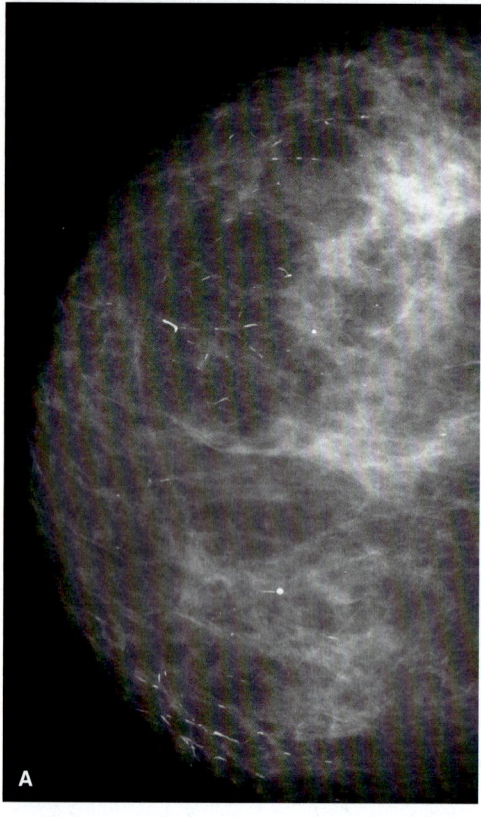
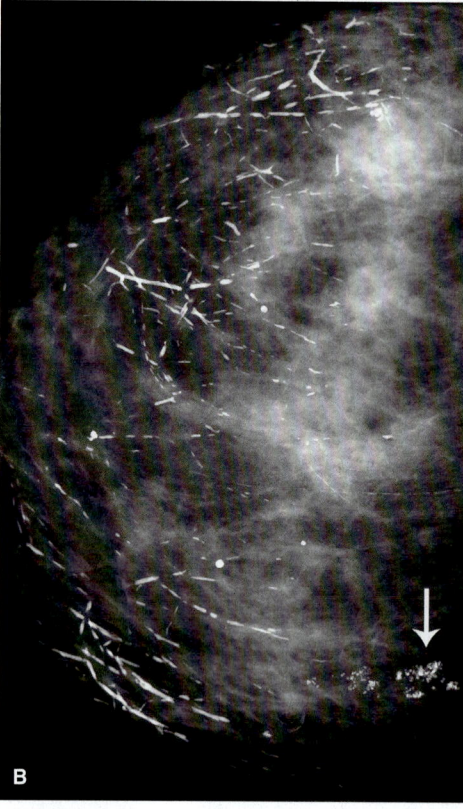

FIG. 6.20 • **Ductal, rod-like calcifications. A:** CC view demonstrating a few rod-like calcifications scattered in the right breast. **B:** CC view 2 years later. Many more dense rod-like calcifications have developed, and the preexisting calcifications are larger and denser. This type of calcification develops bilaterally, some have branch points, and most point toward the nipple. Grouped dystrophic calcifications *(arrow)* are now also noted medially. In these patients, it is easy to be mesmerized by the obviously benign findings. Force yourself to look away and search for the subtleties of a possible cancer among the obviously benign. (From Cardeñosa G. *Breast Imaging [The Core Curriculum Series]*. Philadelphia, PA: Lippincott Williams & Wilkins; 2003.)

with the palpable finding. To mitigate surgical referrals and potentially unnecessary biopsies, the patient and referring physician must be assured that the benign finding correlates with the palpable finding. A subgroup of calcifications occurring in fibroadenomas is fairly distinctive. These calcifications are high-density, "chunky," "coral-like" with jagged edges, some of which form acute angles (Fig. 6.36).

SUTURES

Suture material in the breast can calcify (22,23). These calcifications may be evenly spaced, linear, or curvilinear with smooth borders localized to lumpectomy sites (Fig. 6.37); in some, knots may be apparent. These calcifications appear to be a rare occurrence in the nonirradiated breast. They occur with a higher frequency in women

FIG. 6.21 • **Focal rod-like calcifications.** What is typically a diffuse bilateral process may be focal in some patients. The calcifications are dense, smooth bordered, and no other calcifications are identified in the surrounding tissue. If you have any questions regarding the underlying etiology in these patients, a 6-month follow-up may be helpful in assuring you are not dealing with an atypical presentation of DCIS with central necrosis. BI-RADS 2: Benign finding. (From Cardeñosa G. *Breast Imaging [The Core Curriculum Series]*. Philadelphia, PA: Lippincott Williams & Wilkins; 2003.)

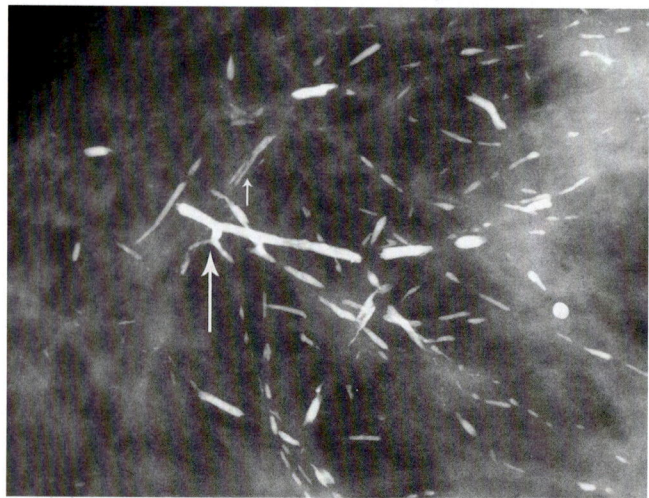

FIG. 6.22 • **Ductal, rod-like calcifications.** Coarse, dense calcifications with smooth borders reflect the attenuated or denuded epithelial lining of the ducts. Branch points may be seen *(long arrow)*. Central lucency *(short arrow)* is noted when the calcifications form periductally. BI-RADS 2: Benign finding. (From Cardeñosa G. *Breast Imaging [The Core Curriculum Series]*. Philadelphia, PA: Lippincott Williams & Wilkins; 2003.)

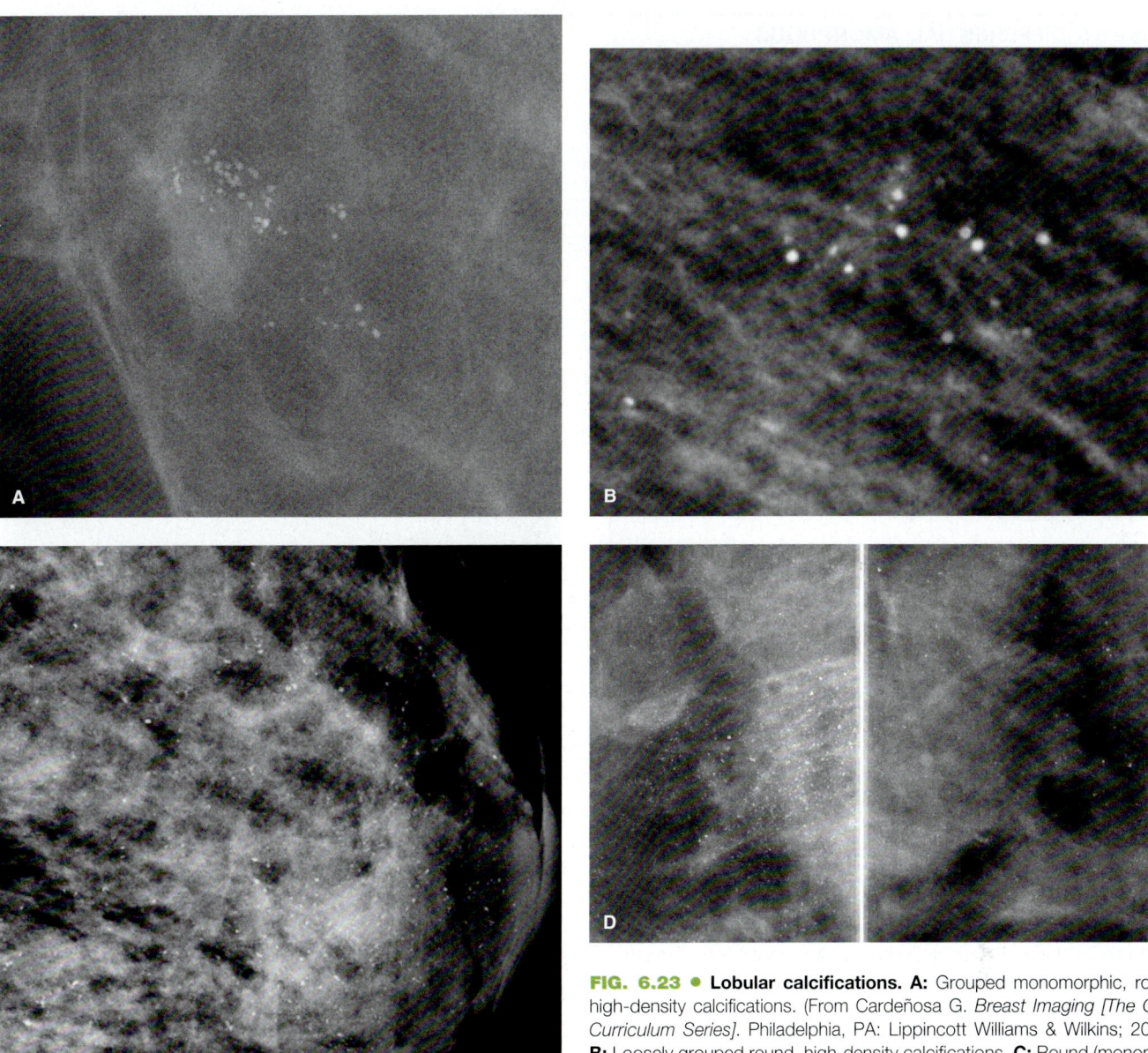

FIG. 6.23 • **Lobular calcifications. A:** Grouped monomorphic, round high-density calcifications. (From Cardeñosa G. *Breast Imaging [The Core Curriculum Series]*. Philadelphia, PA: Lippincott Williams & Wilkins; 2003.) **B:** Loosely grouped round, high-density calcifications. **C:** Round (monomorphic) calcifications are identified diffusely scattered in the dense parenchyma. **D:** MLO views photographically coned to the superior aspect of the image. Round and punctate calcifications are present diffusely scattered bilaterally more in the right breast compared with the left. Again, don't be mesmerized by the obviously benign. Look carefully among the benign for possible significant findings. BI-RADS 2: Benign finding.

following lumpectomy and radiation therapy. It has been postulated that radiation-induced damage and alterations in tissue healing delay the reabsorption of catgut sutures, thereby providing a matrix for the deposition of calcium (23).

PARASITES

Sporadic case reports are available describing the imaging features of parasites localized to the breast. These include filariasis (*Wuchereria bancrofti* and *Brugia malayi*), onchocerciasis (*Onchocerca volvulus*), and loiasis (*Loa loa*), all of which tend to be localized to the subcutaneous tissues, cysticercosis, dracunculosis, and schistosomiasis (24,25). The dead parasites calcify, leading to the development of linear, curvilinear, coiled, lace-like, bead-like, or serpiginous calcifications (Fig. 6.38) in isolation or with an associated soft tissue component (as has been reported for cutaneous myiasis—*Dermatobia hominis*) (26). Trichinosis (*Trichinella spiralis*) involves the pectoral muscles and spares breast tissue (27); fine, monomorphic "pearl-like," punctate calcifications are noted diffusely scattered but limited to the pectoral muscles (Fig. 6.39).

CALCIFICATIONS ASSOCIATED WITH MALIGNANCY

When considering calcifications associated with malignancy, we are primarily talking about proliferative cellular processes occurring in terminal ducts. Ductal carcinoma in situ is cancer arising in the terminal duct lobular units; it is a noninvasive or intraductal disease and

Table 6.5	**DIFFERENTIAL: AMORPHOUS ("SMUDGY") CALCIFICATIONS**

Diffuse

Milk of calcium (amorphous on craniocaudal view only, layer on lateral views)
Sclerosing adenosis
DCIS (commonly low nuclear grade)

Cluster

Sclerosing adenosis
ADH
FEA
Columnar cell change
Fibroadenoma
Papilloma
Fat necrosis
Fibrosis
Mucocele-like lesions
Lobular neoplasia
DCIS

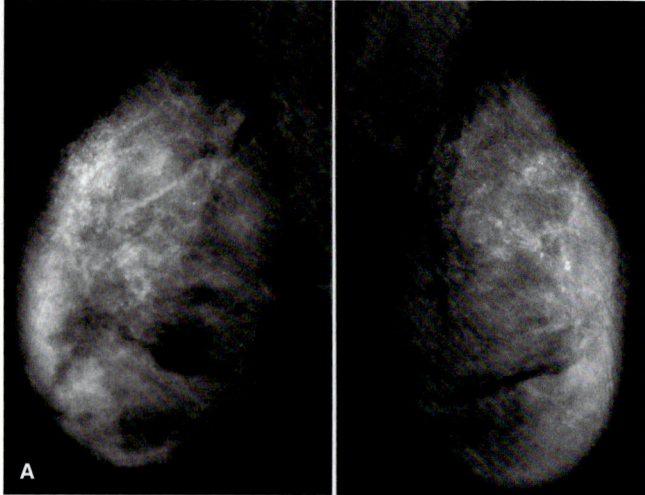

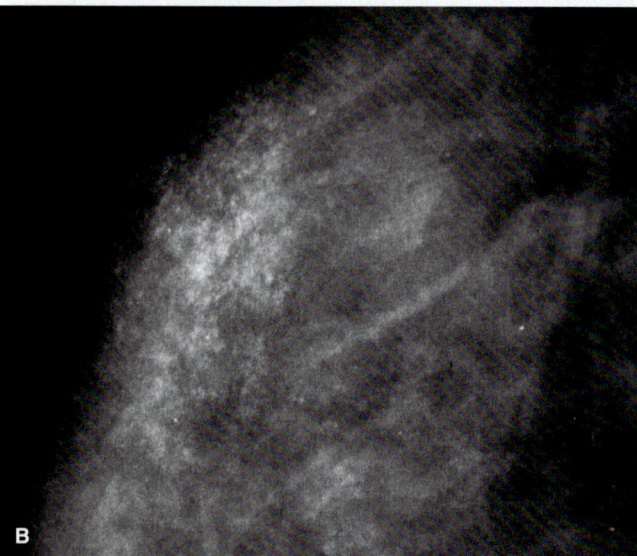

FIG. 6.24 • **Regionally distributed amorphous calcifications. A:** MLO views. Dense tissue with amorphous calcifications regionally distributed in the upper outer (CC views not shown) quadrants bilaterally. **B:** MLO view of the right breast photographically coned to the upper portion of the image. Regionally distributed amorphous calcifications. Given the extensive nature of the findings bilaterally, we manage these patients conservatively with annual follow-up. If any change is perceived, biopsy at the site of the change is done.

should be distinguished from invasive breast cancer. The most common mammographic manifestation of DCIS is calcifications detected in otherwise asymptomatic patients during screening. Rarely, DCIS can present (Table 6.6) as a macrolobulated or spiculated mass (see Figs. 8.20 and 8.21), an area of distortion detected mammographically (see Fig. 8.22), a palpable mass, parenchymal asymmetry (see Figs. 9.27 and 9.28), diffuse parenchymal change (see Figs. 9.20 and 9.21), developing ductal distension (see Figs. 5.38, 9.35, and 9.36), spontaneous nipple discharge (clear, serous or bloody), or Paget disease (see Fig. 9.30) of the nipple (28,29). With the increasing use of magnetic resonance imaging (MRI), mammographically and clinically occult DCIS is being diagnosed following the detection of segmentally distributed, non–mass-like, clumped and linear enhancement (see Fig. 5.38). Currently, MRI may, in fact, be the best method available for detecting DCIS. Additionally, the extent of disease in many patients with mammographically detected DCIS is more accurately demonstrated with MRI (see Fig. 3.16). An increasing number of studies suggest that MRI is more sensitive in detecting and characterizing the extent of DCIS than mammography (30–32).

Until the late 1980s, DCIS was considered a "rare" disease reported in 3% to 5% of all biopsies done for clinical findings (33). Rapid advances in mammographic technique and our ability to detect and characterize calcifications, coupled with increasing numbers of women undergoing screening mammography, have led to dramatic increases in the number of patients diagnosed with DCIS. As the use of breast MRI becomes more prevalent, our ability to detect DCIS has again improved (30–32) significantly.

In screening mammography programs, DCIS represents 22% to 45% of all detected breast cancers (29,34,35). An increase in the number of biopsies done for mammographically detected calcifications has driven the histological descriptions of DCIS, classification schemes, and our overall appreciation for this disease. With the increase in DCIS detection has also come significant controversy as to the biological significance of some of these lesions (31,32,35). However, when discussing DCIS and its significance, it is *imperative* to recognize that DCIS is a heterogeneous disease; not to be all "lumped" in one basket. DCIS is heterogeneous in its imaging and clinical (see Table 6.6) presentations, its histological features and, not surprisingly, its biological behavior. Some forms of DCIS invariably progress to invasion and do so with a rapid time course, while others remain "stable" in the duct for years, regress, or eventually progress into low-grade invasive ductal carcinomas. The daunting challenge we face is determining how to manage patients with some forms of low-grade DCIS appropriately. These are the lesions that may never progress to invasion, and as such, patients may be overtreated (e.g., mastectomy or using radiation therapy after the lumpectomy). This reflects our current inability to distinguish the "insignificant" DCIS lesions from those that recur, invade, and metastasize. It will be interesting to see if the functional information provided by MRI will translate into biological (prognostic) significance (36): Are the DCIS lesions that do not enhance on MRI biologically different from those that demonstrate avid enhancement? And if so, can the MRI findings help us triage patients and tailor treatments more appropriately?

Proliferative cellular processes occurring in the terminal ducts are usually mammographically occult, unless associated with calcifications.

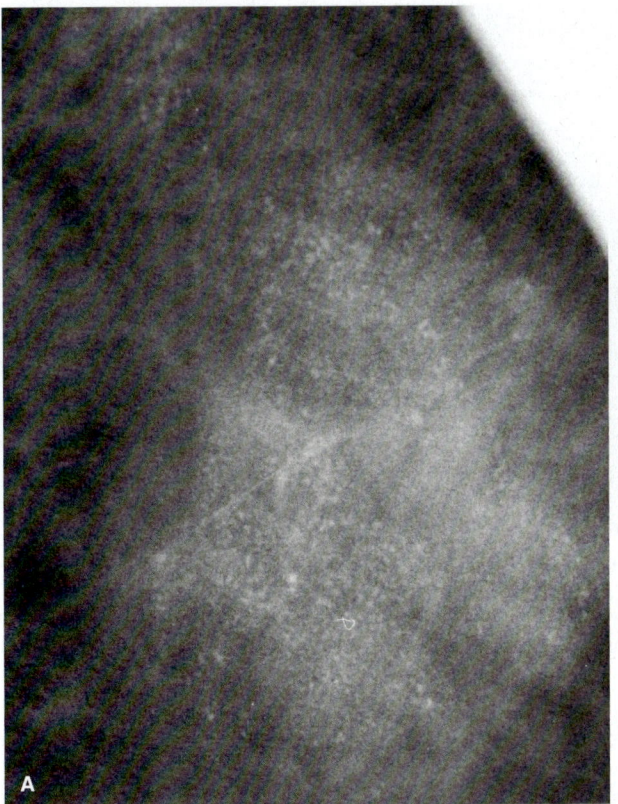
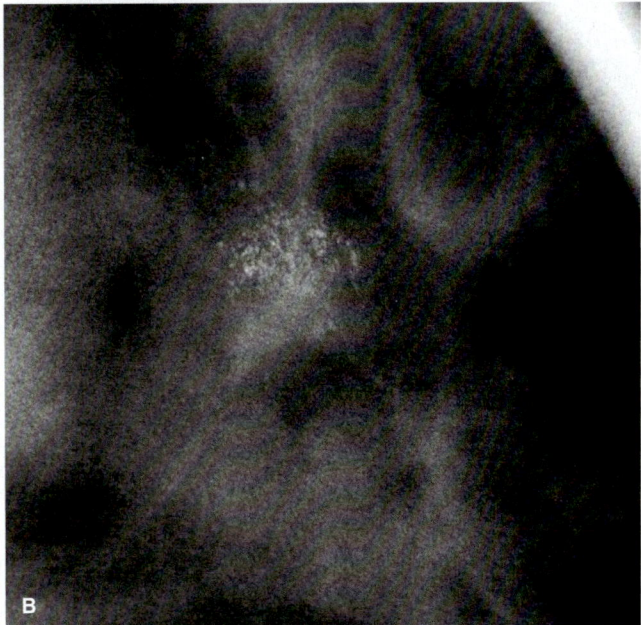
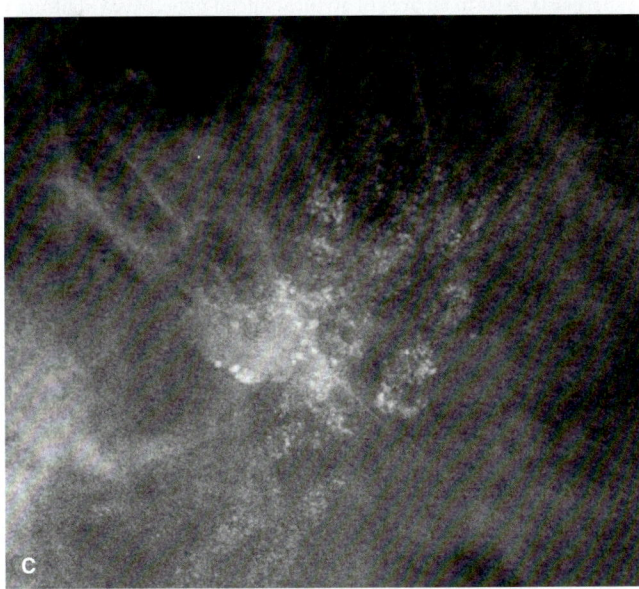

FIG. 6.25 • **Grouped amorphous calcifications. A:** Spot compression magnification view. Amorphous calcifications are present. No linear forms or linear distribution is apparent. In patients with localized amorphous calcifications, we recommend biopsy. BI-RADS 4A: Suspicious abnormality biopsy is indicated. Fibrocystic changes with fibrosis, apocrine metaplasia, and microcalcifications are reported histologically. **B:** Spot compression magnification view. Grouped amorphous calcifications. BI-RADS 4A: Suspicious abnormality biopsy is indicated. FEA is reported on a stereotactically guided biopsy and confirmed on excision. **C:** Spot compression magnification view. Several groups of amorphous calcifications are identified clustered in the right breast. BI-RADS 4A: Suspicious abnormality biopsy is indicated. Low nuclear grade DCIS is diagnosed on core biopsy. Intermediate grade DCIS with extensive FEA is reported on the lumpectomy specimen.

The duct wall is composed of loose connective tissue forming the basement membrane, a discontiguous layer of myoepithelial cells at the base of a contiguous layer of epithelial cells lining the lumen of the duct; a two-cell layer therefore characterizes normal ducts. Hyperplasia refers to an increase in the number of epithelial or myoepithelial cells lining the ducts. It can be qualified by pathologists as mild, moderate, or severe. As the proliferating cells acquire atypical cytologic features, the term atypical ductal hyperplasia (ADH) may be used. It is important, however, to emphasize that the diagnosis of ADH is to some extent subjective and defined differently by pathologists (37). Given the importance of some of the decisions made when a patient is diagnosed with atypia, it behooves radiologists involved in imaging-guided procedures to work closely with the pathologists and have some understanding of their approach to this diagnosis. There is also a growing list of entities described by pathologists, including flat epithelial atypia (FEA), columnar cell change with atypia, and atypical papilloma further confounding management decisions.

On the basis of three dimensional studies of ducts (38) involved with DCIS, biological markers, and associated invasive lesions, consider at least two large subgroups of DCIS: (i) those that appear to "evolve" over time from a spectrum of proliferative processes in the ducts that includes "usual" hyperplasia, ADH, and low nuclear grade DCISs; these processes may have luminal secretions but lack central necrotic debris and (ii) those arising de novo in the duct, characterized by central necrosis and short intraductal phases. The proliferative

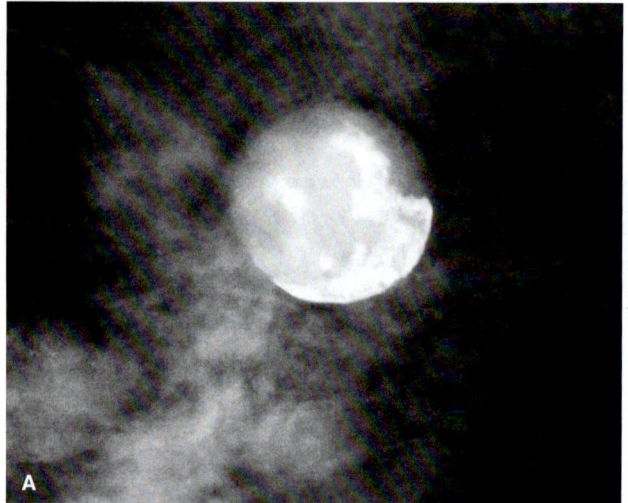
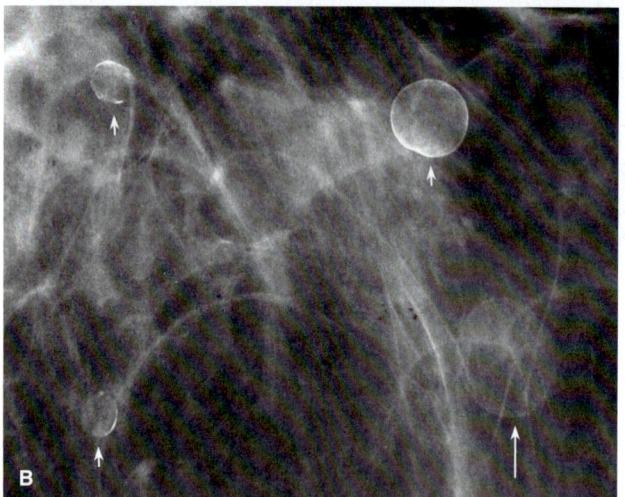

FIG. 6.26 • **Mural calcifications. A:** Dense calcifications developing on the wall of an iso dense round mass. **B:** Multiple oil cysts with rim calcifications at various stages of development *(short arrows)*. An noncalcified oil cyst *(long arrow)* is also present. (From Cardeñosa G. *Breast Imaging [The Core Curriculum Series]*. Philadelphia, PA: Lippincott Williams & Wilkins; 2003.)

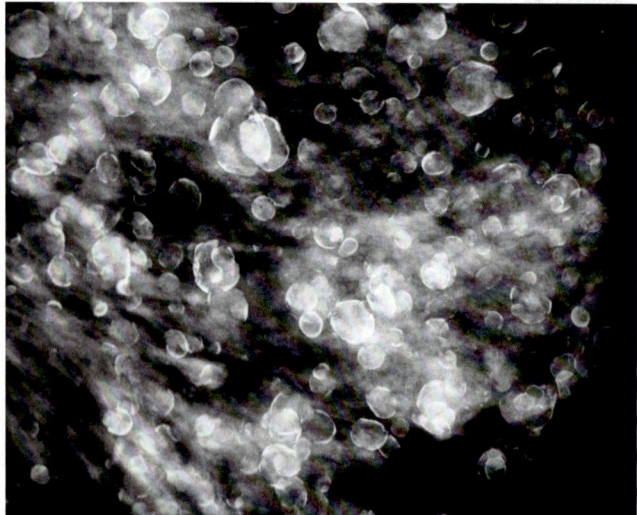

FIG. 6.27 • **Calcifying granulomas.** Many rim- and lucent-centered calcifications in a patient with a history of subcutaneous injections for augmentation.

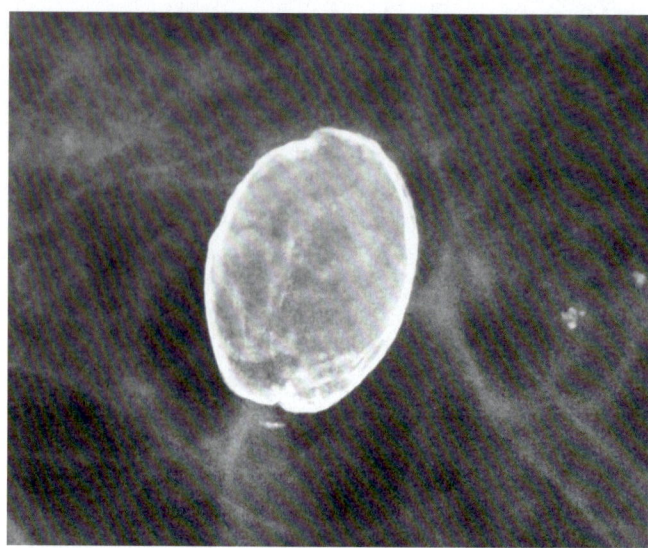

FIG. 6.28 • **Lucent-centered calcifications.** A mass (lucent) with calcifications developing in the wall is identified. Lucent-centered calcifications are thicker than rim calcifications. BI-RADS 2: Benign finding. (From Cardeñosa G. *Breast Imaging [The Core Curriculum Series]*. Philadelphia, PA: Lippincott Williams & Wilkins; 2003.)

processes associated with the first group are in a state of flux and multifocal in the involved ducts. That is, a normal segment of duct may be adjacent to an area of low grade DCIS, next to an area of ductal hyperplasia, next to an area of atypical ductal hyperplasia abutting yet another focus of low nuclear grade DCIS. The calcifications we detect mammographically likely develop in luminal secretions (not necrotic debris) and can therefore develop in association with hyperplasia, ADH, or low-grade DCIS. Since the effects of the proliferative process on the duct lumen overlap, it is not surprising that the mammographic appearance of the calcifications in these different processes is indistinguishable (39). In some patients, but not all, low-grade DCIS likely gives rise to low-grade invasive carcinomas.

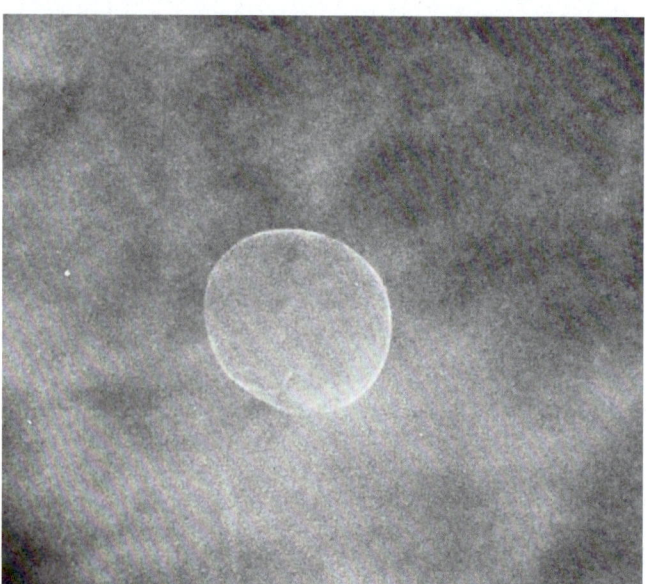

FIG. 6.29 • **Rim calcification.** Thin (<1 mm thick), curvilinear calcification occurring in the wall of an oil cyst. When thicker, the term lucent-centered calcification can be used. BI-RADS 2: benign finding. (From Cardeñosa G. *Breast Imaging [The Core Curriculum Series]*. Philadelphia, PA: Lippincott Williams & Wilkins; 2003.)

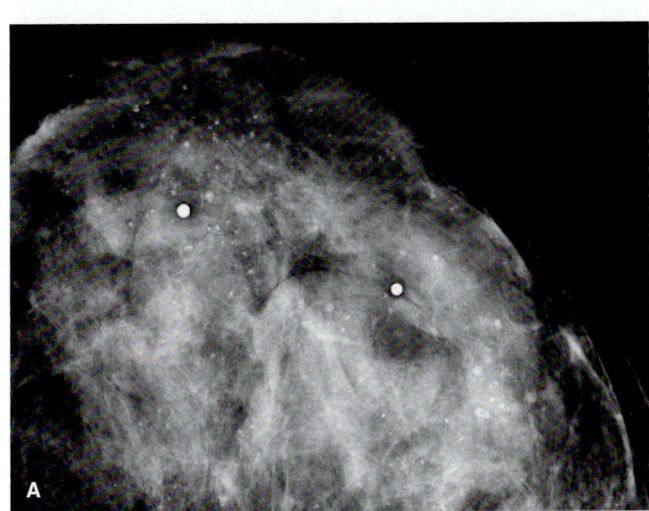
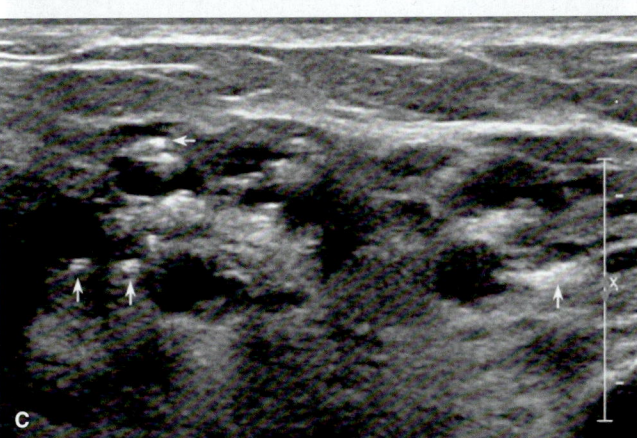
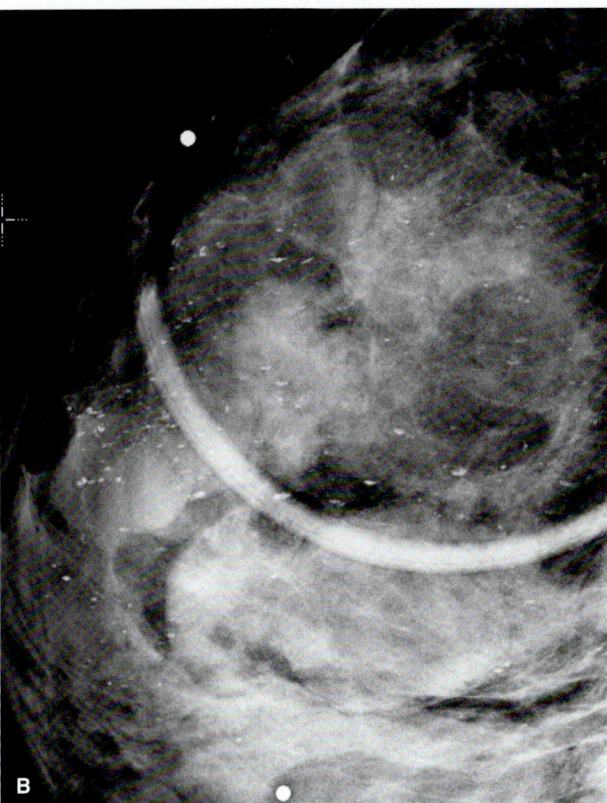

FIG. 6.30 • **Milk of calcium, diffuse. A:** CC view. Rounded "smudgy" areas of calcification with variable density are identified in a patient with dense tissue. **B:** Ninety-degree (LM) lateral spot compression view demonstrates multiple dense, sharply defined, curvilinear calcifications. This differential appearance of the calcifications between CC and 90-degree lateral views is diagnostic of milk of calcium. BI-RADS 2: Benign finding. **C:** Ultrasound. Subcentimeter cysts are identified with associated dependent foci of echogenicity (arrows at some of these), reflecting the calcifications seen mammographically.

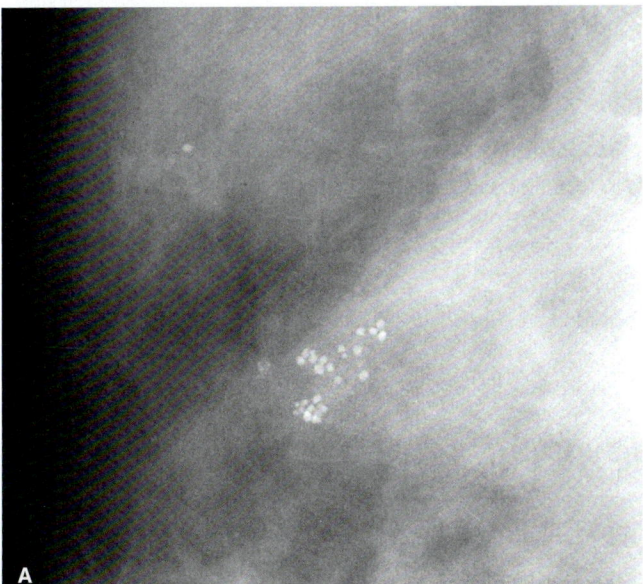
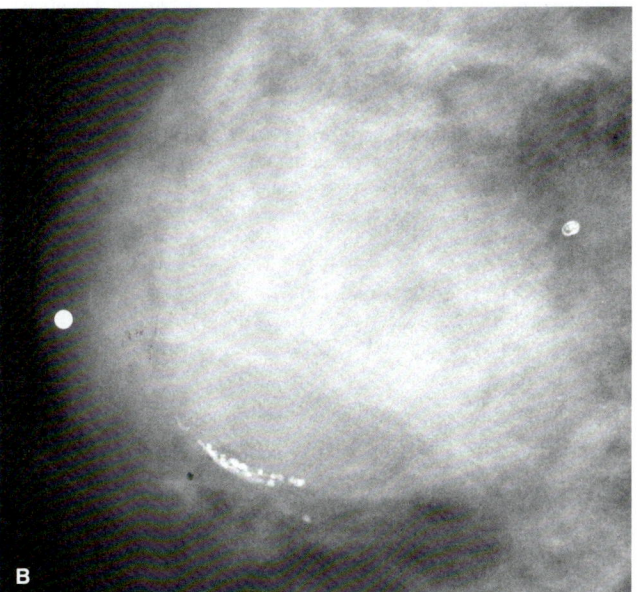

FIG. 6.31 • **Milk (pellets) of calcium. A:** CC view demonstrating grouped round (monomorphic) high-density calcifications. **B:** Ninety-degree (LM) view demonstrates layering of the individual calcifications in what can now be appreciated as a mass (e.g., macrocyst). Given the layering of the calcifications, an ultrasound is not indicated to evaluate the mass; the layering confirms that the mass is fluid-filled. BI-RADS 2: Benign finding. (From Cardeñosa G. *Breast Imaging [The Core Curriculum Series]*. Philadelphia, PA: Lippincott Williams & Wilkins; 2003.)

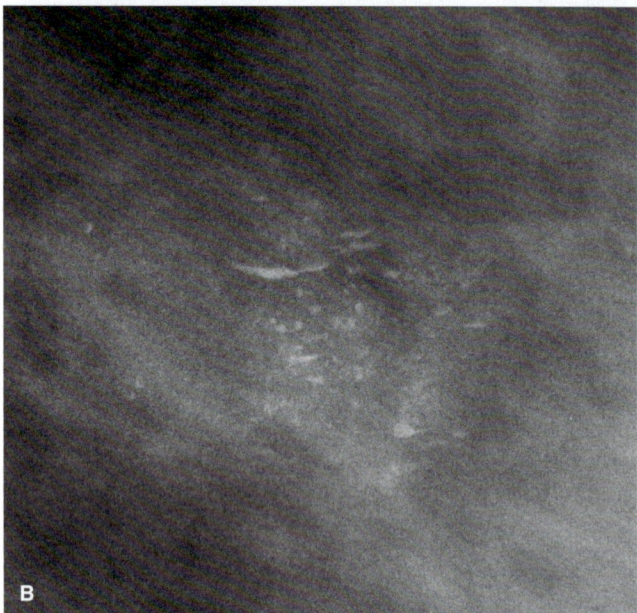

FIG. 6.32 • **Milk of calcium, focal. A:** CC view. Dense tissue and amorphous calcifications mixed with some round and punctate forms. **B:** Ninety-degree (LM) view demonstrates a change in the appearance of the calcifications. Many are now sharply defined, higher in density, and linear (teacups). The differential appearance of these calcifications between CC and oblique or 90-degree lateral views is diagnostic of milk of calcium. No additional evaluation or short interval follow-up is indicated. BI-RADS 2: Benign finding. (From Cardeñosa G. *Breast Imaging [The Core Curriculum Series]*. Philadelphia, PA: Lippincott Williams & Wilkins; 2003.)

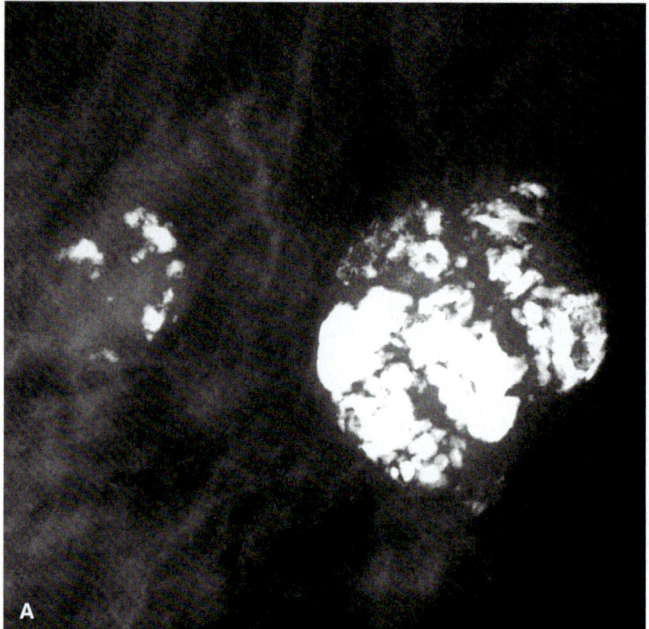

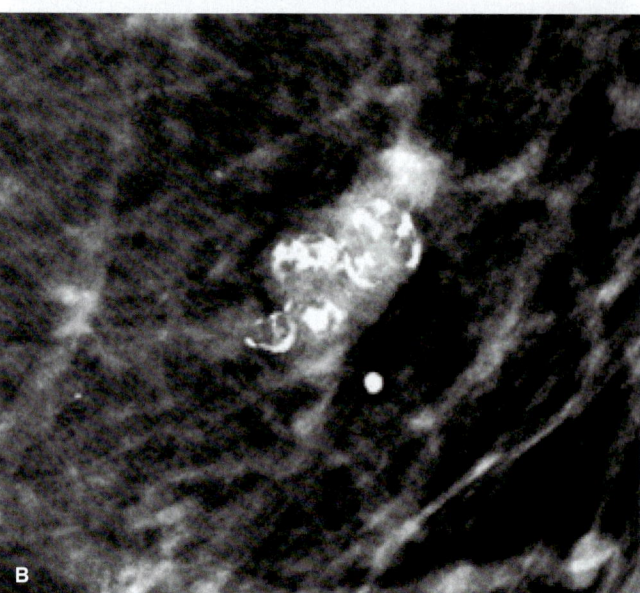

FIG. 6.33 • **Dystrophic calcifications. A:** Dense, coarse dystrophic-type calcifications developing in the hyalinized fibrous stroma of fibroadenomas. These are also referred to as "popcorn" calcifications. (From Cardeñosa G. *Breast Imaging [The Core Curriculum Series]*. Philadelphia, PA: Lippincott Williams & Wilkins; 2003.) **B:** Dense oval mass with "ringlets" of dense coarse curvilinear calcifications; these "hollow" popcorn-type calcifications are typically seen developing in papillomas.

The other major subgroup of DCIS likely arises de novo in the duct rather than evolving from a preexisting process (e.g., low-grade DCIS does *NOT* develop into high-grade DCIS, though they can coexist in a given lesion). These lesions are unifocal and contiguous in the duct, have central necrotic debris, and approximately 85% demonstrate high nuclear grade features. Areas of microinvasion may be apparent. This type of DCIS is thought to become invasive in most, if not all, patients. The progression from intraductal disease to invasive disease may occur rapidly.

Histologically, ducts involved with DCIS are distended compared with normal ducts. Low nuclear grade DCIS is characterized by monomorphic nuclei lacking nucleoli, low mitotic rates (low thymidine labeling rates), cell polarization toward the duct lumen, no cell necrosis or autophagocytosis, and probably a long (in some patient permanent) intraductal phase. The cells can form rigid cribriform spaces, roman bridges, or micropapillary projections (Fig. 6.40A). In some patients, a more solid growth pattern may be seen histologically.

High grade DCIS is characterized by pleomorphic nuclei having multiple nucleoli, high mitotic rates (high thymidine labeling rates), lack of cellular polarization, presence of cell necrosis and autophagocytosis, and a short intraductal phase. Most of these lesions are obligate invaders. The cells circumferentially encroach and narrow the lumen

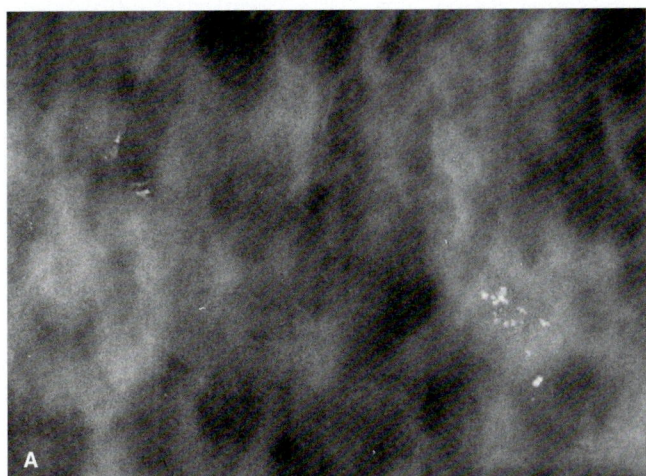
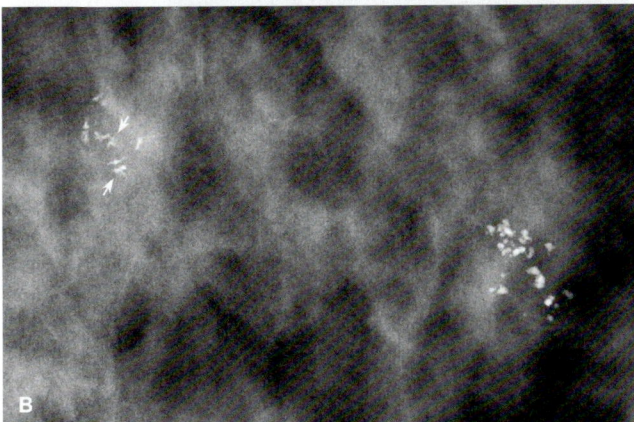

FIG. 6.34 • **Dystrophic calcifications. A:** Two clusters of calcifications are identified. Other similar clusters are noted in the contralateral breast. **B:** Two years following part **A**. Progressive development and coalescing of preexisting calcifications in the hyalinizing fibrous stroma of aging fibroadenomas can be seen without an apparent mass. Note the jagged edges and acute angles *(arrows)* on some of the calcifications. BI-RADS 2: Benign findings. (From Cardeñosa G. *Breast Imaging [The Core Curriculum Series]*. Philadelphia, PA: Lippincott Williams & Wilkins; 2003.)

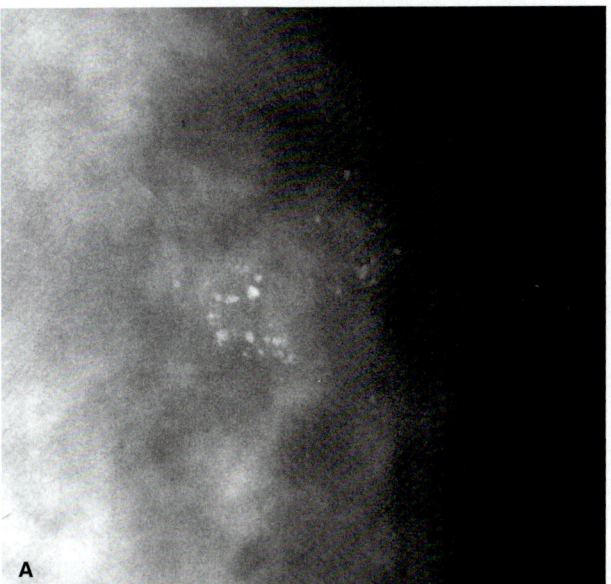
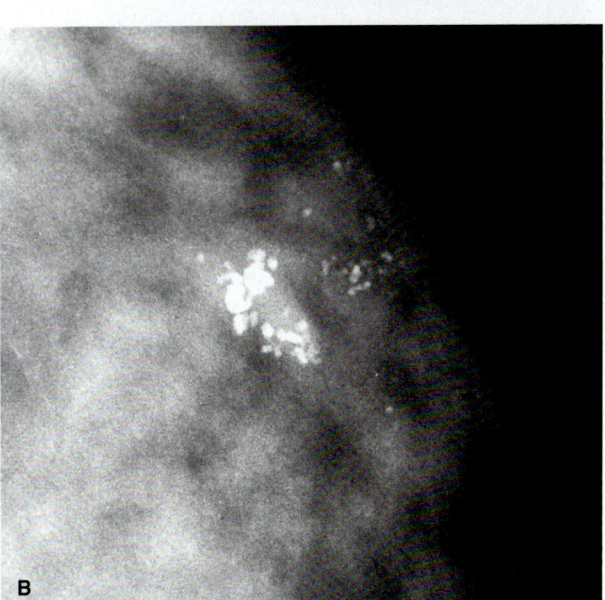

FIG. 6.35 • **Developing dystrophic calcifications. A:** Grouped coarse high-density calcifications with no linear forms or linear distribution. These may be associated with a bilobed mass. **B:** Two and a half years later following image in part **A**. As fibroadenomas hyalinized, they become smaller, denser and, if associated with calcifications, the calcifications may progress and coalesce to become coarse and dense. BI-RADS 2: Benign finding. (From Cardeñosa G. *Breast Imaging [The Core Curriculum Series]*. Philadelphia, PA: Lippincott Williams & Wilkins; 2003.)

of the distended ducts. The lumen contains necrotic cellular debris within which calcifications can form (Fig. 6.40B). In some patients, there is an intense inflammatory reaction surrounding the involved ducts, making it difficult to identify areas of microinvasion. High nuclear grade DCIS lesions are likely to give rise to poorly differentiated, high nuclear grade invasive lesions. These are the types of lesions that we strive to diagnose mammographically. Similarly, one could argue that the lesions with angiogenesis detected on MRI are possibly of more concern, given their ability to grow vessels lacking normal physiologic control mechanisms. Without intervention, these types of DCIS likely progress to invasion; their detection and excision may serve to reduce the likelihood of invasive disease in the future.

The calcifications we detect mammographically, in association with these cellular proliferative processes, develop in luminal secretions or in necrotic cellular debris in the lumen of the distended ducts (40). Calcifications, developing in secretions occurring in the cribriform spaces formed by proliferating cells may include coarse heterogeneous (round, granular) forms (Fig. 6.41A), fine pleomorphic (punctate) forms (Fig. 6.41B), or amorphous (Fig. 6.25C) calcifications of variable densities within a cluster and among clusters. In some patients, linear and segmental distribution of fine pleomorphic (Fig. 6.42A), coarse heterogeneous (Fig. 6.42B), or amorphous calcifications (Fig. 6.5) can be seen; when predominantly round, punctate, and amorphous calcifications are noted in a linear distribution on orthogonal views, it raises our concern for malignancy. When these types of calcifications are associated with DCIS, it is more commonly low or intermediate nuclear grade DCIS; high nuclear grade is diagnosed in a small percentage of patients. Mammographically, we tend to underestimate the extent of these processes. In general, what we see may be the "tip of the iceberg" (41). It is important to emphasize again that the calcifications we see may be in areas of hyperplasia or atypical hyperplasia (Figs. 6.41A and 6.42), and an area of low grade DCIS with no associated calcifications

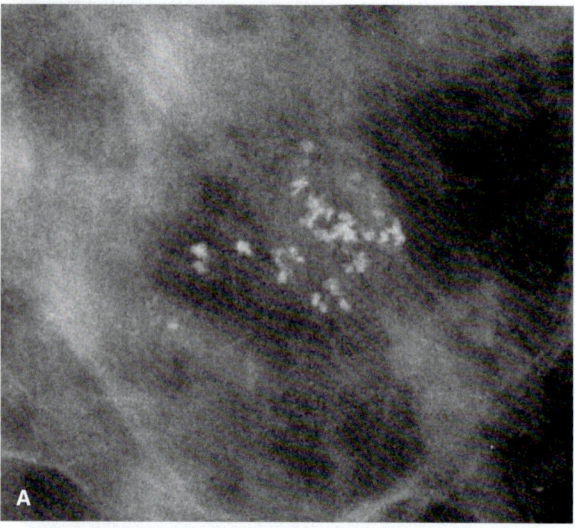
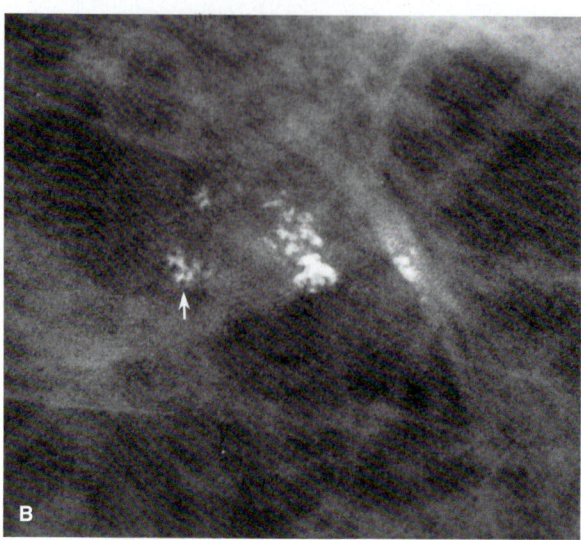
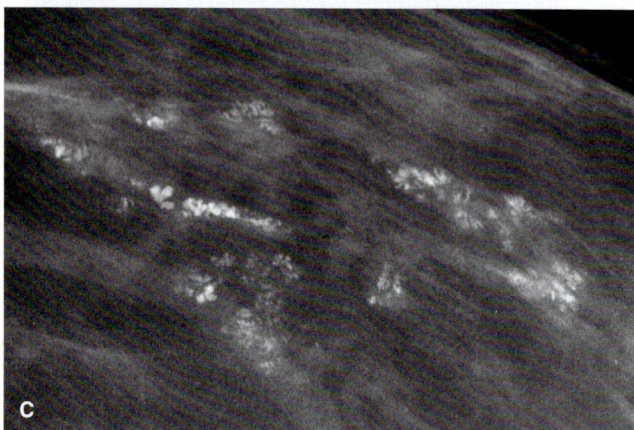

FIG. 6.36 • **Fibroadenomas. A:** Dense, chunky, "coral-like" calcifications with jagged edges and acute angles. These calcifications are fairly distinctive of hyalinizing fibroadenomas. BI-RADS 2: benign finding. **B:** Different patient. High-density chunky, "coral-like" calcifications with jagged edges *(arrow)* are seen developing in hyalinizing fibroadenomas. BI-RADS 2: benign finding. A and B (From Cardeñosa G. *Breast Imaging [The Core Curriculum Series]*. Philadelphia, PA: Lippincott Williams & Wilkins; 2003.) **C:** Different patient. High-density chunky, feathery, and "coral-like" calcifications with jagged edges are seen developing in hyalinizing fibroadenomas. BI-RADS 2: benign finding. Note that in some women calcifications are the only indication of the presence of one or multiple fibroadenomas (e.g., a mass is not seen).

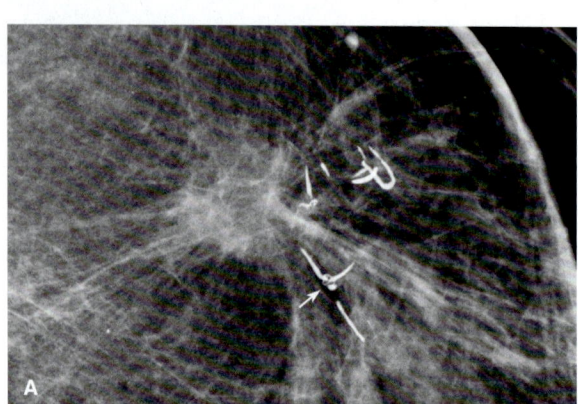
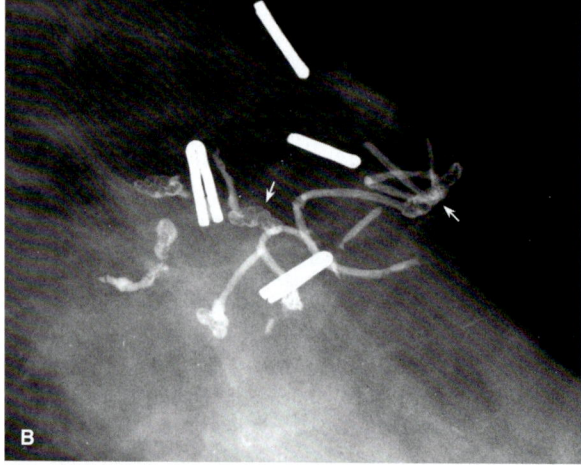

FIG. 6.37 • **Calcification of sutures. A:** Low density mass with spiculated margins and associated skin thickening consistent with fat necrosis at the patient's known lumpectomy site. Dense linear calcifications, one with knot *(arrow)*, are present at the lumpectomy bed consistent with calcifications developing in sutures. **B:** Lumpectomy site with surgical clips (metallic) and calcifications developing in sutures; knots *(arrows)* are apparent in some of the sutures.

Breast Calcifications 163

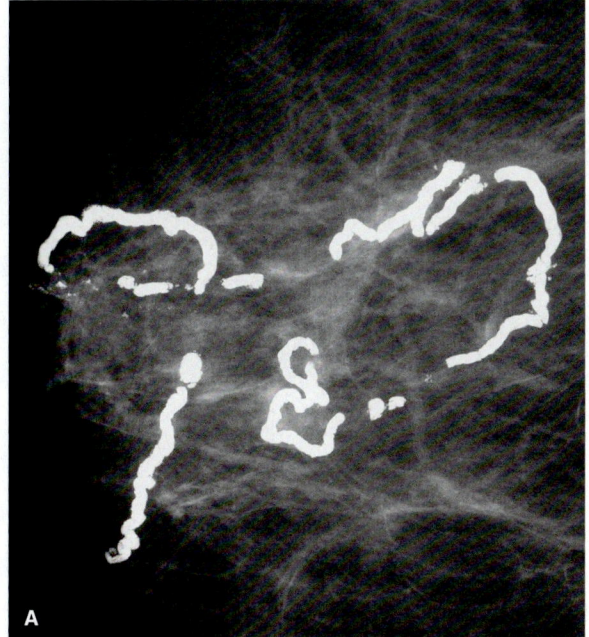

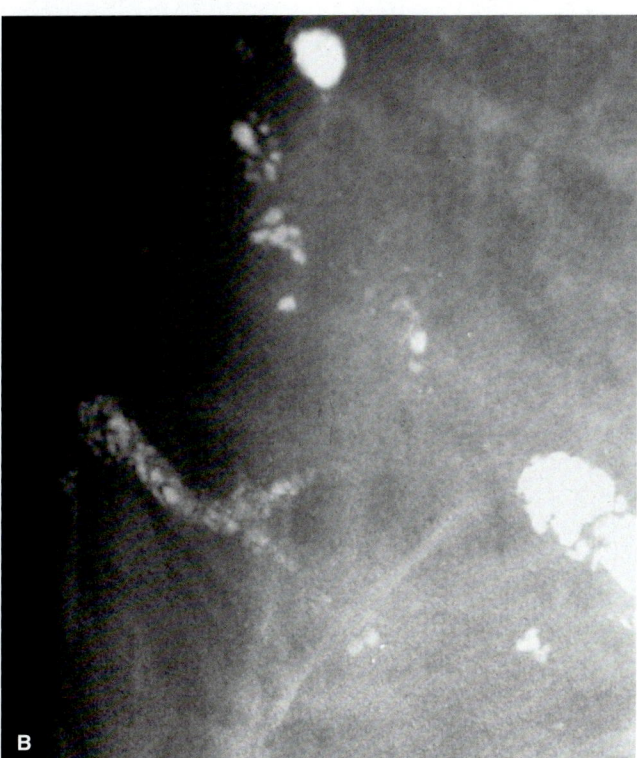

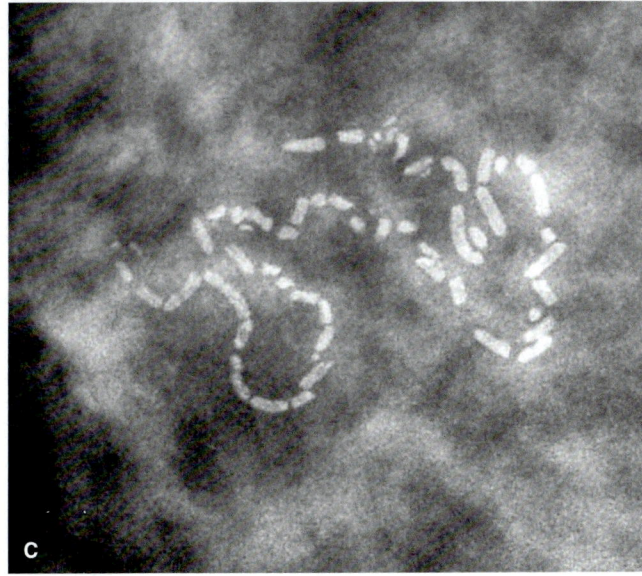

FIG. 6.38 • **Calcified parasites. A:** Dense, coarse, linear, and serpiginous calcifications are seen. **B:** Photographic coned view of the right subareolar area to demonstrate different appearance of the calcifications. The calcifications are coarse, heterogeneous, and pleomorphic, and some are in a linear distribution. **C:** Different patient. Linear, coiled, and serpiginous calcifications are seen in this patient. (From Cardeñosa G. *Breast Imaging [The Core Curriculum Series]*. Philadelphia, PA: Lippincott Williams & Wilkins; 2003.)

is found immediately adjacent to these other benign proliferative processes. When targeting these types of calcifications during imaging-guided biopsies, we need to be aware that there may be an inherent sampling bias so that increasing the numbers of cores obtained to include noncalcified tissue may be appropriate. Targeting the calcifications alone may yield a diagnosis of hyperplasia or atypical ductal hyperplasia (see Chapter 12), yet noncalcified DCIS may be found in the adjacent tissue. Although controversial, excisional biopsy may be preferred in some of these patients to assure adequate sampling and establishing the correct diagnosis.

The types of calcifications that develop in secretions are usually identified in one or multiple clusters (grouped) that may be regional or more diffusely distributed in the breast. Descriptors for the calcifications include amorphous, fine pleomorphic, and coarse heterogeneous calcifications. Differential considerations for grouped fine pleomorphic and coarse heterogeneous calcifications (Fig. 6.43) are listed in Table 6.2 and for amorphous calcifications (Figs. 6.25, 6.42A, 6.44, and 6.45) in Table 6.3. In our experience, depending on comparison with prior studies (e.g., are the calcifications new), location of the cluster in the breast, patient's personal or family history of breast cancer, and the features of the calcifications in orthogonal spot compression magnification views (with no blur), the likelihood of malignancy is under 25%, particularly if there are no linear forms or linear orientation.

Calcifications developing in necrotic cellular debris have a fairly distinctive mammographic appearance. The rapidly proliferating epithelial cells mold these calcifications actively into linear forms with clefts and irregular borders (Figs. 6.2 and 6.4); associated round and punctate calcifications may be seen among the linear calcifications. The calcifications are variable in density within a given lesion and among patients. Focal, segmental, or regional in distribution, they may also have a linear (ductal) orientation and extend to the nipple. Although not pathognomonic of DCIS, in our experience these types of calcifications are associated with malignancy in a significant number of patients; differential considerations (Fig. 6.46) for these types

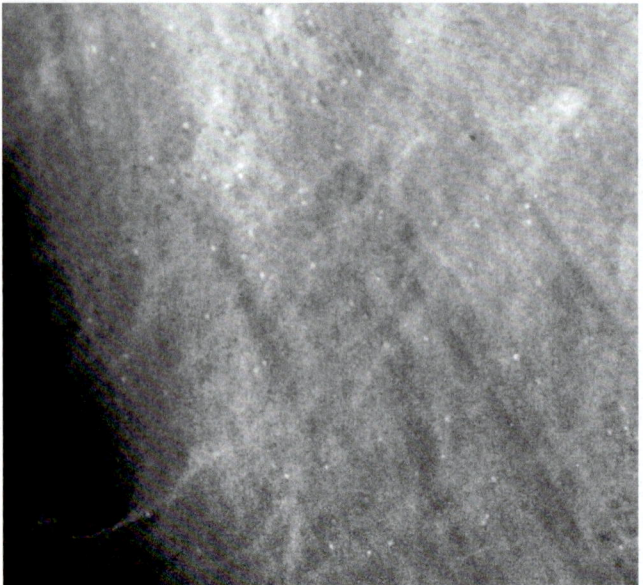

FIG. 6.39 • Calcified parasites. Trichinosis. Monomorphic, punctate calcifications are noted limited to the pectoral muscles (right shown). (From Cardeñosa G. *Breast Imaging [The Core Curriculum Series].* Philadelphia, PA: Lippincott Williams & Wilkins; 2003.)

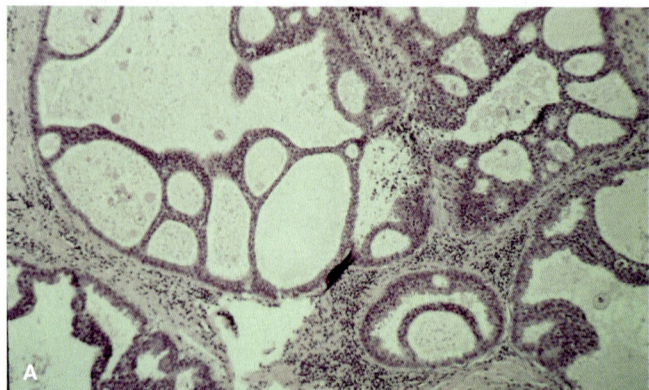

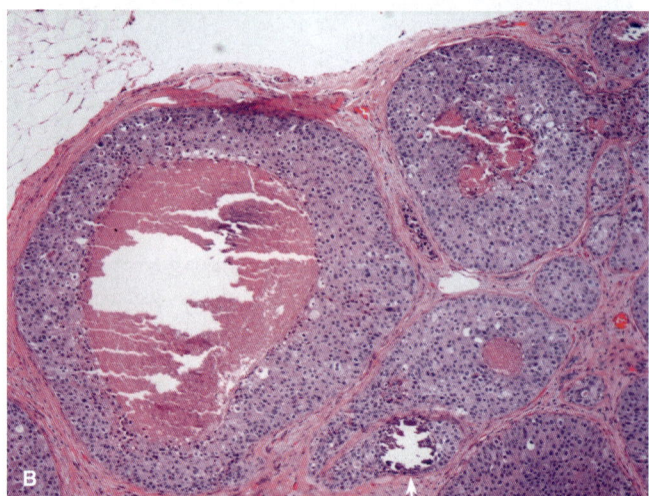

FIG. 6.40 • DCIS, pathology. A: DCIS, low nuclear grade, cribriform and micropapillary types. The ducts are distended. The cells are characterized by monomorphic nuclei-lacking nucleoli, low mitotic rates (low thymidine labeling rates), cell polarization toward the duct lumen, and no cell necrosis or autophagocytosis. Note the rigid variably sized cribriform spaces and roman bridges. **B:** DCIS, high nuclear grade with central necrosis. Multiple adjacent distended ducts in cross section are present. The malignant cells are circumferentially encroaching the duct lumen; they have pleomorphic nuclei with multiple nucleoli, high mitotic rates (high thymidine labeling rates), lack of cellular polarization as well as cell necrosis and autophagocytosis. Necrosis is present centrally in the lumens; a fragment of a calcification *(arrow)* is seen in one of the ducts.

of calcifications are listed in Table 6.1. Biopsy is indicated and care is exercised in establishing imaging and pathology concordance when a benign diagnosis is made on the core samples. In some patients, excisional biopsy may be indicated for confirmation of a benign histology. Targeting this type of calcification with imaging-guided biopsies has a high diagnostic yield. When related to DCIS, the calcifications are molded and in intimate contact with the proliferating cells (Fig. 6.40B).

Lesions characterized by central necrosis tend to be rapidly growing lesions and the calcifications, as reflectors of an ongoing dynamic process, can change rapidly (Fig. 6.47); biopsy is indicated in these patients. In contrast, low-grade processes lacking central necrosis evolve slowly and remain intraductal for longer periods. Appreciable changes in any mammographic findings develop slowly (years). Consequently, we recommend annual follow-up (rather than 6-month follow-up) with comparable magnification views when following patients with clusters of round and punctate calcifications. Increases in the number of round or punctate calcifications in a given cluster, particularly if the cluster is an unusual location, may warrant a biopsy recommendation.

As already mentioned, DCIS was relatively uncommon prior to our ability to detect calcifications on mammography. However, if we accept the premise that invasive ductal carcinoma evolves from intraductal disease, and for as relatively common as DCIS has become following the widespread use of mammography, it is still not as common as one would expect given the number of invasive lesions that have no antecedent, detectable lesion mammographically (31). You can, in fact, suggest that with mammography we underdiagnose DCIS since now, with MRI, our ability to diagnose patients with DCIS is again improved (30–32). Although many of the DCIS lesions detected on MRI are clinically and mammographically occult, they are detectable based on the presence of neovascularity. Consequently, and in contrast to invasive lesions that are considered significant regardless of the detection method, it may be that MRI-detected DCIS or those detected mammographically

Table 6.6 DCIS—PRESENTATIONS

Mammographically

Calcifications (grouped, segmental, or less likely regional)
Mass
Diffuse changes
Parenchymal asymmetry (focal or global)
Distortion
Dilated duct—developing
MRI

Segmentally distributed non–mass-like, clumped and linear enhancement
Clinically

Palpable finding
Nipple discharge (spontaneous)
Paget disease of the nipple

Breast Calcifications 165

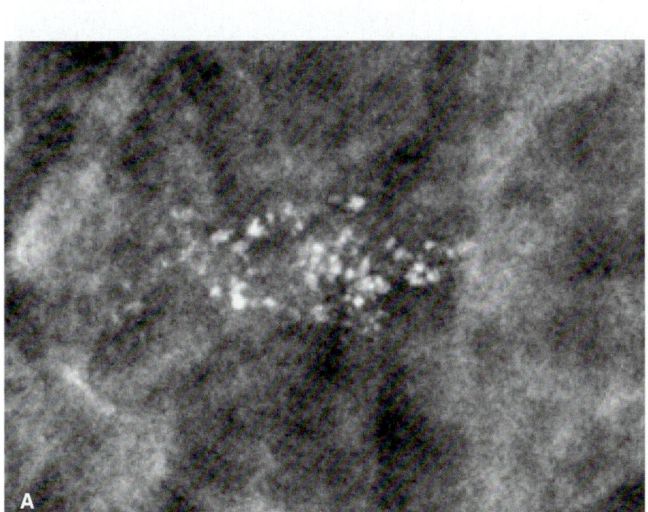
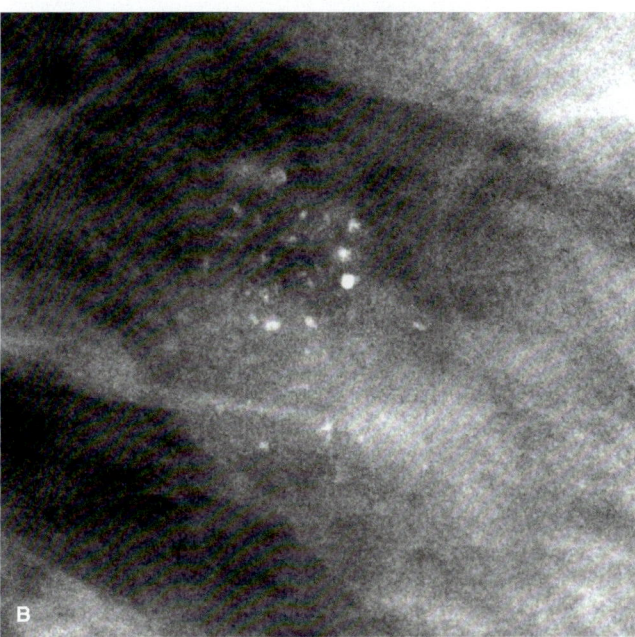

FIG. 6.41 • **DCIS. A:** Grouped coarse heterogeneous calcifications. BI-RADS 4A: Suspicious abnormality, biopsy is indicated. Intermediate nuclear grade DCIS is diagnosed on core biopsy. **B:** Grouped fine pleomorphic calcifications. BI-RADS 4A: Suspicious abnormality, biopsy is indicated. Low nuclear grade DCIS is diagnosed on core biopsy.

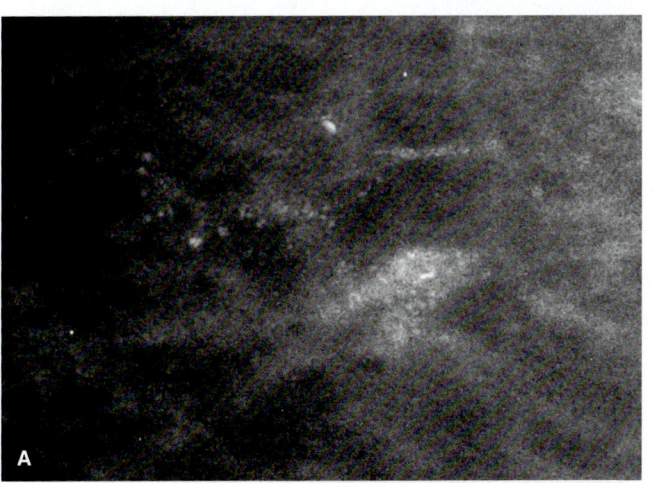
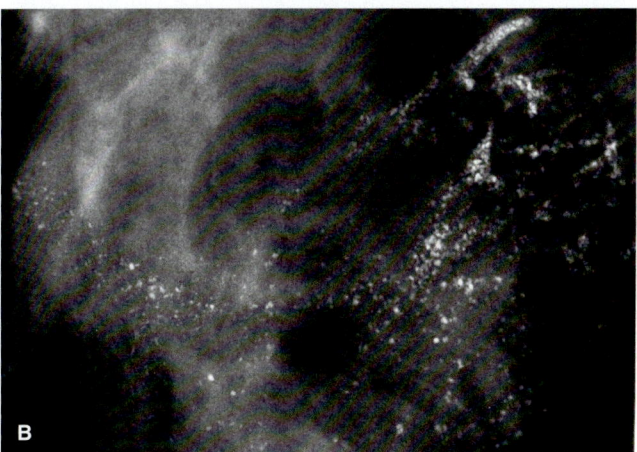
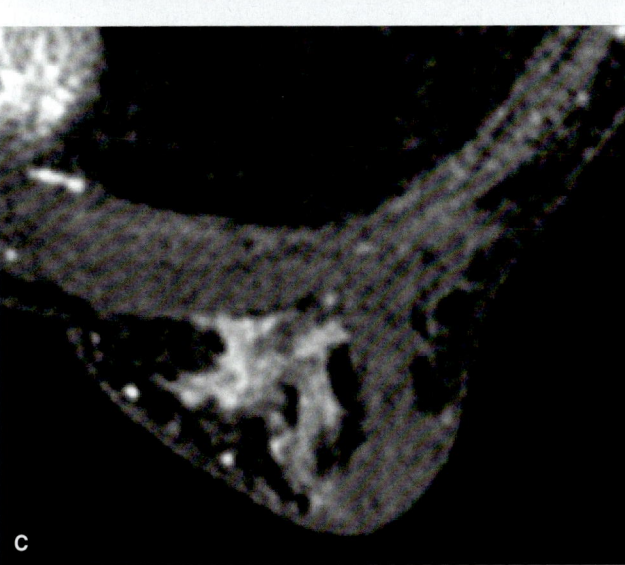

FIG. 6.42 • **Papilloma and DCIS. A:** Fine pleomorphic and amorphous calcifications, some of which demonstrate a linear distribution. BI-RADS 4A: Suspicious abnormality, biopsy is indicated. Papillomas with calcifications associated with the stroma are reported on the cores. **B:** Regional coarse heterogeneous calcifications, most in a linear distribution. BI-RADS 4C: Suspicious abnormality, biopsy is indicated. DCIS, cribriform type is reported on core biopsy. **C:** Axial T1-weighted image of the right breast postcontrast. Heterogeneous non-mass-like enhancement regionally distributed in the lower inner quadrant of the right breast correlating with the calcifications seen in part **B**.

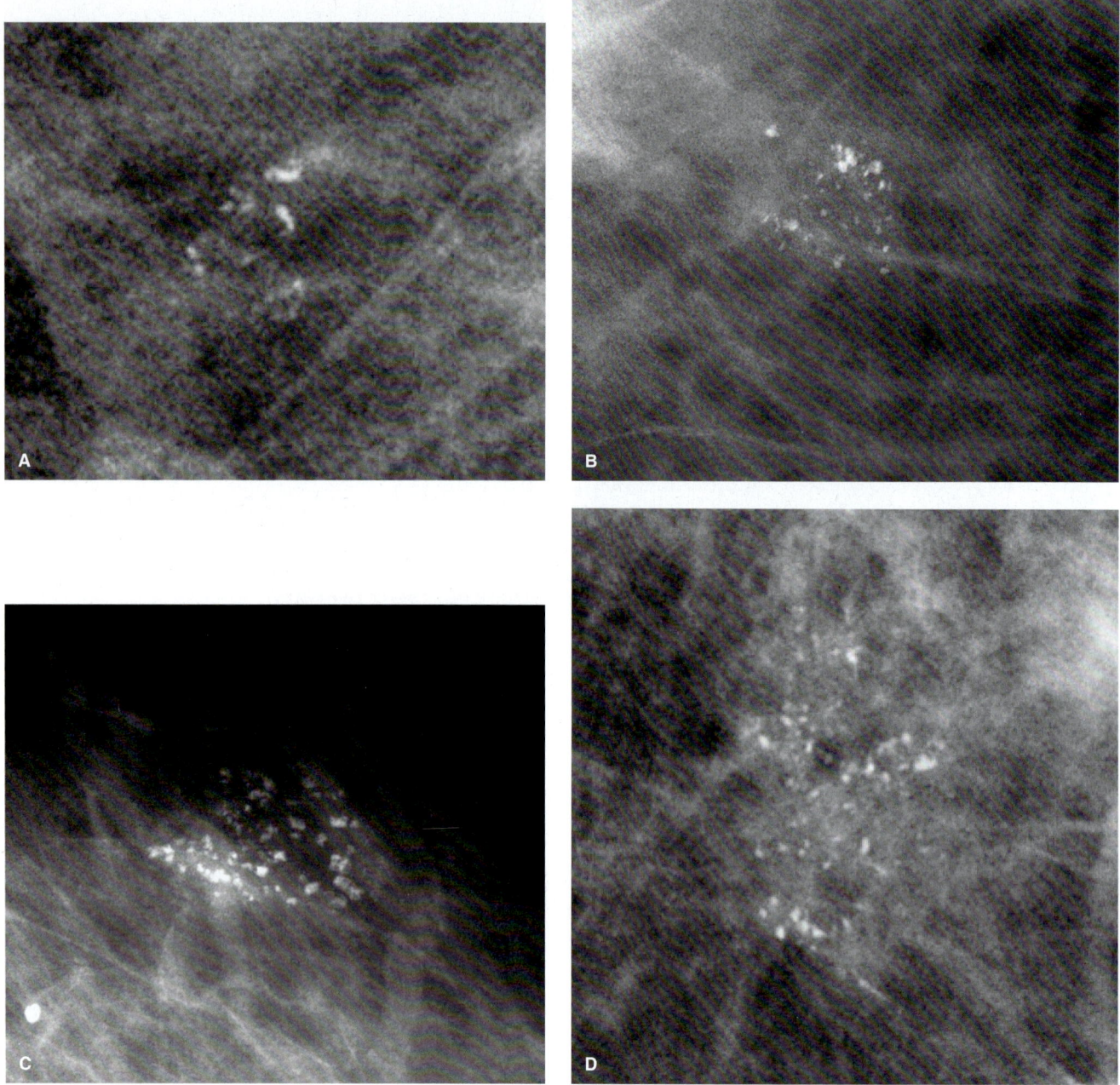

FIG. 6.43 • **Grouped fine pleomorphic and coarse heterogeneous calcifications. A:** Grouped coarse heterogeneous calcifications. BI-RADS 4A: Suspicious abnormality, biopsy is indicated. Fat necrosis with calcifications is diagnosed on core biopsy. **B:** Grouped fine pleomorphic calcifications. BI-RADS 4B: Suspicious abnormality, biopsy is indicated. A fibroadenoma with calcifications is diagnosed on core biopsy. **C:** Grouped coarse heterogeneous calcifications. BI-RADS 4A: Suspicious abnormality, biopsy is indicated. A fibroadenoma with calcifications is diagnosed on core biopsy. **D:** Grouped fine pleomorphic calcifications. Although not the dominant calcification form, linear forms are present. BI-RADS 4C: Suspicious abnormality, biopsy is indicated. DCIS, intermediate, is diagnosed on core biopsy.

associated with enhancement on MRI may have increased clinical significance compared with DCIS having no MRI correlate.

ARTIFACTS, MIMICRY

Artifacts can simulate calcifications and, although usually easy to identify, can sometimes present a challenge. Deodorant (Fig. 6.48A), Desitin (Fig. 6.48B), hair (see Fig. 2.37B), and tattoos can rarely present as high-density particles projecting on the breast parenchyma and simulate breast calcifications. High-density particles reflecting shrapnel from gunshot wounds (Fig. 6.48C) or gold deposited bilaterally in lymph nodes following treatment for rheumatoid arthritis (see Fig. 7.33) may also mimic the appearance of calcifications (42). Meticulous attention to detail and patient preparation can minimize the occurrence of artifacts. If questions persist relative to the presence of underlying calcifications or artifact simulating calcifications, repeat films can be obtained after the potential cause of the artifact has been addressed.

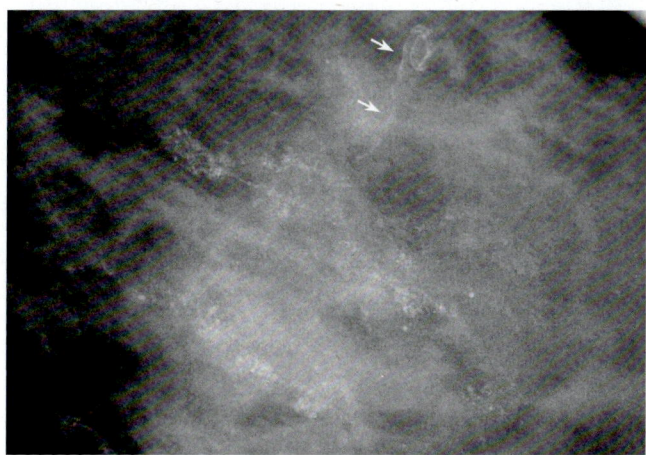

FIG. 6.44 • **Invasive ductal carcinoma and DCIS initially reported as ADH.** Multiple clusters of amorphous calcifications with intervening amorphous calcifications in a linear distribution. Arterial calcification *(arrows)* is also noted. BI-RADS 4C: Suspicious abnormality, biopsy is indicated. ADH is diagnosed on core biopsy. Invasive ductal carcinoma grade I with low-grade DCIS solid cribriform and papillary types is diagnosed on the excisional biopsy.

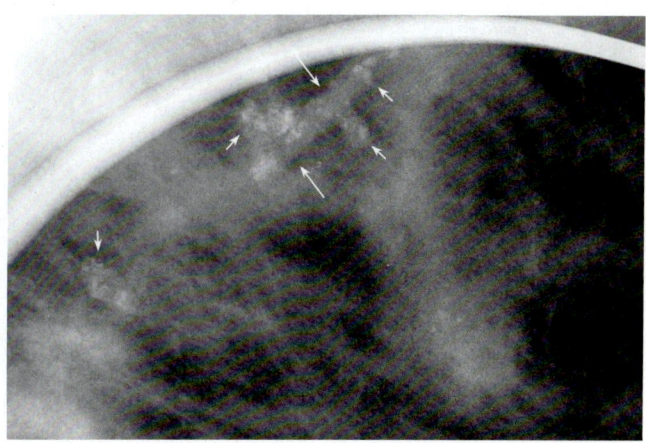

FIG. 6.45 • **Grouped amorphous calcifications in a distended duct, papillomas.** Multiple clusters *(short arrows)* of amorphous calcifications are identified in a dilated tubular structure *(long arrows)* presumed to be a dilated duct. BI-RADS 4B: Suspicious abnormality, biopsy is indicated. Papillomas diagnosed on core biopsy.

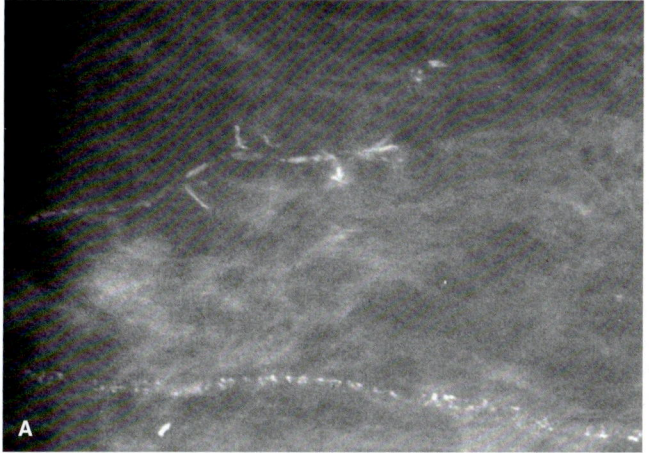

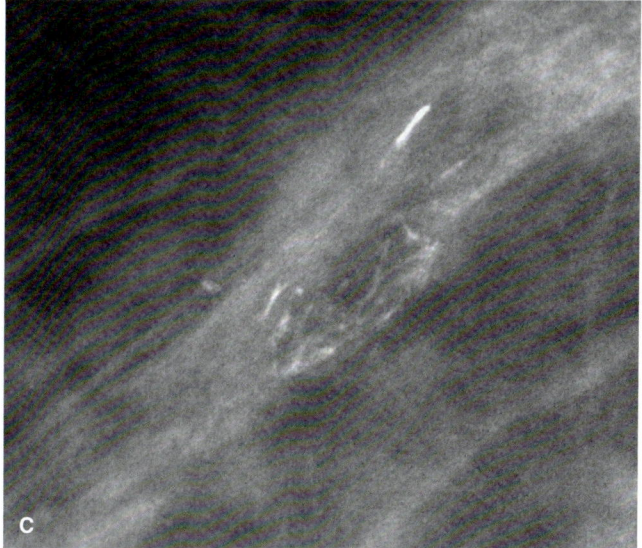

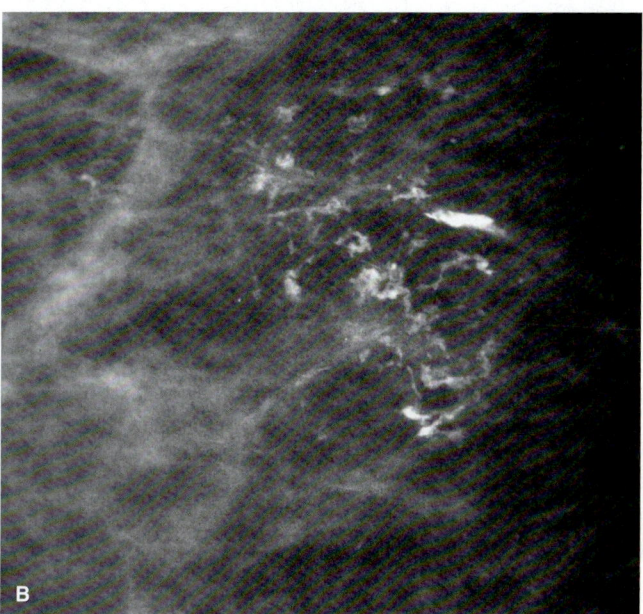

FIG. 6.46 • **Linear calcifications in a linear distribution. A:** Linear calcifications in a linear distribution. Vascular calcifications are also present. BI-RADS 4C: Suspicious abnormality, biopsy is indicated. A fibroadenoma with associated calcifications is diagnosed on core biopsy. **B:** Coarse, linear calcifications in a linear distribution in a patient with dermatomyositis. BI-RADS 2: Benign finding. **C:** Linear calcifications in a linear distribution in a patient who has had a reduction mammoplasty. Although these were thought to likely be benign, a biopsy is done BI-RADS 4A: Suspicious abnormality, biopsy is indicated. Fat necrosis is reported on the core biopsy. **D:** Dense linear calcifications in a linear distribution. BI-RADS 4C: Suspicious abnormality, biopsy is indicated. Fat necrosis with calcifications is diagnosed on core biopsy. **E:** Linear calcifications with variable density, thickness, and branch points. BI-RADS 4C: Suspicious abnormality, biopsy is indicated. ADH is reported on core biopsy. High nuclear grade DCIS is diagnosed on the excisional biopsy. **F:** Linear calcifications in linear distribution as well as fine pleomorphic calcifications in the surrounding tissue. BI-RADS 4C: Suspicious abnormality, biopsy is indicated. DCIS, high-nuclear grade with comedonecrosis and calcifications is reported on the core biopsy and confirmed on the lumpectomy specimen.

(continued)

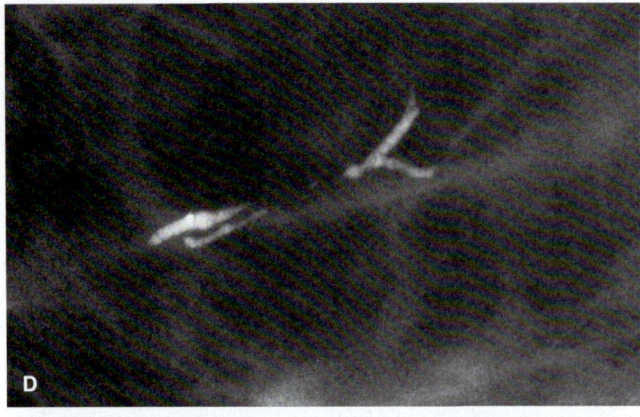
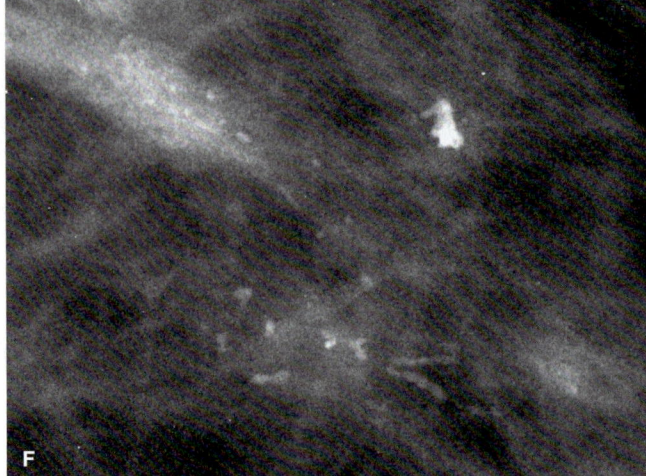
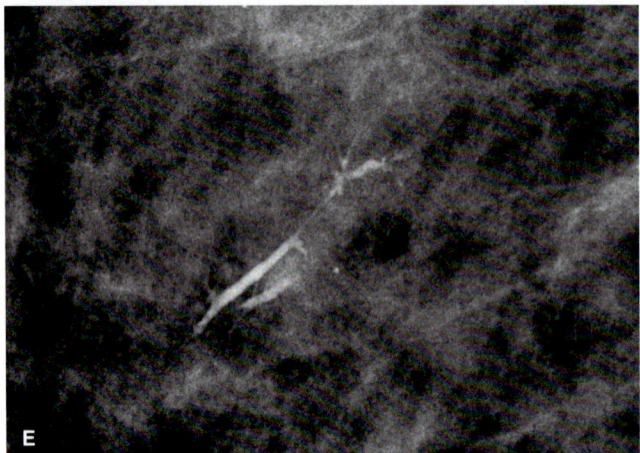

FIG. 6.46 • *(continued)*

ULTRASTRUCTURE

Chemically, breast calcifications are classified into two major types. Type I calcifications are composed of calcium oxalate (weddellite) and occur in association with benign secretory processes and cystic changes. They are colorless and may not be seen on hematoxylin and eosin (H&E) stained tissue. They are, however, visible as birefringent crystals with polarizing microscopy (Fig. 6.49). Type-II calcifications are composed of calcium phosphate crystals (hydroxyapatite) that have been identified in benign and malignant breast tissue and are thought to develop in conjunction with cell necrosis. Type-II calcifications are readily seen on H&E with deeply basophilic staining. They are non-birefringent when viewed with polarizing microscopy (43,44).

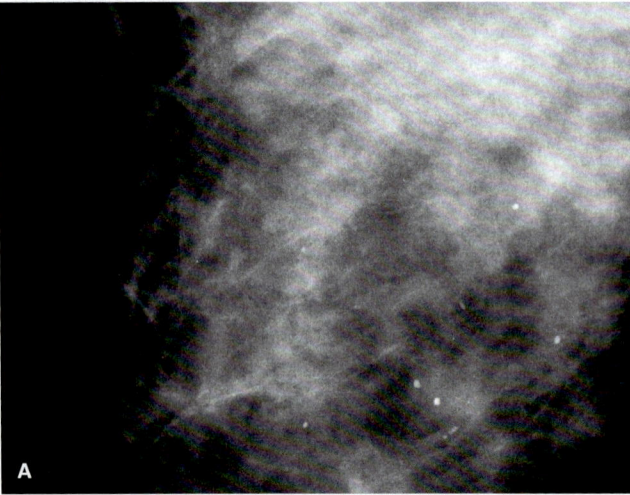
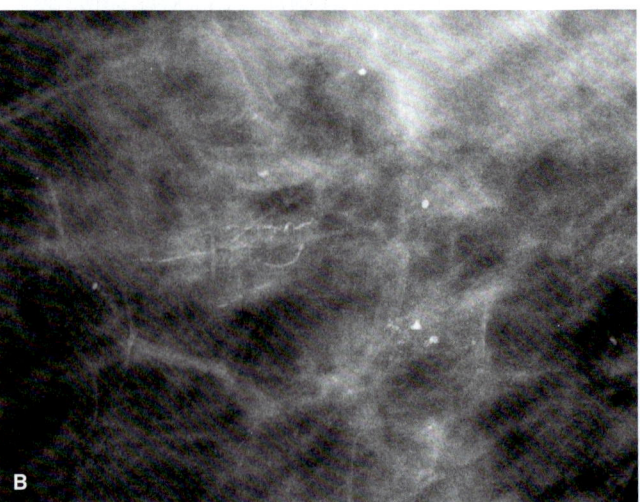

FIG. 6.47 • **DCIS, high nuclear grade with central necrosis. A:** CC view demonstrating scattered round calcifications. **B:** Six months later, new linear calcifications with linear orientation are identified. BI-RADS 4C: Suspicious abnormality, biopsy is indicated.

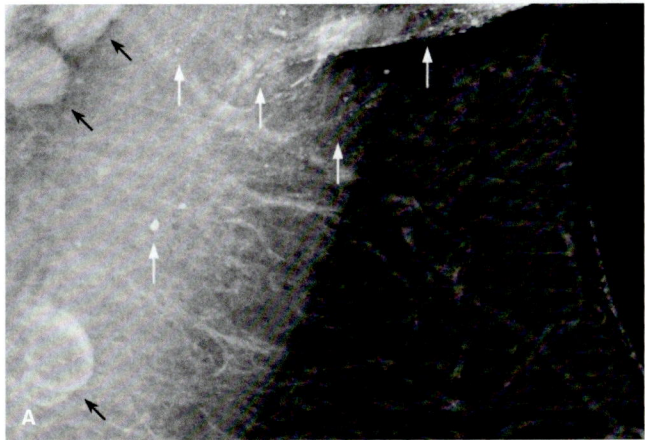
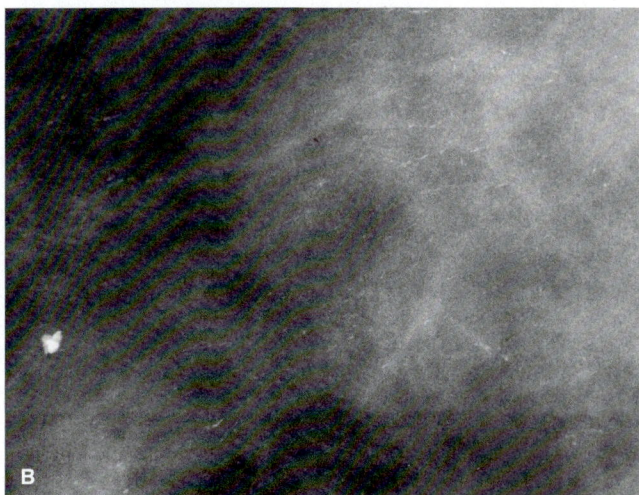
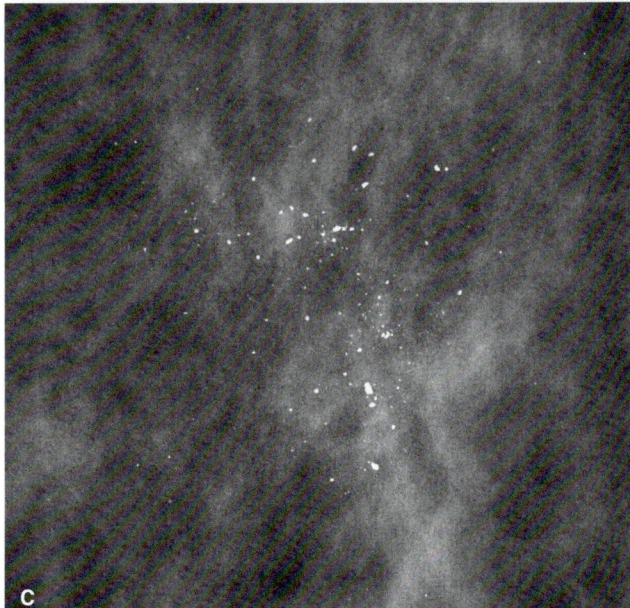

FIG. 6.48 • **Artifacts. A:** Deodorant. MLO view left breast photographically coned to the axilla. Note high-density material *(arrows)*, variable in size and shape, haphazardly distributed on the skin of the left axilla. This is the typical mammographic appearance of some deodorants. Patients should be asked not to wear deodorant for their mammogram appointment, or they can be asked to wipe it off immediately before the images are done. Lymph nodes *(black arrows)* present in the left axilla are partially imaged. **B:** Polymyxin B sulfate (Neosporin) on the skin. Low-density, fine linear material simulating calcifications is noted. Follow-up image after the skin is normal. **C:** Shrapnel. The high density of this artifact is greater than expected for breast calcifications. In some women, a linear distribution of the shrapnel outlines the trajectory of the bullet in the breast. **B** and **C** (From Cardeñosa G. *Breast Imaging [The Core Curriculum Series]*. Philadelphia, PA: Lippincott Williams & Wilkins; 2003.)

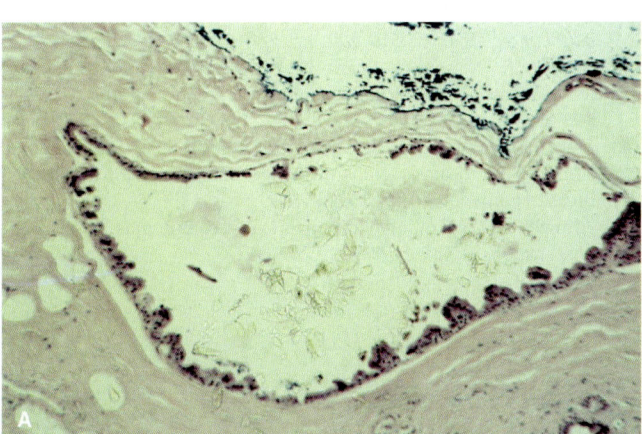
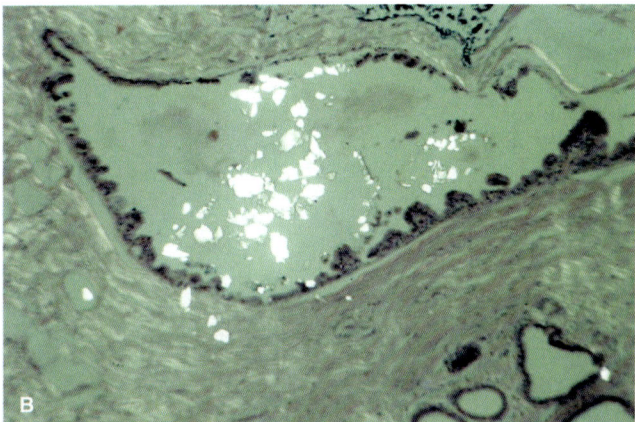

FIG. 6.49 • **Calcium oxalate. A:** A cyst with apocrine metaplasia is seen on H&E–stained slides. **B:** Polarizing microscopy demonstrates the presence of calcium oxalate crystals often found in areas of cystic change. The calcium deposits in the necrotic debris seen with DCIS are readily apparent on H&E and reflect calcium phosphate.

References

1. Bent CK, Bassett LW, D'Orsi CJ, et al. The positive predictive value of BI-RADS microcalcifications descriptors and final assessment categories. *AJR Am J Roentgenol.* 2010;194:1378–1383.
2. Kai KC, Slanetz PJ, Eisenberg RL. Linear breast calcifications. *AJR Am J Roentgenol.* 2012;199:W151–W157.
3. Chen PH, Ghosh ET, Slanetz PJ, et al. Segmental breast calcifications. *AJR Am J Roentgenol.* 2012;199:W532–W542.
4. Demetri-Lewis A, Slanetz PJ, Eisenberg RL. Breast calcifications: the focal group. *AJR Am J Roentgenol.* 2012;198:W325–W343.
5. Berg WA, Arnoldus CL, Teferra E, et al. Biopsy of amorphous breast calcifications: pathologic outcome and yield at stereotactic biopsy. *Radiology.* 2001;221:495–503.
6. Sickles EA, D'Orsi CJ, Bassett LW, et al. ACR BI-RADS® Mammography. In: ACR BI-RADS® Atlas, Breast Imaging Reporting and Data System. Reston, VA, American College of Radiology; 2013.
7. Kopans DB, Meyer JE, Homer MJ, et al. Dermal deposits mistaken for breast calcifications. *Radiology.* 1983;149:592–594.
8. Sickles EA. Breast calcifications: mammographic evaluation. *Radiology.* 1986;160:289–293.
9. Bassett LW. Mammographic analysis of calcifications. *Radiol Clin North Am.* 1992;30:93–105.
10. Moshyedi AC, Puthawala AH, Kurland RJ, et al. Breast arterial calcifications: association with coronary artery disease. *Radiology.* 1995;194:181–183.
11. Iribarren C, Go AS, Tolstykh I, et al. Breast vascular calcification and risk of coronary heart disease, stroke and heart failure. *J Womens Health (Larchmt).* 2004;13:381–389.
12. Fiuza Ferreira EMP, Szejnfeld J, Faintuch S. Correlation between intrammary arterial calcifications and CAD. *Acad Radiol.* 2007;14:144–150.
13. Henkin Y, Abu-Ful A, Shai I, et al. Lack of association between breast arterial calcification seen on mammography and coronary artery disease on angiography. *J Med Screen.* 2003;10:139–142.
14. Zgheib MH, Buchbinder SS, Rafeh NA, et al. Breast arterial calcifications on mammograms do not predict coronary heart disease at coronary angiography. *Radiology.* 2010;254:367–373.
15. Bassett LW, Jackson VP, Jahan R, et al. Chapter 25 Benign Breast Lesions. In: *Diagnosis of Diseases of the Breast.* Philadelphia, PA: WB Saunders Co; 1997:357–443.
16. Asch T, Frey C. Radiographic appearance of mammary duct ectasia with calcification. *N Engl J Med.* 1962;266:86–87.
17. Dixon JM, Anderson TJ, Lumsden AB, et al. Mammary duct ectasia. *Br J Surg.* 1983;70:601–603.
18. MacErlean DP, Nathan BE. Calcification in sclerosing adenosis simulating malignant breast calcification. *Br J Radiol.* 1972;45:944–945.
19. Sickles EA, Abele JS. Milk of calcium within tiny benign breast cysts. *Radiology.* 1981;141:655.
20. Linden SS, Sickles EA. Sedimented calcium in benign breast cysts: full spectrum of mammographic presentation. *AJR Am J Roentgenol.* 1989;152:967–971.
21. Moy L, Slanetz PJ, Yeh DE, et al. The pendant view: an additional projection to confirm the diagnosis of milk of calcium. *AJR Am J Roentgenol.* 2001;177:173–175.
22. Davis SP, Stomper PC, Weidner N, et al. Suture calcification mimicking recurrence in the irradiated breast: a potential pitfall in mammographic evaluation. *Radiology.* 1989;172:247–248.
23. Stacey-Clear A, McCarthy KA, Hall DA, et al. Calcified suture material in the breast after radiation therapy. *Radiology.* 1992;183:207–208.
24. Chow CK, McCarthy JS, Neafie R, et al. Mammography of lymphatic filariasis. *AJR Am J Roentgenol.* 1996;167:1425–1426.
25. Friedman PD, Kalisher L. Case 43: filariasis. *Radiology.* 2002;222:515–517.
26. De Barros N, D'Avila MS, Bauab SP, et al. Cutaneous myiasis of the breast: mammographic and US features—report of five cases. *Radiology.* 2001;218:518–520.
27. Aspesteguia L, Murillo A, Biurrun J, et al. Calcified trichinosis of pectoral muscle: mammographic appearance. *Eur Radiol.* 1995;5:414–416.
28. Stomper PC, Connolly JL, Meyer JE, et al. Clinically occult ductal carcinoma in situ detected with mammography: analysis of 100 cases with radio-pathologic correlation. *Radiology.* 1989;172:235–241.
29. Poplack SP, Wells WA. Ductal carcinoma in situ of the breast: mammographic-pathologic correlation. *AJR Am J Roentgenol.* 1998;170:1543–1549.
30. Raza S, Vallejo M, Chikarmane SA, et al. Pure ductal carcinoma in situ: a range of MRI findings. *AJR Am J Roentgenol.* 2008;191:689–699.
31. Kuhl CK, Schrading S, Bieling HB, et al. MRI for diagnosis of pure ductal carcinoma in situ: a prospective observational study. *Lancet.* 2007;370:485–492.
32. Newstead GM. MR imaging of ductal carcinoma in situ. *Magn Reson Imaging Clin N Am.* 2010;18:225–240.
33. Haagansen CD, ed. *Disease of the Breast.* 3rd ed. Philadelphia, PA: WB Saunders; 1986.
34. Stomper PC, Connolly JL. Ductal carcinoma in situ of the breast: correlation between mammographic calcification and tumor subtype. *AJR Am J Roentgenol.* 1992;159:483–485.
35. Ernster VL, Barclay J, Kerlilowske K, et al. Incidence of and treatment for ductal carcinoma in situ of the breast. *JAMA.* 1996;275:913–918.
36. Kuhl CK. Science to practice: why do purely intraductal cancers enhance on breast MR images? *Radiology.* 2009;253:281–283.
37. Rosai J. Borderline epithelial lesions of the breast. *Am J Surg Pathol.* 1991;15:209–221.
38. Faverly DRG, Burgers L, Bult P, et al. Three-dimensional imaging of mammary ductal carcinoma in situ: clinical implications. *Semin Diagn Pathol.* 1994;11:193–198.
39. Dinkel HP, Gassel AM, Tschammler A. Is the appearance of microcalcifications on mammography useful in predicting histological grade of malignancy in ductal carcinoma in situ? *Br J Radiol.* 2000;73:938–944.
40. Holland R, Hendricks JH. Microcalcifications associated with ductal carcinoma in situ: mammographic-pathologic correlation. *Semin Diagn Pathol.* 1994;11:181–192.
41. Holland R, Hendricks JH, Verbeek AL, et al. Extent, distribution and mammographic/histologic correlations of breast ductal carcinoma in situ. *Lancet.* 1990;336:519–522.
42. Bruwer A, Nelson G, Spark R. Punctate intranodal gold deposits simulating microcalcifications on mammograms. *Radiology.* 1987;163:87–88.
43. Frappart L, Boudeulle M, Boumendil J, et al. Structure and composition of microcalcifications in benign and malignant lesions of the breast. *Hum Pathol.* 1984;15:880–889.
44. Ahmed A. Calcifications in human breast carcinomas: ultrastructural observations. *J Pathol.* 1975;117:247–251.

CHAPTER SELF-ASSESSMENT QUESTIONS

1. Spot compression magnification view of the right breast. MRI is normal. What is indicated?

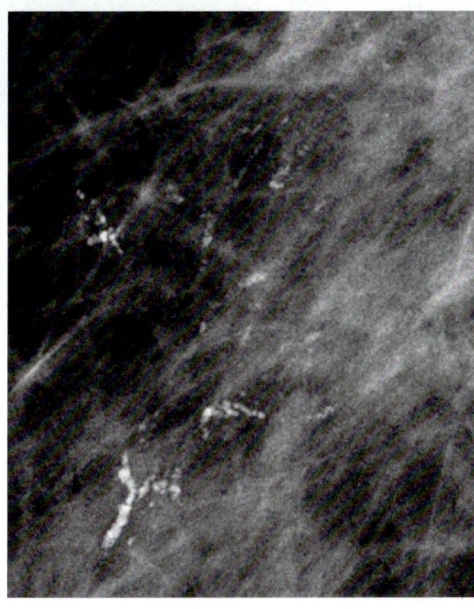

   A. Screening mammography in 1 year
   B. Six-month follow-up with comparable magnification views
   C. Stereotactically guided biopsy
   D. Ultrasound

2. Spot compression magnification views in the mediolateral oblique (below) and craniocaudal (top right) projections. Sclerosing adenosis with microcalcifications is reported on the core biopsies. What is indicated?

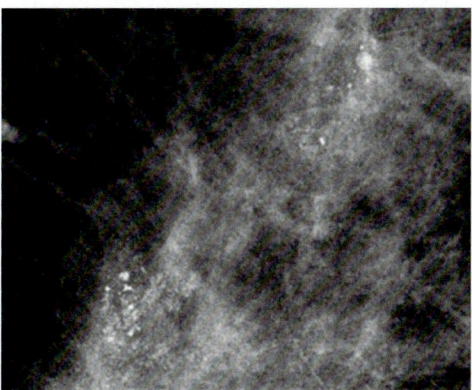

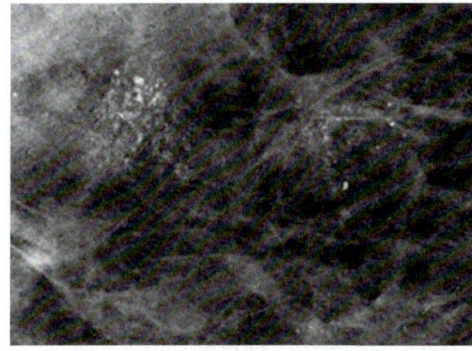

   A. Referral for surgical excision
   B. Magnetic resonance imaging
   C. Six-month follow-up
   D. Screening mammogram in 1 year

Answers to Chapter Self-Assessment Questions

1. C These are segmentally distributed fine linear branching calcifications: BI-RADS 4C. Biopsy is indicated regardless of an MRI correlate. Although some of these may be seen on ultrasound, most will not and as such one or two stereotactically guided biopsies may be indicated to establish the extent of the disease. Ductal carcinoma in situ is diagnosed on core biopsies.

2. D Two adjacent groups of amorphous, round, and punctate calcifications are imaged; no linear forms or linear orientation is apparent. There is no change in the configuration of the calcifications between the craniocaudal and oblique projections (essentially excluding milk of calcium). The differential for these calcifications includes fibrocystic changes (encompasses sclerosing adenosis, fibrosis, hyperplasia, atypical ductal hyperplasia, flat epithelial atypia, columnar cell change with or without atypia), papilloma, fibroadenoma, fat necrosis, mucocele-like lesions, and ductal carcinoma in situ (typically low to intermediate grade). Sclerosing adenosis with associated calcifications is one of the primary considerations and as such the histologic findings are congruent. Magnetic resonance imaging and surgical referral are not appropriate in this patient with benign congruent radiology-pathology findings. In our practice, patients with congruent rad-path results are placed back into the screening population.

Evaluation and Imaging Features of Benign Breast Masses

7

LEARNING OBJECTIVES

1. Patient history to consider when evaluating and considering differentials for a breast mass
2. Evaluation (imaging) algorithm for clinically or mammographically detected breast masses
3. Features of masses to consider and appropriate use of descriptors
4. Differential considerations for round (expansile) masses
5. Differential consideration for masses with spiculated, margins
6. Differential considerations for multiple masses in the breast with similar features
7. Differential considerations for fat containing masses

We place much emphasis on detecting microcalcifications and anguish over their characterization and management, but it is important to recognize that most invasive ductal carcinomas, and virtually all invasive lobular carcinomas, present as a mass. In contrast, when associated with malignancy, microcalcifications usually reflect intraductal, noninvasive breast cancer. Our primary goal with screening mammography is the recognition or perception of a possible mass or distortion related to an underlying mass. Our characterization of masses and management recommendations for patients are predicated on physical examination, spot compression, spot rolled, spot tangential, or spot compression magnification views and breast ultrasound. In some women, what appears to be a mass on screening images is shown to be superimposition of normal glandular tissue and what appears as an innocuous asymmetry is identified as likely malignant with further workup. By integrating patient history, clinical, mammographic, and ultrasound findings, and an understanding of breast histopathology, it is possible to approximate a diagnosis and have significant confidence in the appropriate management recommendations.

Relevant history is reviewed in evaluating and managing women with a breast mass. Women with a personal history of breast cancer or a history of breast cancer involving a first-degree relative (mother, father, sister, brother, daughter, or son) are at increased risk for developing breast cancer. This risk is increased if the relative developed breast cancer premenopausally or had bilateral breast cancer. The age and menopausal status of the patient, use of hormone replacement therapy, and physical findings should be known and factored in the formulation of a differential (Table 7.1).

Table 7.1 **BREAST MASSES: RELEVANT HISTORY**

Personal history of breast (or other malignancies, e.g., ovarian cancer)
Family history of breast cancer
    First-degree relatives
    Premenopausal
    Bilateral
Patient age (incidence of breast cancer increases with advancing age, and differential considerations change depending on age)
Menopausal status (tumor sojourn time is shorter in premenopausal women)
Hormone replacement therapy
Tamoxifen use
Physical findings
    "Lump"
    Focal pain
    Skin dimpling
    Nipple retraction
    Spontaneous nipple discharge
History of cyclical change in primary finding
History of surgical procedures involving the breast
Prior breast biopsy with diagnosis of high-risk marker lesion
    ADH
    Lobular neoplasia (LCIS)

In women over the age of 30 presenting with a focal finding (e.g., "lump," dimpling, focal tenderness), a metallic BB is used to mark the area of concern, and mediolateral oblique (MLO) and craniocaudal (CC) views are obtained bilaterally (1). A spot tangential view of the focal finding is also obtained. Correlative physical examination and ultrasound are usually done. Ultrasound is not absolutely indicated if fatty tissue is imaged corresponding to the site of concern to the patient, and there is no chance that the area of concern has been excluded from the field of view (e.g., if the metallic BB is at the edge of the film, correlative physical examination and ultrasound are always done; see Figs. 3.1 and 3.2).

Physical examination and ultrasound are done in women who are pregnant, lactating, or under 30 years of age and present with a "lump" (see Figs. 4.45 and 4.47). If any concerns persist following this initial evaluation, an MLO may be done to exclude calcifications associated with an intraductal carcinoma that may not be apparent on ultrasound. If an underlying malignancy is suspected, mammographic images are obtained bilaterally to fully evaluate the patient.

As defined by the American College of Radiology Breast Imaging and Reporting Data System (ACR BI-RADS®), a *mass* is a "space-occupying lesion seen in two different projections." This is to be distinguished from *asymmetry*, a term used for "an area of fibroglandular-density tissue that is visible on only one mammographic projection, frequently representing superimposition of normal breast structures" (2). Masses are three-dimensional, have a bulging or convex contour and an abrupt density change at the margin. They may produce architectural distortion and have associated calcifications, skin or nipple changes. Depending on location, size, internal matrix, and surrounding tissue, the mass may be palpable. Asymmetric tissue is planar with a different appearance between projections, scalloped and inhomogeneous with a gradual change in density at the margins. It is usually not palpable (3); palpable asymmetry should be evaluated carefully (see Chapter 9).

Compression, rolled and magnification views done with the round spot compression paddle (see Fig. 3.4A, B) are used to establish the shape, margins, and density of breast masses. *Round, oval,* and *irregular* (if "shape cannot be characterized") are the terms in BI-RADS® to describe the shape of a mass. *Circumscribed, microlobulated, obscured* (margins "hidden by superimposed or adjacent normal tissue"), *indistinct,* and *spiculated* are the terms used to describe the margins of a mass. The x-ray attenuation or density of a mass is described as *high, equal,* or *low* (but not fat-containing) relative to an equal volume of fibroglandular tissue (Table 7.2) (2). Please see Appendix A for the ACR BI-RADS® mammography, US and MRI lexicons. Every rule has an exception; but in general, benign masses have circumscribed or partially circumscribed margins and are low to equal in density. In contrast, malignant lesions have indistinct or spiculated margins, and the expansile (round, oval, lobulated) masses are usually high in density.

Additional features to consider when evaluating masses are listed in Table 7.3. Establishing the presence of associated calcifications and their morphology is helpful in assessing the etiology of a mass. Benign calcifications are usually associated with benign masses (Fig. 7.1). If malignant-appearing calcifications are associated with a mass, invasive ductal carcinoma with an intraductal component is the most likely diagnosis (Figs. 7.2 and 7.3). Likewise, establishing the presence of satellite lesions is helpful (Fig. 7.3). Although maligned, the halo sign is a good indicator of benignity (4–6). The halo sign is narrowly defined as a 1-mm sharp lucency, partially or completely surrounding a mass (Fig. 7.4). Not all masses with a true halo are benign but many are (4,5). The halo sign is probably as good a sign of benignity as spiculation is of malignancy. The halo sign may reflect active changes in the size of the mass (4).

Table 7.2 AMERICAN COLLEGE OF RADIOLOGY, LEXICON DESCRIPTIVE TERMS FOR MASSES

Shape	Margins	Density (Water Density)
Round	Circumscribed	High
Oval	Microlobulated	Low (but not fat-containing)
Irregular	Obscured	Equal
	Indistinct	Fat-containing
	Spiculated	

Sickles EA, D'Orse CJ, Bassett LW, et al. ACR-BIRADS® Mammography. In: ACR-BIRADS® Atlas, *Breast Imaging Reporting and Data System.* Reston, VA, American College of Radiology; 2013.

Table 7.3 MASSES: MAMMOGRAPHIC FEATURES TO CONSIDER

Shape
Margins
Density (low, equal or high density; no fat)
Features of associated calcifications
Effects on surrounding tissue
Architectural distortion
"Halo" sign
Satellite lesions
Multiplicity
Stability (previous films)

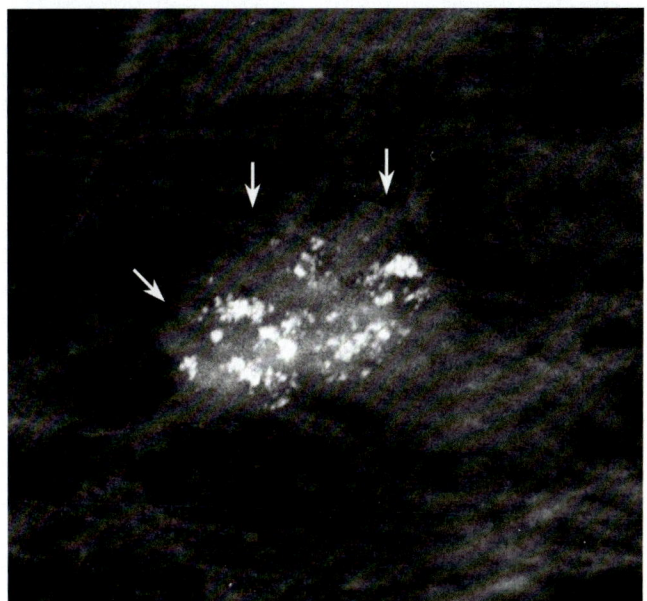

FIG. 7.1 • Fibroadenoma, hyalinizing. Photographically coned image. An isodense oval mass *(arrows)* with indistinct margins and coarse, dense, dystrophic calcifications is imaged on the screening views (only one projection is shown). Although the margins are indistinct, the presence of dystrophic-type calcifications associated with the mass in both projections is consistent with a fibroadenoma undergoing hyalinization and calcification. Masses associated with benign calcifications are usually benign. When benign findings are detected on screening mammography, no additional evaluation is indicated. BI-RADS 2: Benign finding.

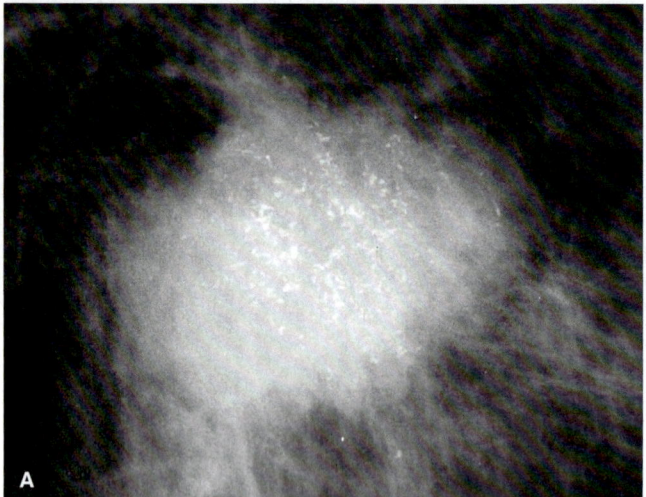

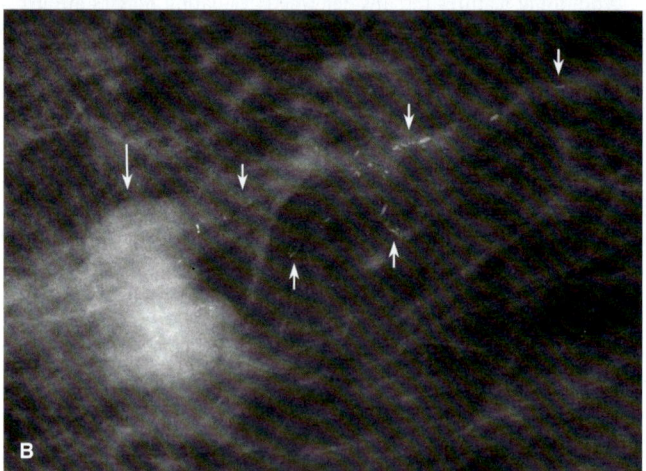

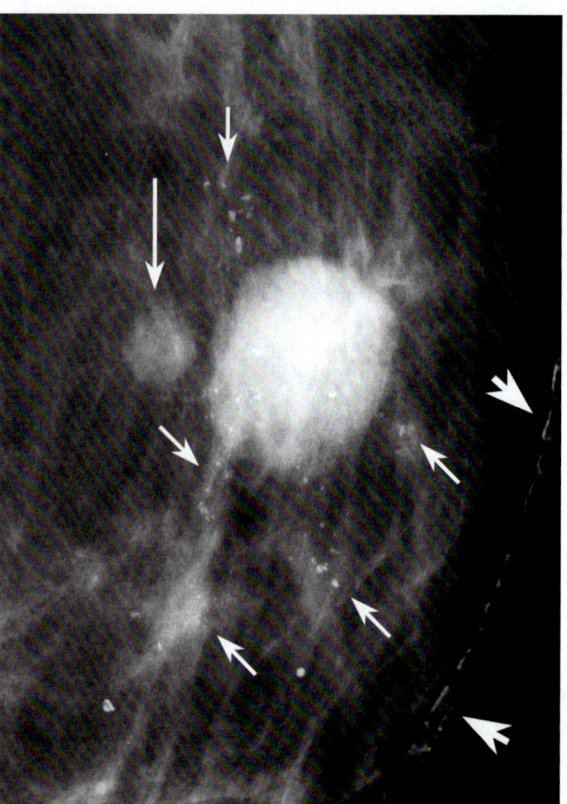

FIG. 7.2 • **Invasive ductal carcinoma, not otherwise specified (NOS), with DCIS. A:** A dense oval mass with indistinct margins and associated malignant-type calcifications is imaged (only one projection is shown). The calcifications are pleomorphic and include linear, round, and punctate forms. Given the density and margins of the mass (expansile, "blow-up" lesion), an invasive ductal carcinoma, high nuclear grade is likely, and the calcifications are consistent with associated DCIS with central necrosis. BI-RADS 5: Highly suggestive of malignancy, biopsy is indicated. **B:** Dense, irregular mass *(long arrow)* with indistinct margins and fine linear calcifications *(short arrows)* extending linearly from the posterior edge of the mass for approximately 3 cm. The mass reflects an invasive ductal carcinoma; the calcifications are consistent with DCIS with central necrosis. At the time of surgery, it is important to excise the mass and all of the calcifications; bracketing this entire area with at least two wires would be appropriate preoperatively. BI-RADS 5: Highly suggestive of malignancy, biopsy is indicated. Palpable or mammographically detected masses with linear-type calcifications most commonly reflect an invasive ductal carcinoma, NOS with associated DCIS.

FIG. 7.3 • **Multifocal, invasive ductal carcinoma, not otherwise specified with DCIS.** Dense, round mass with indistinct margins and fine, pleomorphic calcifications *(short arrows)* extending away from the mass at multiple sites such that invasive ductal carcinoma, high nuclear grade with associated DCIS with central necrosis is the likely diagnosis. A lower density round mass *(long arrow)* is present at the posterior edge of the dominant mass consistent with multifocal disease. BI-RADS 5: Highly suggestive of malignancy. A calcified artery *(short thick arrows)* is incidentally noted in the subcutaneous tissue.

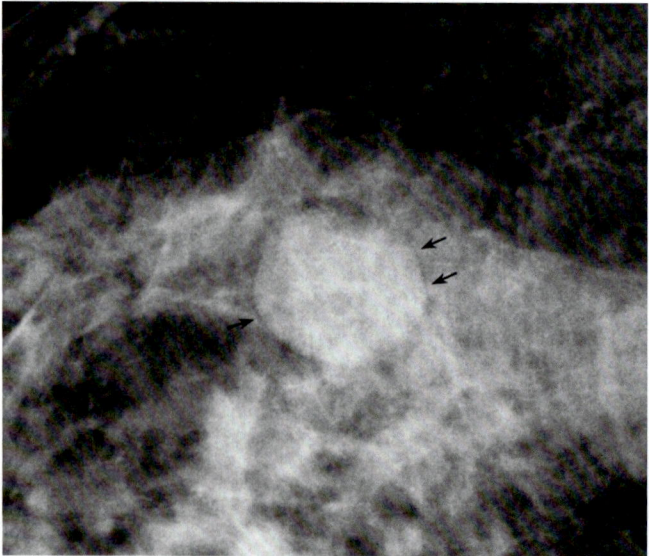

FIG. 7.4 • **"Halo sign," cyst.** A 1-mm sharp lucency *(arrows)* partially outlines this low density mass *(arrows)* with circumscribed margins. Although the halo sign can be seen with malignant masses that are growing rapidly, it is more common with benign masses. A cyst is imaged at this site on ultrasound (not shown). BI-RADS 2: Benign finding.

The presence of multiple masses with similar mammographic features (Fig. 7.5) is suggestive of benignity. However, do not be lulled into a false sense of security by multiplicity. Women with multiple masses can develop breast cancer. It has been reported that since the frequency of cancer development among women not recalled for evaluation of multiple masses and the stage of the cancers diagnosed in these women is no different than that seen in the general screening population, evaluation of multiple masses appears not to be justified (7). Others advocate ultrasound evaluation in these patients (8). Although controversial, our approach to the patient presenting for the first time with multiple

Evaluation and Imaging Features of Benign Breast Masses 175

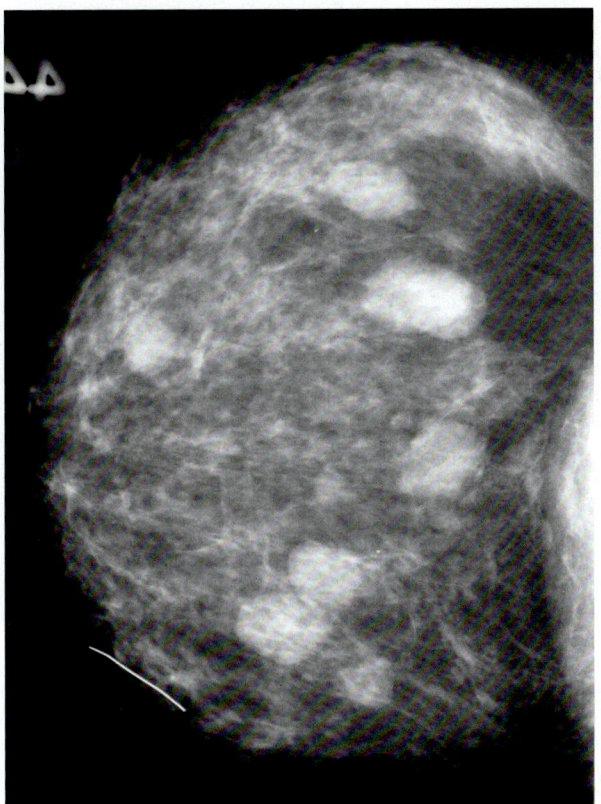

FIG. 7.5 • **Fibroadenomas.** Multiple, isodense, round, or oval masses with circumscribed margins randomly distributed in the right breast. BI-RADS 2: Benign findings.

masses is to evaluate each mass as though it were a single finding. Our decisions are based on physical examination and the mammographic and ultrasound features of the masses evaluated. On subsequent mammograms in these patients we only evaluate new, developing masses. Also, don't let yourself be mesmerized with multiple benign findings, but actively focus your brain away from the obviously benign findings and evaluate the surrounding tissue. Differential considerations for patients presenting with multiple masses is provided in Table 7.4.

Previous films are useful in the evaluation of masses. Although stability is not an absolute sign of benignity, if a mass with benign features (e.g., circumscribed margins, low to isodense) has been present for several years with no change, the likelihood of malignancy is low and recommending a 6-month follow-up is not appropriate. If the mass has features of malignancy (e.g., spiculation, distortion) that are not explained easily (e.g., prior trauma or surgery correlating with the site of the mass) it may represent a low-grade invasive lesion and biopsy is indicated (Fig. 7.6). In selecting prior films for comparison, try to use films from at least 2 years previously if available and, when evaluating a possible finding, look at multiple prior studies to establish slow

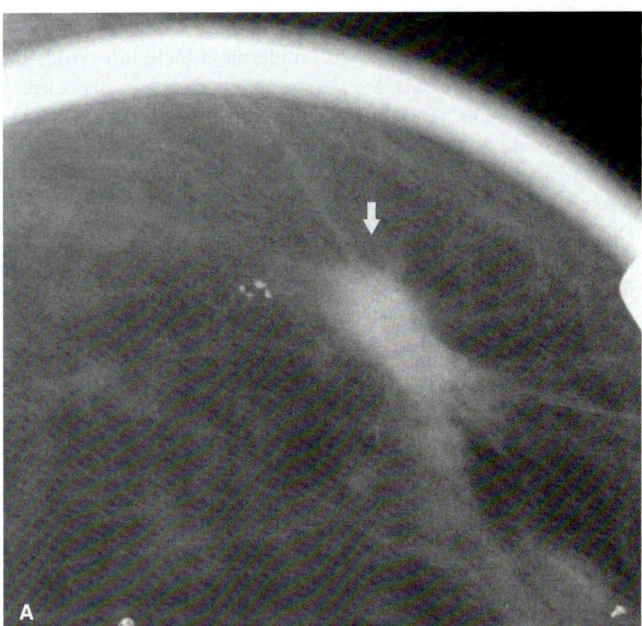

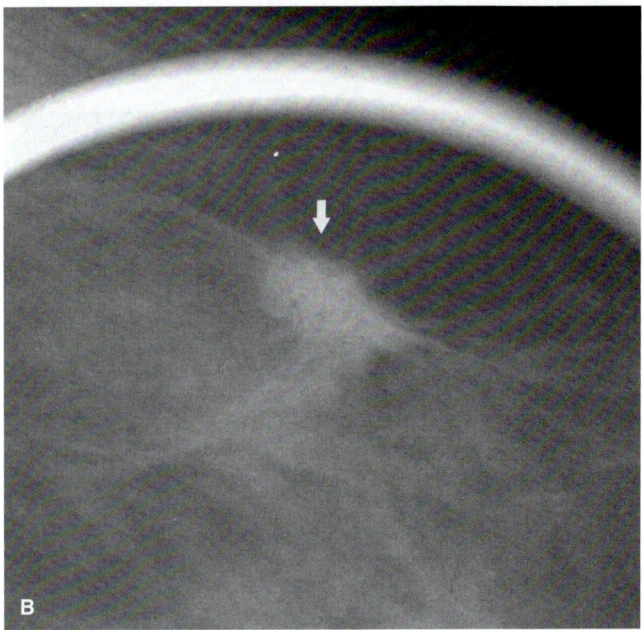

FIG. 7.6 • **Tubular carcinoma. A:** Spot compression view (only one projection shown) of the left breast demonstrates an oval dense mass *(arrow)* with spiculated margins in a 77-year-old patient with a history of a right mastectomy 25 years ago for breast cancer. **B:** Spot compression view, 12 years before the image shown in part **A**. No definite change in the mass *(arrow)* is noted; however, the patient has no history of surgery or trauma to this area. Tubular carcinoma or well-differentiated ductal carcinoma NOS is considered prospectively. BI-RADS 4C: Suspicious abnormality, biopsy is indicated. Tubular carcinoma with associated low nuclear grade DCIS with a cribriform pattern is diagnosed histologically. Sentinel lymph node biopsy is negative. A mass with spiculated margins or distortion that cannot be explained (e.g., trauma or surgery to that specific site) warrants biopsy in spite of stability on the mammogram. (From Cardeñosa G. *Breast Imaging [The Core Curriculum Series]*. Philadelphia, PA: Lippincott Williams & Wilkins; 2003.)

Table 7.4 DIFFERENTIAL: MULTIPLE MASSES WITH SIMILAR FEATURES
Cysts
Fibroadenomas
Lymph nodes
Papillomas
Skin lesions (neurofibromas)
PASH
Invasive ductal carcinoma (multifocal or -centric)
Peripheral papillary carcinomas
Metastatic disease

progression or fluctuation in the finding. Subtle changes may not be apparent from 1 year to the next but may be striking when comparison is made with studies from 2 or 3 years previously (see Fig. 11.9).

SKIN MASSES

Masses on the skin include moles, seborrheic keratosis, accessory nipples, skin tags, sebaceous cysts (epidermoid inclusion cysts), and neurofibromas (9). Keloids may also be noted projecting on the breast parenchyma. Unlike parenchymal masses, a thin lucency (air) may be noted surrounding the margins of the mass that protrude beyond the skin; the lucency is lost where the lesion attaches to the skin (Fig. 7.7). In some women, talc, calcifications, or air outlines the crevices of moles (Fig. 7.8A, B; also see Fig. 6.10). We mark skin lesions with a metallic BB prior to taking films so that we do not call a patient back unnecessarily for a skin lesion.

Sebaceous cysts and epidermoid inclusion cysts are common, often palpable, intradermal masses that may undergo changes in size from one year to the next. They commonly develop in the axilla (Fig. 7.9) or in the lower inner quadrants at the medial most extent of the inframammary fold (Fig. 7.10). On physical examination, sebaceous cysts may cause a smooth skin bulge and the orifice of the gland may be visible as a punctum ("black head"). On palpation, the mass moves with the skin such that you cannot glide skin over the mass. If squeezed, a white, thick, cheesy material that may be malodorous can be expressed from the punctum. When inflamed, localized erythema may be noted and tenderness elicited clinically; incision and drainage may be needed for treatment. However, complete removal of the cyst wall is required, otherwise, these lesions recur. On the mammogram, these masses have

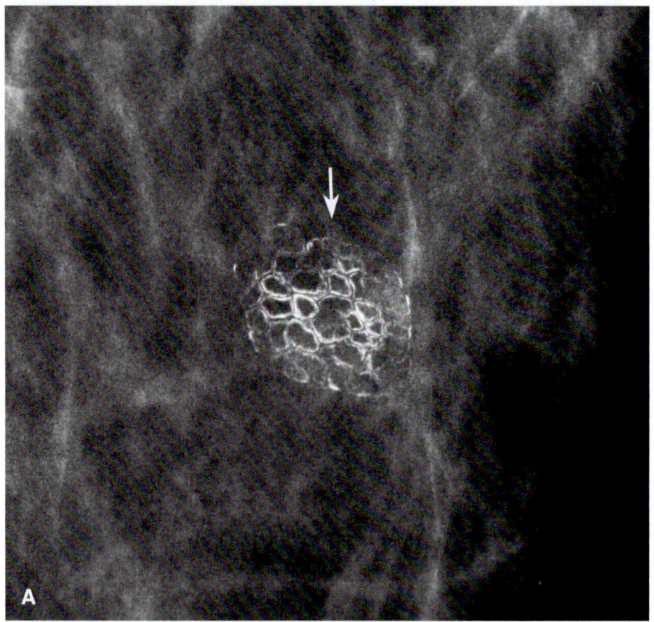

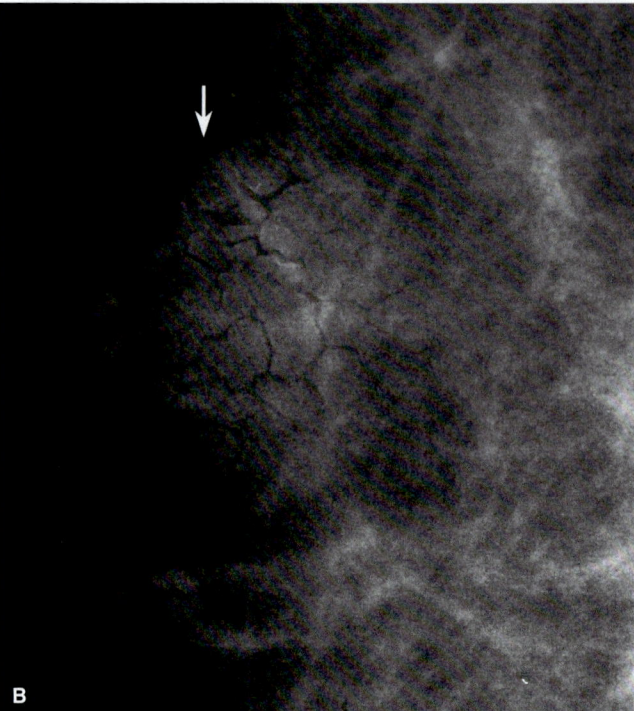

FIG. 7.8 • **Seborrheic keratosis. A:** Seborrheic keratosis *(arrow)* with encrusted high-density material and air outlining the crevices of the lesion. **B:** Seborrheic keratosis *(arrow)* with air outlining the interstices of the mass. BI-RADS 2: Benign finding. Ideally, the technologist should mark and document obvious skin lesions so that callbacks for skin findings are minimized.

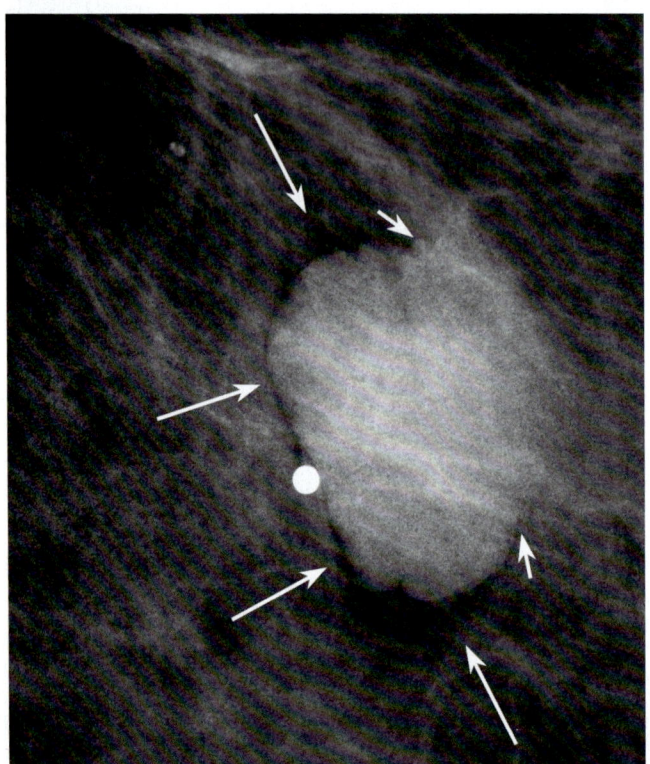

FIG. 7.7 • **Skin lesions.** Lucency (air) surrounding the portion of a lobulated mass that extends beyond the skin. The lucency *(long arrows)* is lost where the mass attaches to the skin *(short arrows)*. Metallic BB is used to mark the skin lesion.

circumscribed margins or, when inflamed, indistinct (Fig. 7.11A) or spiculated (Fig. 7.12A) margins; associated calcifications may be present (Fig. 7.13; also see Fig. 6.9). On spot tangential views, they are localized to the skin (Figs. 7.9B and 7.12B). On ultrasound, an anechoic, hypoechoic, or echogenic mass often with posterior acoustic enhancement may be seen separating the dermal layers (Fig. 7.11C). As the patient is scanned and the transducer is manipulated, the skin track can be identified in some patients (Fig. 7.12B; also see Fig. 4.11).

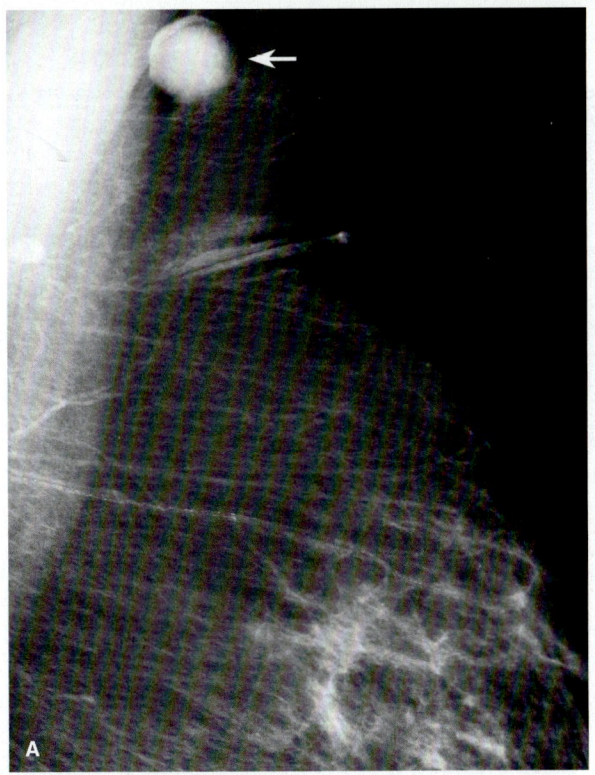
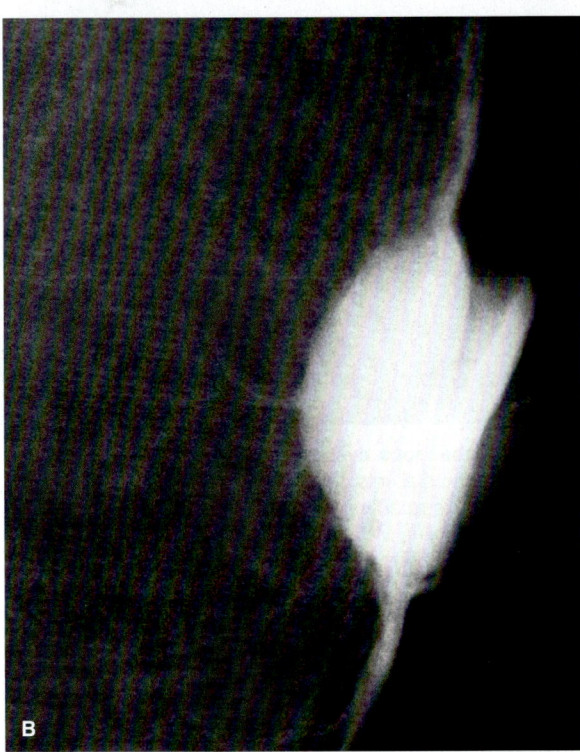
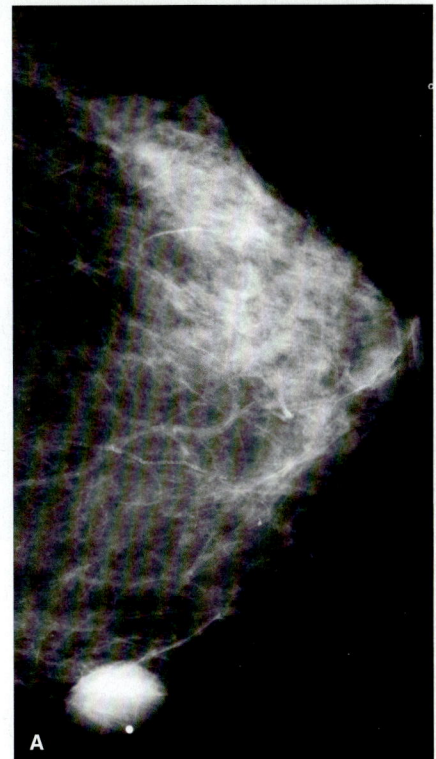
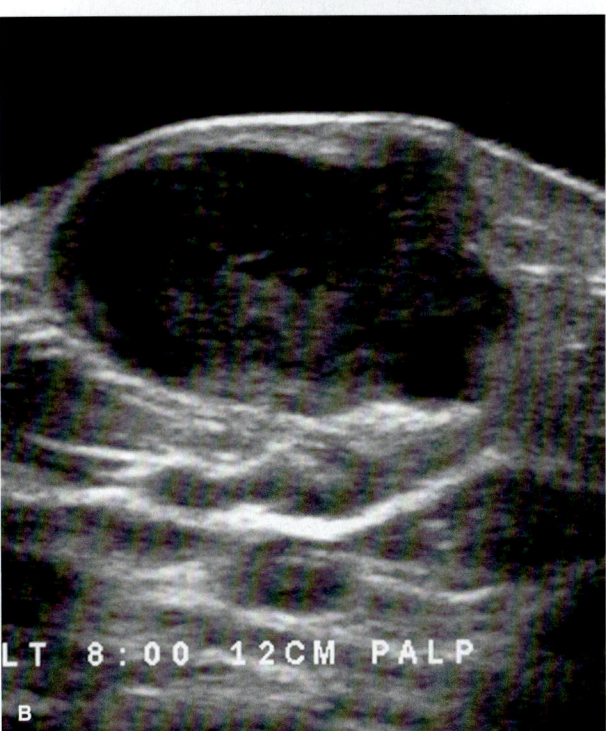

FIG. 7.9 • **Sebaceous cysts. A:** Left MLO view photographically coned to upper aspect of the image. A round, dense mass (arrow) is imaged in the axilla correlating to a "lump" described by the patient. **B:** Spot tangential view. A round dense mass with circumscribed margins is imaged associated with the dermis, focally thickened at this site. This is a nice illustration of how useful the spot tangential can be in localizing lesions to the skin. BI-RADS 2: Benign finding. Sebaceous cysts can occur anywhere on the breast but are most common in the axillae and the medial most extent of the inframammary fold. If on physical examination a punctum is identified and the "lump" moves with the skin, and on the spot tangential view, the lesion is imaged in the skin, no further evaluation or short-interval follow-up is indicated. It is important to reassure the patient of the unequivocally benign etiology of the "lump." If she is symptomatic, surgical referral for complete excision of the cyst wall/lining is appropriate.

FIG. 7.10 • **Sebaceous cyst. A:** Left CC view demonstrates a dense, oval mass with circumscribed margins at the medial most extent of the inframammary fold corresponding to the site of a "lump" described by the patient. The metallic BB marks the site of the palpable finding. **B:** Ultrasound. On visual inspection, a bulge in the contour of the breast is apparent at the site of the clinical finding. On physical examination a hard mass is palpated corresponding to the site of the mammographically described mass. An oval, lobulated complex cystic and solid mass with circumscribed margins and minimal posterior acoustic enhancement disrupting the deep dermal layer and extending into the subcutaneous tissue is imaged corresponding to the clinical and mammographically apparent mass. This is a sebaceous cyst. BI-RADS 2: Benign finding. Given the predilection of some of these lesions for the axillae and medial location along the inframammary fold (bra line), surgical excision is sometimes requested by the patient for symptomatic relief.

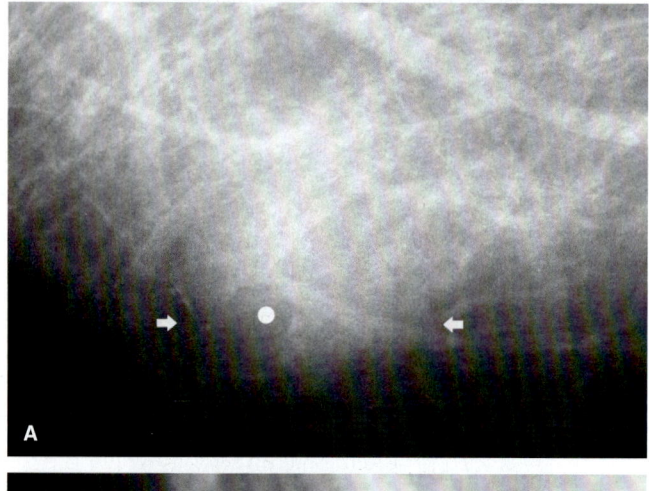
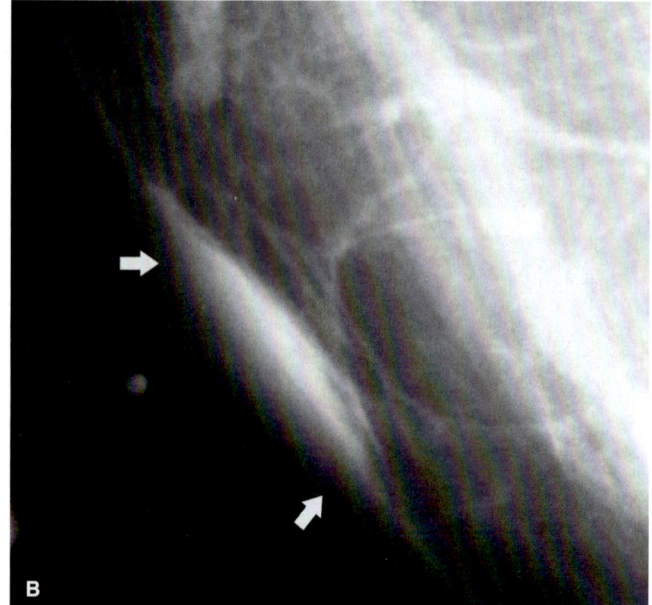
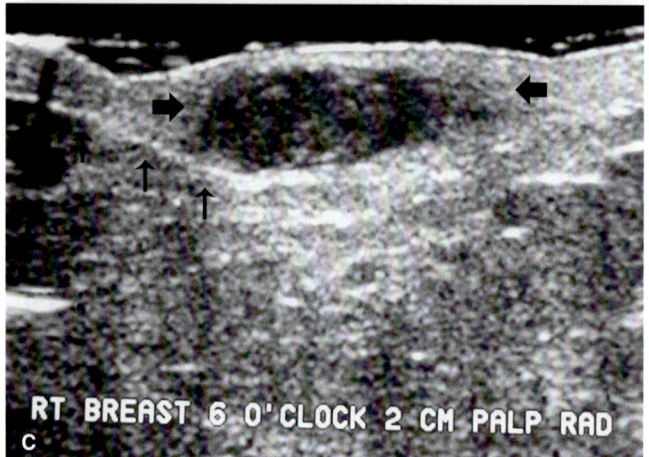

FIG. 7.11 • **Sebaceous cyst. A:** MLO view, photographically coned to the lower aspect of the breast in a patient who presents with a superficial "lump" that is painful. A metallic BB marks the location of the lesion. Increased density *(arrows)* is seen at the site of concern to the patient without a mass. **B:** Spot tangential view places the lesion *(arrows)* in tangent to x-ray beam and effectively localizes the finding to the skin. **C:** A hypoechoic mass *(thick arrows)* is imaged in the dermis. The mass splits the dermal layers such that the deep dermal layer *(long arrows)* is displaced inferiorly. BI-RADS 2: Benign finding. (From Cardeñosa G. *Breast Imaging [The Core Curriculum Series]*. Philadelphia, PA: Lippincott Williams & Wilkins; 2003.)

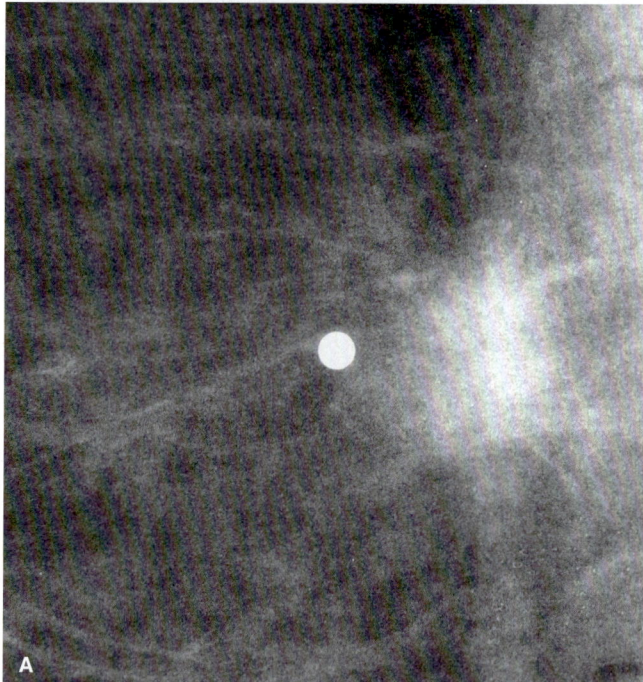
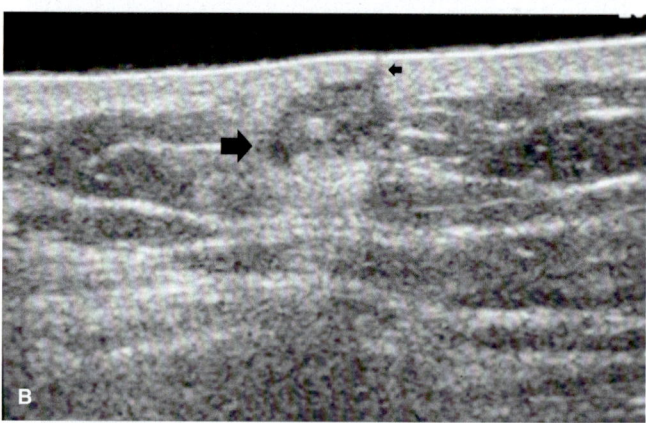

FIG. 7.12 • **Sebaceous cyst. A:** Photographically coned down image in a patient who presents with a "lump" that is painful. An isodense, round mass with spiculated margins is imaged corresponding to the site of concern to the patient. Metallic BB used to mark the "lump" described by the patient. **B:** Ultrasound. A hypoechoic mass *(thick large arrow)* is imaged intradermally corresponding to the area of concern to the patient. A track to the skin surface is noted *(small arrow)*. BI-RADS 2: Benign finding. (From Cardeñosa G. *Breast Imaging [The Core Curriculum Series]*. Philadelphia, PA: Lippincott Williams & Wilkins; 2003.)

As the mass enlarges, the deep dermal layer may not be readily apparent (Fig. 7.10B). With inflammation or associated calcifications, the echotexture may be heterogeneous. These lesions can attain significant sizes such that patients present with discomfort particularly when the sebaceous cyst is in the axilla or along the inframammary fold (e.g., along the bra line). On magnetic resonance imaging (MRI), sebaceous cysts are masses localized to the skin that demonstrate a high T2 signal with no significant enhancement (Fig. 7.14), unless there is associated inflammation.

Keloids are clinically apparent, developing at prior surgical sites. They occur with a higher incidence among Black and Hispanic patients and reflect abnormal wound healing. They are irregular, serpiginous, tubular, or mass-like structures noted at, and extending away from,

Evaluation and Imaging Features of Benign Breast Masses

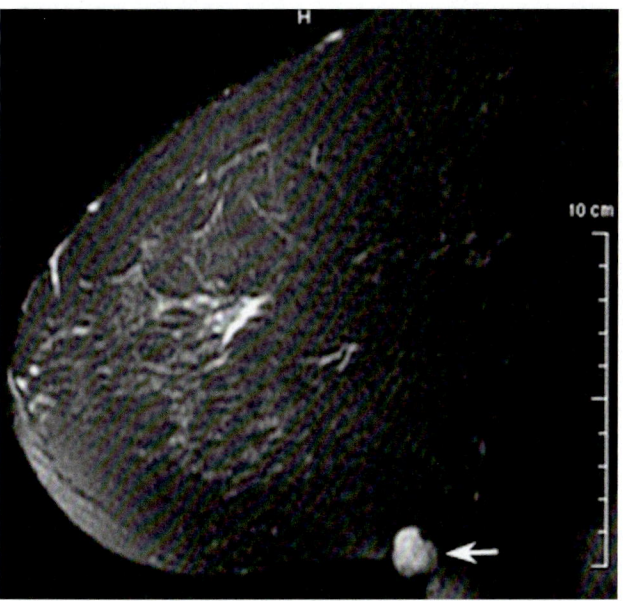

FIG. 7.13 • **Sebaceous cyst with calcifications.** A low to isodense, round mass with circumscribed margins and coarse calcifications internally. BI-RADS 2: Benign finding. Sebaceous cysts can develop calcifications that are commonly coarse, dense, and dystrophic in appearance.

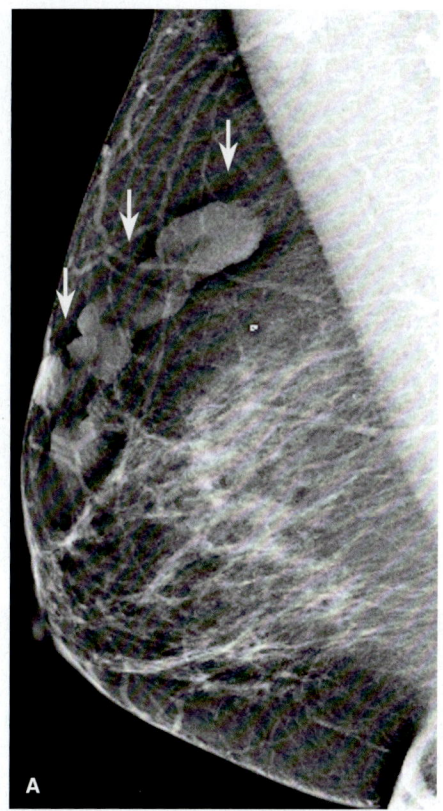

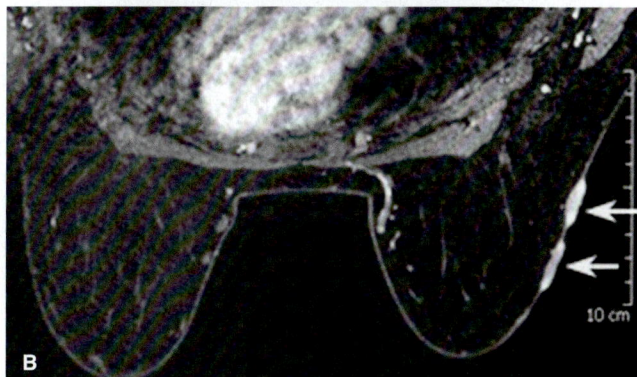

FIG. 7.14 • **Sebaceous cyst.** MRI, sagittal T2 fat-suppressed image of the right breast. A mass *(arrow)* with smooth margins, high T2 signal, and no enhancement (images not shown) is imaged along the inframammary fold associated with the skin consistent with a sebaceous cyst.

FIG. 7.15 • **Keloid. A:** Right MLO view. A wide, tubular, low density, serpiginous structure *(arrows)* with a lucency (air) sharply defining some of the margins is seen involving the superior aspect of the right breast. Focal skin thickening is evident anteriorly at the inferior extent of the keloid. **B:** MRI, axial images postcontrast in the same patient. Masses *(arrows)* with smooth margins are seen associated with the skin. Minimal enhancement is evident on the subtraction images and on kinetic curve evaluation (not shown).

the surgery site. The portion that projects beyond the skin is outlined by air such that a thin radiolucency is apparent mammographically (Fig. 7.15A). On MRI, they can be localized to the dermis and do not usually demonstrate significant enhancement (Fig. 7.15B). Treatment options are variable and include injections (steroids, 5 fluorouracil, interferon, retinoids, and calcium channel blockers) directly into the keloid, surgery, radiation therapy, topical applications of silicone gel, laser, pressure therapy, and cryosurgery. Mixed results are reported for each, and appropriate treatment remains controversial.

Clinically, neurofibromas are readily apparent in patients with neurofibromatosis. There is wide variation in the number, size, and distribution of the lesions on the breasts; however, there is a predilection for the periareolar areas in many patients. Although patients can develop new lesions, and preexisting lesions can increase in size, the rapid growth of a single lesion is of concern and biopsy may be indicated since malignant peripheral nerve sheath tumors may develop in preexisting neurofibromas (Fig. 7.16A). Neurofibromas are noted mammographically as masses that may be lobulated with circumscribed margins and partially or completely outlined by air. Depending on the number of lesions, evaluation of the underlying breast parenchyma may be difficult. Extra care should be used to actively disregard the obvious benign findings in search of a possible unsuspected malignancy in these patients. On ultrasound, a hypoechoic mass with gently lobulated, circumscribed margins and posterior

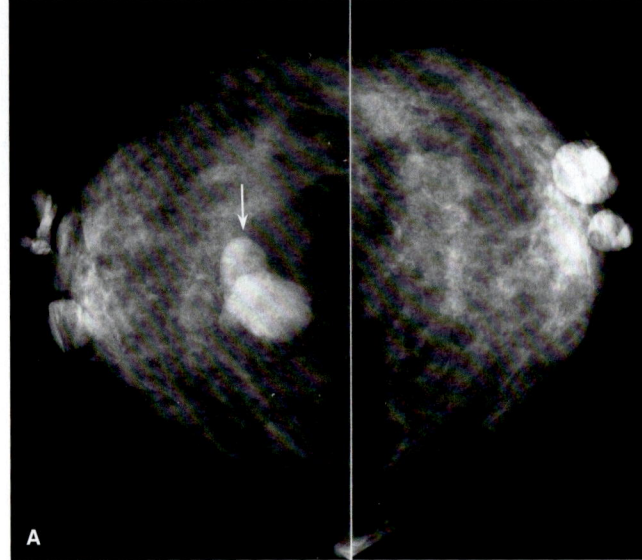
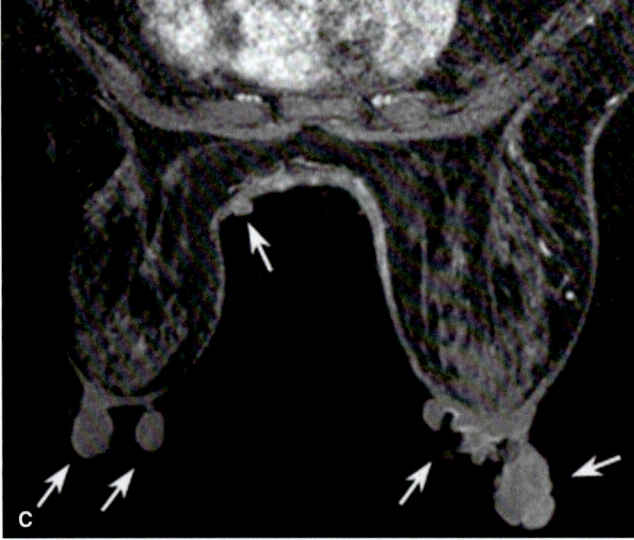
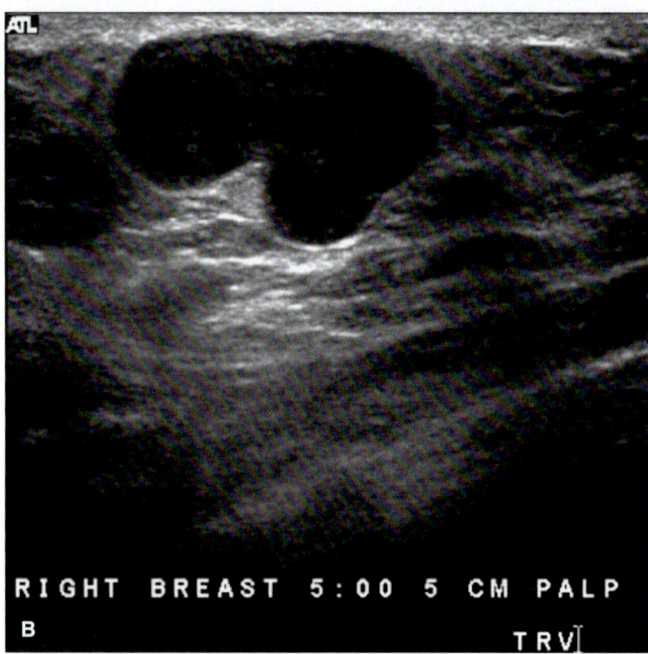

FIG. 7.16 • **Malignant peripheral nerve sheath tumor in a patient with neurofibromatosis. A:** CC views. Multiple neurofibromas are evident bilaterally primarily involving the subareolar areas. Some of the neurofibromas project beyond the breast such that a thin lucency (air) can be seen surrounding the portion of the neurofibroma that extends beyond the skin. A neurofibroma *(arrow)* in the lower central aspect of the right breast posteriorly developed within a year and, as described by the patient, is "getting bigger, fast." **B:** Ultrasound. A hypoechoic, macrolobulated mass with circumscribed margins and posterior acoustic enhancement is imaged in the subcutaneous tissue associated with the deep dermal layer. Because of the progressive change in size, an ultrasound-guided biopsy is done, and a malignant peripheral nerve sheath tumor is diagnosed. **C:** MRI, MIP image. Variably sized neurofibromas *(arrows)* with no enhancement are seen extending beyond the skin anteriorly from the periareolar margin as well as centrally in the cleavage.

acoustic enhancement is imaged in the dermis or in a subcutaneous location (Fig. 7.16B). On MRI, the lesions can be seen extending beyond the borders of the breast and usually demonstrate no significant enhancement (Fig. 7.16C).

An increasing number of patients are being referred to us for the evaluation of cellulitis. In most patients, no underlying etiology is identified; in some, radiation therapy may precede the presentation. Clinically, localized or diffuse erythema is the primary finding, and depending on the amount of inflammation, peau d'orange changes or localized areas of necrosis may be apparent (Fig. 7.17A); significant tenderness is elicited and often precludes a mammogram. The main differential consideration in many of these patients is inflammatory breast carcinoma (IBC). Patients with cellulitis are more likely to have localized findings, be more tender, and respond to antibiotics with no progression or recurrence of symptoms. At presentation, ultrasound is often the starting point because some of these patients do not tolerate the compression required for a mammogram. Ultrasound is helpful in localizing the process to the skin (Fig. 7.17B), excluding the presence of an underlying abscess requiring drainage or other focal parenchymal finding. Axillary lymph nodes may be prominent in patients with cellulitis; however, the lymph nodes retain normal morphologic features in contrast to the grossly abnormal lymph nodes that are seen in many patients with IBC at the time of presentation.

FAT-CONTAINING MASSES

Fat-containing masses in the breast are almost always benign (1–3,5). These masses can be completely fatty (Table 7.5) or mixed in density (Table 7.6). Although ultrasound findings are described for completeness, the diagnosis is established reliably when lucent or mixed-density masses are seen on the mammogram (with some of these lesions, the features on ultrasound may raise concerns inappropriately). It is important to note that, although many of the entities described are commonly fatty or mixed in density, they may also present as water density masses. So you will find an overlap in the differentials provided for each. For example, lymph nodes and fat necrosis are typically considered mixed-density masses, but each may present as a water density mass. Rarely, entities typically presenting as water density masses (including malignancy) may be noted to have lucent areas.

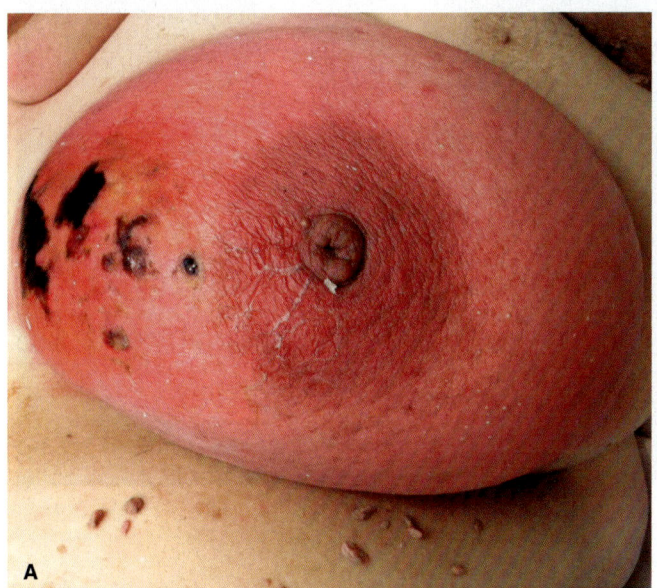
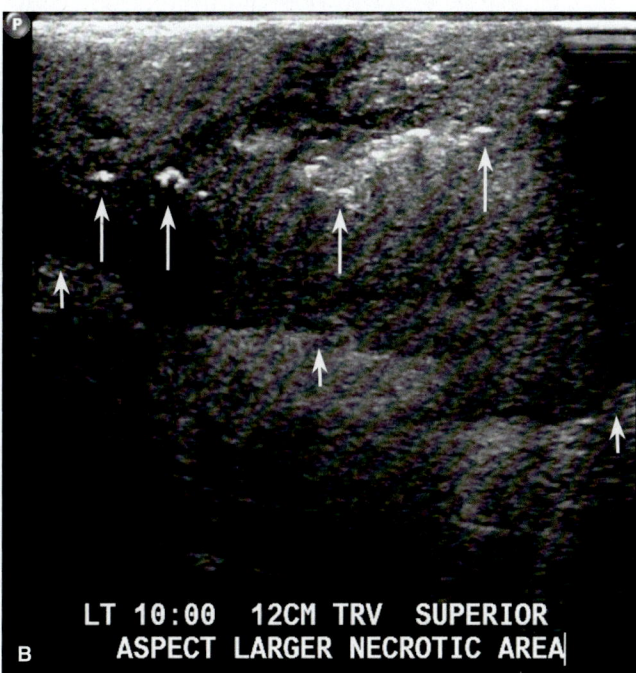

FIG. 7.17 • **Cellulitis, methicillin-resistant** *Staphylococcus aureus* **(MRSA) infection. A:** Patient presents describing a red swollen left breast. The left breast is enlarged and diffusely erythematous with several areas of necrotic skin (eschar) medially. Skin tags are incidentally noted on the upper aspect of the abdominal wall and left axilla. **B:** Ultrasound. The dermis is thickened *(short arrows)*, expands into, but does involve, the parenchyma and demonstrates a heterogeneous echotexture with bright echogenic foci *(long arrows)* possibly reflecting air. This process is limited to the skin and does not extend into the parenchyma; no solid or cystic masses are apparent in the breast tissue. The clinicians are told that the process is limited to the skin and is consistent with a cellulitis. MRSA is cultured; the patient is treated effectively with superficial debridement and IV antibiotics.

Table 7.5 DIFFERENTIAL: FAT DENSITY MASSES (RADIOLUCENT)
Lipoma
Oil cyst
Galactocele

Table 7.6 DIFFERENTIAL: MASSES WITH MIXED DENSITY
Intramammary lymph nodes
Fibroadenolipomas (hamartomas)
Fat necrosis, oil cysts
Galactocele
Postoperative/traumatic fluid collections (hematomas, seromas)

LIPOMA

Patients with a lipoma can be asymptomatic or present with a soft or hard, mobile mass. A radiolucent mass with an expansile circumscribed margin and a thin fibrous capsule are detected in the breast (Fig. 7.18A), or less commonly in the pectoral muscle (Fig. 7.18B), on the mammogram. Although the diagnosis is reliably made on mammographic findings, a mass with circumscribed margins and a homogeneously hypo-, iso-, or hyperechoic echotexture is imaged on ultrasound (see Fig. 4.40A) (10); in some patients, short, curvilinear hyperechoic internal septations may be apparent (Fig. 7.19A). Gentle mass effect can be seen on surrounding structures (Fig. 7.19B). Uncommonly, hemorrhage may occur in preexisting lipomas so that on the mammogram a mixed-density mass (Fig. 7.20A, B) is seen at the site of a preexisting lucent mass. As the hemorrhage resolves, the lucent nature of the mass becomes more apparent on follow-up mammograms; the mass is complex on ultrasound and fluid–fluid levels may be seen (Fig. 7.20C). A mass with the signal characteristics of fat (high T1 and T2 signal, suppressed on fat-suppression images) and no enhancement is incidentally noted on MRIs performed as screening studies in high-risk women or those being evaluated for other breast-related issues (Fig. 7.21). Histologically, these lesions are characterized by the presence of mature lipocytes surrounded by a thin capsule (11,12). If otherwise asymptomatic, no intervention or short-term follow-up is indicated. Rarely, liposarcomatous lesions can present in the breast typically as a rapidly growing mass. The size, age of the patient, and growth pattern should suggest a malignant process. On the mammogram, internal septations may be seen in an otherwise lucent mass and the typically homogenous echotexture on ultrasound may be more heterogeneous (see Fig. 8.50).

OIL CYSTS

Oil cysts are radiolucent, solitary (Fig. 7.22), or multiple (see Fig. 6.26B), uni- or bilateral masses. They vary in size, can progressively decrease, and resolve completely on subsequent mammograms. They are idiopathic or develop in areas of prior trauma or

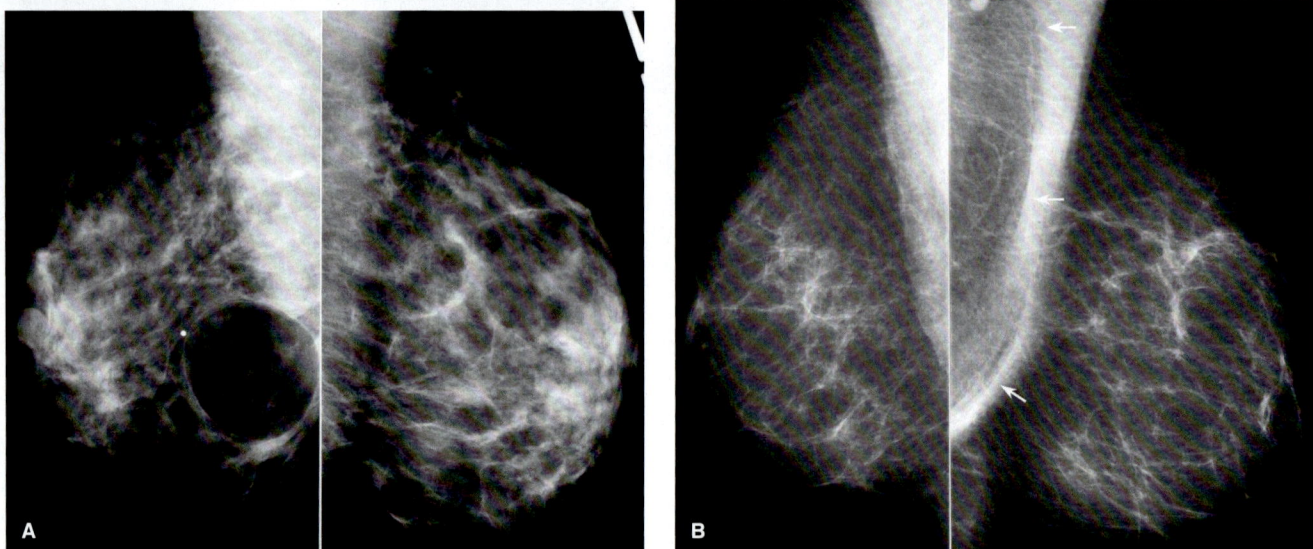

FIG. 7.18 • **Lipomas. A:** MLO views. A round, lucent mass with circumscribed margins is imaged in the right breast corresponding to the site of a "lump" described by the patient. The metallic BB denotes the palpable finding. Lucent masses in the breast are benign, and no further workup is indicated. BI-RADS 2: Benign finding. **B:** MLO views, different patient. An oval, lucent mass (arrows) with circumscribed margins is partially imaged in the left pectoral muscle. The size of the pectoral muscles is asymmetric, resulting in an asymmetric breast size as well. This is an intrapectoral lipoma that requires no additional evaluation. BI-RADS 2: Benign finding.

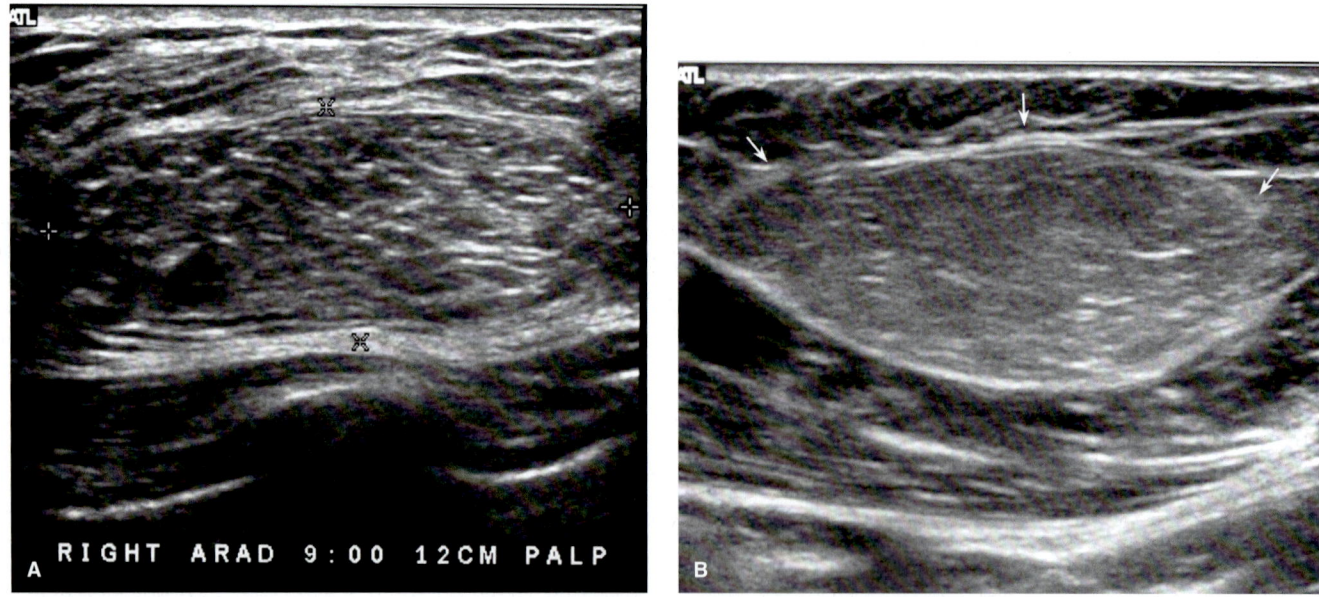

FIG. 7.19 • **Lipomas. A:** Ultrasound. An oval mass (calipers) with heterogeneous internal echotexture, predominantly hyperechoic with short, curvilinear foci of hyperechogenicity is correlated to a soft mobile lucent mass mammographically (mammogram not shown). BI-RADS 2: Benign finding. **B:** Ultrasound, different patient. A homogeneously hyperechoic mass (arrows) with short, curvilinear foci of hyperechogenicity and gentle mass effect on the pectoral muscle. BI-RADS 2: Benign finding.

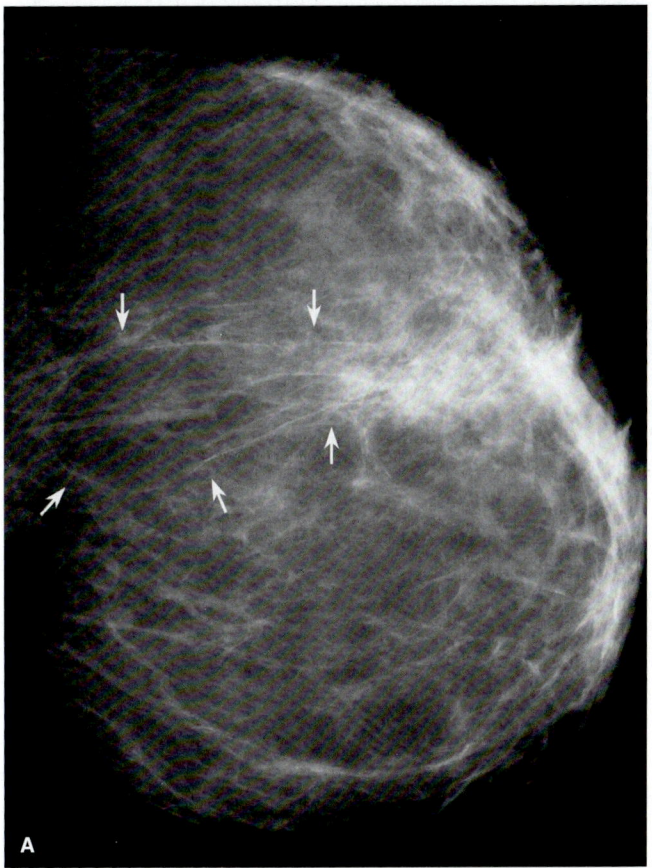
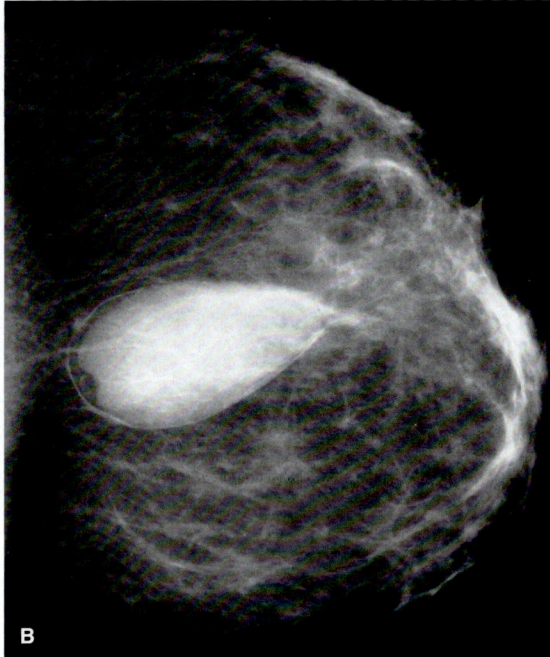
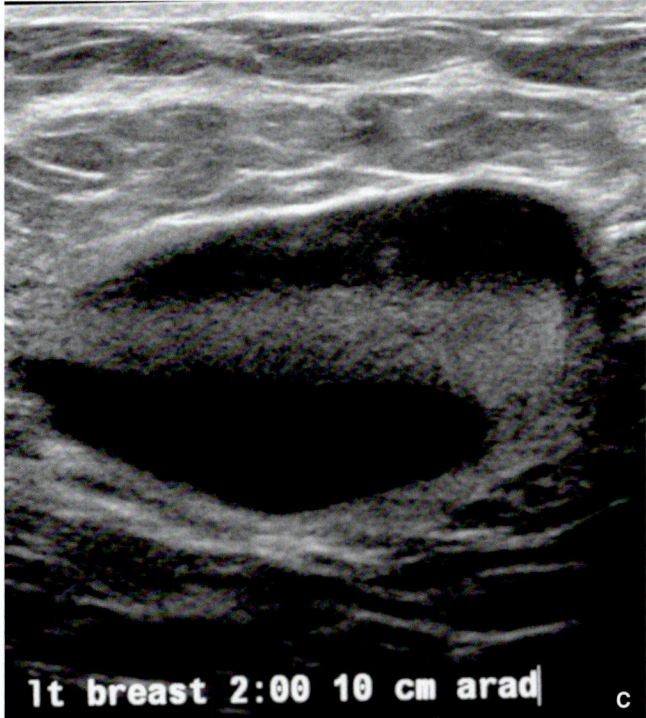

FIG. 7.20 • **Lipoma with hemorrhage. A:** Left CC view. An oval lucent mass *(arrows)* is present centrally in the right breast. **B:** Left CC view following a motor vehicle accident. A mixed-density mass with circumscribed margins is now apparent at the site of the preexisting lipoma. BI-RADS 2: Benign finding. **C:** Ultrasound. A complex cystic mass with a fluid–fluid level is imaged corresponding to the mixed-density mass seen mammographically. Two years following the accident, the internal density had resolved, leaving the preexisting lucent mass.

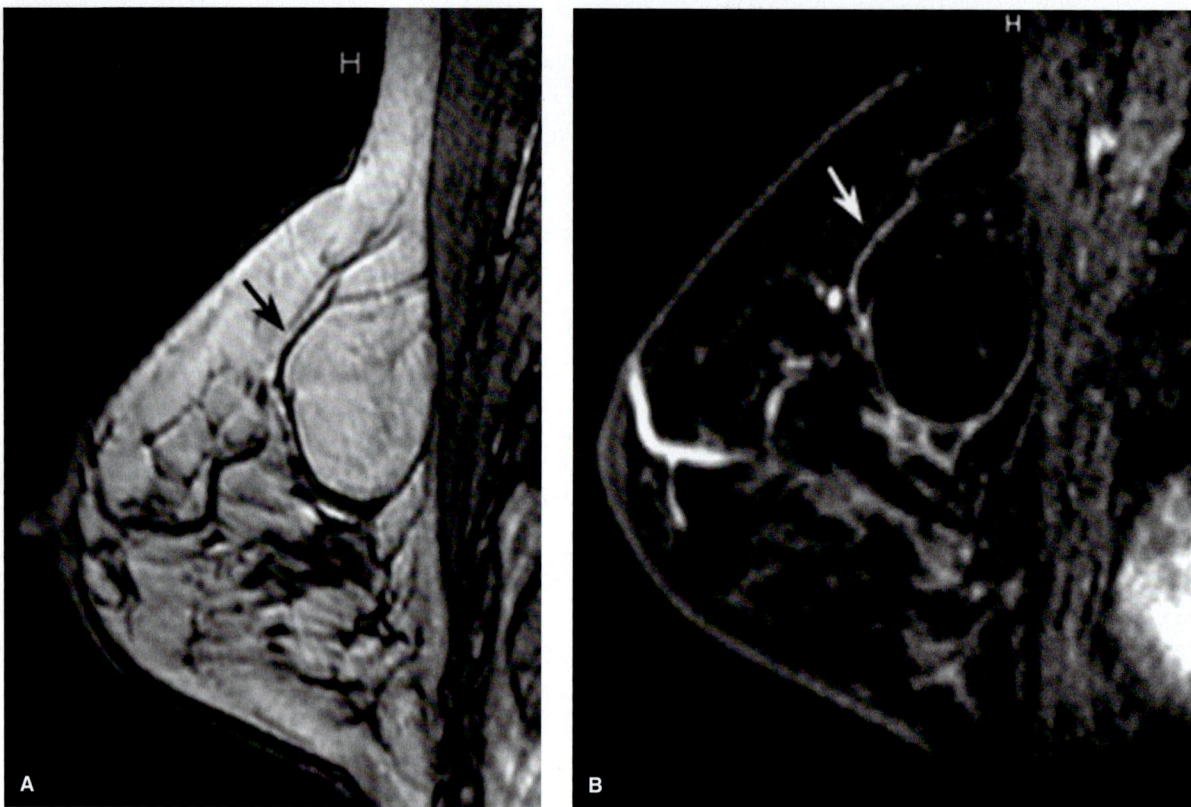

FIG. 7.21 • **Lipoma. A:** MRI, sagittal, T1-weighted, nonfat-suppressed image of the left breast. An oval, fat containing mass (arrow) with circumscribed margins is imaged abutting the right pectoral muscle. **B:** MRI, T1 fat-suppressed sagittal image of the left breast postcontrast. The mass (arrow) is low in signal on the fat-suppressed images and demonstrates minimal enhancement of a thin rim. BI-RADS 2: Benign finding. The MRI was done for screening purposes in a high-risk patient with a personal history of breast cancer.

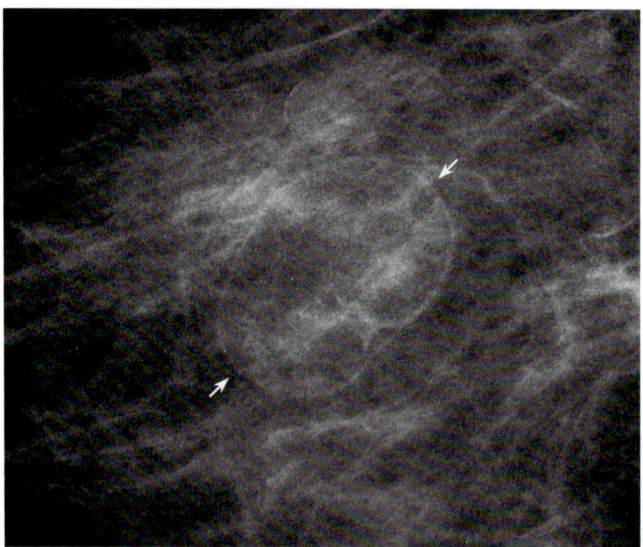

FIG. 7.22 • **Oil cyst.** Oval, lobulated, lucent mass (arrows) with circumscribed margins. BI-RADS 2: Benign findings.

surgery and, in this setting, probably represent an end stage of fat necrosis. Some develop mural calcifications resulting in lucent-centered (or rim) calcifications (see Figs. 6.26B and 6.29A), while in others, the mural calcifications are seen "en-phase" having a coarse, irregular, curvilinear appearance (see Fig. 6.28). In most women, oil cysts are noted incidentally on screening mammography. Some patients may present for diagnostic mammography describing a discrete, hard mass that is correlated with one or multiple oil cysts mammographically. In this situation it is important to assure the patient and referring physician that the palpable finding is an oil cyst requiring no intervention or follow-up. The diagnosis is established on the mammogram (Figs. 7.23 and 7.24) such that ultrasound is rarely indicated. Given the variability in the appearance of oil cysts on ultrasound, the ultrasound features may raise concerns over the benign diagnosis (see Fig. 4.34). They may be anechoic with through-transmission indistinguishable from fluid-containing cysts (Fig. 7.23B). Internal echoes, fluid–fluid levels, septations, and complex cystic masses either predominantly cystic with intracystic or mural solid-appearing components (Fig. 7.24B) or solid with cystic components or they may appear solid (13). On MRI, oil cysts are characterized by circumscribed margins and demonstrate decreased signal on T2-weighted, fat-suppressed images (Fig. 7.25A) and a high signal on T2- and T1-weighted, non–fat-suppressed images. Most oil cysts demonstrate no enhancement (Fig. 7.25B); however, a thin enhancing rim may be apparent in some patients.

In some women, oil cysts may be more appropriately characterized as mixed-density masses (Fig. 7.26) because of thickened, ill-defined, or spiculated margins, or the presence of a round or oval intracystic mass. With a history of trauma or surgery, and if fat (radiolucency) is associated with these masses in orthogonal projections, no intervention or short-term follow-up is warranted regardless of the spiculated margins or associated nodules (see below, fat necrosis).

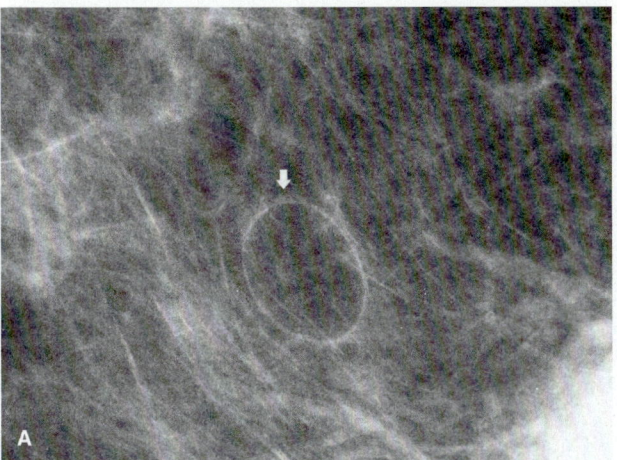
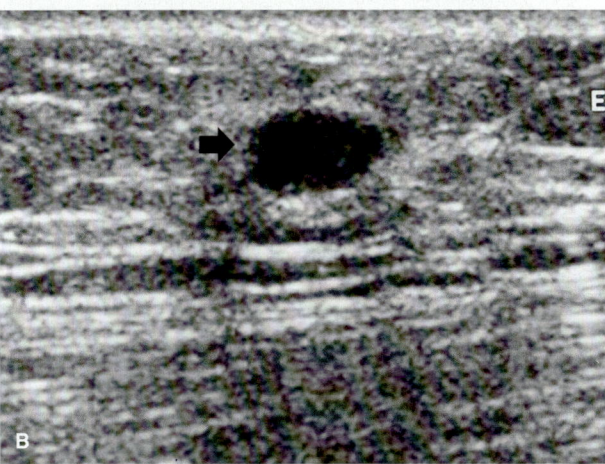

FIG. 7.23 • **Oil cyst. A:** Photographically coned image of the right breast. An oval lucent mass *(arrow)* with circumscribed margins is identified. This is pathognomonic of an oil cyst with the diagnosis reliably established on the mammogram. BI-RADS 2: Benign finding. **B:** Ultrasound. An anechoic mass *(arrow)* with some posterior acoustic enhancement is imaged corresponding to the oil cyst seen on the mammogram. In this patient the ultrasound is not needed to reliably establish a benign diagnosis. (From Cardeñosa G. *Breast Imaging [The Core Curriculum Series]*. Philadelphia, PA: Lippincott Williams & Wilkins; 2003.)

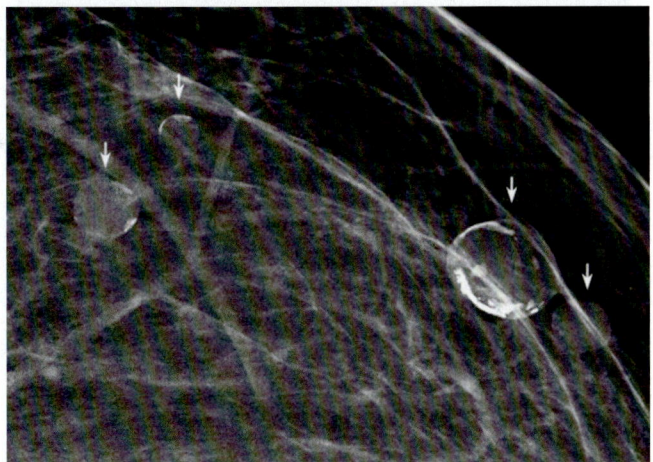

FIG. 7.24 • **Oil cyst. A:** Photographically coned image of the left breast in a patient who presents describing a "lump." The metallic BB at the upper right hand corner of the image denotes the palpable finding. An oval lucent mass *(thick arrow)* with circumscribed margins is imaged corresponding to the palpable finding. Several round lucent masses *(small thick arrows)* are localized within the dominant mass on orthogonal projections (only one shown here). A dystrophic calcification is incidentally noted *(long thin arrow)*. BI-RADS 2: Benign finding. **B:** Ultrasound. A complex cystic mass with mural nodules *(arrows)* is imaged corresponding to the palpable finding and the radiolucent mass seen on the mammogram. The ultrasound findings may raise concerns and differentials that include malignant processes; however, the mammographic findings effectively exclude those entities. In this patient, the ultrasound is not needed to establish a benign diagnosis accurately. (From Cardeñosa G. *Breast Imaging [The Core Curriculum Series]*. Philadelphia, PA: Lippincott Williams & Wilkins; 2003.)

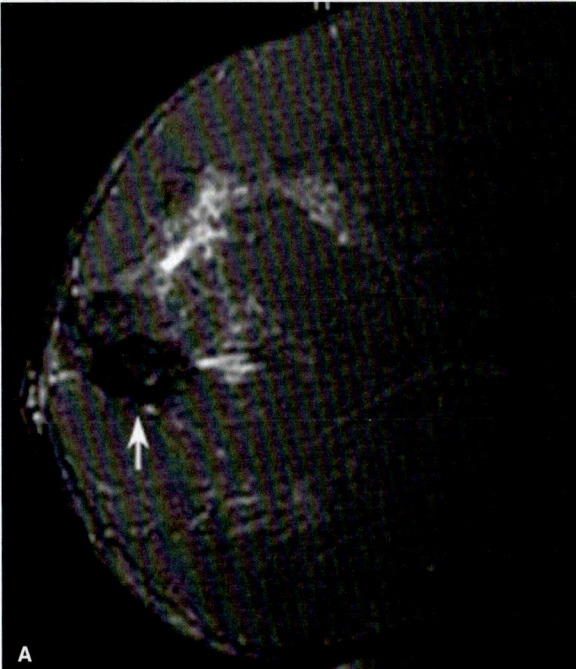
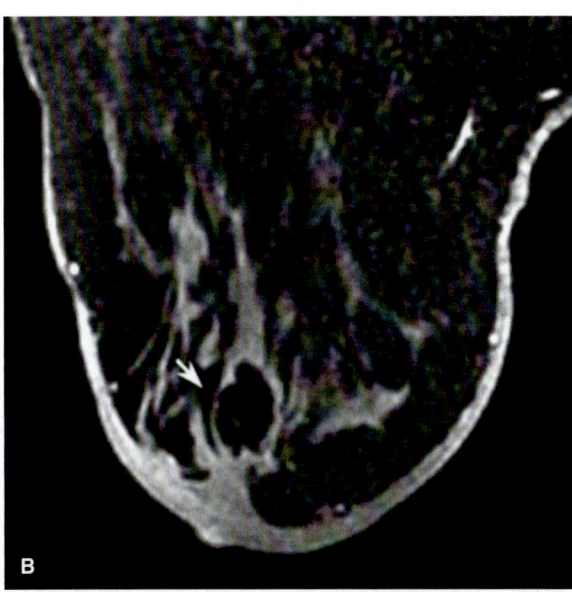

FIG. 7.25 • **Oil cyst. A:** MRI, sagittal T2-weighted fat-suppressed image of the left breast. An oval mass *(arrow)* with fatty tissue internally is imaged in the subareolar areas. **B:** MRI, axial image of the left breast following contrast. A fat-containing mass *(arrow)* with no associated enhancement is imaged at the site of the mass depicted in part **A**.

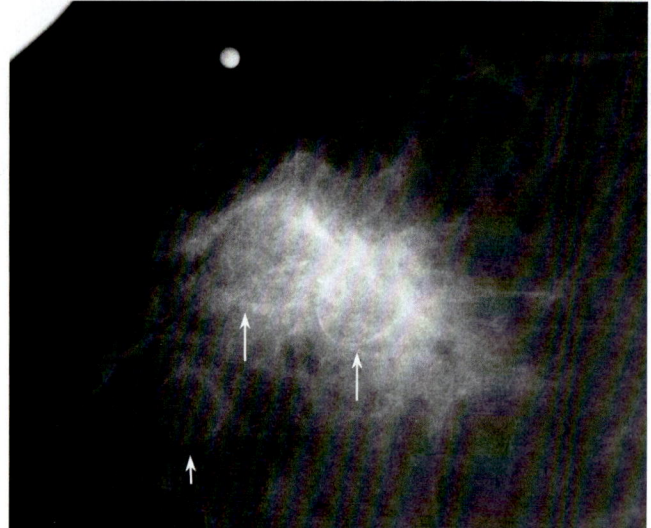

FIG. 7.26 • **Oil cysts.** Spot tangential view done at the site of a new "lump" (metallic BB) described by the patient in the right breast. Two adjacent oil cysts *(long arrows)* with thickened indistinct margins (or is it a mixed-density mass with central lucency?) correlating to the site of the palpable finding. A third oil cyst *(small arrow)* with no surrounding density is present. Note focal skin thickening and associated soft tissue stranding correlating to the location of the oil cysts. The findings are posttraumatic in etiology, and our job is to obtain correlative history to confirm this impression and reassure the patient of the benign etiology of the findings. Even though the margins are indistinct, the presence of fat centrally is sufficient to characterize this as a benign finding. No additional intervention of follow-up is indicated for this finding. BI-RADS 2: Benign finding.

Steatocystoma multiplex is a rare condition with an autosomal dominant mode of inheritance associated with multiple intradermal oil cysts scattered over the body but with a predilection for the trunk and upper extremities (14,15). Although more commonly seen in males, women with this condition may be found to have multiple oil cysts in the breasts bilaterally.

MIXED-DENSITY MASSES

Lymph Nodes

Intramammary and axillary lymph nodes are common and variable in number, size, density, shape, and location (Fig. 7.27). They can fluctuate in size, and in some women can disappear only to reappear on subsequent studies. Keep in mind that on the basis of the positioning of the woman for the MLO views, you may see variable amounts of axillary tissue, and with that, a variation in our ability to evaluate axillary lymph nodes mammographically. Typically, they are round or oval masses of mixed density with circumscribed and sometimes lobulated margins located in the upper outer quadrants posteriorly and in the axillae; however, they can be found anywhere, including, less commonly, the medial quadrants of the breast. The presence of a variably sized fatty hilum either centrally or peripherally is required prior to assuming that a mass in the upper outer quadrant of the breast is a lymph node. Size alone is not used to determine the need for evaluation. We rely on density, margins, contour (bulging) alterations, absence of a fatty hilum, and changes compared with prior studies to determine appropriate management.

On ultrasound, lymph nodes are round or oval hypoechoic masses with circumscribed margins and an area of hyperechogenicity either centrally or peripherally (Fig. 7.28; also see Fig. 4.21). Reactive lymph

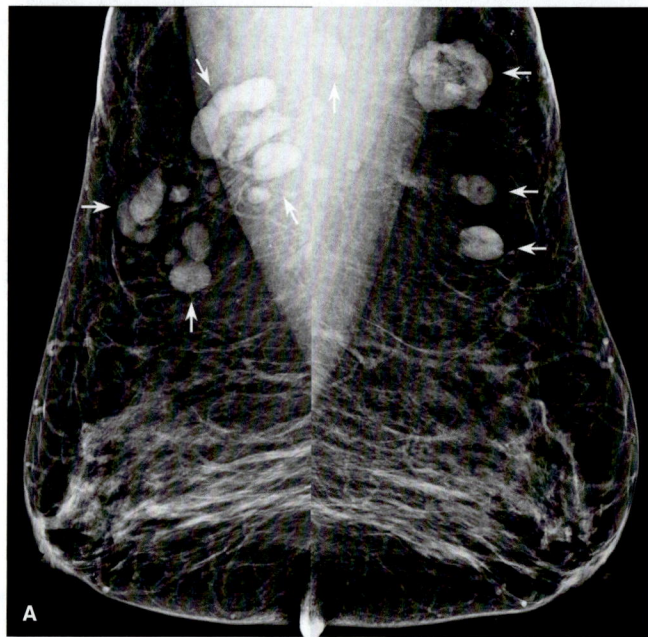

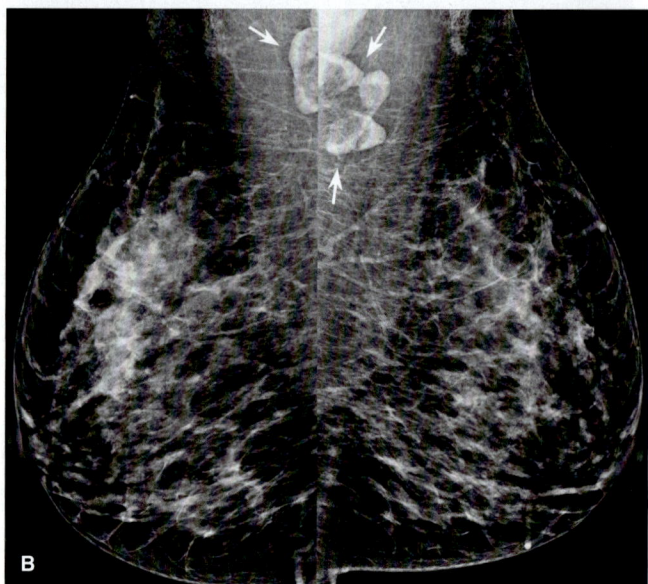

FIG. 7.27 • **Lymph nodes. A:** MLO views. Multiple masses *(arrows)* with circumscribed margins are present in the axillae extending into the parenchyma bilaterally. They are variable in size, shape, and density (within and among patients). Some are mixed in density. **B:** MLO views, different patient. Variably sized, mixed-density masses *(arrows)* in the axillae. It is important to emphasize that size alone is *not* useful in assessing lymph nodes in the axillae.

nodes may demonstrate a symmetric increase in the size and density of the cortex and may or may not retain a fatty hilum. If the fatty hilum is not readily apparent on the mammogram, it may be seen on ultrasound (Fig. 7.28); however, if a fatty hilum is not identified with either modality and the mass is new or enlarging, biopsy is indicated (Fig. 7.29). Although in evaluating lymph nodes it is important to factor in all features including cortical thickening and bulging (16), the echogenicity of the cortex on ultrasound can be a helpful guide. The cortex in patients with an underlying inflammatory process is often iso to slightly hyperechoic, whereas in patients with metastatic breast cancer or lymphoma,

Evaluation and Imaging Features of Benign Breast Masses   187

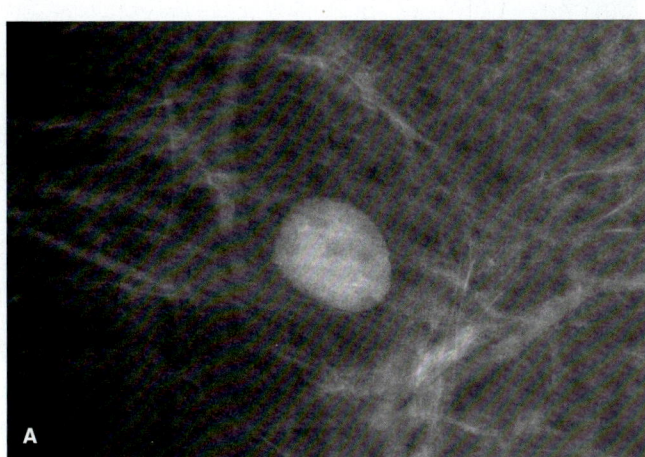 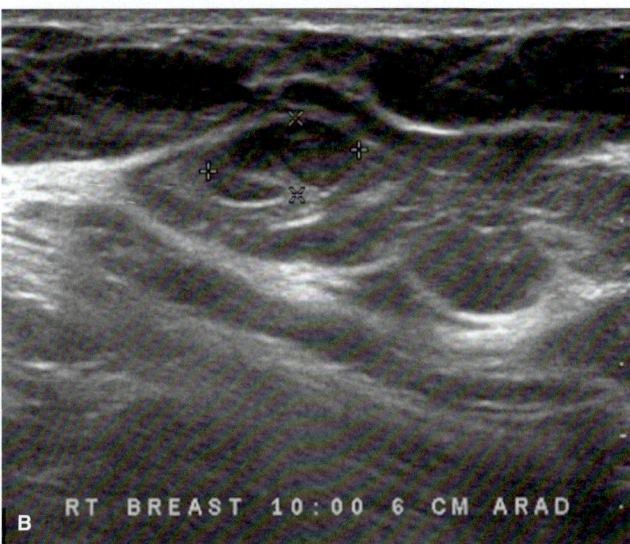

FIG. 7.28 • **Lymph node. A:** Spot compression views (only one is shown) of the upper outer of the right breast demonstrate an oval isodense mass with circumscribed margins. No identifiable fatty component is seen. Additional evaluation with ultrasound is indicated. **B:** Ultrasound. An oval mass *(calipers)* with circumscribed margins and an echogenic fatty hilum is identified along the 10 o'clock axis, 6 cm from the right nipple corresponding to the mass seen mammographically. Note that the cortex is slightly hyperechoic. BI-RADS 2: Benign finding. Although intramammary lymph nodes are most commonly seen in the upper outer quadrants of the breast as in this patient, they can be found anywhere, including the inner quadrants in approximately 5% of women.

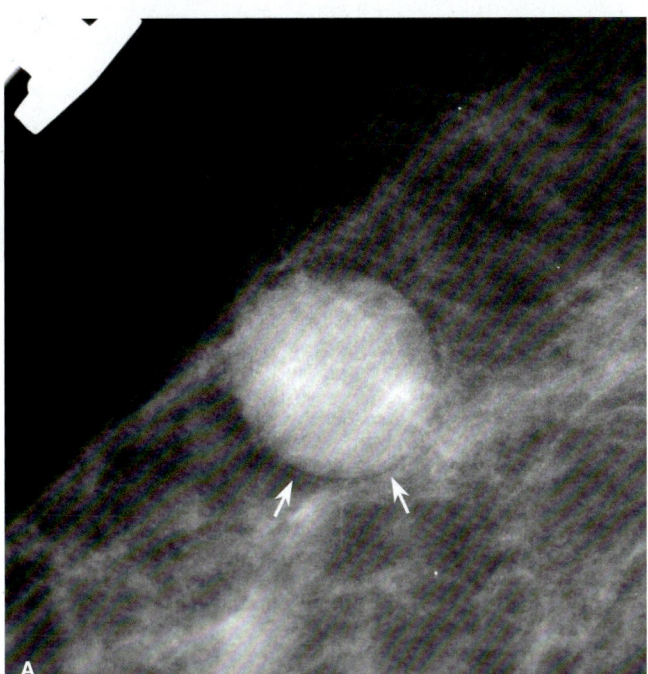 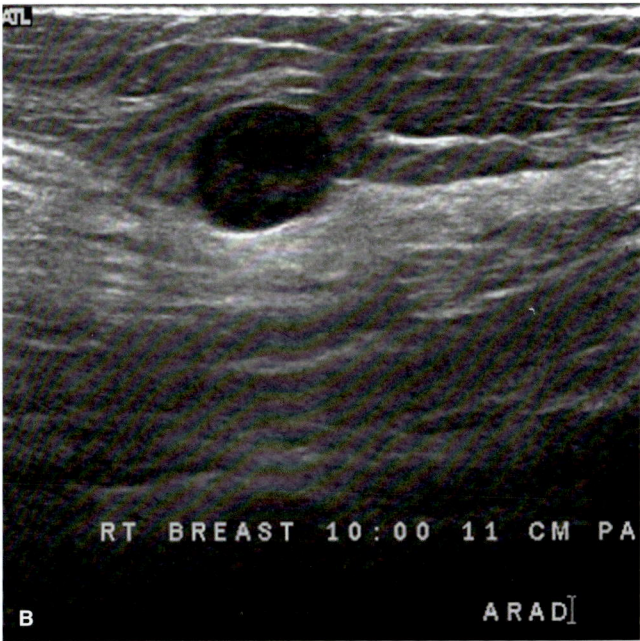

FIG. 7.29 • **Lymph node, reactive. A:** Spot tangential view of a "lump" described by a 70-year-old patient. A round, iso-to dense mass with circumscribed margins is present with an associated partial "halo" *(arrows)*. This mass is not identified on prior studies. Additional evaluation with ultrasound is indicated. **B:** Ultrasound. A round hypoechoic mass with circumscribed margins and minimal posterior acoustic enhancement is imaged correlating to the palpable and mammographically apparent mass. No fatty component is identified with either modality. A new mass that is solid requires biopsy, particularly in a 70-year-old patient. BI-RADS 4B: Suspicious finding, biopsy is indicated. A reactive lymph node is described on the ultrasound-guided core biopsy.

the cortex is often markedly hypoechoic (almost anechoic), the fatty hilum is either attenuated or not present, and there may be posterior acoustic enhancement (see Figs. 4.22, 8.59, through 8.61).

The oval shape and circumscribed margins of lymph nodes described mammographically and on ultrasound are also noted on MRI (see Fig. 5.18). The distribution and relationship to vasculature is readily appreciated on MRI. The extension of lymph nodes from the axilla inferiorly along the midaxillary line is also readily apparent on MRI in some patients (see Fig. 8.61A). The enhancement pattern of lymph nodes is variable but normal lymph nodes commonly demonstrate rapid washin and washout kinetics on the dynamic T1 sequences. Unlike most malignancies, lymph nodes demonstrate an intermediate to high T2 signal. The fatty hilum may have a high signal on T1 non–fat-suppressed sequences and low signal on the fat-suppressed sequences.

On screening mammograms, diffuse increases in the size and density of axillary, and less commonly intramammary, lymph nodes may be identified in some patients. Before undertaking extensive workups it is important to review the patient's history with respect to possible underlying causes of benign lymphadenopathy (Table 7.7) (17). If no underlying etiology is readily identified in the patient's history, the patient is called back and evaluated with spot compression views, physical examination, and ultrasound. On the basis of this evaluation, a core biopsy may be done (Fig. 7.30) to determine the underlying cause of the adenopathy (18).

Gold particles imaged as high density, punctate particles mimicking microcalcifications can be seen bilaterally in the axillary and intramammary lymph nodes of women treated for rheumatoid arthritis with gold (Fig. 7.31) (19). Coarse calcifications occurring in lymph nodes are often related to granulomatous disease and do not require intervention.

In a retrospective 5-year review, Lee et al. (20) reported unilateral enlargement of axillary or intramammary lymph nodes in 0.2% of their patients with otherwise normal mammograms. In their experience, biopsy is indicated in patients with a history of an underlying malignancy if the lymph node enlarges by more than 100% over baseline. If the woman does not have a history of a malignancy, the lymph node enlargement is small, the node is not palpable, and it maintains a benign appearance, they suggest clinical and mammographic follow-up. In the majority of their patients, lymph node enlargement decreased on follow-up studies. Please see Chapter 8 for a more detailed discussion of the imaging features of potentially abnormal lymph nodes.

Fibroadenolipomas (Hamartoma)

Fibroadenolipomas (FAL) or hamartomas are characterized by the presence of a pseudocapsule within which fatty, glandular, and fibrous elements are admixed. This appearance has led some to describe them

Table 7.7 BENIGN CAUSES OF INTRAMAMMARY AND AXILLARY LYMPHADENOPATHY

Lymphoid hyperplasia (acute or chronic inflammation)
Collagen vascular disorders (rheumatoid arthritis, scleroderma, lupus)
Granulomatous disease (sarcoid, tuberculosis)
Human immunodeficiency virus (HIV)
Dermatopathic (exfoliative or atopic dermatitis, psoriasis, infectious rashes)
Silicone adenopathy
Histoplasmosis
Toxoplasmosis (cat scratch)

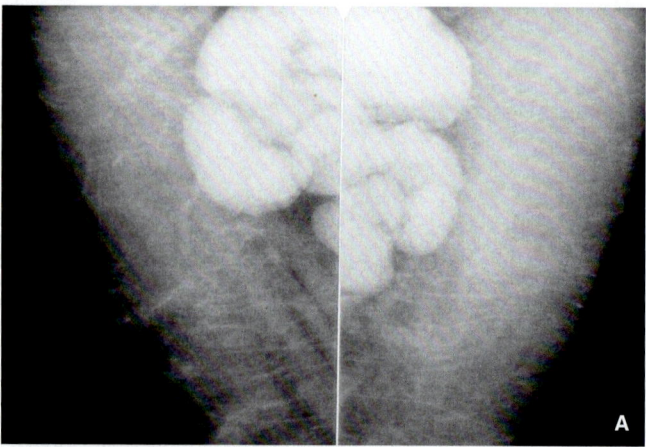
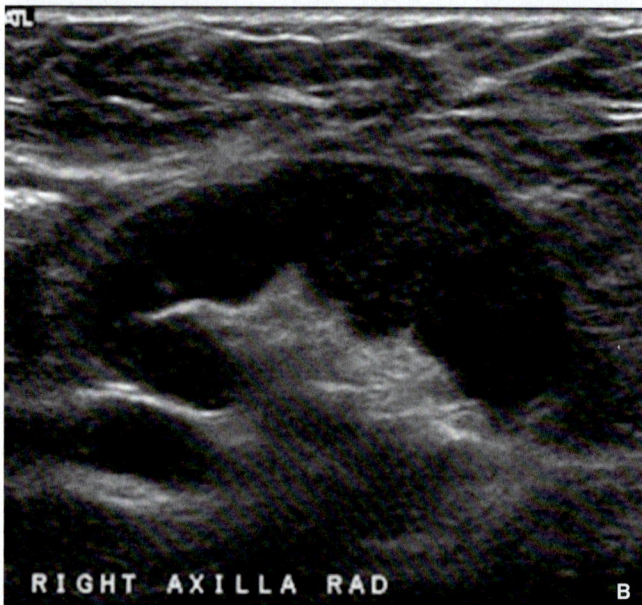

FIG. 7.30 • **Lymph nodes, HIV. A:** MLO views from a screening study photographically coned to the upper portion of the images. Multiple, dense, round, and oval lymph nodes with circumscribed margins are imaged in the axillae. These findings represent a change compared with prior studies in a patient with no significant medical history. BI-RADS 0: Need additional imaging evaluation. **B:** Ultrasound. Multiple lymph nodes are imaged in the axillae; this image of a lymph node in the right axilla is representative of their features. All of the lymph nodes have a fatty hilum and thickened cortices that are iso to slightly hyperechoic but exert no mass effect on the hyperechoic fatty hila. Findings on core biopsy are suggestive of HIV, a diagnosis that is confirmed on blood tests.

as a "breast within a breast" (Fig. 7.32A). The overall density of these lesions is variable depending on the proportions of intermingled fat and glandular tissue. In some women, FAL may enlarge and present as a palpable mass (Fig. 7.33A). Since the lesions are made up of breast tissue, breast cancer of any type can arise in hamartomas (21). Development of pleomorphic calcifications (Fig. 7.34), increasing density, particularly if ill-defined or spiculated in a FAL, should prompt further evaluation and, if indicated, an imaging-guided biopsy. If the patient presents with a palpable mass in an FAL, imaging guidance is helpful in targeting the areas of soft tissue in the FAL; otherwise, false-negatives may result if fatty elements are sampled. On ultrasound, these lesions can be distinguished from the surrounding glandular tissue and have

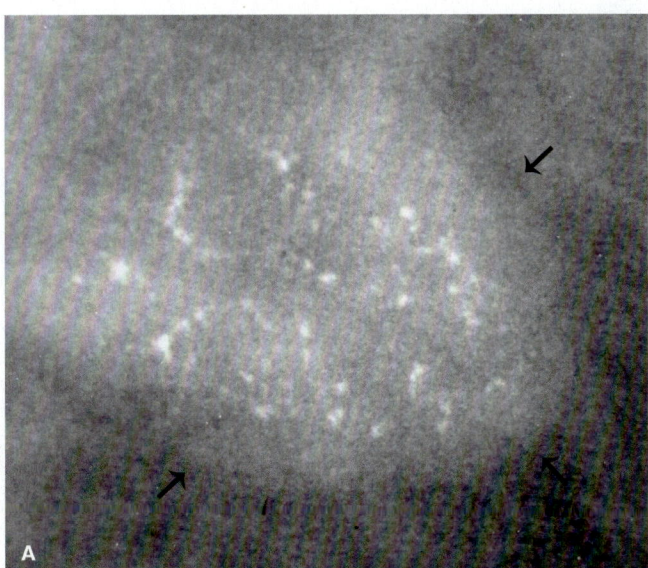
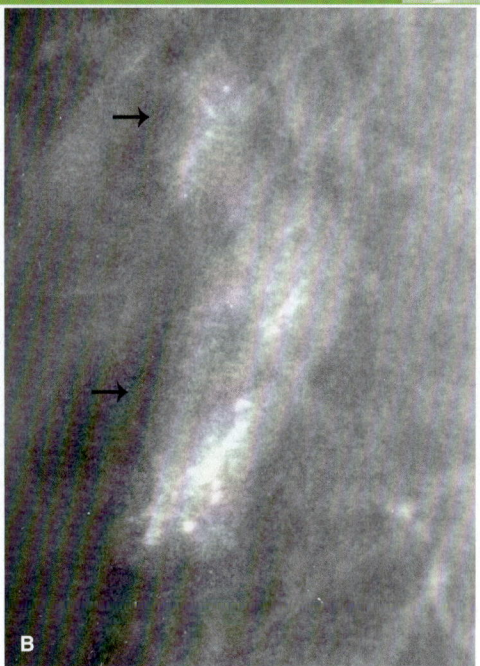

FIG. 7.31 • **Gold deposits. A:** High-density particles in an axillary lymph node *(arrows)* simulate calcifications. This is gold in a patient with rheumatoid arthritis. **B:** Different patient. High-density particles in two axillary lymph nodes *(arrows)*. This is gold in a patient who received gold treatments for rheumatoid arthritis. Gold is typically seen as high-density lace-like particles involving all otherwise morphologically normal intramammary lymph nodes and those in the axillae. (From Cardeñosa G. *Breast Imaging [The Core Curriculum Series]*. Philadelphia, PA: Lippincott Williams & Wilkins; 2003.)

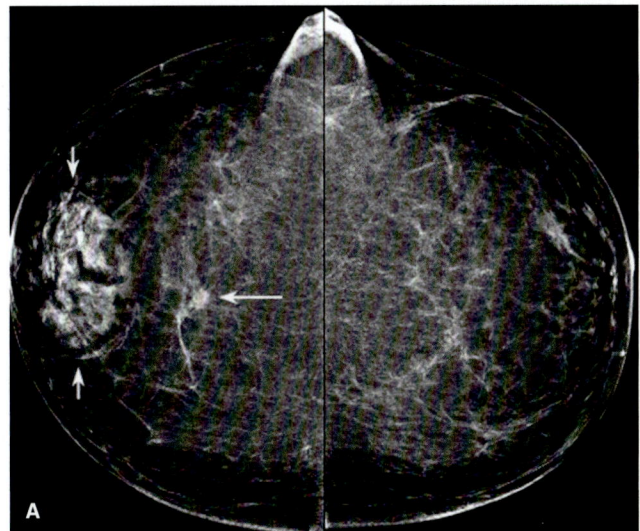
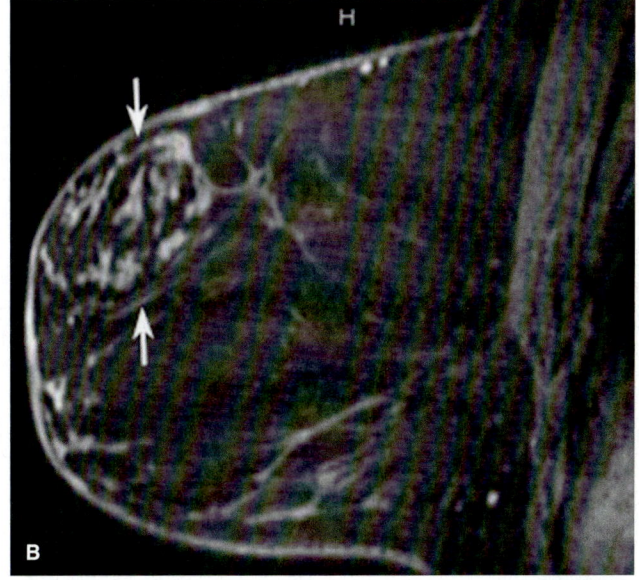
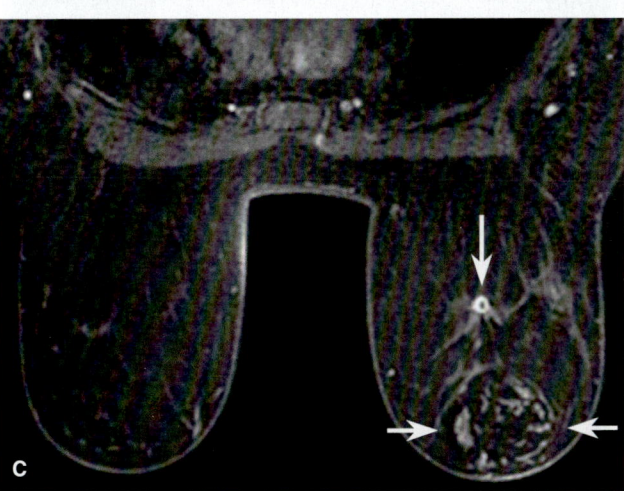

FIG. 7.32 • **Fibroadenolipoma and invasive ductal carcinoma. A:** CC views from a screening study. A mixed-density mass *(short arrows)* is imaged in the right subareolar area. Don't be mesmerized by the obviously benign finding, force your brain to focus away from the benign mass in search of potential cancers. A round mass *(long arrow)* is present approximately 1.5 cm posterior to the fibroadenolipoma. On spot compressions (not shown) it is characterized by spiculated margins; an invasive ductal carcinoma is diagnosed on an ultrasound-guided core biopsy (not shown). **B:** MRI, sagittal T2-weighted fat-suppressed image. The fat signal in the FAL *(arrows)* is suppressed, and the glandular tissue demonstrates intermediate T2 signal. **C:** MRI, axial T1-weighted image post-contrast. A round, rim-enhancing mass *(long arrow)* with circumscribed margins is seen in the central aspect of the right breast correlating with the mass seen mammographically and the site of the patient's known invasive ductal carcinoma. The fibroadenolipoma *(short arrows)* is noted in the right subareolar area. The glandular elements in the FAL are characterized by slow to medium washin and persistent-delayed kinetic curves.

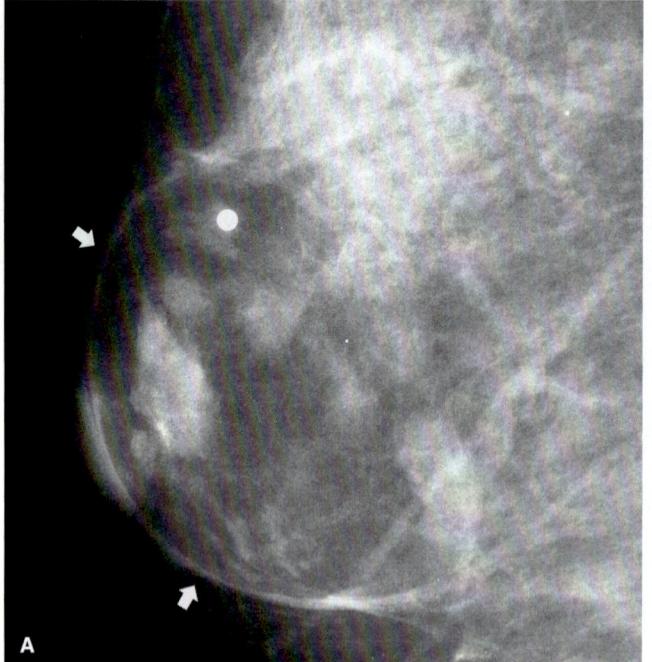
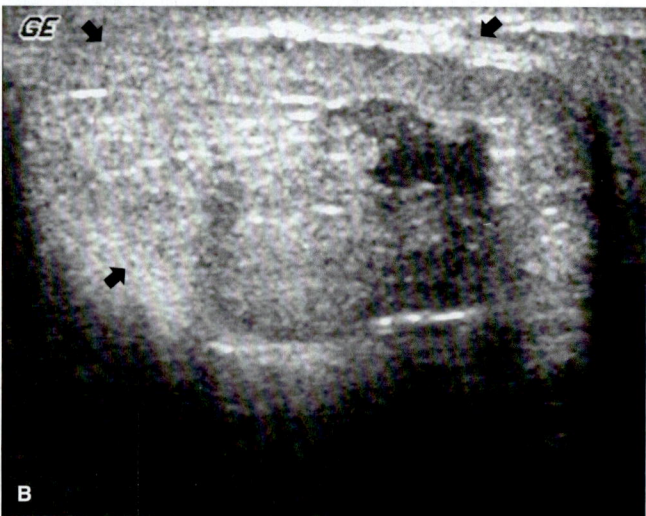

FIG. 7.33 • **Fibroadenolipoma. A:** Photographically coned view of the anterior aspect of the right breast in a patient who presents describing a "lump." A metallic BB denotes the location of the "lump." A fat containing mass is imaged mammographically. Predominantly fatty tissue with some islands of glandular tissue surrounded by a fibrous pseudocapsule *(arrows)* is imaged correlating to the site of the palpable finding. The benign etiology of the finding is made based on the mammographic finding. BI-RADS 2: Benign finding. **B:** An oval hyperechoic mass *(arrows)* with areas of hypoechogenicity is seen on ultrasound correlating to the palpable and mammographically apparent mass. (From Cardeñosa G. *Breast Imaging [The Core Curriculum Series]*. Philadelphia, PA: Lippincott Williams & Wilkins; 2003.)

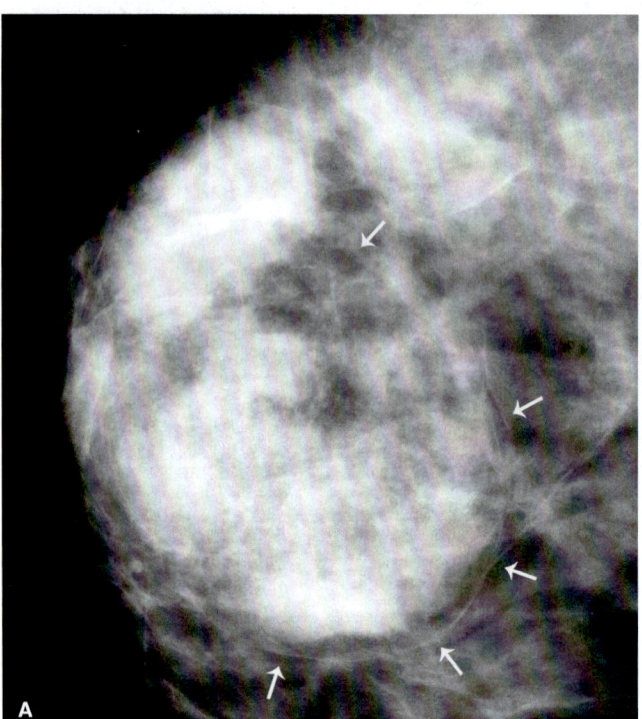
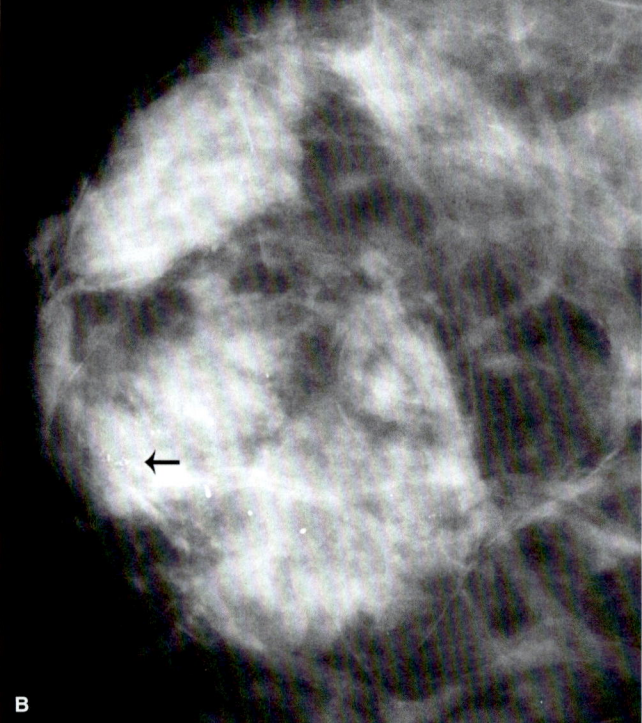

FIG. 7.34 • **Fibroadenolipoma with developing DCIS. A:** Photographically coned view of the anterior aspect of the right breast in a 64-year-old woman who is asymptomatic. A mixed-density mass *(arrows)* with predominantly dense glandular but some intermingled fatty tissue is noted consistent with a hamartoma or FAL. BI-RADS 2: Benign finding. **B:** Subsequent screening mammogram demonstrates calcifications *(arrow)* developing in the FAL. BI-RADS 0: Need additional imaging evaluation. Magnification views are indicated. **C:** Spot compression magnification views (only one projection is shown) demonstrate grouped fine linear calcifications *(arrow)*. BI-RADS 4C: Suspicious abnormality, biopsy is indicated. A stereotactically guided biopsy is done. DCIS, high nuclear grade with central necrosis is diagnosed on the cores. The tissue in FALs is no different than tissue elsewhere in the breasts; it needs to be evaluated as meticulously as glandular tissue elsewhere in the breasts. (From Cardeñosa G. *Breast Imaging [The Core Curriculum Series]*. Philadelphia, PA: Lippincott Williams & Wilkins; 2003.)

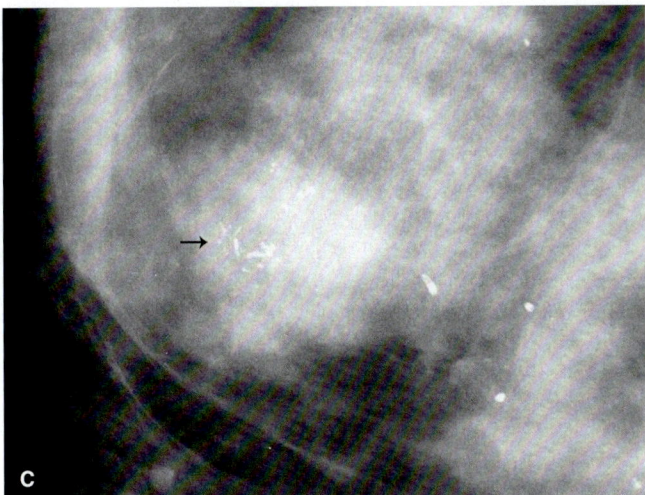

FIG. 7.34 • *(continued)*

a heterogeneous echotexture with admixed areas of hypo- and hyperechogenicity; gentle mass effect may be seen on the surrounding tissue (Fig. 7.33B). On MRI, fatty and glandular elements are isolated within the breast by a thin "pseudocapsule" (Fig. 7.32B). Progressive enhancement of the glandular tissue may be seen on the dynamic sequence (Fig. 7.32C).

Fat Necrosis

Trauma or surgery resulting in the release of fatty substances in the stroma of the breast can lead to an inflammatory response commonly characterized, in the acute setting, by an irregular mass with fatty tissue centrally, spiculated margins and architectural distortion; skin thickening and retraction may be present (Fig. 7.35). Alternatively, a round or oval mass with indistinct margins (Fig. 7.36A), an irregular

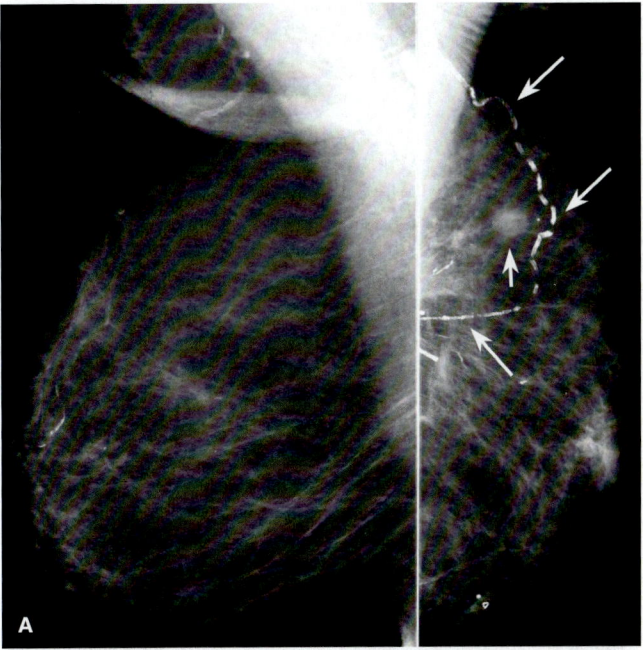

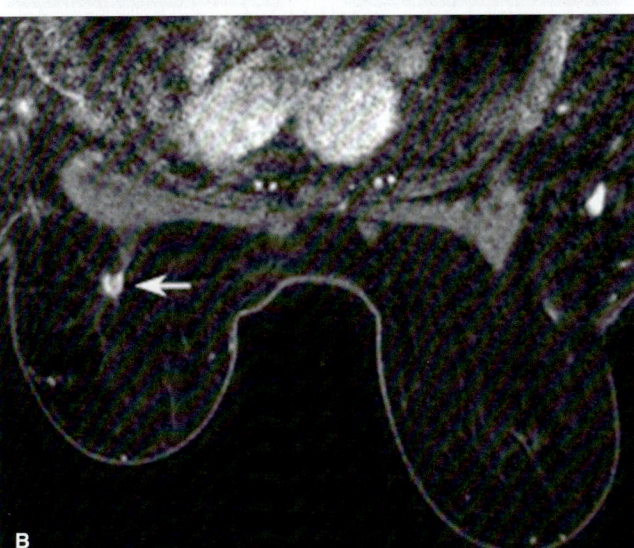

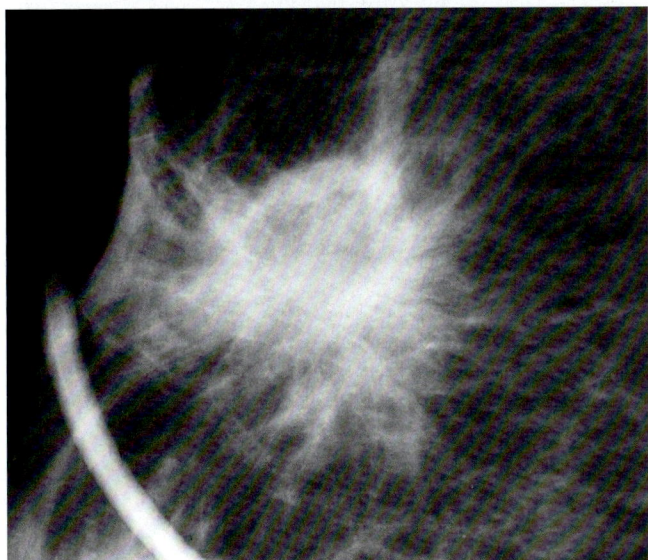

FIG. 7.35 • **Fat necrosis.** Spot tangential view done at a lumpectomy site demonstrates a mixed-density mass, with central lucency, indistinct, and spiculated margins associated with skin thickening and retraction. BI-RADS 2: Benign finding.

FIG. 7.36 • **Fat necrosis. A:** MLO views in a 76-year-old patient with a history of left breast cancer treated with lumpectomy and radiation therapy 12 years ago. The left breast is smaller with distortion posteriorly at the lumpectomy site (metallic clip is seen at edge of image) and progressive asymmetrical calcification *(long arrows)* of the arteries likely a radiation therapy effect. A new round mass *(short arrow)* with indistinct margins is confirmed on spot compression views (not shown) in the superior aspect of the left breast. No internal fatty component is apparent mammographically. **B:** MRI, T1 axial postcontrast image. Oval mass *(arrow)* with peripheral enhancement characterized by rapid washin and washout type kinetic curves corresponding to the mass seen mammographically. Asymmetric breast size is again apparent with the left breast smaller. A homogeneously enhancing lymph node with smooth margins is noted in the right axilla. **C:** MRI, sagittal T2-weighted fat-suppressed image of the left breast. A mass with a low T2 signal consistent with a fat *(arrow)* is imaged at the site of the enhancing mass. Fat necrosis is confirmed on core biopsy. Edematous changes along the pectoral fascia are related to the prior lumpectomy and radiation therapy.

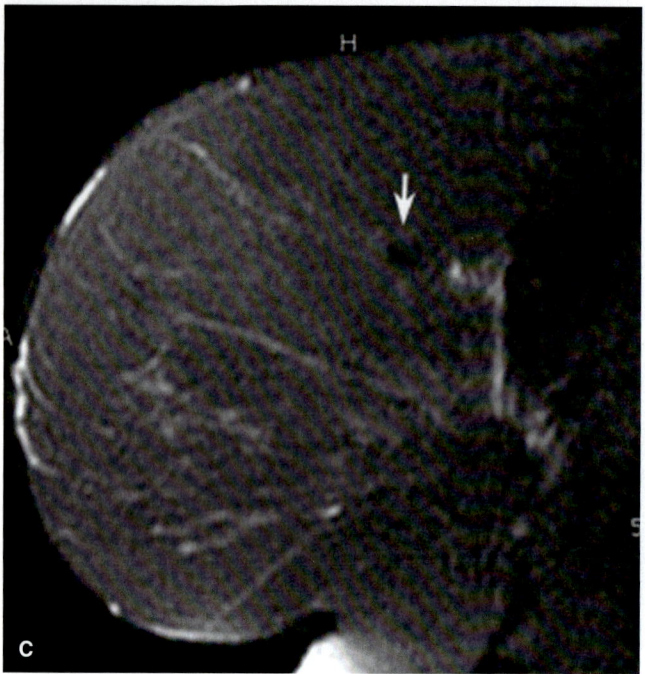

FIG. 7.36 • (continued)

mass with spiculated margins (Fig. 7.37A), a mixed-density mass with indistinct margins, or an irregular area of density (Fig. 7.38A) may be seen. As the inflammatory response subsides, the mammographic and ultrasound features of the lesion usually evolve. In some women, the mixed-density mass with spiculated margins becomes less dense and a fatty center develops; as the ill-defined soft tissue component resolves, a smooth thin walled oil cyst may be all that remains. The progression from dense, mass with spiculated margins to oil cyst is appreciated as films are viewed sequentially (Fig. 7.38B, C). In the intermediate stages, densities or nodules may be seen in the developing oil cyst (Fig. 7.38B, C). As the lesion continues to evolve, dystrophic-type calcifications can develop (Fig. 7.39); however, early in their formation, the calcifications can be linear with irregular margins and pleomorphism indistinguishable from the microcalcifications associated with comedo necrosis in ductal carcinoma in situ (DCIS) (see Figs. 6.43A and 6.46C, D). In other women, fat necrosis resolves completely, with no residual abnormality seen on subsequent studies (22). Less common appearances for fat necrosis include developing parenchymal asymmetry (Fig. 7.40A) or trabecular thickening, forming a fine reticular pattern (Fig. 7.40B).

Soo et al. (23) describe a wide range of ultrasound patterns for fat necrosis. In their experience, a complex mass with echogenic bands that may shift in position as the patient is moved is strongly suggestive of fat necrosis. They also found masses with echogenic mural nodules (Fig. 7.41B) that evolve with time, solid-appearing masses, and anechoic

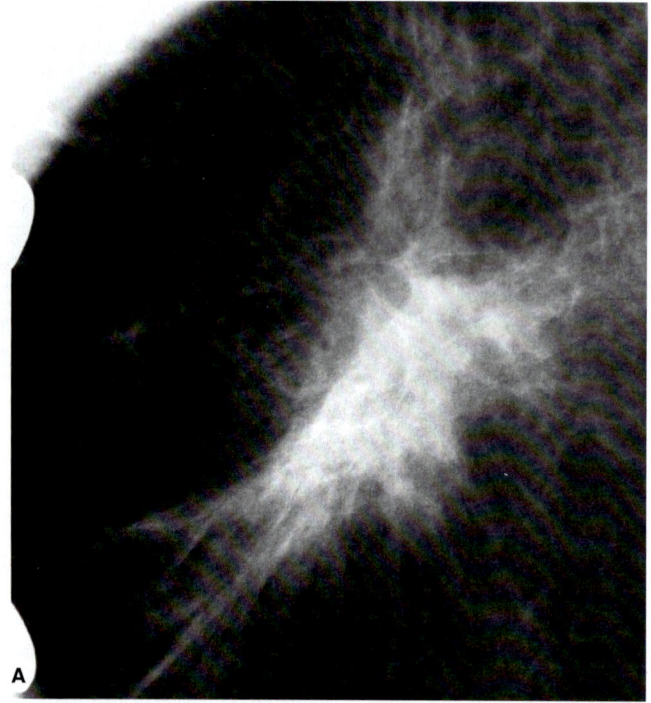

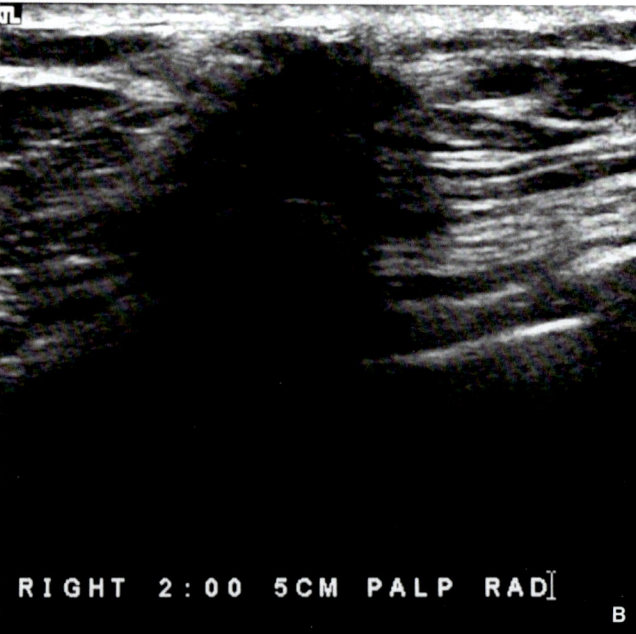

FIG. 7.37 • **Fat necrosis. A:** Spot compression view done to evaluate a screen-detected abnormality. An irregular mass with spiculated margins and distortion is confirmed on the spots (only one projection is shown). **B:** A vertically oriented mass with angular margins and intense shadowing is imaged in the upper inner quadrant of the right breast, zone B corresponding to the mammographic finding. On questioning, the patient recalls having had a fall one year ago with bruising of her right breast. The correlation with the clinical history is critical because otherwise this lesion requires biopsy. It is our contention that the correlation is best established by the breast imager. BI-RADS 2: Benign finding. The mammographic finding has resolved on follow up screening studies.

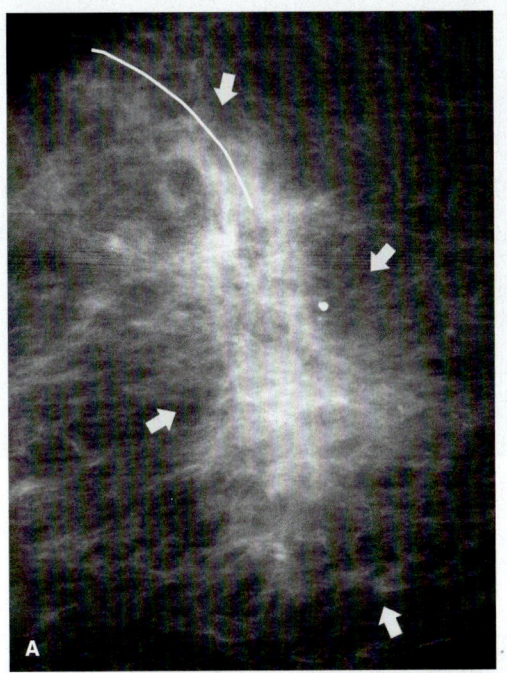
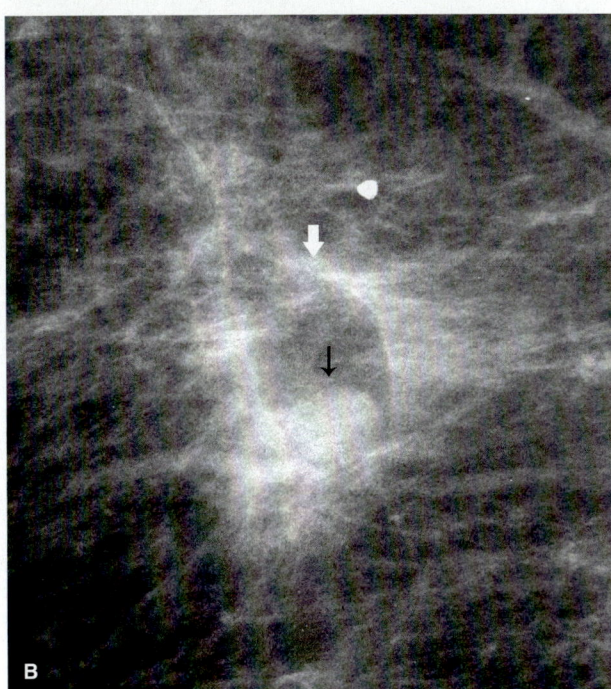
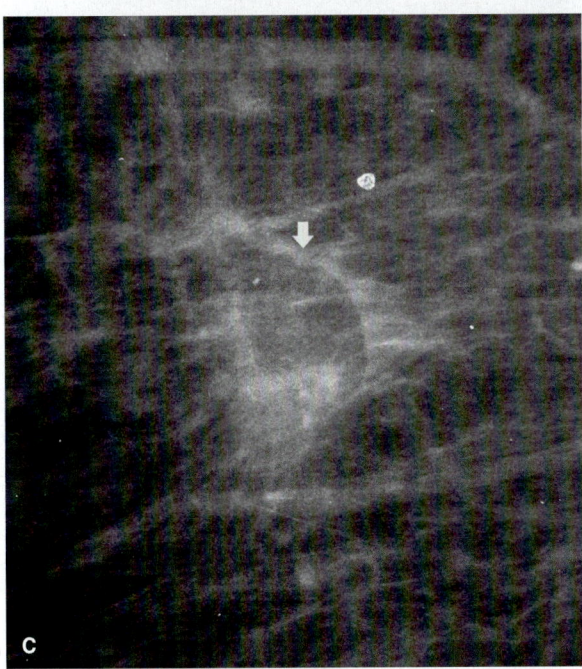

FIG. 7.38 • **Fat necrosis. A:** Photographically coned down view of the left breast demonstrating an ill-defined mixed-density mass *(arrows)* correlating to a prior excisional biopsy site. **B:** Three months later. The mass *(white arrow)* is getting smaller and the central fatty component is increasing. A soft tissue component *(black arrow)* is apparent in the oil cyst. **C:** Four years later. The soft tissue component continues to decrease with only a small amount of residual soft tissue density remaining surrounding the oil cyst. Intracystic nodule is also almost completely resolved. BI-RADS 2: Benign finding. (From Cardeñosa G. *Breast Imaging [The Core Curriculum Series]*. Philadelphia, PA: Lippincott Williams & Wilkins; 2003.)

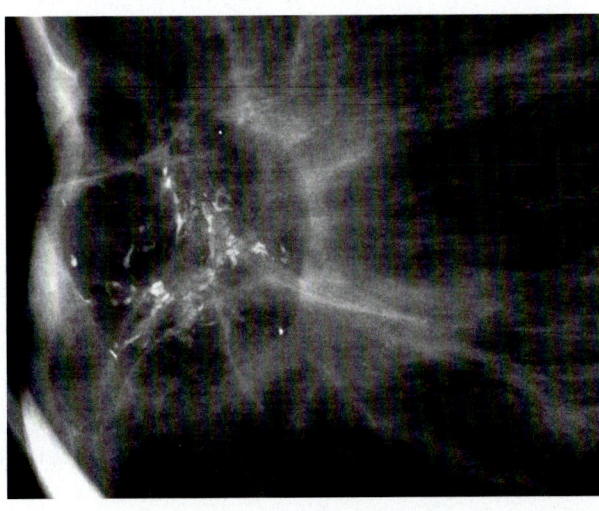

FIG. 7.39 • **Fat necrosis.** Spot compression view demonstrates a mixed-density mass with indistinct and spiculated margins as well as dense, course dystrophic-type calcifications. Localized skin thickening and retraction are also apparent. BI-RADS 2: Benign finding.

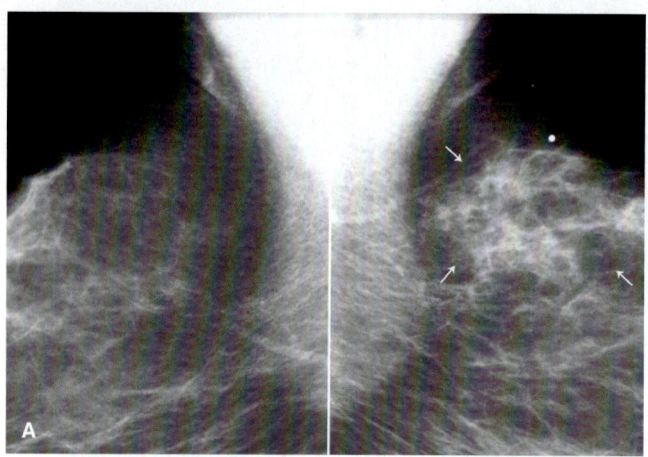
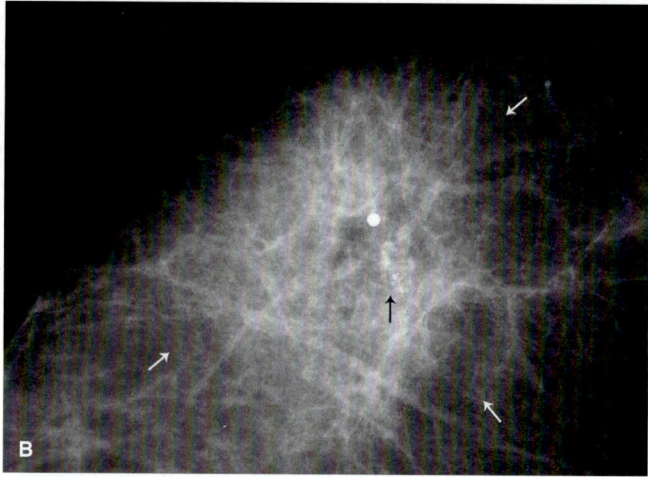

FIG. 7.40 • **Fat necrosis. A:** Palpable area (metallic BB) of parenchymal asymmetry *(arrows)* developing at the site of chest wall trauma. Ultrasound (not shown) demonstrates disruption of normal tissue architecture with diffuse hyperechogenicity and associated small cystic spaces. **B:** Palpable area (metallic BB) of parenchymal asymmetry and prominence of the trabecular markings *(white arrows)* developing at a site of trauma. Some amorphous calcifications are present in this area *(black arrow)*. (From Cardeñosa G. *Breast Imaging [The Core Curriculum Series]*. Philadelphia, PA: Lippincott Williams & Wilkins; 2003.)

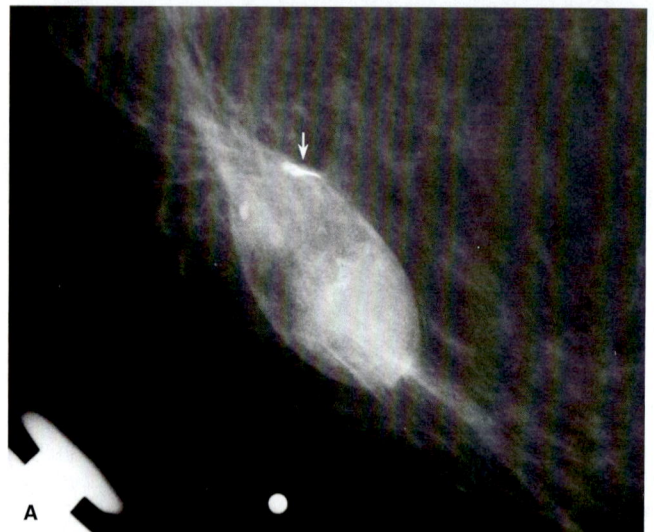
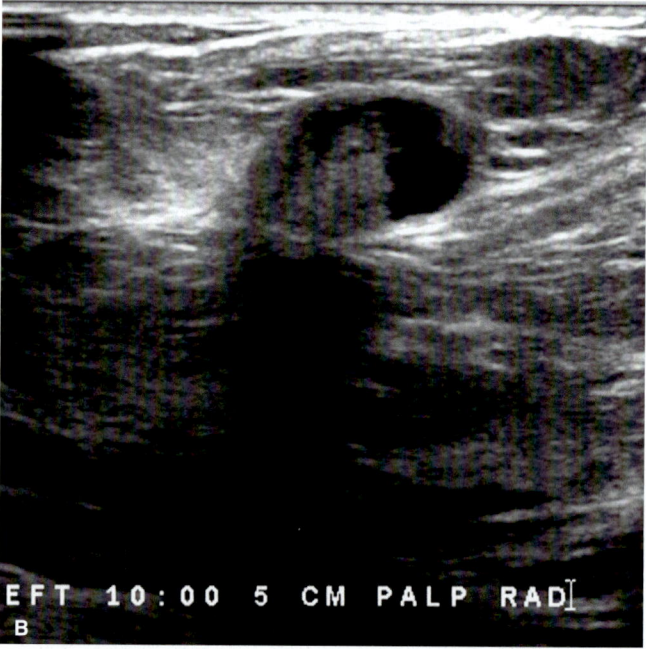
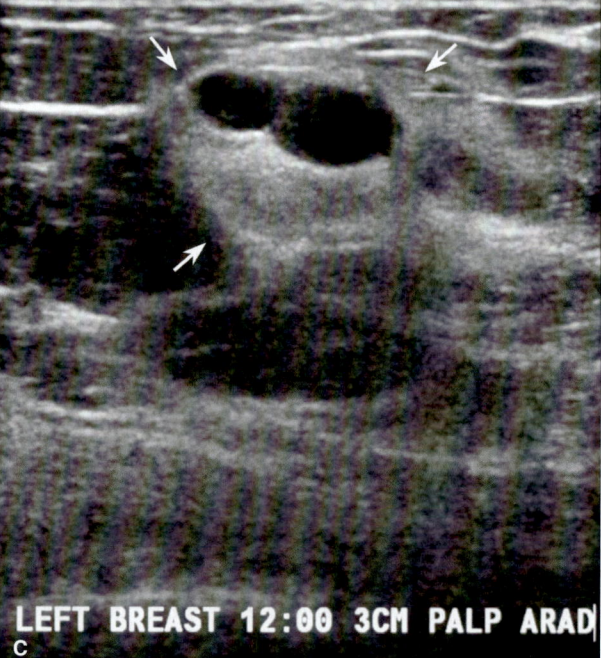

FIG. 7.41 • **Fat necrosis. A:** Spot tangential view done at the site of a "lump" described by the patient in her right breast. Oval, mixed-density or fat containing mass with circumscribed and indistinct margins as well as associated dystrophic calcifications *(arrow)* corresponding to the "lump" described by the patient. The metallic BB is used to denote the site of the "lump." The mass developed at a site of prior trauma. Given the history of trauma, and a correlating mixed-density mass mammographically, no further evaluation or short-interval follow-up is indicated. BI-RADS 2: Benign finding. **B:** Ultrasound. An oval complex cystic and solid mass with mixed shadowing and posterior acoustic enhancement is imaged correlating to the palpable and mammographic finding. **C:** Ultrasound, different patient. A hyperechoic mass *(arrows)* with internal cystic changes and indistinct margins is imaged correlating to the clinical and mammographic finding. Note the disruption of normal tissue planes. Complete resolution of this finding is noted a year later on the screening mammogram.

masses with posterior acoustic enhancement or shadowing (Fig. 7.37B) as manifestations of fat necrosis on ultrasound. In our experience, one of the more common ultrasound features of fat necrosis is an area of hyperechogenicity that may be well- to ill-defined, associated with cystic spaces or small round or oval areas of hypoechogenicity (Fig. 7.41C; also see Fig. 4.36) commonly disrupting tissue planes.

The appearance of fat necrosis on MRI is variable and, as seen with mammography and ultrasound, fat necrosis can mimic breast cancer on MRI (24). Low signal is noted on fat-suppressed T1 and T2 images (Figs. 7.36C and 7.42C) correlating with the fatty component seen mammographically, commonly in a subcutaneous location. The edges of these lesions may demonstrate smooth rim enhancement in the predominantly cystic lesions; however, the rim may be thickened, spiculated, or indistinct. If there is no lipid component, these lesions can simulate cancers morphologically with kinetic curves that can range from slow to rapid initial washin and progressive, plateau, and rapid washout delayed kinetics (Figs. 7.36B and 7.42B).

A history of trauma or surgery and the appearance of the lesion on sequential mammograms provide the assurance needed to characterize these lesions as benign in many patients. Ultrasound is usually not needed for the diagnosis. It is critical to recognize that following biopsy or trauma, mammographic findings peak approximately 4 to 6 months following the event, after which the findings stabilize or slowly resolve as described. Rarely, fat necrosis can develop and increase in size and density years after a biopsy or trauma. Since the mammographic, ultrasound (Fig. 7.43A, B), and MRI (Figs. 7.36B and 7.42B) features of fat necrosis overlap those of cancer, biopsy is indicated in those patients without a history of surgery or trauma correlated to the site of the imaging findings or in those in whom it develops years after the surgery with no apparent cause.

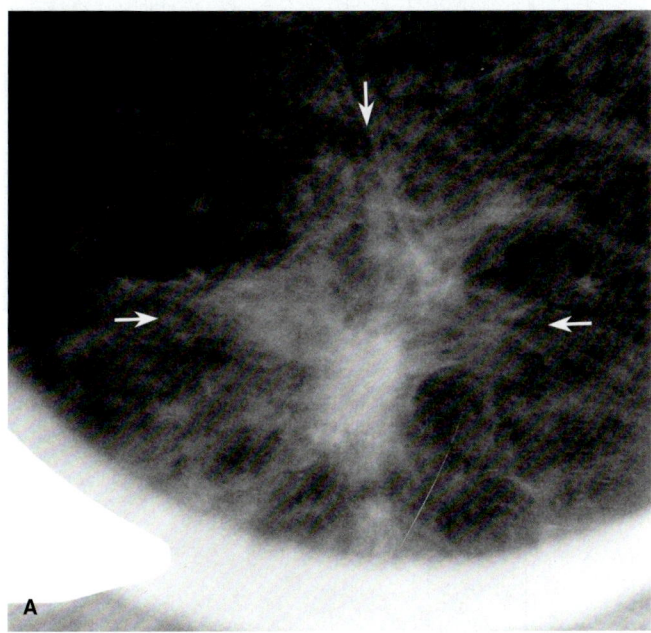

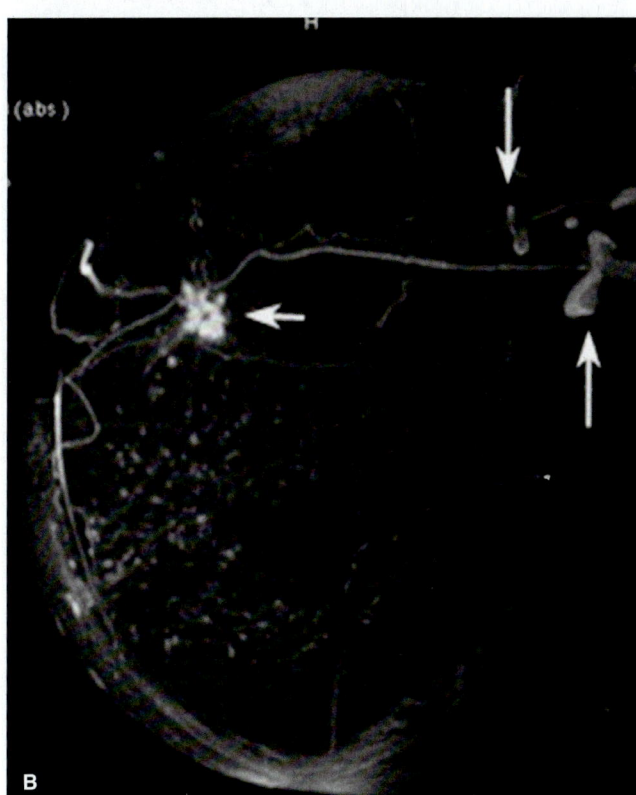

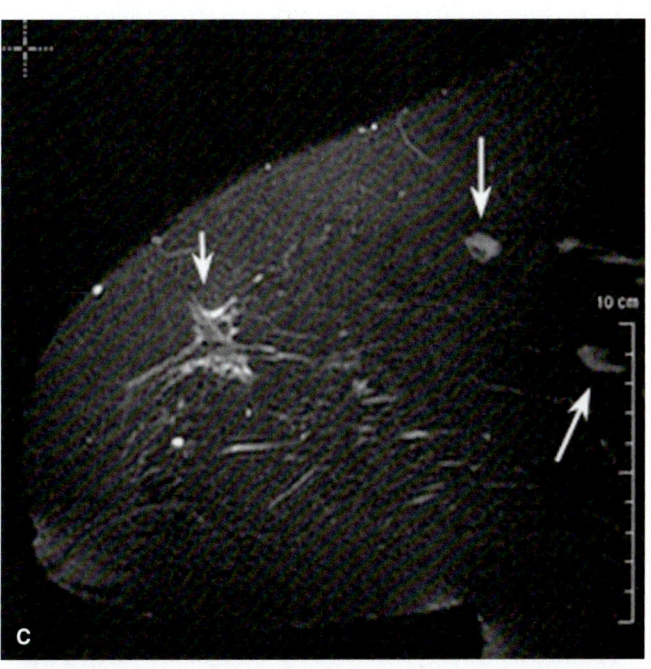

FIG. 7.42 • **Fat necrosis. A:** Spot compression view, right breast. An irregular mass with spiculated margins and associated distortion *(arrows)* is confirmed on the spot compression views (only one projection is shown). No correlative abnormality is identified on ultrasound at the expected location of the mammographic finding. **B:** MRI, sagittal maximum intensity projection image. An irregular mass *(short arrow)* with spiculated margins, distortion, and heterogeneous enhancement characterized by rapid washin and washout kinetic curves corresponding to the mass seen mammographically. Incidentally noted are multiple foci of nonspecific enhancement randomly scattered in the parenchyma and several enhancing lymph nodes *(long arrows)* with retained fatty hila. **C:** MRI, sagittal T2 fat-suppressed image of the right breast. Distortion with central low T2 signal *(short arrow)*, suggestive of fat internally and high T2 signal spiculations is imaged corresponding to the enhancing mass and mammographic finding. Fat necrosis is diagnosed following an MRI-guided biopsy. Note masses *(long arrows)* with high T2 signal and fat-suppressed hila consistent with lymph nodes.

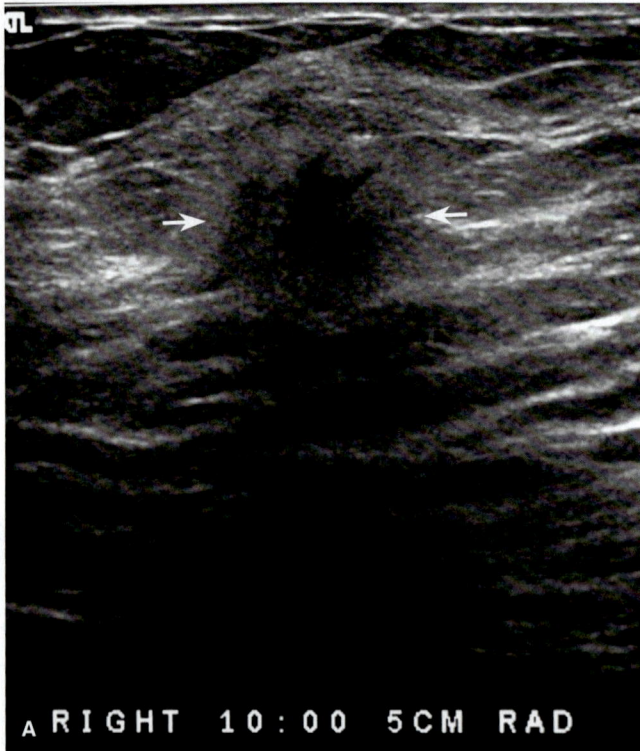
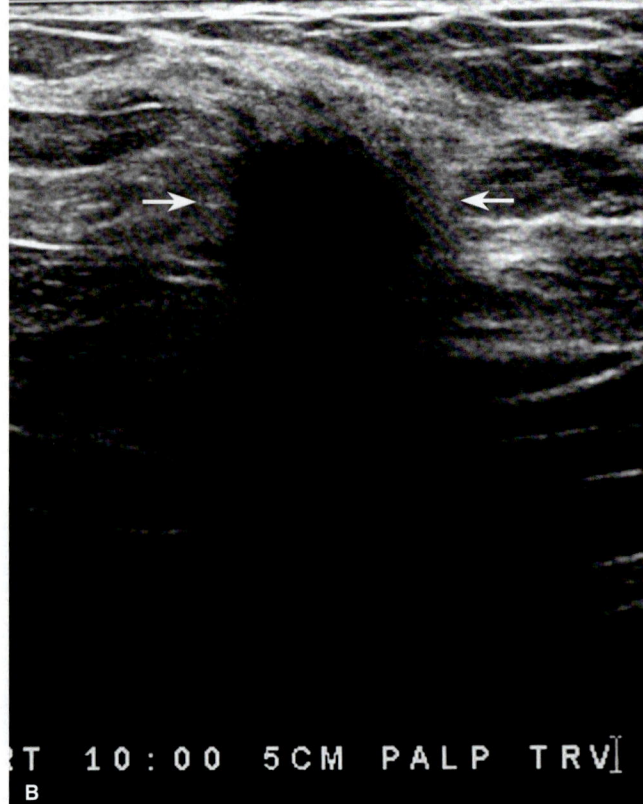
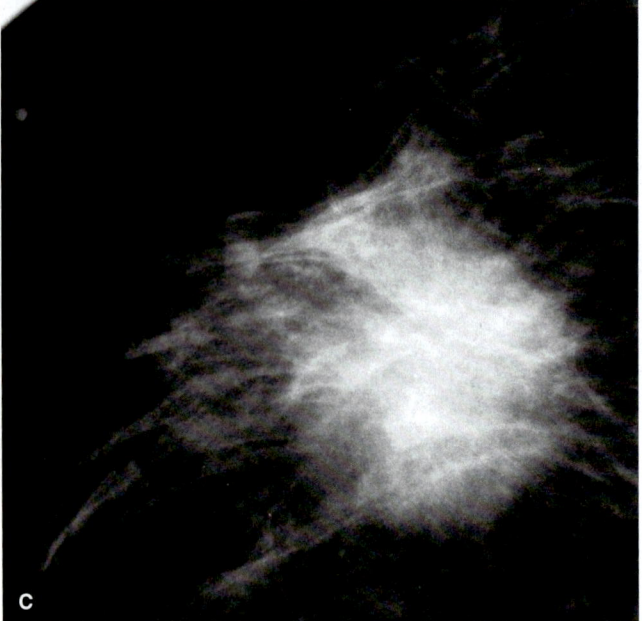

FIG. 7.43 • **Fat necrosis. A:** Ultrasound. Mass *(arrows)* with indistinct and spiculated margins and some shadowing corresponding to a new mass detected mammographically. Fat necrosis is diagnosed following an ultrasound-guided core biopsy. **B:** Ultrasound. One year later. A mass *(arrows)* with angular and spiculated margins, an echogenic rim, and intense shadowing is imaged at the site of the prior biopsy; it is now palpable. **C:** Spot tangential compression view done at the site of the "lump" described by the patient corresponding to the previously biopsied mass shown in parts **A** and **B**. Dense, round mass with indistinct and spiculated margins is imaged corresponding to the site of the palpable finding. The lesion has stabilized on subsequent mammograms.

Histologically, fat necrosis is characterized by acute changes that evolve with time. Initially, fat cell disruption and hemorrhage is followed by hemosiderin deposition, infiltration by variable numbers of histiocytes, plasma cells, and lymphocytes. Chronic, progressive fibrosis develops peripherally surrounding the necrotic fat cells and calcifications (11,12).

WATER DENSITY MASSES

These masses contain no fat. In addition to the shape and marginal features of these masses, consider their density. The density can be described as low, equal to, or increased, compared with the density of an equal volume of breast tissue. Differential considerations for the more common benign and malignant round or oval masses with circumscribed to indistinct margins are provided in Table 7.8. The differential for some of the more common benign and malignant masses with spiculated margins is provided in Table 7.9. Depending on history, clinical presentation, palpable findings, imaging features (mammography and ultrasound), the lists can be more appropriately focused to a given patient and the clinical and imaging features of the mass. The age of a patient is a particularly critical factor when considering an appropriate differential for an individual patient: a developing, solid

Table 7.8 DIFFERENTIAL: ROUND, OVAL (EXPANSILE) WATER DENSITY MASSES

Benign	Malignant
Cyst	Infiltrating ductal carcinoma (NOS)
Sebaceous cyst	
Epidermal inclusion cyst	Mucinous carcinoma
Fibroadenoma	Papillary carcinoma
Complex fibroadenoma	Medullary carcinoma
Tubular adenomas	DCIS
Lactational adenoma	Metastatic disease
Papillomas (solitary, multiple)	Lymphoma
Reactive lymph nodes	
Galactocele	
Postop/traumatic fluid collections	
Abscess	
Phyllodes	
Fat necrosis	
Pseudoangiomatous stromal hyperplasia	
Focal fibrosis	
Sclerosing adenosis	
Granular cell tumor	
Epidermoid inclusion cyst (post reduction)	
Vascular lesions	

mass in a postmenopausal patient raises differential considerations that are different from the considerations for a developing solid mass in a woman in her 30s or early 40s.

CYSTIC BREAST MASSES

Simple and "Complicated" Cysts

Cysts are common breast lesions occurring in women of all ages (13). There is some predilection for the perimenopausal years with a smaller peak of incidence in women in their late 70s and 80s. If women do not take hormone replacement therapy following menopause, cysts usually decrease in size and most resolve spontaneously. Clinically, patients with cysts present with one or several "lumps," focal tenderness,

Table 7.9 DIFFERENTIAL: WATER DENSITY MASSES WITH SPICULATED MARGINS

Benign	Malignant
Fat necrosis (postbiopsy or trauma)	Invasive ductal carcinoma (NOS)
Mastitis	Tubular carcinoma
Focal fibrosis	Invasive lobular carcinoma
Sclerosing adenosis	DCIS
Complex sclerosing lesions (radial scar <1 cm)	Metastatic disease to lymph nodes
Granulomatous disease	
Extra-abdominal desmoid (fibromatosis)	
Granular cell tumor	

or rarely nipple discharge. When the cyst is inflamed, erythema may be present overlying the site of the "lump." Cysts are hormonally responsive and as such fluctuate in size and associated tenderness cyclically, becoming more apparent to the patient in the premenstrual phase of the cycle. In many women, cysts are asymptomatic with a mass or multiple masses detected on screening mammography and characterized with ultrasound as cystic.

Cyst fluid contains a variety of electrolytes, proteins, and hormones (25). On the basis of electrolyte content and cell lining, cysts can be separated into two primary groups. Epithelial-lined cysts are characterized by fluid high in sodium and low in potassium content much like the composition of serum. It has been suggested that these cysts do not often recur following aspiration. Cysts lined with cells demonstrating apocrine metaplasia are characterized by fluid that is low in sodium and high in potassium content. This electrolyte content suggests a more active cellular process leading to the concentration of potassium. It may be that these cysts recur following aspiration more commonly than the epithelial-lined cysts (11,25).

Cysts are variable in their mammographic appearance (13). They can occur singularly (Fig. 7.44A) or as multiple uni- or bilateral masses (Fig. 7.45A) of varying sizes. Commonly, cysts demonstrate a density that can be characterized as being low- to equal (isodense); however, they are sometimes high in density, and although many demonstrate circumscribed margins, some may have obscured (Fig. 7.45A) or indistinct margins. Spiculation or distortion is rare. Calcifications can develop in the wall of cysts (see Fig. 6.26A) or within cysts (milk of calcium). Unless associated with milk of calcium (see Fig. 6.31), most cysts are indistinguishable from other water density masses, including malignancies, and as such, ultrasound is indicated for further evaluation.

On ultrasound, simple cysts are anechoic masses with circumscribed margins, posterior acoustic enhancement, and thin-edge shadows (Figs. 7.44B and 7.45B; also see Fig. 4.23) (13). Reverberation artifact may be seen parallel to the anterior wall of a cyst (see Fig. 4.24). With small cysts deep in the breast, posterior acoustic enhancement may not be seen. The term "complicated" cyst is advocated when describing uncommon ultrasound features of cysts, including the presence of internal echoes that may whorl as gain is increased (e.g., gurgling cysts) (Fig. 7.46; also see Fig. 4.26) or a solid-appearing component (artifact) abruptly interfacing with an anechoic component ("ying-yang" sign) (Fig. 7.46C). To us, these represent variants of simple cysts, and to suggest they are "complicated" is misleading. Aspiration of these "complicated" cysts typically yields fluid that is indistinguishable from that aspirated from "simple" cysts; hemorrhagic cysts are rare. When pus is obtained, it is more appropriate to label the mass as an abscess.

Cysts are variably sized, with a homogeneously high T2 signal, circumscribed margins, and no internal enhancement on MRI. A thin smooth rim of enhancement may be apparent presumably when there is some associated inflammation (Fig. 7.44C, D; also see Fig. 5.17). Fluid–fluid levels may be seen. They are often scattered bilaterally and in some patients intermingled with nonspecific foci of enhancement.

Among our clinical colleagues, the traditional approach to women presenting with a palpable mass has been palpation-guided aspiration. If no fluid is obtained, a mammogram may or may not be ordered and excisional biopsy may be recommended. With the availability of modern ultrasound units, we should challenge this approach. As a starting point, cysts are benign and often multiple and do not need to be aspirated unless the patient is tender or the diagnosis of a cyst is in question on ultrasound. Some clinicians would suggest that patients with a palpable mass want it to go away. This is not the case with most of our

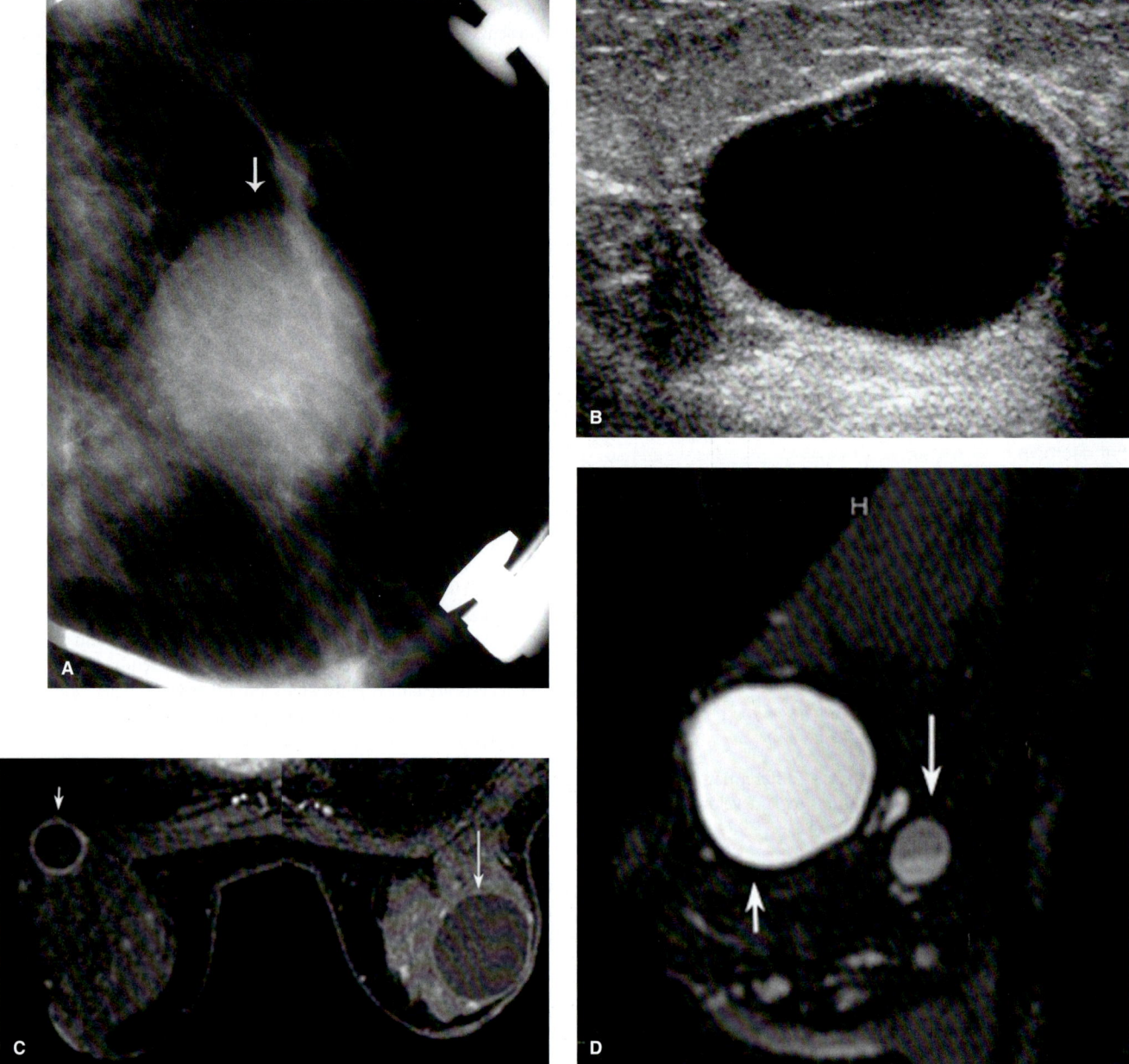

FIG. 7.44 • **Cysts. A:** Spot tangential view done at the site of a "lump" described by the patient. Oval isodense mass with circumscribed margins *(arrow)*. **B:** Ultrasound. Anechoic mass with circumscribed margins and posterior acoustic enhancement. BI-RADS 2: Benign finding. A & B are (From Cardeñosa G. *Breast Imaging [The Core Curriculum Series]*. Philadelphia, PA: Lippincott Williams & Wilkins; 2003.) **C:** MRI, axial T1 postcontrast images, different patient. A rim-enhancing mass with smooth margins and low internal T1 signal and high T2 signal (T2 sequence not shown) is present posterolaterally in the left breast *(short arrow)*; a non-enhancing mass *(long arrow)* with smooth margins, low internal T1 signal, and high T2 signal (see image in part **D**) is also present in the central to lateral aspect of the right breast anteriorly. **D:** MRI, sagittal T2 fat-suppressed image of the right breast. A dominant mass *(short arrow)* with a homogeneously high T2 signal is imaged corresponding to the nonenhancing mass seen on the axial images in the right breast. A second smaller cyst *(long arrow)* with a fluid–fluid level is seen inferior and posterior to the dominant mass. A mass with a high T2 signal is also imaged in the left breast corresponding to the rim-enhancing mass on the axial images (images not shown).

patients. What women want is the reassurance that what they feel is not breast cancer. If this can be done with ultrasound (with the added benefit of evaluating the tissue surrounding the palpable area), aspiration is not needed, particularly since many cysts resolve spontaneously or fluctuate and some recur within days of an aspiration. Second, just because fluid is not obtained during palpation-guided aspiration does not mean the lesion is not a cyst. A thick wall may preclude aspiration. Under ultrasound guidance it is clear that some cysts are pushed away by the advancing needle rather than penetrated. Consequently, the amount of pressure needed to puncture the cyst wall is best judged with imaging guidance. Lastly, attempts to aspirate lesions may limit subsequent mammographic and ultrasound evaluations. It is recommended that mammographic and ultrasound studies be done prior to any interventional procedures.

Evaluation and Imaging Features of Benign Breast Masses

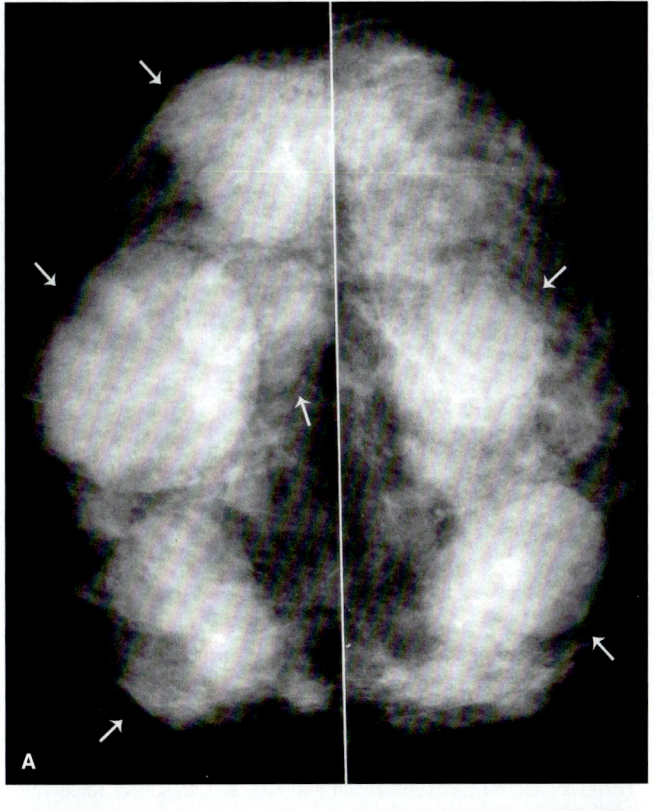
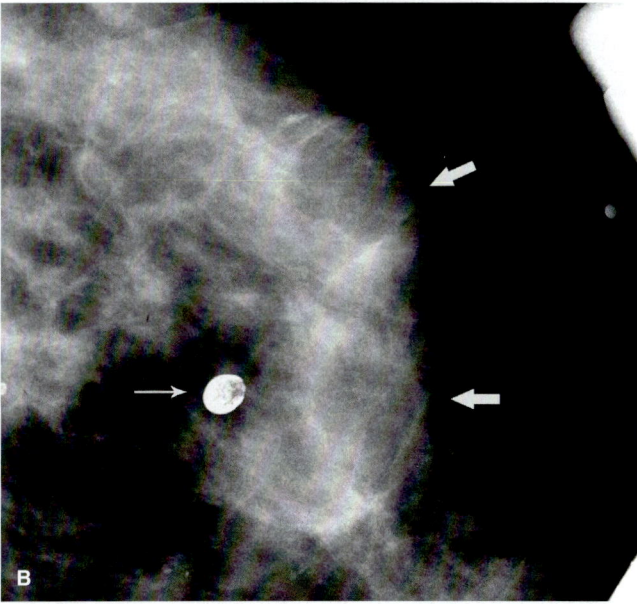
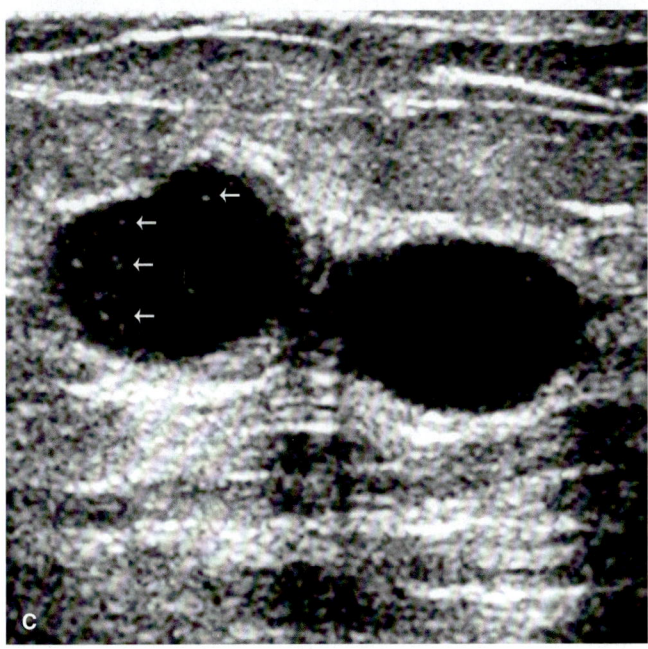

FIG. 7.45 • **Cysts. A:** CC views. Multiple masses *(arrows)* of similar morphology and density are present bilaterally. On ultrasound, multiple cysts are imaged in each breast. BI-RADS 2: Benign finding. **B:** Different patient. Spot tangential view, done at the site of a "lump" described by the patient. Two masses *(thick arrows)* with obscured margins are imaged corresponding to the area of concern to the patient. A lucent centered calcification is also noted *(thin arrow)*. **C:** Ultrasound. Two anechoic masses with posterior acoustic enhancement are imaged corresponding to the palpable mass. A few "floating" echoes are seen in one of the two cysts *(arrows)*. BI-RADS 2: Benign finding. (From Cardeñosa G. *Breast Imaging [The Core Curriculum Series]*. Philadelphia, PA: Lippincott Williams & Wilkins; 2003.)

Clustered Microcysts

With optimal ultrasound equipment and meticulous technique, early cyst development, as acini within a lobule begin to distend, can be seen on ultrasound as a cluster of small anechoic masses separated by thin echogenic septations (Fig. 7.47A,B; also see Fig. 4.25). Posterior acoustic enhancement may be seen (13,26). As the acini continue to distend, they fuse and give rise to larger cysts (Fig. 7.47C). During real-time scanning it is important to evaluate the entire lesion and assure that the septations are all thin. Now comfortable with these ultrasound findings, we are not routinely recommending short-interval follow-up or core biopsy of these areas. However, if there is any question about the correct diagnosis, core biopsy is appropriate (13,27). If a core biopsy is undertaken, these lesions decrease in size and may disappear completely after the first or second pass through the lesion. Histologically, pieces of epithelial and apocrine-lined cysts (apocrine metaplasia) are reported following core biopsy of these areas (Fig. 7.48). Interestingly, on mammography, these lesions may have a predilection for the medial aspect of

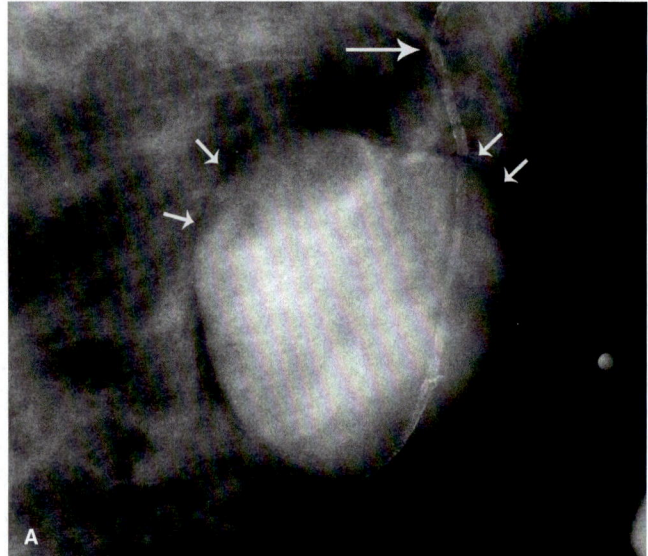
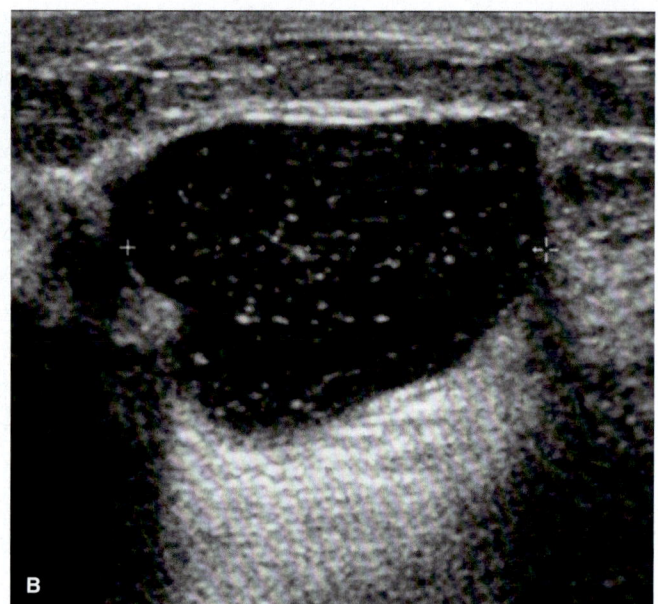
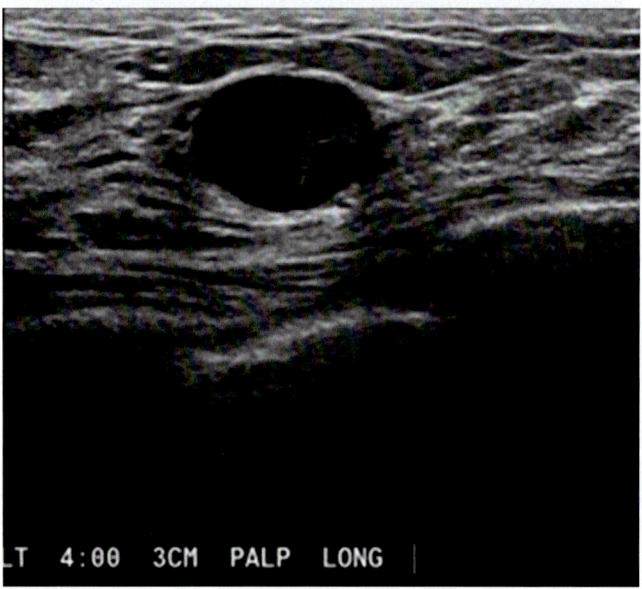

FIG. 7.46 • **Cysts. A:** Spot tangential view, done at the site of a "lump" described by the patient. Oval macrolobulated mass with circumscribed margins and a "halo" *(small arrows)* partially outlining the mass. Incidentally noted is vascular calcification *(large arrow).* **B:** Ultrasound. Mass with circumscribed mass, internal echoes, and posterior acoustic enhancement. During real-time scanning, the internal echoes swirl and shift in position consistent with a cyst ("gurgling"). We do not routinely aspirate this type of cyst unless the patient is symptomatic or another atypical feature is noted. BI-RADS 2: Benign finding. A and B: (From Cardeñosa G. *Breast Imaging [The Core Curriculum Series]*. Philadelphia, PA: Lippincott Williams & Wilkins; 2003.) **C:** Ultrasound, different patient. A mass characterized by an anechoic component and a homogeneous hypoechoic component is imaged. The curvilinear interface between these components is often curved ("ying-yang" sign). In most patients, the internal echoes either dissipate or can be seen going into the needle if the aspiration is watched during real time; no residual solid component is noted post aspiration. If no fluid is obtained or the lesion does not collapse completely, core biopsy is done.

the breast and are often lobulated, low-density masses with circumscribed margins.

Complex Cystic and Solid Masses and Solid Masses with Cystic Spaces

As the heading implies, these are a group of masses that on ultrasound can be characterized as having one of two patterns: predominantly cystic with solid intracystic or mural components or predominantly solid masses with cystic spaces. These masses may be denser than those of simple cysts with margins that may be indistinct on the mammogram. Differential considerations for masses that are predominantly cystic with solid components include a cyst (e.g., the apparent solid component liquefies and is aspirated when aspiration is done), galactocele, abscess, papillary lesions (benign and malignant), fat necrosis, and invasive ductal carcinoma, high nuclear grade with necrosis. The differential for predominantly solid masses with cystic spaces includes postoperative fluid collections, galactocele, abscess, complex fibroadenomas, phyllodes, pseudoangiomatous stromal hyperplasia, papillary lesions, fat necrosis, mucinous carcinomas, invasive ductal carcinomas, high nuclear grade with areas of necrosis, and rarely metastatic disease (melanoma) (13).

Patients with these types of masses require needle biopsy for histological diagnosis (28). In as many as 50% of patients with malignancy, the diagnosis is not reliably established with fluid cytology alone (29–31). In the patients with predominantly cystic masses, our approach is to aspirate as much of the fluid as possible under ultrasound guidance before doing cores of the solid component. If the cystic component of the mass "spills" into the surrounding tissue, as would happen when doing a core without first aspirating, the fluid can generate an aseptic inflammatory reaction that is troublesome to the patient, may take several days to a week or two to resolve, and does not respond well to treatment other than maybe to anti-inflammatory agents. Some authors argue against this approach, suggesting the lesion will no longer be apparent after aspiration. This has not been our experience. If there is a lesion, it is readily apparent following aspiration of the fluid component. Additionally, in the presence of an

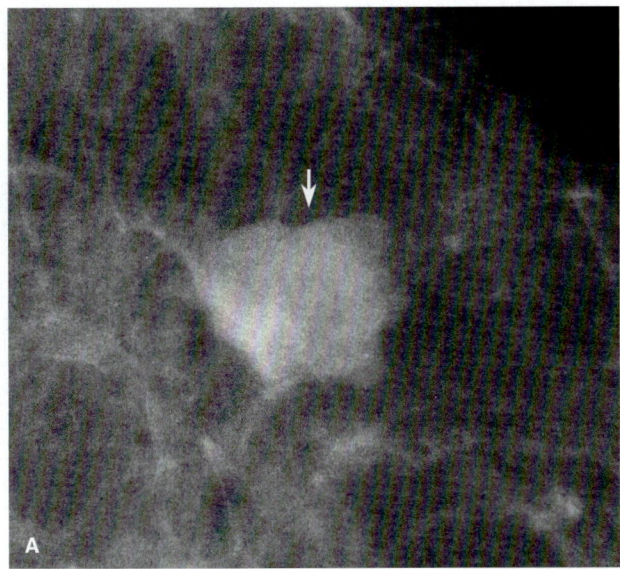
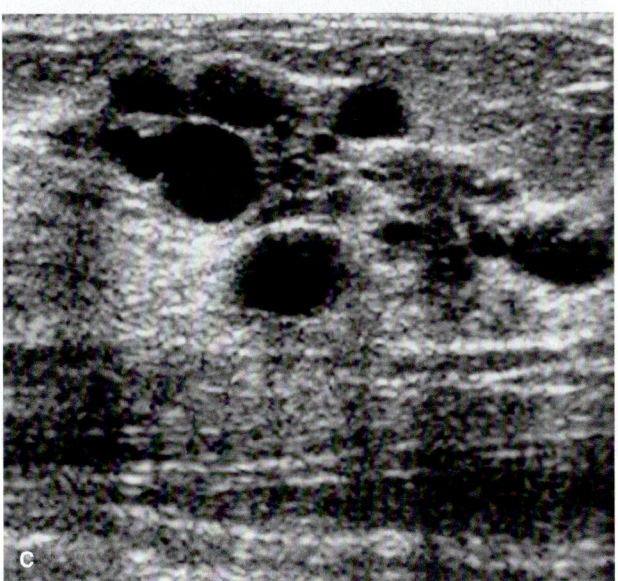
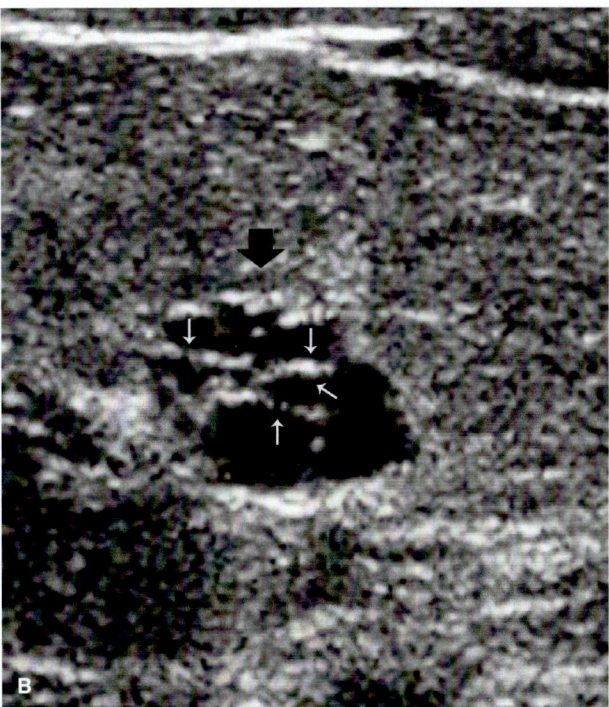

FIG. 7.47 • **Clustered microcysts. A:** Spot compression view of a new, macrolobulated isodense mass *(arrow)* with circumscribed margins. **B:** A cluster of small anechoic round masses *(black arrow)* is imaged on ultrasound. Thin septations *(white arrows)* are seen separating the cysts. It is important that the septations be thin. Adjacent epithelial and apocrine metaplasia-lined cysts are seen histologically. Given our own audit data and experience with the appearance of these lesions, we do not routinely recommend biopsy. If biopsy is undertaken, the lesion decreases or disappears after the first pass that goes through the lesion. **C:** Different patient. As the acini within a lobule continue to distend, individual small, clustered cysts can be imaged associated with a ductal structure centrally. BI-RADS 2: Benign finding. (From Cardeñosa G. *Breast Imaging [The Core Curriculum Series]*. Philadelphia, PA: Lippincott Williams & Wilkins; 2003.)

underlying mass, the fluid re-accumulates rapidly, so the patient can be reevaluated if needed. Since we do the aspiration under real-time ultrasound guidance, in some patients, we can see the seemingly solid components being sucked into the needle. So if the mass collapses completely after aspiration, no biopsy is done. In patients with predominantly solid masses with cystic changes, we do the core biopsy with no aspiration.

ABSCESS

In thinking about abscesses occurring in the breast consider three different patient populations: those presenting during lactation, those with findings limited to the subareolar area, and less commonly, those with peripheral abscesses.

Lactational Abscess

Inflammatory symptoms in women who are breast-feeding are common and typically present in the first 3 months postpartum. The term mastitis is routinely used to encompass subjective presentations of focal inflammation in some patients to more diffuse inflammation

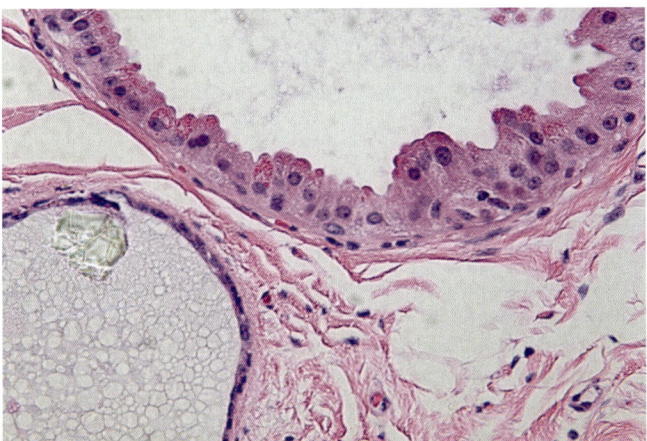

FIG. 7.48 • **Histological section with two adjacent cysts: one with epithelial lining and the other apocrine metaplasia.** The one in the lower left hand aspect of the image demonstrates a flattened epithelial cell lining and a crystal in its lumen. The larger of the two, in the upper aspect of the image, demonstrates lining cells that are cuboidal with apical snouts filled with eosinophilic granules consistent with apocrine metaplasia.

with systemic symptoms and leukocytosis. The reported incidence of lactational mastitis ranges from 3% to 33%, supporting the indiscriminate use of the term mastitis (32). The role of bacterial pathogens and progression to breast abscess formation is unclear; consequently appropriate management and treatment is controversial. Patients are encouraged to continue breast-feeding, and most women are started on antibiotics.

Kvist et al. (32) have reported that women who are breast-feeding have potentially pathogenic bacteria in their breast milk and increasing bacterial counts alone are not a reliable method to establish the need for antibiotic therapy in patients with inflammatory symptoms; many of these women with high bacterial counts are asymptomatic. Although some argue that mastitis should be treated to prevent the eventual formation of an abscess, there is no evidence to support this progression, and patients presenting with an abscess have no history of antecedent or ongoing mastitis.

Patients with inflammatory changes presenting during lactation (mastitis) are managed clinically and not usually imaged. Rarely, when a mass is palpated, imaging may be obtained. When referred for imaging, our evaluation in these patients includes correlative physical examination and ultrasound; mammography is not done routinely. On physical examination, erythema may be noted localized to an area of thickening or overlying a palpable mass; tenderness is elicited on palpation. Lactational abscesses can occur anywhere in the breast. On ultrasound, a complex cystic mass or a "complicated" cyst may be imaged corresponding to the site of the palpable finding (Fig. 7.49); some may be multiloculated (Fig. 7.50). There may be skin thickening and the tissue surrounding the mass may demonstrate increased echogenicity and loss of normal soft tissue planes. Aspiration yields variably thickened, purulent fluid that is submitted for culture and sensitivity. *Staphylococcus aureus* is a common causative agent.

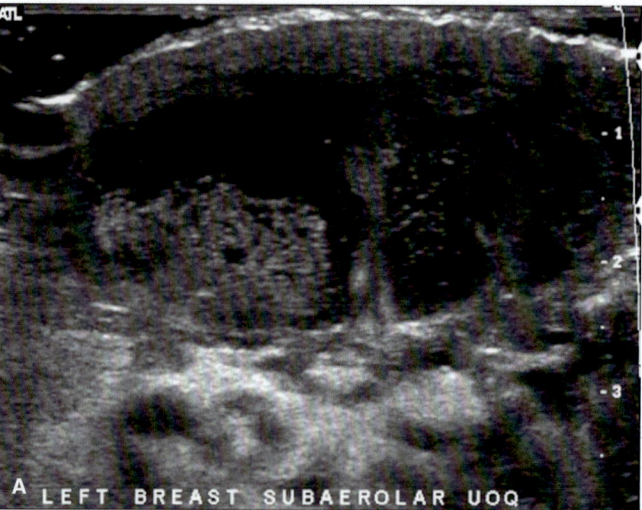
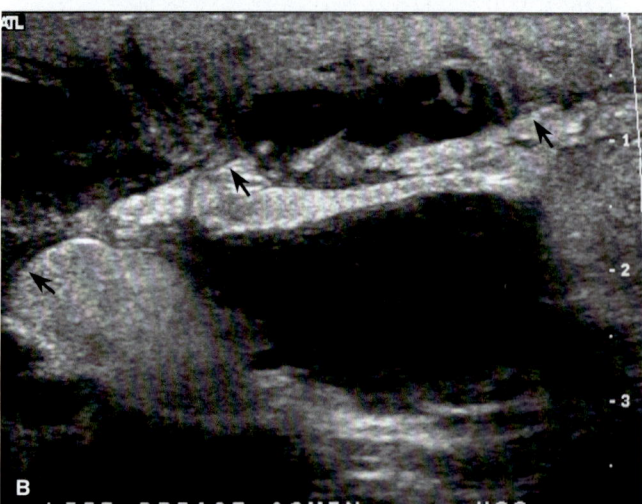

FIG. 7.50 • **Multiloculated lactational abscess. A:** Ultrasound, left subareolar area. A bulge in the contour of the breast is noted on visual inspection of the left breast. A complex cystic and solid mass with posterior acoustic enhancement is imaged extending to involve and thicken the skin. **B:** Representative ultrasound image of the upper outer quadrant (UOQ) of the left breast 6 cm from the nipple demonstrates interconnecting complex cystic and solid masses with extension to the skin *(arrows)*. The echogenicity of the surrounding tissue is increased, and there is complete disruption of normal tissue planes. Given the extent and multiloculated nature of the process, the patient is referred for surgical management.

Subareolar Abscess

This is a distinct entity reportedly occurring more commonly in younger premenopausal women who are heavy smokers. These abscesses are not associated with pregnancy, lactation, or nipple rings. Patients typically present with the rapid onset of pain, erythema, and swelling in the central aspect of the breast (Fig. 7.51A); systemic symptoms may be present in up to 10% of patients. If patients delay seeking treatment, they may spontaneously develop a fistula (Zuska disease) in the periareolar area (Fig. 7.51B). Ipsilateral reactive adenopathy may be noted at the time of presentation (Figs. 7.51C and 7.52A). Approximately 25% of patients recur after surgical management, and some present with an abscess in the contralateral breast. On subsequent presentations, healed fistulas may be seen along the periareolar margin, and the progressive development of horizontal inversion of the nipple may be noted.

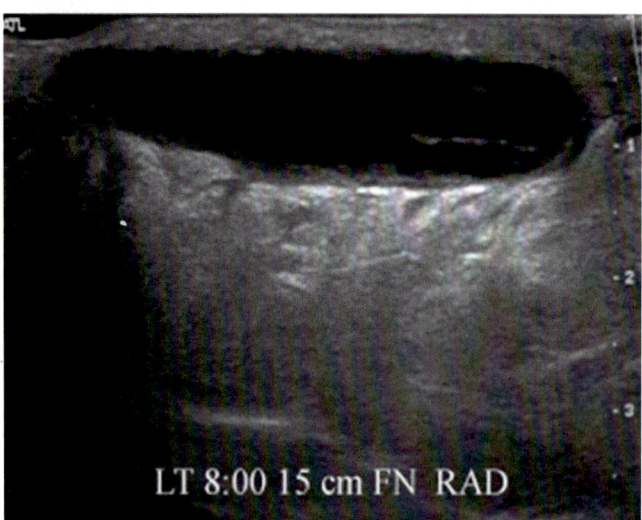

FIG. 7.49 • **Lactational abscess.** Ultrasound. An oval mass that is predominantly cystic with some internal echoes and a thickened wall and posterior acoustic enhancement is imaged in the subcutaneous tissue of the left breast in the lower inner quadrant, 15 cm from the left nipple corresponding to a palpable mass in a patient who is breast-feeding. Skin thickening is present, and there is disruption of normal tissue planes as well as an increase in the overall echogenicity of the surrounding tissue consistent with hyperemia and an ongoing inflammatory process. Ultrasound-guided aspiration is done, yielding purulent fluid submitted for microbiology. The patient is encouraged to continue breast-feeding and treated effectively with one course of antibiotics.

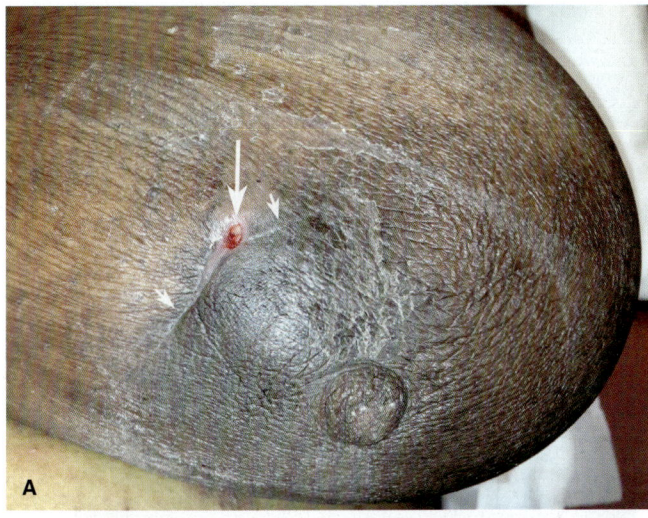
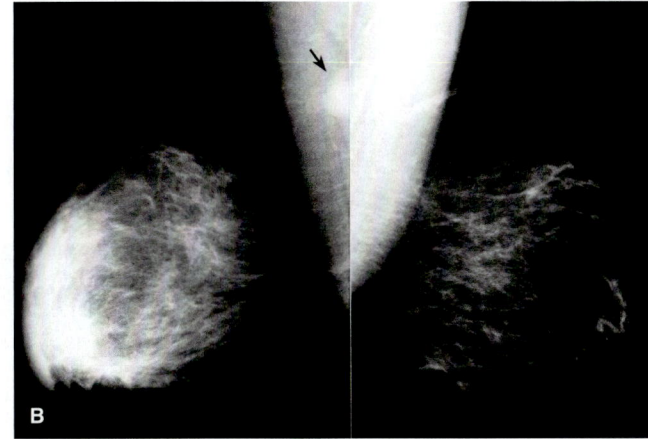
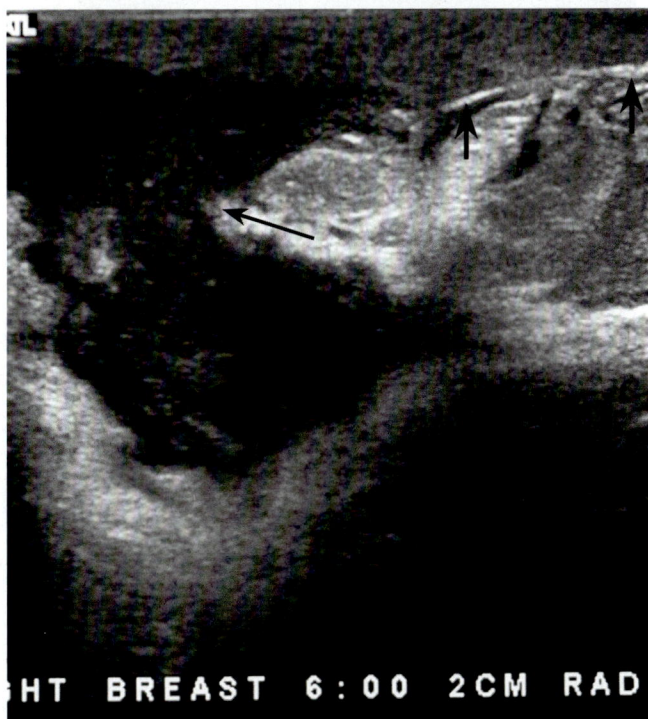

FIG. 7.51 • **Subareolar abscess, fistula formation (Zuska disease), reactive adenopathy. A:** Fistula. Patient presents describing the rapid development of a painful lump, followed a few days later by drainage of malodorous purulent fluid. A contour bulge of the upper outer aspect of the areola is apparent. Subareolar abscesses typically extend to involve the skin and, if left untreated, often drain spontaneously through a fistula *(long arrow)* that, as seen in this patient, forms at the periareolar margin (Zuska disease). Also note that this patient has a healed surgical scar *(small arrows)* in the periareolar area denoting prior surgical drainage of a subareolar abscess. Patients with subareolar abscess are difficult to manage medically and surgically with high recurrence rates. **B:** MLO views in a different patient. The right breast is less compressible. Increased density of the parenchyma is particularly noticeable anteriorly. The trabecular markings are diffusely prominent and one dense lymph node *(arrow)* is partially imaged in the right axilla. **C:** Ultrasound. A complex cystic and solid mass with indistinct margins and posterior enhancement extends to involve and thicken the skin *(short arrows)*. The funnel-shaped extension *(long arrow)* and involvement of the skin is a characteristic finding with this type of abscess. Disruption of normal soft tissue planes and the increased echogenicity of the surrounding tissue are also seen in these patients.

Acutely, tenderness limits the ability of patients to tolerate mammography. Technical factors may need to be adjusted for adequate exposure. Increased density is typically seen in the subareolar area or more diffusely involve the breast. Additional findings include an irregular mass with indistinct or spiculated margins and distortion (Figs. 7.51 and 7.52). Enlarged, dense lymph nodes may be present in the ipsilateral axilla (Figs. 7.51A and 7.52A, D). On ultrasound, a complex cystic mass with variable cystic and seemingly solid components and irregular thickened spiculated margins is imaged in the subareolar area. These fluid collections almost always extend to involve the skin such that a wide tubular-shaped ("funnel"-like) extension to the skin results in a lenticular-like thickening of the skin at the areolar margin (Fig. 7.51C). The surrounding tissue is hyperemic with loss of normal soft tissue planes and increased hyperechogenicity. Magnetic resonance imaging is not usually done in these patients since the diagnosis is established clinically and with mammography and ultrasound. Rim enhancement of the abscess cavity can be seen with high T2 signal centrally; the surrounding tissue is usually edematous (high signal) on T2 images.

Histologically, squamous metaplasia is reported on excised tissue in most of these patients (12). It has been postulated that the metaplastic changes result in obstruction of the central ducts with resultant distension and eventual periductal inflammation. It is the resulting periductal fibrosis from chronic inflammation that likely leads to the horizontal nipple inversion noted in many of the patients with recurrent subareolar abscesses.

Peripheral Abscess

This type of abscess is not related to lactation, can present across the ages, and is not subareolar in location. On physical examination, the breast may be focally erythematous, with localized or generalized peau d'orange changes. A hard mass is palpable and tenderness is elicited. A mass with indistinct margins may be seen mammographically. Increased prominence of the trabecular markings surrounding the mass

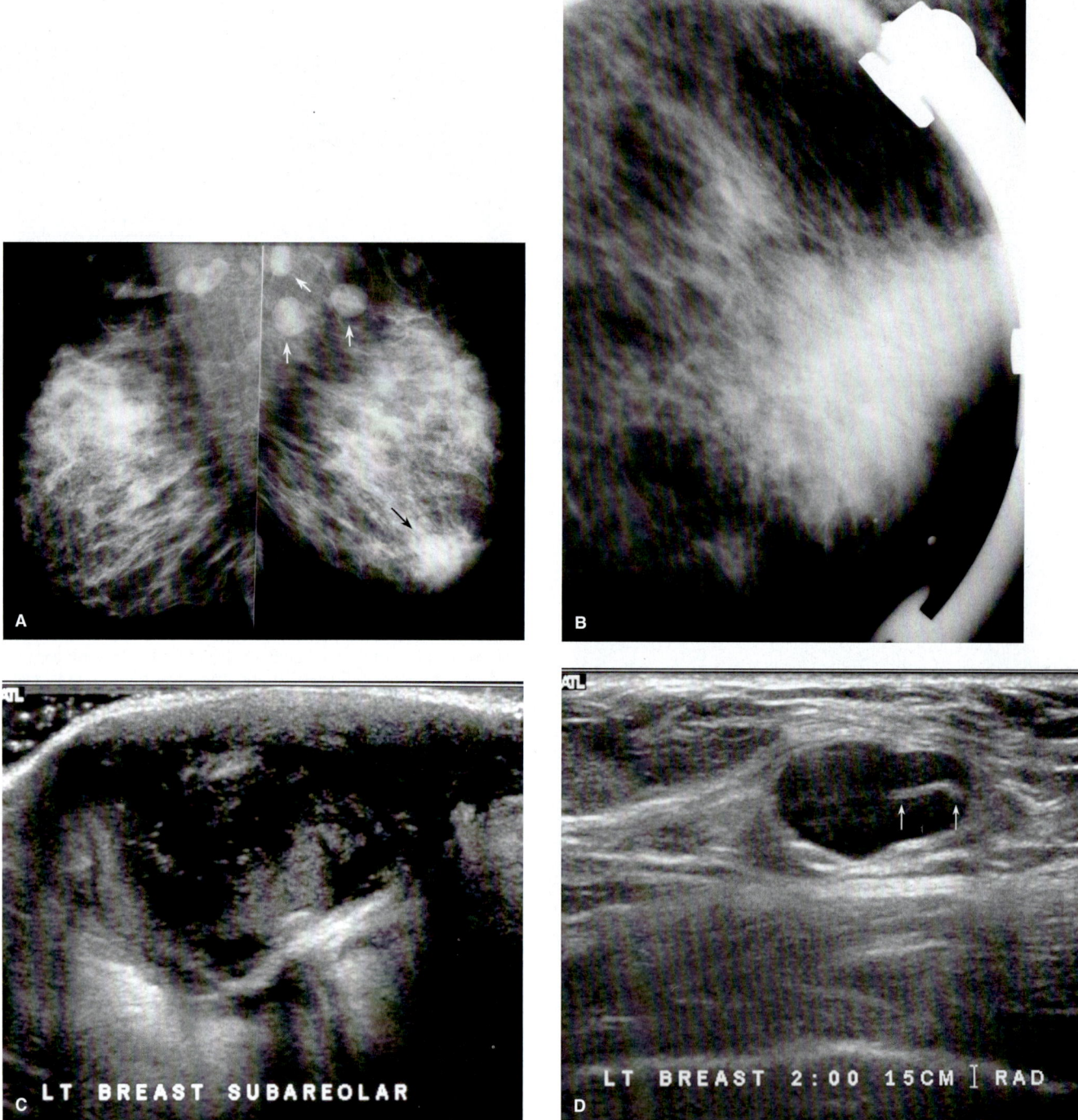

FIG. 7.52 ● **Subareolar abscess with reactive lymphadenopathy. A:** MLO views. Asymmetrically increased density *(black arrow)* with spiculation is present in the left subareolar area. Note prominent axillary lymph nodes *(white arrows)* on the left; lymph node in the right axilla maintains a fatty hilum. **B:** Spot compression view confirms the presence of an irregular mass with indistinct and spiculated margins in the left subareolar area. **C:** Ultrasound. A bulge in the contour of the left subareolar area is apparent on physical examination. A complex cystic and solid mass extending to involve and thicken the skin with a resultant contour abnormality is imaged corresponding to the bulge and the mammographically apparent mass. This mass demonstrates posterior acoustic enhancement and shadowing. The skin involvement is characteristic for subareolar abscesses. **D:** Lymph node in the left axillary tail with a thickened cortical area and thinning (mass effect) of the fatty hilum *(arrows)*. Posterior acoustic enhancement is also noted. Reactive changes reported on core biopsy.

likely reflects the ongoing inflammatory process (Fig. 7.53A). Dense lymph nodes with increased cortical width may be seen in the axilla. A localized complex cystic and solid mass may be imaged on ultrasound correlating to the palpable mass (Fig. 7.53B; also see Fig. 4.51A); depending on the size of the inflammatory process, the ultrasound findings may be less well defined with fluid noted intermingled with the tissue (Fig. 7.54; also see Fig. 4.51B). When the abscess is not well-defined on ultrasound, the diffuse nature of the process can be established by looking for slow movement (e.g., "gurgling") of the fluid as the transducer is held steady over a given area; increasing the gain

Evaluation and Imaging Features of Benign Breast Masses   205

develop in the breast parenchyma. Patients with peripheral abscess may be treated effectively with percutaneous aspiration and oral antibiotics (33). Recurrences are not common.

OTHER FLUID COLLECTIONS

Included in this group are postoperative or traumatic fluid collections (e.g., hematoma) and galactoceles. The mammographic appearance of postoperative fluid collections is variable. Round and oval masses

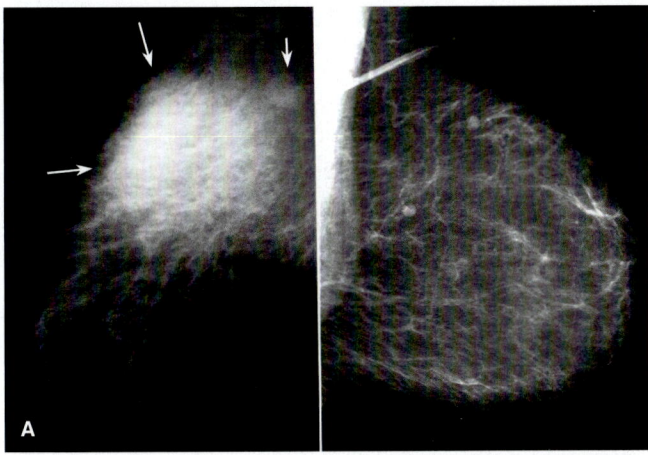
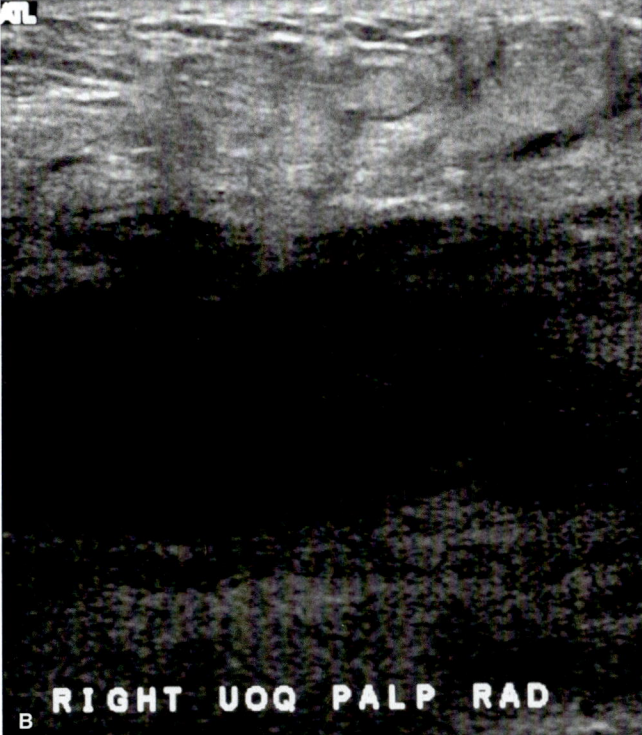

FIG. 7.53 • **Peripheral abscess. A:** MLO views in a 54-year-old patient who presents with a "lump," pain, swelling, and redness in the right breast. Compressibility of the right breast is limited, as evidenced by the sagging breast and uneven exposure (technique used can be checked for confirmation). A dense mass *(long arrows)* with indistinct margins is present superiorly associated with asymmetrically increased trabecular markings in the surrounding tissue. A second smaller, low-density mass *(short arrow)* with a fatty notch at the superior and posterior edge of the dominant mass is a reactive lymph node (ultrasound images of this are not shown). Two morphologically normal intramammary lymph nodes are present in the left breast. **B:** Ultrasound. An oval fluid collection with indistinct margins and irregularly thickened lobulations is imaged in the parenchyma corresponding to the palpable mass in the upper outer quadrant of the right breast. The echogenicity of the superficial tissue is increased with loss of normal tissue planes. Purulent material is aspirated, and beta hemolytic streptococcus is grown in culture. Patient is treated with antibiotics with complete resolution and no recurrence. BI-RADS 2: Benign finding.

may facilitate perception of the "gurgling." Increased echogenicity of the surrounding tissue with loss of normal soft tissue planes is noted consistent with edema and hyperemic changes (Fig. 7.54C). These abscesses are not related to the skin or subcutaneous tissue but rather

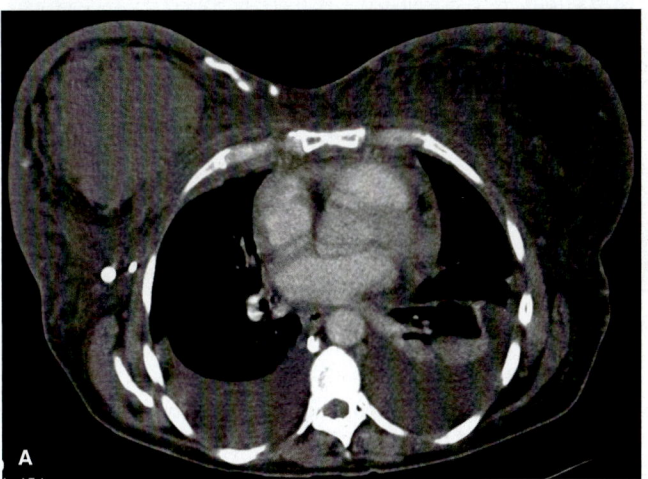
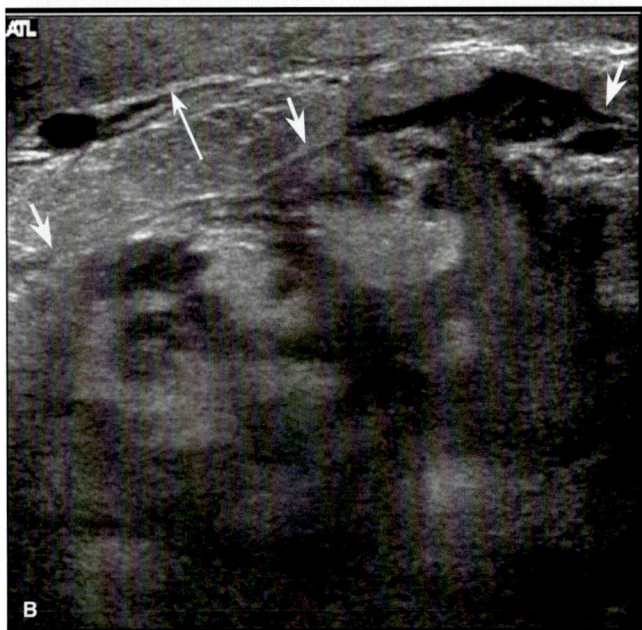

FIG. 7.54 • **Peripheral abscess. A:** CT scan in a 43-year-old patient with a history of fibrosing mediastinitis who presented with a new, painful "lump" in the right breast. Mass encompassing most of the right breast is noted at this scan level. Diffuse skin thickening and trabecular prominence in the breasts as well as bilateral pleural effusions reflecting known mediastinitis. **B:** Ultrasound. A complex fluid collection *(short arrows)* without clearly defined margins is imaged encompassing most of the right breast. During the real-time portion of the study, echoes could be seen "gurgling." A small amount of tissue with increased echogenicity is seen interposed between the fluid collection and the thickened skin *(long arrow)*. **C:** Ultrasound. Increased echogenicity of tissue with obliteration of soft tissue planes indicate edematous and hyperemic changes. Anechoic tubular structures are seen in the subcutaneous tissue, some of which reflect prominent vasculature as demonstrated with Doppler.

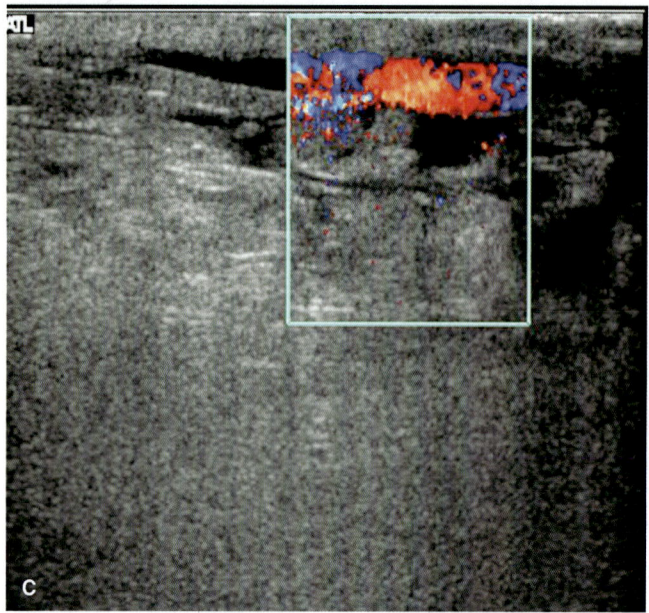

FIG. 7.54 • *(continued)*

with indistinct margins are common. The density of these may be high (see Figs. 11.24 through 11.26); however, given the size of some of these lesions, they are often low to isodense, suggesting a benign etiology (most malignant masses of comparable size are dense). An internal halo may be seen in some postoperative fluid collections (see Fig. 11.25). Hematomas resulting from trauma may appear initially as water density masses. As they liquefy and resolve, a mixed-density (Fig. 7.55; also see Fig. 11.14) or lucent mass may be seen with progressively developing mural calcifications (see Fig. 11.16). Postoperative or traumatic fluid collections can appear as cystic, complex cystic and solid masses or solid masses on ultrasound (see Figs. 4.31, 11.14, and 11.17). Please see Chapter 11 for additional discussion of postlumpectomy fluid collections.

Galactoceles develop in women who are pregnant, lactating, or have stopped lactation within the last 2 to 3 years. A mixed-density mass or water density mass can be seen mammographically. A fluid–fluid level may be apparent on the mammogram and ultrasound. Complex cystic and solid masses, solid-appearing masses, or cysts are seen on ultrasound (Fig. 7.56) with posterior acoustic enhancement or shadowing (see Fig. 4.28).

ADENOMAS (FIBROEPITHELIAL LESIONS)
Fibroadenomas

Fibroadenomas are common lesions particularly in women in their 20s and 30s. In postmenopausal women, fibroadenomas decrease in size and increase in density as a result of hyalinization, and some develop calcifications. With estrogen (ER) replacement therapy these changes may not develop, and preexisting fibroadenomas can enlarge or, uncommonly, develop in postmenopausal women (34). Rarely, one or multiple fibroadenomas develop in patients being treated with cyclosporine A for immunosuppression following cardiac or renal transplantation (Fig. 7.57) (35). Clinically, women with fibroadenomas may present with a hard mobile mass. Since fibroadenomas are hormonally responsive, some patients describe cyclical fluctuation in the size of the mass and associated tenderness.

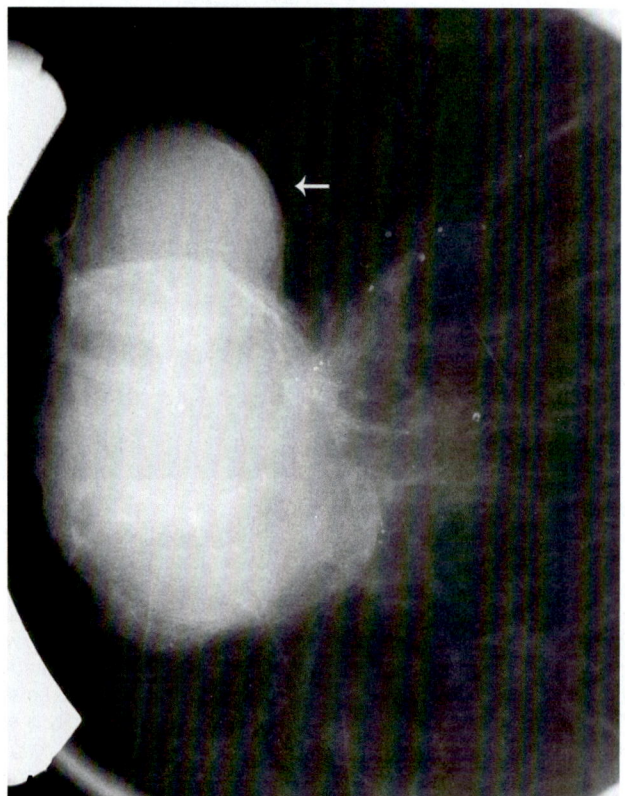

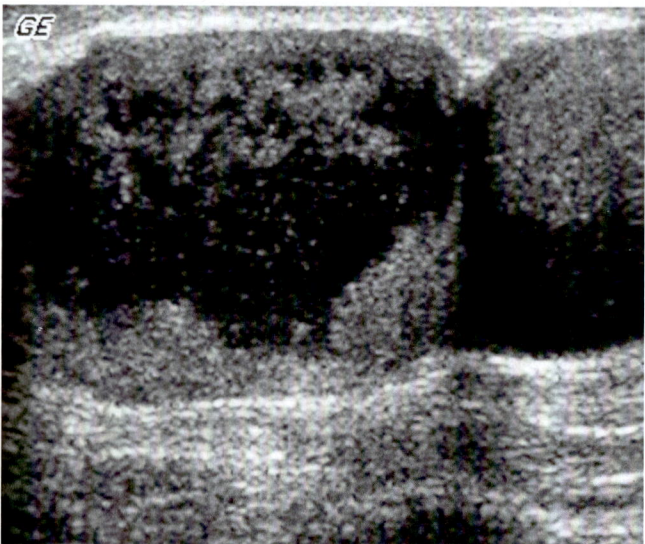

FIG. 7.55 • **Hematoma. A:** Spot compression view of the right subareolar area. Two masses (*arrow*) are noted in the right subareolar area following a car accident several years previously. **B:** Ultrasound. Two masses with heterogeneous echotexture are imaged corresponding to the masses seen mammographically. Thick brown fluid is aspirated with little residual abnormality seen post aspiration. No malignancy or atypia is seen cytologically. (From Cardeñosa G. *Breast Imaging [The Core Curriculum Series]*. Philadelphia, PA: Lippincott Williams & Wilkins; 2003.)

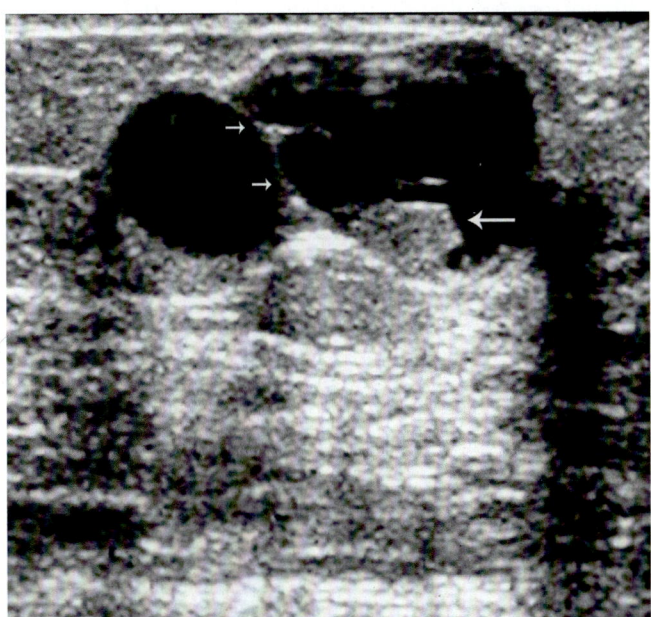

FIG. 7.56 • **Galactocele.** Ultrasound. A patient who is lactating presents with a "lump." A complex cystic and solid mass with posterior acoustic enhancement, septations *(small arrows)*, and a seemingly solid component *(large arrow)* is seen on ultrasound. Thick milky fluid is aspirated with no residual abnormality seen post aspiration. (From Cardeñosa G. *Breast Imaging [The Core Curriculum Series]*. Philadelphia, PA: Lippincott Williams & Wilkins; 2003.)

Round (Fig. 7.57A and 7.58), oval, or macrolobulated masses with circumscribed margins are common mammographic findings in women with fibroadenomas. These lesions may have obscured (Fig. 7.58A) or ill-defined margins; spiculation is rare. On ultrasound, an oval, homogeneously hypoechoic mass (Fig. 7.58C; also Figs. 4.38B, C and 4.52) with circumscribed margins and one or two gentle macrolobulations is the most common finding (24). Internal echogenic fibrous septations may be seen in some fibroadenomas. Posterior acoustic enhancement, particularly in younger patients with myxoid fibroadenomas, may be prominent, while shadowing is common as the lesion undergoes hyalinization. It is important, however, to emphasize that the mammographic and ultrasound appearance of fibroadenomas is variable. Clustered microcalcifications with or without an associated mass can be seen, as can coarse popcorn-type calcifications. Fibroadenomas are variable in size and can enlarge; however, most stop growing after reaching 2 to 3 cm in diameter. Multiple fibroadenomas are reported in approximately 20% of women (34). Giant fibroadenomas, arbitrarily defined as 8 cm or more in size, typically present during adolescence.

On MRI, the appearance of fibroadenomas is also variable (36). In the younger patients with hormone-stimulated fibroadenomas, and depending on the timing of the MRI with respect to their cycle, a mass with high T2 signal (Fig. 7.59A) and enhancement may be imaged. Non-enhancing internal septations may be present (Fig. 7.59B; also see Fig. 5.14). In older women, a mass with circumscribed margins and low T1 and T2 signal as well as no enhancement may be noted correlating to hyalinizing or calcified fibroadenomas (Fig. 7.60).

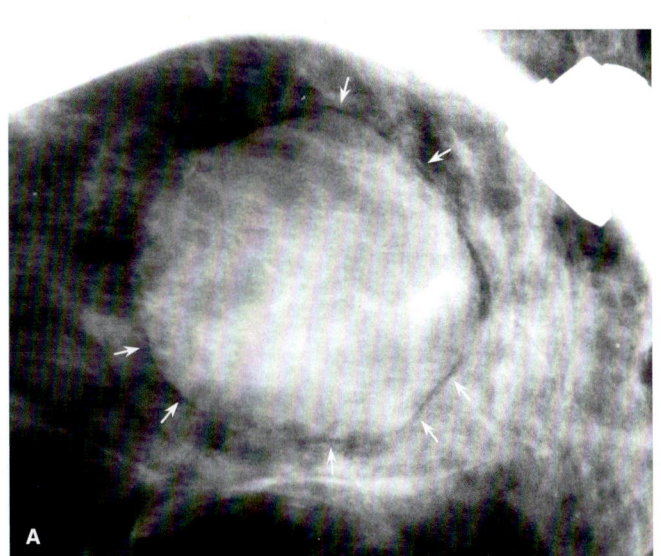
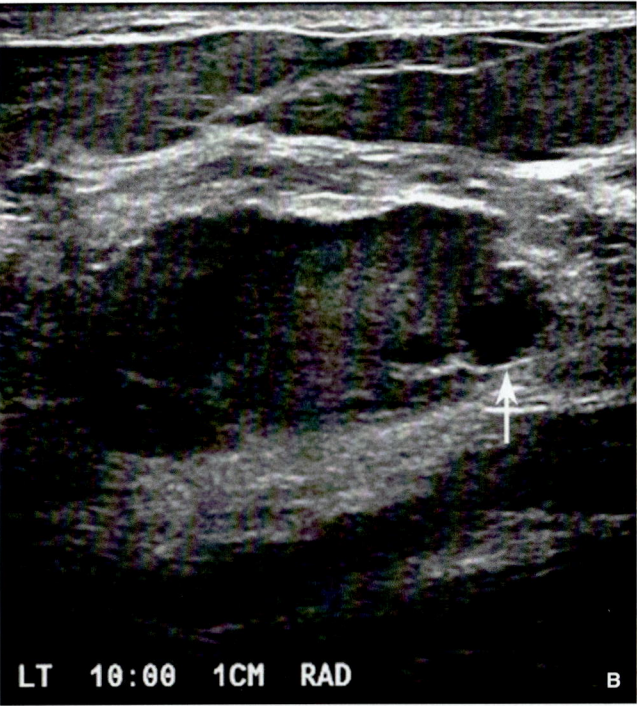

FIG. 7.57 • **Fibroadenoma, cyclosporine induced. A:** Spot compression view. Round, isodense mass with predominantly circumscribed margins and partial "halo" *(arrows)*. This is a new mass in a 46-year-old patient on cyclosporine A. **B:** Ultrasound. A hypoechoic mass with circumscribed margins, posterior acoustic enhancement, and a small cyst *(arrow)* is imaged in the left breast correlating to the mass seen mammographically. BI-RADS 4A: Suspicious abnormality, biopsy is indicated.

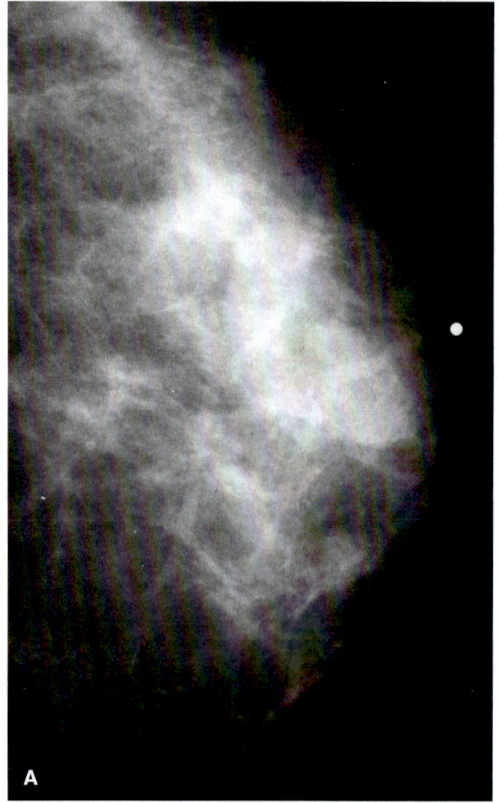
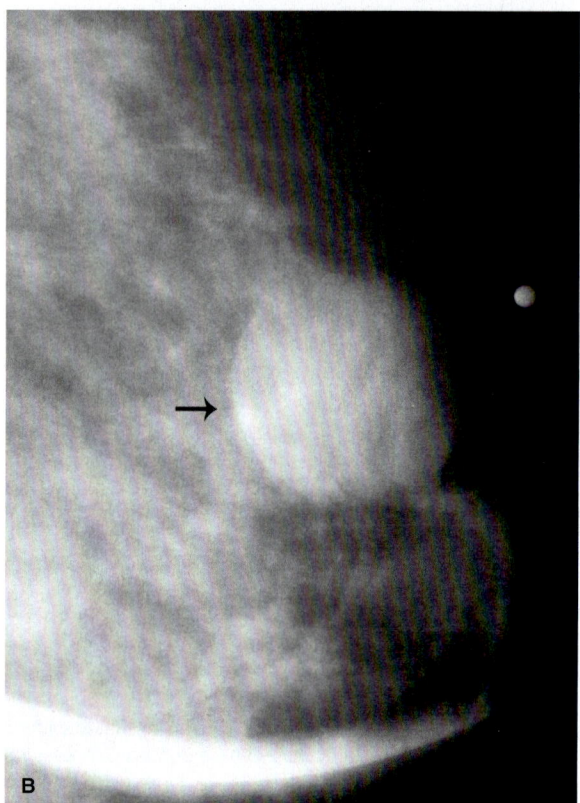
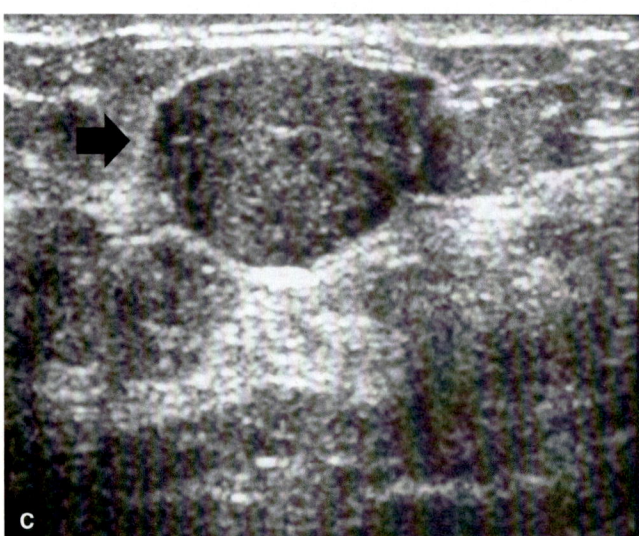

FIG. 7.58 • **Fibroadenoma. A:** CC view photographically coned to the anterior aspect of the left breast in a 39-year-old woman who presents describing a "lump." The metallic BB denotes the palpable finding. Dense glandular tissue obscures the lesion. **B:** Spot tangential view demonstrates a round isodense mass *(arrow)* with circumscribed margins corresponding to the palpable finding. **C:** Ultrasound. An oval hypoechoic mass *(arrow)* with gentle lobulation and posterior acoustic enhancement is imaged corresponding to the clinically and mammographically apparent mass. (From Cardeñosa G. *Breast Imaging [The Core Curriculum Series]*. Philadelphia, PA: Lippincott Williams & Wilkins; 2003.)

Histologically, fibroadenomas are lobulocentric lesions demonstrating proliferative changes involving the stroma and glandular elements. The glandular elements (acini) may be compressed and elongated by the proliferating stroma (intracanalicular); when the proliferating ductal elements are not compressed, the pattern may be described as pericanalicular. The glandular elements and stromal cellularity are prominent in younger patients (Fig. 7.61A) but mitotic figures are rare in the stroma of fibroadenomas. As the patient ages, and hormone levels decrease, epithelial elements decrease, and the stroma undergoes hyalinization (Fig. 7.61B). To establish the diagnosis of a fibroadenoma, epithelial and stromal elements must be present in the tissue submitted for histology (11,12). In the absence of epithelial elements, as may occur in older fibroadenomas, a diagnosis of fibroadenoma may be elusive to establish.

When a patient is diagnosed with a fibroadenoma on core biopsy, we return her to screening; with a congruent diagnosis, we do not obtain 6-month follow-up studies. We also do not recommend excisional biopsy when small increases in the size of core biopsy–proven fibroadenomas are noted on subsequent mammograms. If the pathologist describes a fibroepithelial lesion or a fibroadenoma with stromal cellularity in a woman in her 40s, the findings are discussed directly with the pathologist. If the stromal cellularity is such that the pathologist is concerned about the possibility of a phyllodes tumor, excisional biopsy is indicated.

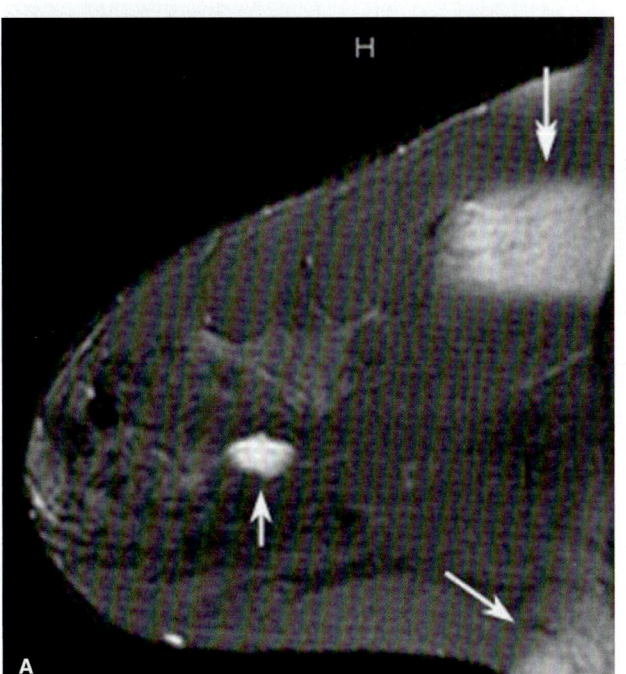
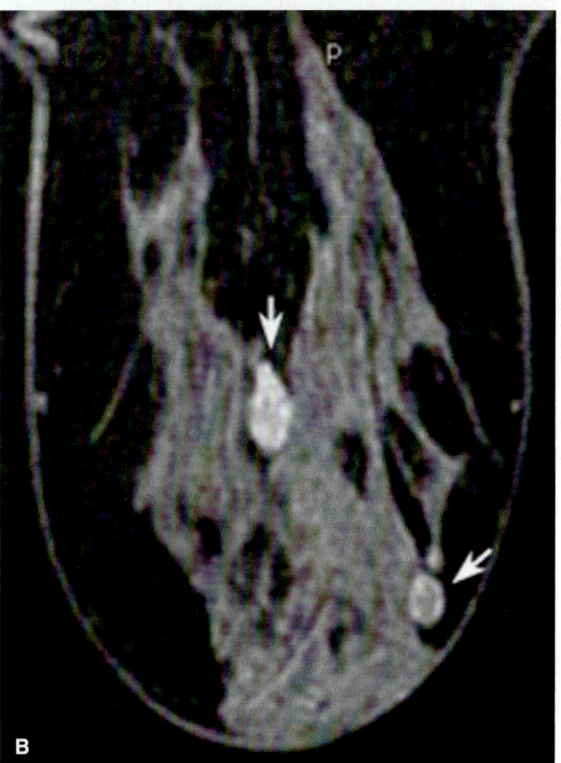

FIG. 7.59 • **Fibroadenoma. A:** MRI, sagittal T2 fat-suppressed image of the right breast. An oval mass *(short arrow)* with circumscribed margins and high T2 signal is imaged centrally in the right breast, zone B. The T2 signal of fibroadenomas is variable. Signal flaring from the proximity of the breast to the coil *(long arrows)* is noted. **B:** MRI, T1-weighted axial image of the right breast, postcontrast. Two oval enhancing masses *(arrows)* with smooth margins and non-enhancing internal septations are imaged in the right breast; the larger of the two, centrally in the breast, zone B, correlates to the mass with high T2 signal shown in part **A**. The imaging features of fibroadenomas are variable depending on the age of the patient. In younger patients, fibroadenomas commonly have a high T2 signal (myxoid) signal and demonstrate enhancement that may be characterized by non-enhancing internal septations; on ultrasound posterior acoustic enhancement may be apparent. As the patient ages, and hormone stimulation on the fibroadenoma decreases, fibroadenomas become denser on the mammogram (hyalinization) and are more likely to have a low T2 signal with no enhancement on MRI and shadowing on ultrasound.

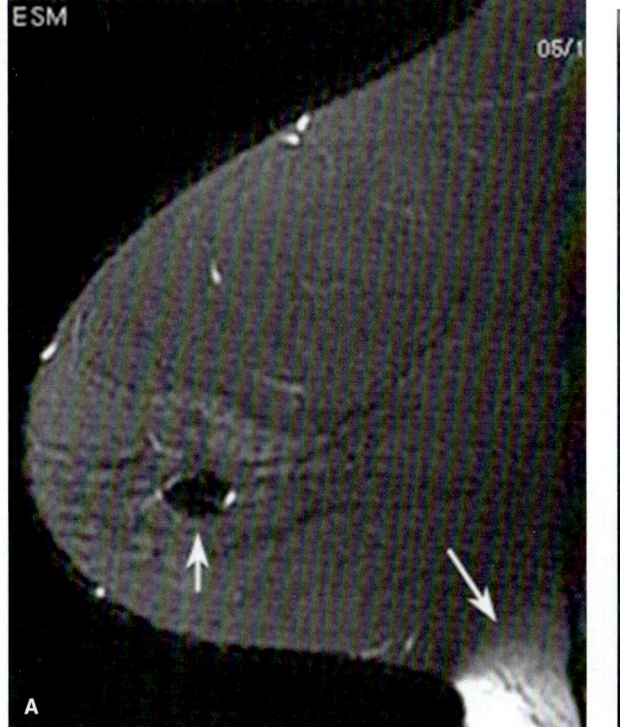
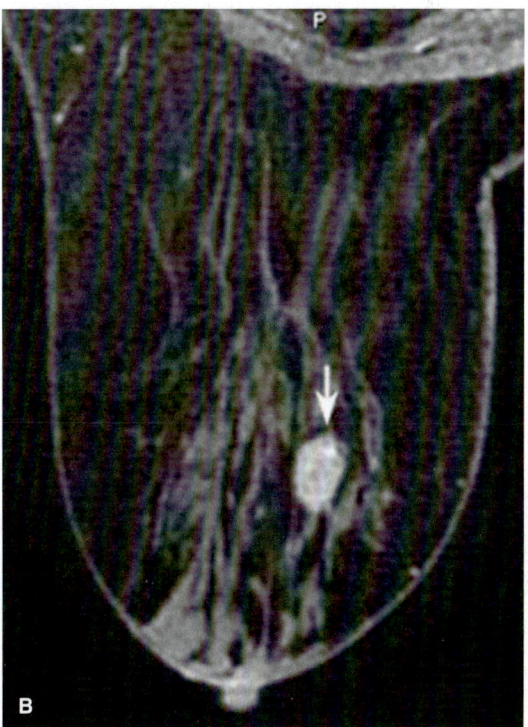

FIG. 7.60 • **Fibroadenoma, hyalinized. A:** MRI, sagittal T2 fat-suppressed image of the left breast. Oval mass *(small arrow)* with circumscribed margins and low T2 signal is imaged in the left breast. Note coil artifact *(long arrow)* at the inframammary fold. **B:** MRI, axial image left breast postcontrast. Oval mass *(arrow)* with circumscribed margins in the central to slightly medial aspect of the left breast, zone B, with no enhancement corresponding to mass shown in part **A**.

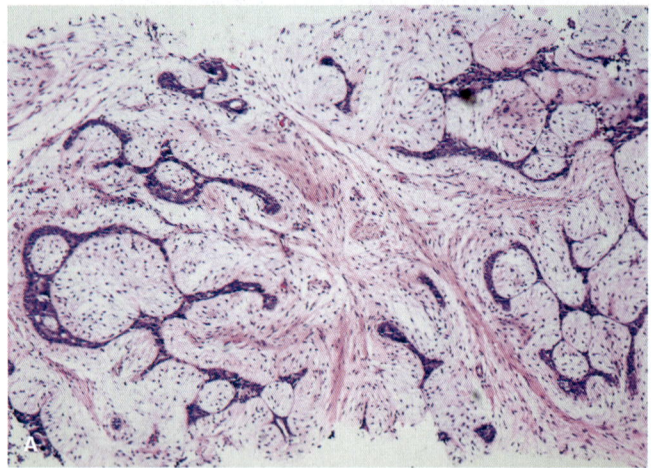

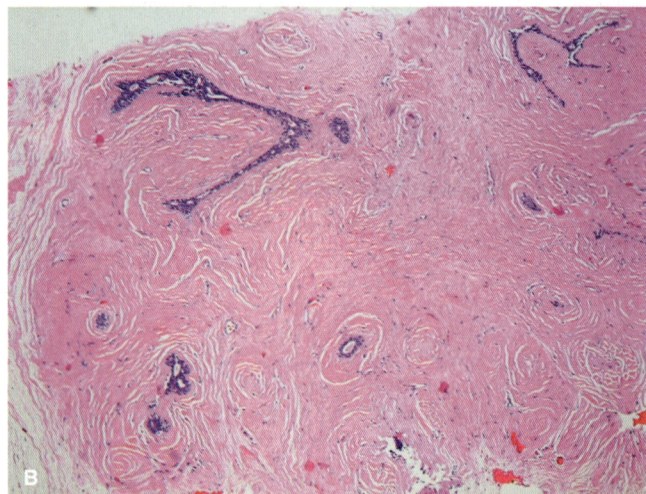

FIG. 7.61 • **Fibroadenomas, pathology. A:** Fibroadenoma diagnosed on core biopsy in a young woman. Cellular stroma compressing and elongating the glandular elements: findings diagnostic of a fibroadenoma (intracanalicular). **B:** Different patient. Hyalinization, limited stromal cellularity, and paucity of epithelial elements are findings that characterize fibroadenomas in postmenopausal women. Epithelial and stromal elements must be present in the tissue for the diagnosis to be established histologically. If epithelial elements are not apparent on the cores, the pathologist is unable to characterize the lesion as a fibroadenoma; dense fibrosis (with hyalinization) may be described without the definitive diagnosis of a fibroadenoma.

Complex Fibroadenoma

A term coined by Dupont et al. (37), it describes fibroadenomas with superimposed fibrocystic changes specifically cysts greater than 3 mm (Fig. 7.62), sclerosing adenosis (Fig. 7.63), epithelial calcifications, and papillary apocrine changes.

In their study, approximately 33% of the fibroadenomas could be classified as complex. These lesions may be associated with an increased risk for the subsequent development of breast cancer. Reportedly, the risk is increased to 3.88× if proliferative changes are present in the stroma surrounding a complex fibroadenoma (CFA) (37).

The imaging features of CFAs are usually indistinguishable from those of fibroadenomas (38). In some patients, however, mammographic and ultrasound findings may suggest the diagnosis of a CFA. Epithelial calcifications may be seen on the mammogram as pleomorphic calcifications including round, punctate, and, less commonly,

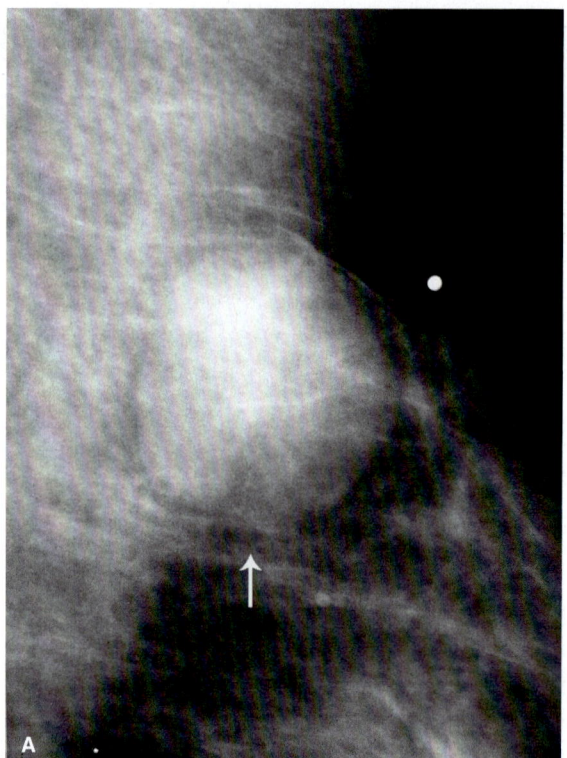

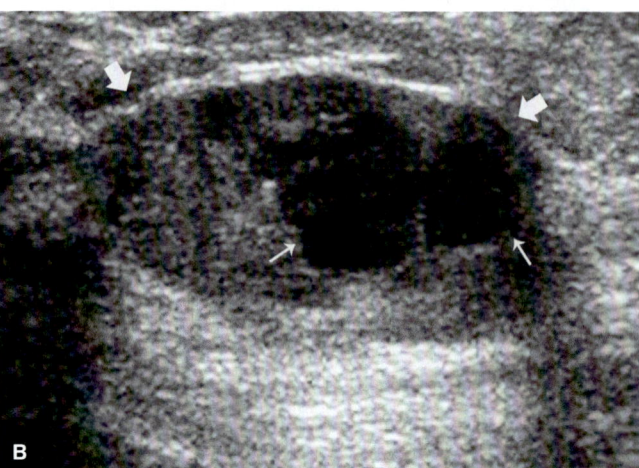

FIG. 7.62 • **Complex fibroadenoma. A:** Left MLO view photographically coned to the upper portion of the image. A round, isodense mass *(arrow)* with circumscribed margins is imaged in a 32-year-old woman who presents describing a "lump." The metallic BB denotes the site of the palpable finding. **B:** Mass *(thick arrows)*, which is predominantly solid with cystic spaces *(thin arrows)* and posterior acoustic enhancement. BI-RADS 4A: Suspicious abnormality, biopsy is indicated. A complex fibroadenoma with cystic changes and epithelial hyperplasia is diagnosed on an ultrasound-guided core biopsy. With a specific diagnosis that is congruent with the imaging findings, the patient is returned to screening (or annual screening mammography is recommended starting at age 40, if the patient is under the ge 40). No excisional biopsy or short-term follow-up is recommended. (From Cardeñosa G. *Breast Imaging [The Core Curriculum Series]*. Philadelphia, PA: Lippincott Williams & Wilkins; 2003.)

linear forms. An associated mass may or may not be seen. Amorphous calcifications (Fig. 7.63A) associated with a mass may reflect the presence of sclerosing adenosis in the fibroadenoma. Lastly, a predominantly solid mass with cystic spaces greater than 3 mm in size

Evaluation and Imaging Features of Benign Breast Masses

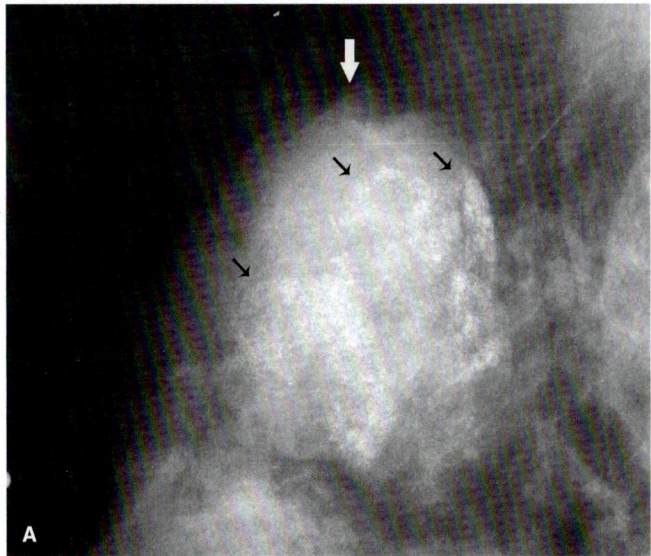

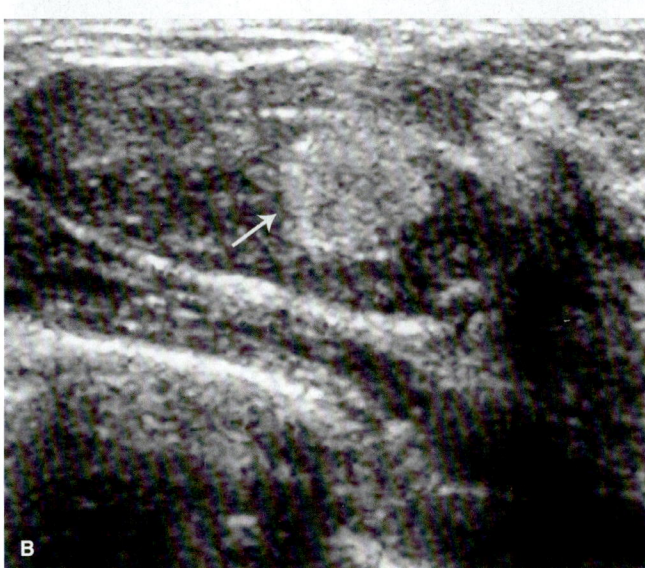

FIG. 7.63 • **Complex fibroadenoma. A:** Right MLO view photographically coned to the upper portion of the image. An oval, dense mass with partially indistinct margins *(white arrow)* and associated amorphous ("smudgy") calcifications *(black arrows)* is imaged at the site of a "lump" described by a 35-year-old woman. **B:** Oval hypoechoic mass with a focal area of hyperechogenicity *(arrow)*. BI-RADS 4B: Suspicious abnormality, biopsy is indicated. A complex fibroadenoma with superimposed sclerosing adenosis is diagnosed on the core biopsy. With a specific diagnosis that is congruent with the imaging findings, the patient is returned to screening. Since this patient is 35, annual screening mammography is recommended starting at age 40. No excisional biopsy or short-term follow-up is recommended. (From Cardeñosa G. *Breast Imaging [The Core Curriculum Series]*. Philadelphia, PA: Lippincott Williams & Wilkins; 2003.)

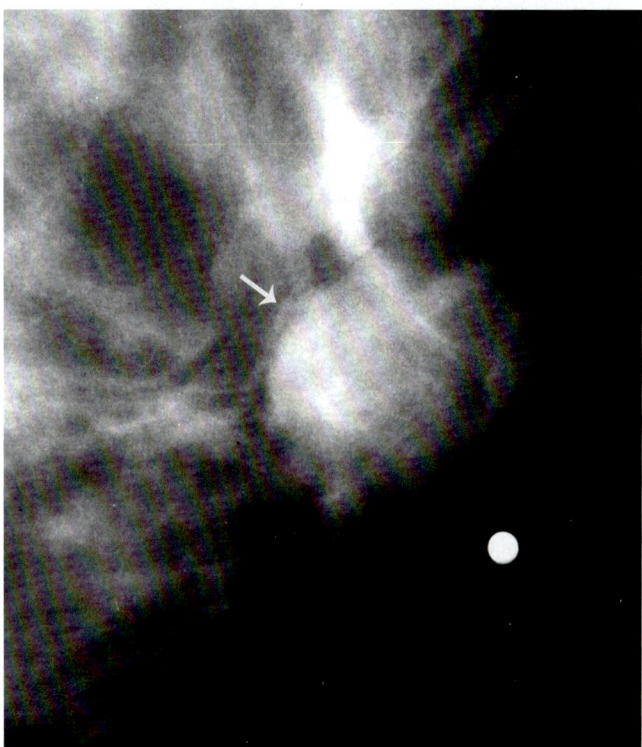

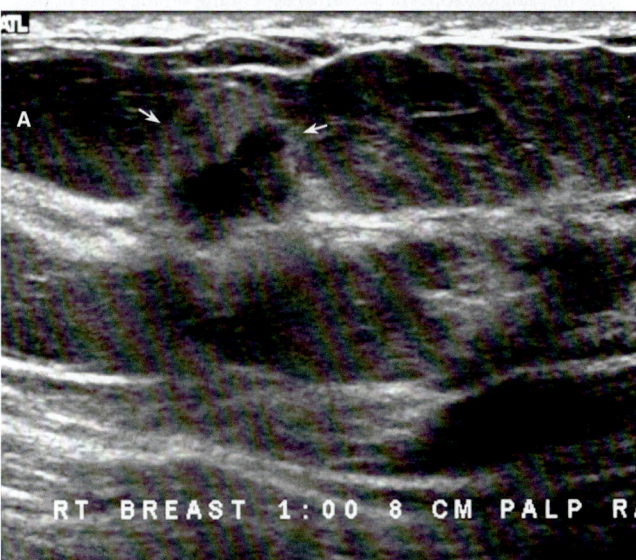

FIG. 7.64 • **Tubular adenoma. A:** A round isodense mass *(arrow)* with circumscribed margins is imaged at the site of a "lump" described by a 58-year-old woman. The metallic BB denotes the palpable finding. An oval mass with heterogeneous echotexture is imaged (not shown) on ultrasound. BI-RADS 4B: Suspicious abnormality, biopsy is indicated. **B:** Ultrasound (different patient). An irregular, vertically oriented mass *(arrows)* with a heterogeneous echo pattern is imaged at the site of a palpable finding in the right breast. BI-RADS 4B: Suspicious abnormality, biopsy is indicated. Tubular adenoma is diagnosed on core biopsy. With a specific diagnosis that is congruent with the imaging findings, the patient is returned to screening. No excisional biopsy or short-term follow-up is recommended.

(Fig. 7.62B; also see Fig. 4.35) may be seen on ultrasound. Since at most, this is a marker lesion for increased risk, we do not recommend excisional biopsy when a CFA is reported on core biopsy. Patients are screened annually.

Tubular Adenoma

Women with tubular adenomas present commonly in their 20s and 30s with palpable mobile masses. The imaging findings are indistinguishable from those described for fibroadenomas. A round (Fig. 7.64A) or oval mass with circumscribed margins is seen on the mammogram. Rarely, the mass may be irregular with indistinct margins (Fig. 7.64B). An oval homogeneously hypoechoic mass is seen on ultrasound (26). Posterior acoustic enhancement may be noted. Clusters of pleomorphic calcifications may also be seen (39). In women presenting with a mass with circumscribed margins, and a diagnosis of tubular adenoma on needle biopsy, we do not recommend excision or short-interval follow-up. The patient is returned to annual screening mammography. These tumors are not premalignant and have no associated increased risk for breast cancer.

Grossly, tubular adenomas lack a true capsule, yet are circumscribed, and separable from the adjacent tissue. Histologically, these tumors are composed of uniformly small, closely packed tubular structures with scant surrounding stroma. A contiguous layer of epithelial and a discontinuous basilar layer of myoepithelial cells line the proliferating tubules reminiscent of normal ducts in the breast (11,12,25). Infarction may be present, but hemorrhage and necrosis are not seen (40).

Lactational Adenoma

The term lactational adenoma is a misnomer since patients with these lesions typically present during the third trimester of pregnancy with a palpable mobile mass. At presentation, patients may describe rapid growth and pain. Because of the age of most patients, and their presentation during pregnancy or lactation, mammograms are not usually done. Macrolobulated, hypoechoic masses with circumscribed margins and posterior acoustic enhancement are among the ultrasound characteristics of lactational adenomas (41). Fibrous bands traversing the lesion or short curvilinear hyperechoic bands and microcystic spaces may be seen (Fig. 7.65).

The histological appearance varies depending on the stage of pregnancy at the time of diagnosis. In women who are less than 6 months pregnant, the tubular structures, unlike those of tubular adenomas, vary in size. The epithelial cells contain cytoplasmic vacuoles and mitotic figures are common. Lesions diagnosed after the second trimester of pregnancy are characterized by alveolar spaces filled with foamy material, variegated shape, and cytoplasmic vacuoles. These lesions may grow rapidly, and infarction with necrosis may occur (11,12,25).

Phyllodes Tumors

Phyllodes tumors are fibroepithelial tumors accounting for less than 1% of all breast neoplasms (11,12,23,42–47). Most are benign; however, metastasis has been reported in 6% to 22% of patients (25). The mean age of patients with phyllodes is 45 years; however, they can occur in patients of all ages. As many as 80% of patients present with a palpable mass, while 20% are detected on screening mammography (42). A dense round or oval mass (Figs. 7.66 and 7.67) that may be lobulated with circumscribed or indistinct margins is the most common mammographic manifestation of phyllodes. Tumors that are larger than 3 cm in size are more likely to have histological features suggestive of malignancy (42). Although these lesions can attain "large" sizes (Fig. 7.66), size alone is no longer used as a diagnostic criterion (Fig. 7.68). Depending on the size of the lesion, phyllodes can range from a round to oval homogeneously hypoechoic mass (Fig. 7.68B) with circumscribed margins to having a more heterogeneous internal matrix (Fig. 7.66B, C) on ultrasound. Hyperechoic bands may be seen, and posterior acoustic enhancement may be prominent. Localized areas of shadowing may be seen in some lesions. Cystic changes may be more common in malignant lesions; however, this cannot be used to distinguish benign from malignant phyllodes. Calcifications are uncommon (8%) and not useful in distinguishing benign from malignant tumors (42). An expansile lobulated mass with circumscribed margins, a heterogeneous T2 signal with areas of high T2 signal on fat-suppressed images, edematous changes in the surrounding tissue, and commonly rapid washin with either plateau or washout delayed kinetic curves are common characteristics on MRI (Fig. 7.67B–D, 7.69C and 7.70B).

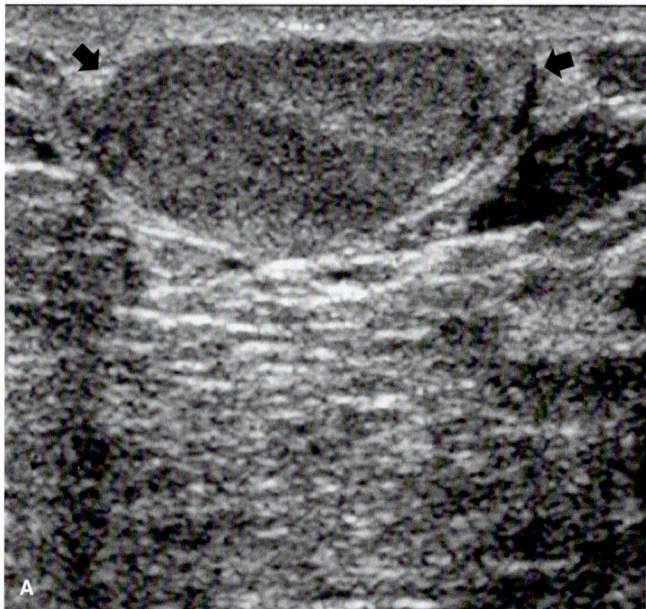
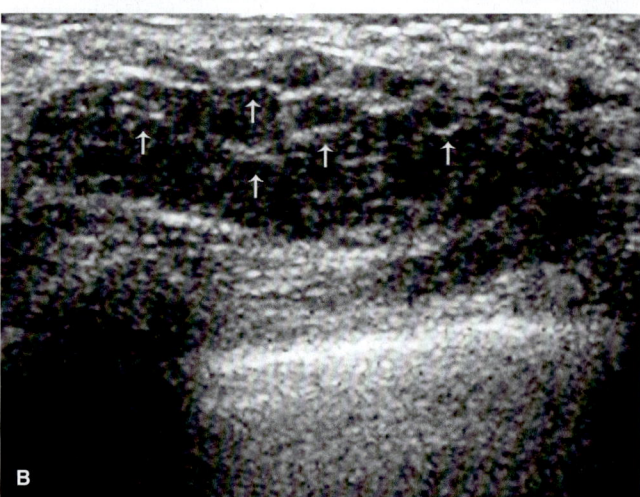

FIG. 7.65 • **Lactational adenomas. A:** Ultrasound. A homogeneously iso to slightly hyperechoic mass *(arrows)* with circumscribed margins and posterior acoustic enhancement is imaged in a 46-year-old woman who presents with a "lump" in the subareolar area during the third trimester of pregnancy. Although a lactational adenoma is suspected on the imaging findings, the patient requested a core biopsy that confirmed the diagnosis. **B:** Ultrasound, in a 33-year-old woman in her second trimester of pregnancy presenting with a "lump" in the right breast. A hypoechoic mass with circumscribed margins, hyperechoic fibrous bands *(arrows)*, and gentle mass effect on the pectoral muscle is imaged at the site of the clinically apparent mass. Although these lesions are called lactational adenomas, patients commonly present during the third trimester of pregnancy. (From Cardeñosa G. *Breast Imaging [The Core Curriculum Series]*. Philadelphia, PA: Lippincott Williams & Wilkins; 2003.)

Histologically, the proliferation and appearance of the epithelial elements in phyllodes tumors and fibroadenomas are similar; the epithelial component in phyllodes is polyclonal. It is the cellularity of the stroma that distinguishes phyllodes from fibroadenomas; the stromal component in phyllodes is monoclonal. Increased cellularity of the stroma and projection of stromal elements into cystic spaces to create a leaflike (phyllodes) pattern characterize phyllodes tumors (11,12,25,43). The criteria used in the classification

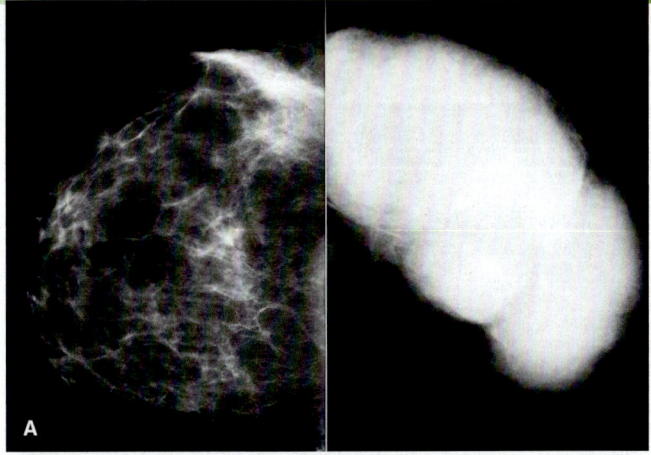
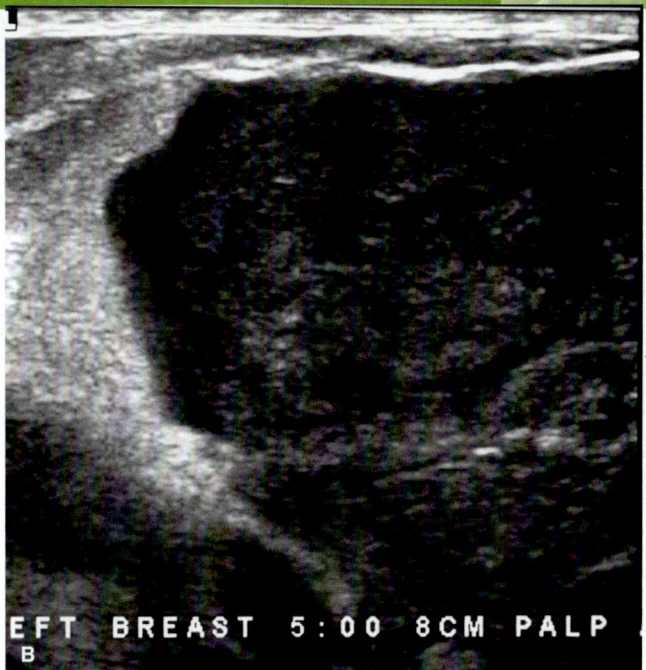
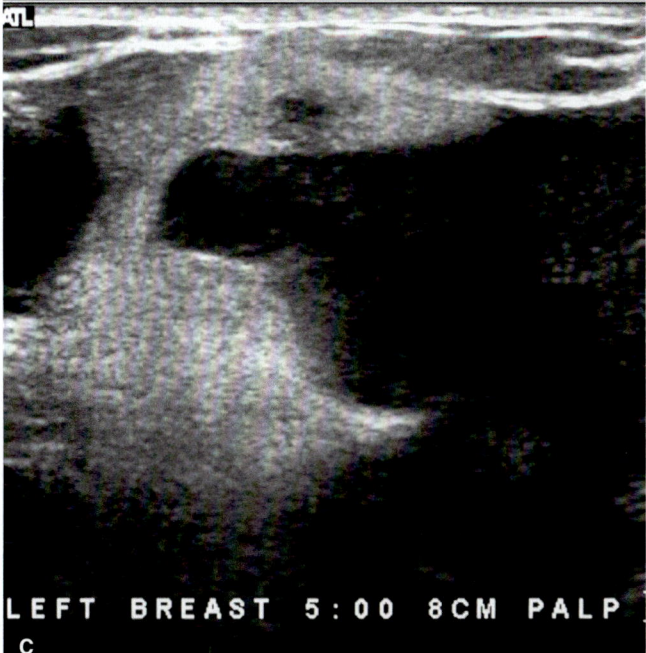

FIG. 7.66 • **Malignant phyllodes tumor with liposarcomatous degeneration. A:** CC views. A dense oval macrolobulated mass is present, almost completely replacing the left breast in a 47-year-old patient. **B:** Ultrasound. Portions of the mass seen mammographically have a relatively homogeneously hypoechoic internal matrix. **C:** Ultrasound. A complex cystic component with surrounding echogenicity is apparent in other portions of this mass. An MRI could not be done in this patient because her left breast did not fit in the breast coil.

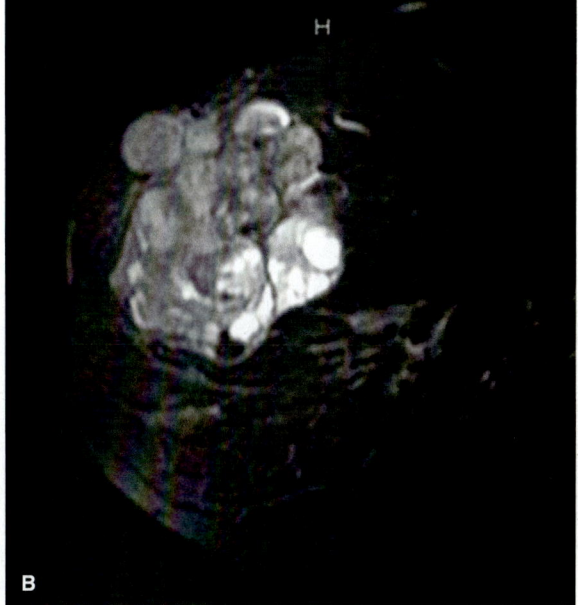
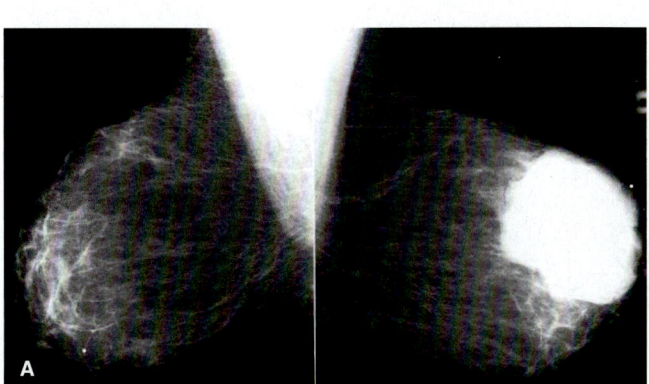

FIG. 7.67 • **Malignant phyllodes tumor, low grade. A:** MLO views. A dense, round, macrolobulated mass is imaged anteriorly correlating to a "lump" described by a 54-year-old patient in her left breast. Metallic BB used to denote site of palpable finding. **B:** MRI, sagittal T2 fat-suppressed image of the left breast. A lobulated mass that demonstrates intermediate T2 signal with localized areas of high T2 signal inferiorly correlates with the mass seen mammographically.

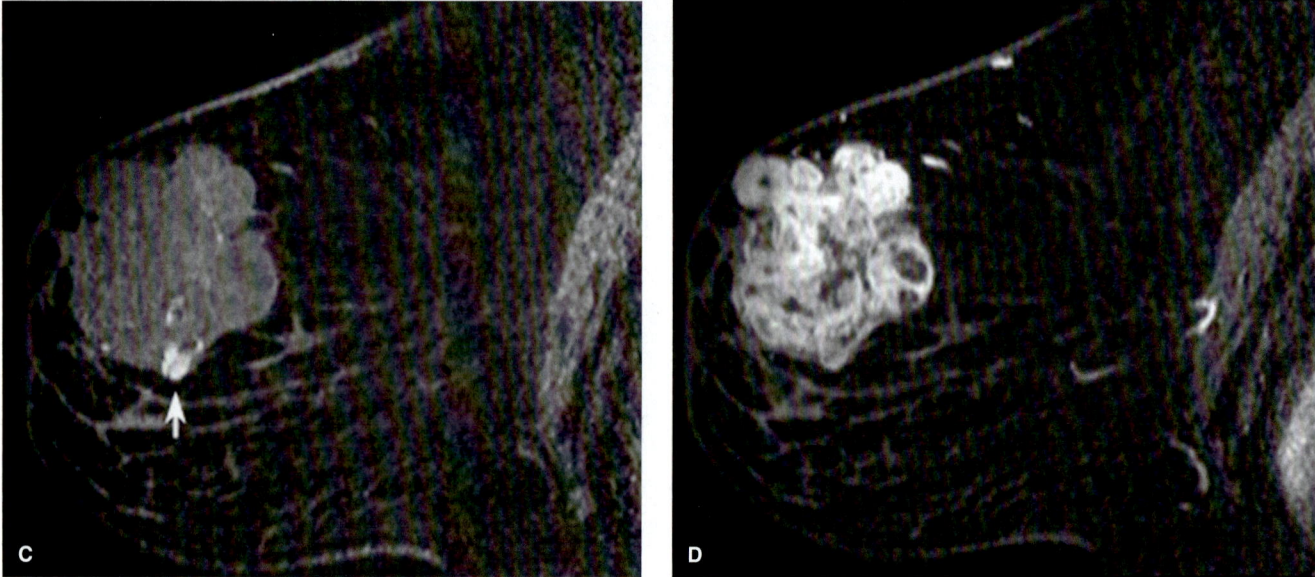

FIG. 7.67 • *(continued)* **C:** MRI, sagittal T1 reconstruction left breast, precontrast. The mass demonstrates intermediate T1 signal intensity with a localized area of high T1 signal *(arrow)* inferiorly. **D:** MRI, sagittal T1 reconstruction left breast postcontrast. Mass with circumscribed, lobulated margins and heterogeneous enhancement with rapid washin and washout type kinetic curves intermingled with plateau-type delayed kinetic curves. Patient had a mastectomy.

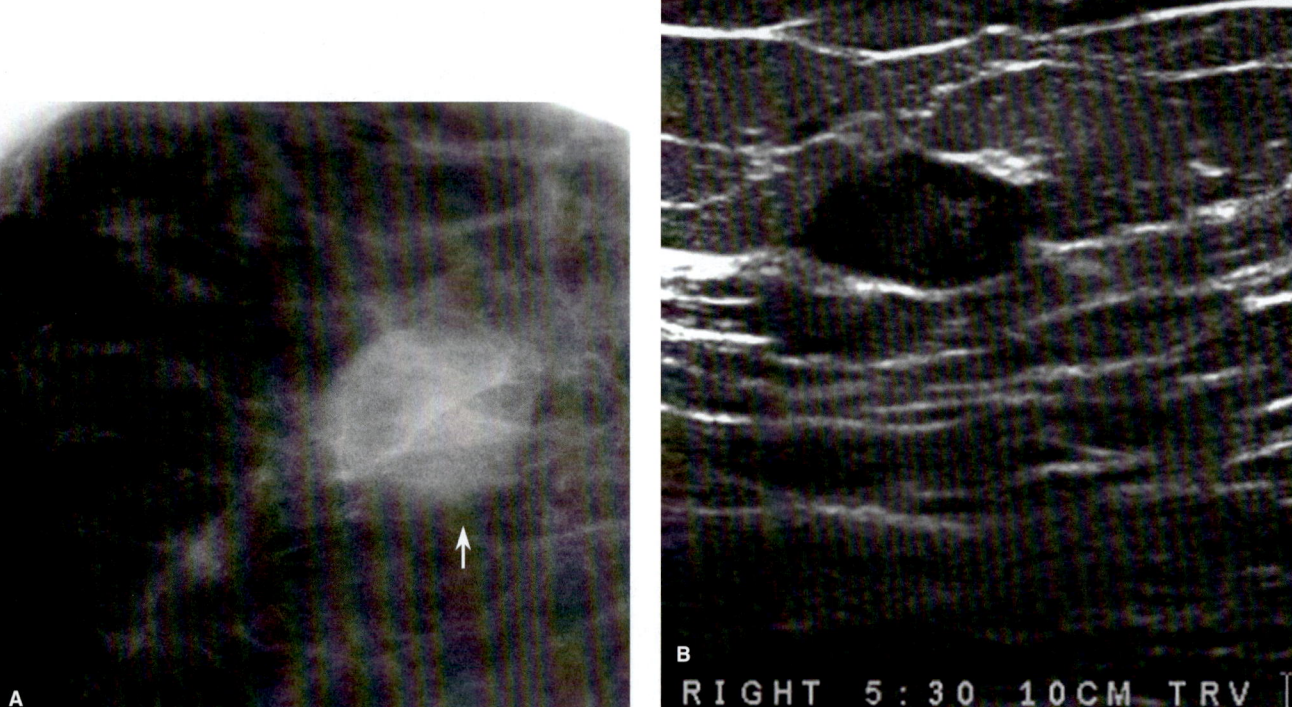

FIG. 7.68 • **Phyllodes tumor, benign. A:** Spot compression view (only one projection shown) of a screen detected mass in a 44-year-old woman demonstrates an isodense round mass with indistinct margins *(arrow)*. **B:** Ultrasound. Oval mass with circumscribed margins is imaged corresponding to the site of the mass detected mammographically. Although a large size used to be a criterion for the diagnosis of phyllodes tumor, with the routine use of screening mammography these lesions are now being diagnosed following detection on screening mammography. A fibroepithelial lesion is reported on the ultrasound-guided core biopsy. Since a phyllodes tumor could not be excluded, an excisional biopsy is done and a low-grade phyllodes tumor is reported on the excisional biopsy.

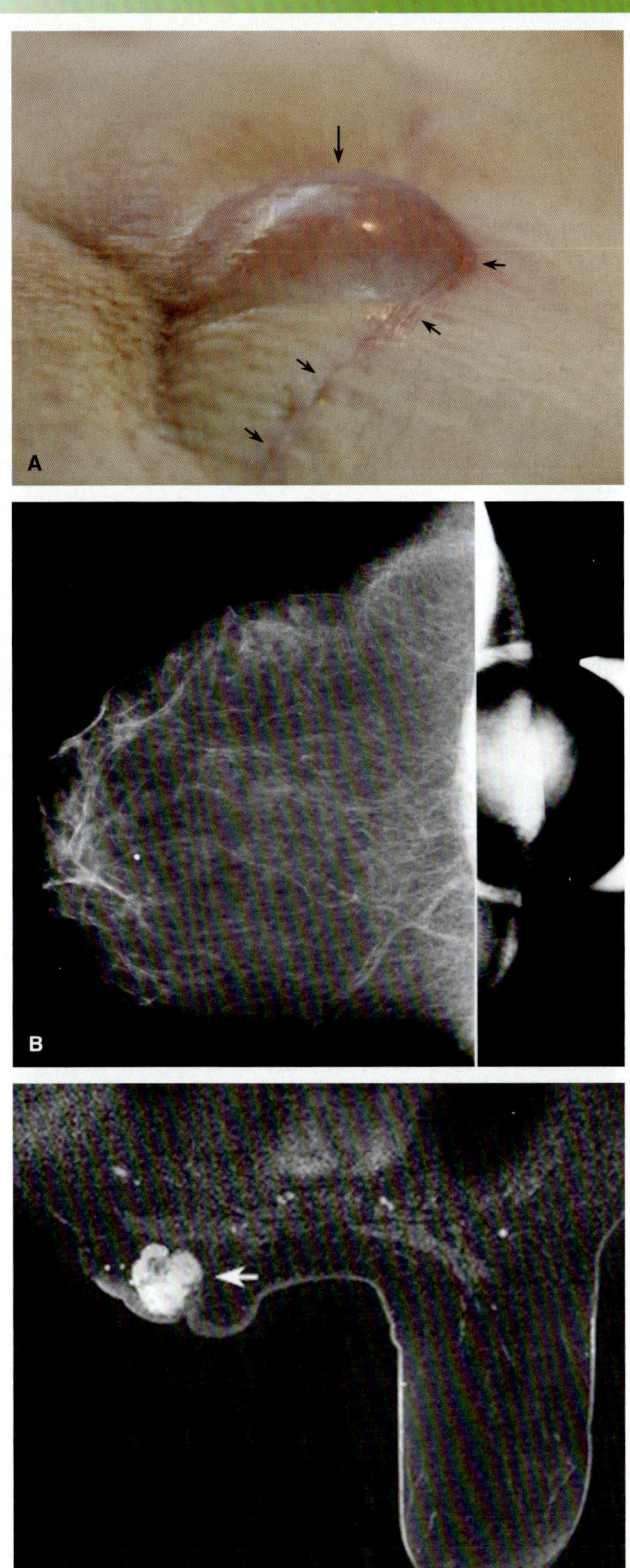

FIG. 7.69 • **Malignant phyllodes tumor, recurrent at mastectomy site. A:** On visual inspection, a protuberant fleshy mass *(long arrow)* with smooth margins is noted associated with the mastectomy scar line *(short arrows)* in a patient who had a mastectomy one year previously for phyllodes tumor (patient images at time of presentation are shown in Fig. 7.67). **B:** Left spot compression view in the CC projection back to back with the right CC view. A dense round mass is imaged at the left mastectomy site. A homogenously hypoechoic mass is imaged on ultrasound (not shown). **C:** Magnetic resonance image, T1 axial postcontrast. A heterogeneously enhancing mass *(arrow)* with lobulation, circumscribed margins, and rapid washin and washout delayed kinetic curves is imaged consistent with local recurrence.

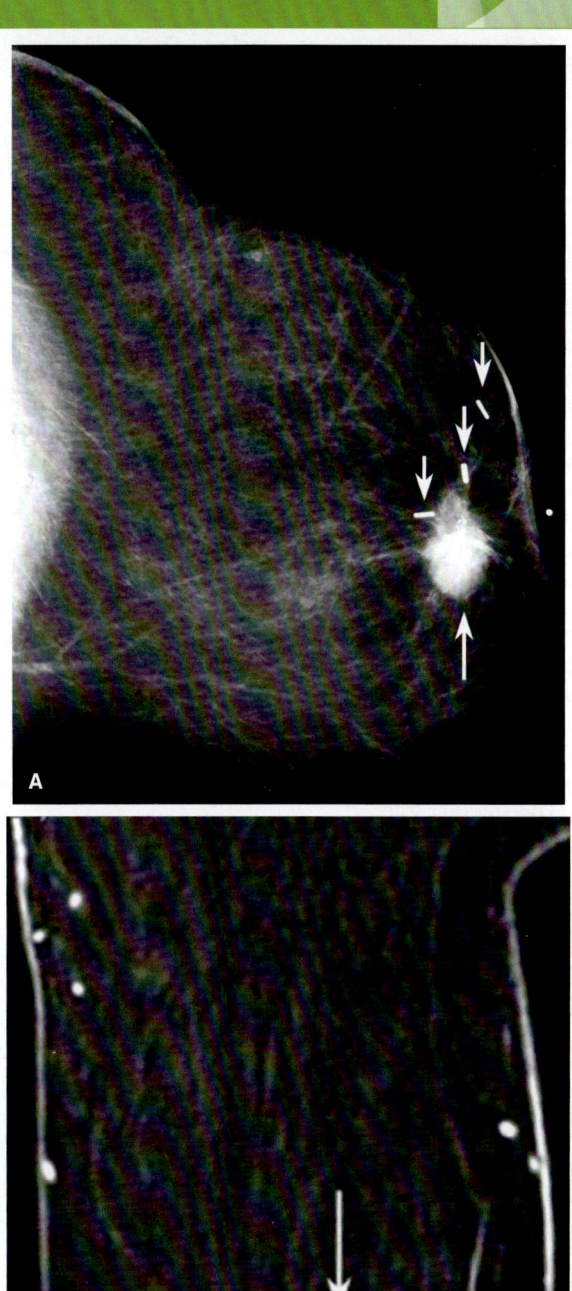

FIG. 7.70 • **Phyllodes tumor, recurrent. A:** Left CC view in a patient who had a lumpectomy with negative margins 6 years previously for a malignant phyllodes tumor with rhabdomyosarcomatous differentiation. A new dense oval mass *(long arrow)* with indistinct and spiculated margins is present at the lumpectomy site. Surgical clips *(small arrows)* are present denoting the lumpectomy site. **B:** MRI, T1 axial image of the left breast postcontrast. The lumpectomy site is characterized by the presence of a non-enhancing mass *(small arrow)* with spiculated margins and central signal void. A rim-enhancing mass *(long arrow)* corresponding to the dense mass seen mammographically is noted arising from the posteromedial margin of the lumpectomy site consistent with a recurrence. A high-grade malignant phyllodes tumor with at least one site of squamous cell carcinoma in situ is reported on the ultrasound-guided core biopsy (not shown).

of phyllodes tumors as benign or malignant have varied. Border characteristics (infiltrative vs. expansile), cellular atypism, mitotic activity and stromal cellularity, and overgrowth are used currently. Defined margins, no cytological atypia, and fewer than five mitoses per high power field characterize benign tumors. Features suggestive of malignancy include microscopically invasive margins, areas of stromal overgrowth, stromal hypercellularity with atypism, and prominent mitotic activity (more than five mitoses per high power field) (11,12,25,42–47). Given the presence of heterologous components (bone, cartilage, smooth muscle, and fat) in the stroma of some phyllodes tumors, a variety of associated sarcomatous lesions have been described, including osteosarcoma, liposarcomas, fibrosarcomas, leiomyosarcomas, and rhabdomyosarcomas (11,12,25,42–47).

Management of these lesions requires complete surgical excision. Mastectomy may be indicated in women with malignant phyllodes. When metastases occur they are hematogenous, and, as such, axillary nodal dissections are not done unless clinically abnormal lymph nodes are palpated. Local recurrences reported in as many as 20% of patients are usually related to incomplete surgical excisions. The role of radiotherapy and systemic therapy remain unclear (48). Recurrences are usually clinically apparent as a mass developing at the lumpectomy or mastectomy site (Fig. 7.69) but may also be detected on follow-up mammograms (Fig. 7.70).

SOLITARY PAPILLOMA

These lesions develop in subsegmental ducts. Women with solitary papillomas commonly present with spontaneous nipple discharge. In these patients, ductography (see Chapter 12) is helpful in establishing the presence, number, and location of lesions (49). Mammographic findings (31–54) in patients with papillomas include a dilated subareolar duct (see Figs. 9.33 and 9.34), round or oval (Fig. 7.71A), less commonly, irregular (Fig. 7.72A) mass with circumscribed, indistinct, obscured (Fig. 7.73A) or spiculated (Fig. 7.74) margins, mass with an associated focally dilated duct (Fig. 7.75), cluster of punctate calcifications (see Fig. 6.42A and 6.45) or coarse, curvilinear ("hollow popcorns") calcifications that may be localized to a dilated duct (see Fig. 9.34).

In patients presenting with nipple discharge, intraductal lesions may be identified on ultrasound, particularly if the lesion is close to the nipple and the duct is dilated (see Fig. 4.17). A complex cystic and solid mass (Fig. 7.71C) is the most common ultrasound finding in patients with papillomas (50–54). These are usually cystic with solid components (see Fig. 4.30 and 4.31) or less commonly, predominantly solid with cystic changes (see Fig. 4.32). In some lesions a duct may be seen extending from the mass toward the nipple and sometimes away from the nipple. If a pneumocystogram is done following aspiration, the lesion can be outlined by air (see Fig. 12.14F). A homogeneously hypoechoic mass indistinguishable from other solid masses may also

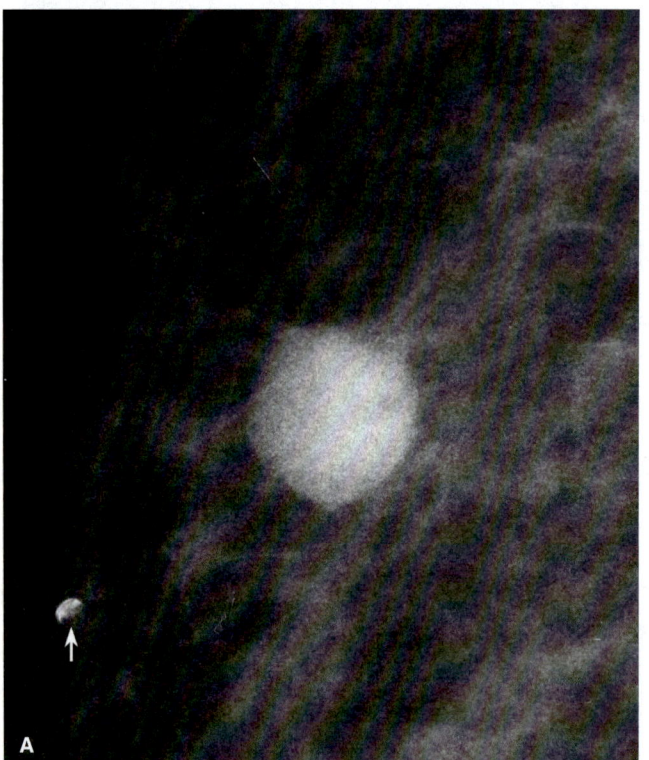
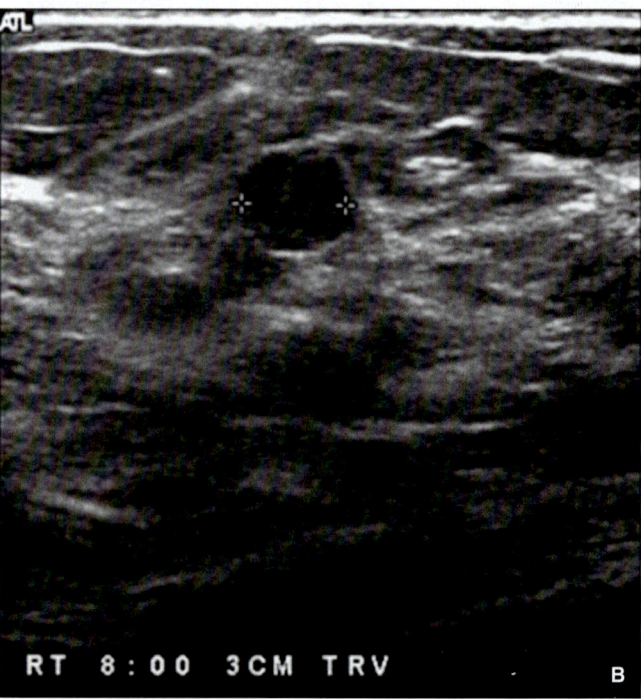

FIG. 7.71 • Papillomas. **A:** Spot compression view, right breast. An isodense, round mass with circumscribed margins is imaged on the spot compression views (only one is shown). A dystrophic-type calcification *(arrow)* is also present on this image. **B:** Ultrasound. A round hypoechoic mass *(calipers)* with circumscribed margins and bright back wall is imaged correlating to the finding seen on the mammogram. Compared with her prior studies, this represents a new finding, and, as such a biopsy is indicated. BI-RADS 4A: Suspicious abnormality, biopsy is indicated. If the patient had no prior studies for comparison, this mass could be followed in 6 months as a BI-RADS 3: probable benign finding; this, provided the patient is comfortable with a plan for follow-up. **C:** Ultrasound. Different patient. Complex cystic and solid mass is imaged corresponding to a dense, round mass with circumscribed margins and a partial halo seen on spot compression views (not shown).

be seen (Fig. 7.76B). Given the cystic component in many of these lesions, it is not surprising that they can fluctuate in size.

On MRI, many of these lesions are masses that demonstrate circumscribed margins and homogeneous enhancement characterized by rapid washin and washout delayed kinetics. Some have components with a high T2 signal (Fig. 7.72C–E) and in others a relationship to ductal structures may be demonstrated (Fig. 7.72E) (51–54).

Papillary lesions of the breast are a diverse group of lesions that include solitary intraductal papillomas and multiple peripheral papillomas, both of which may be further characterized by the presence of atypia or DCIS arising in the papilloma as well as intraductal (intracystic) papillary carcinomas that may or may not be invasive. Accurate classification of these lesions and the determination of invasion in intraductal papillary carcinomas pose a challenge for the pathologist. The absence of myoepithelial cells in a papillary lesion indicates malignancy; however, the presence of these cells does not completely exclude an intraductal papillary carcinoma since myoepithelial cells may be seen sporadically in the fronds of intraductal papillary carcinomas (see Chapter 8 and Fig. 8.38) (11,12,25,55,56).

Papillomas are small friable tumors with an epithelial lining contiguous with that of the duct and therefore characterized by the presence

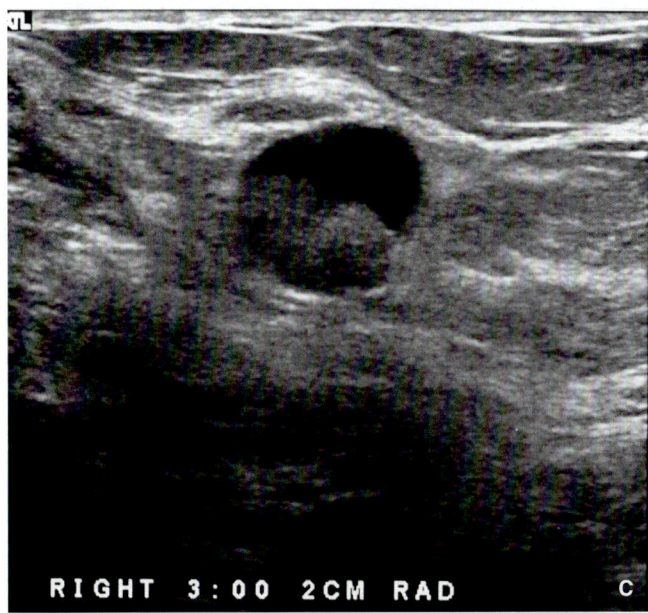

FIG. 7.71 • (continued)

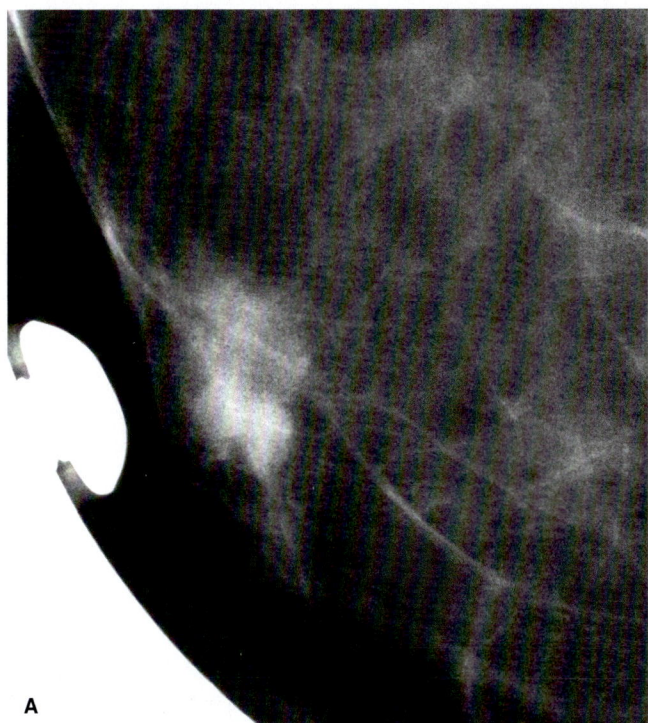

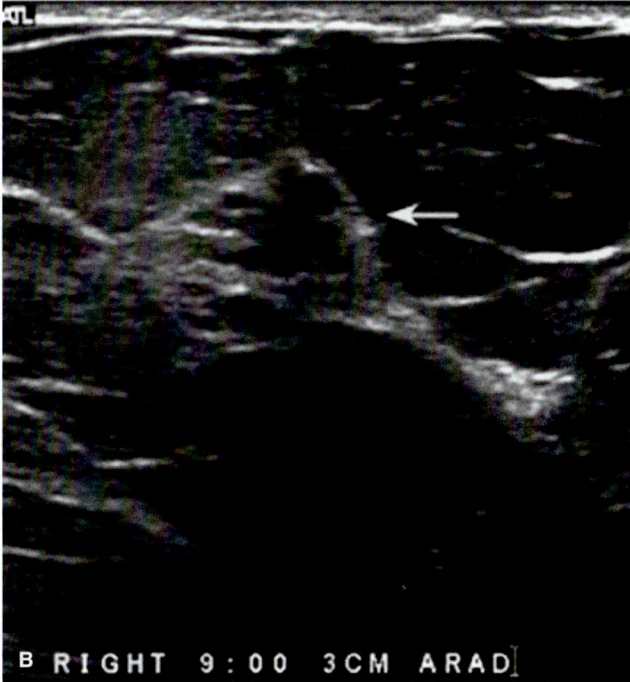

FIG. 7.72 • **Papilloma. A:** Spot compression view of the right breast. An irregular mass with indistinct margins is confirmed at the site of a screen-detected abnormality. **B:** Ultrasound. A lobulated hypoechoic mass *(arrow)* with indistinct margins is imaged on ultrasound correlating to the finding seen on the mammogram. **C:** MRI, T1 axial image of the right breast postcontrast. Irregular mass *(long arrow)* with heterogeneous enhancement characterized by rapid washin and washout kinetic curves medially in the right breast corresponding to the mass seen mammographically. Coil artifact *(short arrow)* is seen posteromedially. **D:** MRI, sagittal T2 fat-suppressed image of right breast. An irregular mass *(short arrow)* with intermediate-to-high T2 signal is noted corresponding to the mass shown in **A**, **B**, and **C**. Coil-related artifact *(long arrow)* is seen inferiorly. **E:** MRI, sagittal T2 fat-suppressed image of left breast in a different patient. A filling defect *(short arrows)* is seen in a dilated fluid-filled (high T2 signal) duct. Coil-related artifact *(long arrow)* is noted inferiorly. On the contrast-enhanced images (not shown), the filling defect enhances with rapid washin and washout kinetic curves. An intraductal mass is seen on ultrasound (not shown) and a papilloma is confirmed on excisional biopsy. Nipple marker (vitamin E tablet) is noted as a round high-T2 signal area anteriorly.

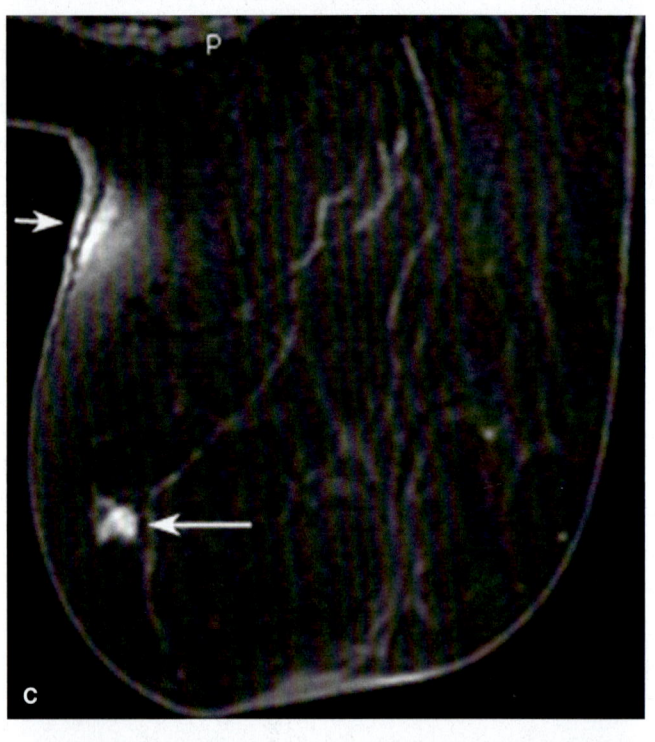
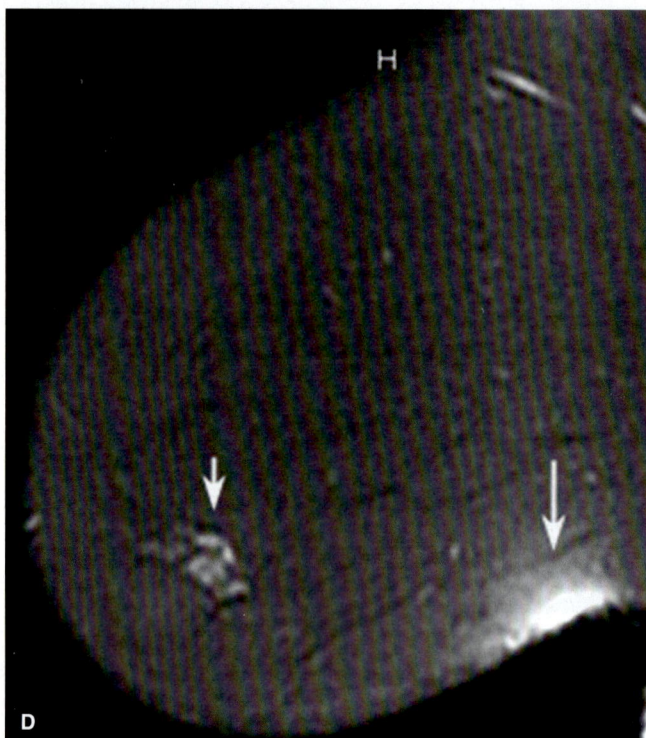
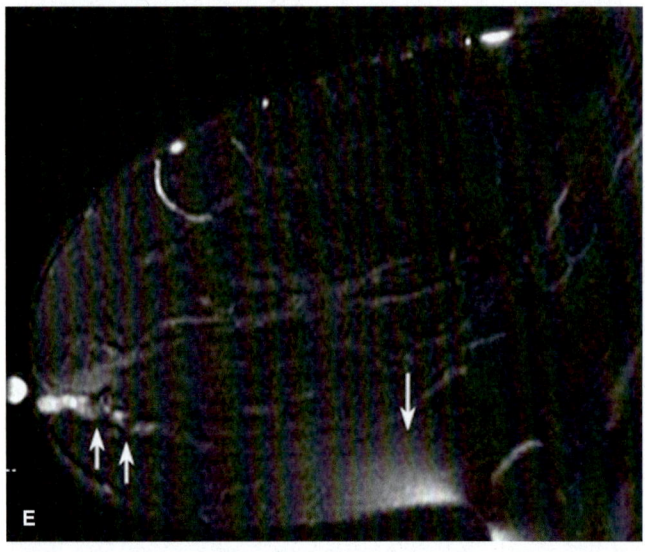

FIG. 7.72 • *(continued)*

of a contiguous layer of epithelial cells and a discontinuous basilar layer of myoepithelial cells. The presence of a central fibrovascular core distinguishes these lesions from epithelial hyperplasia with papillary changes (papillomatosis) (11,12,23,55,56).

MULTIPLE PAPILLOMAS

Multiple papillomas develop in the terminal ducts. Histologically, these lesions are identical to solitary papillomas. Spontaneous nipple discharge is the presenting symptom in approximately 20% of women with multiple peripheral papillomas (50). The other patients are usually asymptomatic with findings detected on screening mammography. A lobulated mass, multiple peripheral masses of varying sizes (Figs. 7.76A and 7.77A), or clusters of punctate calcifications uni- or bilaterally are the mammographic findings in women with peripheral papillomas (31). Multiple solid masses or a combination of intracystic, intraductal, and solid masses may be seen (Figs. 7.76B and 7.77B; also see Figs. 4.31, 4.32 and 4.33) on ultrasound. These lesions are considered as marker lesions in that atypical ductal hyperplasia (ADH), DCIS typically low nuclear grade, lobular neoplasia, and invasive ductal carcinoma, low grade may be found in the tissue surrounding multiple peripheral papillomas in as many as 45% of patients. Given the potential significance of these lesions, if the pathologists you work with use the term papillomatosis, make sure you know how they define the term: for some, papillomatosis is used when describing patients with multiple peripheral papillomas (e.g., lesions having a central fibrovascular core), whereas others use the term when describing papillary hyperplasia (e.g., papillary proliferations with no central fibrovascular core).

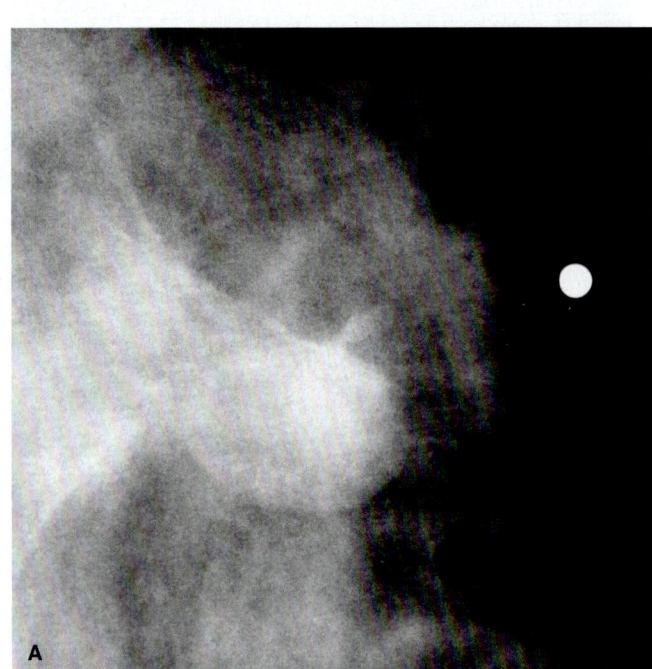
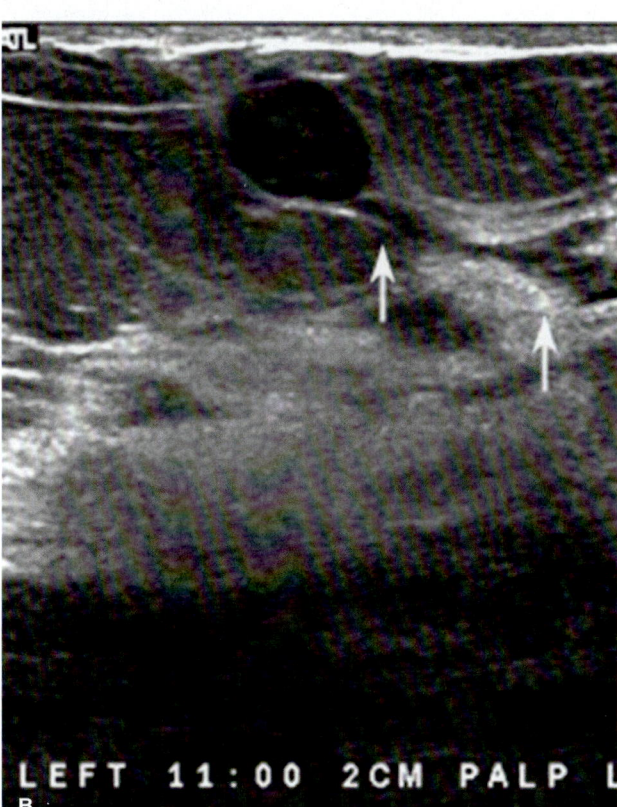

FIG. 7.73 • **Papilloma. A:** Spot tangential view in a patient who presents describing a "lump" in her left breast. An oval, dense mass with circumscribed margins is imaged corresponding to the "lump" described by the patient. Metallic BB used to mark palpable finding. **B:** Ultrasound. An oval mass with circumscribed margins and ductal extension *(arrows)* is imaged corresponding to the clinically and mammographically apparent mass. Although this was thought to be a papilloma, biopsy is done. BI-RADS 4A: Suspicious abnormality, biopsy is indicated.

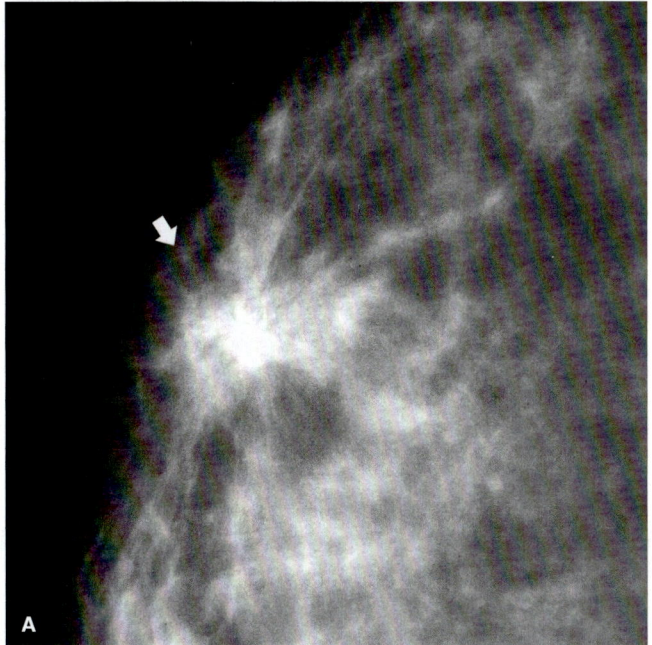
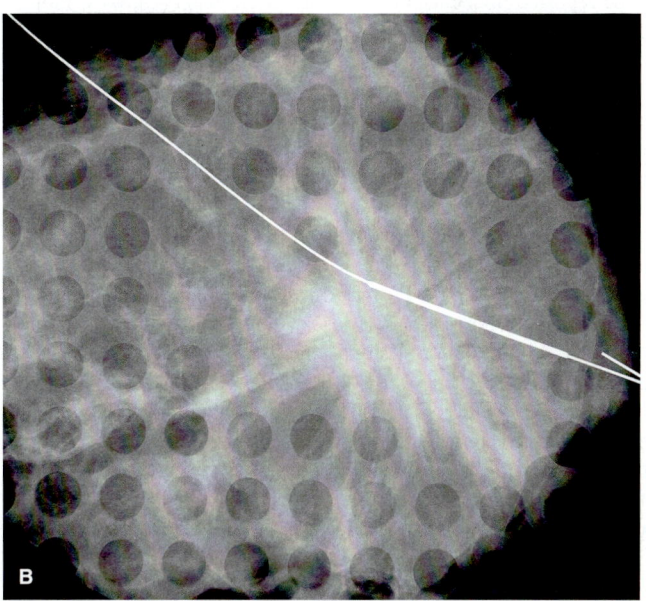

FIG. 7.74 • **Papilloma. A:** Photographically coned image of the right breast. A mass with spiculated margins *(arrow)* is present. BI-RADS 4C: Sclerosing intraductal papilloma with florid hyperplasia is reported on core biopsy. Given a mass with spiculated margins, the pathology on the core biopsy was felt to be incongruent; excisional biopsy is recommended. **B:** Specimen radiograph. Mass with spiculated margins is confirmed in the specimen. A sclerosing papilloma with focal areas of ADH is diagnosed on the excisional biopsy. (From Cardeñosa G. *Breast Imaging [The Core Curriculum Series]*. Philadelphia, PA: Lippincott Williams & Wilkins; 2003.)

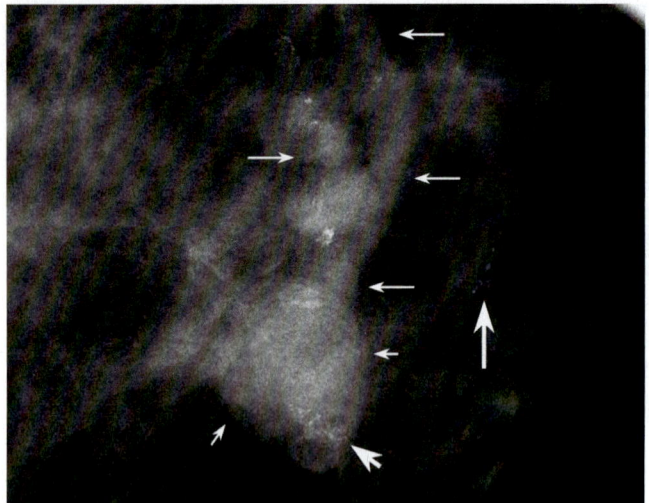

FIG. 7.75 • **Papilloma.** Spot compression view of the left breast. A round mass *(small arrows)* with circumscribed margins, associated ductal structures *(long thin arrows)*, and amorphous calcifications *(short thick arrow)* is imaged corresponding to a screen-detected abnormality. Coarse calcifications are present associated with the ductal structures, and a cluster of round and punctate calcifications is also noted in the tissue adjacent to the mass *(long thick arrow)*; this cluster of calcifications is unchanged from prior studies.

FOCAL FIBROSIS

Clinically, focal fibrosis is usually diagnosed in premenopausal women presenting with a hard, discrete mass on physical examination. Various terms have been used including focal breast fibrosis, breast fibrosis, breast sclerosis, fibrous mastopathy, and fibrous tumor. Theories on pathogenesis include selective hormonal stimulation of the fibroelastic tissue of the breast, a normal involutional change, or the end result of an inflammatory process (12).

The reported incidence of focal fibrosis on imaging-guided biopsies ranges from 2.1% to 15% (57,58). On mammography, an oval or round mass with circumscribed (Fig. 7.78) to partially obscured to indistinct margins (Figs. 7.79) is the most common finding reported in as many as 72% of women diagnosed with this entity. A developing area of asymmetric density, an architectural distortion, or a spiculated mass are less common imaging findings (57–61).

On ultrasound a hypoechoic mass with circumscribed, lobulated, or indistinct margins is the most common finding (Fig. 7.78B). In some patients, the mass is isoechoic or centrally echogenic with a hypoechoic rim (Fig. 7.79B). Posterior acoustic enhancement or shadowing has been reported in 17% to 21% and 14% to 40% of lesions respectively; 44% to 68% of lesions demonstrate neither of these two features (57–60).

The diagnosis of focal fibrosis following an imaging-guided biopsy can be considered congruent with the imaging findings provided targeting of the lesion is accurate and the lesion under question does not have features highly suggestive of malignancy (e.g., spiculation). Repeat core biopsy or excisional biopsy is appropriate for lesions with imaging features highly suggestive of malignancy.

Histologically, there is proliferation of the fibrous stroma with a decrease or obliteration of ductal and lobular elements. This process may be localized to the perilobular or interlobular stroma, or it may involve both. Vascular structures and nerves are sparse, and no perivascular or perilobular inflammatory infiltrate is seen (11). Review of pathology in some patients with an initial diagnosis of stromal fibrosis or fibrous tumors may demonstrate that pseudoangiomatous stromal hyperplasia is a more appropriate diagnosis (62). It is our contention that in

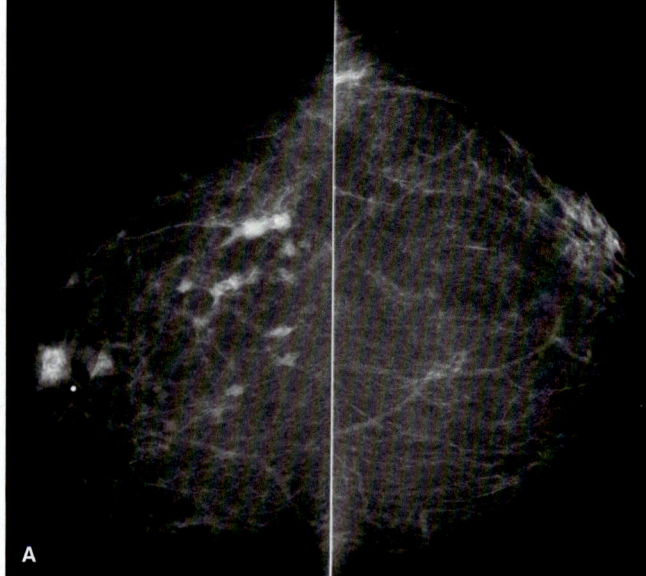

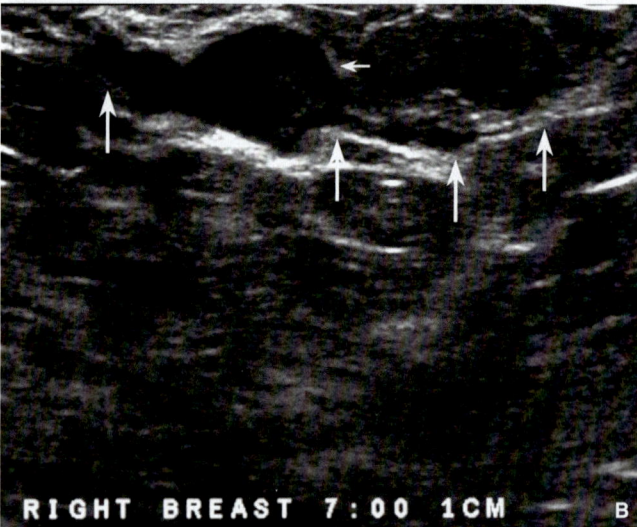

FIG. 7.76 • **Multiple papillomas. A:** CC views in a patient who presents describing a "lump" in the right breast. The metallic BB denotes the location of the palpable finding anteriorly in the right breast. A round high-density mass is imaged corresponding to the palpable finding. Multiple other masses of varying sizes are imaged in the lower central aspect of the right breast extending from the subareolar area to the posterior aspect of the right breast. **B:** Ultrasound. A round mass *(short arrow)* is seen focally distending a ductal structure *(long arrows)*; these findings are consistent with a papillary lesion. This is one of several masses imaged on ultrasound in this patient in the lower central aspect of the right breast. Mammographic and ultrasound findings are consistent with multiple peripheral papillomas.

some patients, areas of focal fibrosis are burned out fibroadenomas lacking the epithelial elements needed for the diagnosis.

DIABETIC MASTOPATHY

This is an uncommon entity usually reported in premenopausal women (63); however, it can also be seen in men (64). Significantly, these patients have a history of long-standing, juvenile-onset insulin-dependent diabetes; at the time of presentation with breast symptoms, many of these patients have other diabetes-related complications, including retinopathy, nephropathy, and neuropathy. This entity has

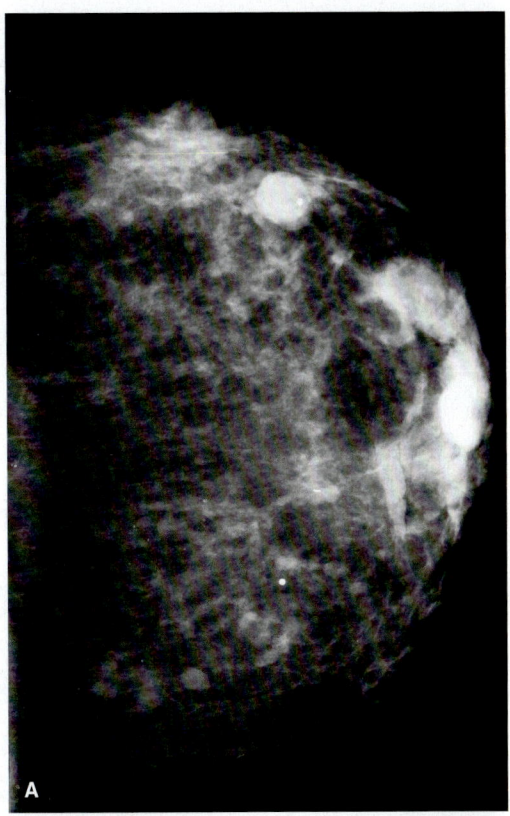
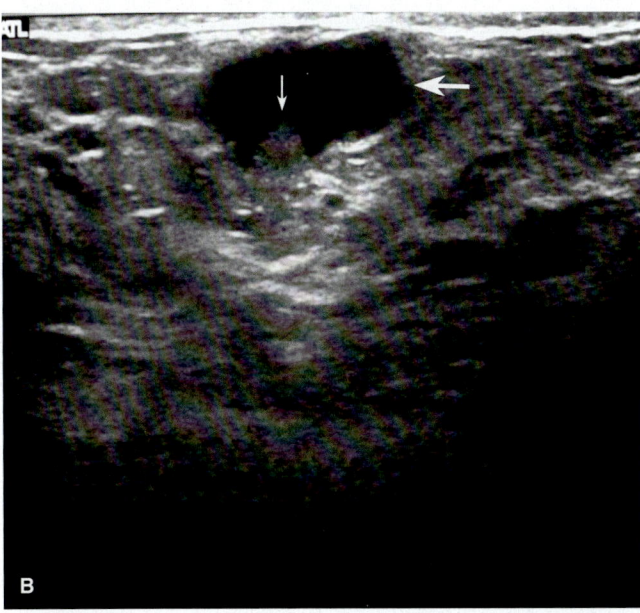
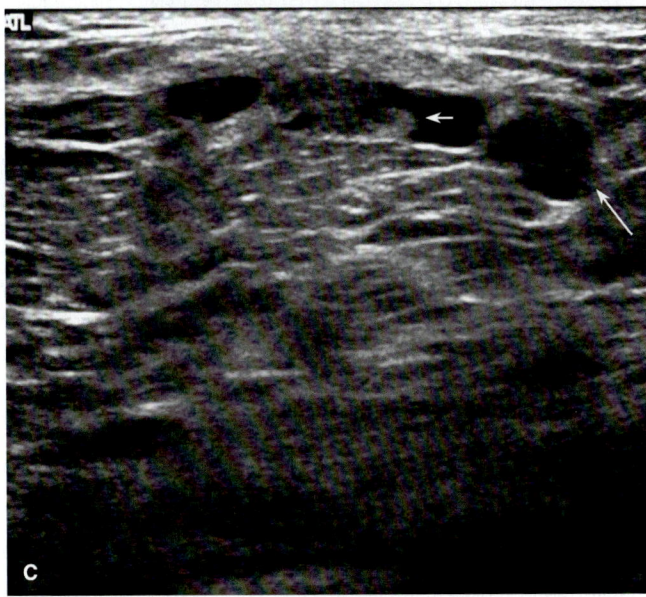

FIG. 7.77 • **Multiple papillomas. A:** Left CC view. Many masses of varying sizes, shapes, and densities are present throughout the left breast. This is a common mammographic presentation for patients with multiple peripheral papillomas. **B:** Ultrasound. Predominantly cystic mass *(large arrow)* with a solid mural nodule *(small arrow)* and posterior acoustic enhancement is one of several different ultrasound appearances for the masses imaged mammographically in this patient. **C:** Ultrasound. In another area of the breast, a dilated duct with an intraductal mass *(short arrow)* and a complex cystic and solid mass *(long arrow)* are imaged. During the real-time portion of the study, this mass could not be connected to the adjacent dilated duct. This patient illustrates the variability in the ultrasound appearance of papillomas.

also been reported in type-2 diabetics and those with thyroid disease. Patients present describing a "lump." On physical examination, firm sometimes ill-defined masses that are mobile and variable are size are palpated in these patients; the mass is not usually tender. Synchronous or metachronous breast lesions are common. This is a self-limited condition that may regress spontaneously.

Reported imaging findings include dense tissue on the mammogram, a mass with obscured or indistinct margins, and intense posterior acoustic shadowing on ultrasound (Fig. 7.80). Although many of these patients are young, vascular calcifications may be present (63). In the appropriate clinical and histological context, core biopsy can reliably establish the diagnosis.

Dense fibrosis characterized by thick bundles of collagen with keloidal features and peri- ductal, lobular, and vascular inflammatory infiltrates are the histological hallmarks of diabetic mastopathy. An autoimmune etiology has been proposed for this condition. It has been suggested that glycosylation and abnormal cross-linking of collagen somehow impedes degradation (11,12).

PSEUDOANGIOMATOUS STROMAL HYPERPLASIA

The clinicopathological spectrum of pseudoangiomatous stromal hyperplasia (PASH) ranges from an incidental microscopic change

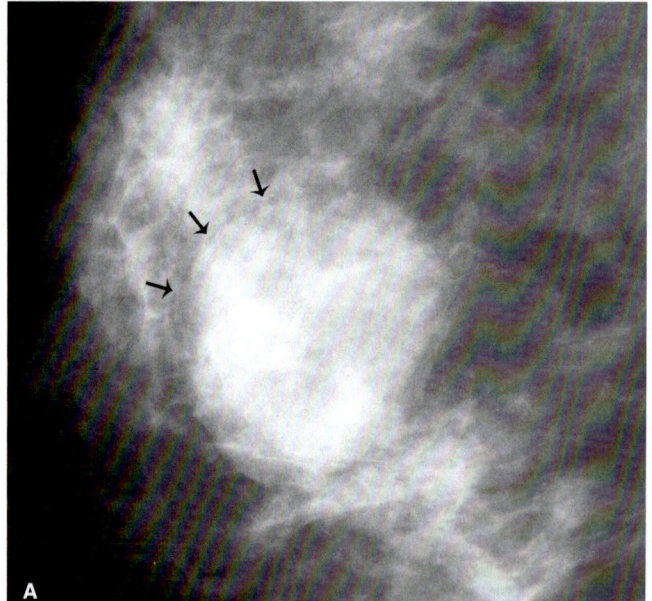

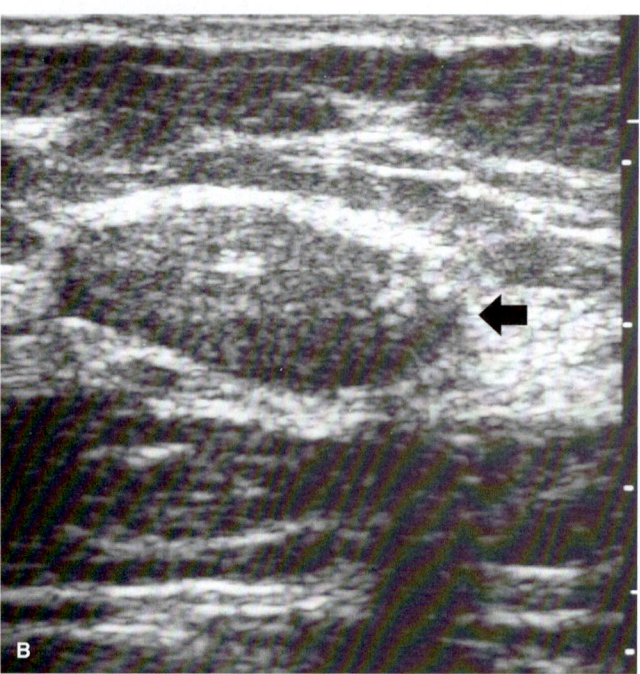

FIG. 7.78 ● **Focal fibrosis. A:** A round isodense mass with circumscribed margins and a partial halo *(arrows)*; screen-detected. **B:** Oval hypoechoic mass *(arrow)* with circumscribed margins and round internal areas of hyperechogenicity. Appearance on mammography and ultrasound simulates that of a fibroadenoma. The assessment category depends on what prior studies show. If this mass is new, or has increased in size, biopsy is indicated. If this mass is stable, no intervention is warranted. If no prior studies are available, and in consultation with the patient, this could be classified as a BI-RADS 3 with follow-up ultrasound done in 6 months to establish stability. (From Cardeñosa G. *Breast Imaging [The Core Curriculum Series]*. Philadelphia, PA: Lippincott Williams & Wilkins; 2003.)

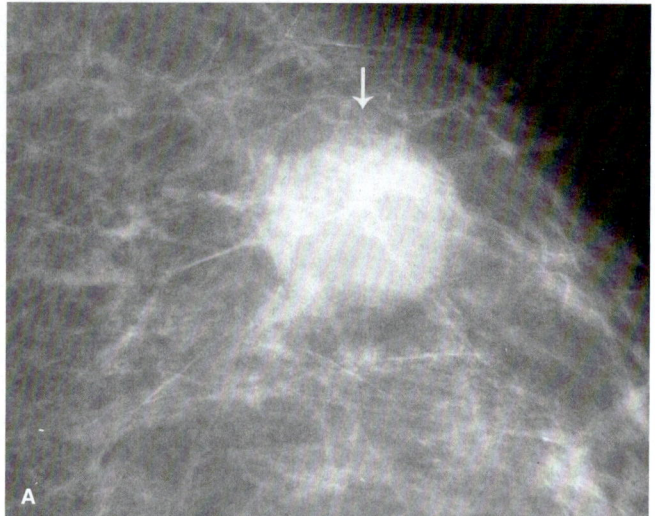

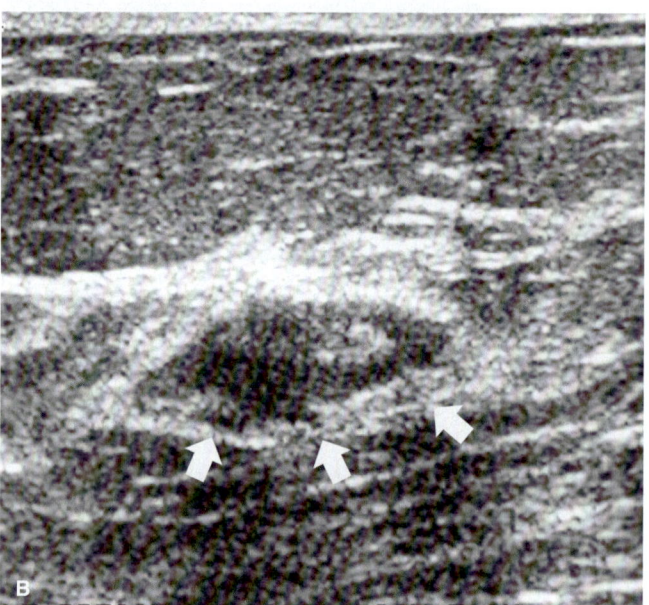

FIG. 7.79 ● **Focal fibrosis. A:** Round isodense mass *(arrow)* with indistinct and spiculated margins. **B:** Ultrasound. Oval hypoechoic mass with associated areas of hyperechogenicity. Margins are irregular and possibly spiculated *(arrows)*. BI-RADS 4B: Suspicious abnormality, biopsy is indicated. (From Cardeñosa G. *Breast Imaging [The Core Curriculum Series]*. Philadelphia, PA: Lippincott Williams & Wilkins; 2003.)

reported as a focal lesion in as many as 23% of breast biopsy specimens to, less commonly, a mass detected mammographically or clinically (65). Multifocality has been reported in as many as 60% of patients (12). Symptomatic patients presenting with a firm, mobile, nontender mass are typically premenopausal or postmenopausal women on hormone replacement therapy. Rarely, PASH can present with asymmetric breast enlargement and tenderness in patients as young as 15 (66) as well as the rapid development of bilateral breast enlargement (67). In males, PASH has been reported as an incidental component of gynecomastia in close to 50% of patients (see Fig. 10.10). These lesions are typically progesterone receptor-positive and estrogen receptor-negative. A hormonal etiology has been suggested as an exaggerated response of myofibroblasts to hormone stimulation, particularly progesterone. This lesion does not increase the risk for subsequent breast cancer (68).

A noncalcified mass with circumscribed to indistinct margins (Figs. 7.81A, 7.82A, and 7.83A) and rarely spiculation is the typical mammographic presentation of PASH. An oval hypoechoic mass with circumscribed (Fig. 7.81B), less commonly, indistinct margins

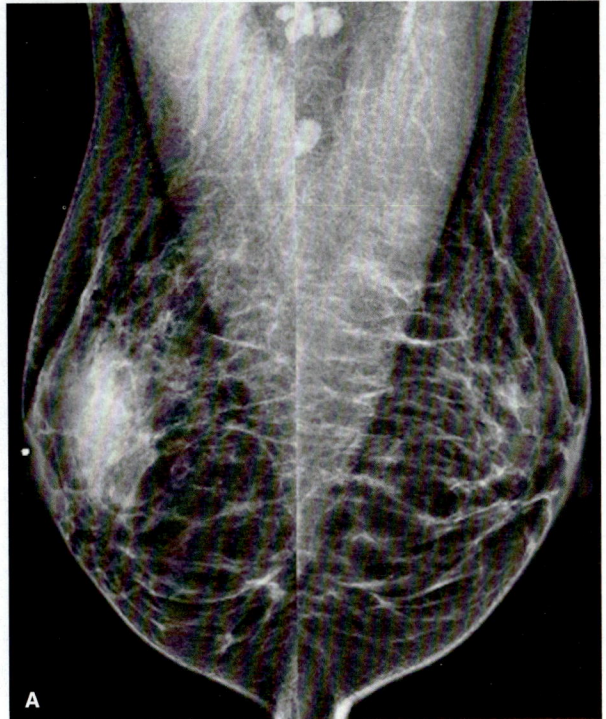
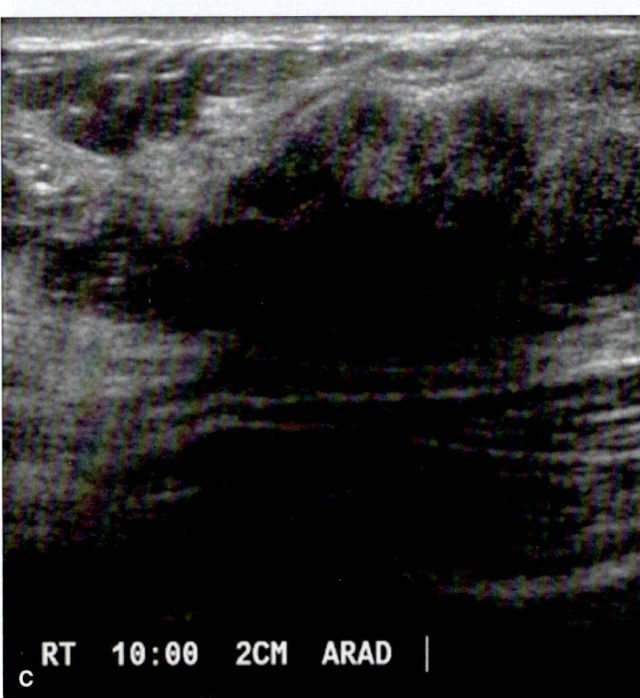
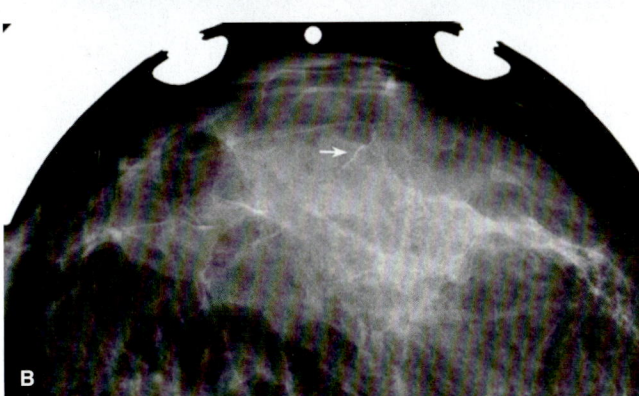

FIG. 7.80 • **Diabetic fibrous mastopathy. A:** MLO views in a 30-year-old patient who presents describing a "lump" detected by her physician. The metallic BB denotes the site of the palpable finding. **B:** Spot tangential view done at the site of the palpable finding confirms the presence of asymmetric glandular tissue with scalloping and gradual transition in density. It is helpful in that arterial calcification *(arrow)* is noted. In a 30-year-old, arterial calcification is unusual unless the patient has diabetes. **C:** Ultrasound. On physical examination, a hard mobile mass is palpated in the right subareolar area. On ultrasound, an irregular mass with shadowing is imaged corresponding to the palpable area. During the ultrasound study, it is confirmed that the patient has been an insulin-dependent diabetic since age 9. BI-RADS 4A: Suspicious abnormality, biopsy is indicated. Diabetic fibrous mastopathy is diagnosed on core biopsy.

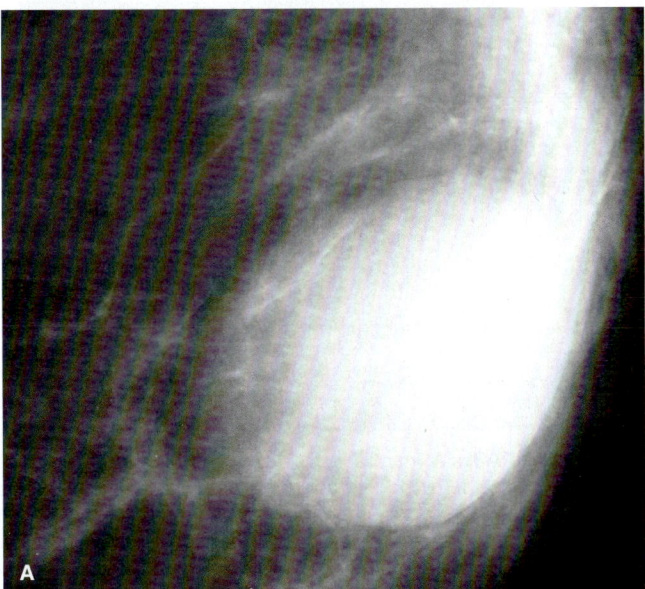
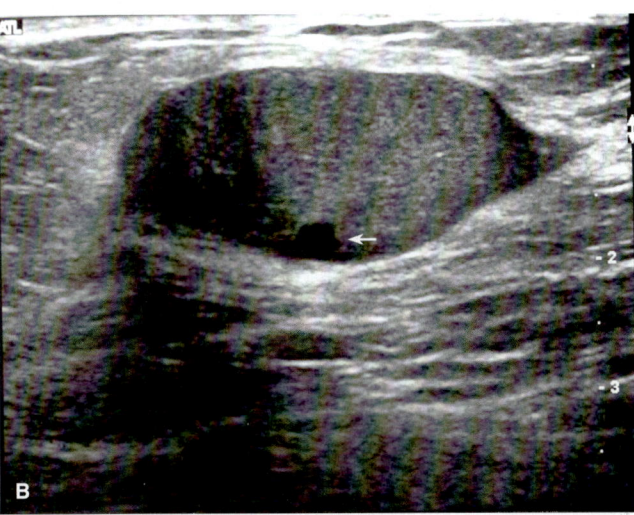

FIG. 7.81 • **PASH. A:** Left CC view, photographically coned to the anterior aspect of the breast. An oval dense mass with circumscribed, indistinct, and obscured margins is imaged medially in the left breast. **B:** Ultrasound. Oval mass with heterogeneous echotexture, circumscribed margins, a cystic component *(arrow)*, and mostly posterior acoustic enhancement is imaged in the left breast corresponding to the mass seen mammographically. Given an increase in size compared with prior studies (not shown), an excisional biopsy is done confirming a diagnosis of PASH obtained previously on needle biopsy.

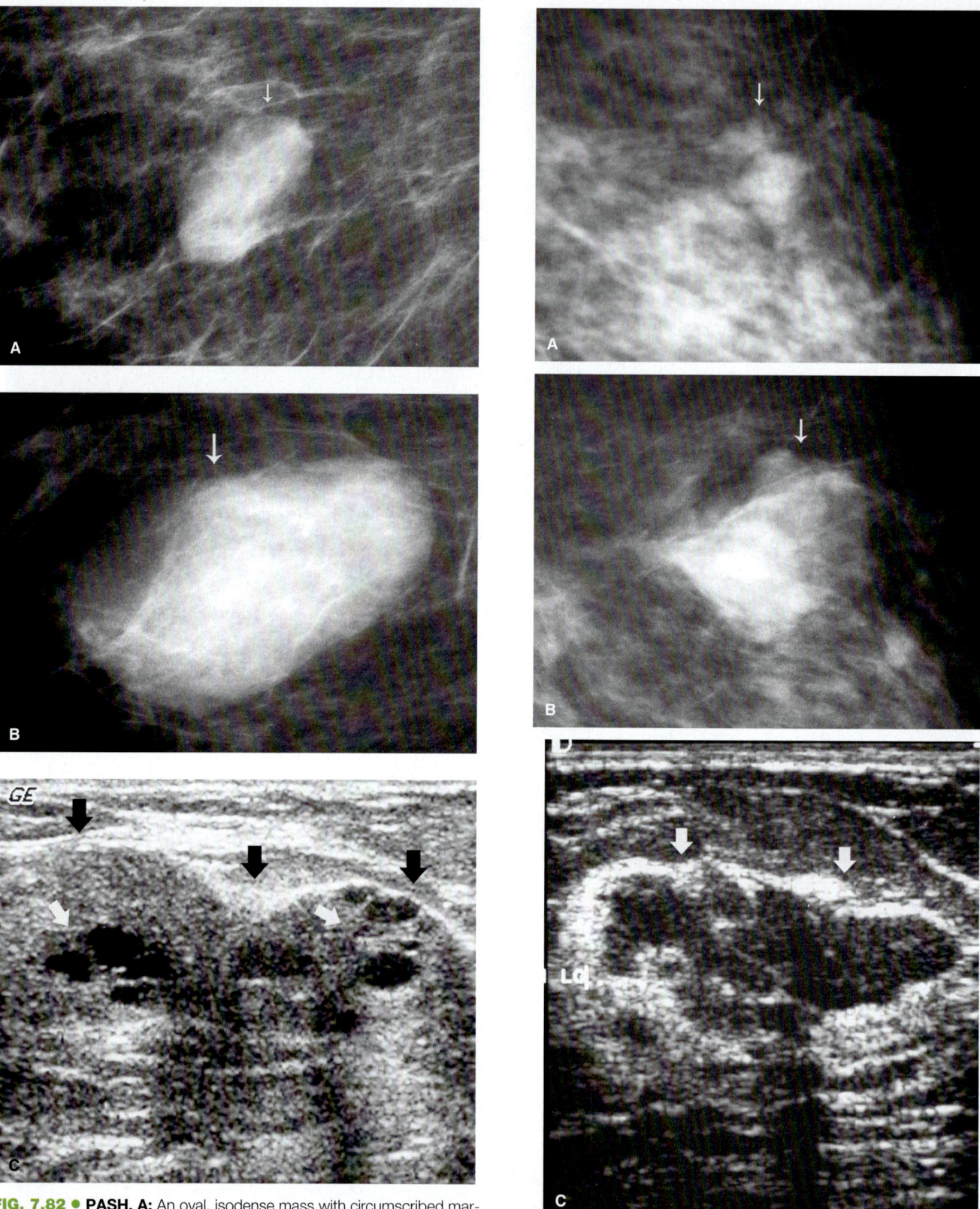

FIG. 7.82 • **PASH. A:** An oval, isodense mass with circumscribed margins *(arrow)*. PASH is diagnosed on needle biopsy. **B:** Three years following needle biopsy: oval isodense mass *(arrow)* with circumscribed mass has increased in size compared with the prior study. **C:** Ultrasound. A macrolobulated mass *(black arrows)* within which two clusters of cystic spaces *(white arrows)* are imaged on ultrasound correlating to the mass seen on the mammogram. PASH is confirmed on excisional biopsy. (From Cardeñosa G. *Breast Imaging [The Core Curriculum Series]*. Philadelphia, PA: Lippincott Williams & Wilkins; 2003.)

FIG. 7.83 • **PASH. A:** Irregular, lobulated mass *(arrow)* in the left breast. PASH is described following wire localization and excisional biopsy. Specimen radiograph (not shown) shows the lesion in the specimen and appropriately localized for the pathologist. **B:** An irregular mass *(arrow)* with indistinct margins is seen 4 years after the excisional biopsy at the prior excisional biopsy site. PASH is diagnosed on core biopsy with features similar to those seen in the biopsy from 4 years previously. **C:** Macrolobulated hypoechoic mass *(arrows)* with fibrous septations and focal areas of shadowing. A hyperechoic rim is seen partially outlining the mass. (From Cardeñosa G. *Breast Imaging [The Core Curriculum Series]*. Philadelphia, PA: Lippincott Williams & Wilkins; 2003.)

is seen on ultrasound; rarely, these lesions are iso to hyperechoic (69–71). Cystic spaces may be seen in the lesion (Figs. 7.81B and 7.82C) as can acoustic enhancement, rarely shadowing. These lesions can enlarge over time (Fig. 7.82) or, less commonly, may recur after excision (Fig. 7.83). A diagnosis of PASH following an imaging-guided biopsy is considered congruent with the imaging findings provided targeting of the lesion is accurate and the lesion under question does not have features highly suggestive of malignancy (e.g., spiculation). Repeat core biopsy or excisional biopsy is appropriate for lesions with imaging features highly suggestive of malignancy. On MRI, these lesions demonstrate variable T1 and T2 signal characteristics. Persistent-type kinetic curves are typical. In patients with diffuse breast enlargement, edematous changes of the parenchyma are seen on T2 images intermingled with progressively enhancing tissue (72,73).

Histologically, PASH may be mistaken rarely for a low-grade angiosarcoma. In PASH, disruption and separation of collagen fibers in the intralobular stroma create a pattern of anastomosing slit-like (capillary-like) spaces that are incompletely lined by spindle myofibroblasts lacking a basement membrane. Mucopolysaccharides occupy the pseudovascular spaces. In angiosarcomas, the lumina are open, lined by endothelial cells, and contain red blood cells. The pleomorphism, mitotic activity, and necrosis reported in angiosarcomas are not seen in PASH. Also, factor VIII, an endothelial specific marker, is not identified in PASH, nor are these lesions cytokeratin positive; however, reactivity for CD34 and muscle actin is seen (11,12,25,66).

COMPLEX SCLEROSING LESIONS (RADIAL SCAR)

The etiology of these lesions is unknown. They are not, however, related to prior trauma or surgery. It has been suggested that complex sclerosing lesions (CSLs) may be related to an inflammatory process or to ischemia and infarction occurring in areas of proliferative change (74). Radial scars are distinctive histological lesions seen commonly by pathologists as an incidental finding in breast tissue. By definition, these lesions measure less than 1 cm in size and are therefore not usually identified on a mammogram. Complex sclerosing lesions have histological features similar to those of radial scars; however, these lesions measure more than 1 cm in size (11,12). These lesions are not as common as radial scars. Most of the lesions detected on a mammogram are larger than 1 cm in size and as such represent CSLs.

When clinical and imaging findings are considered, the presence of a CSL can sometimes be suggested prospectively. Architectural distortion with fat in the center of the lesion and minimal if any central mass formation, long curving spicules, and a differential appearance of the lesion on orthogonal views (e.g., lesion is more evident in one projection compared to the orthogonal view) are the hallmark (Figs. 7.84 and 7.85) (5,75–85) findings of CSLs mammographically. Calcifications may be seen in as many as 37% of patients with CSLs (76). Although these lesions are often 1.5 to 3 cm in size, the physical examination in these patients is usually normal. Invasive ductal carcinomas that measure 1.5 to 3 cm in size are typically palpable, and the palpable abnormality feels larger than the lesion seen mammographically (e.g., the "Leborgne" sign: invasive ductal carcinoma palpate larger than suggested on imaging).

Cohen and Sferlazza (77) reported that radial scars are often seen on ultrasound and have greater conspicuity on ultrasound when compared with mammography. Our own experience with ultrasound in these patients is that it is not as helpful as mammography and physical examination. In our hands, many of these lesions are subtle on ultrasound and when imaged are hypoechoic with variable amounts of

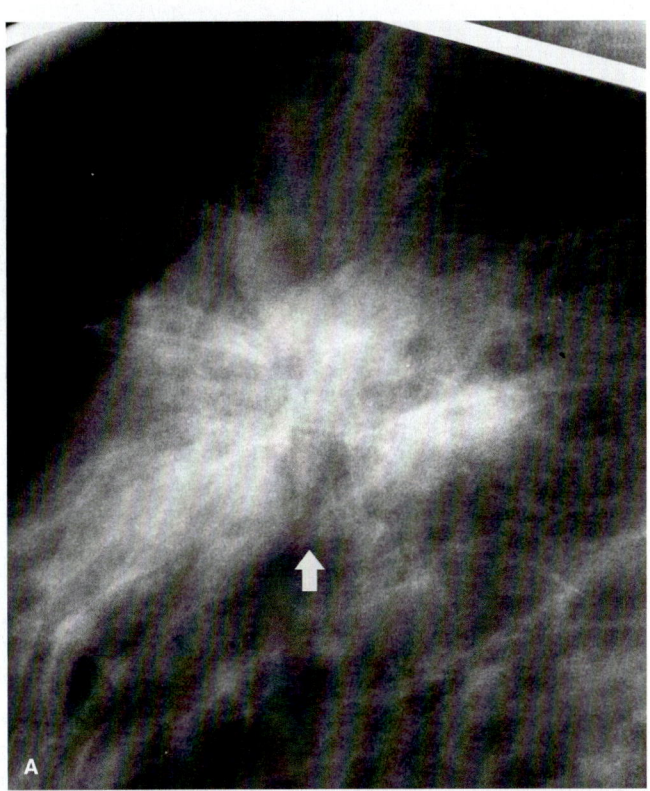

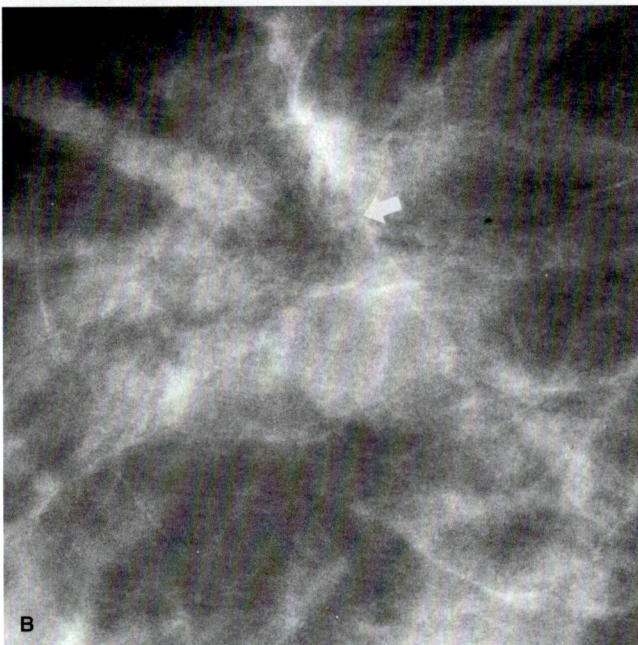

FIG. 7.84 • **CSL. A:** Double spot compression magnification, MLO projection. Distortion with radiolucency centrally and fatty tissue outlining long spicules *(arrow)* is present. **B:** Double spot compression magnification, CC projection. Distortion is less conspicuous but still visible *(arrow)* with central radiolucency and long spicules. BI-RADS 4B: Suspicious abnormality biopsy is indicated. (From Cardeñosa G. *Breast Imaging [The Core Curriculum Series]*. Philadelphia, PA: Lippincott Williams & Wilkins; 2003.)

shadowing (Fig. 7.85C) and may only be seen in one orientation of the transducer and not confirmed easily as the transducer is rotated over the area of concern. The MRI appearance of CSLs is at this time not well-described.

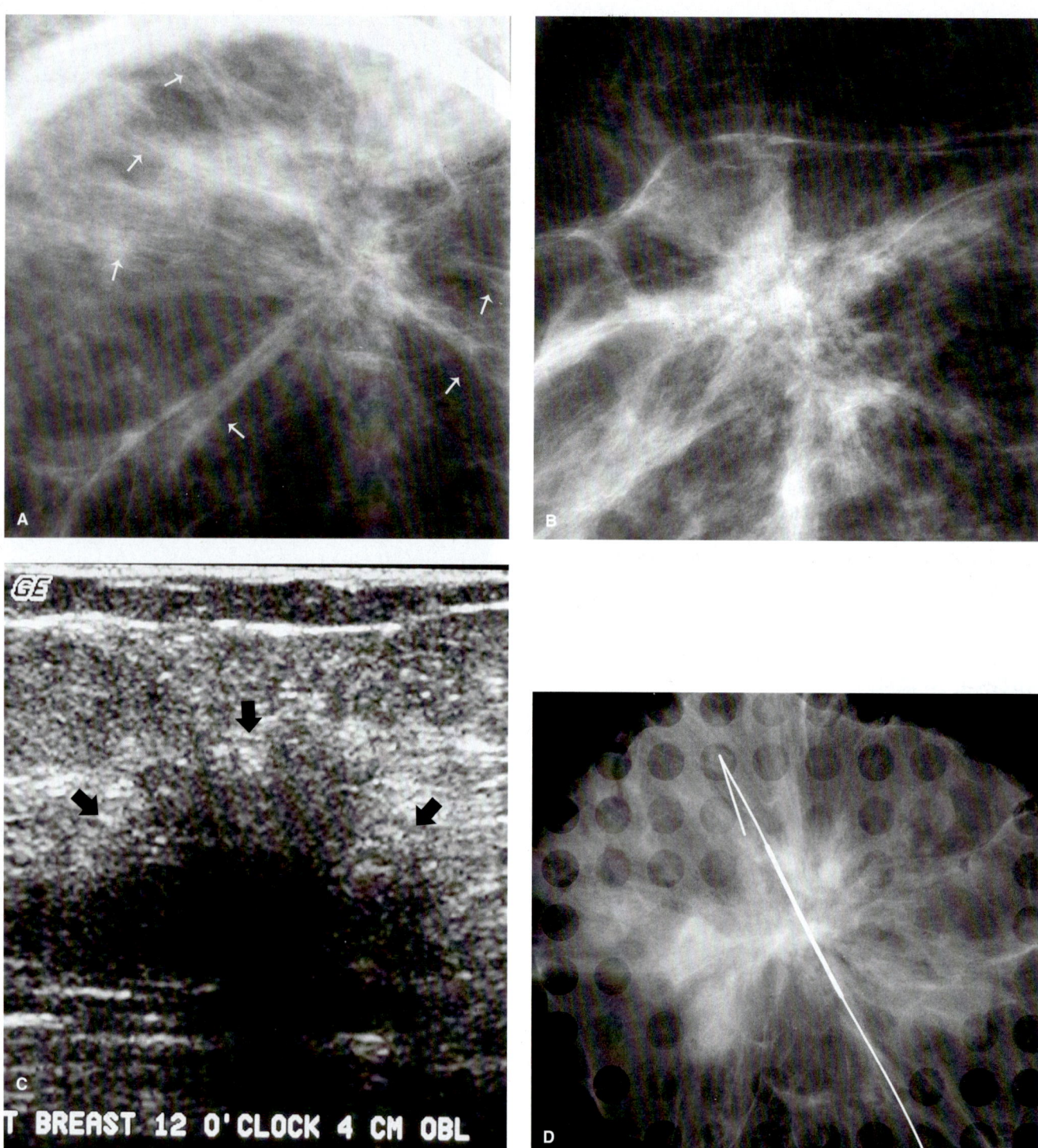

FIG. 7.85 • **CSL. A:** Double spot compression magnification, MLO view. Distortion characterized by central lucency and long spicules *(arrows)* is confirmed. **B:** Double spot compression magnification, CC projection. Distortion with central lucency and long spicules is also imaged in this projection. Notice the differences in the appearance of this lesion on the two projections. These are thought to be planar lesions and therefore more apparent in one projection than the other. **C:** Ultrasound. An irregular mass with indistinct and spiculated margins as well as shadowing *(arrows)* is imaged at the expected location of the lesion. No palpable abnormality is appreciated as the lesion is scanned. **D:** Specimen radiograph demonstrating distortion and long spicules. (From Cardeñosa G. *Breast Imaging [The Core Curriculum Series]*. Philadelphia, PA: Lippincott Williams & Wilkins; 2003.)

The management of CSLs remains controversial (84,85). Some advocate excisional biopsy when a CSL is suspected prospectively on the basis of imaging findings and excisional biopsy following a diagnosis of a CSL on an imaging-guided core biopsy. Others advocate imaging-guided core biopsy of these lesions with no excision required if the lesion is not associated with ADH, the biopsy include at least 12 specimens and when the mammographic findings are reconciled with the histologic findings (84). There are three related issues to consider (83–85): (i) Is the pathologist able to reliably distinguish CSLs from tubular carcinomas (it is also sometimes difficult to distinguish from sclerosing adenosis; however, since this is also a benign lesion, this potential misdiagnosis can be viewed as not significant)? (ii) In a woman with a spiculated mass and distortion, can we accept the diagnosis of radial scar or CSL following core biopsy? (iii) Are these lesions associated with other lesions such as ADH, lobular neoplasia, low nuclear grade DCIS, and tubular carcinomas often enough to warrant excision in all patients? We continue to take a conservative approach to women with a CSL detected mammographically with the findings described earlier, and distinguish these patients from those with incidentally noted radial scars on biopsies done for unrelated findings. If a CSL is suspected on the basis of imaging findings, we are still currently recommending excisional biopsy, and, if we do a core biopsy on a lesion and the diagnosis is a CSL, we recommend excisional biopsy. Approximately 33% of our patients with CSLs are found to have a risk marker lesion (ADH, lobular carcinoma in situ [LCIS], multiple papillomas) or a malignancy (DCIS, low nuclear grade or tubular carcinoma) at the time of excision.

SCLEROSING ADENOSIS

Most women with sclerosing adenosis are asymptomatic with a cluster of either round and punctate or amorphous calcifications detected on a screening mammogram. Rarely, sclerosing adenosis can present with a clinically or mammographically detected mass (Fig. 7.86).

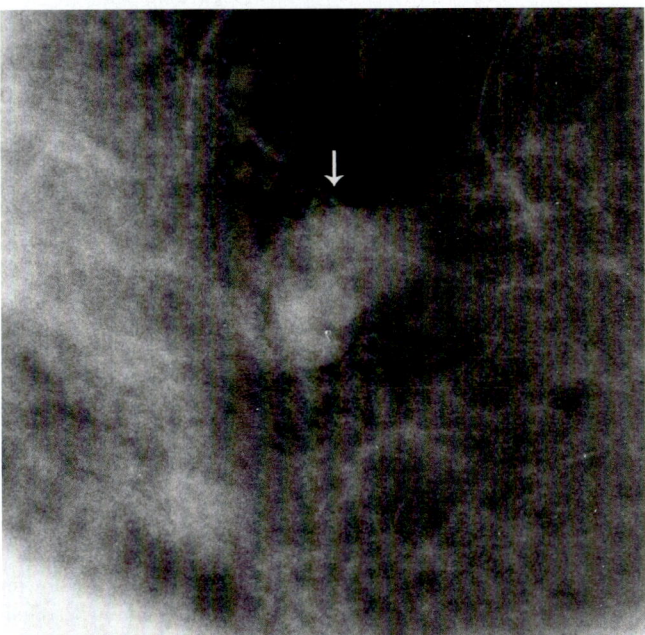

FIG. 7.86 • **Sclerosing adenosis.** Oval, low-density mass *(arrow)* with partially circumscribed margins detected on a screening mammography. (From Cardeñosa G. *Breast Imaging [The Core Curriculum Series]*. Philadelphia, PA: Lippincott Williams & Wilkins; 2003.)

The masses can be round to irregular, with circumscribed to spiculated margins mammographically; associated distortion or calcifications may be seen.

This is a lobulocentric lesion characterized by the proliferation of acini and surrounding intralobular stroma. The acinar spaces can be compressed and elongated by the proliferating stroma. These lesions can sometimes be mistaken for tubular carcinomas. In sclerosing adenosis the lumens of the glands are flattened or elongated, and there is a two-cell layer (epithelium and myoepithelium) lining the acini. In contrast, the glands in tubular carcinomas are round, uniform, and angulated and no myoepithelial cells are seen lining the proliferating glands (11,12,25).

EXTRA-ABDOMINAL DESMOID (FIBROMATOSIS)

These are rare benign stromal tumors representing less than 0.2% of all breast tumors (11,12). Though most commonly reported in women, they have also been reported in men. They occur sporadically but have been reported associated with Gardner syndrome, as well as following trauma or surgery (breast reduction, augmentation) in other patients. Fibromatosis in the breast does not appear to be related to pregnancy (unlike the reported association of abdominal desmoids and pregnancy). These tumors are benign but can be locally aggressive lesions, and, as such, wide surgical excision is considered the primary line of therapy. In approximately 20% of patients, fibromatosis recurs locally within the first 5 years. Radiation therapy, as an alternative therapy, reportedly increases the likelihood of local control and has been used to treat recurrent lesions. Some reports are emerging describing systematic therapy. Interestingly, although these lesions are typically ER/PR-negative, antiestrogens (tamoxifen) alone or in combination with nonsteroidal inflammatory agents have been used with some regression reported in size (86).

Patients can present with a palpable mass that may cause skin dimpling or retraction. A round, oval, or irregular mass with indistinct or spiculated margins (Fig. 787A) that may be close to the pectoral muscle is seen on the mammogram; rarely the lesion presents as an area of distortion (87). A hypoechoic mass (Figs. 7.87B and 7.88A) with variable amounts of shadowing is seen on ultrasound (88). Imaging features on MRI are nonspecific (87,89). They are variable in T2 signal, reflecting myxoid (high T2) and fibrotic (low T2 signal) areas. Fibromatosis commonly demonstrates a benign progressive pattern of enhancement (Fig. 7.88B) in some patients; however, they can have rapid washin and washout or plateau-type kinetic curves. MRI is particularly helpful in establishing pectoral muscle and chest wall invasion. Histologically, spindle cells (fibroblasts and myofibroblasts) and collagen infiltrate the stroma; the spindle cells show no nuclear pleomorphism or mitotic activity.

GRANULAR CELL TUMORS

Granular cell tumors (GCTs) most commonly arise in the head, neck, and tongue, but can present in the breast in approximately 5% of patients (90–93). Less than 1% of all of these tumors are malignant. They are thought to be of peripheral nerve, Schwann cell origin (11,12). In the breast they are almost always diagnosed in premenopausal women but have also been reported in men. They have a predilection for the upper inner quadrant of the breast (possibly related to the cutaneous sensory territory of the supraclavicular nerve) and can involve skin, subcutaneous tissue, and the pectoral fascia (90–93). Multifocality has been reported in some patients. The treatment of choice for these

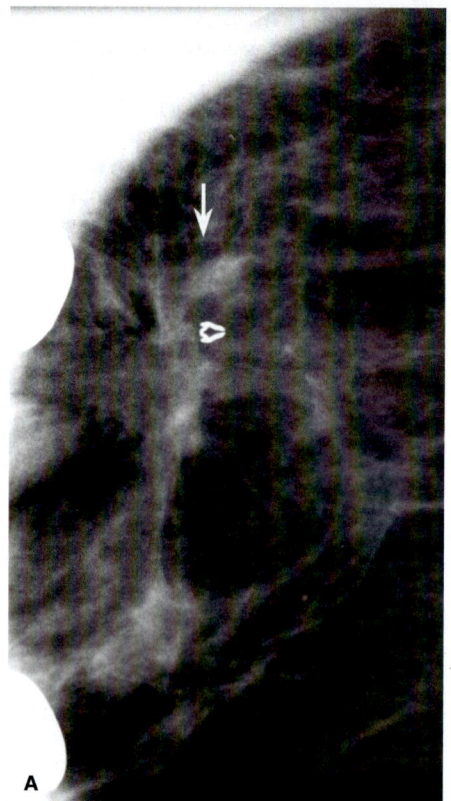

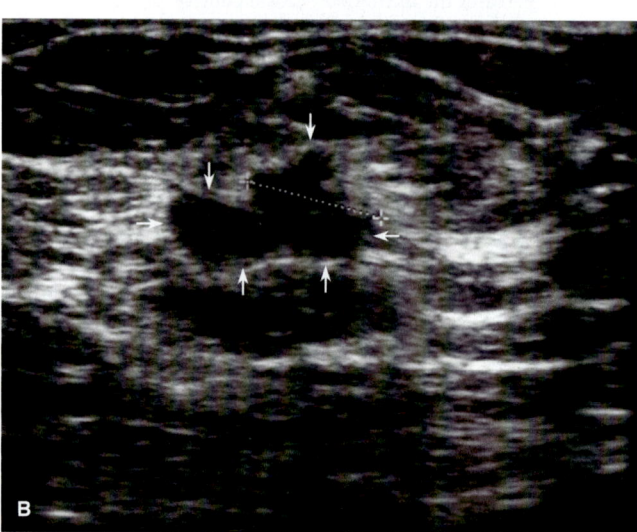

FIG. 7.87 • **Extra-abdominal desmoid (fibromatosis). A:** Spot compression view, left breast. A low-density mass *(arrow)* with spiculated margins and associated distortion is imaged; a biopsy clip is present. **B:** Ultrasound. An irregular mass *(arrows)* with angular margins and no posterior acoustic features (e.g., no enhancement or shadowing) is imaged in the left breast corresponding to the finding on the mammogram.

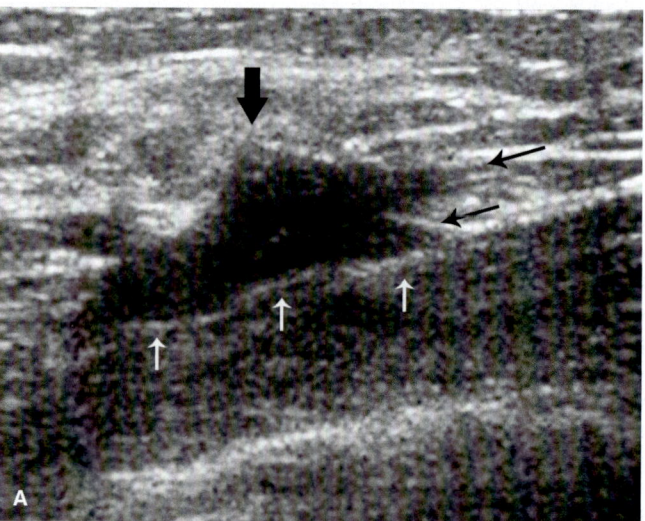

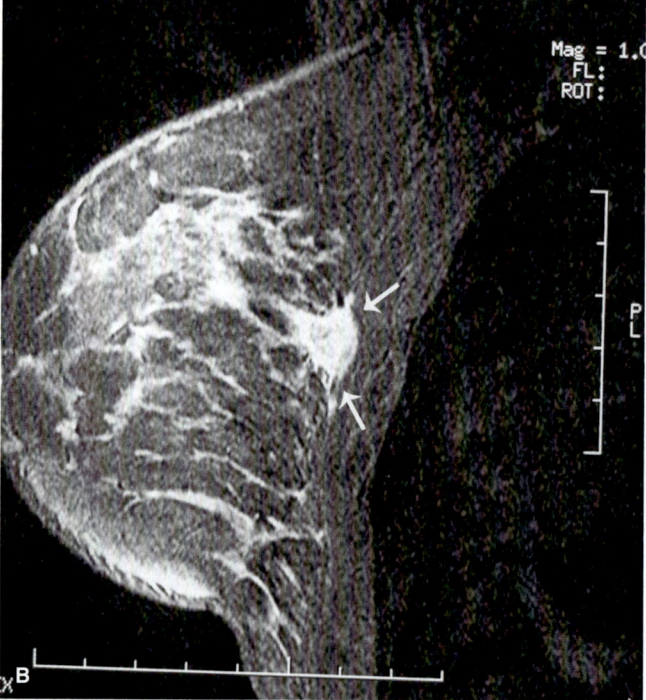

FIG. 7.88 • **Extra-abdominal desmoid (fibromatosis). A:** Ultrasound. An irregular mass *(thick black arrow)* with spiculation *(thin black arrows)* abutting the deep pectoral fascia *(white arrows)* is imaged corresponding to a tender palpable mass in a 23-year-old patient. Dense glandular tissue with no discrete lesion is seen on the spot tangential view (not shown). **B:** MRI, T1 sagittal image postcontrast. Irregular mass with heterogeneous enhancement and spiculated margins abutting the pectoral muscle *(arrows)* is imaged corresponding to the clinical and ultrasound finding. Wide local excisions are critical in reducing the likelihood of local recurrences. (From Cardeñosa G. Breast Imaging [The Core Curriculum Series]. Philadelphia, PA: Lippincott Williams & Wilkins; 2003.)

lesions is wide surgical excision, particularly since local recurrences have been described following incomplete resections.

Patients can present with a palpable mass, and if in the subcutaneous tissue, skin dimpling. Irregular, round, or oval masses with circumscribed, indistinct (Fig. 7.89), or spiculated (Fig. 7.90) margins are seen mammographically (92). Calcifications are not typically seen. On ultrasound, these lesions are variable in appearance, including hypoechoic masses with variable amounts of shadowing as well as masses with a heterogeneous echo pattern and hyperechoic rims (90,92). Magnetic resonance imaging in these lesions is particularly helpful in assessing the extent of disease as well as in the evaluation of the contralateral breast. Although there are scattered reports of the MRI appearance of these lesions in the breast (91,93), GCTs in other body parts demonstrate variable T2 signal (ranging from low to

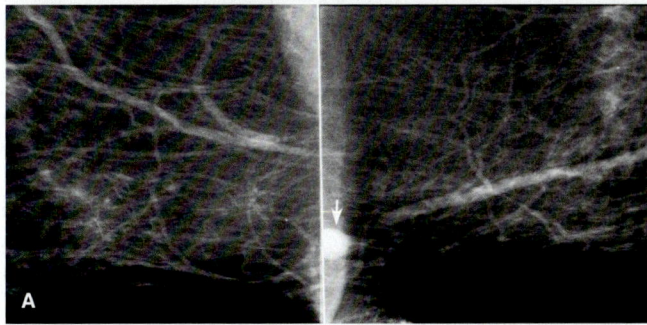

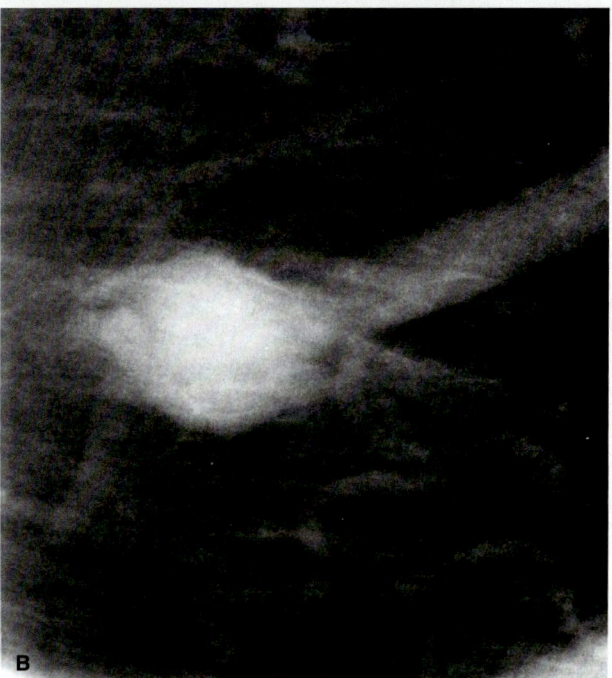

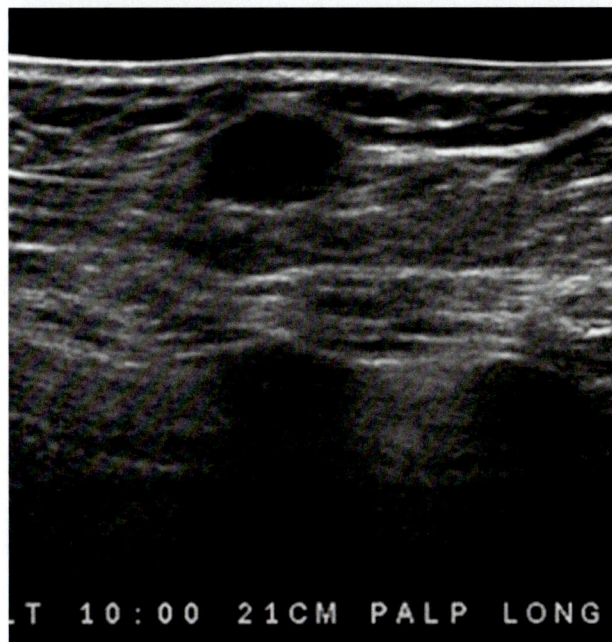

FIG. 7.89 • **Granular cell tumor. A:** CC views photographically coned to the posteromedial tissue. A dense mass *(arrow)* is partially imaged posteriorly on the left CC view, seemingly superimposed on the pectoral muscle. BI-RADS 0: Need additional imaging evaluation. The patient is called back. **B:** Spot compression view of the left breast, CC projection (spot in MLO projection is not shown). A dense round mass with indistinct margins is confirmed in the upper inner quadrant of the left breast separate from the pectoral muscle on the spot views. **C:** A round mass with indistinct margins and no posterior acoustic features (e.g., no enhancement or shadowing) is imaged corresponding to the mammographic finding. During the ultrasound, the mass could be palpated easily. BI-RADS 4B: Suspicious finding, biopsy is indicated.

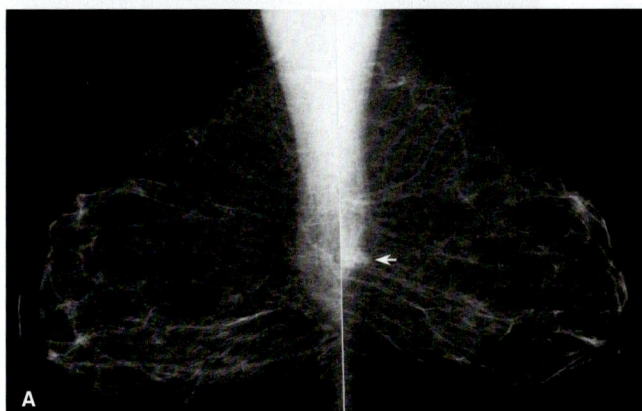

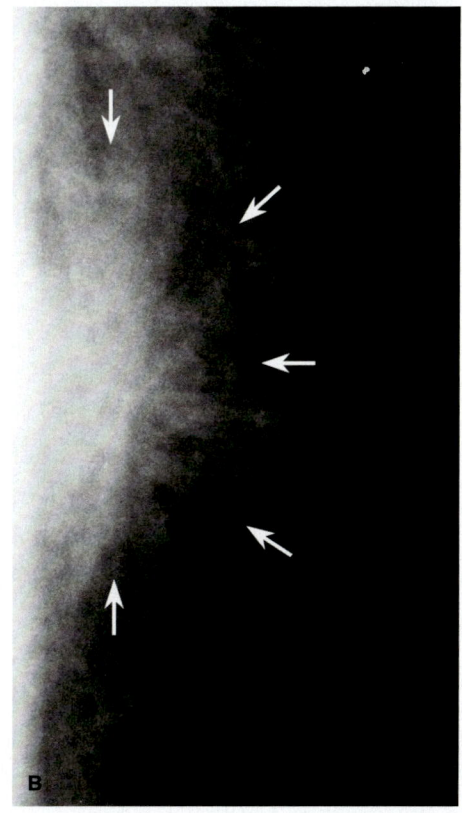

FIG. 7.90 • **Granular cell tumor. A:** MLO views, screening study. A possible mass *(arrow)* with spiculated margins is imaged at the edge of the left pectoral muscle. A similar finding could be seen on the CC view posteromedially (not shown). BI-RADS 0: Need additional imaging evaluation. The patient is called back. **B:** Spot compression view, MLO projection. A mass *(arrows)* with spiculated margins is partially imaged on the spot compression views (spot in CC projection is not shown). **C:** MRI, axial T2-weighted image. Mass *(arrow)* with spiculated margins and low T2 signal is imaged embedded in the left pectoral muscle. Incidentally noted is a small amount of pleural fluid on the right. **D:** MRI, sagittal T1 reconstruction of the left breast postcontrast. Mass with heterogeneous enhancement and spiculated margins is imaged in the lower aspect of the left pectoral muscle anteriorly correlating with mammographic findings. **E:** Pathology demonstrates cells with eosinophilic granules in the cytoplasm surrounded by skeletal muscle.

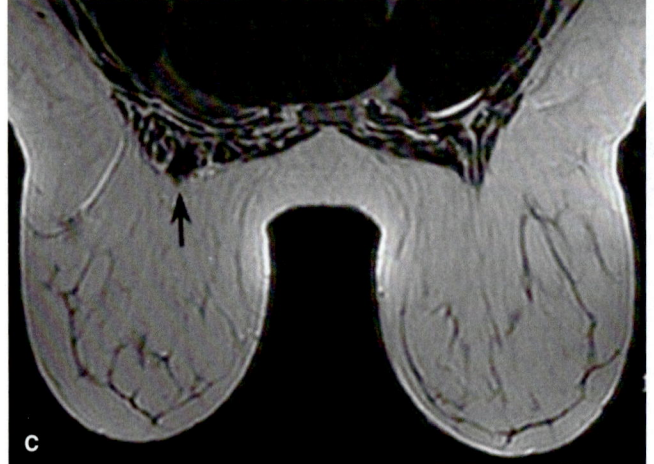

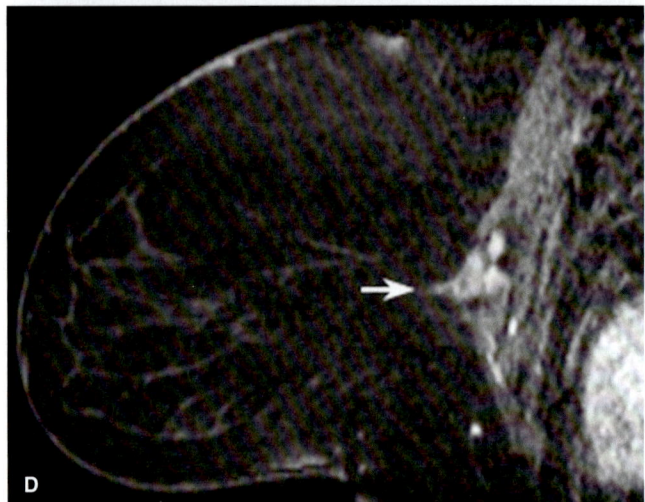

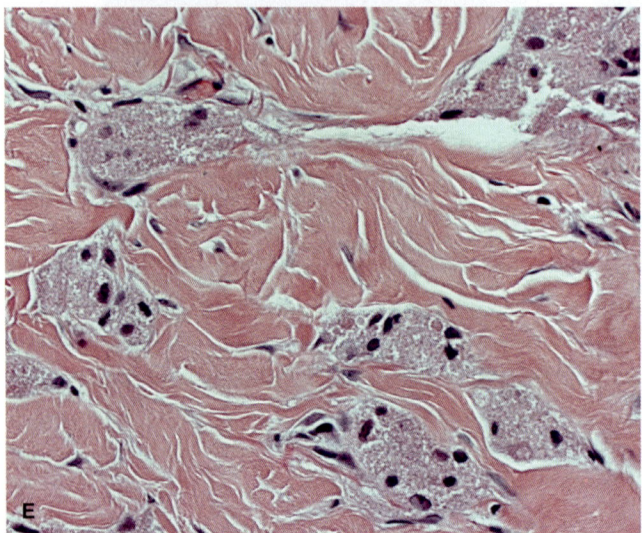

FIG. 7.90 • *(continued)*

high) and low-to-intermediate T1 signal. Rim enhancement may be seen and plateau- or persistent-type kinetic curves may predominate.

Histologically, compact polygonal cells containing abundant eosinophilic granules in the cytoplasm characterize granular tumors (Fig. 7.90E); the granules are periodic acid–Schiff positive, diastase resistant (11,12). These cells show no epithelial markers, are ER/PR-negative, and contain no mucin. They stain positive for S100, CD68, carcinoembryonic antigen (CEA), and are reactive for vimentin (12). Peripherally, focal areas of a lymphoplasmacytic infiltration and rarely nerve bundles may be seen. Although most of these tumors are well defined and localized, a more infiltrative pattern may be seen.

BENIGN VASCULAR LESIONS

A variety of benign vascular lesions may be seen arising in breast tissue. These include hemangiomas (perilobular, cavernous, capillary), angiomas, and venous hemangiomas. A round or oval mass (Figs. 7.91 and 7.92) is the most common finding mammographically; in some patients, punctate calcifications in isolation of a mass may be seen. On ultrasound the masses may be hyperechoic or contain hyperechoic foci within them. Histologically, the differentiation of these lesions from angiosarcomas is critical and may be difficult to establish on core samples. Excisional biopsy and evaluation of the entire lesion is indicated in most patients (12).

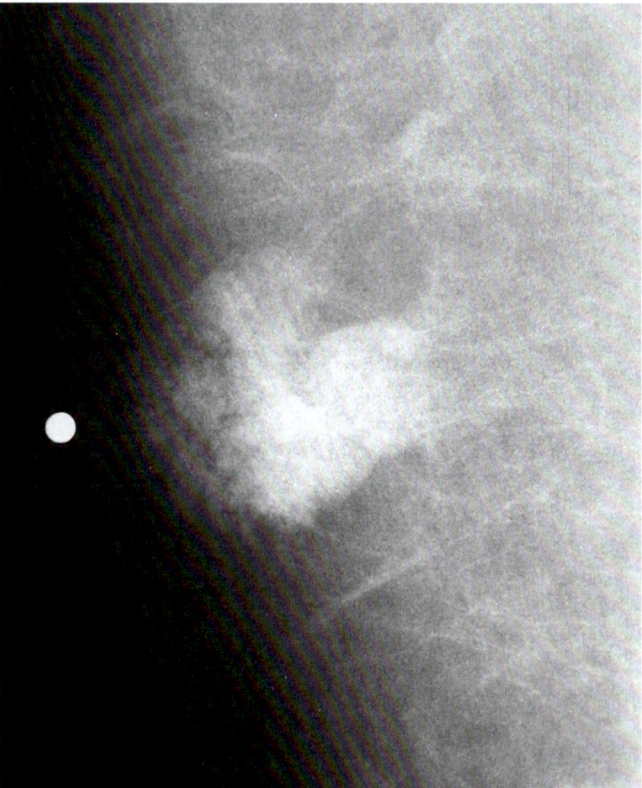

FIG. 7.91 • **Angiolipoma.** Spot tangential compression view demonstrates an irregular mass ("cloud-like") corresponding to a "lump" described by the patient in the right breast. The metallic BB denotes the site of the palpable finding. An oval mass with heterogeneous echotexture and focal areas of hyperechogenicity is imaged on ultrasound (not shown) corresponding to the palpable finding. BI-RADS 4B: Suspicious abnormality, biopsy is indicated. (From Cardeñosa G. *Breast Imaging [The Core Curriculum Series]*. Philadelphia, PA: Lippincott Williams & Wilkins; 2003.)

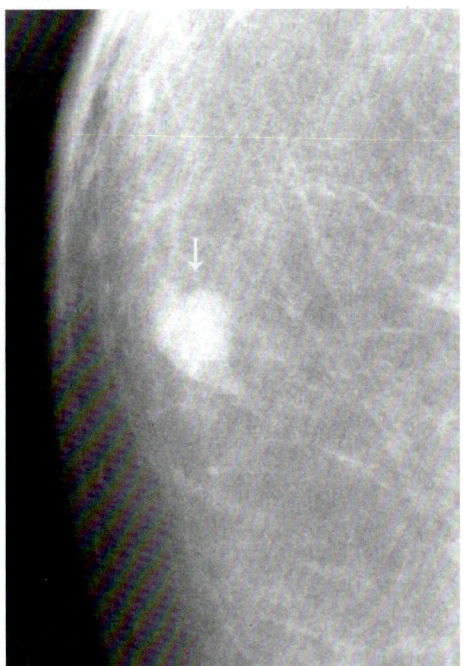

FIG. 7.92 • **Hemangioma.** Spot compression view of a screen-detected mass (arrow) in a 71-year-old woman. An irregular dense mass (arrow) with indistinct margins is confirmed on spot compression views (only one is shown). A mass with a heterogeneous echotexture is imaged corresponding to the area of mammographic concern. A central area of hypoechogenicity is almost completely surrounded by a thick rim of hyperechogenicity (not shown). BI-RADS 4C: Suspicious abnormality, biopsy is indicated. (From Cardeñosa G. *Breast Imaging [The Core Curriculum Series]*. Philadelphia, PA: Lippincott Williams & Wilkins; 2003.)

References

1. Evans WP. Breast masses: appropriate evaluation. *Radiol Clin North Am*. 1995;33:1085–1108.
2. Sickles EA, D'Orsi CJ, Bassett LW, et al. ACR BI-RADS® Mammography. In: ACR BI-RADS® Atlas, *Breast Imaging Reporting and Data System*. Reston, VA, American College of Radiology; 2013.
3. Feig SA. Breast masses: mammographic and sonographic evaluation. *Radiol Clin North Am*. 1992;30:67–92.
4. Cupples TE, Eklund GW, Cardenosa G. Mammographic halo sign revisited. *Radiology*. 1996;199:105–108.
5. Tabar L, Dean PB. *Teaching Atlas of Mammography*. 4th ed. New York, NY: Thieme; 2011.
6. Swann CA, Kopans DB, Koerner FC, et al. The halo sign and malignant breast lesions. *AJR Am J Roentgenol*. 1987;149:1145–1147.
7. Leung JWT, Sickles EA. Multiple bilateral masses detected on screening mammography: assessment of need for recall imaging. *AJR Am J Roentgenol*. 2000;175:23–29.
8. Mendelson EB, Tobin CE. Critical pathways in using breast US. *Radiographics*. 1995;15:935–945.
9. Giess CS, Raza S, Birdwell RL. Distinguishing breast skin lesions from superficial breast parenchymal lesions: diagnostic criteria, imaging characteristics and pitfalls. *Radiographics*. 2011;31:1959–1972.
10. Fornage BD, Tassin GB. Sonographic appearance of superficial soft tissue lipomas. *J Clin Ultrasound*. 1991;19:215–220.
11. Tavassoli FA. *Pathology of the Breast*. 2nd ed. New York, NY: McGraw Hill; 1999.
12. Rosen PP. *Rosen's Breast Pathology*. 3rd ed. Philadelphia, PA: Lippincott Williams & Wilkins; 2008.
13. Berg WA, Sechtin AG, Marques H, et al. Cystic breast masses and the ACRIN 6666 experience. *Radiol Clin North Am*. 2010;48:931–987.
14. Pollack AH, Kuerer HM. Steatocystoma multiplex: appearance at mammography. *Radiology*. 1991;180:836–838.
15. Mester J, Darwish M, Deshmukh SM. Steatocystoma multiplex of the breast: mammographic and sonography findings. *AJR Am J Roentgenol*. 1998;170:115–116.
16. Bedi DG, Krishnamurthy R, Krishnamurthy S, et al. Cortical morphologic features of axillary lymph nodes as a predictor of metastasis in breast cancer: in vitro sonographic study. *AJR Am J Roentgenol*. 2008;191:646–652.
17. Leibman AJ, Wong R. Findings on mammography in the axilla. *AJR Am J Roentgenol*. 1997;169:1385–1390.
18. Walsh R, Kornguth PJ, Soo MS, et al. Axillary lymph nodes: mammographic, pathologic and clinical correlation. *AJR Am J Roentgenol*. 1997;168:33–38.
19. Bruwer A, Nelson G, Spark R. Punctate intranodal gold deposits simulating microcalcifications on mammograms. *Radiology*. 1987;163:87–88.
20. Lee CH, Giurescu ME, Philpotts LE, et al. Clinical importance of unilaterally enlarging lymph nodes on otherwise normal mammograms. *Radiology*. 1997;203:329–334.
21. Mester J, Simmons RM, Vazquez MF, et al. In situ and infiltrating ductal carcinoma arising in a breast hamartoma. *AJR Am J Roentgenol*. 2000;175:64–66.
22. Hogge JP, Robinson RE, Magnant CM, et al. The mammographic spectrum of fat necrosis in the breast. *Radiographics*. 1995;15:1347–1356.
23. Soo MS, Kornguth PJ, Hertzberg BS. Fat necrosis in the breast: sonographic features. *Radiology*. 1998;206:261–269.
24. Daly CP, Jaeger B, David DS. Variable appearance of fat necrosis on breast MRI. *AJR Am J Roentgenol*. 2008;191:1374–1380.
25. Elston CW, Ellis IO, eds. *The Breast*. 3rd ed. Edinburgh, UK: Churchill Livingstone; 1998.
26. Warner JK, Kumar D, Berg WA. Apocrine metaplasia: mammographic and sonographic appearances. *AJR Am J Roentgenol*. 1998;170:1375–1379.
27. Berg WA. Sonographically depicted breast clustered microcysts: is follow-up appropriate. *AJR Am J Roentgenol*. 2005;185:952–959.
28. Doshi DJ, March DE, Crisi GM, et al. Complex cystic breast masses: diagnostic approach and imaging-pathologic correlation. *Radiographics*. 2007;27:S53–S64.
29. Ciatto S, Cariaggi P, Bulgaresi P. The value of routine cytologic examination of breast cyst fluids. *Acta Cytol*. 1987;31:301–304.
30. Smith DN, Kaelin CM, Korbin CD, et al. Impalpable breast cysts: utility of cytologic examination of fluid obtained with radiologically guided aspiration. *Radiology*. 1997;204:149–151.
31. Hindle WH, Arias RD, Florentine B, et al. Lack of utility in clinical practice of cytologic examination of nonbloody cyst fluid from palpable breast cysts. *Am J Obstet Gynecol*. 2000;182:1300–1305.
32. Kvist L, Larsson BW, Hall-Lord ML, et al. The role of bacteria in lactational mastitis and some considerations of the use of antibiotic treatment. *Int Breastfeed J*. 2008;3:6.
33. Trop I, Dugas A, David J, et al. Breast abscess: evidence-based algorithms for diagnosis, management and follow-up. *Radiographics*. 2011;31:1683–1699.
34. Fornage BD, Lorigan JG, Andrey E. Fibroadenomas of the breast: sonographic appearance. *Radiology*. 1989;172:671–675.
35. Weinstein SP, Orel SG, Collazzo L, et al. Cyclosporine A-induced fibroadenomas of the breast: report of five cases. *Radiology*. 2001;220:465–468.
36. Wurdinger A, Herzog AB, Fischer DR, et al. Differentiation of phyllodes breast tumors from fibroadenomas on MRI. *AJR Am J Roentgenol*. 2005;185:1317–1321.
37. Dupont WD, Page DL, Parl FF, et al. Long-term risk of breast cancer in women with fibroadenoma. *N Engl J Med*. 1994;331:10–15.
38. Sklair-Levy M, Sella T, Alweiss T, et al. Incidence and management of complex fibroadenomas. *AJR Am J Roentgenol*. 2008;190:214–218.
39. Soo MS, Dash M, Bentley R, et al. Tubular adenomas of the breast: imaging findings with histologic correlation. *AJR Am J Roentgenol*. 2000;174:757–761.
40. Salemis NS, Gemenetzis G, Gregorios K, et al. Tubular adenoma of the breast: a rare presentation and review of the literature. *J Clin Med Res*. 2012;4:84–87.

41. Sumkin JH, Perrone AM, Harris KM, et al. Lactating adenoma: US features and literature review. *Radiology*. 1998;206:271.
42. Liberman L, Bonaccio E, Hamele-Bena D, et al. Benign and malignant phyllodes tumors: mammographic and sonographic findings. *Radiology*. 1996;198:121–124.
43. Parker SJ, Harries SA. Phyllodes tumours. *Postgrad Med J*. 2001;77:428–435.
44. Czumm JM, Sanders LM, Titus JM, et al. Breast imaging case of the day (phyllodes). *Radiographics*. 1997;17:448.
45. Singhal V, Chintamani, Cosgrove JM. Osteogenic sarcoma of the breast arising in a cystosarcoma phyllodes: a case report and review of the literature. *J Med Case Reports*. 2011;5:293.
46. Krishnamurthy J. Osseous differentiation in cystosarcoma phyllodes—diagnosed by fine needle aspiration cytology. *J Cytol*. 2010;27:149–151.
47. Balaji R, Ramachandran KN. Magnetic resonance imaging of a benign phyllodes tumor of the breast. *Breast Care (Basel)*. 2009;4:189–191.
48. Reimer T. Management of rare histological types of breast tumours. *Breast Care (Basel)*. 2008;3:190–196.
49. Cardenosa G, Doudna C, Eklund GW. Ductography of the breast: technique and findings. *AJR Am J Roentgenol*. 1994;162:1081–1087.
50. Cardenosa G, Eklund GW. Benign papillary neoplasms of the breast: mammographic findings. *Radiology*. 1991;181:751–755.
51. Muttarak M, Lerttumnongtum P, Chaiwun B, et al. Spectrum of papillary lesions of the breast: clinical, imaging and pathologic correlation. *AJR Am J Roentgenol*. 2008;191:700–707.
52. Eiada R, Chong J, Kulkarni S, et al. Papillary lesions of the breast: MRI, ultrasound and mammographic appearance. *AJR Am J Roentgenol*. 2012;198:264–271.
53. Zhu Y, Zhang S, Liu P, et al. Solitary intraductal papillomas of the breast: MRI features and differentiation from small invasive ductal carcinomas. *AJR Am J Roentgenol*. 2012;199:936–942.
54. Brookes MJ, Bourke AG. Radiological appearances of papillary breast lesions. *Clin Radiol*. 2008;63:1265–1273.
55. Mulligan AM, O'Malley FP. Papillary lesions of the breast. *Adv Anat Pathol*. 2007;14:108–119.
56. Ibarra JA. Papillary lesions of the breast. *Breast J*. 2006;12:237–251.
57. Venta LA, Wiley EL, Gabriel H, et al. Imaging features of focal breast fibrosis: mammographic-pathologic correlation of noncalcified breast lesions. *AJR Am J Roentgenol*. 1999;173:309–316.
58. Rosen EL, Soo MS, Bentley RC. Focal fibrosis: a common breast lesion diagnosed at imaging-guided core biopsy. *AJR Am J Roentgenol*. 1999;173:1657–1662.
59. Harvey SC, Denison CM, Lester SC, et al. Fibrous nodules found at large-core needle biopsy of the breast: imaging features. *Radiology*. 1999;211:535–540.
60. Revelon G, Sherman ME, Gatewood OMB, et al. Focal fibrosis of the breast: imaging characteristics and histopathological correlation. *Radiology*. 2000;216:255–259.
61. Sklair-Levy M, Samuels TH, Catzavelos C, et al. Stromal fibrosis of the breast. *AJR Am J Roentgenol*. 2001;177:573–577.
62. Piccoli CW, Feig SA, Palazzo JP. Developing asymmetric density. *Radiology*. 1999;211:111–117.
63. Logan WW, Hoffman NY. Diabetic fibrous breast disease. *Radiology*. 1989;172:667–670.
64. Weinstein SP, Conant EF, Orel SG, et al. Diabetic mastopathy in men: imaging findings in two patients. *Radiology*. 2001;219:797–799.
65. Ibrahim RE, Sciotto CG, Weidner N. Pseudoangiomatous hyperplasia of mammary stroma: some observations regarding its clinicopathologic spectrum. *Cancer*. 1989;63:1154.
66. Teh HS, Chiang S-H, Leung JWT, et al. Rapidly enlarging tumoral pseudoangiomatous stromal hyperplasia in a 15-year-old patient. *J Ultrasound Med*. 2007;26:1101–1106.
67. Ryu EM, Whang IY, Chang ED. Rapidly growing bilateral pseudoangiomatous stromal hyperplasia of the breast. *Korean J Radiol*. 2010;11:355–358.
68. Degnim AC, Frost M, Radisky D, et al. Pseudoangiomatous stromal hyperplasia and breast cancer risk. *Ann Surg Oncol*. 2010;17:3269–3277.
69. Cohen MA, Morris EA, Rosen PP, et al. Pseudoangiomatous stromal hyperplasia: mammographic, sonographic and clinical patterns. *Radiology*. 1996;198:117–120.
70. Polger MR, Denison CM, Lester S, et al. Pseudoangiomatous stromal hyperplasia: mammographic and sonographic appearances. *AJR Am J Roentgenol*. 1996;166:349–352.
71. Mercado CL, Naidrich SA, Hamele-Bena D, et al. Pseudoangiomatous stromal hyperplasia of the breast: sonographic features with histopathologic correlation. *Breast J*. 2004;10:427–432.
72. Solomou E, Kraniotis P, Patriarcheas G. A case of a giant pseudoangiomatous stromal hyperplasia of the breast: magnetic resonance imaging findings. *Rare Tumors*. 2012;4:e23.
73. Baskin H, Layfield L, Morrell G. MRI appearance of pseudoangiomatous stromal hyperplasia causing asymmetric breast enlargement. *Breast J*. 2007;13:203–210.
74. Sewell CW. Pathology of benign and malignant breast disorders. *Radiol Clin North Am*. 1995;33:1067–1080.
75. Mitnick JS, Vasquez MF, Harris MN, et al. Differentiation of radial scar from scirrhous carcinoma of the breast: mammographic-pathologic correlation. *Radiology*. 1989;173:697–700.
76. Greenstein-Orel S, Evers K, Yeh IT, et al. Radial scar with microcalcification: radiologic-pathologic correlation. *Radiology*. 1992;183:479–482.
77. Adler DD, Helvie MA, Oberman HA, et al. Radial sclerosing lesion of the breast: mammographic features. *Radiology*. 1990;176:737–740.
78. Ciatto S, Morrone D, Catarzi S, et al. Radial scar of the breast: review of 38 consecutive mammographic diagnoses. *Radiology*. 1985;187:757–760.
79. Cohen MA, Sferlazza SJ. Role of sonography in evaluation of radial scars of the breast. *AJR Am J Roentgenol*. 2000;174:1075–1078.
80. Frouge C, Tristant H, Guinebretiere JM, et al. Mammographic lesions suggestive of radial scars: microscopic findings in 40 cases. *Radiology*. 1995;195:623.
81. Nielsen M, Christesen L, Andersen J. Radial scars in women with breast cancer. *Cancer*. 1987;59:1019.
82. Linnell F, Ljungberg O, Andersen I. Breast carcinoma: aspects of early stages, progression and related problems. *Acta Pathol Microbiol Scand Suppl*. 1980;272:1.
83. Jacobs TW, Byrne E, Colditz G, et al. Radial scars in benign breast biopsy specimens and the risk of breast cancer. *N Engl J Med*. 1999;340:430–436.
84. Brenner RJ, Jackman RJ, Parker SH, et al. Percutaneous core needle biopsy of radial scars of the breast: when is excision necessary? *AJR Am J Roentgenol*. 2002;179:1179–1184.
85. Linda A, Zuiani C, Furlan A, et al. Radial scars without atypia diagnosed at imaging-guided needle biopsy: how often is associated malignancy found at subsequent surgical excision and do mammography and sonography predict which lesions are malignant? *AJR Am J Roentgenol*. 2010;194:1148–1151.
86. Plaza MJ, Yepes M. Breast fibromatosis response to tamoxifen: dynamic MRI findings and review of the current treatment options. *J Radiol Case Rep*. 2012;6:16–23.
87. Glazebrook KN, Reynolds CA. Mammary fibromatosis. *AJR Am J Roentgenol*. 2009;193:856–860.
88. Leibman AJ, Kossoff MB. Sonographic features of fibromatosis of the breast. *J Ultrasound Med*. 1991;10:43–45.
89. Nakazone T, Satoh T, Hamamoto T, et al. Dynamic MRI of fibromatosis of the breast. *AJR Am J Roentgenol*. 2003;181:1718–1719.
90. Aoyama K, Kamio T, Seshimo A, et al. Granular cell tumors: a report of six cases. *World J Surg Oncol*. 2012;10:204.
91. Scaranelo AM, Bukhanov K, Crystal P, et al. Granular cell tumour of the breast: MRI findings and review of the literature. *Br J Radiol*. 2007;80:970–974.
92. Yang WT, Edeiken-Monroe B, Sneige N, et al. Sonographic and mammographic appearance of granular cell tumors. *J Clin Ultrasound*. 2006;34:153–160.
93. Maki DD, Horne D, Damore LJ, et al. Magnetic resonance imaging of granular cell tumor of the breast. *Clin Imaging*. 2009;33:395–397.

CHAPTER SELF-ASSESSMENT QUESTIONS

1. Diagnostic mammogram (top and middle) and spot tangential view (bottom) in a 35-year-old patient describing a "lump" in the right breast. What is indicated?

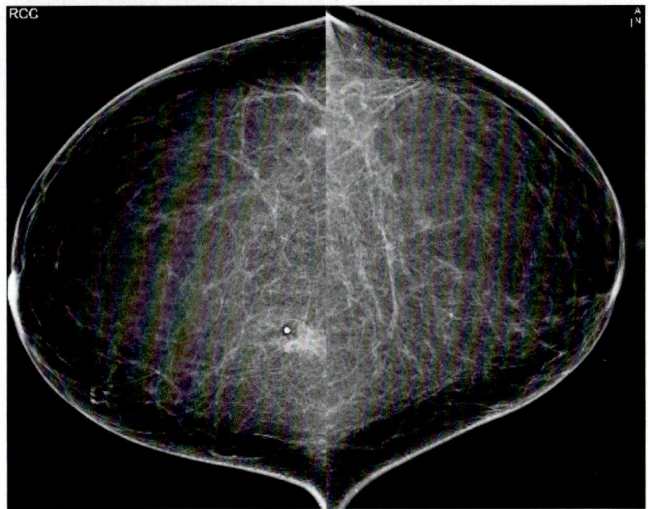
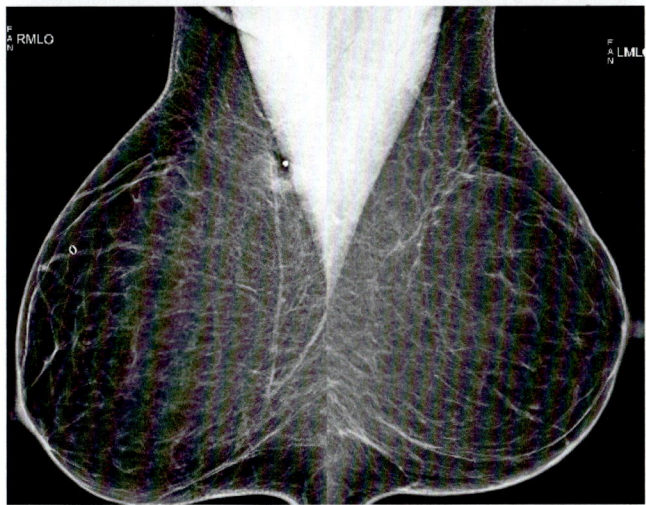
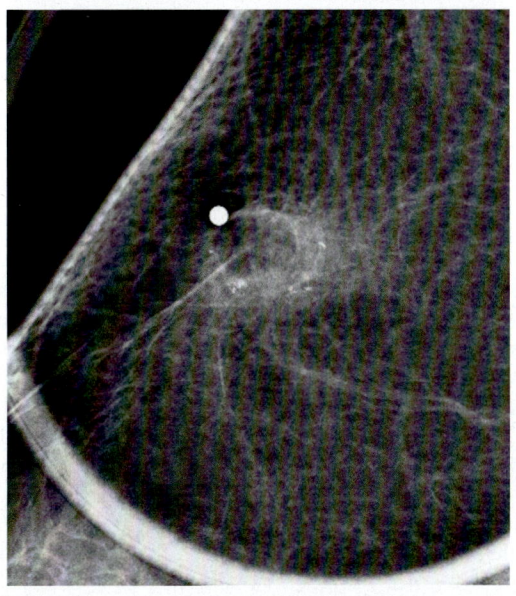

A. Annual screening mammography starting at age 40
B. Ultrasound of the right breast
C. Biopsy of the palpable finding
D. Six-month follow-up

2. Representative ultrasound image from a study in a 36-year-old patient presenting with a "lump" in the left breast. What might you want to ask her about?

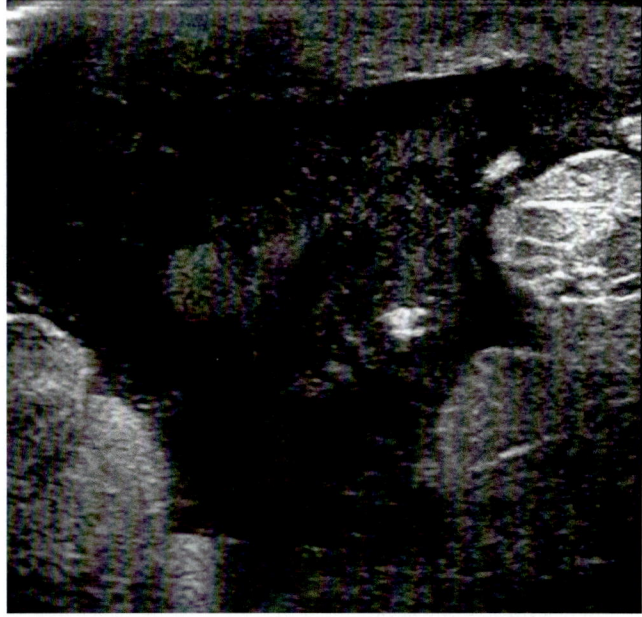

A. BRCA status
B. Nipple rings
C. Breast-feeding
D. Smoking

Answers to Chapter Self-Assessment Questions

1. A In this patient, the spot tangential view is quite useful. An oil cyst with developing mural calcifications is imaged associated with surrounding indistinct soft tissue. No additional imaging, intervention, or short-term follow-up is indicated. The patient should be reassured that what she is feeling is benign, likely related to prior trauma and encouraged to start annual screening mammography at age 40.

2. D A "funnel"-shaped complex fluid collection is imaged extending from thickened skin into the breast parenchyma. The finding is consistent with a subareolar abscess. These occur more commonly in patients with a significant smoking history and are not related to pregnancy or nipple rings. The BRCA status of the patient is not a consideration in this entity. These patients have a high incidence of recurrence even after surgical drainage and major duct excision, and approximately 25% of patients will present at different times with bilateral subareolar abscesses. Central horizontal nipple inversion may be seen in patients with recurrent abscesses. Patients need to be warned about the possibility of developing a fistula at the periareolar margin (Zuska disease) with spontaneous drainage of purulent, malodorous fluid.

Evaluation and Imaging Features of Malignant Breast Masses

8

LEARNING OBJECTIVES

1. Invasive ductal carcinoma, not otherwise specified (NOS)
   - Clinical features
   - Imaging features
   - Histology
2. Extensive intraductal component (EIC)
   - Definition
3. Ductal carcinoma in situ (DCIS)
4. Tubular carcinoma
   - Clinical features
   - Imaging features
   - Histology
5. Mucinous carcinoma
   - Clinical features
   - Imaging features
   - Histology
6. Medullary carcinoma
   - Clinical features
   - Imaging features
   - Histology
7. Papillary carcinoma
   - Clinical features
   - Imaging features
   - Histology
8. Metaplastic carcinoma
   - Clinical features
   - Imaging features
   - Histology
9. Invasive lobular carcinoma
   - Clinical features
   - Imaging features
   - Histology
10. Lymphoma
    - Clinical features
    - Imaging features
    - Histology
11. Sarcomas
    - Primary
    - Radiation related
12. Metastatic disease to the breast
13. Metastatic disease to intramammary and axillary lymph nodes

The focus of this chapter is on breast cancers that present with a mass detected on physical examination or with imaging. Invasive ductal carcinoma NOS is the most common type of breast cancer followed in frequency by invasive lobular carcinoma. Also discussed are relatively common variants of invasive ductal carcinoma including tubular, mucinous, papillary, medullary, and metaplastic carcinomas. It is important to emphasize, however, that there are additional variants of invasive ductal carcinoma that, because of their rarity, are beyond the scope of this book and not discussed. They include squamous, apocrine, adenoid cystic, secretory, neuroendocrine, cystic hypersecretory, cribriform, small cell, lipid rich, glycogen rich, and invasive micropapillary carcinomas (1,2).

INVASIVE DUCTAL CARCINOMA

Invasive ductal carcinoma NOS, or no special type, is the most common type of breast cancer representing 65% to 75% of mammary carcinomas (1,2). Depending on the size of the lesion, size of the breast, and proximity of the lesion to the skin, patients can present with a hard, fixed, palpable mass that may cause skin thickening and retraction (Fig. 8.1). If the cancer is in the subareolar area, patients may describe progressive flattening of the nipple, nipple deviation, inversion, or retraction (Fig. 8.2) or changes in the periareolar area (Fig. 8.3). When more advanced, the patient may present with skin ulceration (Fig. 8.4), a mass that protrudes or fungates through the skin (Fig. 8.5), more

Evaluation and Imaging Features of Malignant Breast Masses   235

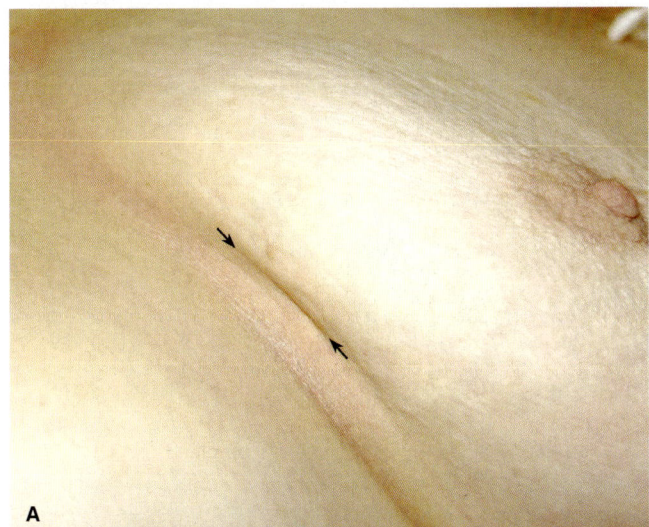

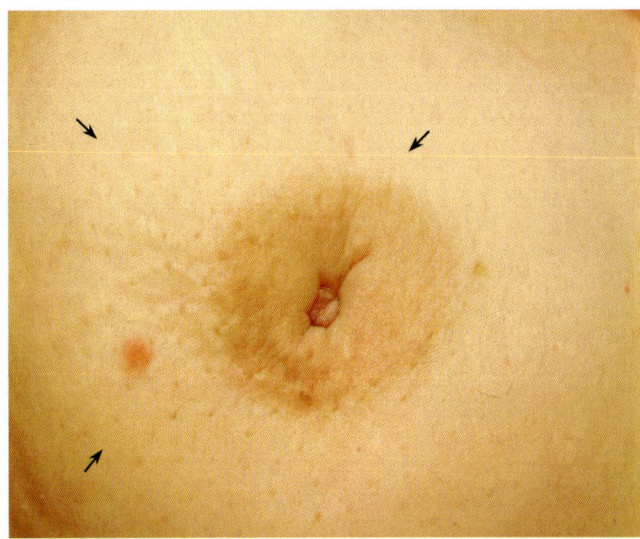

FIG. 8.2 • **Nipple inversion and retraction, focal peau d'orange.** Nipple inversion and retraction with slight lateral deviation as well as localized peau d'orange changes *(arrows)* extending from the areolar margin into the upper outer quadrant of the right breast in a patient with invasive ductal carcinoma. Skin in the lower inner quadrant is normal.

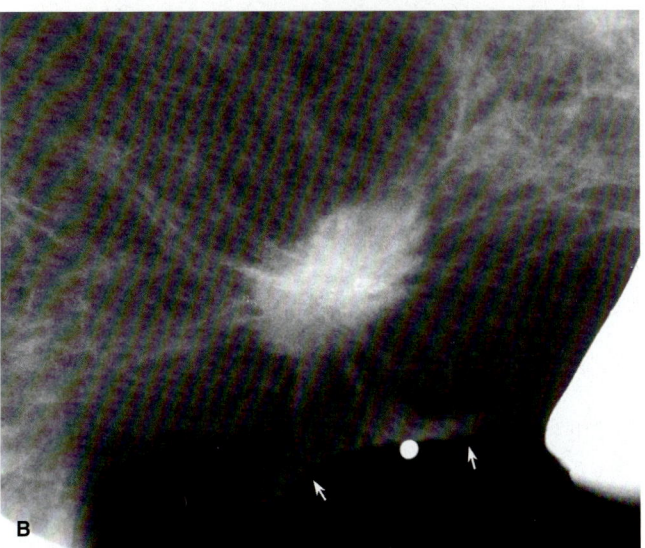

FIG. 8.1 • **Skin dimpling, invasive ductal carcinoma, NOS, well-differentiated. A:** This 77-year-old patient presents with dimpling *(arrows)* just above the inframammary fold on the left. In some patients, dimpling becomes apparent during positioning and as compression is applied; the technologist is in a unique position to identify skin and nipple changes; any observation should be documented so that the information is available to the interpreting radiologist. **B:** Spot tangential view at site of skin dimpling. An iso dense oval mass with spiculated margins and associated skin thickening and retraction *(arrows)* is correlated to the site of clinical concern. (From Cardeñosa G. *Breast Imaging [The Core Curriculum Series]*. Philadelphia, PA: Lippincott Williams & Wilkins; 2003.)

detected clinically or symptoms have developed. A mass with spiculated margins (Figs. 8.1B and 8.8) is one of the most common presentations in asymptomatic women. Less frequently, invasive ductal carcinoma presents as a round (Fig. 8.9), oval (Fig. 8.10), or irregular mass with indistinct margins, less often, circumscribed margins. Although cancers are more commonly iso to high in density, some are low in density, and as such, the density of a mass alone cannot be used to distinguish benign from malignant masses. Likewise, size

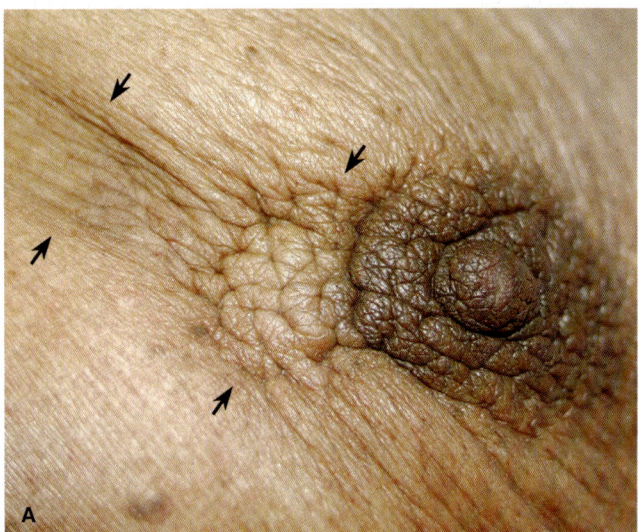

FIG. 8.3 • **Skin dimpling and retraction, invasive ductal carcinoma NOS, moderately differentiated. A:** Thickening, dimpling, and retraction of the skin *(arrows)* extending peripherally from the upper central margin of the left areola in a 90-year-old patient. Note slight deviation of the nipple. **B:** Spot compression view, left breast. A dense, round mass with ill-defined and spiculated margins, associated skin thickening, and retraction *(arrows)* is imaged adjacent to the left nipple *(N)*. The metallic BB is used to denote the area of clinical concern. Extensive arterial calcification is present. (From Cardeñosa G. *Breast Imaging [The Core Curriculum Series]*. Philadelphia, PA: Lippincott Williams & Wilkins; 2003.)

diffuse breast deformity and ulcerations, (Fig. 8.6) or areas of necrotic tissue focally or more diffusely involving the breast (Fig. 8.7). Localized or more diffuse edematous or erythematous changes (peau d'orange) may be apparent; skin nodules reflecting metastatic disease may be seen in patients with locally advanced breast cancer (Fig. 8.6A). Rarely, patients present with spontaneous nipple discharge, and less than 1% of patients present with metastatic disease to the axilla but no clinically or mammographically detectable primary breast lesion. As discussed in Chapter 5, magnetic resonance imaging (MRI; see Fig. 5.27) is useful in depicting the primary lesion in the breast in this group of patients (3).

With the increasing use of screening mammography, patients with invasive ductal carcinomas are diagnosed before signs of cancer are

(continued)

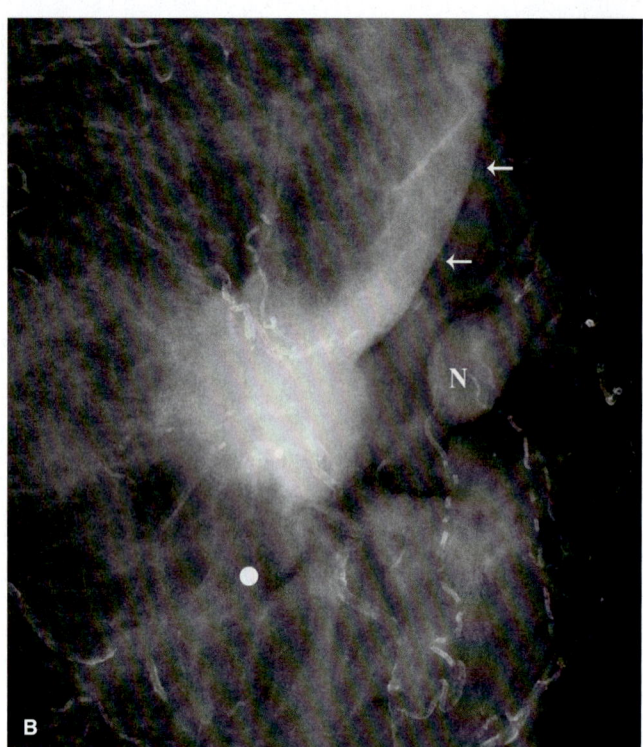

FIG. 8.3 • *(continued)*

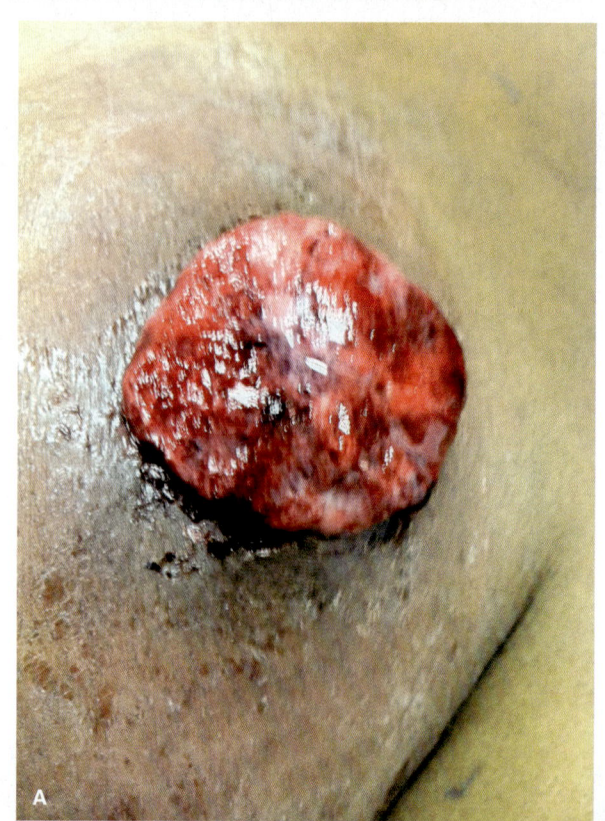

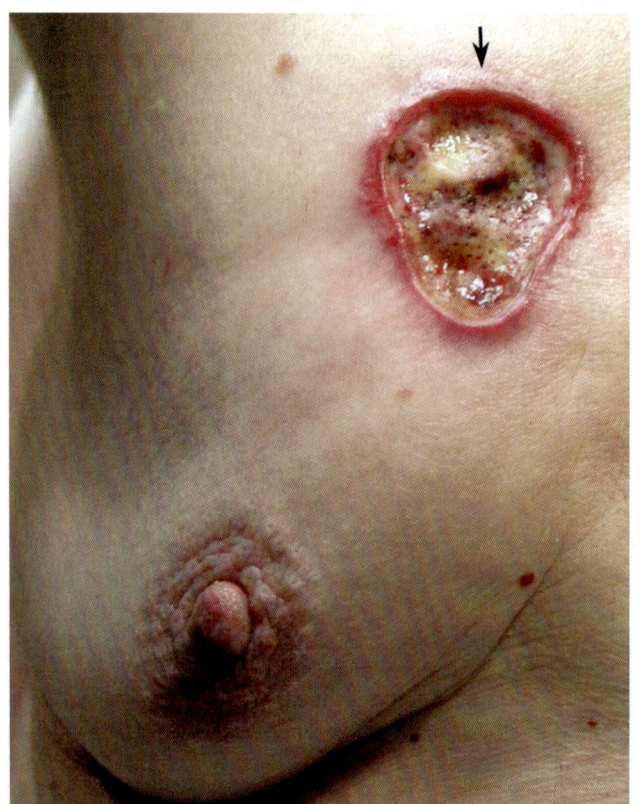

FIG. 8.4 • **Skin ulceration, invasive ductal carcinoma NOS, moderately differentiated.** Skin ulceration *(arrow)* with surrounding erythema is present in the upper inner quadrant of the right breast in a 78-year-old patient with an underlying hard fixed mass on palpation. (From Cardeñosa G. *Breast Imaging [The Core Curriculum Series]*. Philadelphia, PA: Lippincott Williams & Wilkins; 2003.)

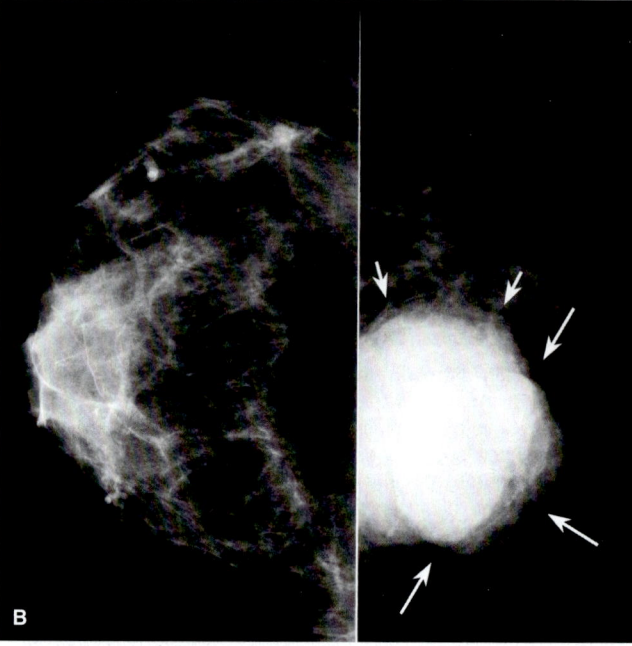

FIG. 8.5 • **Fungating mass, invasive ductal carcinoma NOS, high nuclear grade. A:** A fungating, necrotic mass is evident in the upper inner quadrant of the left breast in a 54-year-old patient. **B:** Craniocaudal (CC) views. A dense, round mass with indistinct margins posteriorly *(short arrows)* is partially imaged medially in the left breast; the portion of the mass that extends beyond the skin *(long arrows)* is outlined by air and therefore appears circumscribed. **C:** MRI, T1-weighted sagittal reconstruction of the left breast post-contrast. An irregular mass *(short arrows)* with heterogeneous enhancement and central necrosis *(long arrow)* is imaged protruding from the upper inner quadrant of the left breast. Diffuse skin thickening and edematous changes are also apparent in the subcutaneous tissue. Following neoadjuvant therapy, residual non-enhancing soft tissue is imaged on MRI (see Fig. 5.29B) at the site of the original tumor; no residual malignancy is evident at the time of the mastectomy (e.g., complete pathological response [cPR]) and no metastatic disease is identified in two sentinel lymph nodes.

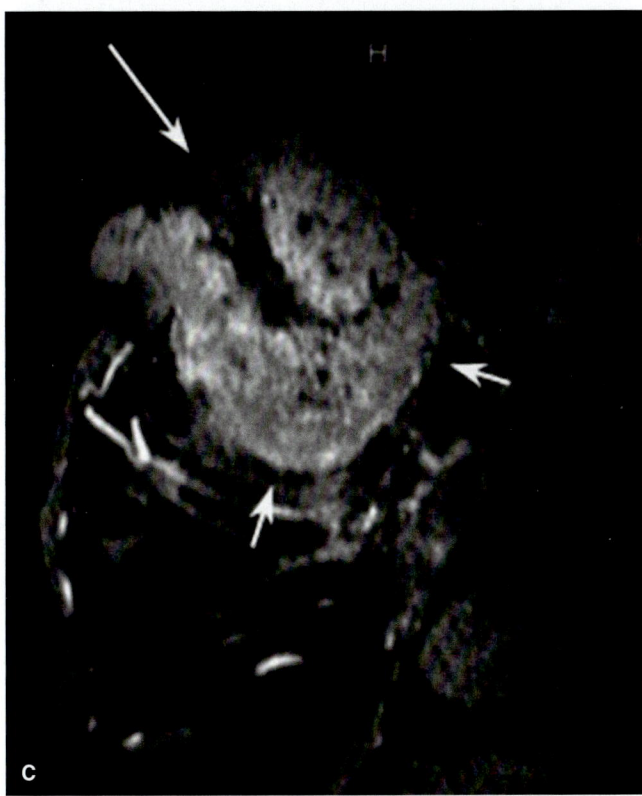

FIG. 8.5 • *(continued)*

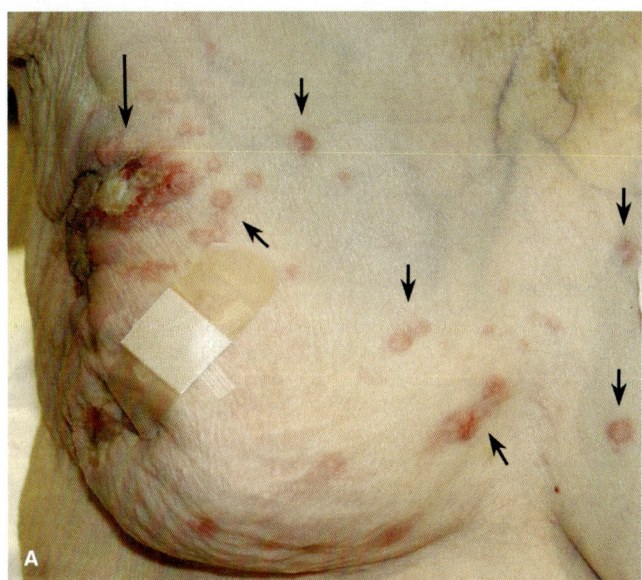

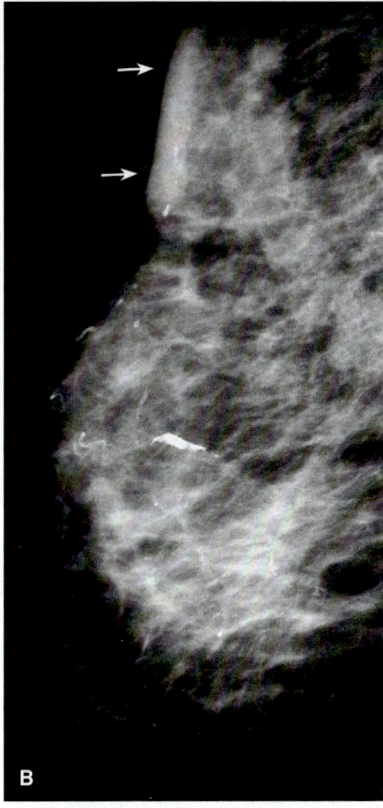

FIG. 8.6 • Skin ulceration, metastatic disease to skin, invasive ductal carcinoma NOS, poorly differentiated. **A:** Deformed right breast in a 97-year-old patient presenting with locally advanced breast cancer. The right breast is smaller, with skin thickening and several areas of ulceration *(long arrow)* laterally as well as lateral displacement of the nipple areolar complex. Raised, erythematous nodules *(short arrows)* on the right breast and medially in the left breast represent skin metastases. **B:** Right mediolateral oblique (MLO) view demonstrating a diffusely abnormal right breast with decreased compressibility as well as skin and trabecular thickening. Skin thickening is particularly prominent at the site of ulceration *(arrows)*. Some of the mammographic findings may be attributable to ipsilateral axillary adenopathy with resulting lymphatic obstruction. (From Cardeñosa G. *Breast Imaging [The Core Curriculum Series]*. Philadelphia, PA: Lippincott Williams & Wilkins; 2003.)

alone is not a reliable criterion in distinguishing benign from malignant masses.

Additional mammographic presentations for invasive ductal carcinoma include focal parenchymal asymmetry (Fig. 8.11), distortion (Fig. 8.12), or diffuse changes (Fig. 8.13; also see Figs. 9.14 through 9.16). All of the presentations may be found in isolation or in combination (e.g., a mass with associated distortion). They may also be associated with malignant-type calcifications that often reflect the presence of intraductal disease. It is important to describe the calcifications particularly when they extend away from the primary finding. If the calcifications are in tissue extending a distance from the mass, a separate biopsy of the calcifications may be appropriate to establish the extent of disease accurately. In planning preoperative wire localizations in these patients, bracketing may be needed to include the area of the calcifications (Fig. 8.14; also see Figs. 7.2B and 7.3).

Breast cancers occur anywhere in the breast but are reportedly more common in the upper outer quadrants. The upper inner quadrants and subareolar area are the next most common sites for the development of breast cancer. Kopans and coworkers (4) have described a predilection for cancer to develop at the periphery of the glandular tissue just deep to the subcutaneous fat or in the glandular tissue interfacing with retroglandular fat. Stacey-Clear et al. (4) reported that in women under the age of 50, more than 70% of cancers develop in this peripheral zone. Since accessory nipples and glandular tissue (see Fig. 9.23) can be found in some women along the milk lines extending bilaterally from the axillae to the groins, breast cancer can rarely develop outside of the breast proper along these milk lines.

In many women, the mammographic features of the mass (e.g., mass with spiculated margins in a patient with no history of trauma or surgery, or a round mass with linear, casting-type calcifications) are such that an ultrasound may not add additional information with

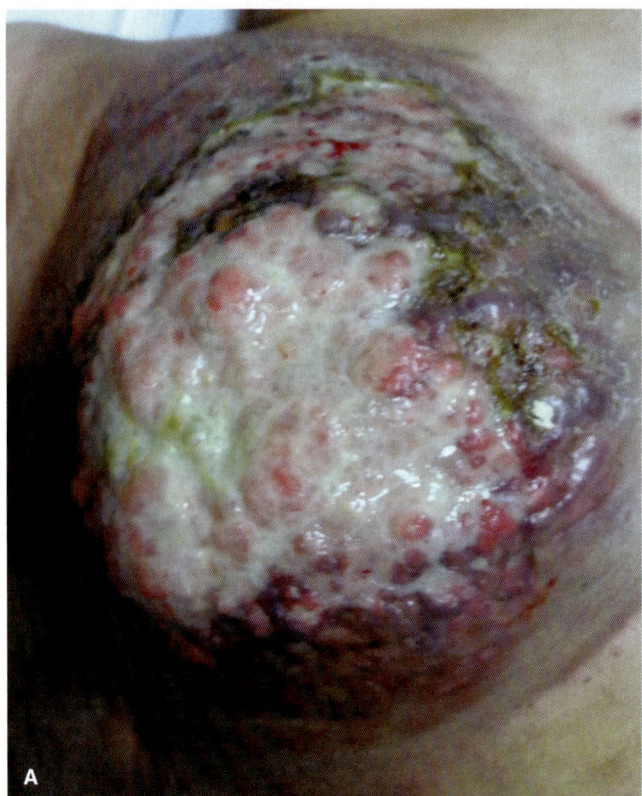

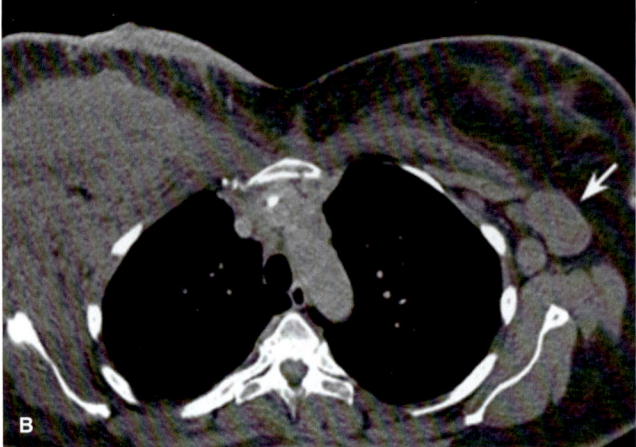

FIG. 8.7 • **Necrotic breast, invasive ductal carcinoma NOS, locally advanced with metastatic disease to the contralateral axilla. A:** The right breast is necrotic and completely replaced by a locally advanced breast cancer in a 50-year-old patient. No nipple areolar complex is evident with necrosis extending into the subclavicular area and the midaxillary line. Hard masses are palpated in the contralateral (left) axilla. **B:** CT scan image demonstrating a mass almost completely replacing the right breast with involvement of the skin, as well as the pectoralis and anterior serratus muscles; axillary adenopathy is present bilaterally but because of patient positioning, it is only seen in the left axilla *(arrow)* on this image.

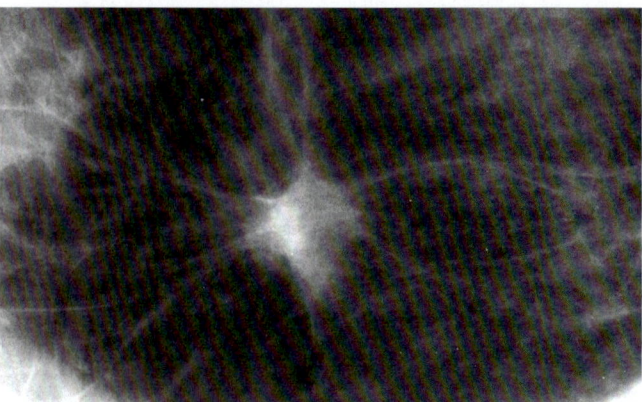

FIG. 8.8 • **Invasive ductal carcinoma NOS, low nuclear grade, and DCIS, cribriform pattern.** Spot compression view, right breast CC projection in a 51-year-old patient. Round iso dense mass with spiculated margins. This is a common mammographic presentation for invasive ductal carcinoma. BI-RADS 4C: Suspicious abnormality; biopsy is indicated. When the mass has spiculated margins, it is more commonly a low- to intermediate-grade invasive lesion (e.g., infiltrative pattern). When low-grade invasive lesions have associated DCIS, it is typically low- to intermediate-grade DCIS. In this patient, the tumor is estrogen- and progesterone-positive and HER2/neu-negative. The sentinel lymph node (LN) biopsy (0/3 LNs) is negative.

respect to the mass. The management for the patient is based on the mammographic findings. In these patients, ultrasound is done to help direct the imaging-guided biopsy and to scan the remainder of the breast, ipsilateral axilla, and the contralateral breast for additional disease. In other patients, however, ultrasound is helpful and compliments mammography in characterizing the primary lesion. For example, in a patient with a mass in whom a cyst is a realistic possibility, the appropriate management for the patient is based on the ultrasound findings (e.g., the BI-RADS for the mammogram alone would be BI-RADS 0: Need additional imaging evaluation). Likewise, as discussed in Chapters 3 and 4, when a patient presents with a palpable finding and dense tissue is seen on spot compression or spot tangential views done at the site of clinical concern, or if there is a possibility that a lesion has been excluded from the field of view, ultrasound is critical in helping characterize the palpable abnormality (Fig. 8.15; also see Figs. 3.1, 3.2, 4.46, and 10.18). On the ultrasound, normal glandular tissue, a cyst, or a solid mass may be imaged corresponding to the palpable finding. The patient's management will, in large part, depend on the physical findings and ultrasound features of the palpable area. Marked hypoechogenicity, spiculation, microlobulation, vertical orientation, angular margins, a thickened echogenic rim, calcifications, extension of tumor into ducts extending toward the nipple, and branching of tumor away from the nipple with variable amounts of shadowing are findings on ultrasound (see Figs. 4.39 through 4.43) associated with malignant lesions (5). In patients with predominantly fatty tissue, less commonly glandular tissue, the ultrasound study may be normal because the lesion is isoechoic to the surrounding tissue (Fig. 8.15D).

It is important to recognize that patients with breast cancer have a higher risk of concurrent ipsilateral or bilateral breast cancer, or developing subsequent breast cancer. The presence of multiple lesions at the time of diagnosis is something that has been described by pathologists for years and is now also evident when breast MRIs are done routinely in patients with known breast cancer. *Multifocal* lesions are defined as multiple cancers occurring in the same quadrant (Figs. 8.9C and 8.16). *Multicentric* cancers are those occurring in different quadrants of the involved breast, or if more than 5 cm apart in the same quadrant (Fig. 8.13; also see Figs. 2.50, 5.21, and 5.22). Bilateral cancers are *synchronous* when diagnosed at the same time (Fig. 8.17; also see Figs. 2.51 and 5.23) or within 6 months of each other, and *metachronous* (Fig. 8.18; also see Fig. 2.47 and 10.11) when they occur bilaterally at different times (diagnosed more than 6 months apart). The reported

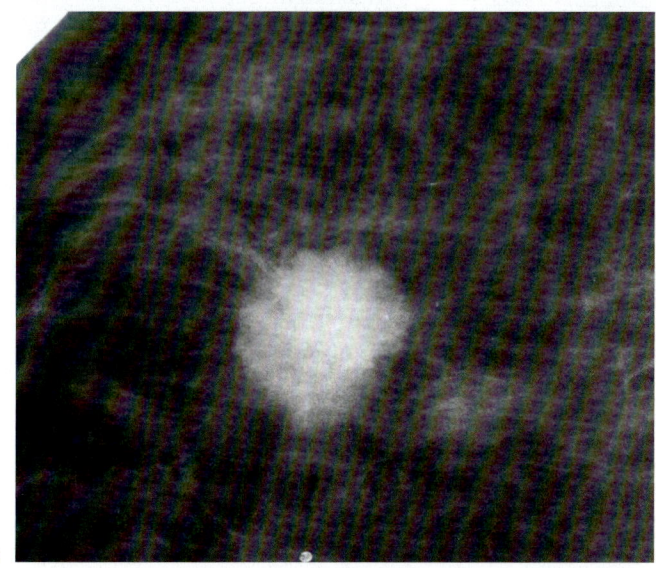
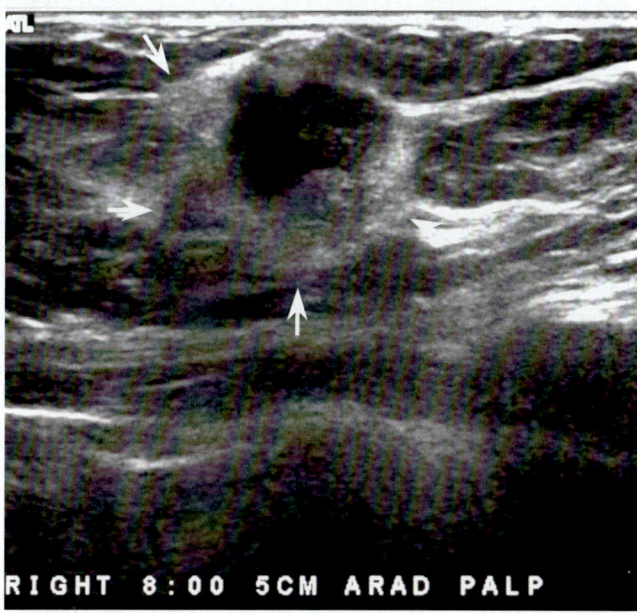
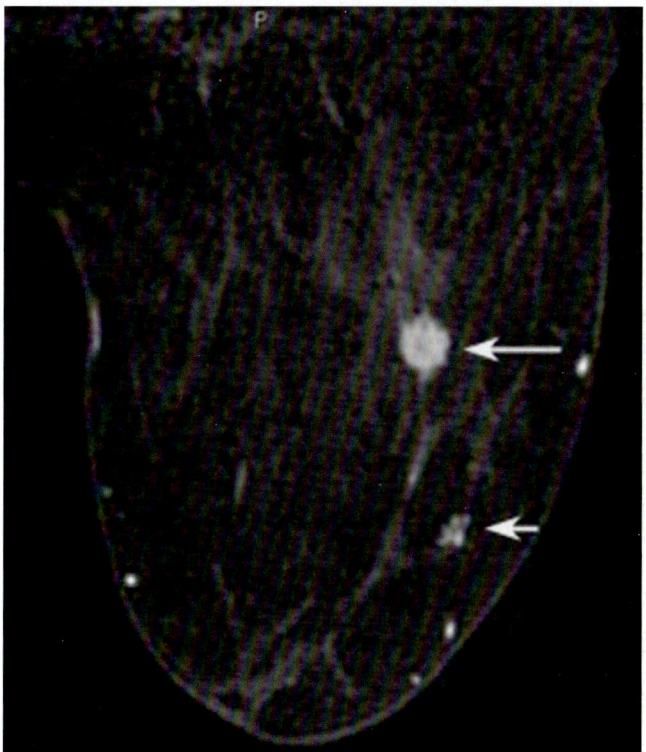

FIG. 8.9 • **Invasive ductal carcinoma NOS, intermediate grade with extensive DCIS intermediate nuclear grade (EIC). A:** Spot compression view, right breast CC projection in a 65-year-old patient. A dense round mass with microlobulated margins as well as a few punctate calcifications is present. **B:** Ultrasound. A mass *(arrows)* with a heterogeneous echotexture is imaged correlating to the mammographically detected mass. Echogenic foci in the mass are thought to represent calcifications. BI-RADS 4C: Suspicious abnormality; biopsy is indicated. Please note that although this patient has a screen-detected abnormality, the lesion is palpable at the time of the focused ultrasound *(PALP)*. When the patient is positioned for the ultrasound and palpation is done as the patient is scanned, many screen-detected cancers can be palpated. An invasive ductal carcinoma, intermediate nuclear grade is diagnosed on core biopsy. It is estrogen and progesterone receptor-positive and HER2/neu-negative. **C:** MRI, axial T1-weighted image of the right breast post-contrast. A round mass *(long arrow)* with lobulated margins and heterogeneous enhancement characterized predominantly by rapid wash-in and wash-out kinetic curves is correlated to the mass detected mammographically and the site of the patient's known invasive ductal carcinoma. Focal, non-mass–like heterogeneous enhancement *(short arrow)* is detected anterolaterally in the right breast, 2.8 cm anterior to the known site of invasive disease. DCIS, solid and cribriform types, low nuclear grade is diagnosed on an MRI-guided biopsy of this site. The sentinel lymph node biopsy is positive, and as such a full axillary dissection is done (1/16 positive LNs). An extensive intraductal component is described at the time of the patient's lumpectomy. As illustrated by this patient and discussed in Chapter 5, additional sites of disease (multifocal, multicentric, and bilateral) are detected routinely on MRI's in patients with a new breast cancer diagnosis.

frequency of multifocality varies depending on study design and meticulousness of histological evaluation, and may be as high as 33% to 50% (6,7). The described frequency of synchronous lesions is 0.1% to 2% compared with 1% to 12% for metachronous lesions. In the general population, 0.1% of women per year are expected to develop breast cancer. In comparison, the frequency of developing a second breast cancer among patients with a history of breast cancer is 0.53% to 0.8% per year (7). Nielsen and colleagues (8) reported on 86 women with a diagnosis of invasive ductal carcinoma in whom at autopsy invasive and in situ lesions were identified in the contralateral breast in 33% and 35% of patients, respectively. In a separate study, done by the same investigators on an age-matched population, autopsy results identified 14 patients with in situ lesions and only 1 patient with invasive cancer among 77 women with no history of breast cancer (9).

In analyzing masses and considering an appropriate differential for possible malignant etiologies the age of the patient, any physical findings and the imaging features of the lesion are helpful. Many of our patients presenting with a round high-density mass (expansile margins, or "blow up" lesions) on the mammogram, and marked hypoechogenicity, cystic spaces (see Fig. 4.37), and posterior acoustic enhancement on ultrasound, are diagnosed with poorly differentiated, rapidly growing invasive ductal carcinomas, NOS (see Table 7.8 for differential considerations). In the younger patients (pre-menopausal), these lesions may represent interval cancers (cancers presenting between screening

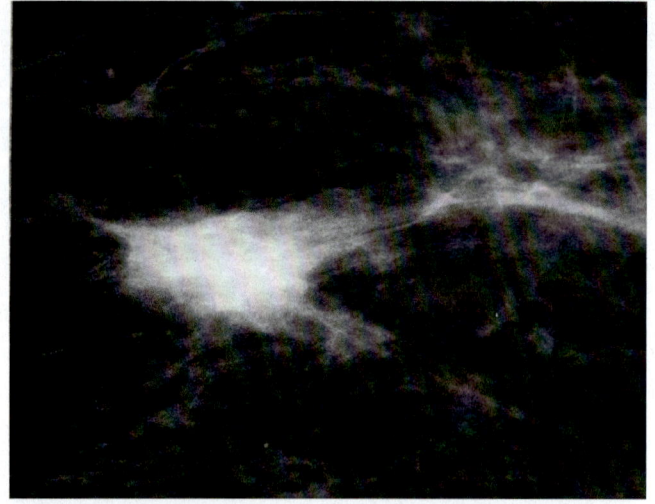

A

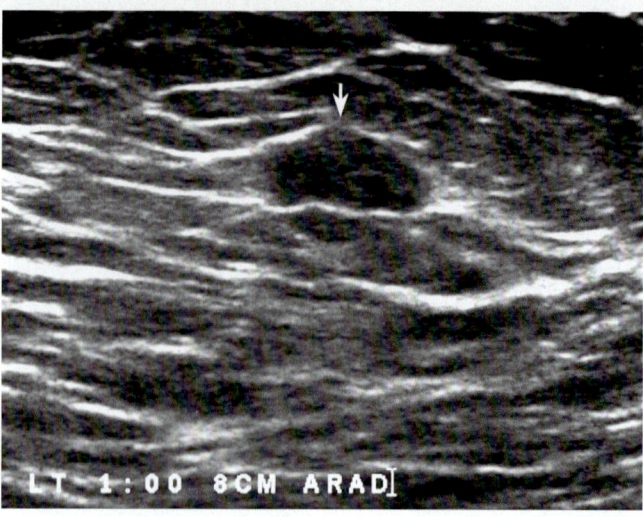

B

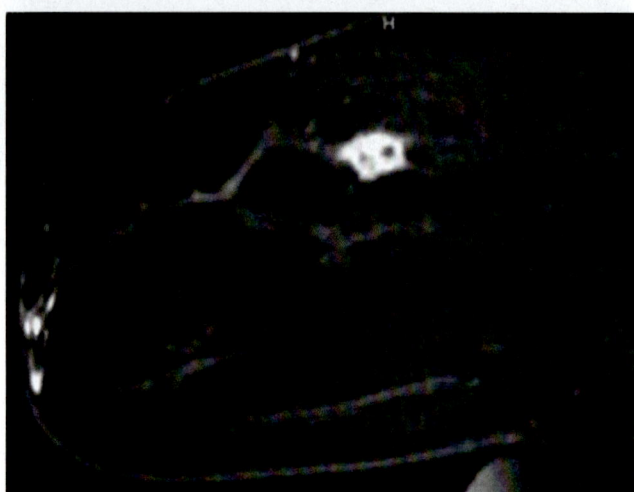

C

FIG. 8.10 • Invasive ductal carcinoma NOS, high nuclear grade.
A: Spot compression view, left breast MLO projection in a 65-year-old patient. Oval, high-density mass with indistinct margins is confirmed in the left breast. **B:** Ultrasound. An oval hypoechoic, horizontally oriented mass (arrow) is imaged in the left breast correlating to the mass identified mammographically. At the time of the ultrasound, this mass could not be palpated. Given the patient's age and the mammographic features of this lesion, biopsy is done. BI-RADS 4C: Suspicious abnormality; biopsy is indicated. An invasive ductal carcinoma high nuclear grade is reported on the cores. The tumor is estrogen and progesterone receptor-negative, HER2/neu-positive. **C:** MRI, T1-weighted sagittal reconstruction of the left breast post-contrast. An oval mass with irregular and spiculated margins and heterogeneous enhancement is imaged corresponding to the site of the patient's known malignancy. No other lesions are identified in either breast. The histology is confirmed at the time of lumpectomy. The sentinel LN biopsy is negative (0/3 LNs).

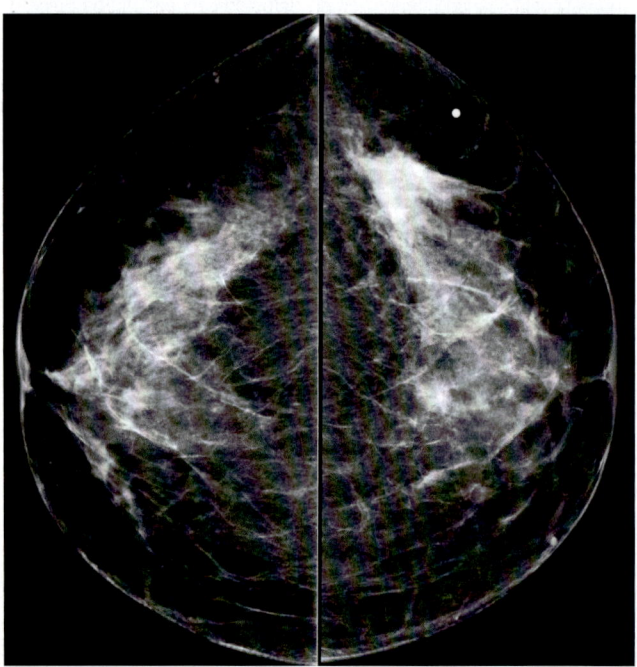

A

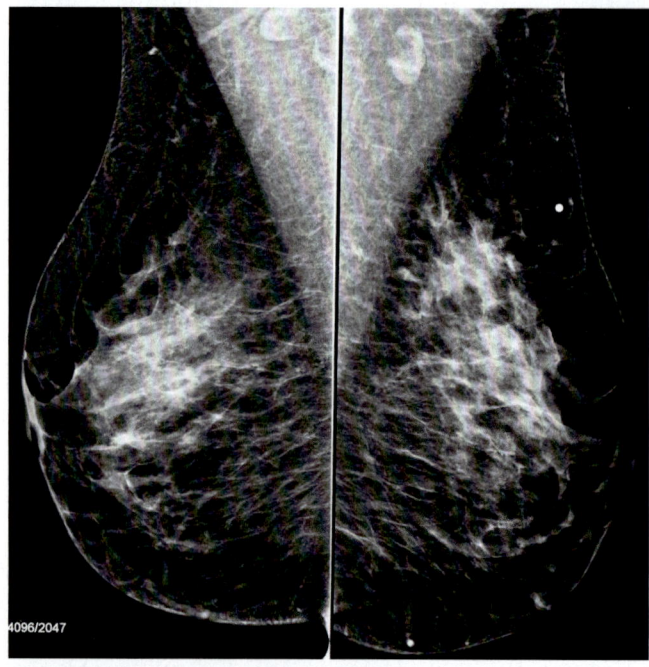

B

FIG. 8.11 • Palpable asymmetry, invasive ductal carcinoma, NOS intermediate nuclear grade. CC **(A)** and MLO **(B)** views in a 47-year-old patient. Parenchymal asymmetry is imaged in the upper outer quadrant of the left breast corresponding to a "lump" (metallic BB) described by the patient; at least on the CC, the area of asymmetry is the densest portion of the mammogram. Note morphologically normal-appearing lymph nodes in the axillae. Palpable parenchymal asymmetry requires evaluation with spot compression view (not shown), correlative physical examination, and ultrasound. The tumor in this patient is estrogen and progesterone receptor-positive, HER2/neu-negative. The sentinel lymph node (LN) biopsy is negative (0/2LNs).

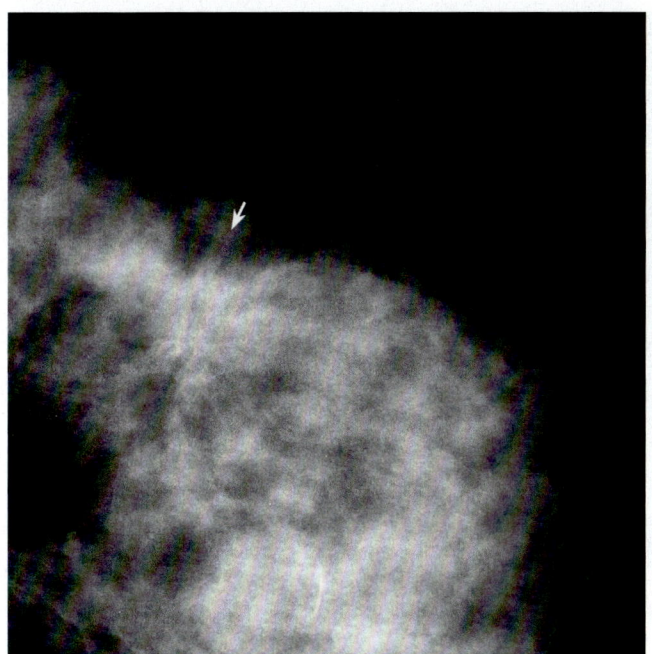

FIG. 8.12 • **Invasive ductal carcinoma NOS, intermediate grade.** CC view photographically coned to the lateral aspect of the left breast, screening study in a 52-year-old woman. Distortion *(arrow)* is noted laterally in the left breast. Confirmed on orthogonal spot compression views (not shown). The only thing that might prevent a biopsy with this type of finding (e.g., distortion, spiculation) is a history of prior surgery localized to this site. BI-RADS 4C: Suspicious abnormality; biopsy is indicated. Diagnosis of invasive ductal carcinoma intermediate nuclear grade is established on an ultrasound-guided core biopsy. (From Cardeñosa G. *Breast Imaging [The Core Curriculum Series]*. Philadelphia, PA: Lippincott Williams & Wilkins; 2003.)

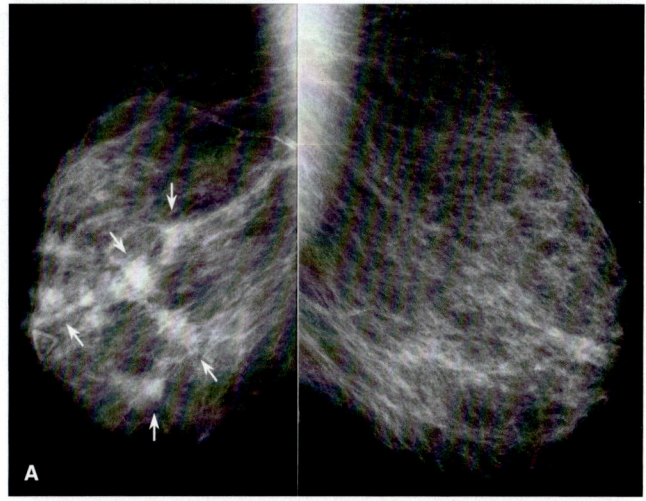

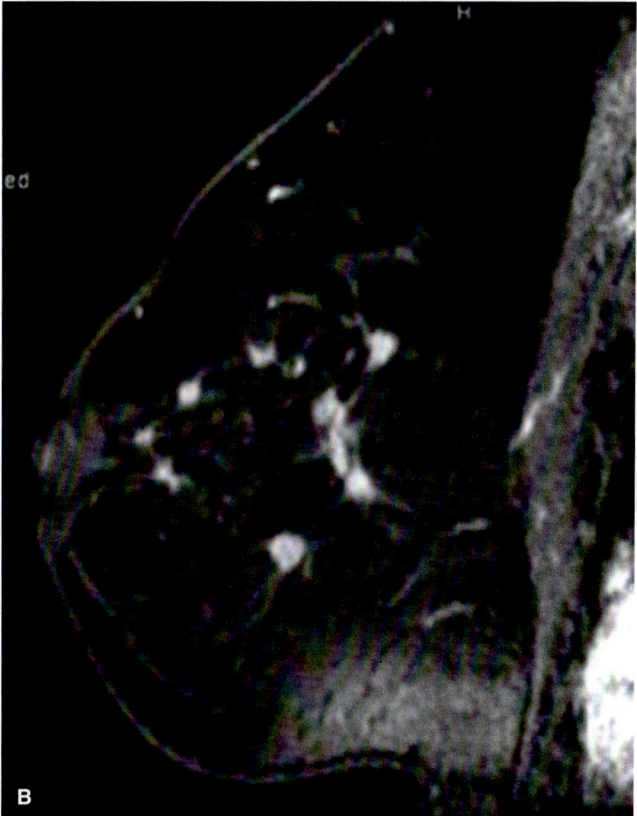

FIG. 8.13 • **Multifocal and multicentric invasive ductal carcinoma, NOS intermediate nuclear grade with micropapillary features.** **A:** MLO views in a 72-year-old patient presenting with a "lump" anteriorly (radiopaque triangular marker). As compared to her prior studies (not shown), the right breast is now smaller with diffuse prominence of the trabecular markings and multiple masses *(arrows)*. BI-RADS 4C: Suspicious abnormality; biopsy is indicated. In this patient, the two masses furthest apart are biopsied to establish the extent the disease. **B:** MRI, T1-weighted sagittal reconstruction of the right breast postcontrast. Multiple masses with spiculated margins and heterogeneous enhancement, are imaged encompassing multiple quadrants in the breast (not all the masses are included at this scan plane). Nipple retraction is also noted on the MRI. The lesions are estrogen and progesterone receptor-positive, HER2/neu-negative. Signal flaring is noted in the area of the inframammary fold.

studies) and are often triple-negative lesions (estrogen and progesterone receptor-negative, HER2/neu-negative) (Fig. 8.19). The triple-negative cancers are also reportedly more common in African American patients (10,11). On physical examination, these lesions are often seemingly larger than the lesion seen on mammography or ultrasound (Leborgne law). If there is associated intraductal disease, it is usually characterized by central necrosis such that linear calcifications may be seen mammographically. In patients with an "expansile" mass, it is appropriate to consider some of the more common invasive ductal subtypes including medullary, mucinous, papillary, and metaplastic carcinomas. Medullary carcinomas are more common in younger premenopausal patients and may present as interval cancers. Mucinous and papillary carcinomas are slower growing (less likely to be interval cancers) and more common in post-menopausal women. On ultrasound, mucinous carcinoma may be difficult to identify because it is often iso to slightly hyperechoic, and papillary carcinomas are usually a complex cystic mass in the subareolar area. Except for the pleomorphic variant (rare), invasive lobular carcinoma rarely presents as a round mass and as such it is usually not included in the differential for round masses.

In considering the differential for malignancies presenting with masses that have spiculated margins (see Table 7.9 for differential considerations), invasive ductal carcinoma NOS is the most likely, and many of these are low to intermediate grade. If associated intraductal disease (DCIS) is present, it is not typically characterized by central necrosis; it is often low to intermediate grade such that, if there are calcifications, they are likely to be predominantly fine pleomorphic including round, punctate, and amorphous forms. Of the

FIG. 8.14 • **Invasive ductal carcinoma, low nuclear grade with associated DCIS.** Spot compression view, MLO projection in 63-year-old patient. An iso dense mass *(long arrows)* with spiculated margins is present. Fine pleomorphic (round and punctate) calcifications *(short arrows)* are noted extending away from the mass with some of the calcifications demonstrating a linear distribution. BI-RADS 4C: Suspicious abnormality; biopsy is indicated. In taking care of this patient, biopsies are done of the mass and the anterior-most extent of the calcifications, thereby establishing the extent of the disease. If the patient wants conservative therapy, bracketing the mass and calcifications with two wires is important preoperatively. Likewise, alerting the pathologist to the location of the calcifications away from the primary finding on the specimen radiograph is critical in establishing an accurate diagnosis and extent of disease. In this patient, synchronous DCIS is diagnosed on MRI (not shown) in the contralateral breast.

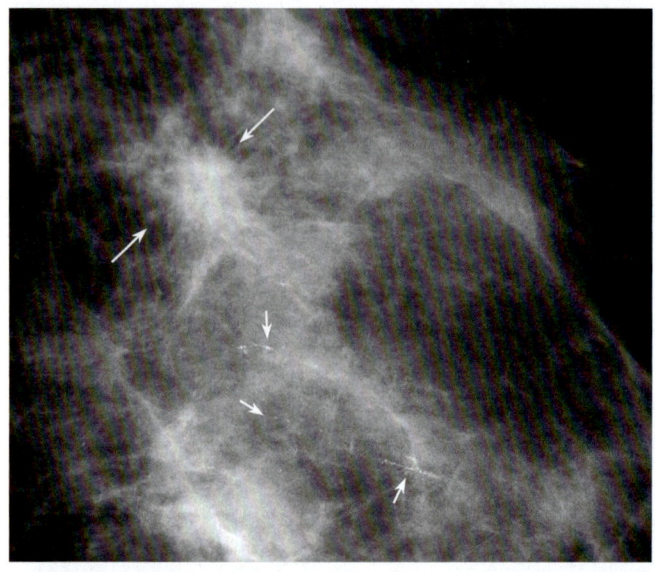

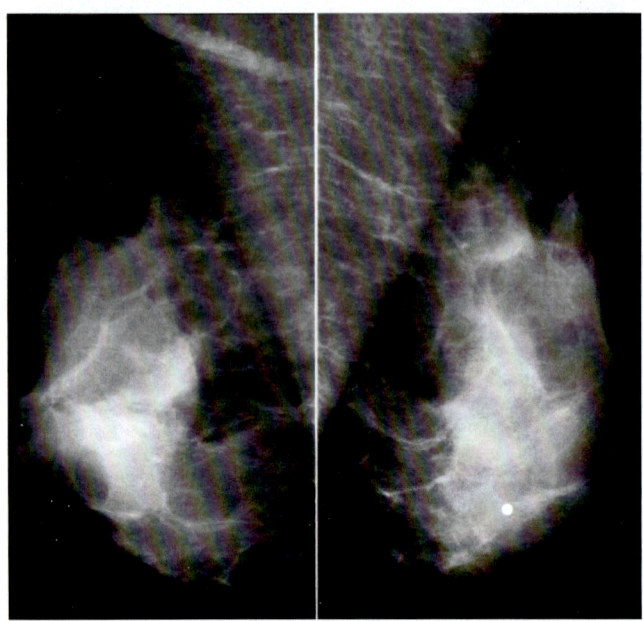

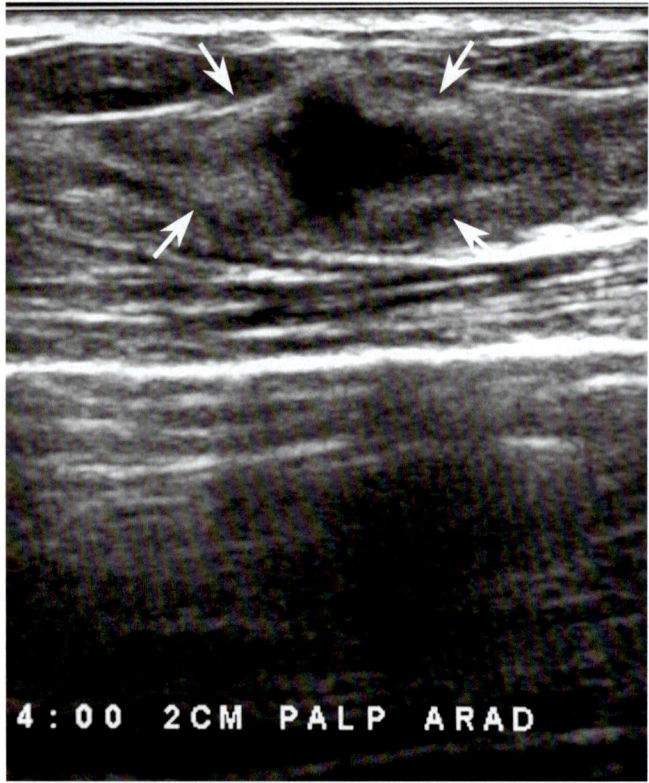

A B

FIG. 8.15 • **Invasive ductal carcinoma, NOS. A:** MLO views in a 37-year-old patient who presents describing a "lump" in her left breast. The metallic BB marks the site of the palpable finding. Dense tissue is imaged at the site of concern on all images (CC and spot tangential views not shown). **B:** Ultrasound. An irregular, vertically oriented, markedly hypoechoic mass *(arrows)* with angular margins and a thickened and irregular echogenic rim is imaged in the lower outer quadrant of the left breast corresponding to a discrete, fixed hard mass *(PALP)*. BI-RADS 4C: Suspicious finding; biopsy is indicated. This BI-RADS is based on the clinical and ultrasound findings, not the mammogram (which in this patient is normal). The evaluation of a patient with dense tissue mammographically corresponding to a site of concern is incomplete without correlative physical examination and an ultrasound. The diagnosis in this patient is established after an ultrasound-guided biopsy. **C:** MRI, T1-weighted sagittal reconstruction of the left breast post-contrast. A homogeneously enhancing irregular mass *(long arrow)* with smooth margins is imaged in the lower outer quadrant of the left breast zone B. Clumped and linear enhancement *(short arrow)* is identified extending anteriorly from the mass for approximately 2 cm consistent with associated DCIS. **D:** CC view of the right breast photographically coned to medial quadrants in a different patient. An oval dense mass *(arrow)* with indistinct margins is identified in the right breast. The features of this mass are confirmed on spot compression views (not shown). Seemingly normal tissue is seen on ultrasound at the expected location for this mass. Since no cyst is imaged, it is presumed that the mass seen mammographically is solid and isoechoic with surrounding tissue. Given the mammographic features (new, medial location, margins), a stereotactically guided biopsy is done to establish the diagnosis of invasive ductal carcinoma, poorly differentiated. BI-RADS 4C: Suspicious finding; biopsy is indicated.

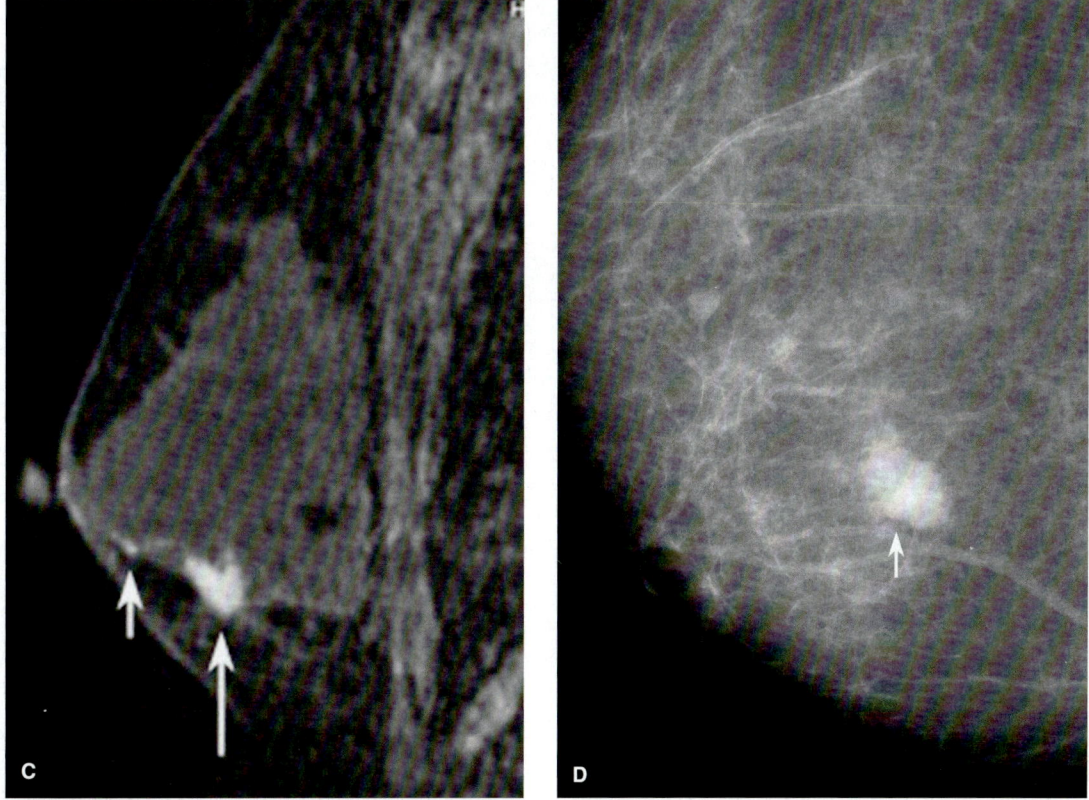

FIG. 8.15 • (continued)

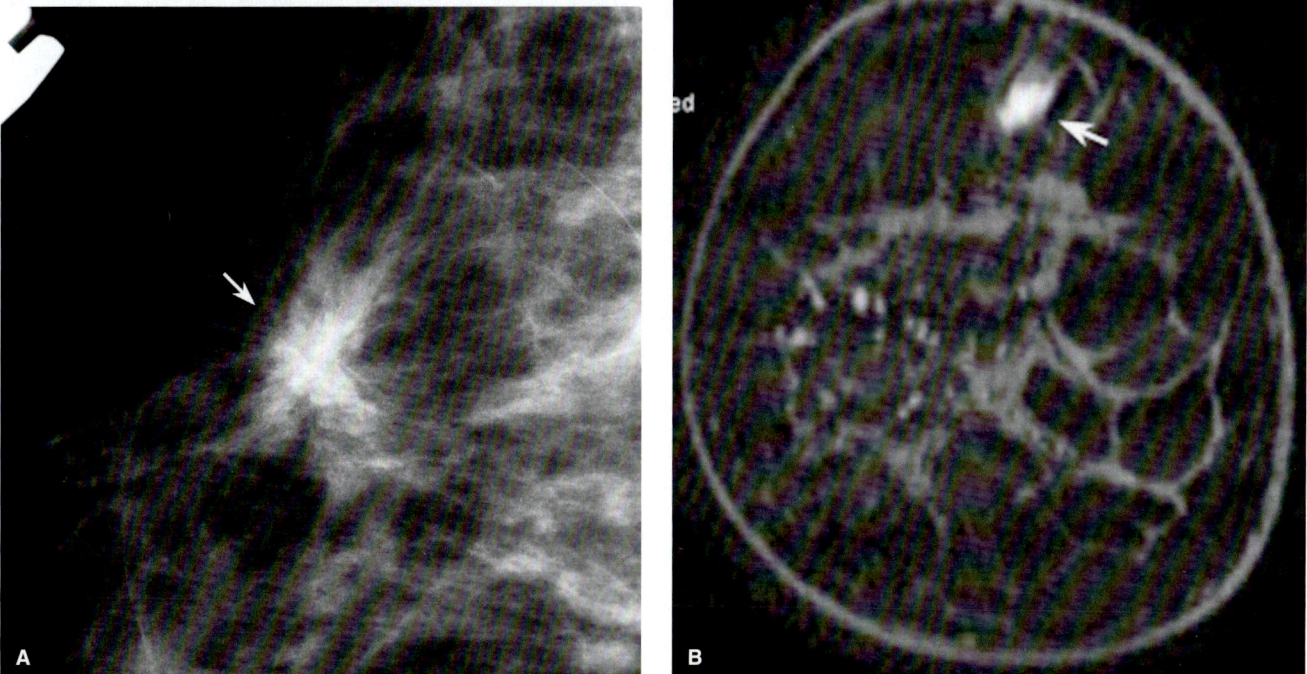

FIG. 8.16 • **Multifocal, invasive ductal carcinoma NOS, intermediate grade. A:** Spot compression view, right breast MLO projection done to further evaluate possible distortion noted on the screening mammogram in a 76-year-old woman. A dense irregular mass *(arrow)* with spiculated margins and associated distortion is confirmed on orthogonal spot compression views (only one projection is shown). BI-RADS 4C: Suspicious abnormality; biopsy is indicated. Ultrasound-guided biopsy (not shown) is done to establish the suspected diagnosis. **B:** MRI, T1-weighted coronal reconstruction, right breast pre-contrast. An oval mass with high T1 signal *(arrow)* is seen superiorly in the right breast prior to the contrast bolus consistent with a biopsy-related hematoma. **C:** MRI, T1-weighted coronal reconstruction, right breast post-contrast. Three enhancing masses are identified on the MRI. The largest of these *(long arrow)* demonstrates spiculated margins and heterogeneous enhancement and corresponds to the mass identified mammographically and the site of the patient's known invasive ductal carcinoma. Two smaller ("satellites") more homogeneously enhancing masses *(short arrows)* are seen in close proximity to the primary lesion. Three foci of invasive ductal carcinoma are confirmed at the time of the patient's lumpectomy. In comparison with the pre-contrast image shown in part **B**, the hematoma shows no enhancement.

(continued)

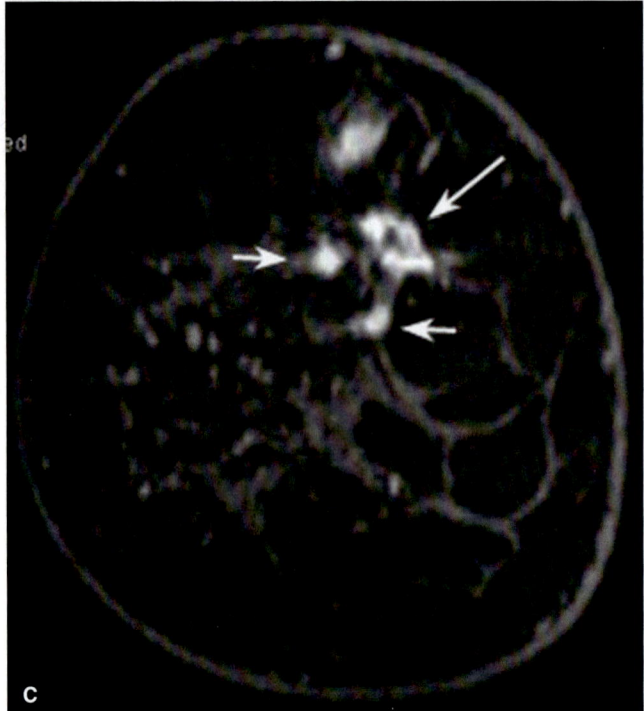

FIG. 8.16 • (continued)

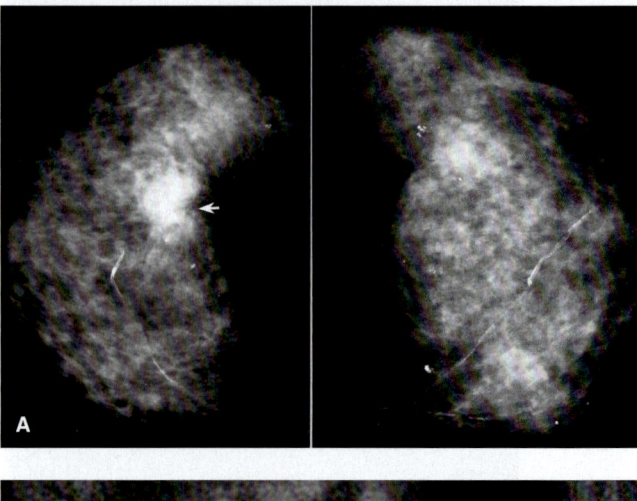

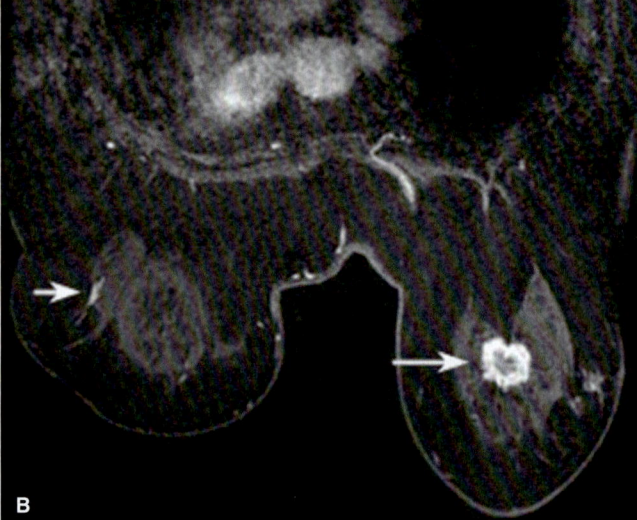

FIG. 8.17 • **Synchronous lesions, invasive ductal carcinoma NOS intermediate grade in the right breast and DCIS (extensive), intermediate grade in the left breast. A:** CC views in a 72-year-old woman. Dense breast parenchyma is present with arterial calcification and dystrophic-type calcifications scattered bilaterally (**left** more than **right**). A dense, round mass with indistinct and spiculated margins is present at the glandular tissue–retroglandular fat interface in the right breast. Note also that this is the densest area in this patient's mammogram. A hypoechoic mass with internal echoes consistent with calcifications, indistinct, spiculated and angular margins, and shadowing is imaged on ultrasound (not shown) corresponding to the mass seen mammographically in the right breast. Although this is a screen-detected abnormality, a hard immobile mass is palpated at the time of the ultrasound. **B:** MRI, axial T1-weighted image post-contrast. A mass (long arrow) with thickened, irregular rim enhancement and spiculated margins is imaged in the right breast at the site of patient's known cancer. Focal non-mass–like linear enhancement (short arrow) is noted in the left breast laterally in zone B. DCIS intermediate grade is diagnosed on an MRI-guided biopsy. The findings are confirmed at the time of bilateral lumpectomies. The DCIS in the left breast is described as extensive; however, no invasion is identified.

more common invasive ductal subtypes, tubular carcinoma is the only one that typically presents as one or several small masses with spiculated margins and is more common in pre-menopausal women. Invasive lobular carcinoma is also included in this differential since a mass with spiculated margins is the most common presentation for this type of tumor; patients with invasive lobular are often older post-menopausal women.

In patients with known invasive breast primaries, we routinely scan the ipsilateral axilla (see discussion at the end of this chapter). Ultrasound evaluation of the ipsilateral axilla in patients with a probable malignancy can be useful because it provides access to an area that may be difficult to evaluate on the mammogram. If a suspicious lymph node is identified, a core biopsy or fine needle aspiration is done at the time of biopsy of the primary breast lesion. Patients identified with metastatic disease bypass sentinel lymph node biopsy and go on to have full axillary dissections at the time of the lumpectomy. Alternatively, depending on the size of the primary, patients with positive axillary lymph nodes at the time of presentation may be treated with neo-adjuvant therapy prior to any surgery.

Histologically, invasive ductal carcinomas NOS demonstrate variable growth patterns (infiltrative, expansile), cellular morphology, and no special features. Several grading systems are available based on tubule formation, nuclear morphology, and mitotic activity. Estrogen receptors are reportedly positive in 55% to 72% of lesions; however, poorly differentiated lesions are less likely to have estrogen receptors. Progesterone receptors occur in 33% to 70% of lesions, and approximately 15% of lesions are estrogen receptor-positive and progesterone receptor-negative (1,2,7). HER2/neu (ERBB2) is an epidermal growth factor receptor (type 2) that may be present in some breast cancers. The ERBB2 gene is amplified in approximately 25% of all breast cancers as well as some ovarian cancers and amplification is almost always associated with overexpression. The amplification of this gene in breast cancers is associated with a bad prognosis such that patients have an increased rate of metastasis as well as decreases in time to recurrence and overall survival. Trastuzumab (Herceptin) is used in the treatment of patients with HER2/neu-positive tumors (1).

EXTENSIVE INTRADUCTAL COMPONENT

Patients with invasive ductal carcinomas and extensive areas of associated intraductal carcinoma were initially thought to have a worse

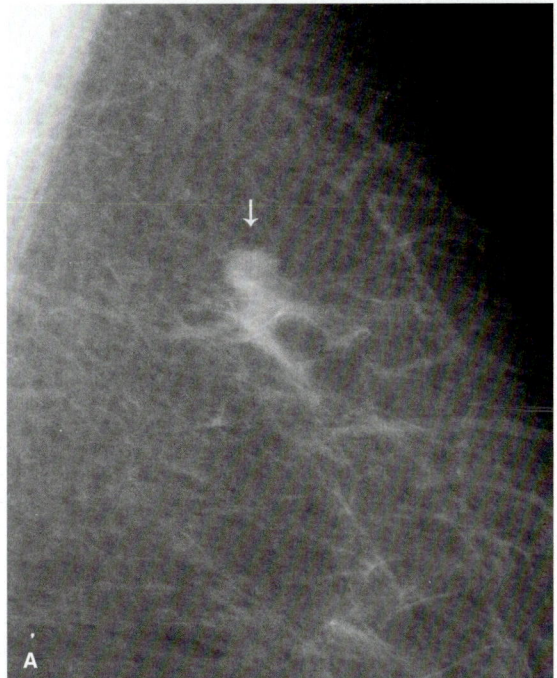
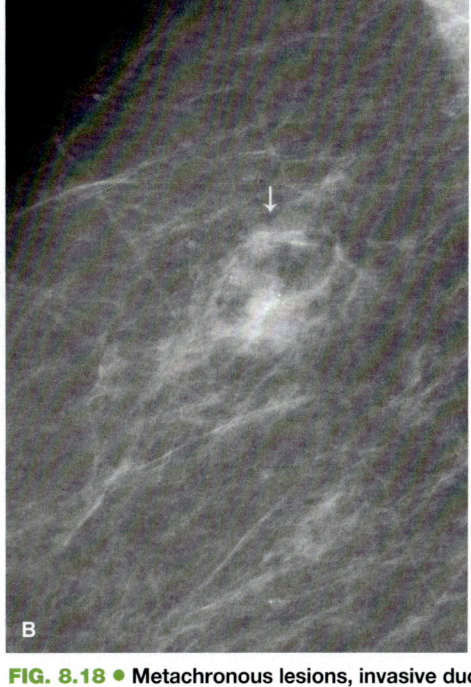
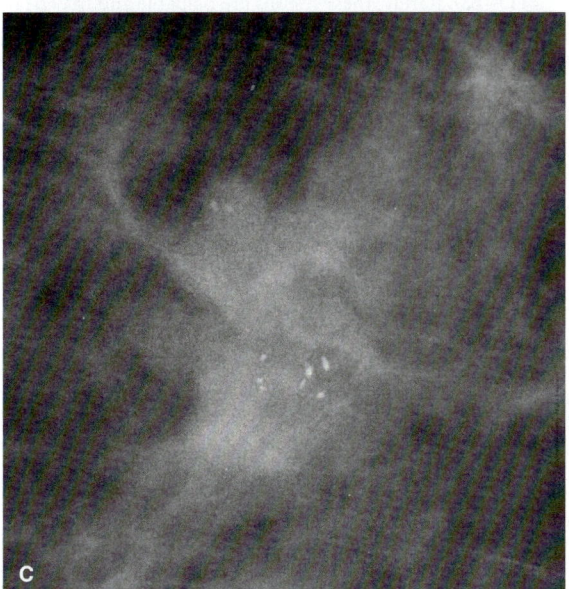

FIG. 8.18 • **Metachronous lesions, invasive ductal carcinoma, NOS. A:** MLO view, left breast photographically coned to the upper portion of the image. An irregular iso dense mass *(arrow)* with indistinct margins is detected on the screening study. Invasive ductal carcinoma is diagnosed following imaging-guided biopsy. **B:** MLO view, right breast, 3 years following "A" photographically coned to the upper portion of the image. A developing density *(arrow)* with possible calcifications is seen superiorly in the right breast. BI-RADS 0: Need additional imaging evaluation. **C:** Double spot compression magnification views (only MLO projection is shown) confirm the presence of an irregular iso dense mass with associated calcifications. In patients with a history of breast cancer, aggressively pursue any perceived changes in the contralateral breast. In this patient, the second lesion is arising in tissue, is irregular, and has associated DCIS consistent with a second primary rather than metastatic disease from the contralateral breast (metastatic disease often presents as one or several round or oval masses, and typically does not have associated DCIS). (From Cardeñosa G. *Breast Imaging [The Core Curriculum Series]*. Philadelphia, PA: Lippincott Williams & Wilkins; 2003.)

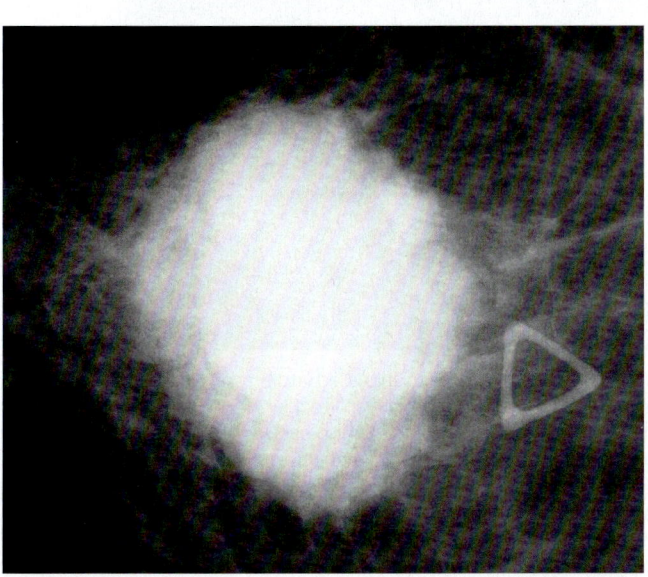

FIG. 8.19 • **Invasive ductal carcinoma NOS, high nuclear grade.** Dense, round, mass with microlobulated, indistinct margins corresponding to a "lump" described by the patient in her left breast (triangular opacity used to denote the palpable finding). This is a rapidly developing expansile ("blow up") lesion in a 48-year-old pre-menopausal woman. Not surprisingly, it is a triple-negative (estrogen and progesterone receptor, HER2/neu-negative), poorly differentiated invasive ductal carcinoma.

prognosis, and were described as having a higher incidence of local recurrence following conservative treatment. This is probably related to incomplete resection of the lesion and residual disease in the breast (12). When patients with lesions having EIC are adequately resected, prognosis is not significantly different from that of women with lesions lacking EIC (13,14). When malignant-type calcifications, or clumped and linear enhancement on MRI, are seen extending for a distance away from a clinically or mammographically detected mass (Fig. 8.14; also see Figs. 7.2B, 7.3, and 3.16), it is important to alert the surgeon and pathologist with respect to the extent of disease and adequately bracket the area at the time of surgery so that the intraductal disease is resected with the invasive component. MRI is the best modality available in detecting and characterizing the extent of EIC (e.g., DCIS is underdiagnosed and the extent underestimated on mammography). Definitions of EIC have varied. Currently, EIC is diagnosed when DCIS constitutes 25% or more of the invasive tumor, or when DCIS is present within and extends beyond (Fig. 8.9C and 8.14) the invasive component (1,2,7,15).

DUCTAL CARCINOMA IN SITU

As discussed in Chapter 6, DCIS is now most commonly diagnosed in asymptomatic women following the detection of calcifications on screening mammograms or the identification of clumped and linear enhancement following MRI. Prior to the widespread use of screening mammography, however, DCIS was uncommon and constituted less than 5% of all breast cancers; patients presented with a palpable mass, spontaneous nipple discharge, or Paget disease of the nipple (16). Although uncommon (so much so that DCIS is rarely included in the differential of an uncalcified, mammographically detected mass), DCIS can be detected as an uncalcified, round, oval, irregular or microlobulated, mass with partially circumscribed (Fig. 8.20) or spiculated margins (Fig. 8.21), distortion (Fig. 8.22), developing ductal distension (see Figs. 5.38, 9.35, and 9.36), parenchymal asymmetry (see Figs. 9.27 and 9.28), or diffuse change (see Figs. 9.20 and 9.21 and Table 6.6 for DCIS presentations). These findings are attributable to the presence of distended, cancer-containing ducts, in aggregate, and an associated periductal inflammatory process. Histologically, central necrosis may be present.

TUBULAR CARCINOMA

Tubular carcinomas are uncommon lesions representing less than 2% of all breast cancers and commonly diagnosed in women in their late 40s. These are a subtype of invasive ductal carcinoma with well-differentiated features. The pure form of tubular carcinoma is almost always ER/PR-positive, HER2/neu-negative, and associated with an excellent prognosis, and yet approximately 10% of patients are found to have axillary metastasis at the time of diagnosis (1).

Mammographically, tubular carcinomas are commonly diagnosed as one or more small (<1 cm), iso- to low-density masses with spiculated margins (Fig. 8.23) or distortion in asymptomatic women (17–22). Rarely, these lesions are palpable and may be mammographically occult. Associated fine pleomorphic calcifications including amorphous, round, and punctate forms (Fig. 8.24) may be present since low nuclear grade DCIS lacking central necrosis is reported in as many as 65% of patients with tubular carcinomas. An irregular hypoechoic mass with spiculated, angular margins and shadowing is the most common presentation for tubular carcinomas on ultrasound. Rarely, these tumors may be more round in appearance (Fig. 8.25). On MRI, tubular carcinomas can demonstrate rapid wash-in and wash-out kinetics; however, rarely these lesions may demonstrate little if any

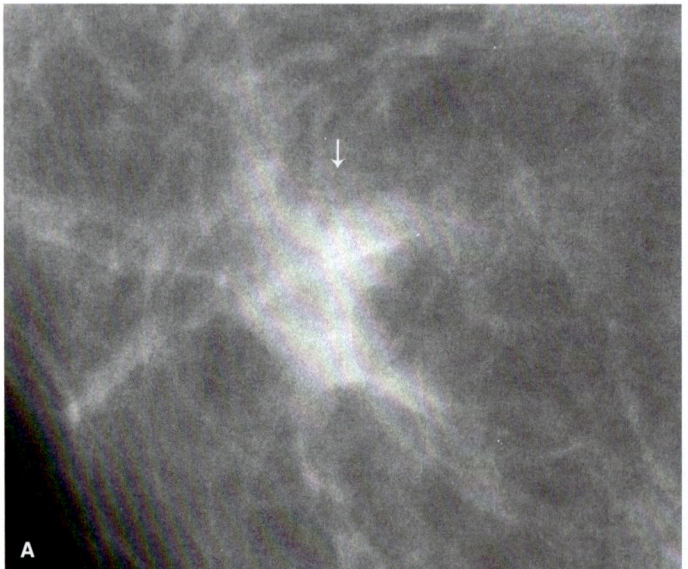
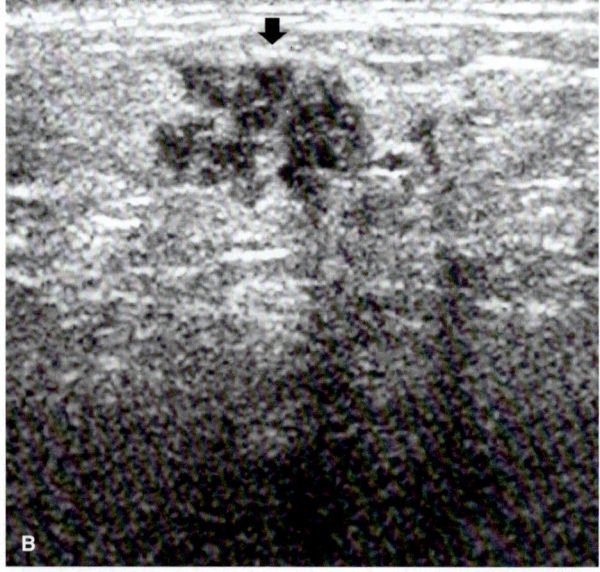

FIG. 8.20 • **Multifocal, DCIS high nuclear grade. A:** Spot compression view, in a 73-year-old patient called back from screening for a mass in the right breast. The spot compression views (only one is shown) demonstrate an irregular low-density lobulated mass *(arrow)* with circumscribed and indistinct margins in the medial aspect of the right breast. **B:** An irregular mass *(arrow)* with heterogeneous echotexture and angular margins is imaged in the upper inner quadrant of the right breast corresponding to the area of mammographic concern. BI-RADS 4C: Suspicious abnormality; biopsy is indicated. Ultrasound-guided core biopsy is done. Diagnosis of DCIS with no associated invasive disease is confirmed on excisional biopsy. Rarely, DCIS presents with a mass and no associated calcifications. (From Cardeñosa G. *Breast Imaging [The Core Curriculum Series]*. Philadelphia, PA: Lippincott Williams & Wilkins; 2003.)

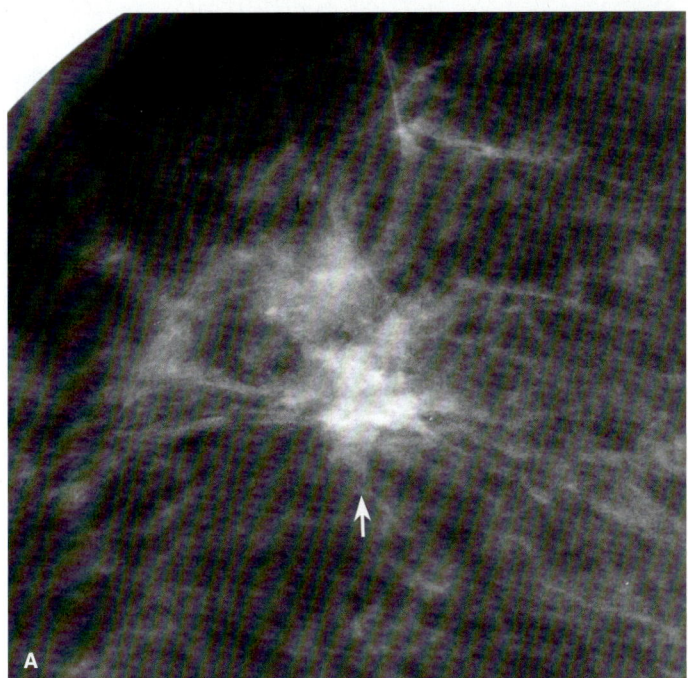
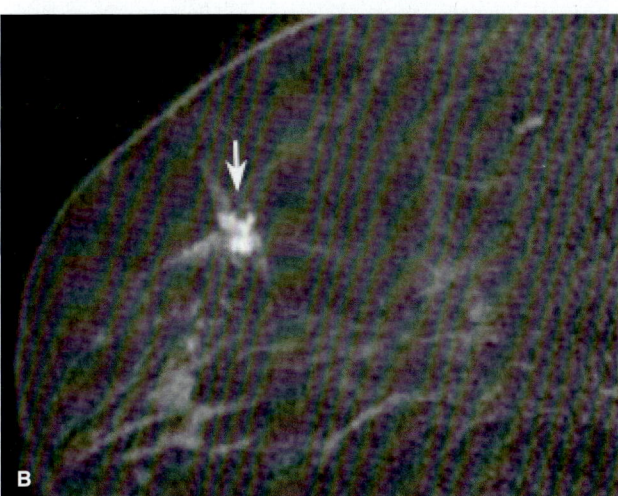

FIG. 8.21 • **DCIS, high nuclear grade with central necrosis. A:** Spot compression view, right MLO projection in a 63-year-old patient confirms the presence of an irregular iso dense mass *(arrow)* with spiculated margins and associated distortion. Screen-detected abnormality. BI-RADS 4C: Suspicious abnormality; biopsy is indicated. Because no abnormality is identified on ultrasound at the expected location for this finding, a stereotactically guided biopsy is done. "Scant breast parenchyma with fibrocystic changes" is reported on the cores. What do you think? These results are not congruent with the imaging findings. **B:** MRI, sagittal maximum intensity projection of the right breast. An irregular mass *(short arrow)* with spiculated margins, heterogeneous enhancement, and associated distortion is imaged corresponding to the mammographic finding. DCIS, high nuclear grade is diagnosed on an MRI-guided core biopsy (see Fig. 12.37G for biopsy image). Morphologically normal-appearing lymph nodes are noted in the right axilla *(long arrows)*. The diagnosis of DCIS with no associated invasive disease is confirmed on excision. Although this patient was diagnosed accurately following the MRI biopsy, it is important to emphasize that, if the MRI had been normal at the site of the mammographic finding, a repeat stereotactically guided biopsy or an excisional biopsy would be indicated for the mammographic finding.

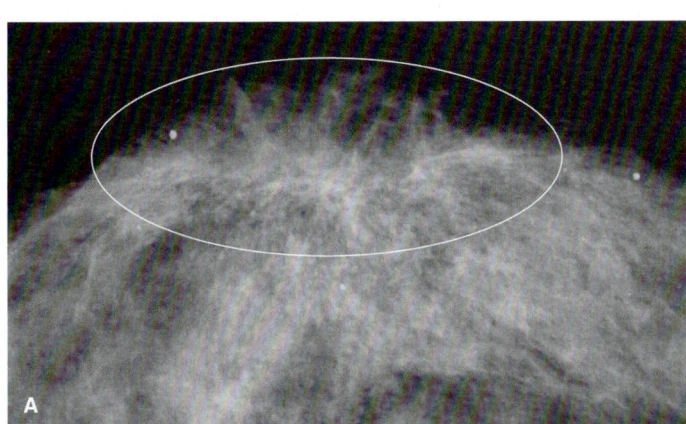
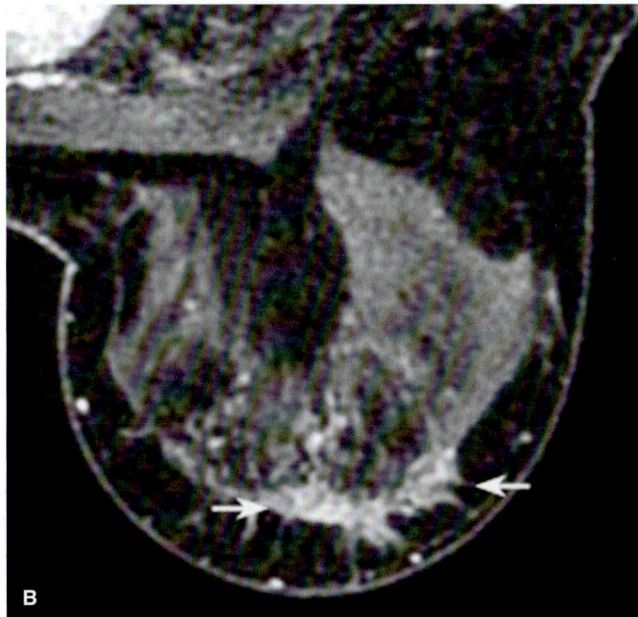

FIG. 8.22 • **Distortion, extensive DCIS, intermediate nuclear grade, cribriform and solid patterns. A:** CC view right breast photographically coned to the anterior aspect of the breast. Distortion *(within oval)* of the tissue is identified involving the subareolar area of the right breast. **B:** MRI, axial T1-weighted image of the right breast post-contrast. Non-mass–like *(arrows)* heterogeneous, enhancement is present along the anterior edge of the glandular tissue corresponding to the area of distortion identified mammographically. DCIS is confirmed at the time of definitive surgery. Given the extent of disease noted on the imaging studies, a sentinel lymph node (LN) biopsy is done and reported as negative (0/2 LNs).

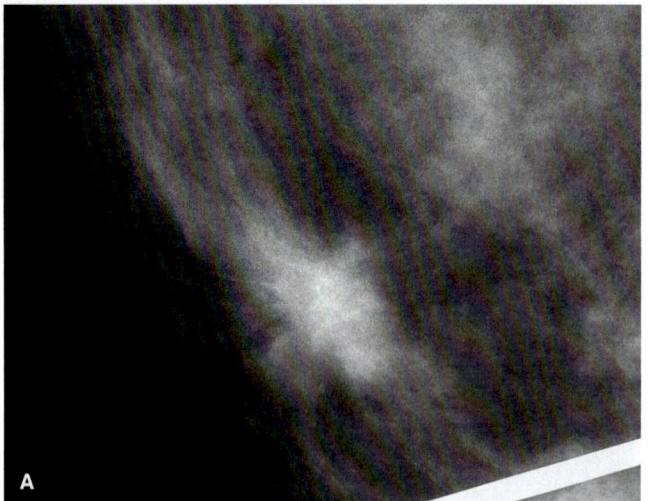
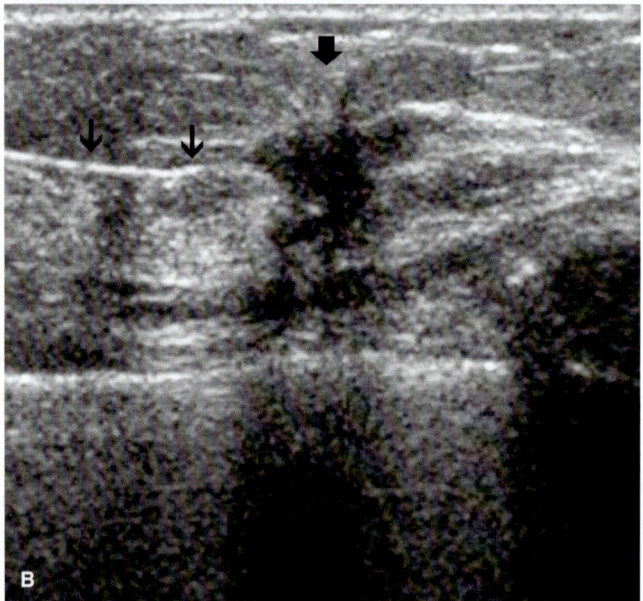

FIG. 8.23 • **Tubular carcinoma. A:** Spot compression magnification view in the medial aspect of the right breast demonstrates an irregular iso dense mass with spiculated margins but no associated calcifications. BI-RADS 4C: Suspicious abnormality; biopsy is indicated. **B:** Ultrasound. Vertically oriented, irregular hypoechoic mass *(thick arrow)* with spiculation, angular margins, shadowing, and disruption of ligaments *(thin arrows)* is imaged correlating to the mammographic finding. Imaging-guided core biopsy diagnosis is confirmed at the time of the lumpectomy. (From Cardeñosa G. *Breast Imaging [The Core Curriculum Series]*. Philadelphia, PA: Lippincott Williams & Wilkins; 2003.)

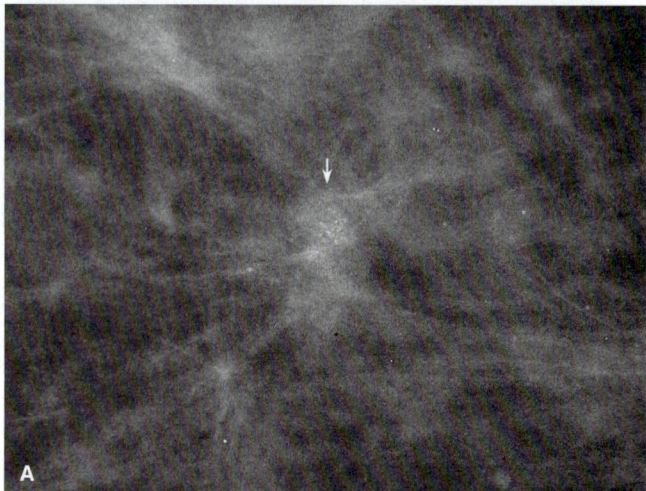
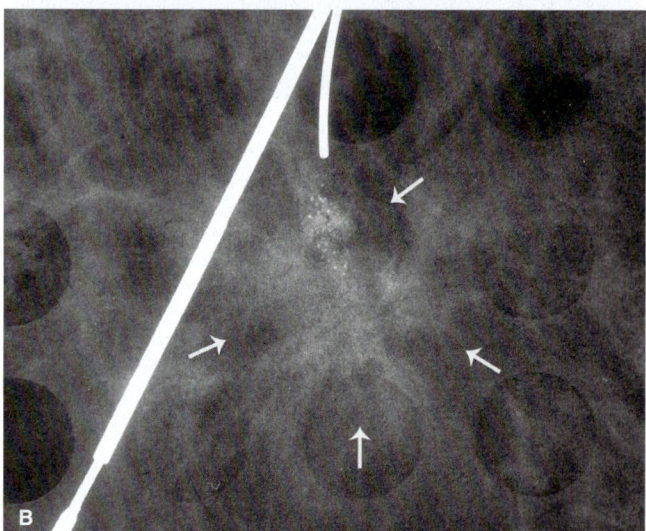

FIG. 8.24 • **Tubular carcinoma with associated DCIS low nuclear grade (cribriform). A:** Spot compression magnification view confirms the presence of an irregular low-density mass *(arrow)* with spiculated margins, associated distortion, and fine pleomorphic calcifications. BI-RADS 4C: Suspicious abnormality; biopsy is indicated. **B:** Specimen radiography demonstrates a low-density mass with spiculated margins, distortion, and calcifications *(arrows)*. Localization wire is partially imaged. (From Cardeñosa G. *Breast Imaging [The Core Curriculum Series]*. Philadelphia, PA: Lippincott Williams & Wilkins; 2003.)

enhancement (e.g., false-negative MRI). As with mammography and ultrasound, tubular carcinomas are typically small irregular masses with spiculated margins having heterogeneous less commonly homogenous enhancement; rarely, they may be more round and oval with circumscribed margins (Fig. 8.25A).

Histologically, there is proliferation of angulated, oval, and elongated tubules lined with a single epithelial cell layer. The proliferating tubules are distinguished from normal ducts by the absence of myoepithelial cells. Pathologists may use special stains (e.g., p63) to establish the absence of myoepithelial cells and confirm the diagnosis (see additional discussion in papillary carcinoma section). Histologically, these lesions need to be distinguished from sclerosing adenosis and complex sclerosing lesions, both of which demonstrate myoepithelial cells. Mitoses are uncommon (1,2).

MUCINOUS CARCINOMA

Mucinous carcinomas are a subtype of invasive ductal carcinoma, and can be further subdivided into pure and mixed forms (mucinous and invasive ductal NOS components) (23,24). In the pure form, mucinous carcinomas represent approximately 2% of all breast cancers and, although they can present at any age, at least the pure forms, are reportedly more common in older post-menopausal women. Estrogen and progesterone receptors have been reported to be positive in 91% to 94% and 79% to 81% of patients with pure mucinous carcinomas, respectively (25). The reported incidence of axillary metastases ranges from 2% to 14% in pure mucinous carcinomas and

Evaluation and Imaging Features of Malignant Breast Masses

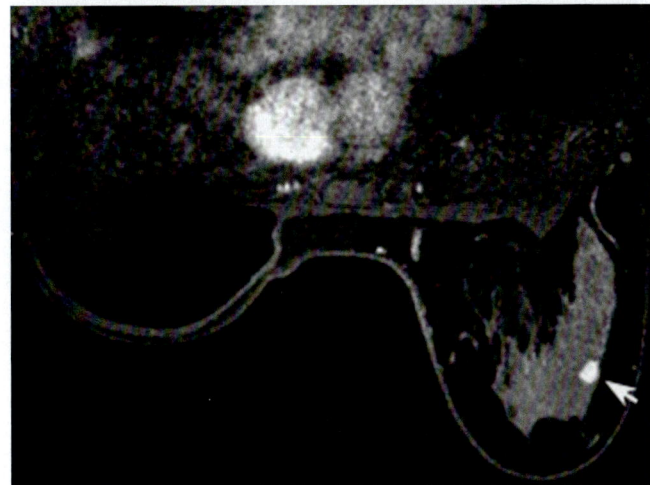

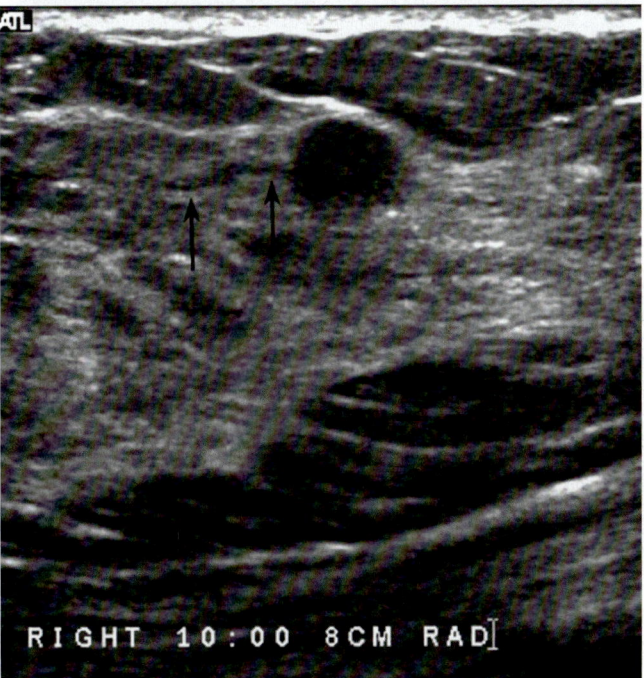

FIG. 8.25 • **Tubular carcinoma. A:** MRI axial T1-weighted image post-contrast. This is a screening MRI in a high-risk, 46-year-old woman with a history of a left mastectomy and implant reconstruction for breast cancer 2 years previously. A round homogeneously enhancing mass *(arrow)* with circumscribed margins is imaged at the fat-glandular interface laterally in the right breast. BI-RADS 4B: Suspicious abnormality; biopsy is indicated. Dense tissue is imaged mammographically on the right. Patient is called back for ultrasound evaluation. If no correlative abnormality is identified on ultrasound, an MRI-guided biopsy is indicated. **B:** Ultrasound. A hypoechoic round mass with indistinct margins and ductal extension *(arrows)* is identified corresponding to the MRI-detected mass. Ultrasound-guided biopsy is done to establish the diagnosis of tubular carcinoma. This diagnosis is confirmed at the time of definitive surgery.

45% to 64% in patients with mixed forms (25). Although it has been suggested that axillary dissection may not be needed in women with pure mucinous carcinoma, this is not generally accepted (25,26). Reported factors increasing the likelihood of axillary disease in patients with pure mucinous carcinoma include younger age at the time of diagnosis, aneuploidy, high nuclear grade, and negative estrogen receptor status. The influence of size on the likelihood of metastatic disease is controversial: some reports describe a direct correlation between tumor size and positive lymph nodes, others do not (25).

Patients can present with a palpable mass (Fig. 8.26) or, if asymptomatic, a round (Fig. 8.27) or oval mass with circumscribed to indistinct margins (Fig. 8.28); the mixed forms are more likely to be irregular in shape (24,27–30). Many of these lesions are slow-growing and as such may be seen on prior studies. Minimal increases in size and loss of marginal definition in a small round mass in an older patient should suggest the diagnosis of mucinous carcinoma. The diagnosis is further suggested if on ultrasound, an iso- to slightly hyperechoic mass with defined margins and variable amounts of posterior enhancement is imaged correlating to the mass seen mammographically. Their tendency to be iso- to slightly hyperechoic (Figs. 8.26B, 8.27B and 8.28C) makes detection on ultrasound challenging such that meticulous ultrasound technique is often required. Less commonly, mucinous carcinomas are hypoechoic or have a heterogeneous echotexture (Fig. 8.29) that may demonstrate variable amounts or shadowing. Rarely, a complex cystic mass is seen (Fig. 8.30).

On MRI, pure mucinous carcinomas are characterized by a high T2 signal (close to that of water), a reflection of the mucinous component of these lesions (Figs. 8.26D, 8.27C, 8.28C; also see Fig. 5.16); degeneration, necrosis, fibrosis, hemorrhage, or calcification may alter the T2-signal intensity (24,30). The T1 signal of these lesions is variable pre-contrast. Gradual enhancement (persistent-type kinetic curve) is typical; however, it appears that with increases in the cellularity of the described cell aggregates (see below), heterogeneous and intense rim enhancement is seen on early phase images (Figs. 8.26D, 8.27D and 8.28D). Some of the larger lesions may demonstrate non-enhancing septations (Fig. 8.26D) that are dark on T2 (similar to findings sometimes seen in patients with fibroadenomas and phyllodes) (24,30).

Grossly, core samples and the cut surface of these lesions are distinctly gelatinous and glistening in appearance (Fig. 8.31A, B). Histologically, mucinous carcinomas are characterized by cancer cell aggregates floating in extracellular pools of mucin (Fig. 8.31C). The aggregates vary from dense to sparse cellularity, and fibrous septae may be seen separating the pools of mucin. Some mucinous carcinomas have associated low- to intermediate-grade DCIS lacking central necrosis; however, associated DCIS is not usually a prominent feature. Necrosis is uncommon (1,2).

MEDULLARY CARCINOMA

Medullary carcinomas are a subtype of invasive ductal carcinoma. The reported incidence is variable secondary to an overdiagnosis of this tumor type (31). When strict histological criteria are followed, these tumors represent less than 2% of breast cancers. Medullary carcinomas present as round or oval masses with circumscribed to indistinct margins (Fig. 8.32A). On ultrasound they are moderately to markedly hypoechoic with indistinct margins (Fig. 8.32B); in some patients, posterior acoustic enhancement is noted (31,32). They may be palpable, and can be characterized by rapid growth rates, at times presenting in young women as interval cancers. The MRI features of these lesions are similar to those described for invasive ductal carcinomas NOS (33,34).

Histologically, nests of large, high-grade epithelial cells with scant surrounding stroma form a syncytial pattern. Nuclei are pleomorphic and there is a high mitotic rate. A significant lymphocytic and plasma cell infiltrate is present surrounding the lesions. Associated DCIS may be seen at the periphery of these lesions. Areas of necrosis may be present as the rapid growth of the tumor outstrips the vascular supply. Most of medullary carcinomas are triple-negative tumors (estrogen and progesterone receptor-negative, HER2/neu-negative) (1,2).

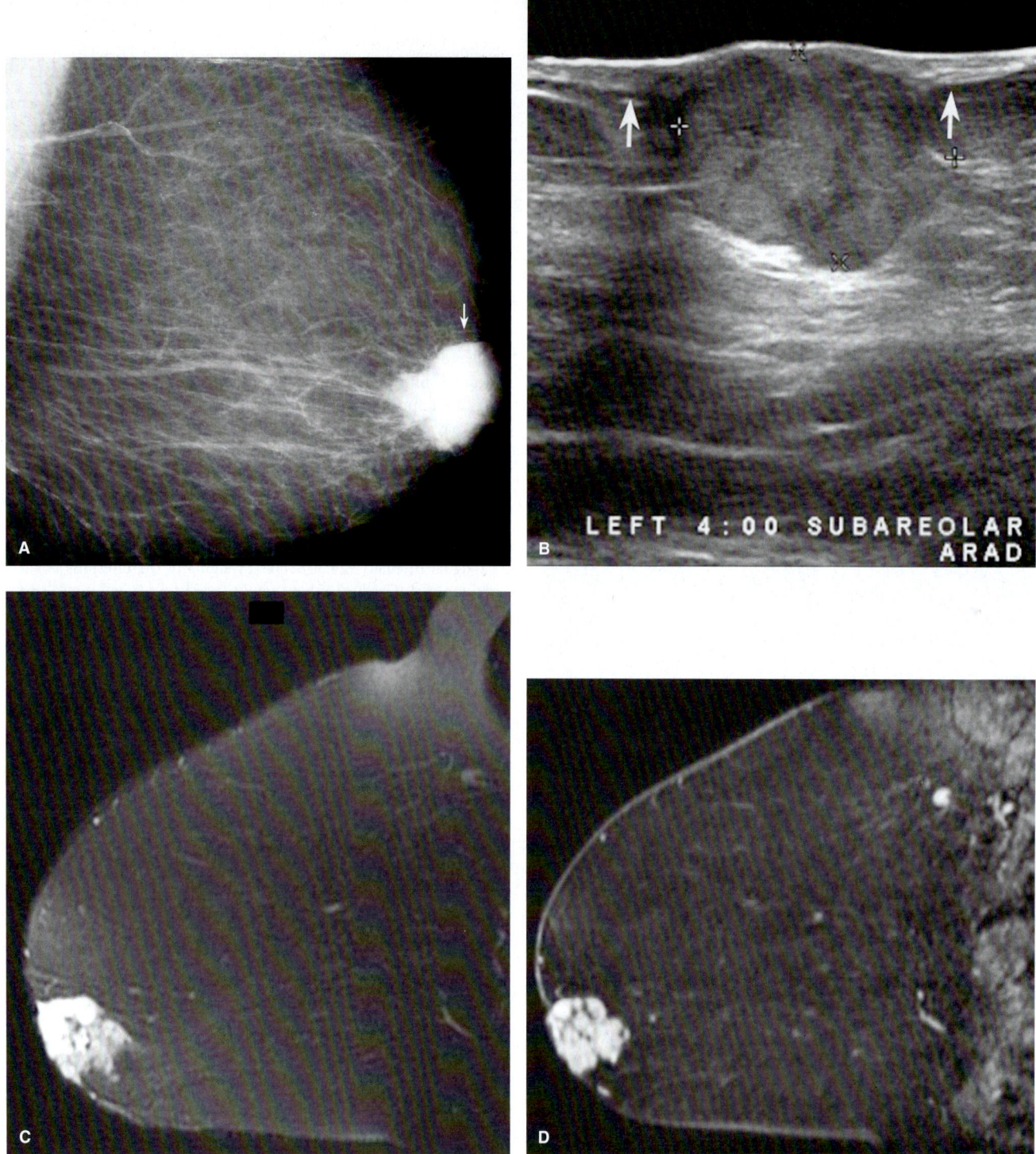

FIG. 8.26 • **Mucinous carcinoma. A:** MLO view of the left breast photographically coned to the anterior aspect of the breast in a 70-year-old patient presenting with a "lump." An irregular dense mass *(arrow)* is imaged superficially in the subareolar area of the left breast corresponding to the palpable finding. **B:** Ultrasound. An iso to hyperechoic round mass (calipers) with posterior acoustic enhancement causing a slight contour (bulge) abnormality is imaged at the site of the palpable and mammographic finding. Ill-defined, irregular thin linear bands of relative hypoechogenicity are noted coursing though the mass. The deep dermal layer *(arrows)* appears disrupted such that skin involvement may be present. Although not pathognomonic, the echogenicity of this mass should raise the possibility of a mucinous carcinoma. BI-RADS 4C: Suspicious abnormality; biopsy is indicated. **C:** MRI, sagittal T2-weighted fat suppressed image of the left breast. A mass with circumscribed margins and predominantly high but heterogeneous T2 signal is imaged in the left subareolar area. **D:** MRI, T1-weighted sagittal reconstruction of the left breast, post-contrast. Heterogeneously enhancing mass with non-enhancing internal septations is imaged in the left subareolar area. Although a homogeneously high T2 signal is usually considered a feature of benign lesions (cysts, young fibroadenomas, lymph nodes), areas of intermediate-to-high (heterogeneous) T2 signal can be seen in mucinous, papillary, and metaplastic carcinomas, necrotic areas in high-grade invasive ductal carcinomas NOS, and phyllodes tumors. This patient's tumor is estrogen receptor-positive, progesterone receptor-negative, and HER2/neu-negative.

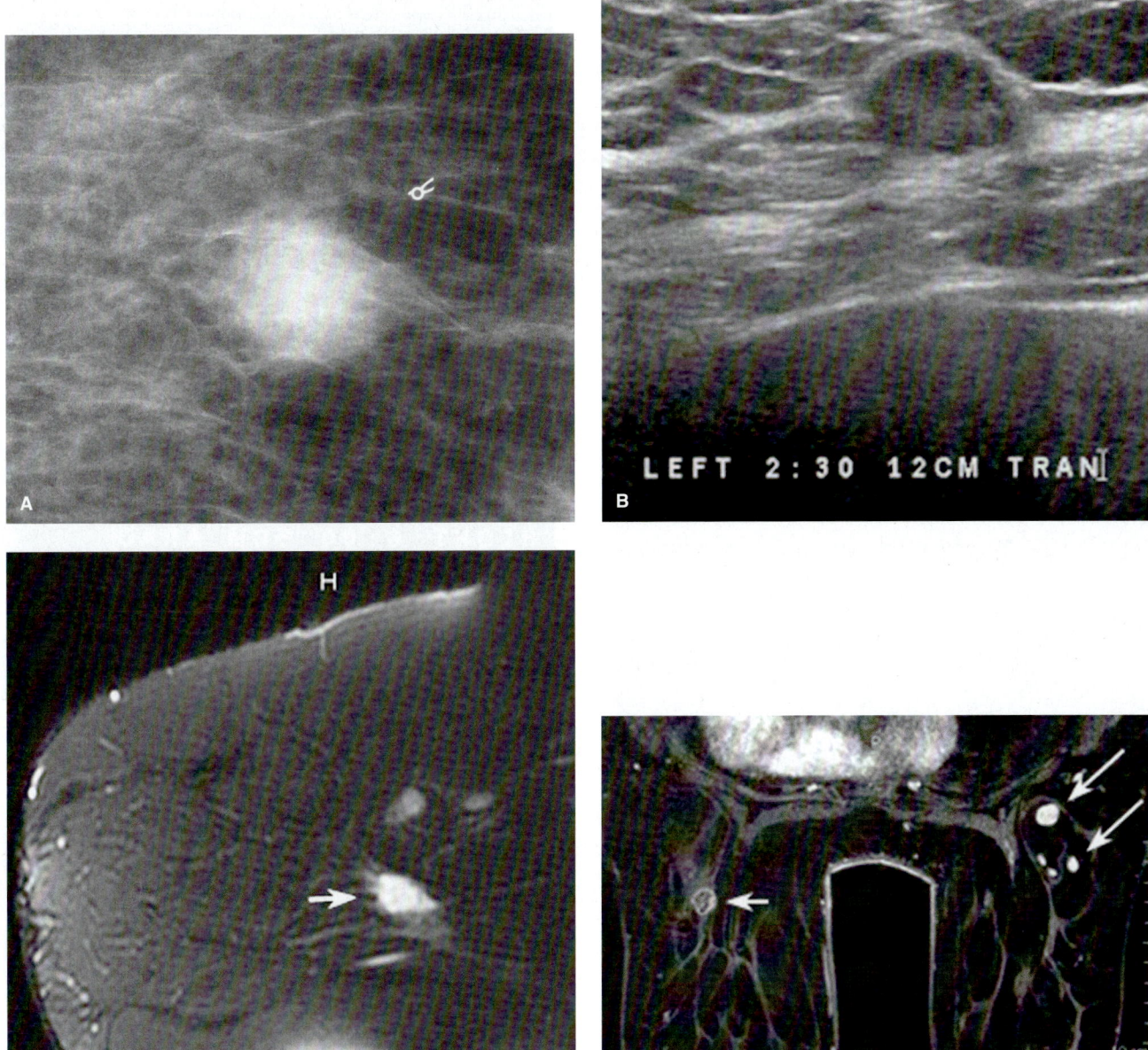

FIG. 8.27 • **Mucinous carcinoma. A:** Spot compression view, MLO projection done to evaluate a screen-detected mass in a 64-year-old patient. An iso dense round mass with indistinct margins is present in the left breast. Incidentally noted is a *biopsy clip* in close proximity to the mass. **B:** Ultrasound. A horizontally oriented, iso-to-slightly hyperechoic mass with an echogenic rim is imaged in the left breast correlating to the mass seen mammographically. BI-RADS 4C: Suspicious abnormality; biopsy is indicated. **C:** MRI, sagittal T2-weighted fat-suppressed image of the left breast. A mass *(arrow)* with high (heterogeneous) T2 signal is imaged in the left breast posteriorly corresponding to the site of the patient's known mucinous carcinoma (e.g., mass detected mammographically). Two oval masses with intermediate T2 signal superior to the mass are lymph nodes. Coil-related artifact (signal flaring) is noted primarily in the area of the inframammary fold. **D:** MRI, T1-weighted axial image post-contrast. A rim-enhancing mass *(short arrow)* is imaged in the central to slightly lateral aspect of the left breast posteriorly correlating to the mass with high T2 signal shown in part **C**. The mammography, ultrasound, and MRI findings in a 64-year-old patient are highly suggestive of mucinous carcinoma. Note several homogeneously enhancing lymph nodes *(long arrows)* posterolaterally in the right breast; these are morphologically normal when viewed in sagittal and coronal reconstructions (not shown). This patient's mucinous carcinoma is estrogen and progesterone receptor-positive, HER2/neu-negative, and the sentinel lymph node (LN) biopsy is negative (0/5 LNs).

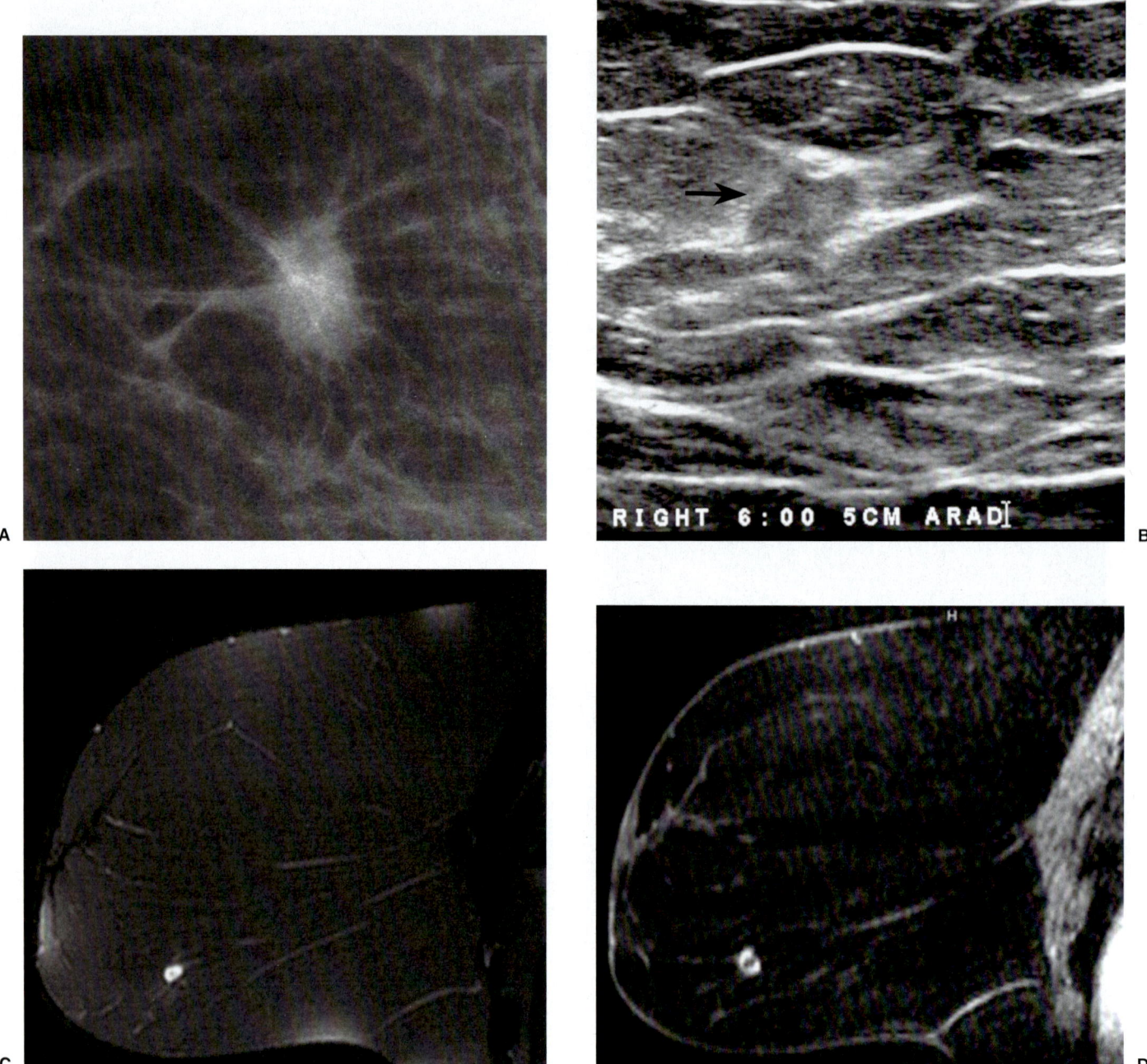

FIG. 8.28 • **Mucinous carcinoma. A:** Spot compression view done to evaluate a screen-detected mass in a 69-year-old patient. A low-density oval mass with indistinct and spiculated margins is confirmed in the right breast on the spot compression views (only one is shown). **B:** Ultrasound. A horizontally oriented oval hyperechoic mass *(arrow)* with gentle macrolobulation is imaged on ultrasound corresponding to the mammographic finding. BI-RADS 4C: Suspicious abnormality; biopsy is indicated. The mammography and ultrasound features of this mass in a 69-year-old patient are highly suggestive of mucinous carcinoma. **C:** MRI, sagittal T2-weighted fat-suppressed image of the right breast. A mass with high T2 signal is imaged in the inferior aspect of the right breast. **D:** MRI, T1-weighted sagittal reconstruction of the right breast, post-contrast. A mass with rim enhancement is imaged corresponding to mass with high T2 signal shown in part **C**. Kinetic curves demonstrate rapid wash-in with rapid wash-out of contrast. This patient's tumor is estrogen and progesterone receptor-positive, HER2/neu-negative, and the sentinel lymph node (LN) biopsy is negative (0/1 LN).

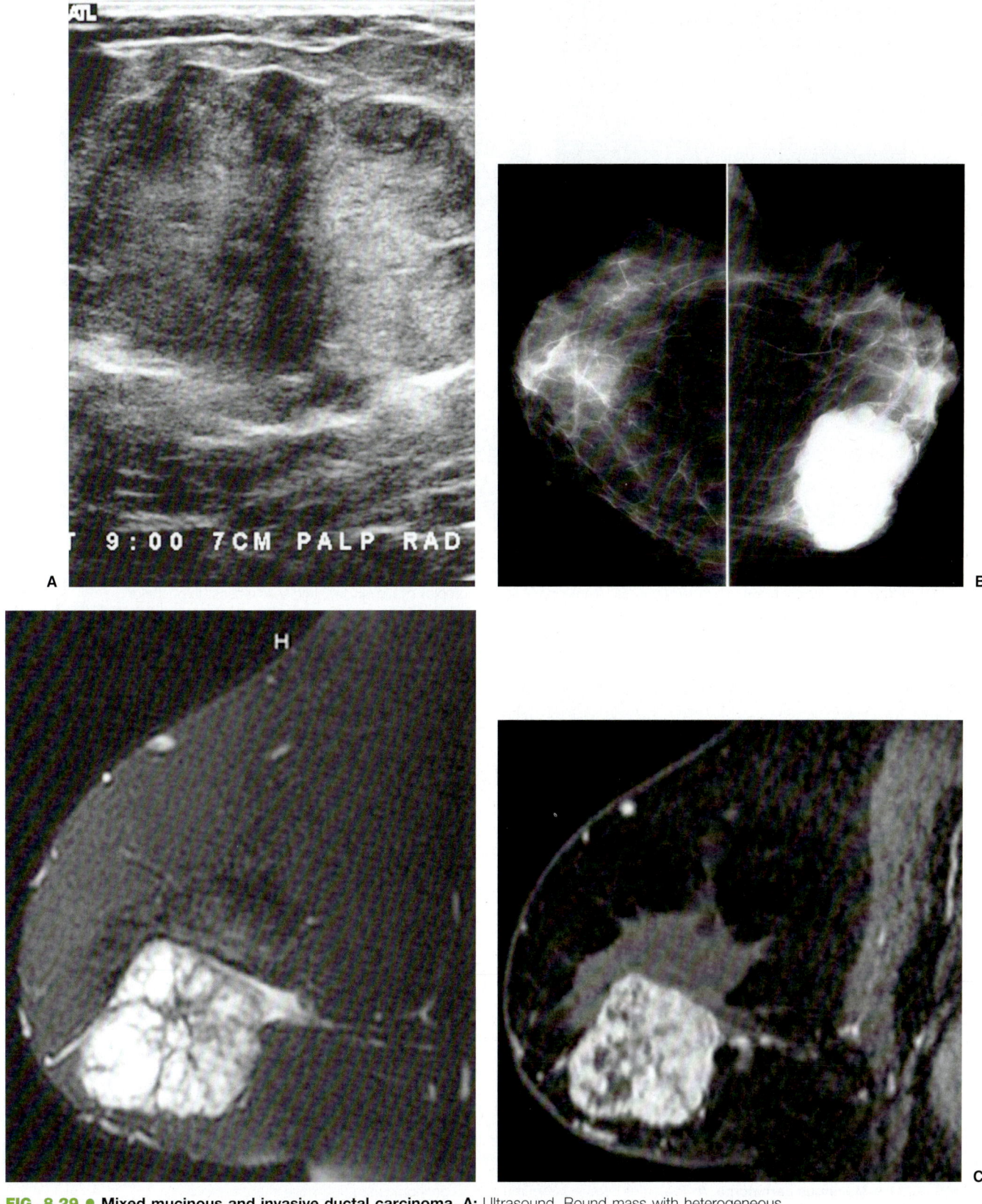

FIG. 8.29 • **Mixed mucinous and invasive ductal carcinoma. A:** Ultrasound. Round mass with heterogeneous echotexture and posterior acoustic enhancement is imaged corresponding to a palpable mass in a 56-year-old patient. **B:** CC views. A dense mass with circumscribed macrolobulated margins is present medially in the left breast corresponding to the mass shown in part **A**. **C:** MRI, sagittal T2-weighted fat-suppressed image of the left breast. A round mass with areas of intermediate and high T2 signal is imaged in the left breast corresponding to the mass shown in parts **A** and **B**. Internal low T2 signal septations are also noted. **D:** MRI, sagittal T1-weighted reconstruction of the left breast post-contrast. The mass demonstrates heterogeneous internal enhancement with predominantly rapid wash-in and wash-out kinetic curves and circumscribed lobulated margins. The tumor is estrogen receptor-positive, progesterone receptor-negative, and HER2/neu-negative.

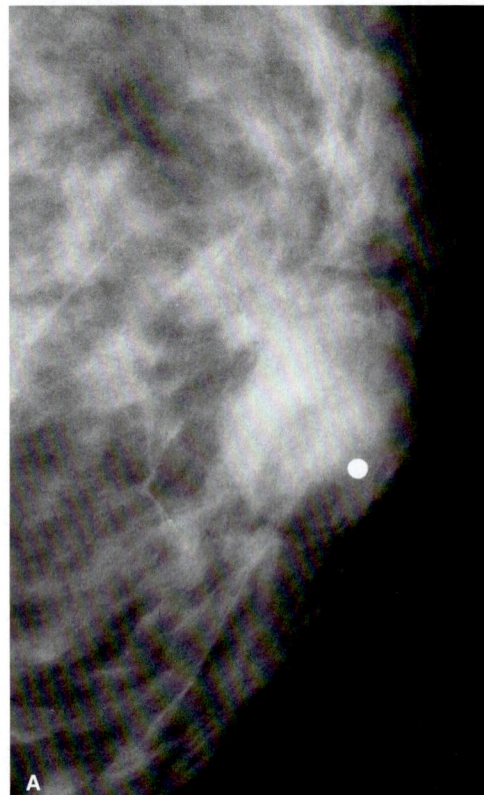
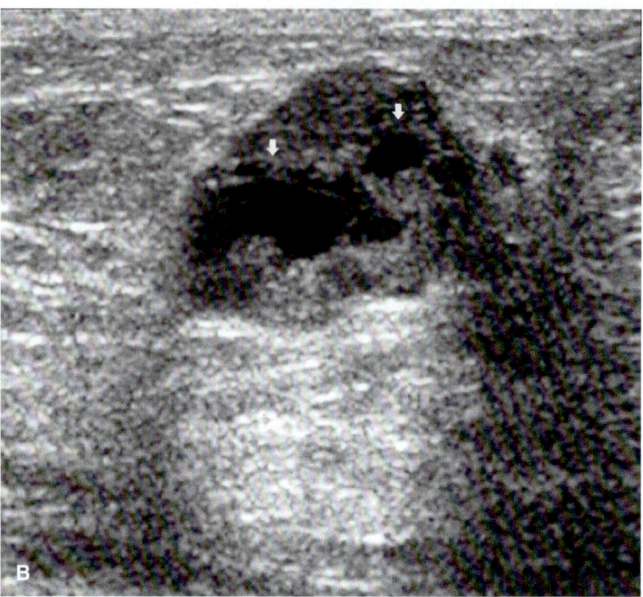

FIG. 8.30 • **Mucinous carcinoma. A:** An iso dense round mass with circumscribed margins is imaged in the subareolar area of the left breast in a 78-year-old woman presenting with a "lump"; in retrospect, this can be seen on a study done 2 years previously (now larger). **B:** Ultrasound. A round complex cystic *(arrows)* and solid mass with posterior acoustic enhancement is imaged corresponding to the palpable finding and the mass seen mammographically. Imaging-guided core biopsy is done to establish the diagnosis.

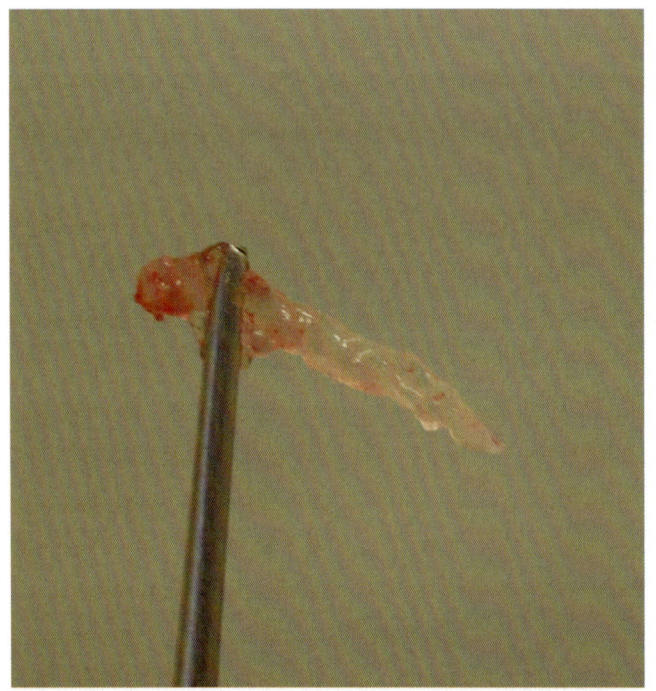
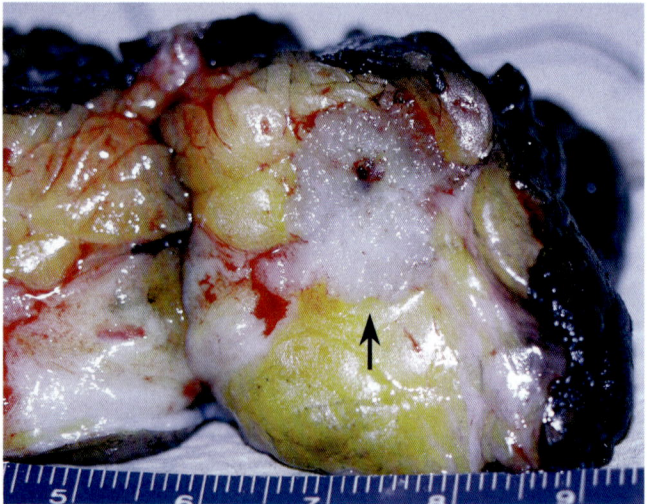

FIG. 8.31 • **Mucinous carcinoma. A:** The cores obtained from mucinous carcinomas are distinctive in appearance with a glistening gelatinous appearance. **B:** Grossly on cross-section, a microlobulated mass *(arrow)* with a gelatinous consistency is seen. A 0.2-cm focus of hemorrhage in the upper aspect of the mass reflects a core biopsy site. The surface of the specimen is black because it has been immersed in India ink; this is used to establish the proximity of the tumor to the margins. **C:** Histologically, mucinous carcinomas are characterized by nests of malignant cells *(short arrows)* floating in pools of mucin separated by thin fibrovascular septae *(long arrows)*. The cellularity of the nests is variable in a given lesion and between lesions; some have used this variability in cellularity and amount of extracellular mucin to explain the various imaging characteristics of mucinous carcinomas.

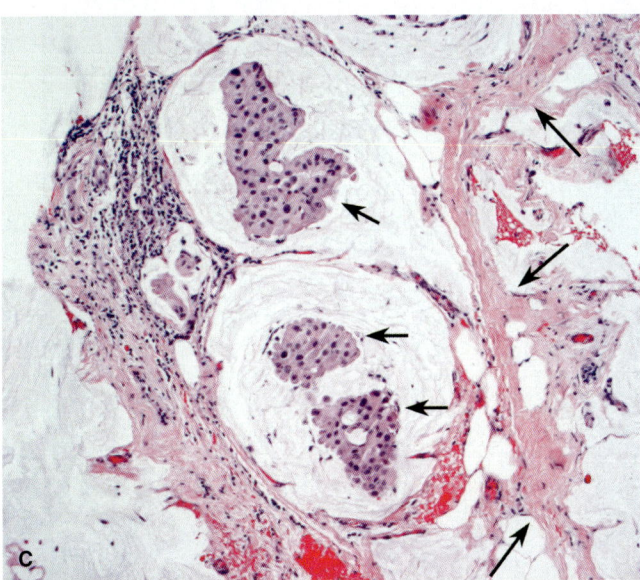

FIG. 8.31 • (continued)

PAPILLARY CARCINOMA

These lesions represent approximately 1% to 2% of all breast cancers and are more common in older post-menopausal women who present describing a palpable mass or nipple discharge. Like papillomas, these lesions can be solitary, usually central in location, or multifocal and peripheral in location. In women with solitary papillary carcinomas, the mass is often subareolar in location and may cause nipple displacement and skin stretching. Patients may have associated nipple discharge. Mammographically, one of two presentation patterns may be seen. Solitary papillary carcinomas are common in the subareolar area presenting as a dense round, oval or macrolobulated mass with circumscribed (expansile) margins (Figs. 8.33A and 8.34A). A complex cystic and solid mass (Fig. 8.33B) is the most common ultrasound feature in patients presenting with a subareolar mass (35,36). Alternatively, multiple peripheral papillary carcinomas present as multiple round, oval, or macrolobulated masses of varying sizes and densities with circumscribed to indistinct margins (Fig. 8.35). On ultrasound, the peripheral lesions are often solid (Fig. 8.36) and indistinguishable from any other solid mass; however, complex cystic and solid masses may also be seen (Fig. 8.37). The appearance of these lesions on MRI is also variable. An enhancing mass with margins that range from circumscribed to spiculated, a high T2 signal component, or an association with a dilated duct may all be seen (Figs. 8.34B–D, 8.36B–D, and 8.37D, E). Rapid to medium wash-in and wash-out or plateau-type kinetic curves are seen commonly with these lesions (37–39).

Malignant papillary tumors are a complex group of lesions, variably defined by pathologists and characterized by confusing terminology. Included are DCIS arising in a papilloma, papillary DCIS (Fig. 8.34), intraductal papillary carcinoma (CA) (e.g., intracystic or encapsulated papillary CA), solid papillary CA, invasive carcinoma arising in an intracystic papillary CA (Figs. 8.36 and 8.37), and invasive papillary

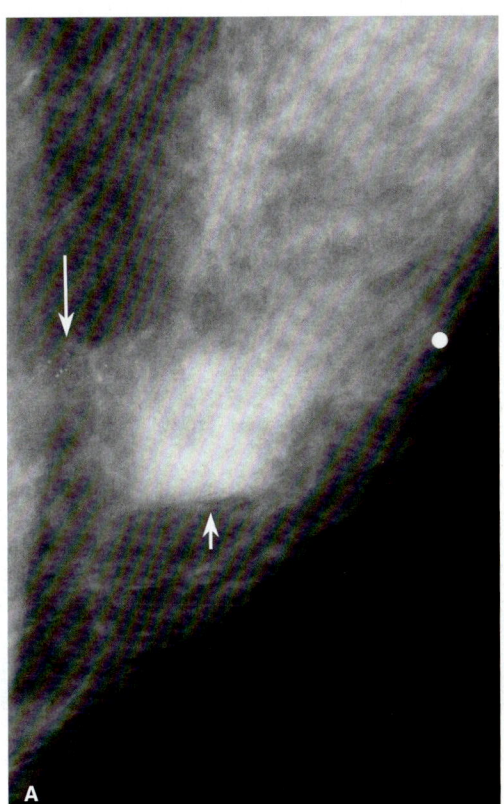
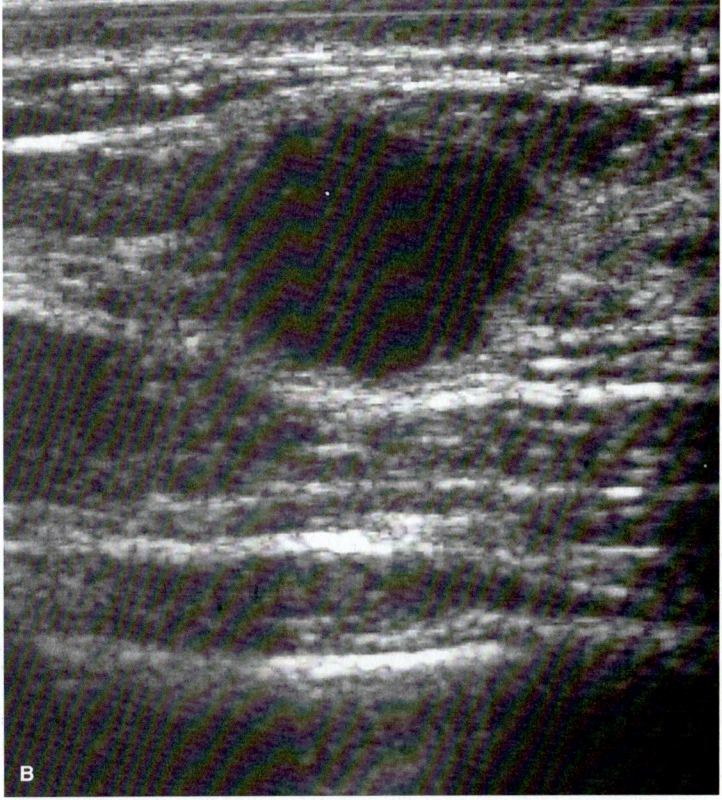

FIG. 8.32 • **Medullary carcinoma with adjacent DCIS. A:** CC view photographically coned to the inner aspect of the left breast in a 40-year-old patient presenting with a "lump." The metallic BB marks area of concern to the patient. A round iso dense mass (short arrow) with indistinct margins is imaged corresponding to the area of clinical concern. Associated punctate calcifications are noted (long arrow). **B:** Ultrasound. Round, markedly hypoechoic mass with indistinct, angular margins and minimal posterior acoustic enhancement is imaged corresponding to the clinically and mammographically apparent mass. BI-RADS 4C: Suspicious abnormality; biopsy is indicated. (From Cardeñosa G. *Breast Imaging [The Core Curriculum Series]*. Philadelphia, PA: Lippincott Williams & Wilkins; 2003.)

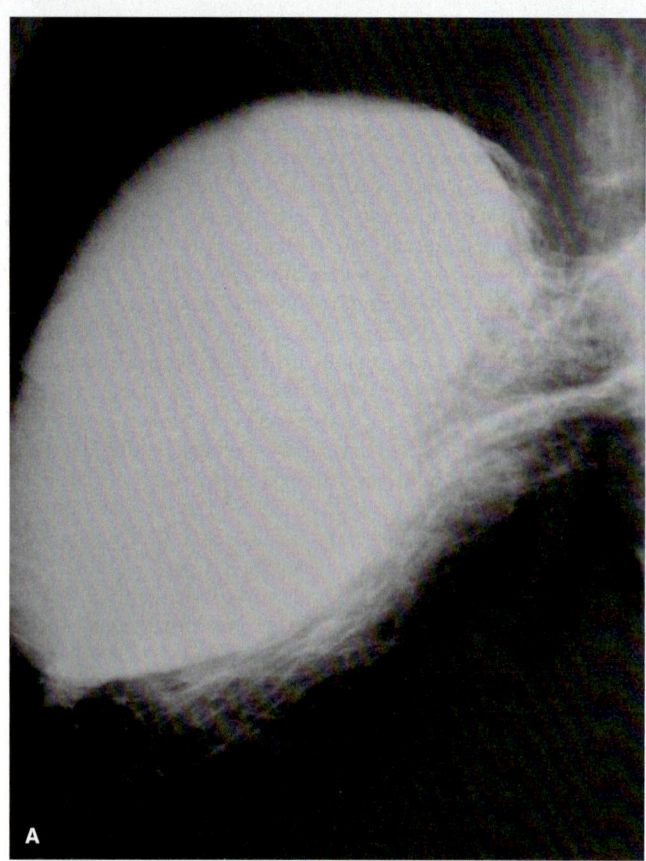
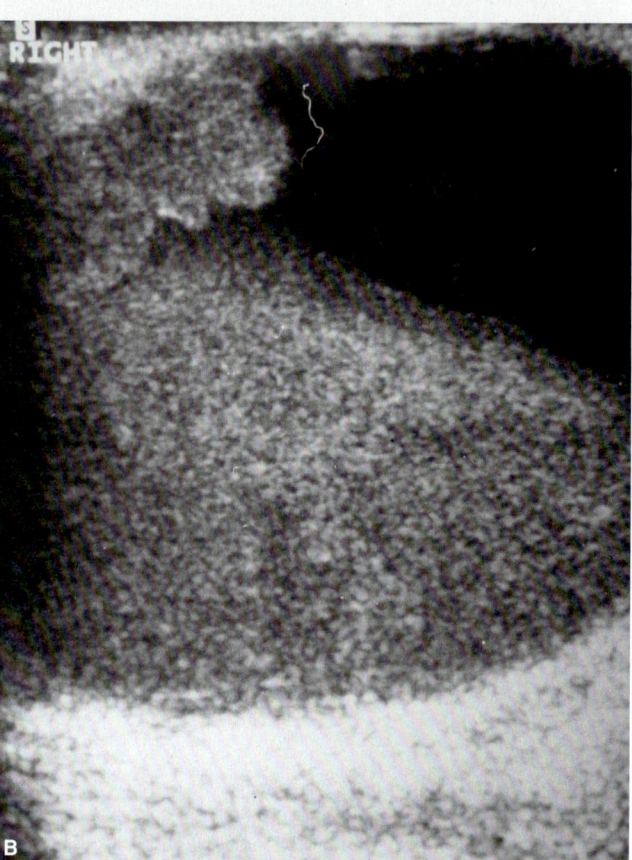

FIG. 8.33 • **Papillary carcinoma. A:** MLO view in a patient presenting with a palpable mass that is smoothly protuberant; overlying skin thinning and stretching with a fading ecchymosis are noted on physical examination. No nipple discharge is elicited. An oval, high-density mass with circumscribed margins is imaged in the right breast. In an attempt to adequately penetrate (expose) the mass, the remainder of the breast parenchyma is "burned" out. **B:** A complex cystic and solid mass with posterior acoustic enhancement is imaged corresponding to the palpable mass. Given the size of the lesion, it is not possible to include all of it in one image. Hemorrhagic fluid is often obtained when the cystic component is aspirated; however, in approximately 50% of patients, the diagnosis is *not* established on the fluid aspirate alone; core biopsy through the solid component is needed to reliably establish a diagnosis. (From Cardeñosa G. *Breast Imaging [The Core Curriculum Series]*. Philadelphia, PA: Lippincott Williams & Wilkins; 2003.)

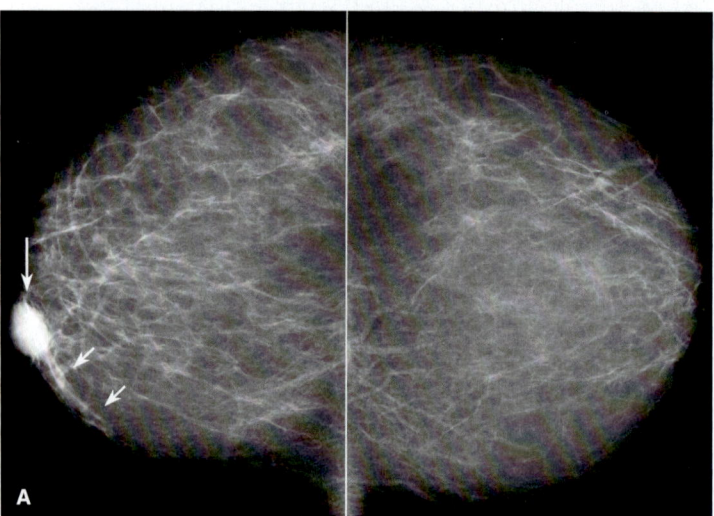
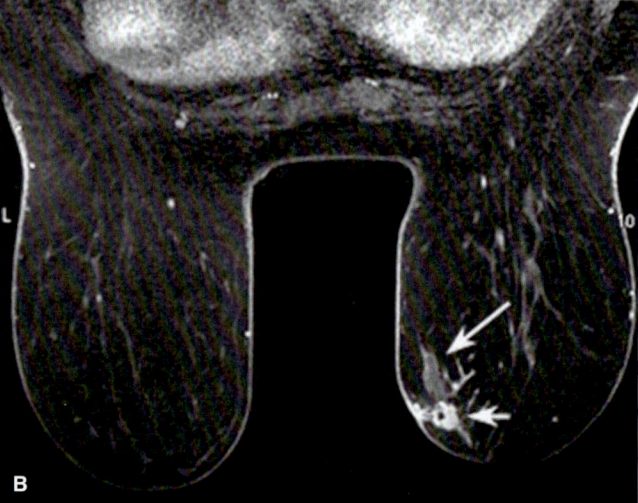

FIG. 8.34 • **Papillary DCIS, intermediate grade forming a mass. A:** CC views in a 62-year-old patient. A dense, round mass *(long arrow)* with circumscribed margins and an associated ductal structure *(short arrows)* confirmed on spot compression views (not shown) is identified in the right subareolar area. **B:** MRI, axial T1-weighted image post-contrast. A heterogeneously enhancing mass *(short arrow)* with circumscribed margins and an associated non-enhancing dilated duct *(long arrow)* extending posteromedially from the mass are imaged in the right subareolar area corresponding to the mass seen mammographically. **C:** MRI, sagittal T2-weighted fat-suppressed image of the right breast. Mass *(arrow)* with heterogeneous but predominantly high T2 signal is imaged corresponding to the enhancing mass seen on the image shown in part **B**. Associated dilated duct is not seen on this scan plane. **D:** MRI, sagittal T2-weighted fat-suppressed image of the right breast. Dilated fluid-filled (high T2 signal) ductal structure *(arrows)* extending posterior from the mass (mass on a different scan plane is shown in part **C**).

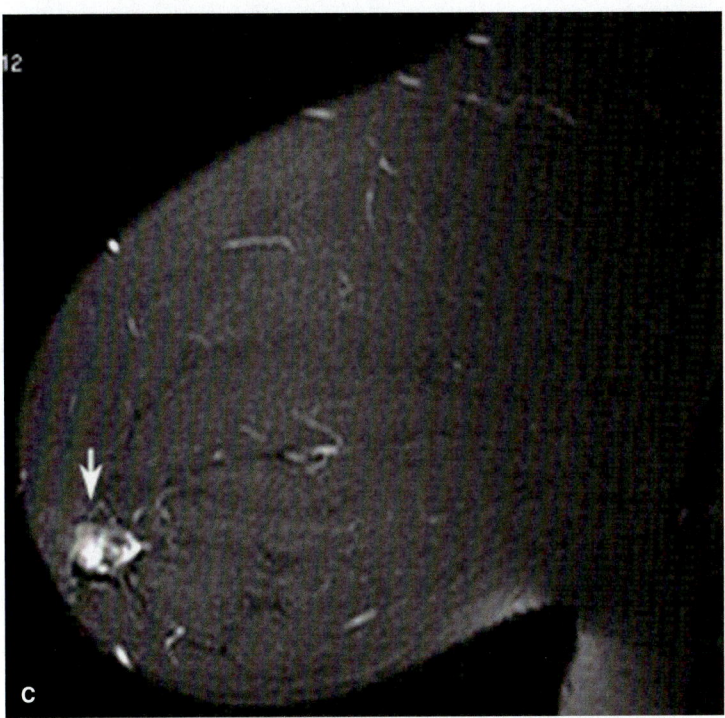
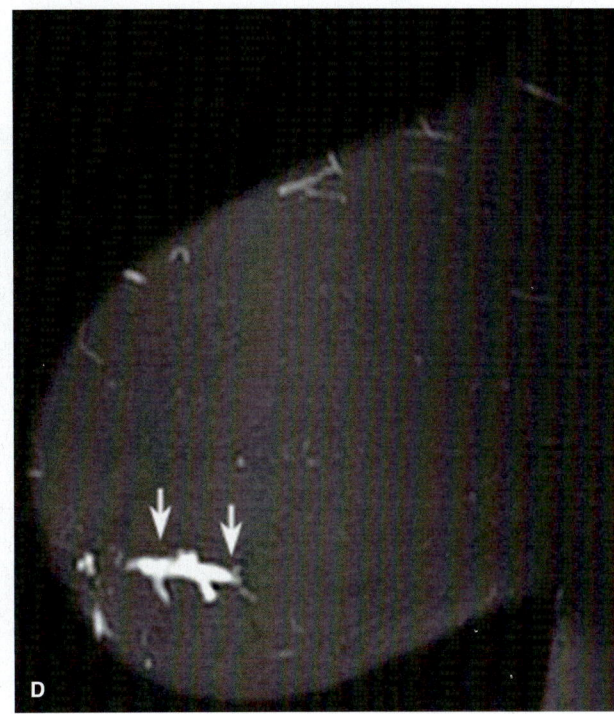

FIG. 8.34 • *(continued)*

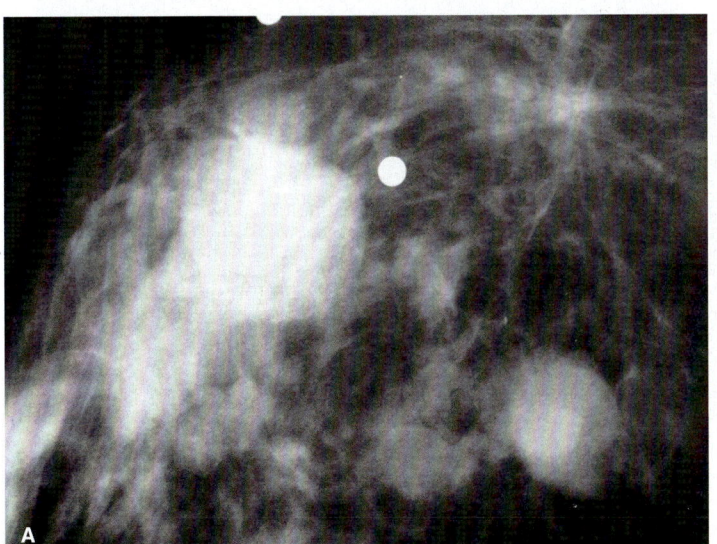
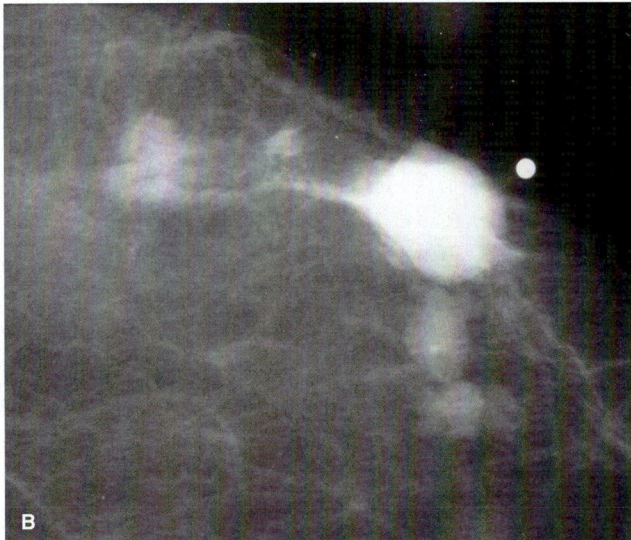

FIG. 8.35 • **Multiple peripheral papillary carcinomas in two different patients. A:** CC projection of the right breast photographically coned to the lateral aspect of the breast. Multiple iso- to high-density round masses with indistinct margins are identified in a 69-year-old patient presenting with a palpable mass in the right breast. The metallic BB marks the site of the palpable finding. Solid masses are imaged on ultrasound (not shown) corresponding to the clinical and mammographically apparent masses. **B:** Left CC view of the left breast photographically coned to the lateral aspect of the breast in a 74-year-old patient presenting with a palpable mass in the left breast. The metallic BB marks the site of the palpable finding. The palpable mass is round and high in density with indistinct margins. Four low-density masses with indistinct margins are noted in the surrounding tissue. Solid masses are imaged on ultrasound (not shown) corresponding to the clinically and mammographically apparent masses. (From Cardeñosa G. *Breast Imaging [The Core Curriculum Series]*. Philadelphia, PA: Lippincott Williams & Wilkins; 2003.)

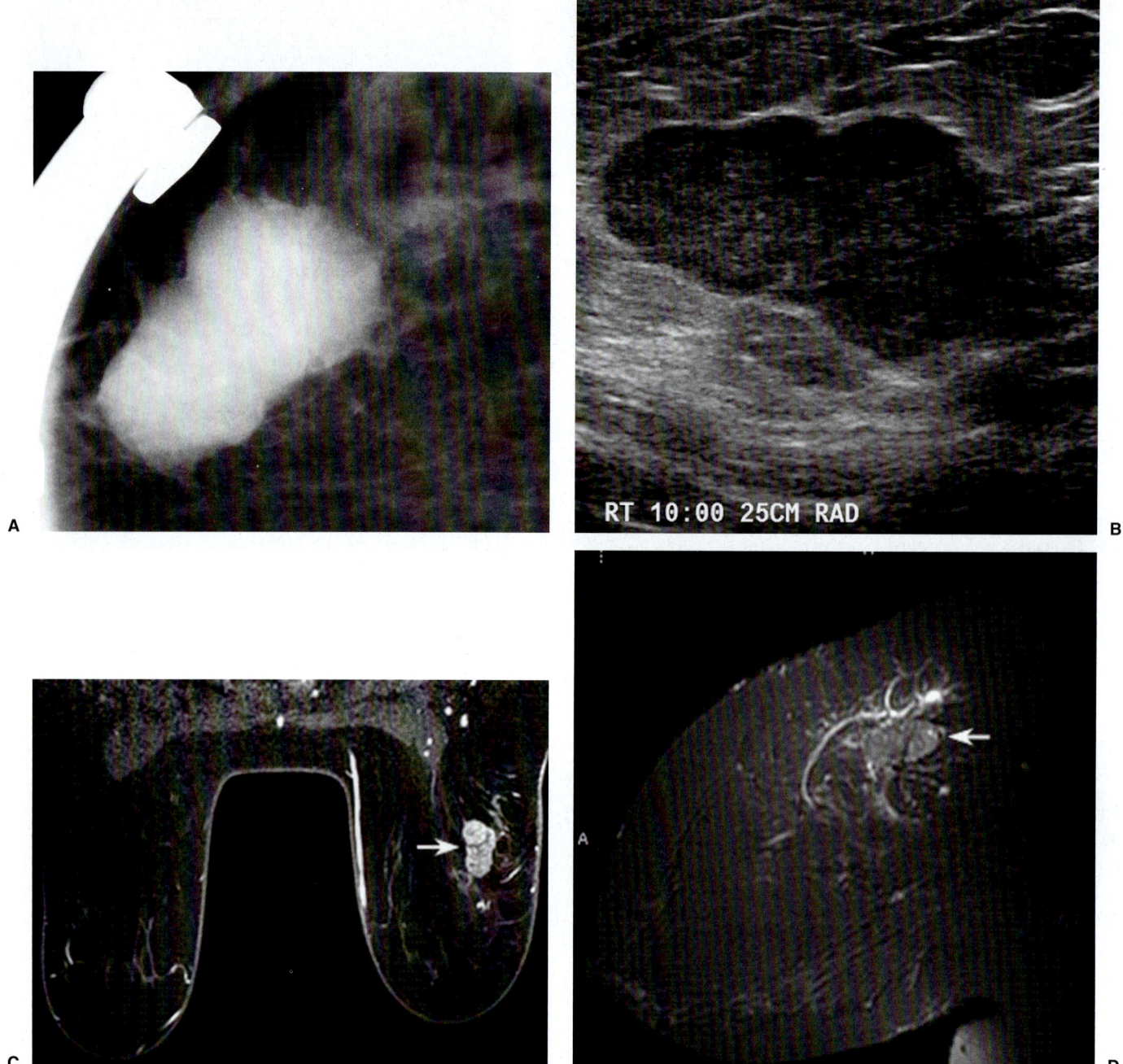

FIG. 8.36 • **Intracystic papillary carcinoma with invasive ductal carcinoma. A:** Spot compression view in the MLO projection done for evaluation of a screen-detected mass in the upper outer quadrant of the right breast posteriorly in a 59-year-old patient. The mass is high in density, lobulated with circumscribed margins. **B:** Ultrasound. A hypoechoic oval mass with gentle lobulations, mostly circumscribed margins, and posterior acoustic enhancement is imaged in the right breast corresponding to the mass described mammographically. **C:** MRI, T1-weighted axial image post-contrast and **D:** MRI, sagittal T2-weighted fat suppressed image of the right breast. A lobulated mass *(arrows)* with circumscribed margins, heterogeneous enhancement, and non-enhancing internal septations is imaged in the upper outer quadrant of the right breast posteriorly. MRI, sagittal T2-weighted fat suppressed image of the right breast. This mass *(arrow)* demonstrates an intermediate T2 signal with minimal surrounding edema. The lesion is estrogen receptor/progesterone receptor-positive, HER2/neu-negative, and the sentinel lymph node (LN) biopsy is negative (0/2 LNs).

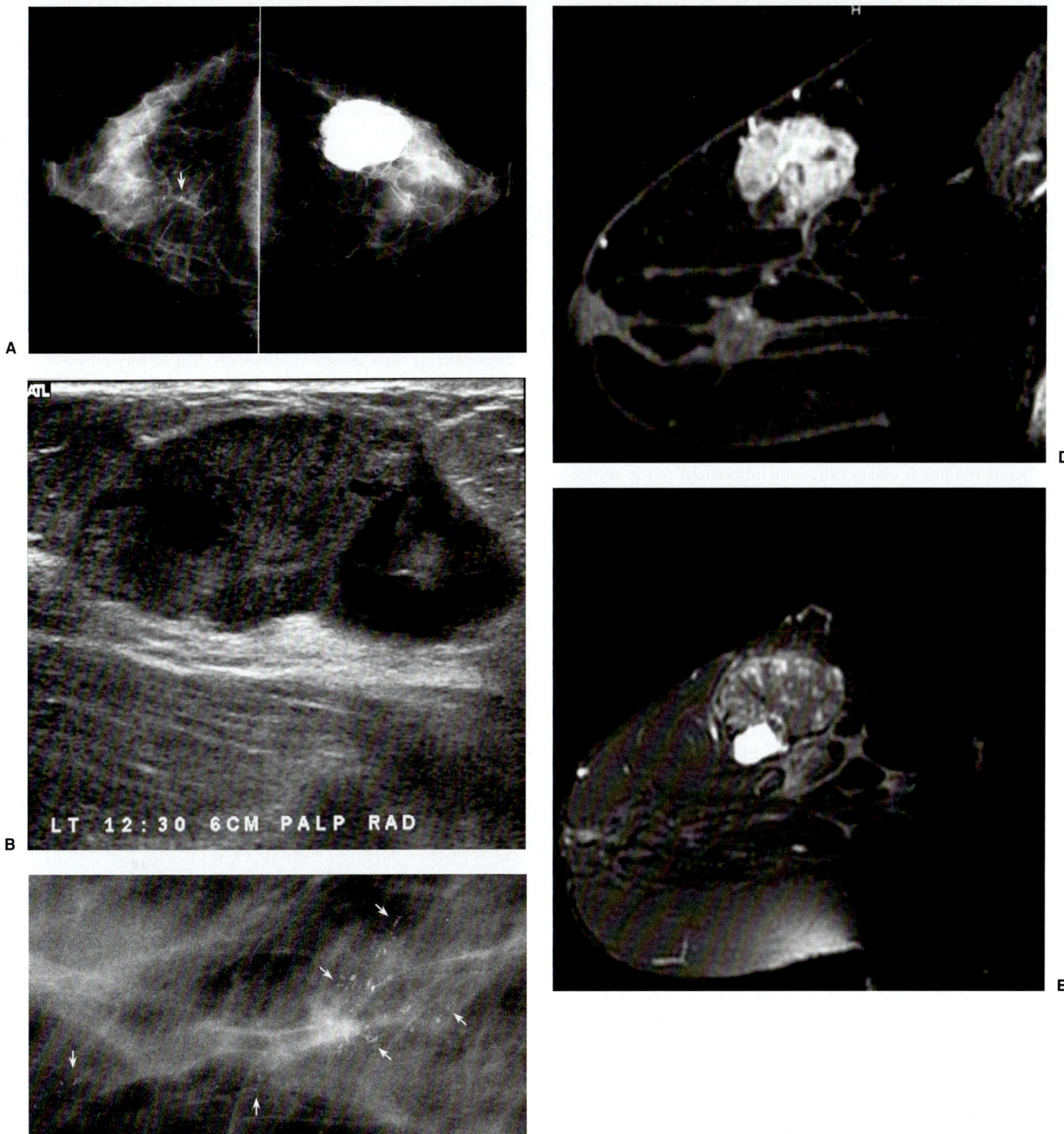

FIG. 8.37 • Synchronous cancers. Papillary carcinoma predominantly in situ with foci of invasive disease in the left breast and DCIS solid and cribriform types with central necrosis in the right breast. **A:** CC views in a 62-year-old patient presenting with a "lump" in the left breast for 3 months. A dense, oval mass with indistinct and lobulated margins is imaged corresponding to the palpable finding. When your brain is focused on a clinically and mammographically apparent mass, it is imperative that you force yourself to evaluate the remainder of the tissue in the left breast as well as the contralateral side. In this patient, a cluster of calcifications *(arrow)* is present in the retroareolar aspect of the right breast in zone B. **B:** Ultrasound. A complex cystic mass that is predominantly solid with cystic components and posterior acoustic enhancement is imaged corresponding to the clinically and mammographically apparent mass in the left breast. **C:** Spot compression magnification view, right breast. Fine pleomorphic calcifications including round, punctate, amorphous, and linear forms *(arrows)* in a segmental distribution are imaged in the right breast. DCIS is diagnosed on a stereotactically guided biopsy of the calcifications. **D:** MRI, sagittal T1-weighted reconstruction of the left breast, post-contrast. A mass with lobulated, circumscrbied margins and heterogeneous internal enhancement is imaged corresponding to the mass in the left breast. **E:** MRI, sagittal T2-weighted fat-suppressed image of the left breast. The T2 signal of the mass is variable with portions demonstrating intermediate and others, high T2 signal. Coil artifact (signal flaring) is noted inferiorly.

carcinoma. Accurate classification of these lesions and the determination of invasion in intraductal papillary carcinomas pose a challenge for the pathologist (40–45).

Histologically, encapsulated papillary CAs demonstrate an arborescent, frond-like proliferation of low-grade epithelial elements with a central fibrovascular core completely contained in a dilated duct. The absence of myoepithelial cells in the papillary lesion indicates malignancy (Fig. 8.38); however, the presence of these cells does not completely exclude an intraductal papillary carcinoma since myoepithelial cells may be seen sporadically in the fronds of intraductal papillary carcinomas. Also considered by some authors in the classification of these lesions is the absence of myoepithelial cells in the wall of the cystically dilated duct surrounding the encysted papillary proliferation (40–45).

Solid papillary carcinomas are characterized by circumscribed nodules of proliferating low-grade homogenous cells packing a dilated duct that lacks myoepithelial cells commonly in the central aspect of the breast. Many are further characterized by the presence of neuroendocrine features as well as extra- and intracellular mucin such that some authors have suggested these lesions may represent precursors of mucinous carcinoma (46).

Although "malignant" papillary lesions are considered to be noninvasive, some have postulated that these are "pushing border" or "expansile" indolent variants of invasive ductal carcinoma. Some actually do demonstrate stromal invasion. The invasive component is usually indistinguishable from invasive ductal carcinoma NOS; less commonly, it may demonstrate a papillary growth pattern.

Papillary lesions are characteristically friable and as such the seeding of epithelial cells into the surrounding stroma, adjacent lymphatic channels (47), and subsequent transport of displaced epithelium into the axillary lymph nodes (48) following needle biopsies is a recognized phenomenon (40–42). This can compound the challenge of accurately characterizing these lesions histologically. The history of recent needle instrumentation, altered red blood cells, inflammatory changes, and a lack of a desmoplastic reaction surrounding the displaced cells can be used to recognize displacement from invasion. Evaluating the edge of the lesion away from areas of recent instrumentation is also recommended (41).

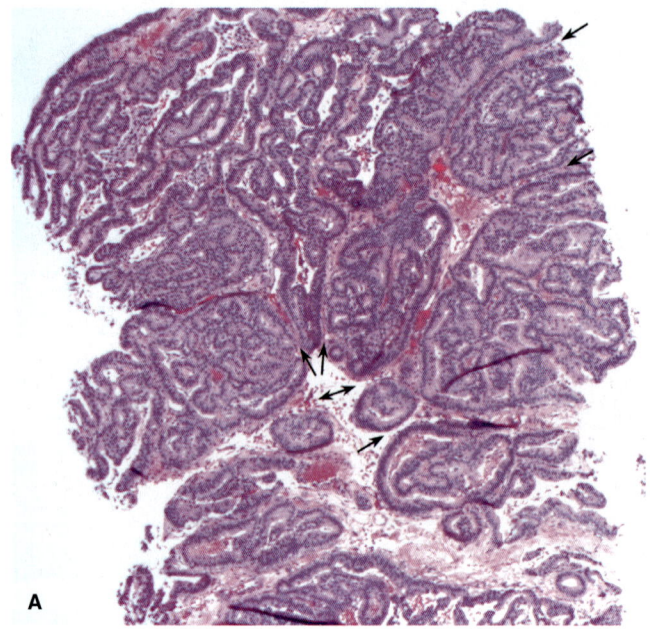
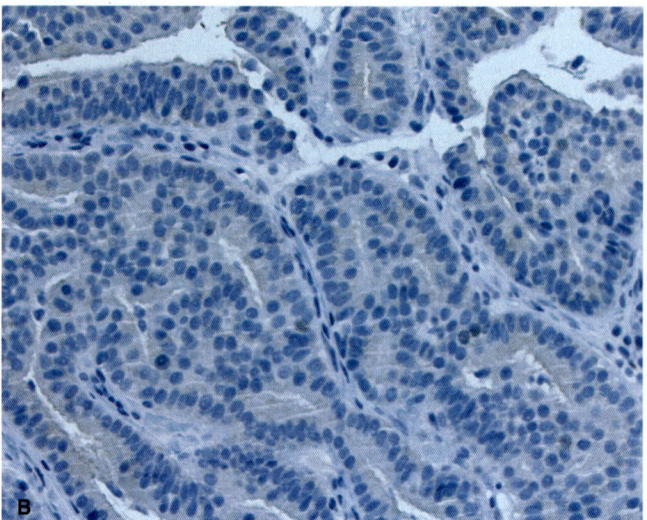
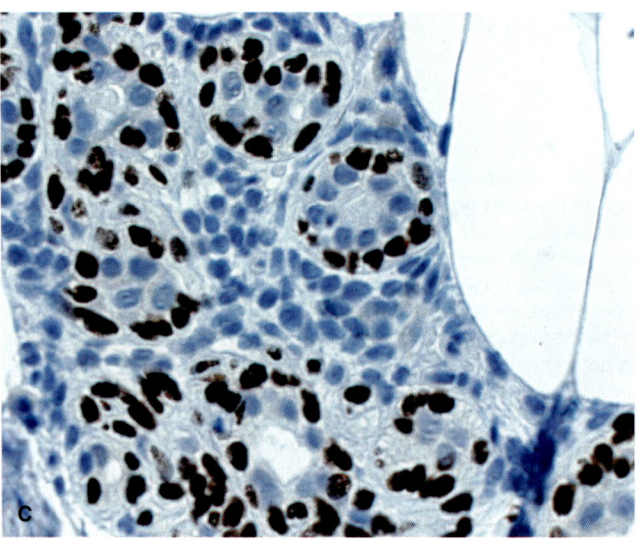

FIG. 8.38 • **Pathology, papillary carcinoma. A:** Low power (4×) of a core biopsy. Frond-like proliferation of epithelial elements with central fibrovascular cores *(arrows)* is apparent on this core. Even at higher power (not shown), no myoepithelial cells could be identified. **B:** Special stain (p63) (20×) confirming the absence of myoepithelial cells. **C:** For comparison, section (20×) through normal breast tissue demonstrating ducts with a contiguous epithelial cell lining and discontiguous intensely staining (brown with p63) myoepithelial cells at the base of the ducts. Absence of the myoepithelial cells is what distinguishes papillary carcinomas from papillomas (and tubular carcinomas from normal ductal structures and benign lesions such as sclerosing adenosis).

Papillary carcinomas should not be confused with invasive micropapillary carcinomas. Clinically and histologically distinct, micropapillary carcinomas are characterized by an aggressive behavior, propensity for lymphovascular space involvement, and positive lymph nodes at the time of diagnosis. Proliferating pseudopapillary structures with no fibrovascular cores are identified histologically in clear empty spaces (41,42,49).

METAPLASTIC CARCINOMA

This invasive ductal subtype represents less than 5% of all breast cancers and is characterized by rapid growth and a poorer prognosis. The patients may present describing a rapidly growing mass or the mass may be detected on screening mammography. Metaplastic carcinomas are typically estrogen and progesterone receptor and HER2/neu-negative (e.g., triple-negative), and although lymphatic metastases are reported in 8% to 40% of patients at the time of presentation, they can also metastasize hematogenously to lung and bone (1,2,50–52).

These tumors are characterized by variable features on mammography including high density, round, oval, or irregular masses with circumscribed (Fig. 8.39A), obscured, indistinct (Fig. 8.40A), or spiculated margins. Calcifications are not a prominent feature, but when present, are typically a mixture of amorphous, round, and punctate forms. Rarely, when there is osseous differentiation, a dense osseous structure (trabecula) may be apparent in the mass. The ultrasound features of metaplastic carcinomas are also variable. These lesions can present as heterogeneous, hypoechoic (Figs. 8.39B and 8.40B), or complex cystic and solid masses with posterior acoustic enhancement. On MRI, an intermediate to increased T2 signal and iso intense to hypointense T1 signal are common. Heterogeneous and rim-enhancement patterns are the two most common appearances on the dynamic sequences. Kinetic curves may be variable; however, rapid wash-in with plateau or wash-out delayed curves predominate (50–52).

Histologically, metaplastic carcinomas are heterogeneous and include glandular (epithelial) elements and non-glandular mesenchymal components that are possibly a reflection of metaplasia involving the myoepithelial cells. Focal squamous metaplasia in an invasive ductal carcinoma is one of the more common features of these lesions. Other tumors demonstrate cohesive sheets of spindle cells such that differentiation from fibromatosis or fibrosarcoma may be difficult. An associated inflammatory reaction is almost always present leading some to mistake the diagnosis. In some patients, metaplastic carcinomas are characterized by matrix formation, cartilaginous or osseous being the more common components described. Carcinosarcoma and osteoclastic giant cells are much less common. In some patients, the tumor demonstrates a mixture of these components (1). The prognosis for these lesions is likely related to the stage at the time of diagnosis and not necessarily to the histologic features of the metaplastic component(s).

INVASIVE LOBULAR CARCINOMA

Invasive lobular carcinoma represents approximately 10% of all breast cancers; it constitutes less than 2% of all breast cancers in women under the age of 35 and 11% in women over the age of 75 (1). It may be

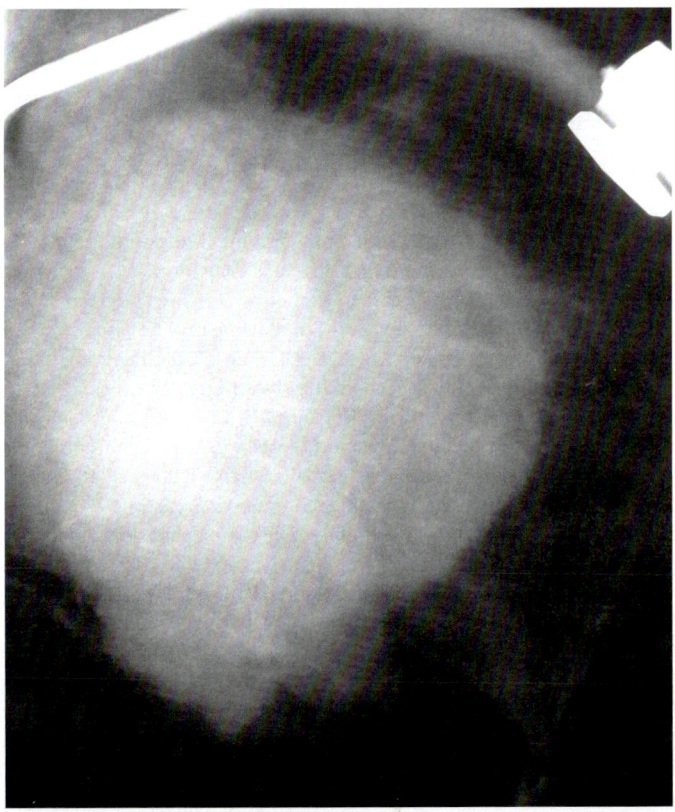
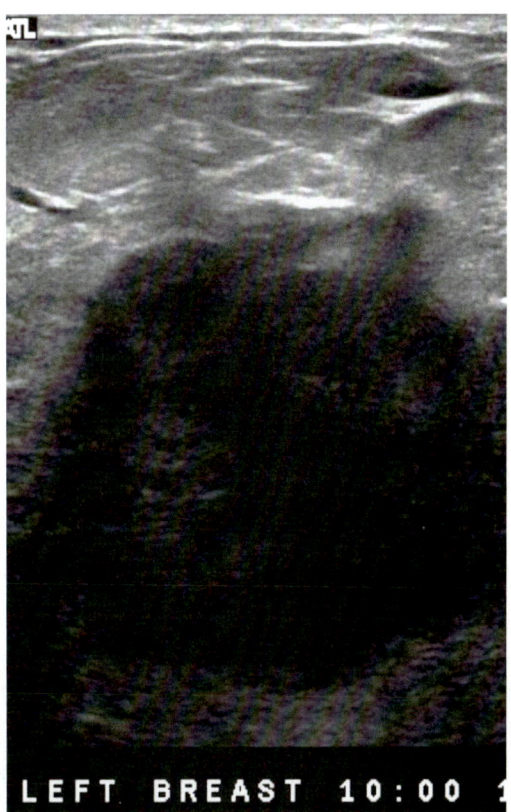

FIG. 8.39 • Metaplastic carcinoma. **A:** Spot compression view in a 34-year-old patient presenting with a "lump" in the left breast. A high-density round mass with circumscribed microlobulated margins is partially imaged at the site of the palpable finding. **B:** Ultrasound. A markedly hypoechoic round mass is imaged correlating to the clinically and mammographically apparent mass. At the time of mastectomy, a metaplastic matrix-producing carcinoma is described. It is estrogen and progesterone receptor-negative, HER2/neu-negative with a negative sentinel lymph node (LN) biopsy (0/4 LNs).

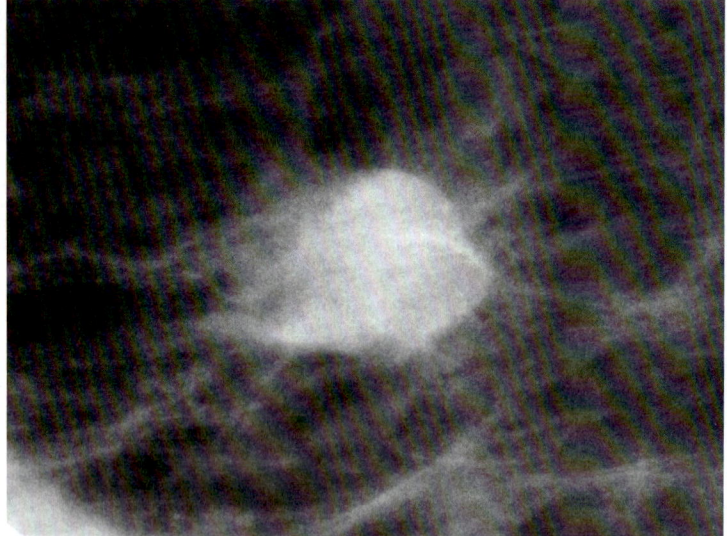 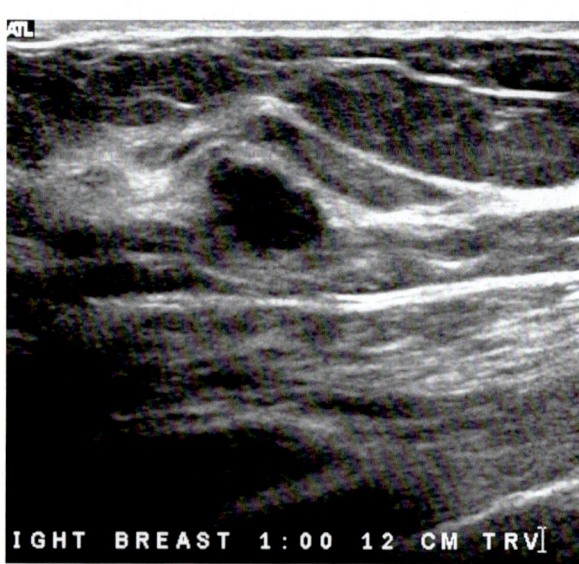

FIG. 8.40 • **Metaplastic carcinoma. A:** Spot compression view done to evaluate a screen-detected mass in the right breast of a 60-year-old patient. An iso dense round mass with indistinct margins is confirmed on the spot compression views (only one projection is shown). **B:** Ultrasound. An irregular hypoechoic mass with angular margins is imaged in the right breast corresponding to the mammographic abnormality. BI-RADS 4C: Suspicious abnormality; biopsy is indicated. A fibroepithial lesion with a papilloma is described on the ultrasound-guided core biopsy. The patient is referred for excisional biopsy. A metaplastic carcinoma with spindle and squamous features arising in the background of a sclerosed papilloma is diagnosed on the excisional biopsy. The lesion is estrogen and progesterone receptor-negative, HER2/neu-negative, and the sentinel lymph node (LN) biopsy (0/2 LNs) is negative.

that the incidence of invasive lobular carcinomas in pre-menopausal women is increasing. The sensitivity of detecting invasive lobular carcinomas using mammography and ultrasound is lower than that for invasive ductal carcinomas; reported false-negative rates of interpretation range from 19% to 43% (53–55). In our experience, 66% of patients with invasive lobular carcinoma are symptomatic at the time of presentation and 41% have positive axillary lymph nodes. Bilateral disease is seen in as many as 28% of patients. Many of these tumors (up to 92%) are estrogen receptor-positive (1,2), with more variability in the progesterone receptor status.

The diagnosis of invasive lobular carcinoma may be elusive at every step: clinically, mammographically, and histologically. The tissue may be thickened such that its consistency is different from that of surrounding tissue or the corresponding region in the contralateral breast. In some patients, the size of the breasts may be asymmetric.

In our experience, the mammographic presentation of invasive lobular carcinoma is variable and parallels what has been described in the literature (54–60). One or multiple masses with spiculated margins (Figs. 8.41 and 8.42) is seen in 40% of our patients, asymmetric densities (Fig. 8.43) in 16%, architectural distortion (Figs. 8.44 and 8.45) in 15%, and diffuse trabecular abnormalities leading to either a shrinking (see Figs. 9.18 and 9.19) or an enlarging breast in 11% of patients. Since these lesions appear to be planar, invasive lobular carcinoma may be more apparent in one projection, often the CC view, and subtle or difficult to see on the orthogonal view (Fig. 8.45); this observation also applies to the conspicuity of the lesion in ultrasound and MRI. A round mass is seen in less than 5% of patients with invasive lobular carcinoma. Although some authors have reported that some invasive lobular carcinomas present with calcifications, in our experience, calcifications do not occur in invasive lobular carcinomas. The malignant cells do not usually form any nests or spaces within which calcifications can develop. The malignant cells invade individually rather than as nests of cells. When biopsies are done for calcifications, the invasive lobular carcinoma is an incidental unsuspected finding and the calcifications are found in benign processes including sclerosing adenosis, fibrocystic changes, and fibroadenomas. In approximately 3% of patients with invasive lobular carcinoma, the mammogram is reportedly normal, and even when present, the mammographic findings often underestimate the extent of disease (Fig. 8.46). MRI may more accurately predict the size and extent of disease in women with invasive lobular carcinoma.

On ultrasound, significant shadowing may be associated with invasive lobular carcinomas (Figs. 8.41B and 8.43C). Alternatively, a vertically oriented hypoechoic mass with angular, spiculated, indistinct margins and shadowing (Figs. 8.42B, C, 8.44C, and 8.46C) or a hypoechoic, lobulated mass may be seen (60,61). Commonly, the lesion seen on ultrasound appears smaller than what is palpated.

Most invasive lobular carcinomas demonstrate enhancement on MRI with rapid wash-in and wash-out or persistent-type delayed kinetic curves (Figs. 8.45 and 8.46). The extent of disease is often better delineated on MRI and the presence of multifocal (Fig. 8.42D), multicentric (Fig. 8.46), bilateral (synchronous) disease can be established on MRI (Fig. 8.45). (60,62,63).

Although there are variants, most lobular carcinomas are characterized by the migration of individual, small cells (Fig. 8.47) through the stroma, with little associated reaction or scirrhous change histologically. The cells can simulate lymphocytes, thereby making the pathological diagnosis difficult in some patients. Lobular neoplasia (a.k.a. lobular carcinoma in situ = LCIS) is found extensively involving the tissue in 41% of our post-menopausal patients with invasive lobular carcinoma. As discussed in Chapter 9, LCIS may represent more of a precursor lesion in some patients rather than just a marker lesion with no malignant potential.

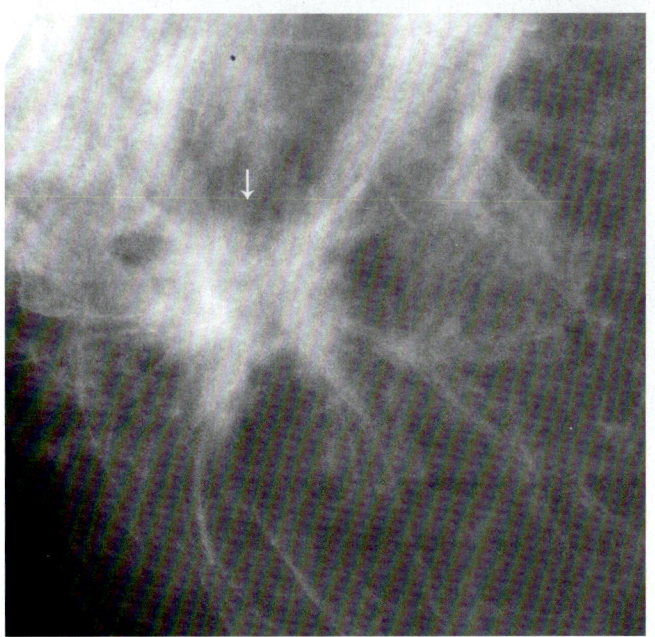
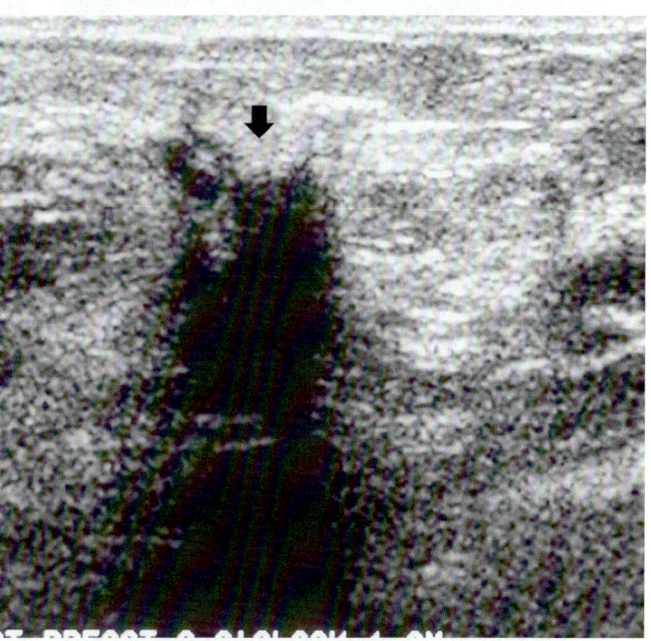

FIG. 8.41 • **Invasive lobular carcinoma. A:** Spot compression view demonstrates an irregular, low-to-iso dense mass *(arrow)* with spiculated margins corresponding to a "lump" described by a 42-year-old patient in her right breast. **B:** Ultrasound. Irregular, vertically oriented mass *(arrow)* with indistinct and angular margins as well as intense shadowing is imaged corresponding to the clinically and mammographically apparent mass. (From Cardeñosa G. *Breast Imaging [The Core Curriculum Series]*. Philadelphia, PA: Lippincott Williams & Wilkins; 2003.)

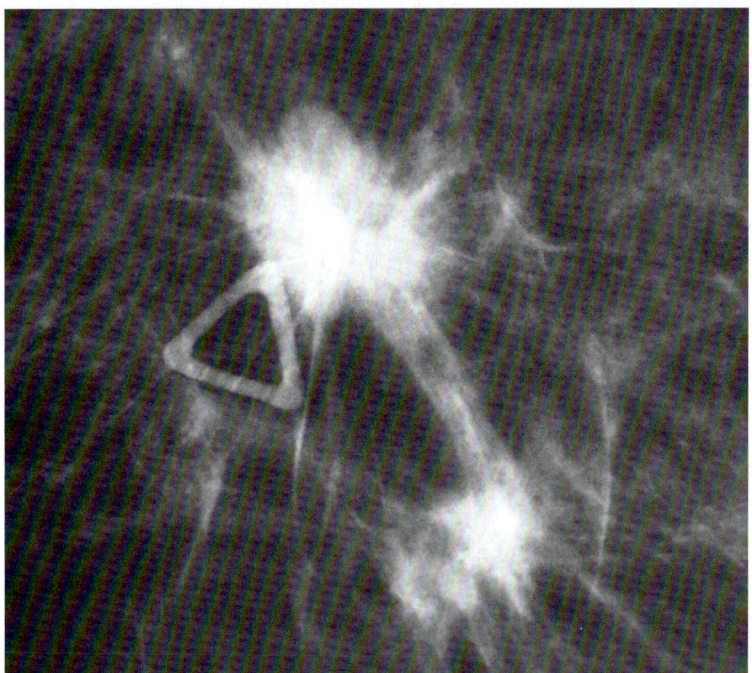
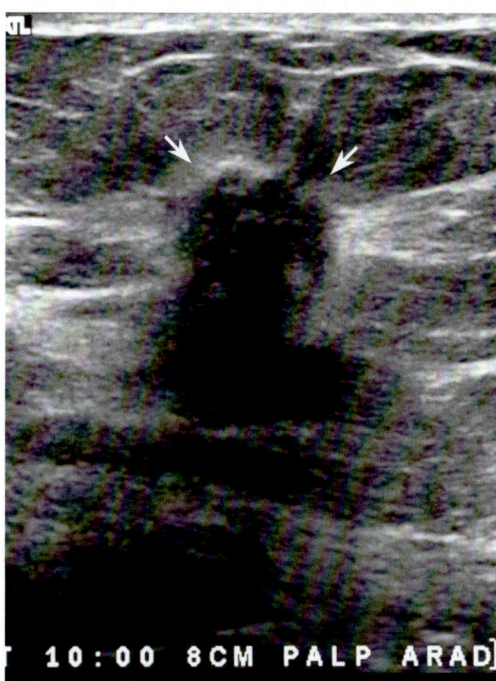

FIG. 8.42 • **Multifocal, invasive lobular carcinoma with DCIS and LCIS. A:** Spot compression view in a 48-year-old patient presenting with a "lump" in her right breast. Two irregular iso dense masses with spiculated margins are imaged, the largest correlating with the triangular marker used to denote a palpable finding. **B:** Ultrasound. Round, hypoechoic mass *(arrows)* with spiculated and angular margins, an echogenic rim, and shadowing is imaged in the right breast. This correlates to the palpable *(PALP)* mass. **C:** Ultrasound. A vertically oriented, irregular, hypoechoic mass *(arrows)* with spiculated and angular margins and shadowing is imaged corresponding to the second mass seen mammographically. This is not palpable. **D:** MRI, T1-weighted sagittal reconstruction of the right breast post-contrast. The masses *(short arrows)* demonstrate heterogeneous enhancement with spiculated margins; non-mass–like linear enhancement *(long arrow)* is noted extending anteriorly from the superior mass. Histologically, the smaller of the two masses is an invasive lobular carcinoma. The clinically apparent and larger of the two masses is predominantly invasive lobular carcinoma; however, there are areas where the lesion is mixed (e.g., invasive lobular and ductal). DCIS is also described and LCIS is noted throughout the surrounding tissue. Both lesions are estrogen/progesterone-positive, HER2/neu-negative. The sentinel lymph node is positive and as such a full axillary dissection is done yielding 2 lymph nodes with metastatic disease out of the 22 sampled. Extracapsular extension is noted affecting one of the positive lymph nodes.

(continued)

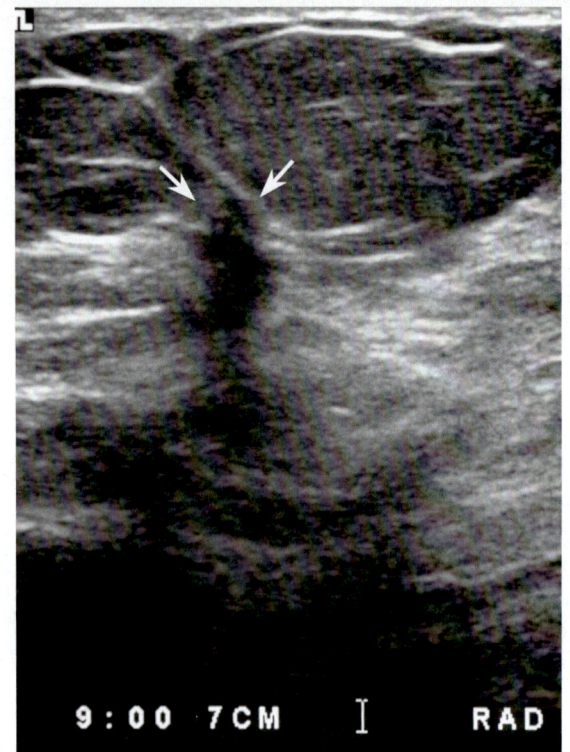
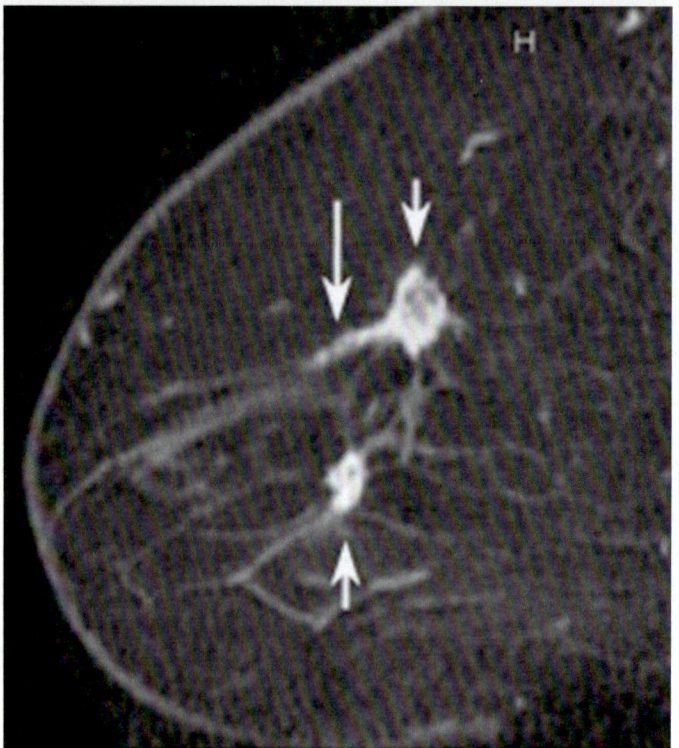

FIG. 8.42 • *(continued)*

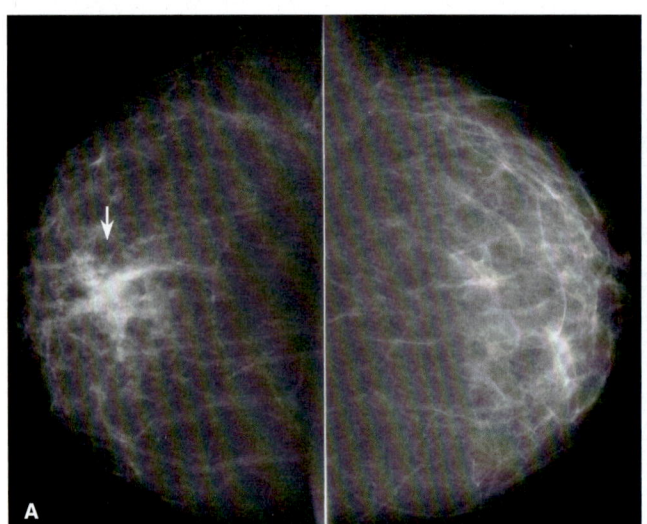

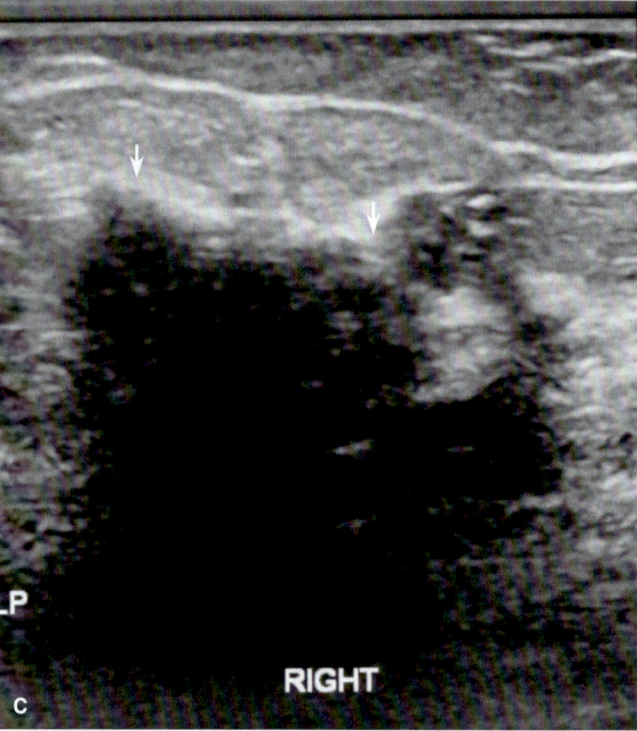

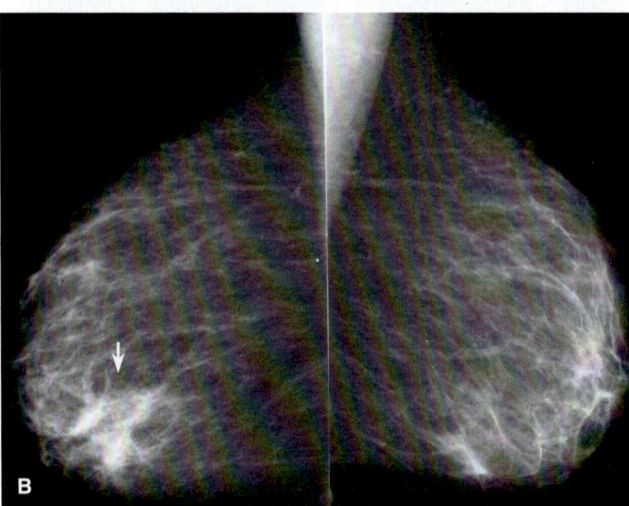

FIG. 8.43 • **Invasive lobular carcinoma.** CC **(A)** and MLO **(B)** views in a 45-year-old patient. Focal parenchymal asymmetry *(arrows)* is present in the lower central aspect of the right breast anteriorly. **C:** Ultrasound. On physical examination, a hard mass is palpated inferiorly in the right breast corresponding to the site of the parenchymal asymmetry. An irregular mass *(arrows)* with angular margins and intense shadowing is imaged at the palpable site corresponding to the asymmetry seen on the mammogram. An abnormal lymph node (not shown) is also identified in the right axilla with metastatic disease diagnosed on core biopsy. BI-RADS 4C: Suspicious abnormality; biopsy is indicated. In addition to the invasive lobular carcinoma, extensive LCIS is reported in the mastectomy specimen and metastatic disease is diagnosed in six of nine axillary lymph nodes. The tumor is estrogen and progesterone-positive, HER2/neu-negative.

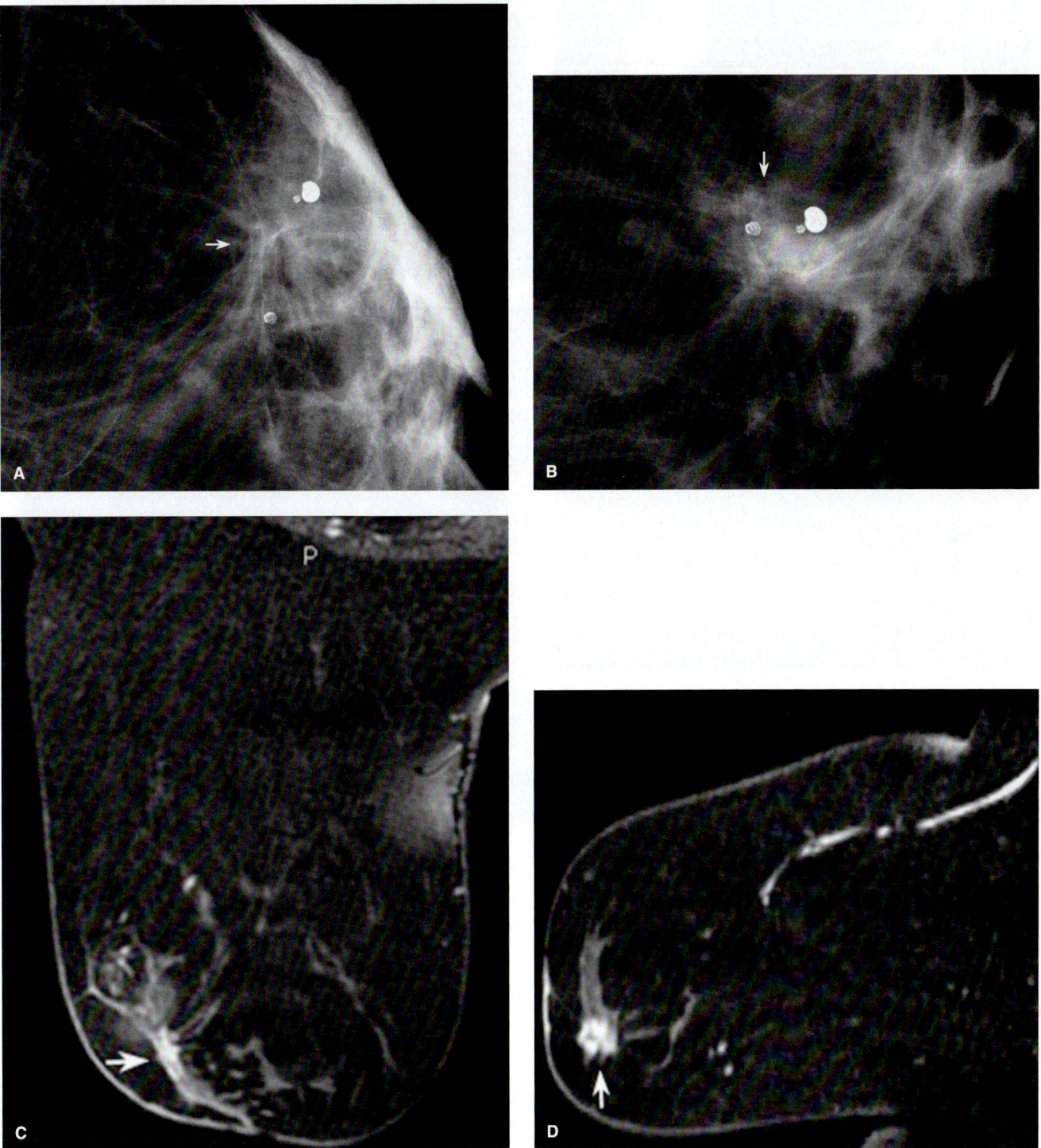

FIG. 8.44 • **Invasive lobular carcinoma.** CC **(A)** and MLO **(B)** views photographically coned to a screen-detected abnormality in a 54-year-old patient. A low-density area of distortion and spiculation *(arrow)* is noted in the CC projection anterolaterally in the left breast. This area is more mass-like *(arrow)* on the oblique view. A vertically oriented markedly hypoechoic mass with angular margins and some shadowing is imaged on ultrasound (not shown) in the left breast corresponding to the mammographic finding. BI-RADS 4C: Suspicious abnormality; biopsy is indicated. **C:** MRI, T1-weighted axial image of the left breast post-contrast. **D:** MRI, T1-weighted sagittal reconstruction of the left breast post-contrast. The mass demonstrates heterogeneous internal enhancement and spiculated margins. The observation made mammographically is also apparent on MRI; the mass *(arrow)* is best seen and appears more mass-like in the sagittal projection in part **D**. The mass *(arrow)* is subtle and more difficult to characterize on the axial images (e.g., equivalent to the CC projection). It is thought that invasive lobular carcinoma demonstrates a planar growth pattern; consequently, it is common for it to be more conspicuous in one of the two orthogonal projections. This lesion is estrogen receptor-positive, progesterone receptor weakly positive, and HER2/neu-negative. The sentinel lymph node (LN) biopsy is negative (0/1 LN).

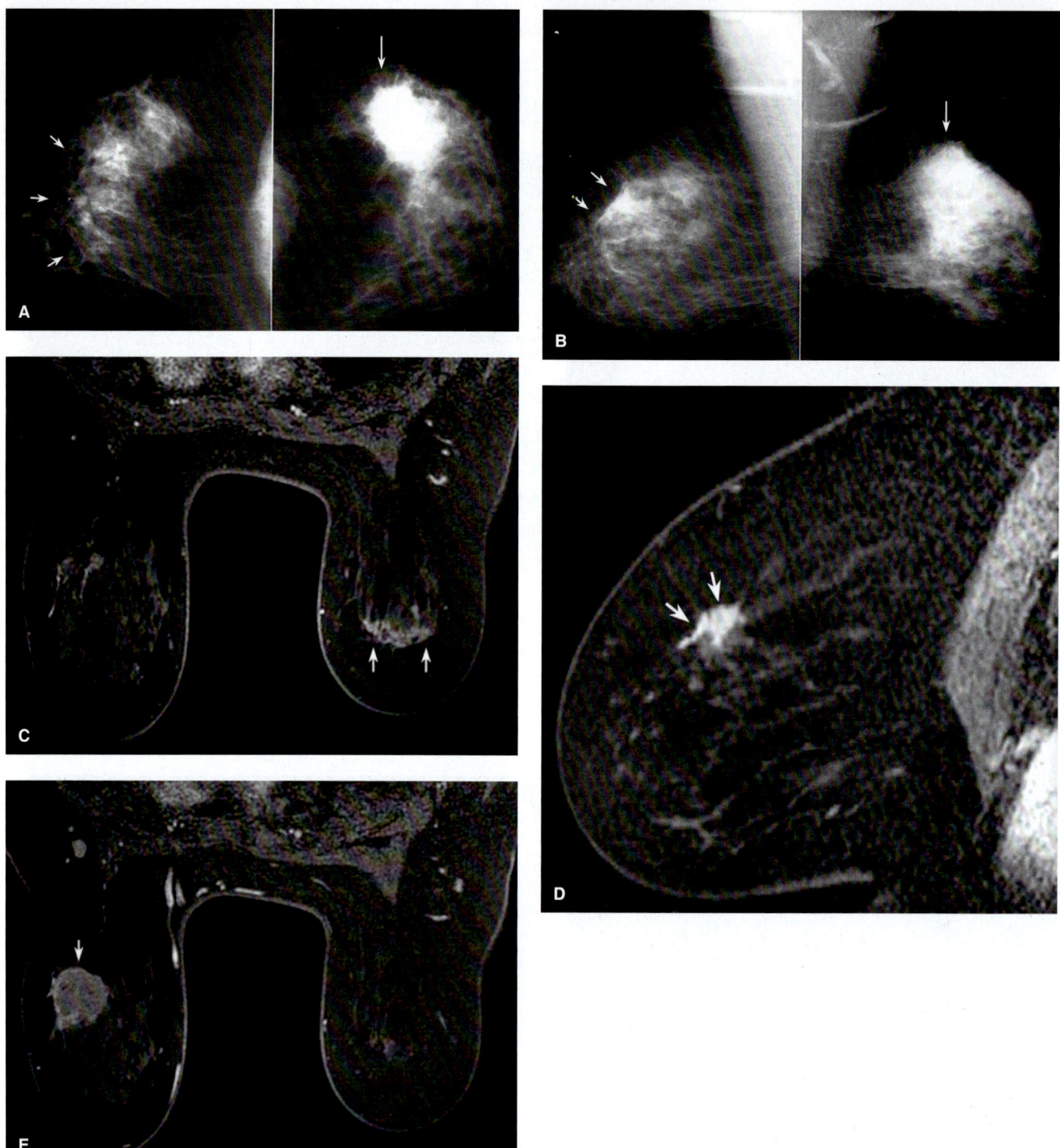

FIG. 8.45 • **Synchronous lesions: invasive lobular carcinoma right breast, invasive ductal carcinoma left breast.** CC **(A)** and MLO **(B)** views in a 63-year-old patient. Your eye is likely drawn to the dense mass *(long arrow)* in the left breast best seen on the CC view. Remember, when faced with an obvious finding, force yourself to evaluate the remaining tissue in that breast as well as the contralateral side, and specifically look for some of the more subtle presentations of cancer including distortion. In evaluating the images of the right breast carefully, you should note distortion anteriorly on the CC view *(short arrows)* and an area of "rigid" tissue with increased density *(short arrows)* on the MLO view. **C:** MRI, T1-weighted axial image post-contrast. Non-mass–like enhancement *(arrows)* of the tissue in the right breast anteriorly matches the area of distortion noted on the CC views. **D:** MRI, T1-weighted sagittal reconstruction of the right breast, post-contrast. Non-mass–like enhancement *(arrows)* is noted superiorly in the right breast comparable to what is seen on the MLO view. This plaque-like (planar) growth appearance is one of the characteristics of invasive lobular carcinoma. The finding is often better seen and more prominent in one projection compared with the other. **E:** MRI, T1-weighted axial image post-contrast at a different scan plane than that shown in part **C** demonstrates the mass *(arrow)* in the left breast. The mass is characterized by lobulated, irregular margins and heterogeneous enhancement. Histologically, an invasive lobular carcinoma is described in the right breast and invasive ductal carcinoma, high grade, is diagnosed in the left breast. Two lymph nodes in the right axilla are positive for metastatic disease; the sentinel lymph node biopsy on the left is negative. The invasive ductal carcinoma is triple-negative. This patient illustrates nicely some of the differences in the imaging presentations between invasive ductal and lobular carcinomas.

Evaluation and Imaging Features of Malignant Breast Masses   267

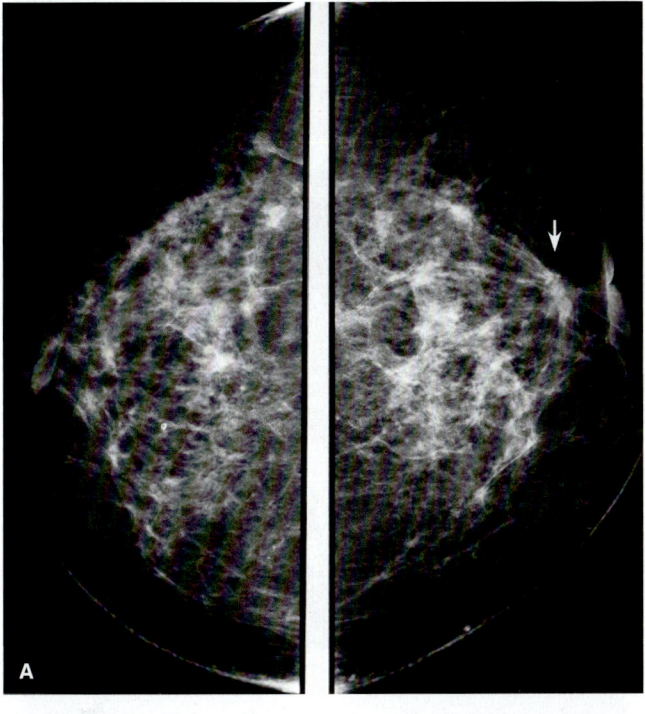

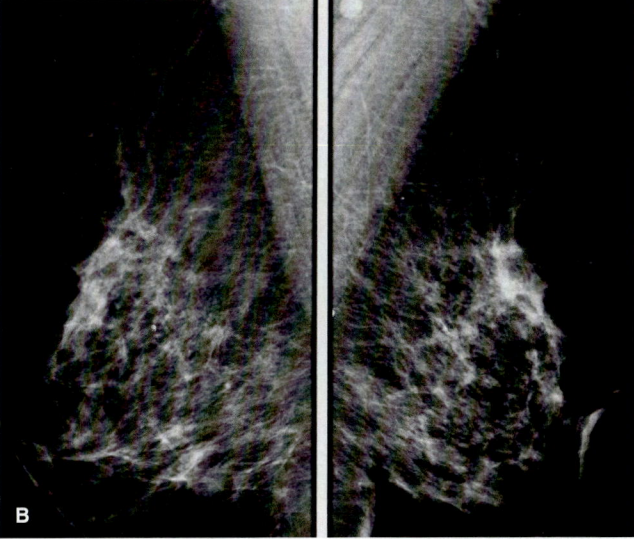

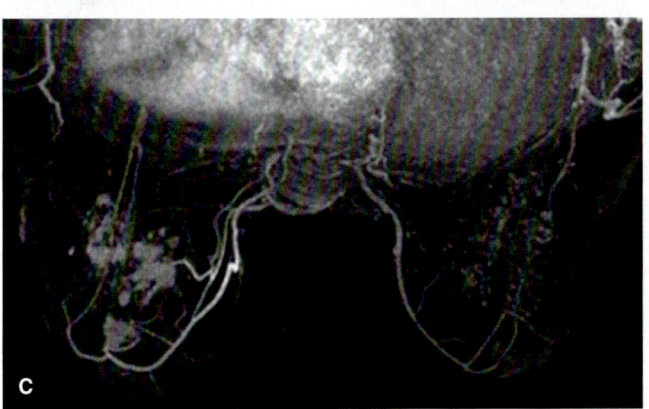

FIG. 8.46 • **Multicentric invasive lobular carcinoma.** CC **(A)** and MLO **(B)** views in a 62-year-old patient. A mass (arrow) with spiculated margins is present in the left subareolar area best on the CC view. Nipple thickening and retraction is apparent in both projections and a new finding compared with prior studies (not shown). A vertically oriented hypoechoic mass with an echogenic rim is imaged on ultrasound (not shown) corresponding to the mass seen mammographically. BI-RADS 4C: Suspicious abnormality; biopsy is indicated. An invasive lobular carcinoma is diagnosed on the ultrasound-guided core biopsy. **C:** MRI, maximum-intensity projection image. Multiple masses with homogeneous enhancement and spiculated margins are noted predominantly involving the upper central and lateral aspects of the left breast. Multicentric invasive lobular carcinoma with extensive LCIS is reported on the mastectomy specimen; estrogen and progesterone receptor-positive, HER2/neu-negative with one of four lymph nodes positive for micrometastatic disease. Multifocality, multicentricity, and bilateral disease are relatively common in patients with invasive lobular carcinoma.

The metastatic pattern for invasive lobular carcinomas may be distinctive in some patients. Unlike invasive ductal carcinomas that tend to metastasize to solid organs including liver, lungs, bones, and brain, invasive lobular carcinomas may simulate ovarian carcinomas in their behavior. Studding of peritoneal and pleural surfaces is seen with the development of ascites and pleural effusions; involvement of the leptomeninges, uterus, ovaries, and stomach can also occur (64).

LYMPHOMA

Primary breast lymphoma represents approximately 0.04% to 0.5% of all breast malignancies. Lymphoma is considered primary to the breast when the breast is the first or major site of involvement and, exclusive of ipsilateral axillary lymph node involvement, there is no lymphoma elsewhere. Ipsilateral axillary lymph node involvement is acceptable, provided the breast and axillary lymph node lesions are diagnosed simultaneously (65). More commonly, lymphomas involve the breast secondarily. Patients may present with a palpable finding. Alternatively, one (Fig. 8.48) or more masses with circumscribed to indistinct margins are detected mammographically, or rarely, as discussed in Chapter 9, parenchymal asymmetry (see Fig. 9.29) or diffuse changes (see Fig. 9.22). Calcifications are

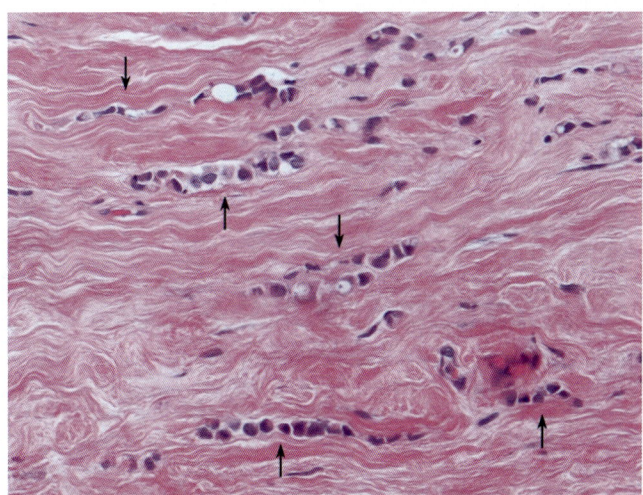

FIG. 8.47 • **Pathology.** Histologically, individual, small relatively monomorphic cells invading the stroma in a single file (arrows) characterize invasive lobular carcinoma. In contrast, nests of cells invading and disrupting surrounding tissue and normal structures characterize invasive ductal carcinoma.

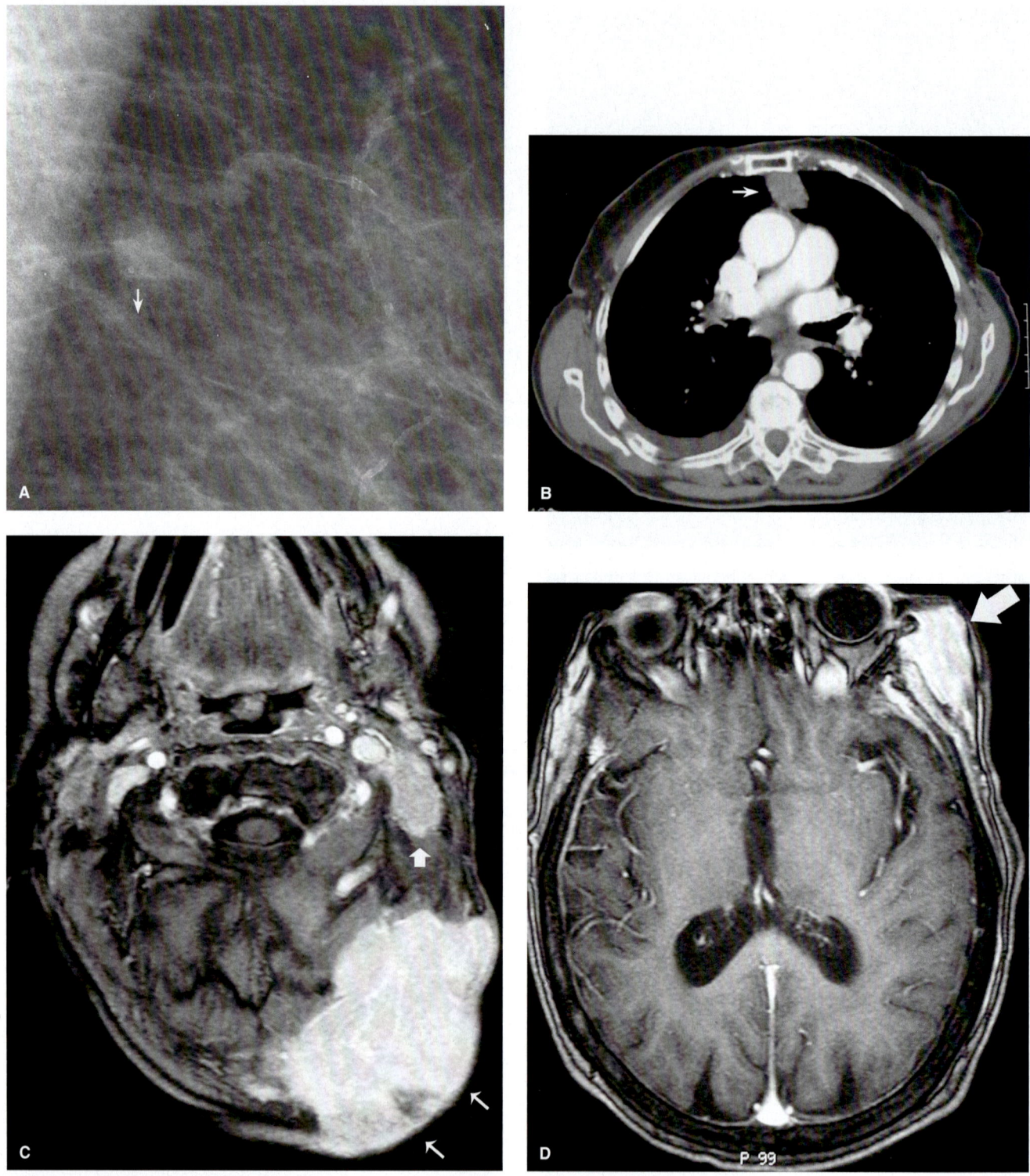

FIG. 8.48 • **Primary breast lymphoma. A:** MLO view in an 80-year-old patient photographically coned to upper aspect of the breast. A low-density oval mass *(arrow)* with indistinct margins is detected mammographically in the upper inner quadrant of the left breast. Arterial calcification is present. Low-grade lymphoma is diagnosed on an excisional biopsy of the mass. Patient has no history of lymphoma and all staging studies done at this time are normal. **B:** CT scan, 2 years following the diagnosis shows a small pleural effusion on the right and anterior mediastinal adenopathy *(arrow)*. **C:** MRI demonstrates a scalp mass *(thin arrows)* and adenopathy *(thick arrow)* adjacent to left jugular vein. **D:** Additionally, a soft tissue mass *(arrow)* is present lateral to the left orbit. Biopsy of the scalp mass is reported as consistent with recurrent lymphoma. A diffuse, large, B-cell–type lymphoma is described. (From Cardeñosa G. *Breast Imaging [The Core Curriculum Series]*. Philadelphia, PA: Lippincott Williams & Wilkins; 2003.)

uncommon. At the time of presentation, axillary nodes are involved in 30% to 40% of patients (1,2). Bilateral disease is uncommon. Night sweats, fever, and weight loss have been reported in 6% to 20% of patients (1).

Two different patient populations have been described with primary breast lymphomas. In the first group, patients present during pregnancy or lactation with rapid, bilateral breast enlargement. In this group of patients, it is usually a Burkitt-type lymphoma with ovarian and CNS involvement and a poor prognosis. The second group of patients presents over a wider age spectrum with unilateral breast involvement, and an underlying histology of a diffuse large cell lymphoma of the B-cell type. Primary breast lymphoma is treated like other extranodal lymphomas. After a histological diagnosis, patients are staged and radiation and chemotherapy are used (65).

SARCOMAS

Malignancies involving the stromal tissues of the breast represent a heterogeneous group of lesions that are rare. Included in this group of lesions are malignant phyllodes tumor (see Figs. 7.66 through 7.69), stromal sarcoma, fibrosarcoma, malignant fibrous histiocytoma, carcinosarcoma, granulocytic sarcoma (chloroma), leiomyosarcoma (Fig. 8.49), liposarcoma (Fig. 8.50), and angiosarcomas (Fig. 8.51). Patients commonly present with a mass that may have circumscribed (Fig. 8.52) margins. On ultrasound, a solid mass with a heterogeneous echotexture and enhancement or shadowing may be seen. Alternatively, a complex cystic and solid mass may be imaged. Axillary lymph nodes are usually not involved since these lesion spread hematogenously (66–68). The MRI features of these lesions are not well-described.

A separate and rare group of patients to consider with sarcomatous lesions are those who present following radiation therapy (see Figs. 11.21 and 11.22). In these patients, the sarcomas are likely radiation-induced and can develop in the skin (e.g., cutaneous angiosarcomas), breast parenchyma, or the soft tissues surrounding the breast (e.g., chest wall, upper abdomen) that were included in the radiation field or exposed to scattered radiation (69,70).

METASTATIC DISEASE TO THE BREASTS

The most common metastatic lesion to the breast is from the contralateral breast through lymphatic channels on the anterior chest wall. Patients present with erythema involving the medial quadrants of the breast; some have nodules that may be ulcerative, associated with the erythema (Fig. 8.6A). There may be relative sparing of the skin overlying the sternum (Fig. 8.53).

Extramammary metastases are usually hematogenous and represent 1% to 3% of all breast lesions (71). Hematopoietic and lymphoreticular lesions such as leukemia and lymphoma (Fig. 8.54), melanoma, lung, ovary (Figs. 8.55 and 8.56), renal, bladder, colon, stomach, and cervix have been reported. Single or multiple masses may be palpated. Very rarely, lung carcinomas can extent through the chest wall to involve the breast secondarily (Fig. 8.57).

Mammographically, single (Figs. 8.56A) or multiple (Fig. 8.55A) uni- or bilateral masses (Fig. 8.54A) are identified. The masses are usually round or oval with circumscribed, less commonly, indistinct margins. Solid hypoechoic masses with variable echotextures are seen on ultrasound. Since some of these lesions grow fairly rapidly, posterior acoustic enhancement may be apparent, as can cystic spaces reflecting areas of necrosis.

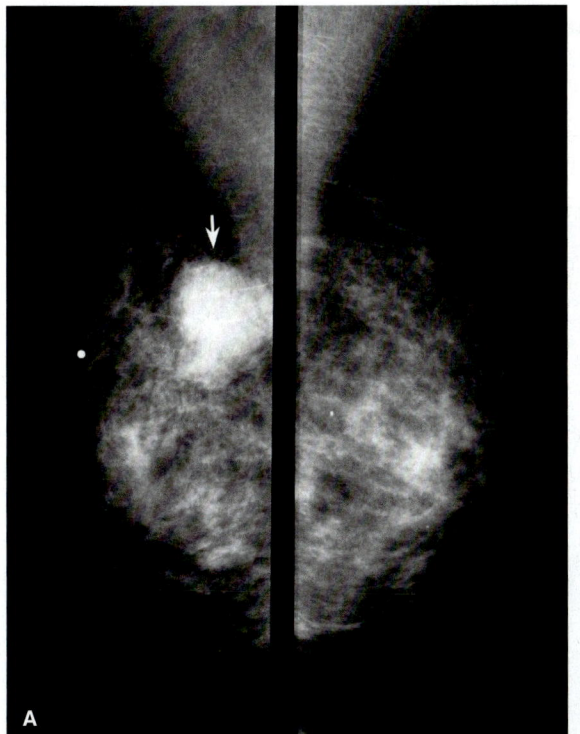
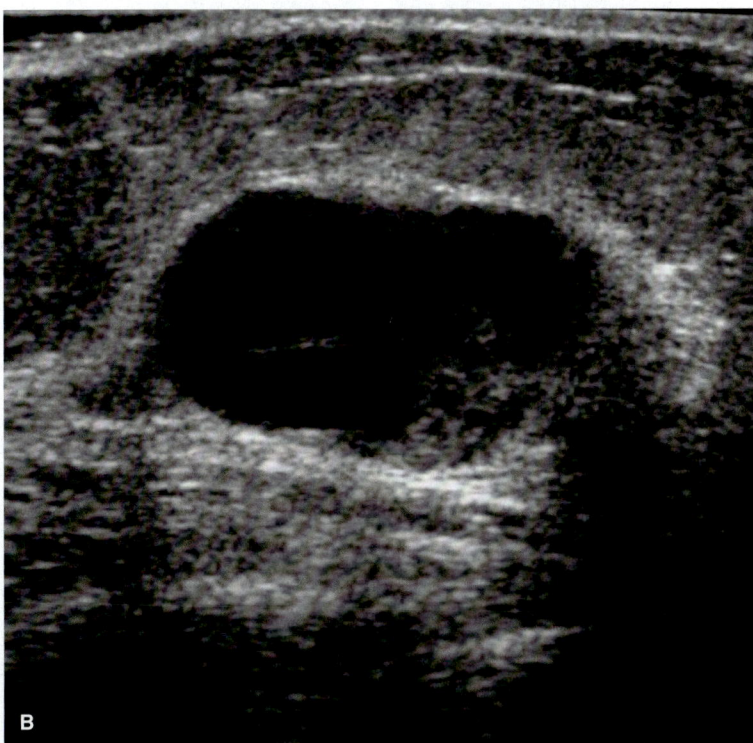

FIG. 8.49 • **Leiomyosarcoma. A:** MLO views in a 54-year-old patient with a "lump." The metallic BB marks the location of the palpable finding. A dense mass *(arrow)* is imaged in the upper central aspect of the right breast posteriorly. **B:** Ultrasound. A complex cystic and solid mass with posterior acoustic enhancement is imaged in the right breast corresponding to the palpable finding. BI-RADS 4C: Suspicious abnormality; biopsy is indicated.

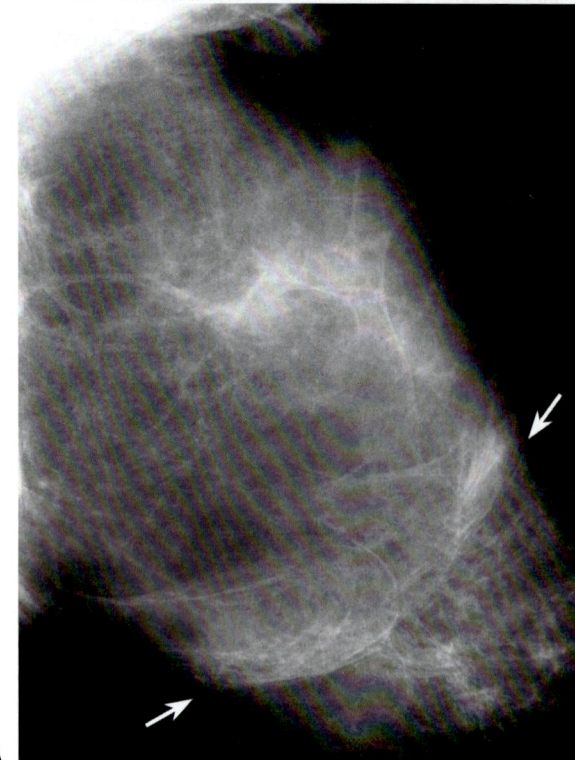
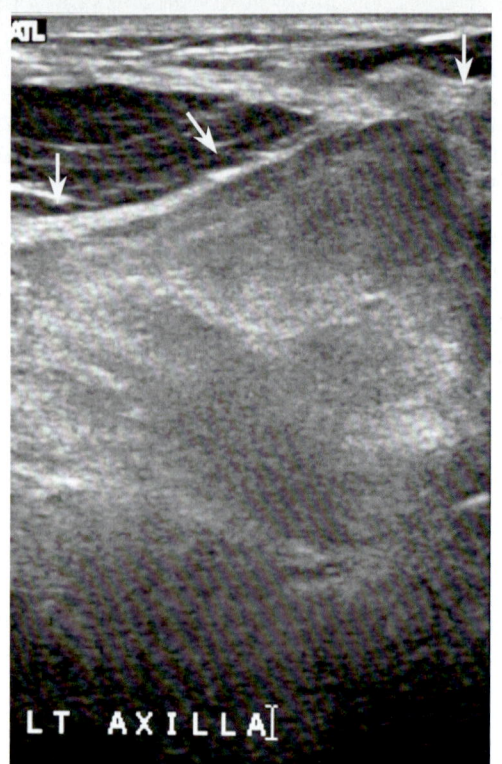
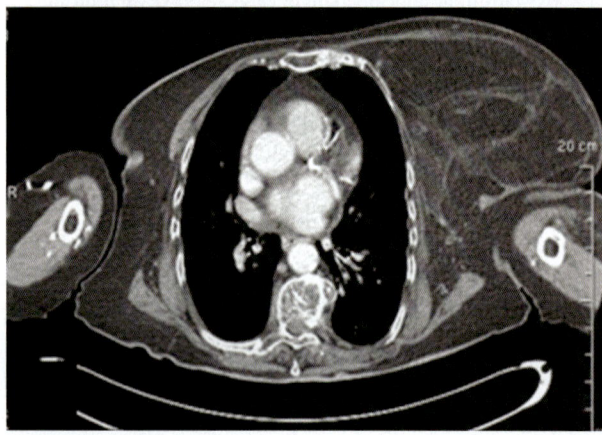

FIG. 8.50 • **Liposarcoma. A:** Left MLO view. A predominantly fatty mass is present extending into the axilla and displacing breast parenchyma anteriorly; the transition between tumor and normal breast tissue is apparent *(arrows)*. Efforts to position the breast to include more pectoral muscle proved unsuccessful. **B:** Ultrasound. A predominantly hyperechoic but heterogeneous mass *(arrows)* is imaged throughout the upper aspect of the left breast extending into the axilla and superiorly to the subclavicular area. Given the size and the infiltrative pattern of the mass it is not possible to image the lesion completely on any one image. **C:** CT scan. The lesion is predominantly fatty with internal septations, expands the left breast and extends into the axilla.

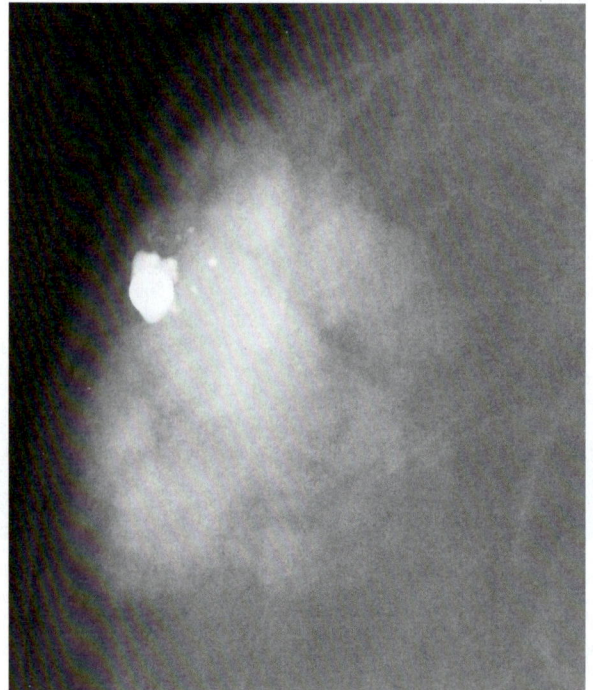

FIG. 8.51 • **Angiosarcoma.** Spot tangential view. A macrolobulated mass with variable density, indistinct margins, and "cloud-like" appearance sometimes seen with vascular lesions is imaged at the site of a palpable finding. Associated coarse calcifications. Some patients with angiosarcomas will have a bruit and a bluish discoloration overlying lesion. (From Cardeñosa G. *Breast Imaging [The Core Curriculum Series]*. Philadelphia, PA: Lippincott Williams & Wilkins; 2003.)

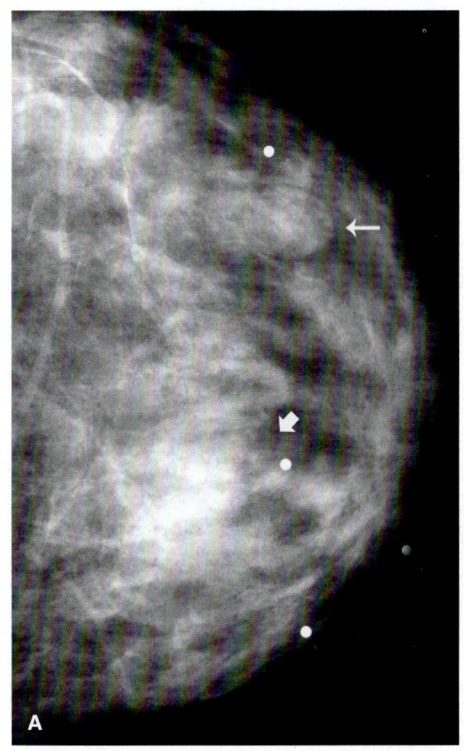
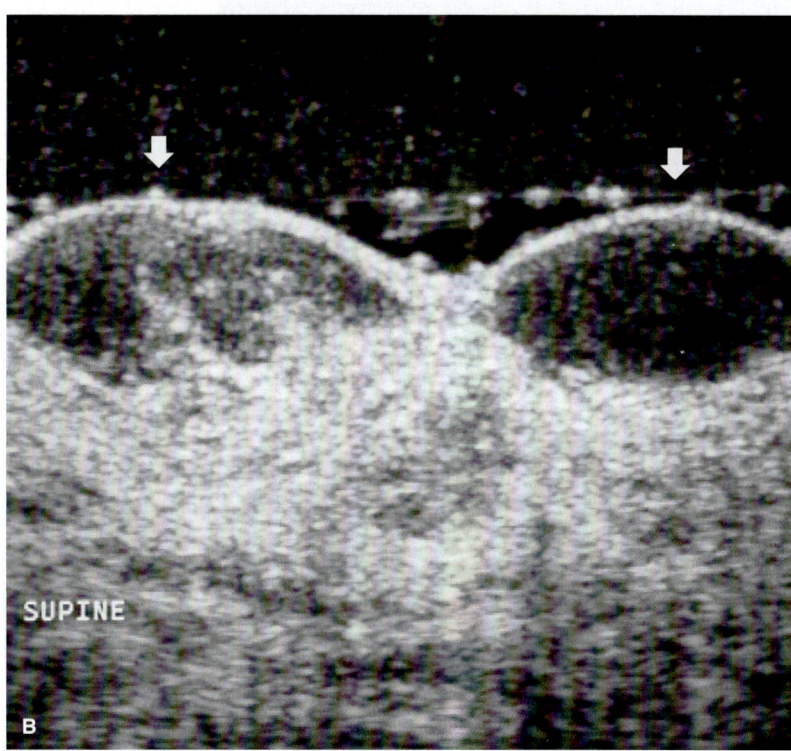
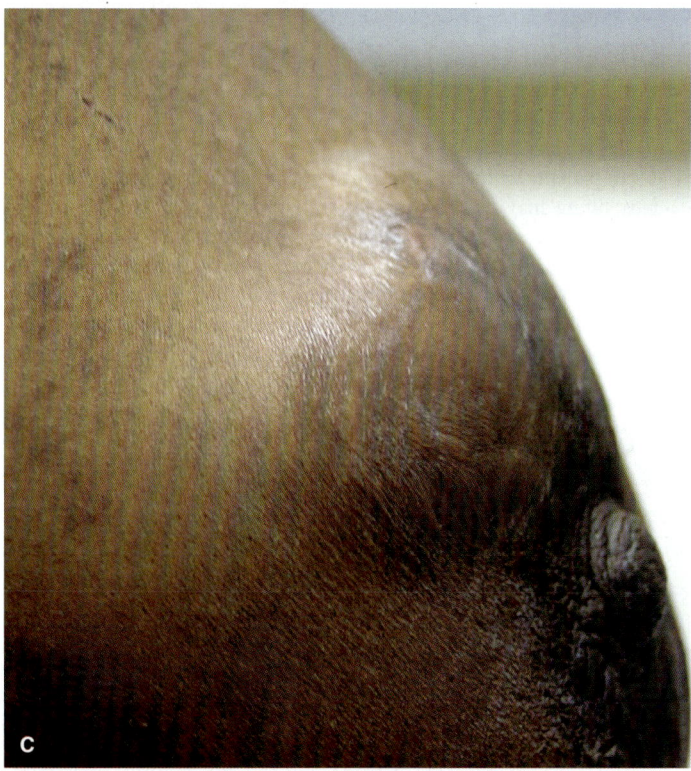

FIG. 8.52 • **Dermatofibrosarcoma protuberans with eventual fibrosarcomatous transformation. A:** Left CC view in a 31-year-old patient with multiple "lumps." Low- to iso- dense mass *(thin arrow)* with circumscribed margins corresponding to one of the palpable areas. Fibroadenoma diagnosed following excisional biopsy of this lesion. No definite mass noted at second palpable site *(thick arrow)*. **B:** Ultrasound using standoff pad to evaluate inner quadrant lesions. Two oval masses *(arrows)* with circumscribed margins causing a bulge in the contour of the breast. It is not possible to determine if these lesions are arising in the breast or the skin. Dermatofibrosarcoma protuberans is diagnosed on the excisional biopsy. Although wider excision was strongly recommended, patient declined further evaluation. **C:** Lateral view of the patient 21 months after image in part **A**. A mass is visible in the upper inner quadrant of the left breast (at the site of the prior biopsy). The patient presents because of significant tenderness associated with the mass. **D:** Left CC view. An oval iso dense mass with circumscribed margins is imaged mammographically corresponding to area of clinical concern. **E:** Ultrasound. An oval mass with heterogeneous echotexture and posterior acoustic enhancement is imaged corresponding to the clinically and mammographically apparent mass. Biopsy at this time shows sarcoma (fibrosarcomatous variant) arising in a dermatofibrosarcoma protuberans. (From Cardeñosa G. *Breast Imaging [The Core Curriculum Series]*. Philadelphia, PA: Lippincott Williams & Wilkins; 2003.)

(continued)

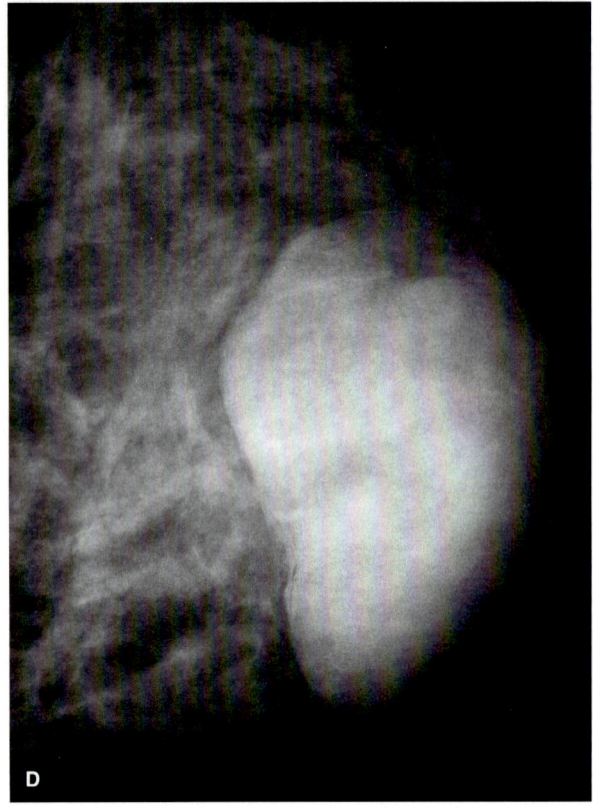
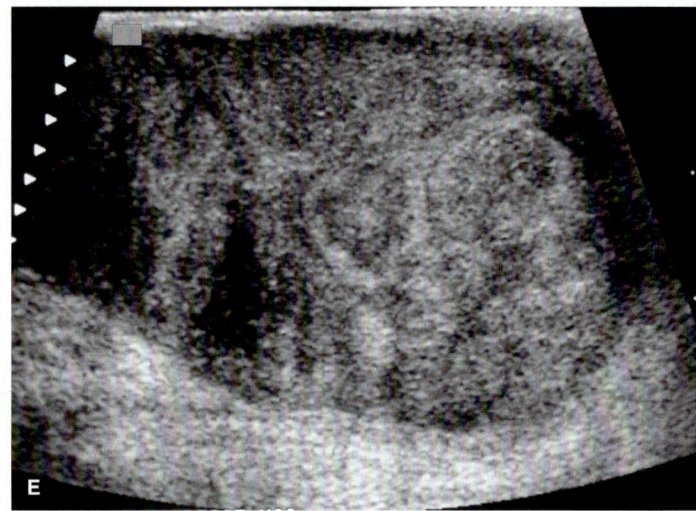

FIG. 8.52 • (continued)

METASTATIC DISEASE TO INTRAMAMMARY AND AXILLARY LYMPH NODES

Metastatic disease to intramammary and axillary lymph nodes is usually related to an underlying ipsilateral breast cancer or uncommonly contralateral breast cancer. Mammographically, detection of lymph nodes particularly in the axilla is variable and dependent on patient positioning (72). From one year to the next, more or less axillary tissue may be included on the oblique views and as such care must be exercised in considering what is perceived as a change. Provided axillary lymph nodes are included on the mammogram, and if comparison films are available, the affected intramammary or axillary node(s) is often enlarged, the fatty hilum is attenuated or absent, and the cortex is thickened and dense (Fig. 8.58). In most patients, the margins of the lymph node remain circumscribed less commonly indistinct or spiculated (72–75).

Ultrasound is a better tool to evaluate the axilla. As mentioned previously, depending on patient positioning, lymph nodes may not be imaged on the mammogram, and as such, the axilla of patients presenting with breast cancer, or those describing a palpable mass in the axilla, should be evaluated with ultrasound. With respect to axillary lymph nodes, we do not use size as a criterion for establishing the need for biopsy but rather rely on mammographic changes if these can be ascertained or their ultrasound features. If a mass with a hyperechoic fatty hilum is imaged in the axilla, we describe it as a lymph node and focus our attention on the relationship of the cortex to the fatty hilum: is there mass effect (Fig. 8.58C) or is the fatty hilum attenuated? With respect to the cortex, we specifically consider its width, contour, and echogenicity. A thickened, markedly hypoechoic cortex with bulging (Fig. 8.59) or mass effect on the fatty hilum (Fig. 8.58C) in a patient with breast cancer suggests the presence of metastatic disease (76,77). In our experience, the echogenicity of the cortex is particularly helpful. In patients in whom the cortex is thickened and bulging, as the echogenicity of the cortex increases, the likelihood of metastatic disease decreases. Hyperechoic cortices are more commonly seen in patients with inflammatory processes while the cortex of lymph nodes in patients with metastatic breast cancer or lymphoma is usually hypoechoic to almost anechoic.

In patients with complete replacement of the node with tumor, the fatty hilum may not be apparent and a markedly hypoechoic (nearly anechoic) mass with posterior acoustic enhancement is imaged in the axilla (Fig. 8.60). Keep in mind that cysts do not occur in the axilla and only rarely do patients with prior sentinel lymph node biopsy or a full axillary dissection present with a postoperative fluid collection in the axilla. Consequently, a non-vascular mass with marked hypoechogenicity

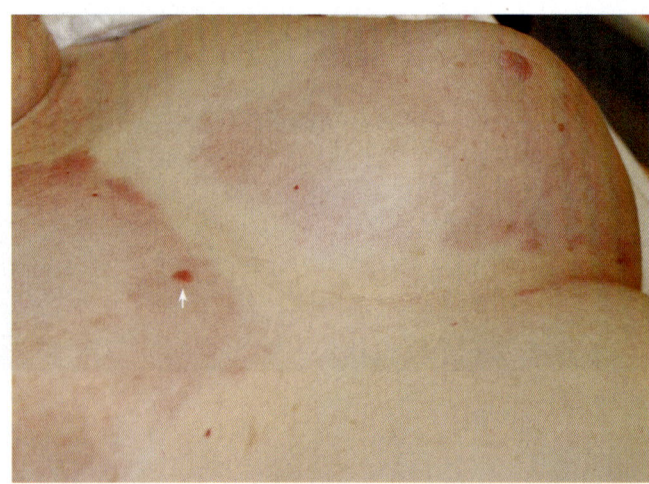

FIG. 8.53 • **Skin metastasis.** Confluent erythematous changes involving the inner quadrants bilaterally with relative sparing of the skin overlying the sternum. At least one raised erythematous nodule (arrow) is noted in the lower inner quadrant on the right.

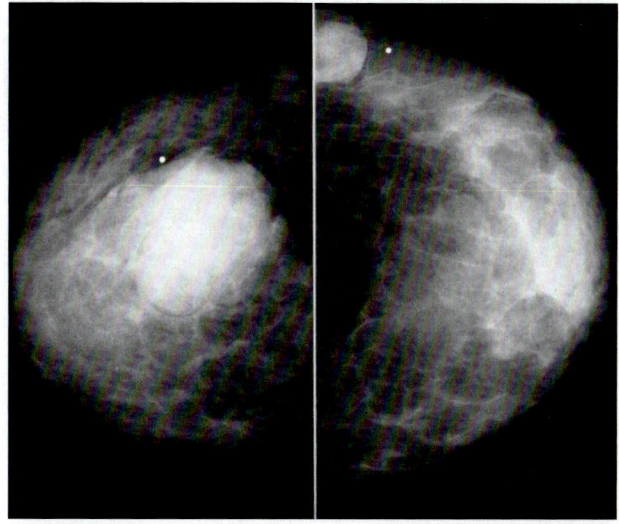

A

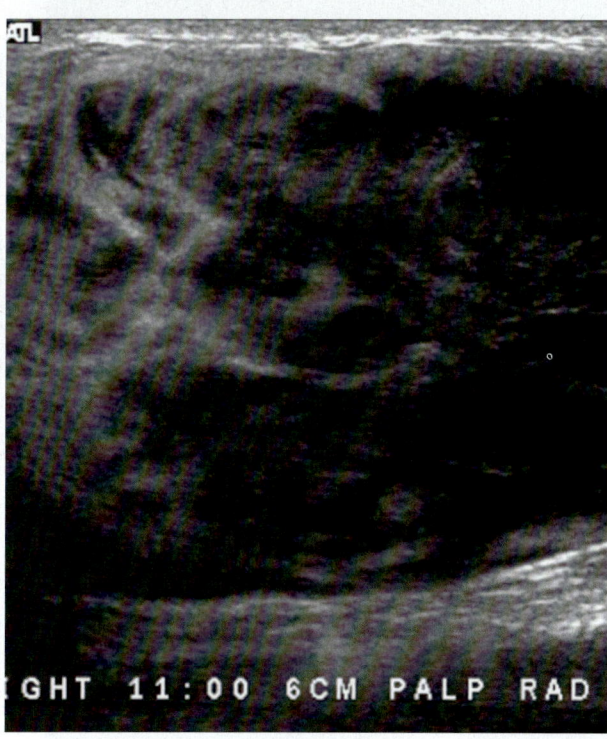

B

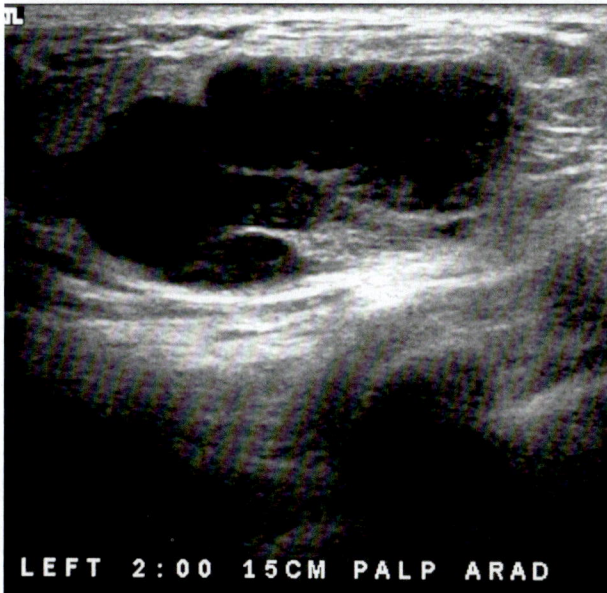

C

FIG. 8.54 • **Metastatic lymphoma, bilaterally. A:** CC views. A dense, round mass with circumscribed macrolobulated margins (a "halo" is seen partially surrounding the mass) is imaged in the right breast, and an oval low-density mass with circumscribed margins is partially imaged posterolaterally in the left breast. The metallic BBs are used to denote the palpable findings in this 40-year-old patient. **B:** Ultrasound. A mass with a heterogeneous echotexture and posterior acoustic enhancement is partially imaged corresponding to the palpable mass in the right breast. **C:** Ultrasound. An oval mass with eccentric echogenicity and a markedly hypoechoic cortical region is imaged corresponding to the mass seen on the mammogram in the left breast. This represents an abnormal intramammary lymph node. Malignant large B-cell lymphoma metastatic to the breast is diagnosed following ultrasound-guided core biopsies.

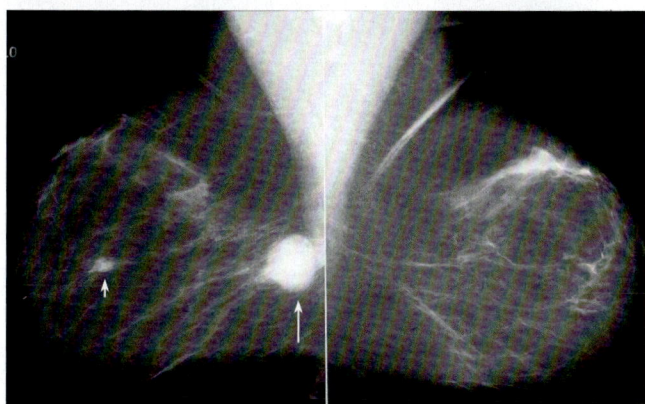

A

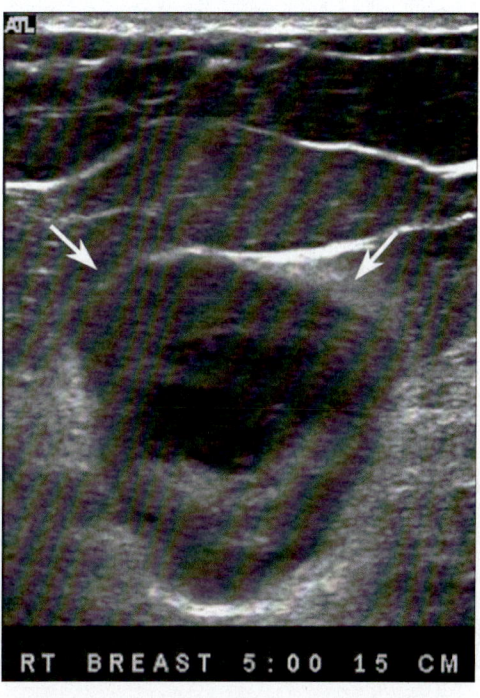

B

FIG. 8.55 • **Metastatic invasive carcinoma high grade with necrosis consistent with metastatic disease from ovarian primary (anaplastic ovarian CA). A:** MLO views in a 42-year-old patient. A round, high density mass *(long arrow)* is imaged in the lower inner quadrant of the right breast posteriorly. A second oval iso dense mass *(short arrow)* is present anteriorly. **B:** Ultrasound. A complex cystic and solid mass *(arrows)* with posterior acoustic enhancement is imaged on ultrasound corresponding to the larger mass seen mammographically. The smaller mass has similar features on ultrasound (not shown). BI-RADS 4C: Suspicious abnormality; biopsy is indicated.

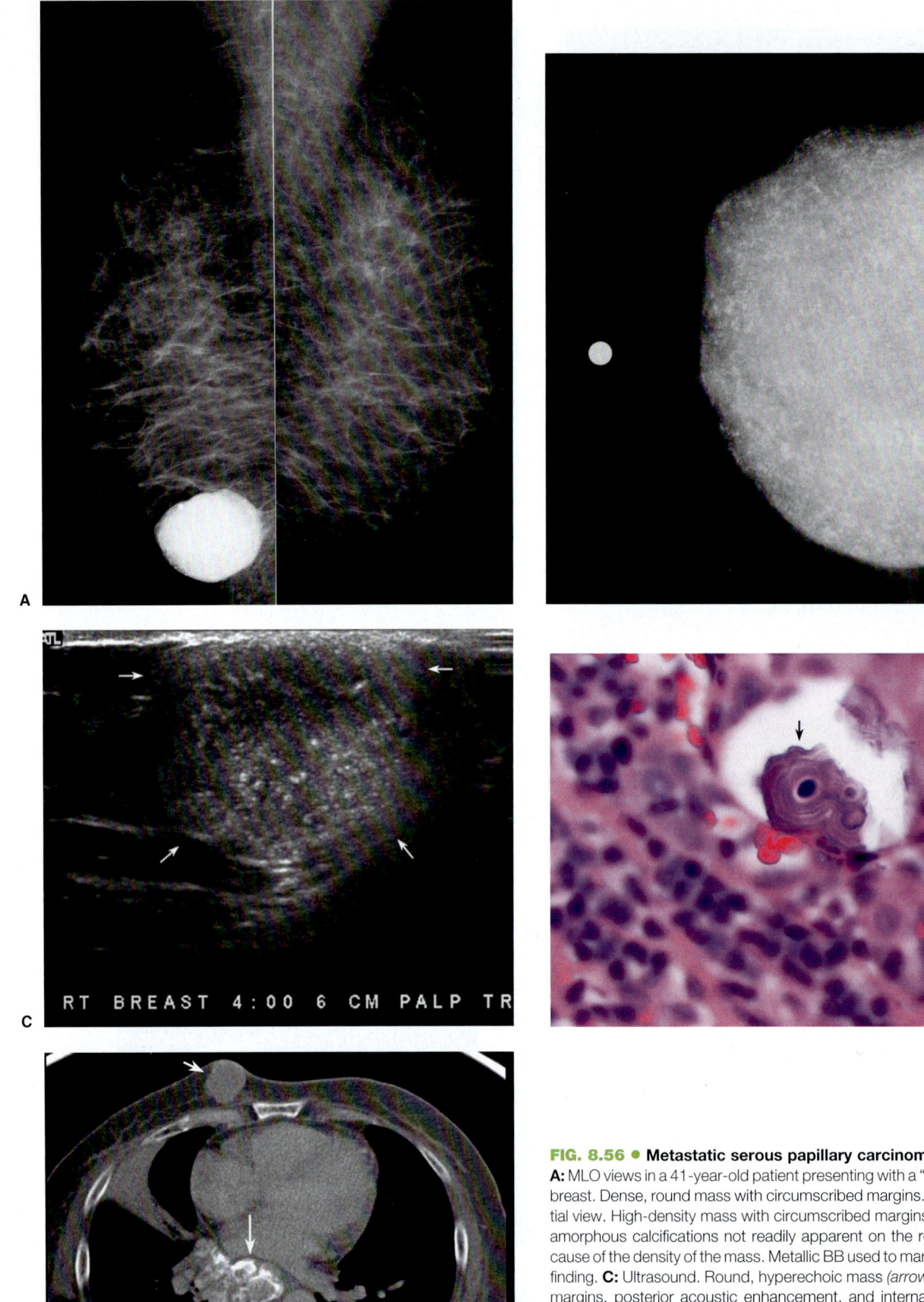

FIG. 8.56 • **Metastatic serous papillary carcinoma of the ovary.**
A: MLO views in a 41-year-old patient presenting with a "lump" in the right breast. Dense, round mass with circumscribed margins. **B:** Spot tangential view. High-density mass with circumscribed margins and associated amorphous calcifications not readily apparent on the routine views because of the density of the mass. Metallic BB used to mark site of palpable finding. **C:** Ultrasound. Round, hyperechoic mass *(arrows)* with indistinct margins, posterior acoustic enhancement, and internal echogenic foci consistent with the calcifications seen on the mammogram. BI-RADS 4C: Suspicious abnormality; biopsy is indicated. Ultrasound-guided biopsy is done to establish the diagnosis. **D:** Psammoma bodies *(arrow)* are described corresponding to the amorphous calcifications seen on the mammogram and ultrasound. **E:** Chest CT scan image at the level of the breast mass *(short arrow)* also demonstrates calcified mediastinal adenopathy *(long arrow)* and resulting collapse of the right middle lobe.

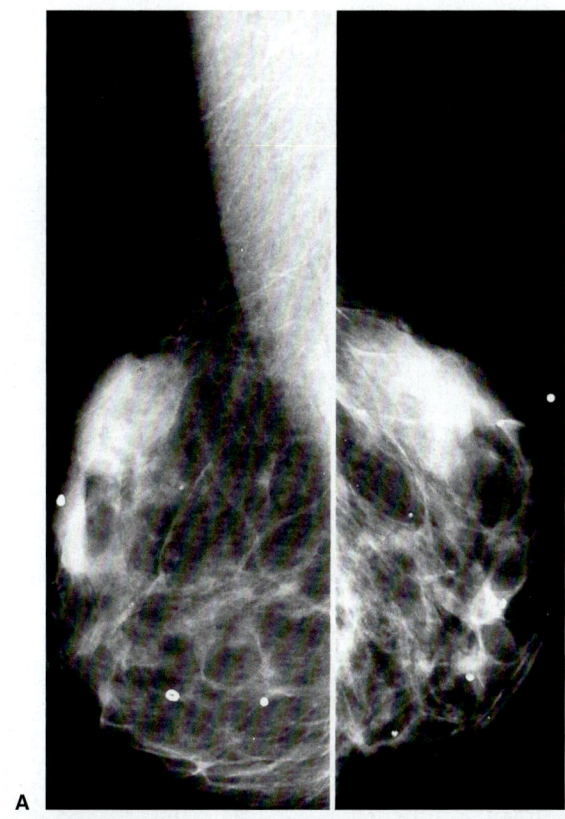
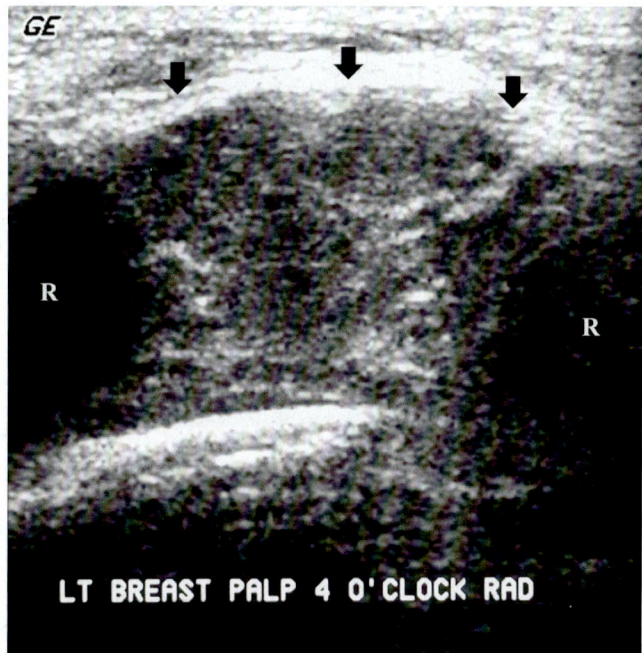
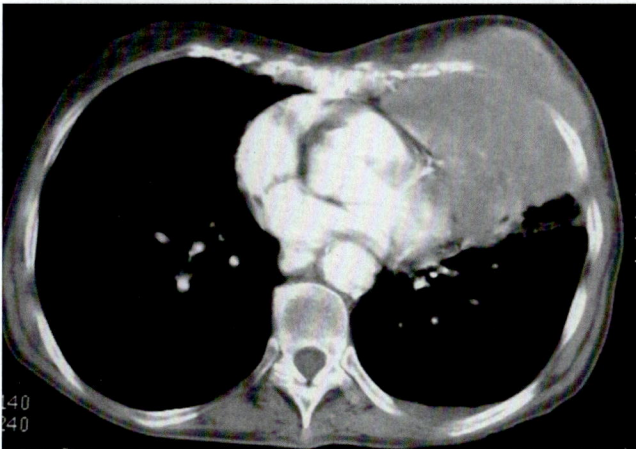

FIG. 8.57 • **Lung cancer, extending into breast. A:** MLO views in a 73-year-old patient presenting with a mass in the lower outer quadrant of the left breast. Metallic BB is used to denote palpable finding. Although multiple attempts are made to include more tissue and pectoral muscle on the left, these are unsuccessful. Other than the positioning issues, no gross abnormality is apparent. **B:** Ultrasound. A mass *(arrows)* is imaged between the ribs *(R)*. The site of origin for the mass is difficult to establish on ultrasound. Core biopsy suggested small cell histology. **C:** Chest CT scan demonstrates lung cancer extending into the left breast. From Cardeñosa G. *Breast Imaging [The Core Curriculum Series]*. Philadelphia, PA: Lippincott Williams & Wilkins; 2003.)

and posterior acoustic enhancement (simulating a cyst) imaged on ultrasound in the axilla is abnormal and may warrant biopsy. When no fatty hilum is identified on ultrasound, it may be unclear if the mass represents a replaced lymph node, or possibly a primary lesion, so we are dependent on the location of the mass: is the mass in the axilla or could it be in axillary tail breast tissue? Histologically, if no lymphoid elements or DCIS are identified on a core biopsy from a mass in the axilla, it is often impossible for the pathologist to differentiate metastatic disease from a primary lesion. If DCIS is seen, the sampled lesion is unlikely to represent metastatic disease and more likely to be a primary lesion. Conversely, if lymphoid elements are identified, metastatic disease is likely. The pathologist is dependent on an accurate description of the location of the lesion being sampled and the impression of the radiologist.

The anatomic variability in the location of lymph nodes can be appreciated on magnetic resonance. Depending on tissue mobility, lymph nodes are sometimes noted extending inferiorly from the axilla along the mid-axillary line (Fig. 8.61). As with mammography and ultrasound, the shape of normal lymph nodes is variable, the margins are often circumscribed, T2 signal is intermediate to high, and the enhancement is often homogeneous with rapid wash-in and wash-out kinetics. Abnormal lymph nodes may be enlarged with indistinct margins, variable T2 signal (often low), and a more heterogeneous, stippled enhancement pattern. MRI also readily enables identification of abnormal internal mammary lymph nodes (see Fig. 5.24).

As mentioned previously, patients with metastatic disease to intramammary or axillary lymph nodes at the time of presentation will bypass sentinel lymph node biopsy and have a full axillary dissection or, with increasing frequency, neo-adjuvant therapy prior to surgery. Also, when an abnormal intramammary lymph node is identified and found to be positive for metastatic disease, we wire localize the positive intramammary lymph node preoperatively since these are not routinely excised during sentinel lymph node biopsy or axillary dissections.

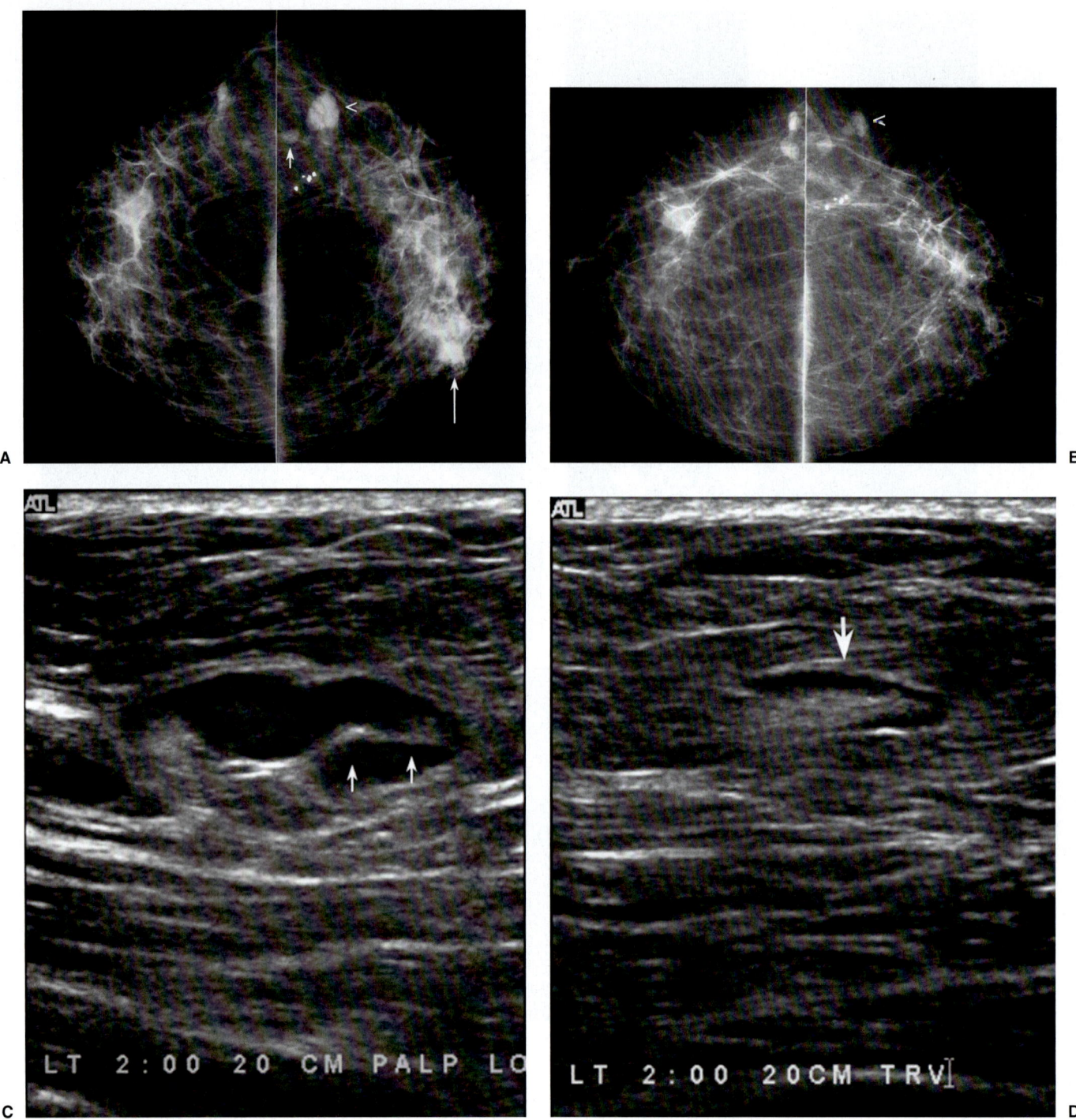

FIG. 8.58 • **Multifocal invasive ductal carcinoma with metastatic disease to an intramammary lymph node.**
A: CC views in a 68-year-old patient. **B:** Comparison CC views 1 year earlier. The patient has developed two masses *(long arrow)* in the medial aspect of the left breast (spot compression views and ultrasound are not shown), diagnosed as invasive ductal carcinoma on needle biopsy. Also note the change in one of two pre-existing intramammary lymph nodes in the lateral aspect of the breast posteriorly. The node *(arrow head)* is now enlarged, is denser, and the fatty hilum is not readily apparent mammographically; the second slightly more posterior lymph node *(short arrow* in image **A**) is low in density and remains unchanged compared with the prior study. Intramammary lymph nodes posterolaterally in the right breast also remain unchanged. **C:** Ultrasound of the larger intramammary lymph node on the left demonstrates a lymph node with eccentric hyperechogenicity and a hypoechoic cortex that is thickened and exerts mass effect on the fatty hilum such that the fatty hilum is attenuated *(arrows)*. Needle biopsy confirms metastatic disease. **D:** Ultrasound. In the tissue adjacent to the lymph node shown in part **C**, a morphologically normal-appearing lymph node is identified corresponding to the more posterior lymph node seen on the mammogram. This is a morphologically normal-appearing lymph node with a prominent fatty hilum ("plump") and a thin surrounding cortex *(arrow)*. **E:** MRI, T1-weighted sagittal reconstruction of the left breast post-contrast. The lymph node demonstrates superior cortical bulging *(arrow)* and heterogeneous enhancement. Vascular structure is imaged entering the hilar region.

Evaluation and Imaging Features of Malignant Breast Masses   277

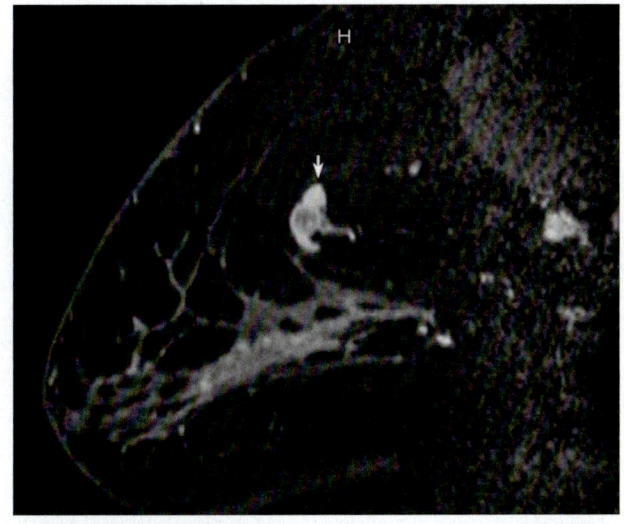

FIG. 8.58 • (continued)

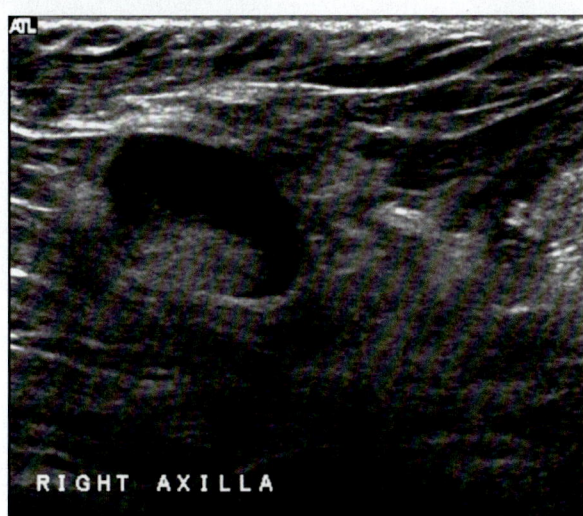

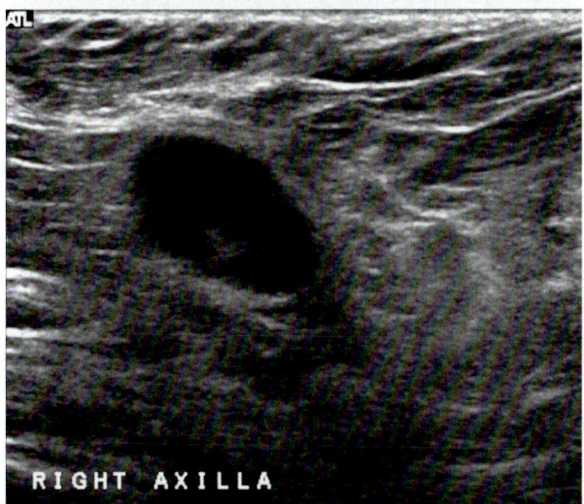

FIG. 8.59 • **Invasive ductal carcinoma, metastatic to a right axillary lymph node. A:** Ultrasound. An oval mass with an eccentric fatty hilum and surrounding hypoechoic ("plump") cortex; at this scan plane, the fatty hilum appears normal. **B:** Ultrasound. As the lymph node is scanned away from the hilum, a cortical bulge is noted superiorly and laterally to the fatty hilum; also note marked hypoechogenicity of the cortex. Metastatic disease is confirmed on ultrasound-guided core biopsy. In these patients, the cortical bulge is targeted for the core biopsy.

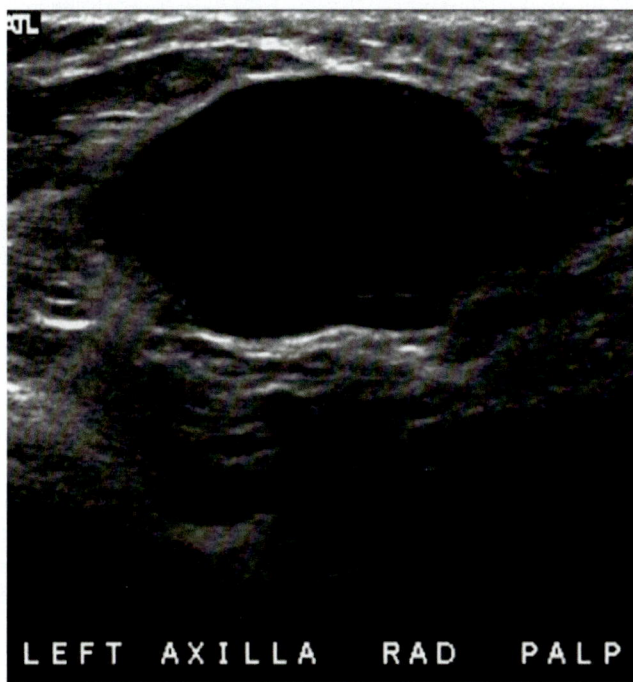

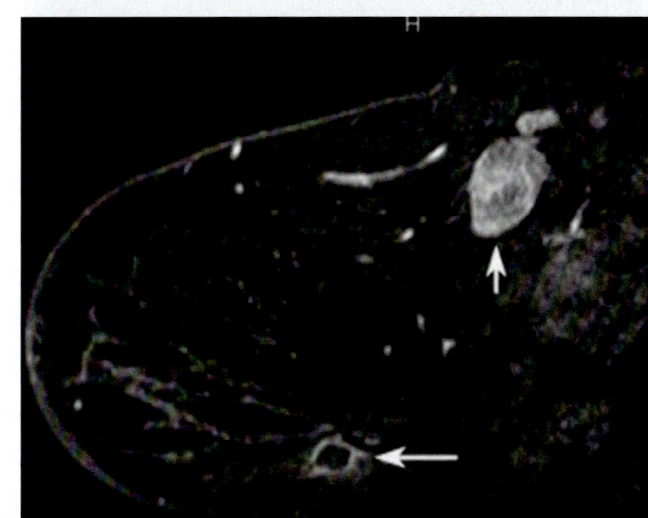

FIG. 8.60 • **Invasive ductal carcinoma, metastatic to a left axillary lymph node. A:** Ultrasound. Oval markedly hypoechoic mass with circumscribed margins and posterior acoustic enhancement. Suspected metastatic disease is confirmed on an ultrasound-guided biopsy. **B:** MRI, T1-weighted sagittal reconstruction of the left breast post-contrast. Oval heterogeneously enhancing mass (short arrow) with circumscribed margins is imaged corresponding to the mass shown in **A**. Rim-enhancing mass (long arrow) is imaged inferiorly in the left breast corresponding to one of two sites of malignancy in this patient.

Lymphoproliferative disorders including lymphoma (Fig. 8.62) and leukemia can also involve intramammary or axillary lymph nodes. Likewise, metastasis from non-breast primaries including melanoma (see Fig. 3.2), lung, and ovarian cancer (Fig. 8.63) can involve axillary lymph nodes (41–45). Rarely, unsuspected malignancies are detected because of enlarged lymph nodes (Fig. 8.62; also see Fig. 5.27). Although pleomorphic calcifications related to metastatic breast cancer have been reported, this is unusual and may reflect the presence of tumor necrosis from a breast primary (Fig. 8.64) or calcifications related to psammoma bodies from ovarian (78) or thyroid primaries (Fig. 8.63).

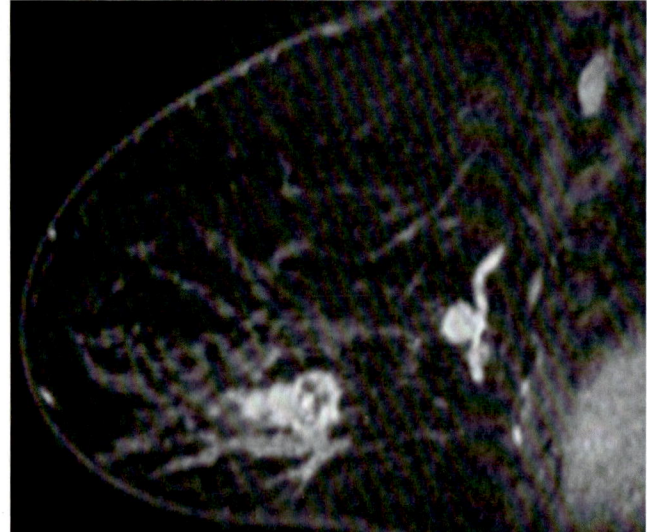
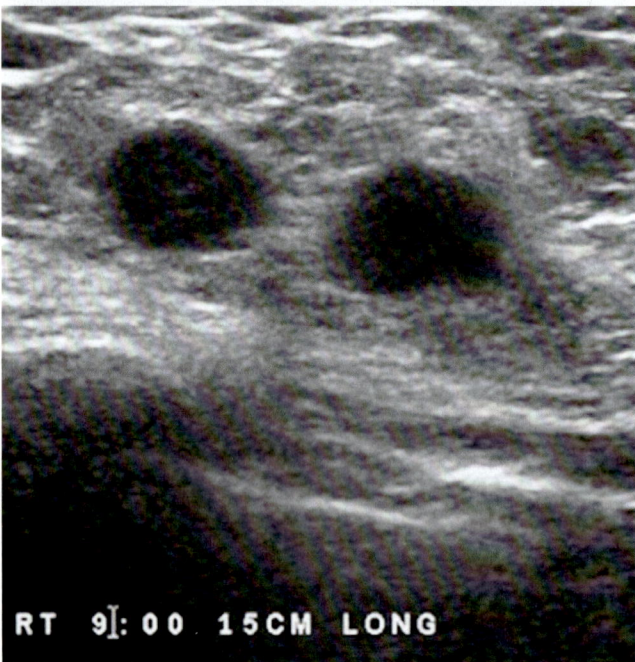

FIG. 8.61 • **Metastatic disease to lymph nodes detected along the mid-axillary line on MRI. A:** MRI, T1-weighted sagittal reconstruction of the right breast, post-contrast. A mass with heterogeneous enhancement, circumscribed margins, and an associated vascular structure is imaged posterolaterally in the right breast. A second similar mass is imaged on a scan a few millimeters lateral to this scan plane. The patient's primary tumor is seen inferiorly with rim and central enhancement, irregular margins, and non-mass–like enhancement extending anteriorly for approximately 2 cm (see Fig. 5.3 for a coronal reconstruction of this tumor). The MRI in this 51-year-old patient was done for staging purposes; an invasive ductal carcinoma was diagnosed in the right breast on an ultrasound-guided biopsy. Morphologically normal lymph nodes were imaged in the right axilla on the ultrasound done at the time of the original evaluation. **B:** Ultrasound. Using the MRI as a guide, the patient is re-scanned along the mid-axillary line. Two nearly anechoic masses with indistinct margins are imaged along the 9 o'clock axis, 15 cm from the right nipple. Ultrasound-guided biopsy confirms suspected metastatic disease. In evaluating for metastatic disease we are now routinely scanning the axilla and coming inferiorly along the mid-axillary line.

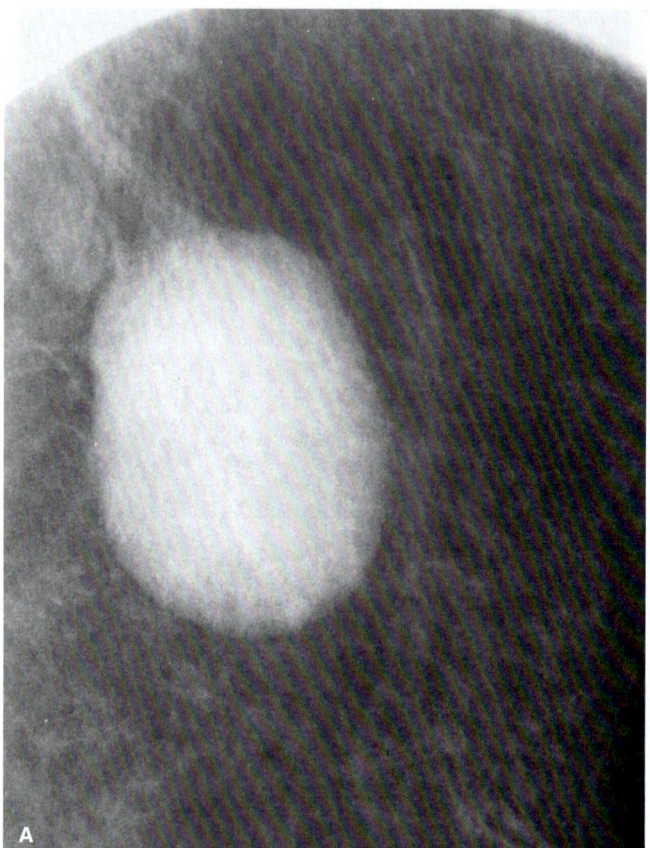
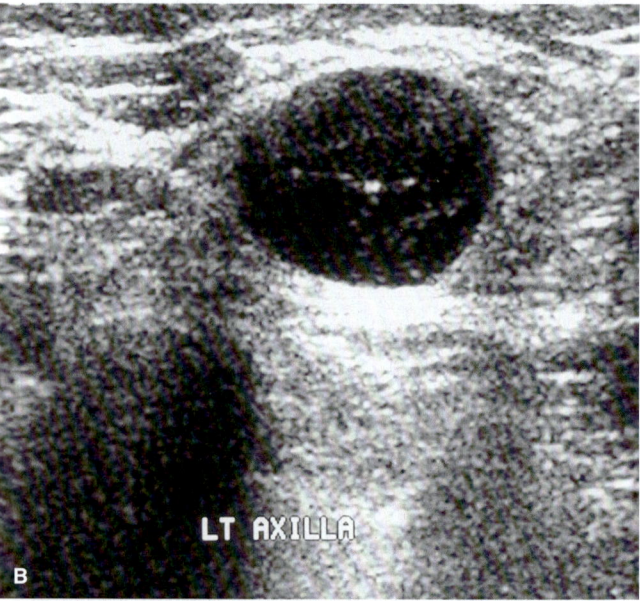

FIG. 8.62 • **Follicular center cell lymphoma grade III (large cell). A:** Spot compression view of the left axilla in a 74-year-old patient presenting with new enlarged lymph nodes in the left axilla. An oval iso dense mass with circumscribed margins is imaged in the left axilla. No fatty hilum is seen. **B:** A round markedly hypoechoic mass with posterior acoustic enhancement is imaged in the left axilla corresponding to a palpable finding. No fatty hilum is identified. Additional enlarged lymph nodes are palpated in left aspect of the neck and two masses are present in the scalp. BI-RADS 4C: Suspicious abnormality; biopsy is indicated. (From Cardeñosa G. *Breast Imaging [The Core Curriculum Series]*. Philadelphia, PA: Lippincott Williams & Wilkins; 2003.)

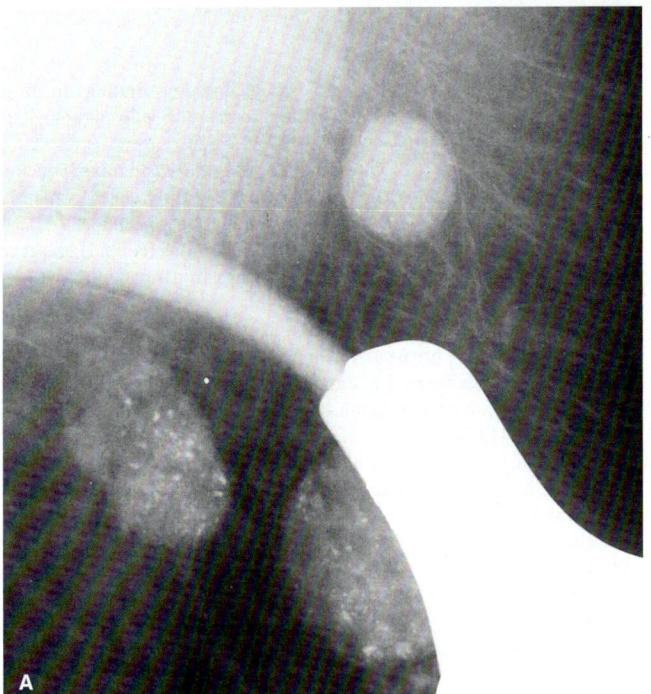
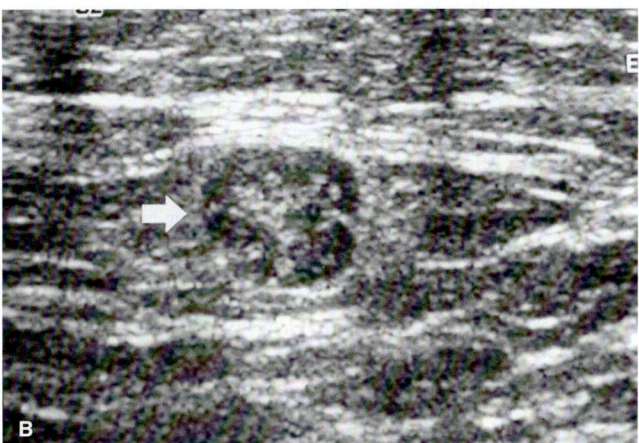

FIG. 8.63 • **Metastatic papillary carcinoma with psammoma bodies. A:** Spot compression view of the left axilla. Enlarged axillary lymph nodes with calcifications are noted on the screening mammogram in a 71-year-old patient (screening images not shown). Three masses with circumscribed margins and fine pleomorphic (round, punctate, and amorphous) calcifications are present. **B:** A hypoechoic mass with foci of hyperechogenicity consistent with calcifications is imaged on ultrasound *(arrow)*. Metastatic papillary carcinoma with psammoma bodies is reported on the ultrasound-guided core biopsy; features suggest gynecologic serous papillary carcinoma or primary serous carcinoma of the peritoneum. (From Cardeñosa G. *Breast Imaging [The Core Curriculum Series]*. Philadelphia, PA: Lippincott Williams & Wilkins; 2003.)

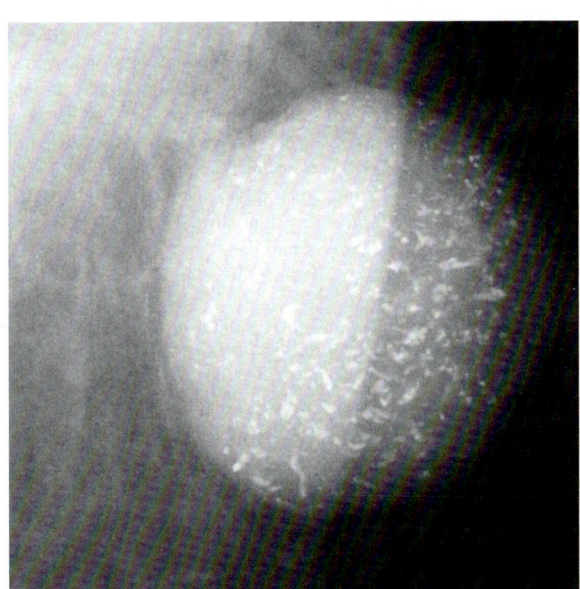
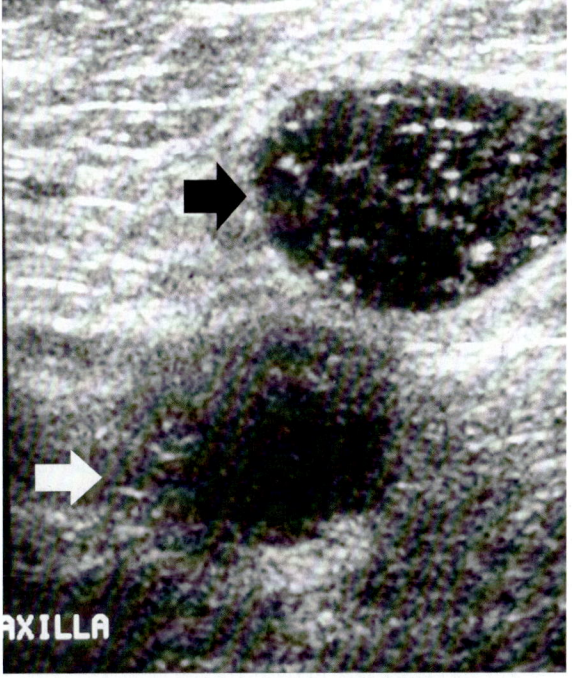

FIG. 8.64 • **Metastatic breast cancer from the contralateral breast. A:** MLO view of the left axilla photographically coned to the upper portion of the image in a 50-year-old patient with a contralateral mastectomy (right breast) for inflammatory carcinoma 2 years previously. Round iso dense mass with circumscribed margins and pleomorphic calcifications. Differential considerations include metastasis from the contralateral cancer or a new primary in the left breast with associated DCIS. **B:** Ultrasound. Two masses are imaged in the left axilla. One of these has hyperechogenic foci consistent with the calcifications seen on the mammogram *(black arrow)*. A second round hypoechoic mass with a nearly anechoic center *(white arrow)* and indistinct margins is imaged deeper in the axilla. An ultrasound-guided needle biopsy of the calcified mass is done. Metastatic breast cancer (similar features to contralateral inflammatory carcinoma) with calcifications in areas of necrosis is diagnosed histologically. No DCIS is seen. Also, note that the mass is arising high in the axillary tail of the breast with no surrounding tissue; this is consistent with metastatic disease (as opposed to a second primary). (From Cardeñosa G. *Breast Imaging [The Core Curriculum Series]*. Philadelphia, PA: Lippincott Williams & Wilkins; 2003.)

References

1. Rosen PP. *Rosen's Breast Pathology*. 3rd ed. Philadelphia, PA: Lippincott Williams & Wilkins; 2008.
2. Tavassoli FA. *Pathology of the Breast*. 2nd ed. New York, NY: McGraw Hill; 1999.
3. Orel SG, Weinstein SP, Schnall MD, et al. Breast MR imaging in patients with axillary node metastases and unknown primary malignancy. *Radiology*. 1999;212:543–549.
4. Stacey-Clear A, McCarthy KA, Hall DA, et al. Observations on the location of breast cancer in women under fifty. *Radiology*. 1993;186:677–680.
5. Stavros AT, Thickman D, Rapp CL, et al. Solid breast nodules: use of sonography to distinguish benign and malignant lesions. *Radiology*. 1995;196:123–134.
6. Tinnemans JGM, Wobbes T, van der Sluis RF. Multicentricity in nonpalpable breast carcinoma and its implications for treatment. *Am J Surg*. 1986;151:334–338.
7. Donegan WL, Spratt JS. *Cancer of the Breast*. 5th ed. Philadelphia, PA: WB Saunders; 2002.
8. Nielsen M, Christensen L, Andersen J. Contralateral cancerous breast lesions in women with clinical invasive breast carcinoma. *Cancer*. 1986;57:897–903.
9. Nielsen M, Christensen L, Andersen J. Precancerous and cancerous breast lesions during lifetime and at autopsy. *Cancer*. 1984;54:612–615.
10. Blaichman J, Marcus JC, Alsaadi T, et al. Sonographic appearance of invasive ductal carcinoma of the breast according to histologic grade. *AJR Am J Roentgenol*. 2012;199:W402–W408.
11. Dogan BE, Gonzalez-Angulo AM, Gilcrease M, et al. Multimodality imaging of triple receptor-negative tumors with mammography, ultrasound and MRI. *AJR Am J Roentgenol*. 2010;194:1160–1166.
12. Bakha EA, Ellis IO. Triple negative/basal-like breast cancer: review. *Pathology*. 2009;41:40–47.
13. Holland R, Connolly JL, Gelman R, et al. The presence of an extensive intraductal component following a limited excision correlates with prominent residual disease in the remainder of the breast. *J Clin Oncol*. 1990;8:113–118.
14. Schnitt SJ, Connolly JL, Khettry U, et al. Pathologic findings on reexcision of the primary site in breast cancer patients considered for treatment by primary radiation therapy. *Cancer*. 1987;59:675.
15. Gage I, Schnitt SJ, Nixon AJ. Pathologic margin involvement and the risk of recurrence in patients treated with breast conserving therapy. *Cancer*. 1996;78:1921.
16. Harris JR, Lippman ME, Morrow M, et al., eds. *Disease of the Breast*. 2nd ed. Philadelphia, PA: Lippincott Williams & Wilkins; 2000.
17. Haagensen CD. *Diseases of the Breast*. 3rd ed. Philadelphia, PA: WB Saunders; 1986.
18. Leibman AJ, Lewis M, Kruse B. Tubular carcinoma of the breast: mammographic appearance. *AJR Am J Roentgenol*. 1993;160:263–265.
19. Helvie MA, Paramagul C, Oberman HA, et al. Invasive tubular carcinoma: imaging features and clinical detection. *Invest Radiol*. 1993;28:202–207.
20. Elson BC, Helvie MA, Frank TS, et al. Tubular carcinoma of the breast: mode of presentation, mammographic appearance and frequency of nodal metastases. *AJR Am J Roentgenol*. 1993;161:1173–1176.
21. Sheppard DG, Whitman GJ, Huynh PT, et al. Tubular carcinoma of the breast: mammographic and sonographic features. *AJR Am J Roentgenol*. 2000;174:253–257.
22. Mitnick JS, Gianutsos R, Pollack AH, et al. Tubular carcinoma of the breast: sensitivity of diagnostic techniques and correlation with histopathology. *AJR Am J Roentgenol*. 1999;172:319–323.
23. Shin HJ, Kim HH, Kim SM, et al. Pure and mixed tubular carcinoma of the breast: mammographic and sonographic differential features. *Korean J Radiol*. 2007;8:103–110.
24. Monzawa S, Yokokawa M, Sakuma T, et al. Mucinous carcinoma of the breast: MRI features of pure and mixed forms with histopathologic correlation. *AJR Am J Roentgenol*. 2009;192:W125–W131.
25. Bae SY, Choi MY, Cho DH, et al. Mucinous carcinoma of the breast in comparison with invasive ductal carcinoma: clinicopathologic characteristics and prognosis. *J Breast Cancer*. 2011;14:308–313.
26. Reimer T. Management of rare histological types of breast tumours. *Breast Care (Basel)*. 2008;3:190–196.
27. Conant EF, Dillon RL, Palazzo J, et al. Imaging findings in mucin-containing carcinomas of the breast: correlation with pathologic features. *AJR Am J Roentgenol*. 1994;163:821–824.
28. Wilson TE, Helvie MA, Oberman HA, et al. Pure and mixed mucinous carcinoma of the breast: pathologic basis for differences in mammographic appearance. *AJR Am J Roentgenol*. 1995;165:285–289.
29. Cardenosa G, Doudna C, Eklund GW. Mucinous (colloid) breast cancer: clinical and mammographic findings in 10 patients. *AJR Am J Roentgenol*. 1994;162:1077–1079.
30. Kawashima M, Tamake Y, Nonaka T, et al. MR imaging of mucinous carcinoma of the breast. *AJR Am J Roentgenol*. 2002;179:179–183.
31. Liberman L, LaTrenta LR, Samli B, et al. Overdiagnosis of medullary carcinoma: a mammographic-pathologic correlative study. *Radiology*. 1996;201:443–446.
32. Meyer JE, Amin E, Lindfors KK, et al. Medullary carcinoma of the breast: mammographic and US appearance. *Radiology*. 1989;170:79–82.
33. Tominaga J, Hama H, Kimura N, et al. MR imaging of medullary carcinoma of the breast. *Eur J Radiol*. 2009;70:525–529.
34. Jeong SJ, Lim HS, Lee SH, et al. Medullary carcinoma of breast: MRI findings. *AJR Am J Roentgenol*. 2012;198:W482–W487.
35. Schneider JA. Invasive papillary breast carcinoma: mammographic and sonographic appearance. *Radiology*. 1989;171:377–379.
36. Soo MS, Williford ME, Walsh R, et al. Papillary carcinoma of the breast: imaging findings. *AJR Am J Roentgenol*. 1995;164:321–326.
37. Muttarak M, Lerttumnongtum P, Chaiwun B, et al. Spectrum of papillary lesions of the breast: clinical, imaging, and pathologic correlation. *AJR Am J Roentgenol*. 2008;191:700–707.
38. Eiada R, Chong J, Kulkarni S, et al. Papillary lesions of the breast: MRI, ultrasound and mammographic appearance. *AJR Am J Roentgenol*. 2012;198:264–271.
39. Brookes MJ, Bourke AG. Radiological appearances of papillary breast lesions. *Clin Radiol*. 2008;63:1265–1273.
40. Mulligan AM, O'Malley FP. Papillary lesions of the breast. *Adv Anat Pathol*. 2007;14:108–119.
41. Ibarra JA. Papillary lesions of the breast. *Breast J*. 2006;12:237–251.
42. Ueng SH, Mezzetti T, Tavassoli FA. Papillary neoplasms of the breast: a review. *Arch Pathol Lab Med*. 2009;133:893–907.
43. Benkaddour YA, Hasnaoui SE, Fichtalli K, et al. Intracystic papillary carcinoma of the breast: report of three cases and literature review. *Case Rep Obstet Gynecol*. 2012;202:979563.
44. Grabowski J, Salzsteing SL, Sadler GR, et al. Intracystic papillary carcinoma: a review of 917 cases. *Cancer*. 2008;113:916–920.
45. Pal SK, Lau SK, Kruper L, et al. Papillary carcinoma of the breast: an overview. *Breast Cancer Res Treat*. 2010;122:637–645.
46. Saremian J, Rosa M. Solid papillary carcinoma of the breast: a pathologically and clinically distinct breast tumor. *Arch Pathol Lab Med*. 2012;136:1308–1311.
47. Nagi C, Bleiweiss I, Jaffer S. Epithelial displacement in breast lesions. *Arch Pathol Lab Med*. 2005;129:1465–1469.
48. Bleiweiss IJ, Nagi CS, Jaffer S. Axillary sentinel lymph nodes can be falsely positive due to iatrogenic displacement and transport of benign epithelial cells in patients with breast carcinoma. *J Clin Oncol*. 2006;24:2013–2018.
49. Yun SU, Choi BB, Shu KS, et al. Imaging findings of invasive micropapillary carcinoma of the breast. *J Breast Cancer*. 2012;15:57–84.
50. Choi BB, Shu KS. Metaplastic carcinoma of the breast: multimodality imaging and histopathologic assessment. *Acta Radiol*. 2012;53:5–11.
51. Leddy R, Irshad A, Rumboldt T, et al. Review of metaplastic carcinoma of the breast: imaging findings and pathologic features. *J Clin Imaging Sci*. 2012;2:21.
52. Yang WT, Hennessy B, Broglio K, et al. Imaging differences in metaplastic and invasive ductal carcinomas of the breast. *AJR Am J Roentgenol*. 2007;189:1288–1293.
53. Gisvold JJ. Imaging of the breast: techniques and results. *Mayo Clin Proc*. 1990;65:56–66.
54. Krecke KN, Gisvold JJ. Invasive lobular carcinoma of the breast: mammographic findings and extent of disease at diagnosis in 184 patients. *AJR Am J Roentgenol*. 1993;161:957–960.

55. Hilleren DJ, Anderson IT, Lindholm K, et al. Invasive lobular carcinoma: mammographic findings in a 10 year experience. *Radiology*. 1991;178:149–154.
56. Le Gal M, Ollivier L, Assclain B, et al. Mammographic features of 455 invasive lobular carcinomas. *Radiology*. 1992;185:705–708.
57. Newstead GM, Baute PB, Toth HK. Invasive lobular and ductal carcinoma: mammographic findings and stage at diagnosis. *Radiology*. 1992;184:623–627.
58. Harvey JA, Fechner RE, Moore MM. Apparent ipsilateral decrease in breast size at mammography: a sign of infiltrating lobular carcinoma. *Radiology*. 2000;214:883–889.
59. Evans WP, Burhenne LJW, Louba L, et al. Invasive lobular carcinoma of the breast: mammographic characteristics and computer-aided detection. *Radiology*. 2002;225:182–189.
60. Lopez JK, Bassett LW. Invasive lobular carcinoma of the breast: spectrum of mammographic, US and MR imaging findings. *Radiographics*. 2009;29:165–176.
61. Butler RS, Venta LA, Wiley EL, et al. Sonographic evaluation of infiltrating lobular carcinoma. *AJR Am J Roentgenol*. 1999;172:325–330.
62. Qayyum A, Birdwell RL, Daniel BL, et al. MR imaging features of infiltrating lobular carcinoma of the breast: histopathologic correlation. *AJR Am J Roentgenol*. 2002;178:1227–1232.
63. Weinstein SP, Orel SG, Heller R, et al. MR imaging of the breast in patients with invasive lobular carcinoma. *AJR Am J Roentgenol*. 2001;176:399–406.
64. Winston CB, Hadar O, Teitcher JB, et al. Metastatic lobular carcinoma of the breast: patterns of spread in the chest abdomen and pelvis on CT. *AJR Am J Roentgenol*. 2000;175:795–800.
65. Brogi E, Harris NL. Lymphomas of the breast: pathology and clinical behavior. *Semin Oncol*. 1999;26:357–364.
66. Liberman LL, Dershaw DD, Kaufman RJ, et al. Angiosarcoma of the breast. *Radiology*. 1992;183:649–654.
67. Yang WT, Hennessy BTJ, Dryden MJ, et al. Mammary angiosarcomas: imaging findings in 24 years. *Radiology*. 2007;242:725–734.
68. Glazebrook KN, Magut MJ, Reynolds C. Angiosarcoma of the breast. *AJR Am J Roentgenol*. 2008;190:533–538.
69. Yi A, Kim HK, Shin HJ, et al. Radiation induced complications after breast cancer radiation therapy: a pictorial review of multimodality imaging findings. *Korean J Radiol*. 2009;10:496–507.
70. Noh JM, Huh SJ, Choi DH, et al. Two cases of post-radiation sarcoma after breast cancer treatment. *J Breast Cancer*. 2012;15:364–370.
71. Lee AHS. The histological diagnosis of metastases to the breast from extramammary malignancies. *J Clin Pathol*. 2007;60:1333–1341.
72. Leibman AJ, Wong R. Findings on mammography in the axilla. *AJR Am J Roentgenol*. 1997;169:1385–1390.
73. Yang WT, Metreweli, Lam PKW, et al. Benign and malignant breast masses and axillary nodes: evaluation with echo-enhanced color power doppler US. *Radiology*. 2001;220:795–802.
74. Murphy TJ, Mowad CM, Feig SA, et al. Breast imaging case of the day (dermatopathic lymphadenopathy). *Radiographics*. 1998;18:536–539.
75. Zack JR, Trevisan SG, Gupta M. Primary breast lymphoma originating in a benign intramammary lymph node. *AJR Am J Roentgenol*. 2001;177:177–178.
76. Bedi DG, Krishnamurthy R, Krishnamurthy S, et al. Cortical morphologic features of axillary lymph nodes as a predictor of metastasis in breast cancer: in vitro sonographic study. *AJR Am J Roentgenol*. 2008;191:646–652.
77. Abe H, Schmidt RA, Kulkarni K, et al. Axillary lymph nodes suspicious for breast cancer metastasis: sampling with US-guided 14-gauge core-needle biopsy—clinical experience in 100 patients. *Radiology*. 2009;250:41–49.
78. Singer C, Blankstein E, Koenigsberg T, et al. Mammographic appearance of axillary lymph node calcification in patients with metastatic ovarian carcinoma. *AJR Am J Roentgenol*. 2001;176:1437–1440.

CHAPTER SELF-ASSESSMENT QUESTIONS

1. Representative spot compression view (left) and ultrasound image (right) in a 73-year-old woman called back for additional evaluation of a mass in the left breast. What is the most likely diagnosis?

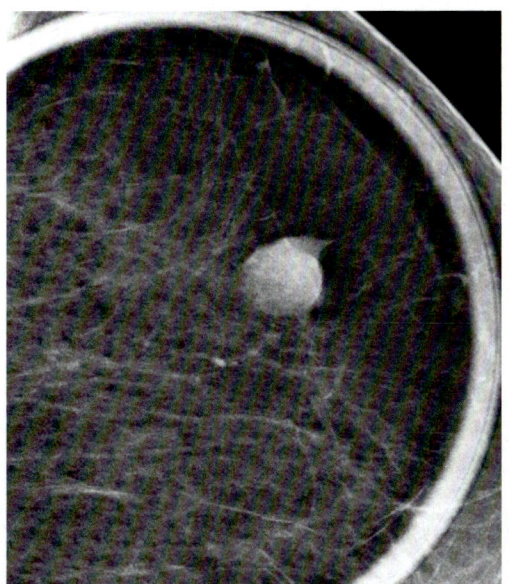
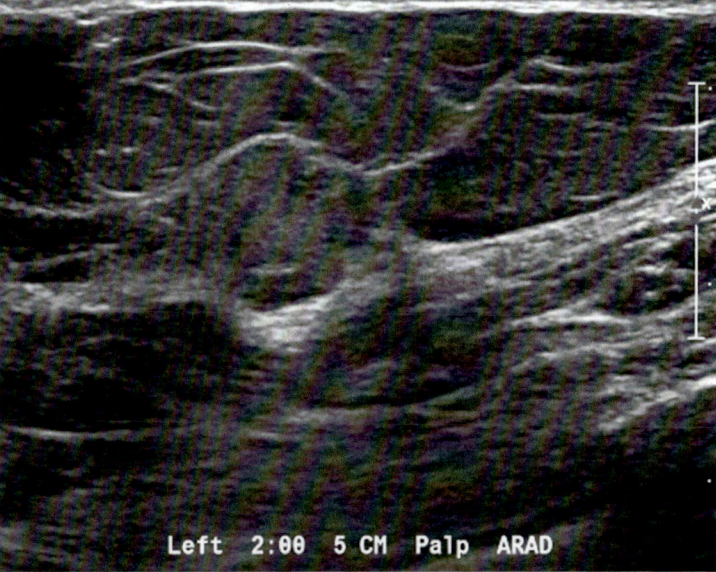

   A. Invasive ductal carcinoma, not otherwise specified
   B. Mucinous carcinoma
   C. Tubular carcinoma
   D. Invasive lobular carcinoma

2. Mediolateral oblique views (top) and representative image from a right breast ultrasound (bottom). This tumor is likely to be:

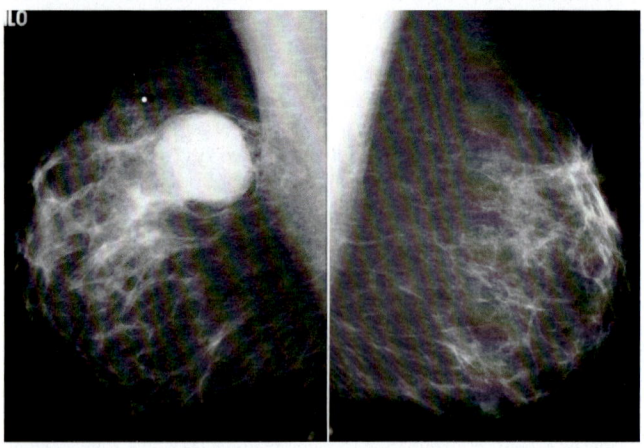

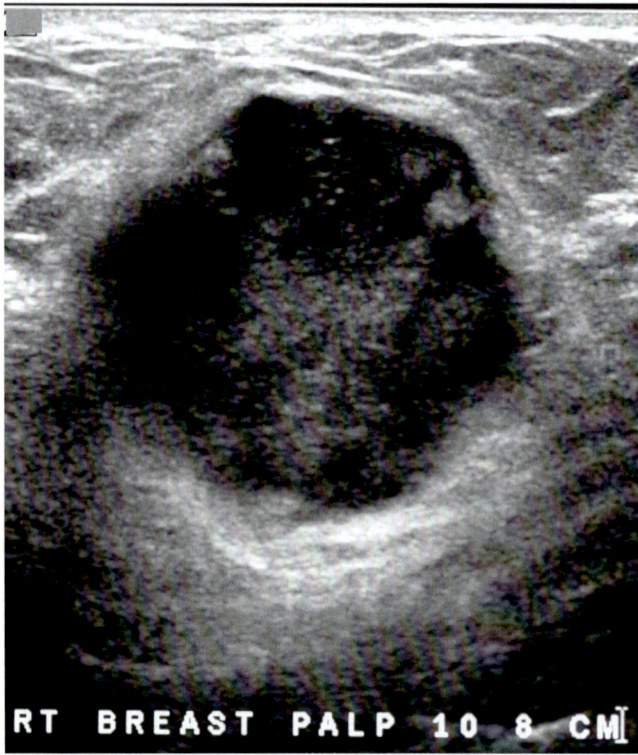

A. Estrogen (ER) and progesterone (PR) receptor positive, Her2-neu positive
B. ER/PR negative, Her2-neu negative
C. ER/PR positive, Her2-neu negative
D. ER/PR negative, Her2-neu positive

Answers to Chapter Self-Assessment Questions

1. B Mucinous carcinoma is the leading consideration in a 73-year-old woman presenting with a round mass with circumscribed margins that is nearly iso to slightly hyperechoic on ultrasound. Invasive ductal carcinomas not otherwise specified are usually hypoechoic, with indistinct margins and overall more conspicuous on ultrasound. Tubular carcinomas are typically small (<1 cm) irregular masses with spiculated margins; on ultrasound these are often associated with distortion and shadowing. Tubular carcinomas are also reportedly more common in premenopausal patients. Invasive lobular carcinoma rarely presents as a round mass with circumscribed margins; a mass with spiculated margins, developing parenchymal asymmetry and distortion are the most common mammographic findings in women with invasive lobular carcinoma. On ultrasound, a mass with spiculated margins as well as associated distortion and intense shadowing are the common findings in patients with invasive lobular carcinoma.

2. B A dense round (expansile) mass with indistinct margins is seen mammographically. On ultrasound, the mass is characterized by a heterogeneous echotexture and posterior acoustic enhancement. An invasive ductal carcinoma, not otherwise specified should be suspected in patients presenting with rapidly developing expansile ("blow up") masses, particularly if the patient is premenopausal. These tumors are often Her2-neu as well as estrogen and progesterone receptor negative (triple negative tumors).

Miscellaneous Mammographic Findings

9

LEARNING OBJECTIVES

1. Diffuse changes in the breasts on mammography, ultrasound, and magnetic resonance imaging (MRI)
2. Benign causes of diffuse changes in the breast
3. Malignant causes of diffuse changes in the breast
4. Inflammatory breast cancer versus locally advanced breast cancer
5. Descriptors for parenchymal asymmetry
6. Differential consideration for parenchymal asymmetry
7. Clinical, imaging, and histological findings in Paget disease
8. Lobular neoplasia: risk marker or precursor?
9. Controversies regarding the management of patients of lobular neoplasia
10. Approach to the management of patients with a solitary dilated duct
11. Dilated vasculature
12. Clinical and imaging findings in patients with Mondor disease

DIFFUSE BREAST CHANGES

Changes that affect the breasts diffusely can be difficult to perceive on a mammogram, particularly if the process is bilateral and evolving slowly. In reviewing mammograms, prepare your brain to perceive these changes by specifically asking yourself: Are the breasts symmetric in size and density? Is there prominence of the trabecular markings? Is there a contrast difference between the breasts? How thick are the breasts (cm of compression), and is compressibility different between the breasts? What technical factors were used for the exposure, and are they different for one view or side compared with the other(s)? Have the technical factors changed from one year to the next? Comparison with prior films can be helpful if studies are viewed in sequence. Diffuse changes are characterized by increases in the overall density of the breast parenchyma, thickening of the trabecular pattern ("Kerley B lines"), and skin thickening. In some women, increases or decreases (shrinking) in the perceived size of the breast accompany these changes. On digital images, the conspicuity of the skin is such that skin thickening can be detected easily. The overall compressibility of the breast may be decreased, and the techniques needed to penetrate the thickened skin, and possibly edematous tissue, increase. As kVp is increased to penetrate the tissue adequately, contrast decreases.

Skin thickening is appreciated readily on ultrasound, though it may require the use of a standoff pad: The hypoechoic central band of the skin increases in width. The deep hyperechoic stripe may not be apparent or appears disrupted. Anastomosing lymphatic channels seen as hypo- to anechoic thin tubular structures may be identified just deep to the deep hyperechoic stripe of the skin. Flow may be seen in some of these structures with Doppler. Associated disruption of the normal breast architecture, loss of normal tissue planes, increases in tissue echogenicity, and, in some patients, focal findings may also be seen on ultrasound. During real-time scanning, pitting edema may be noted related to the pressure applied on the breast with the transducer.

On physical examination, peau d'orange changes reflecting edema may be apparent diffusely involving the breast or, less commonly, localized to the dependent portion of the breast. Depending on the underlying cause of the diffuse change, additional findings including erythema, ecchymotic areas, and increased warmth of the affected breast, variable amounts of tenderness may be elicited. Benign and malignant causes of diffuse breast changes (1–3) are listed in Table 9.1.

Radiation Therapy Effect

Radiation therapy (XRT) is probably one of the most common benign causes of diffuse changes in the breast. It is typically unilateral, limited to the treated breast. On physical examination, the breast is "tanned"; there may be associated tenderness, and surgical changes are present at the lumpectomy site and, commonly, the axilla. Distortion, spiculation, and metallic clips at the lumpectomy site accompany skin and trabecular thickening (Fig. 9.1); similar findings may be seen in the axilla, reflecting the sentinel lymph node (SLN) biopsy site. Diffuse changes are typically seen in the acute setting and slowly resolve over the first 2 years following completion of the radiation therapy. Residual skin thickening is seen in 20% to 40% of patients 2 years after the lumpectomy (4–6). Increases in density, combined with trabecular and skin thickening, that develop after the first 2 years following radiation therapy need to be evaluated carefully, and may warrant an MRI and biopsy, to exclude recurrent disease. Interestingly, even though the affected breast is less compressible and a higher kVp is needed to penetrate the two layers of thickened skin, in many patients, contrast may be perceived as increased on the affected side.

Table 9.1 DIFFERENTIAL: DIFFUSE BREAST CHANGES	
Benign	Malignant
Radiation therapy	Invasive ductal carcinoma (locally advanced)
Fluid overload	Invasive lobular carcinoma (shrinking or enlarging breast)
Cardiac etiology (CHF)	
Renal disease	Inflammatory carcinoma (infiltrating ductal carcinoma)
Dialysis catheter shunt	DCIS
Trauma	Recurrence after conservative breast cancer treatment
Mastitis	Lymphoma
Hormone replacement therapy	
Axillary adenopathy with lymphatic obstruction	
Superior vena cava obstruction (SVC syndrome)	
PASH (rare)	
Granulomatous mastitis (rare)	
Giant cell arteritis (rare)	
Scleroderma (rare)	

In addition to localized findings at the lumpectomy site (nonenhancing soft tissue or a mass with distortion), skin thickening and variable amounts of edema (see Figs. 11.30C and 11.33C, D) are seen on MRI acutely; the radiated breast is often relatively "quiescent" compared with the contralateral normal breast for years following XRT (Fig. 9.2; also see Fig. 5.11).

Fluid Overload

Patients with fluid overload (congestive heart failure, end-stage renal disease) can present with bilateral (Fig. 9.3), less commonly unilateral (Fig. 9.4), prominence of the trabecular markings and skin thickening (Fig. 9.3B). More recently, we have seen a number of patients with dialysis catheter shunts in an arm presenting with unilateral changes diffusely involving the ipsilateral breast (Fig. 9.5). Obtaining technically acceptable images with no blurring is made more difficult in some of these patients because of shortness of breath. Peripheral edema and shortness of breath may be apparent clinically. Patients may describe some tenderness, particularly with compression. With successful treatment of the underlying etiology, the peripheral edema and changes noted in the breasts can resolve rapidly. If the patient is lying preferentially on one side for long periods of time, the edema may be more pronounced or limited to the dependent breast. With significant congestive heart failure, the periareolar region can become quite dense on the mammogram (Fig. 9.6); this is a finding we have not seen with too many other conditions.

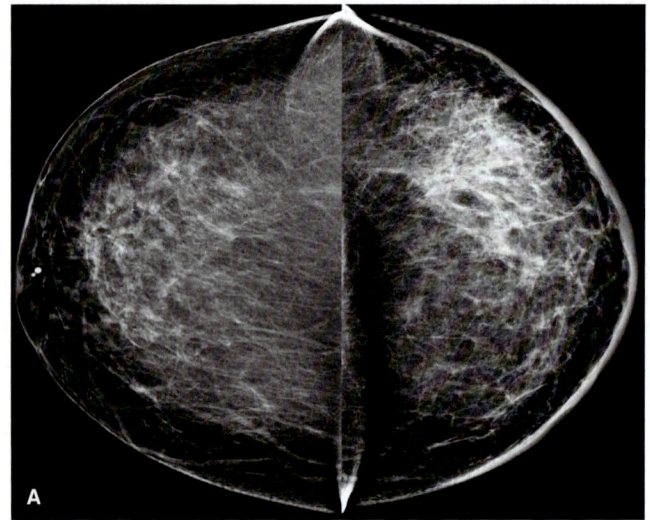
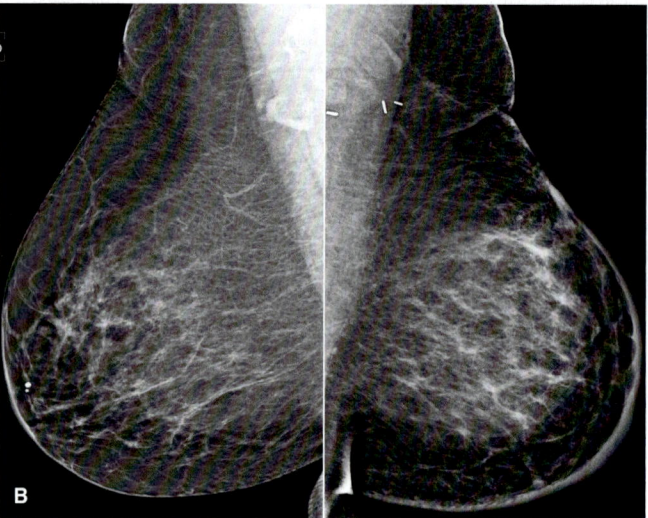
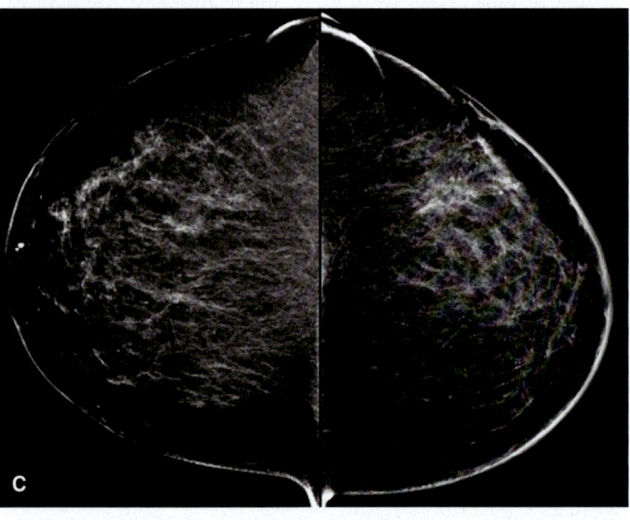

FIG. 9.1 • **Radiation therapy effect.** Craniocaudal (CC) **(A)** and Mediolateral oblique (MLO) **(B)** views in a 55-year-old woman 7 months following completion of radiation therapy. The left breast is smaller and characterized by increased density, diffuse prominence of the trabecular and skin thickening, as well as surgical clips in the lower aspect of the axilla. Notice the increased contrast of the left breast. Morphologically normal-appearing lymph nodes are noted in the axillae. **C:** CC views 1 year following those shown in part **A**, 19 months following the completion of radiation therapy. The asymmetry in breast size is less apparent. The overall density of the left breast is decreasing, as is the prominence of the trabecular markings and skin thickening. A small area of distortion and focal skin retraction persist at the lumpectomy site.

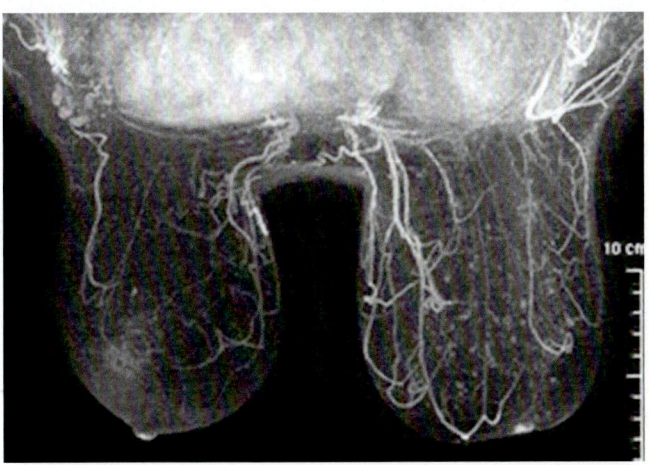

FIG. 9.2 • **Radiation therapy effect.** Magnetic resonance imaging maximum-intensity projection image. Do you notice any difference between the breasts? In this patient, the right breast is larger with scattered foci of nonspecific enhancement and prominent venous structures. The left breast is smaller and quiescent following lumpectomy and radiation therapy. Although not shown, nonenhancing increased soft tissue, distortion, and focal skin retraction are present at the lumpectomy site in the left breast.

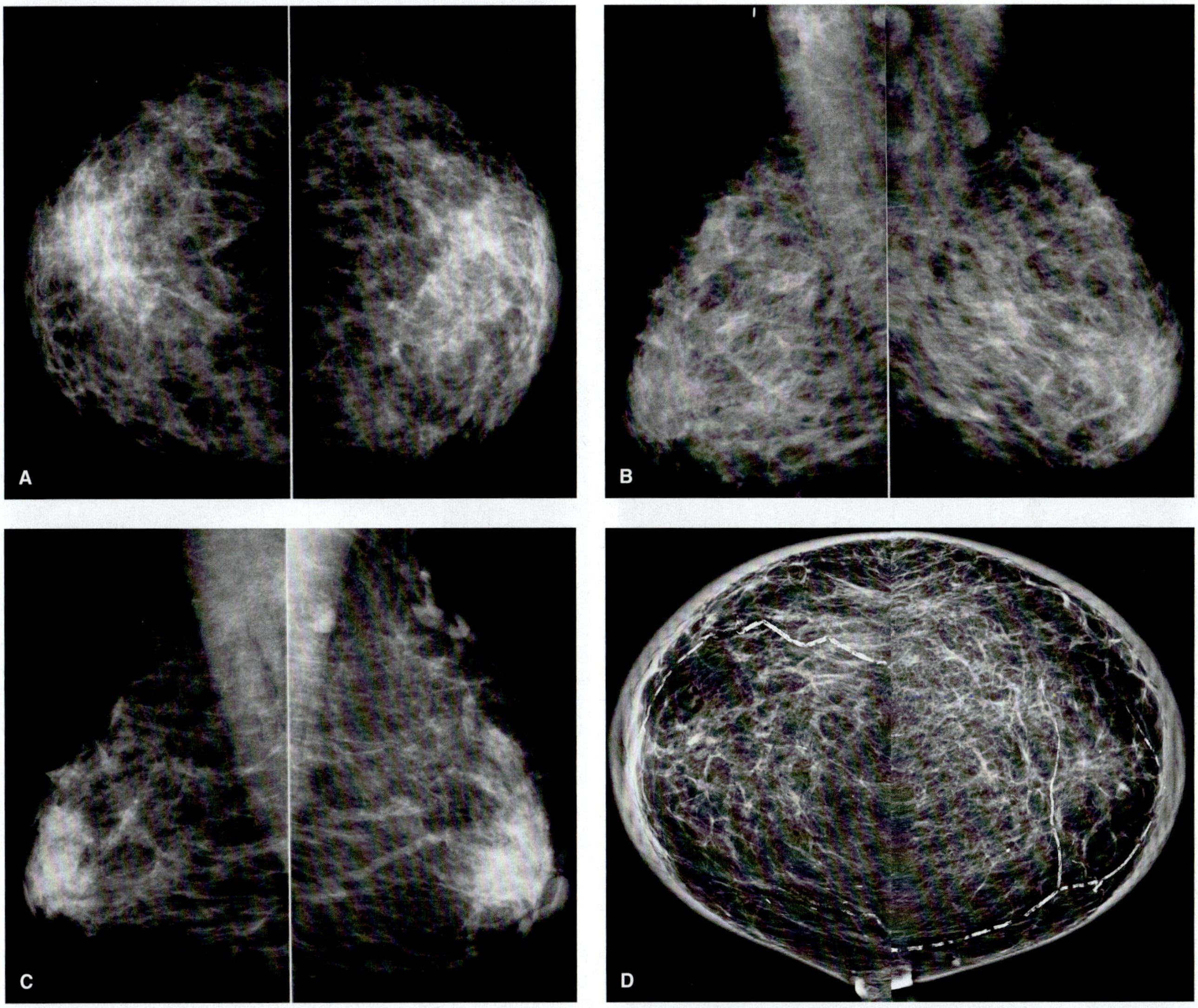

FIG. 9.3 • **Fluid overload.** CC **(A)** and MLO **(B)** views on a 39-year-old patient with end-stage renal disease on dialysis. The density of the breasts is increased, and there is marked prominence of the trabecular markings. This is best demonstrated on the oblique views with trabecular markings superimposed on the pectoral muscles (Kerley B lines). **C:** Previous MLO views in the same patient for comparison. When the process is diffuse and bilateral, it can be difficult to perceive the described changes. It is incumbent upon the interpreting radiologist to consider the possibility of diffuse change, review technical factors, and confirm the observations by reviewing the patient's history, and, if available, comparing with prior studies (going back to the earliest studies available). **D:** CC views in a 61-year-old patient with congestive heart failure. The trabecular markings are thickened bilaterally with diffuse skin thickening readily appreciated on the digital images. Dense arterial calcifications are present bilaterally.

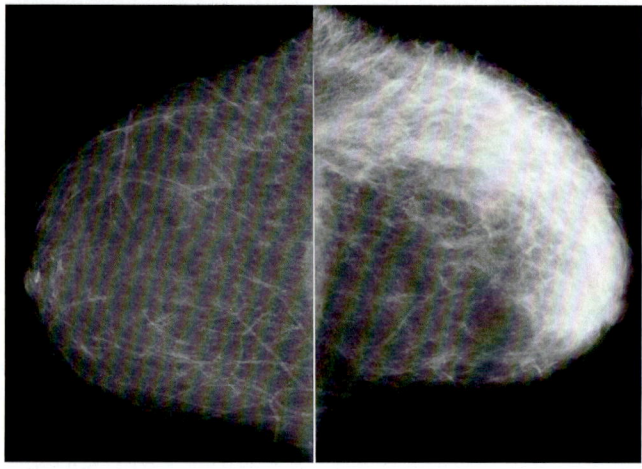

FIG. 9.4 • **Fluid overload.** CC views. Diffuse prominence of the trabecular markings and increased density is noted involving the left breast in a patient with a history of atrial fibrillation and diastolic congestive heart failure. In patients with fluid overload, the changes are usually bilateral; however, they may develop unilaterally if the patient preferentially lies on one side. When asymmetric, diffuse changes are more easily perceived.

Skin thickening, anastomosing lymphatic channels, and hyperemia are identified on ultrasound. Additionally, increased echogenicity of the tissue and disruption of normal soft tissue planes may be localized to the dependent portions of the breasts or may diffusely involve the breasts (Fig. 9.5B, C).

Trauma

Diffuse changes can be seen after significant trauma to the breasts, commonly following a motor vehicle accident with air bag deployment or a major fall. The changes may be unilateral or bilateral. These patients typically do not present in the acute setting but rather months (12–18 months) after the accident describing thickening, heaviness, skin changes, and pain in the affected breast. In addition to diffuse increases in density, prominence of the trabecular markings (Fig. 9.7A, B; also see Fig. 11.15) and possible skin thickening seen on the mammogram, fat necrosis and oil cysts with varying degrees of increased, irregular surrounding density and distortion as well as associated calcifications may be present (Fig. 9.7C). Skin thickening, loss of normal soft tissue planes with increased echogenicity of the tissue, and localized findings including complex cystic and solid masses may be identified on ultrasound (Fig. 9.7D). The extent and speed with which these changes resolve vary from patient to patient. See Chapter 11 for additional comments on trauma to the breast.

Mastitis

Patients with acute bacterial mastitis present with diffuse breast tenderness that may preclude an adequate mammogram because the patient is unable to tolerate significant compression. On physical examination, the affected breast is erythematous and warmer than the contralateral breast. If the patient tolerates the mammogram, diffuse increases in the density of the breast (Fig. 9.8A; also see Fig. 4.49A), prominence of the trabecular marking (Fig. 9.9A), skin thickening, and loss of compressibility may be present. On ultrasound, skin thickening may not be a prominent feature; however, increased echogenicity of the tissue with loss of normal soft tissue planes, hyperemia, and dilated lymphatics

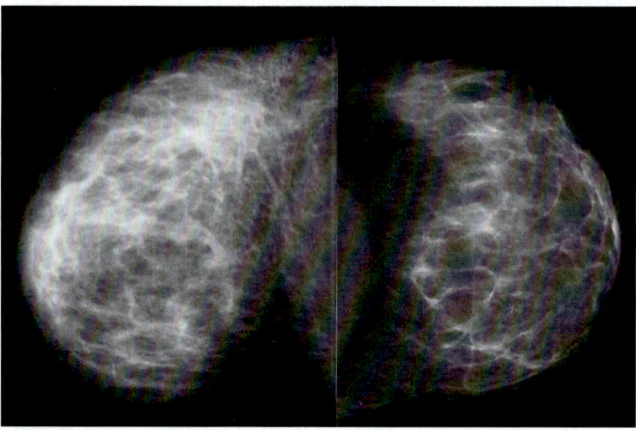

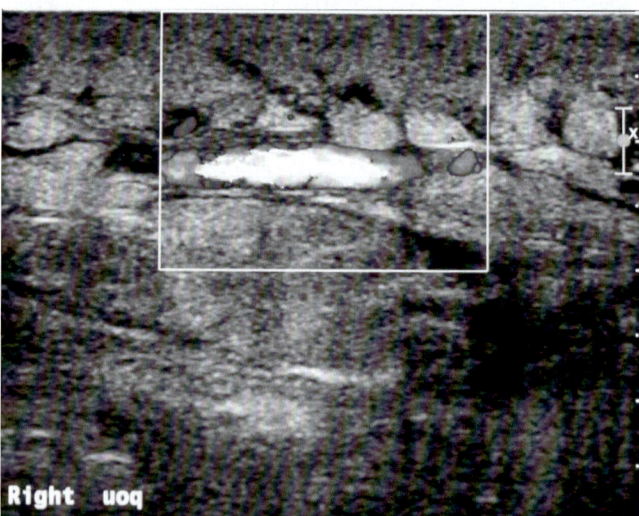

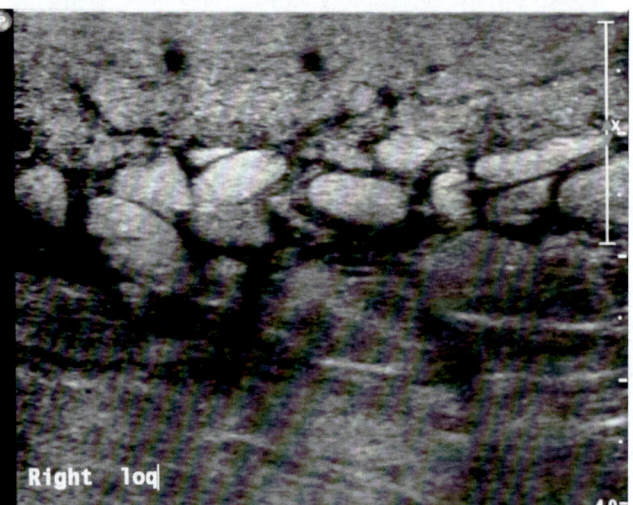

FIG. 9.5 • **Fluid overload. A:** CC views. The patient presents with an increase in the size of her right breast following placement of a dialysis catheter shunt in her right arm. The right breast is larger than the left and demonstrates increased density and diffuse prominence of the trabecular markings. Note the loss of contrast related to the decreased compressibility and increased kVp needed to obtain an adequate exposure. **B** and **C:** Representative ultrasound images of the upper *(uoq)* and lower outer *(loq)* quadrants of the right breast. Skin thickening and anastomosing lymphatic channels are readily apparent in the subcutaneous tissue. Normal soft tissue planes are disrupted, and the echogenicity of the tissue is increased. When Doppler is turned on, flow can be appreciated in some of the larger tubular structures in the upper outer quadrant of the breast.

Miscellaneous Mammographic Findings

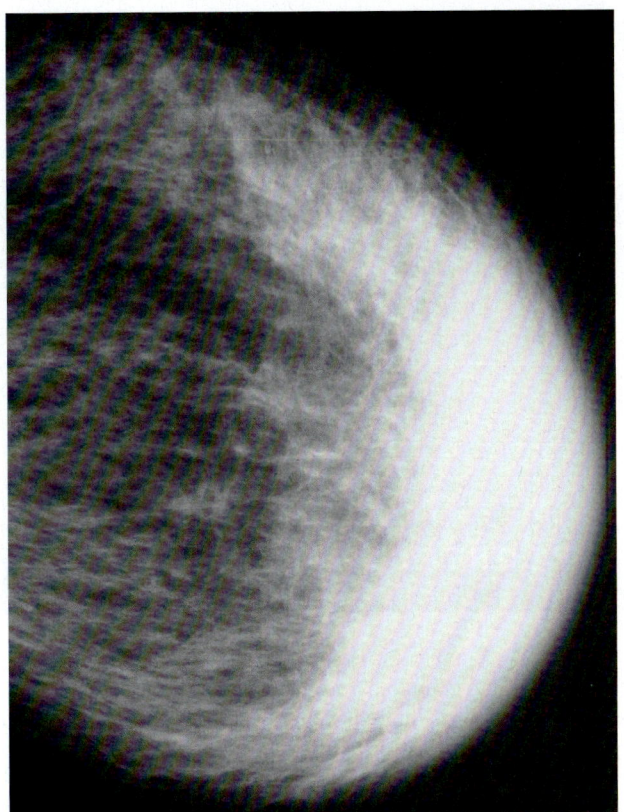

FIG. 9.6 • **Congestive heart failure.** Left CC view in an 89-year-old patient with left breast swelling. Increased density, diffuse trabecular thickening, and marked thickness and density in the periareolar region and anterior portion of the breast are present. Findings are bilateral but less pronounced on the right (not shown). (From Cardeñosa G. *Breast Imaging [The Core Curriculum Series]*. Philadelphia, PA: Lippincott Williams & Wilkins; 2003.)

may be seen (Figs. 9.8B and 9.9B). Mastitis is relatively common in patients who are lactating; however, it can develop in women of all ages, some of whom may have a history of diabetes. An antibiotic that covers aerobic and anaerobic organisms is used in patients who are not lactating. We follow these patients closely to assure that an abscess requiring drainage does not develop and that there is complete resolution of the symptoms and findings following antibiotic therapy. Some patients require two courses of antibiotics for complete resolution.

Axillary or Central Venous Obstruction

In more than 80% of patients, complete or partial obstruction of the superior vena cava is caused by superior mediastinal tumors, including adenocarcinoma of the lung, lymphoma, thyroid carcinoma, thymomas, and teratomas. Less common causes include chronic fibrotic mediastinitis that is idiopathic or secondary to tuberculosis, histoplasmosis, or drugs (e.g., methysergide); thrombophlebitis related to indwelling central venous catheters or pacemaker wires; aortic arch aneurysms and constrictive pericarditis. Symptoms include swelling of the neck and face, headaches, visual disturbances, and obstructive venous drainage of the head, neck, and upper extremities. Facial flushing and dilatation of anterior chest wall veins secondary to collateral flow may develop. Diffuse breast changes and dilated venous structures may be seen mammographically in these patients, more commonly involving the right breast; however, it can be a bilateral process. With a similar mechanism, axillary adenopathy with lymphatic obstruction can lead to diffuse breast changes limited to the ipsilateral breast.

Granulomatous Mastitis

Granulomatous mastitis is an uncommon cause of diffuse changes in the breast usually unilateral, though there are reports of bilateral involvement. Clinically, patients present with a mass that may be tender or, less commonly, diffuse breast tenderness in the absence of focal findings; rarely, they develop fistulas. Patients are relatively young, and in many, the disease presents within 6 years of pregnancy. The etiology

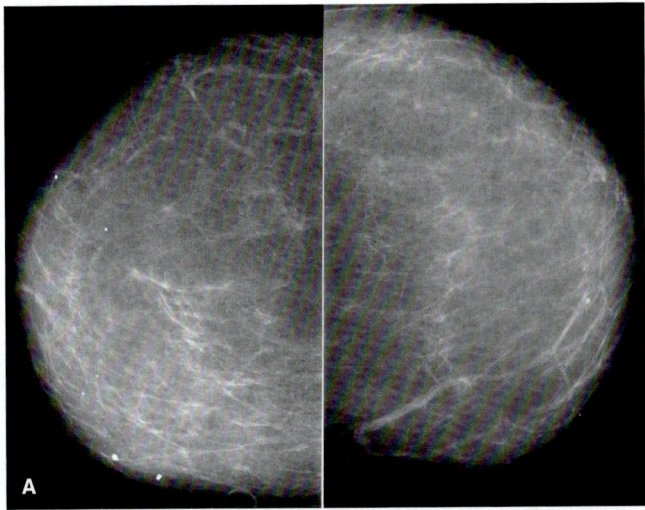 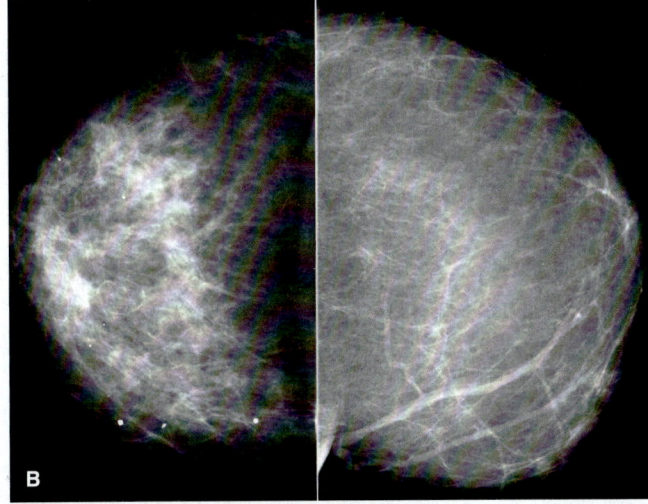

FIG. 9.7 • **Trauma. A:** CC views. A predominantly fatty pattern is present. Other than scattered dense, coarse dystrophic-type calcifications in the right breast, no abnormalities are identified. **B:** CC views 13 months following a motor vehicle accident with air bag deployment. As compared with the prior study, the right breast is smaller, and the trabecular markings are diffusely increased. **C:** Image photographically coned to the anterior aspect of the right breast. Distortion *(large arrow)* and oil cysts *(small arrows)*, some with mural calcifications, are readily apparent, which, in conjunction with the diffuse changes, should suggest the likelihood of trauma. The job of the interpreting radiologist is to make all of the observations, postulate possible theories for the findings, and, in conjunction with a physical examination, review the patient's pertinent history. In this patient, it is important to specifically ask about trauma. The patient may not associate the changes with an event that happened more than 1 year ago. **D:** Representative ultrasound image demonstrating disruption of normal tissue planes, minimally increased tissue echogenicity, and complex cystic and solid masses some with shadowing correlating with oil cysts seen mammographically.

(continued)

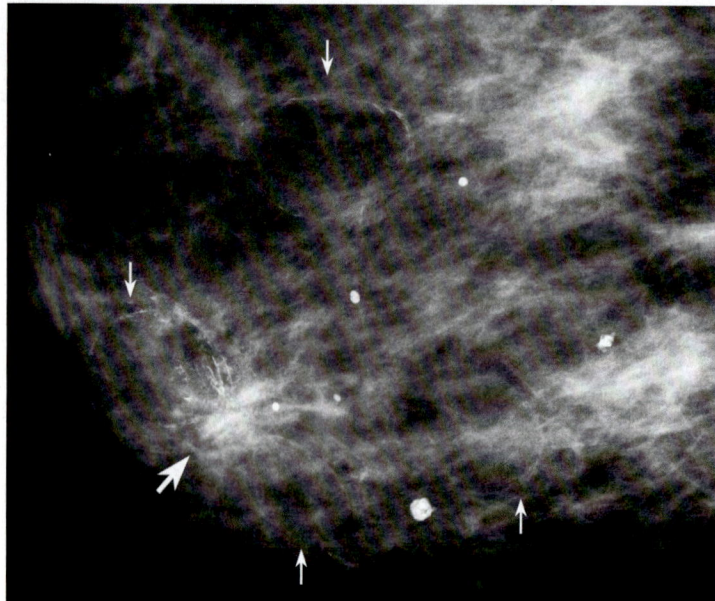
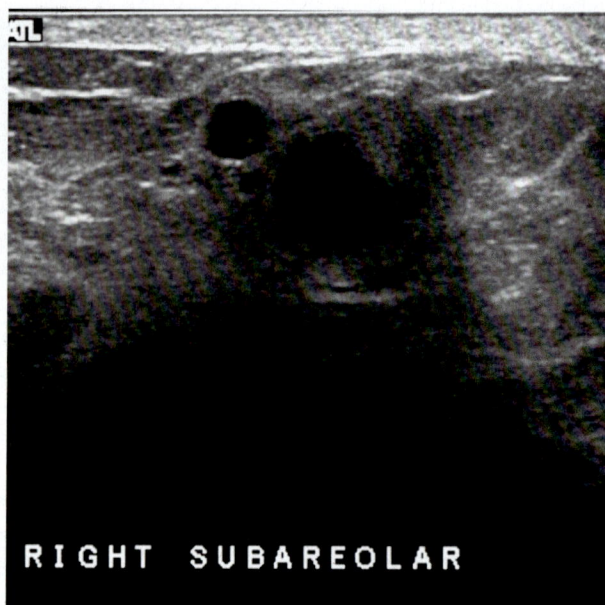

FIG. 9.7 • *(continued)*

is unknown; however, some have suggested an autoimmune reaction to extravasated lobular secretions, undetected organisms, or the use of oral contraceptives (7–10). In addition to diffuse changes in the affected breast (Fig. 9.10; also see Fig. 4.50), other reported mammographic findings include one or multiple masses, or areas of parenchymal asymmetry (11,12). On ultrasound, findings in granulomatous mastitis include multiple relatively circumscribed lesions with a tubular configuration or irregular hypoechoic lesions with shadowing. The findings on MRI are also nonspecific and include heterogeneously enhancing masses with indistinct margins, homogeneously enhancing nodules, or rim-enhancing masses, reflecting abscess formation. Kinetic curve analysis is nonspecific with variability among lesions. Reactive lymphadenopathy can be seen with all imaging modalities (12).

Histologically, granulomatous mastitis is characterized by non-caseating granulomas limited to the perilobular regions; no microorganisms are identified in the tissue (7,8,11). It is a diagnosis of exclusion since granulomatous disease in the breast may also be reported in patients with sarcoid, Wegener granulomatosis, tuberculosis, diabetes, or connective tissue disorders. The treatment of patients with granulomatous mastitis remains controversial and not always effective. Some advocate the use of steroids after the possibility of an underlying bacterial etiology has been eliminated, while others have reported using methotrexate. Surgery alone has also been used with mixed results in that the disease may recur. A combination of steroids and surgery may be a more appropriate approach (13).

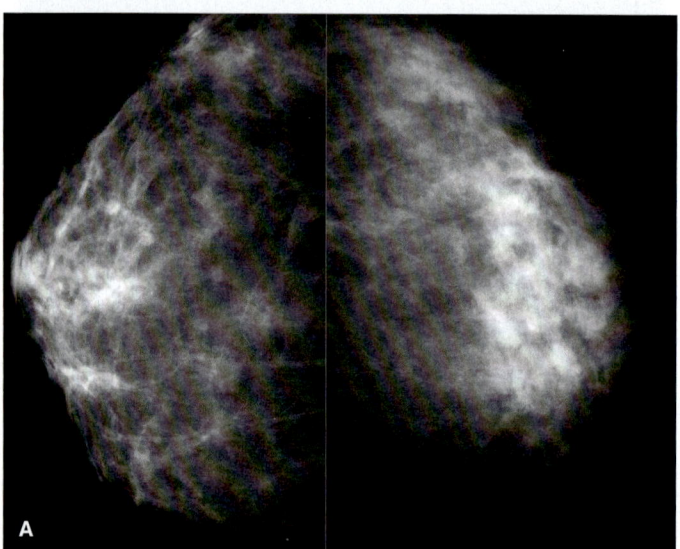
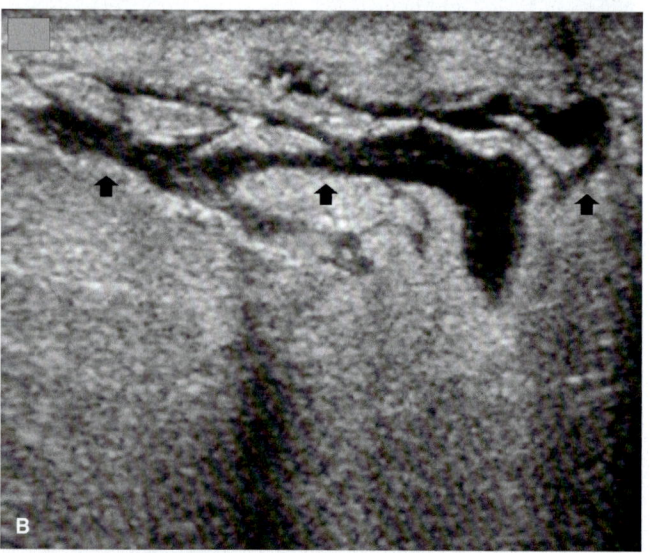

FIG. 9.8 • **Acute bacterial mastitis. A:** Right (kVp = 26, mAs = 68, compression = 4 cm) and left CC views (kVp = 34, mAs = 143, compression = 7 cm) in a patient with diabetes presenting with rapid onset of breast pain on the left with swelling and redness. The left breast is less compressible than the right, and the density of the breast is increased; both of these may in part be related to the patient's inability to tolerate compression. As kV is increased to obtain an adequate exposure on the left, contrast decreases. **B:** Ultrasound. Skin thickening with loss of the echogenic deep dermal layer and dilated lymphatic channels *(arrows)* are seen throughout all four quadrants. The echogenicity of the tissue is increased with loss of normal soft tissue planes, likely reflecting edematous changes. Pus is obtained during surgical excision and drainage. (From Cardeñosa G. *Breast Imaging [The Core Curriculum Series]*. Philadelphia, PA: Lippincott Williams & Wilkins; 2003.)

Miscellaneous Mammographic Findings

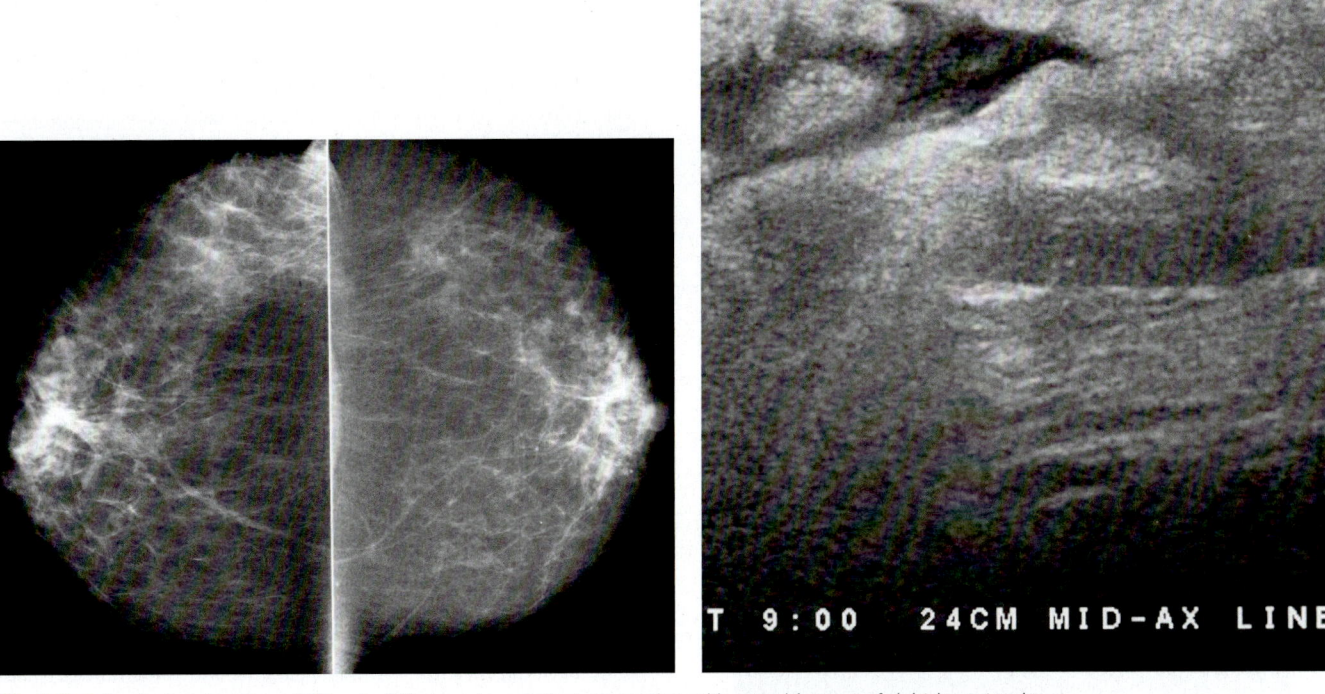

FIG. 9.9 • **Acute bacterial mastitis. A:** CC views in a patient presenting with a rapid onset of right breast pain, swelling, and redness extending into the axilla and midaxillary line. The trabecular makings are increased laterally in the right breast extending to the edge of the film. **B:** Ultrasound. Loss of normal soft tissue planes and increased tissue echogenicity is noted in the lateral central aspect of the breast with extension of the parenchymal process to the midaxillary line along the 9 o'clock axis. In addition to the increased echogenicity of the tissue at this site, a localized irregular pocket of fluid is seen in the subcutaneous tissue with associated skin thickening. The patient is successfully managed with intravenous and subsequently oral antibiotics.

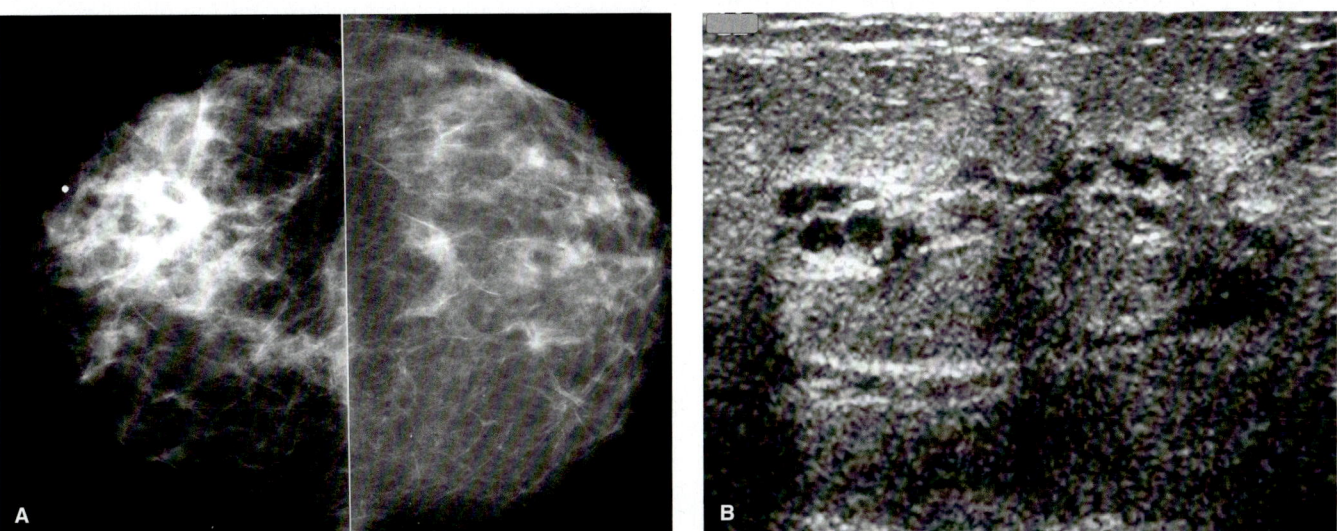

FIG. 9.10 • **Granulomatous mastitis. A:** MLO views in a 52-year-old patient who presents describing swelling and hardness of her right breast for 1 month with some resolution of the tenderness and erythema following a trial of antibiotics. Screening mammogram 8 months previously is normal. The right breast is less compressible and appears smaller than the left. The overall density of the right breast is increased compared with that of the left with higher technical factors (kVp and mAs) needed for an exposure on the right compared with the left. The patient is diagnosed with granulomatous mastitis following core biopsy and surgical excision. **B:** Ultrasound. The breast is diffusely abnormal with disruption of normal tissue planes, areas of hyperechogenicity, and tubular, serpiginous hypoechoic structures. **C:** Right MLO view obtained 5 months following views shown in **A**. The breast is normal in appearance with technical factors comparable to those used for exposures of the left breast. After the surgical resection, symptoms resolved. (From Cardeñosa G. *Breast Imaging [The Core Curriculum Series]*. Philadelphia, PA: Lippincott Williams & Wilkins; 2003.)

(continued)

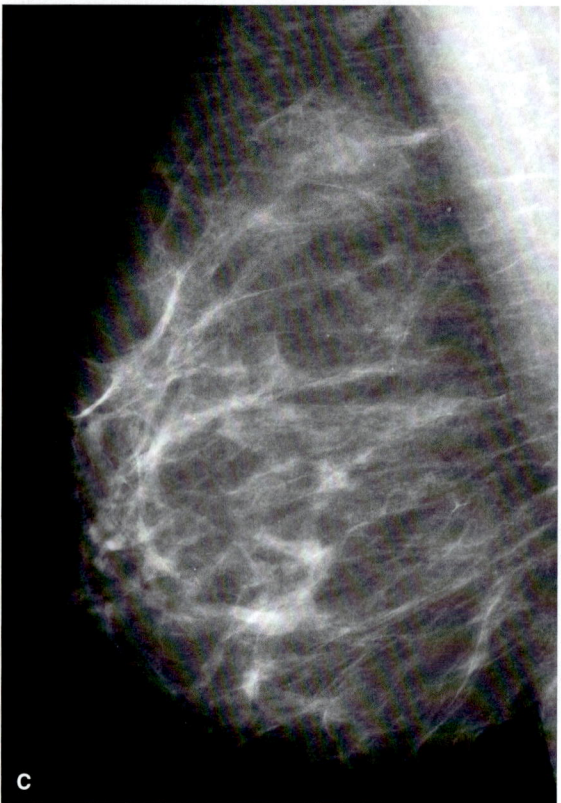

FIG. 9.10 • *(continued)*

Arteritis

Giant cell or temporal arteritis is another rare cause of diffuse changes in the breast (Fig. 9.11). It may be a uni- or bilateral process, and biopsies usually demonstrate granulomatous inflammatory changes surrounding the arteries (7). This is a systemic panarteritis involving medium- and large-sized vessels in patients over the age of 50. The temporal arteries and other extracranial branches of the carotid artery

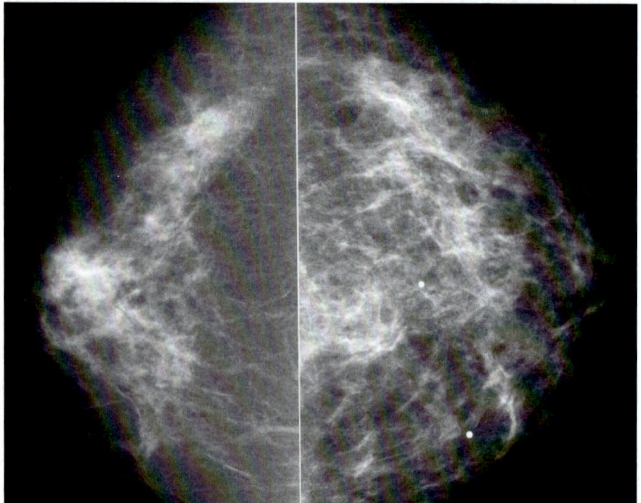

FIG. 9.11 • **Prominent vasculitis consistent with giant cell arteritis.** CC views in a 70-year-old patient with diffuse left breast tenderness and swelling. Left breast appears larger than right. Diffuse prominence of the trabecular markings noted involving the left breast. Diagnosis made on excisional biopsy. (From Cardeñosa G. *Breast Imaging [The Core Curriculum Series]*. Philadelphia, PA: Lippincott Williams & Wilkins; 2003.)

are usually involved. Patients present with headaches, scalp tenderness, visual symptoms, jaw claudication, throat pain, and asymmetry of arm pulses. If blindness occurs, it is often irreversible. Patients have an elevated sedimentation rate with a normal white blood cell count, and approximately 50% have associated polymyalgia rheumatica. Elevated doses of prednisone are used in the treatment of symptoms and are helpful in minimizing visual disturbances.

Inflammatory Breast Cancer and Locally Advanced Breast Cancer

Inflammatory breast cancer (IBC) is characterized by a distinct clinicopathological presentation (14). It needs to be distinguished from locally advanced (neglected) breast cancer that, late in the course of the disease, can mimic some of the clinical findings described for IBC (15).

IBC is an uncommon, aggressive form of breast cancer that constitutes approximately 1% of all breast cancers; it is a stage IIIB cancer at the time of presentation. The diagnosis of inflammatory carcinoma is made on the basis of clinical findings (14). Unlike patients with locally advanced breast cancer in whom signs and symptoms may have been present for 6 months or more, patients with IBC describe the rapid onset of breast warmth, erythema involving at least one-third of the breast, and edema (14–16). As implied by its name, inflammatory carcinoma simulates mastitis in its presentation; however, the involved breast is not usually as tender as that seen in women with a diffuse acute bacterial mastitis. Although patients with inflammatory carcinoma may improve initially on antibiotics, the symptoms persist and eventually worsen.

Histologically, inflammatory carcinomas are usually poorly differentiated invasive ductal carcinomas characterized by tumor emboli in dilated dermal lymphatics and a lymphocytic reaction surrounding dilated vasculature in the dermis. These histological findings are found in approximately 80% of the patients with the clinical diagnosis of inflammatory carcinoma. The histological findings associated with inflammatory carcinoma are found in approximately 4% of patients who do not have the described clinical findings (7,8); the histologic finding of tumor emboli in dilated subdermal lymphatics in the absence of clinical signs and symptoms of IBC should not be used to diagnose patients with IBC (e.g., the diagnosis of IBC is made clinically).

The affected breast is commonly larger and less compressible than the normal breast such that adequate exposure may be difficult to obtain (cm of compression, kVp, and mAs are higher than those used on the contralateral breast) in some patients. Increased breast size, skin thickening, and diffuse increases in the density of the parenchyma are the most common findings (Fig. 9.12) on mammography. Localized findings including a mass, architectural distortion, calcifications, and focal or global asymmetry may be identified in as many as 80% of patients (17–19). On the mammogram, axillary adenopathy has been reported in as many as 58% of patients at the time of presentation. On ultrasound, skin thickening, dilated lymphatics, disruption of normal breast architecture, and increased tissue echogenicity are commonly seen (17–19). In some patients, a focal finding including a mass, distortion, or calcifications may be detected. Ultrasound is also useful in the evaluation of the axilla with abnormal nodes reportedly detected in as many as 93% of patients with IBC (Fig. 9.13). If the appropriate areas are scanned with ultrasound, internal mammary as well as infra- and supraclavicular adenopathy may be detected with ultrasound in as many as 50% of patients (17). As mentioned previously, it is imperative that an effort be made clinically to distinguish patients with IBC from those that may have a locally advanced breast cancer with secondary skin involvement (18) (Figs. 9.14 through 9.16). If signs and symptoms are long-standing (>6 months), and no increased warmth, erythema, and peau d'orange changes (or if only one of these is present) are noted

Miscellaneous Mammographic Findings

involving the affected breast, it is more appropriate to consider the diagnosis of a locally advanced breast cancer and not inflammatory carcinoma.

Magnetic resonance imaging is particularly helpful in identifying a primary breast lesion as well as multifocal and –centric disease in patients with IBC. The affected breast is larger, and may be deformed with diffuse skin thickening and enhancement in more than 95% of all patients. Regional and internal mammary adenopathy can be identified as well as chest wall and pectoral muscle involvement. The detection of an underlying breast lesion is best done with MRI and ultrasound in 100% and 95% of patients, respectively (17). Mammography is reportedly the least sensitive with primary breast lesions being detected in 80% of patients (17).

Patients with IBC are treated aggressively with neoadjuvant chemotherapy for systemic disease followed by surgery and radiation therapy for local control. With anthracycline-based regimes followed by local therapy, 5- and 10-year survival rates of 40% and 33%, respectively, have been reported. The addition of taxanes is associated with higher survival rates as well as higher complete pathological responses (cPR) at the time of mastectomy. In patients with HER2/neu-positive tumors, treatment for 1 year with trastuzumab reportedly increases the likelihood of cPR and disease-free survival (20). After neoadjuvant therapy, a modified radical mastectomy with a full axillary dissection is the preferred surgical approach since SLN biopsy is reportedly not reliable in patients with IBC. Given the high incidence of local regional recurrence following adjuvant therapy and surgery, radiation therapy that encompasses the supraclavicular and internal mammary lymph node chains is recommended.

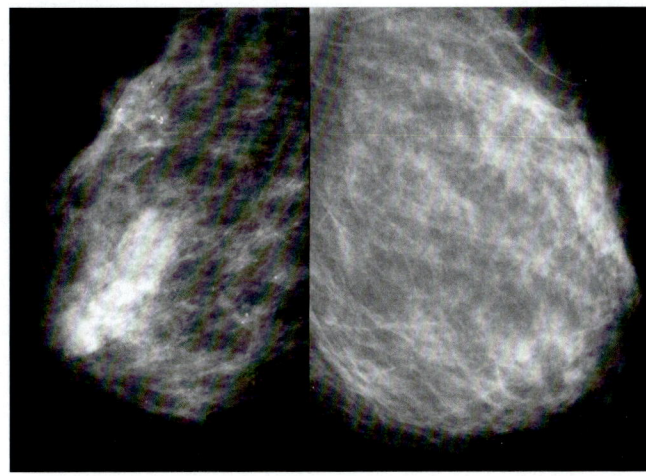

FIG. 9.12 • **Inflammatory carcinoma.** MLO views photographically coned to the anterior aspect of the breasts in a 49-year-old patient presenting with the rapid onset of erythema and edema involving the right breast; minimal tenderness (technique used for right MLO: kVp = 30, mAs = 295, compression = 8.1 cm; technique used for left MLO: kVp = 29, mAs = 122, compression = 6.4 cm). The compressibility of the right breast is decreased, and it appears smaller than the left. Increased density, thickening of the trabecular pattern and skin (seen with bright light) is apparent. Enlarged and dense axillary lymph nodes (not shown) are identified in the axilla on the right MLO view. (From Cardeñosa G. *Breast Imaging [The Core Curriculum Series]*. Philadelphia, PA: Lippincott Williams & Wilkins; 2003.)

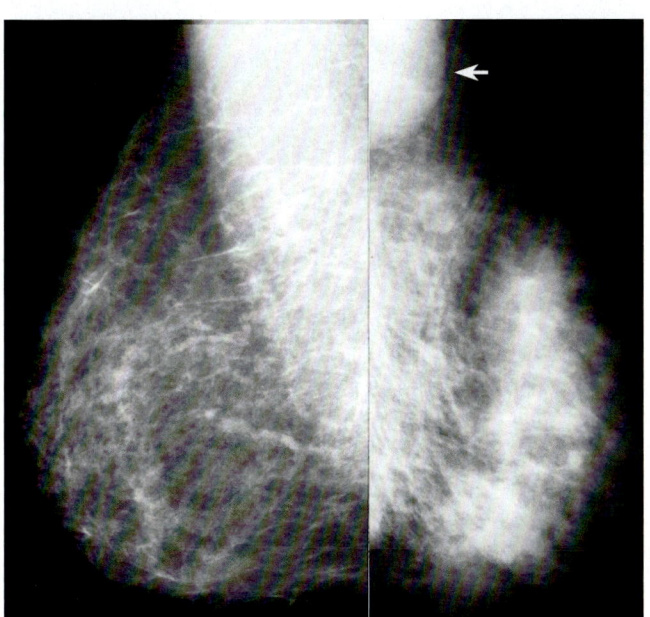
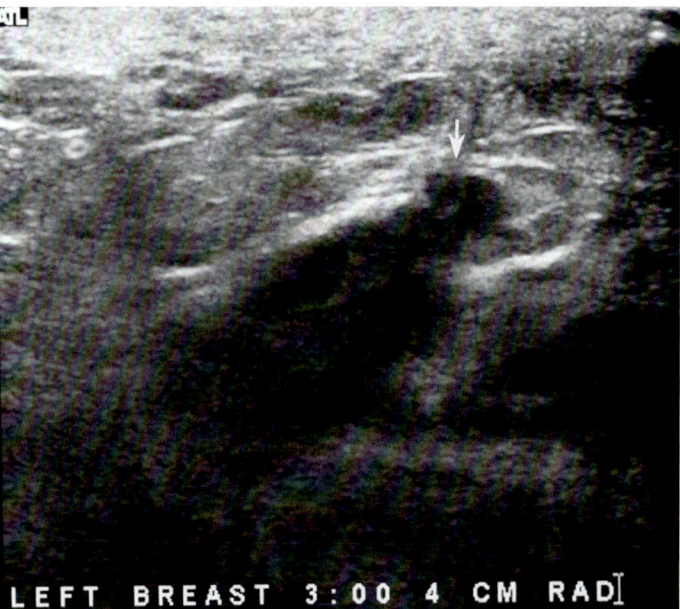

FIG. 9.13 • **Inflammatory carcinoma. A:** MLO views. The patient presents describing the rapid onset of redness, skin changes, and heaviness of the left breast. The left breast appears smaller with diffusely increased density and trabecular markings (Kerley B lines overlying pectoral muscle). A mass is also apparent in the left axilla *(arrow)*. **B:** Ultrasound, left breast. On physical examination, the left breast is thicker and warmer than the right with diffuse erythema and peau d'orange changes. The skin also appears stretched and glistens. As the left breast is scanned, normal tissue planes are not apparent, and skin thickening is noted. An irregular mass *(arrow)* is identified laterally, and enlarged lymph nodes are imaged (not shown) in the axilla. Core biopsies of the mass and one of the axillary lymph nodes are done. Invasive ductal carcinoma, high nuclear grade with metastatic disease to a left axillary lymph node is reported. **C:** CT scan image. Axillary adenopathy *(thick arrow)*, diffuse skin thickening involving the left breast and collateral vessels *(thin arrows)* medially in the area of the cleavage are imaged at this position. **D:** CT scan image. Left breast is thicker and firmer with diffuse skin thickening. At this level, an abnormal internal mammary lymph node *(arrow)* is apparent on the left.

(continued)

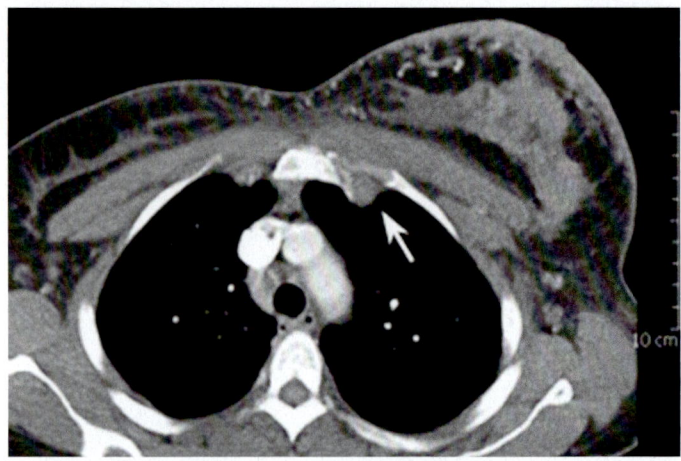

FIG. 9.13 • *(continued)*

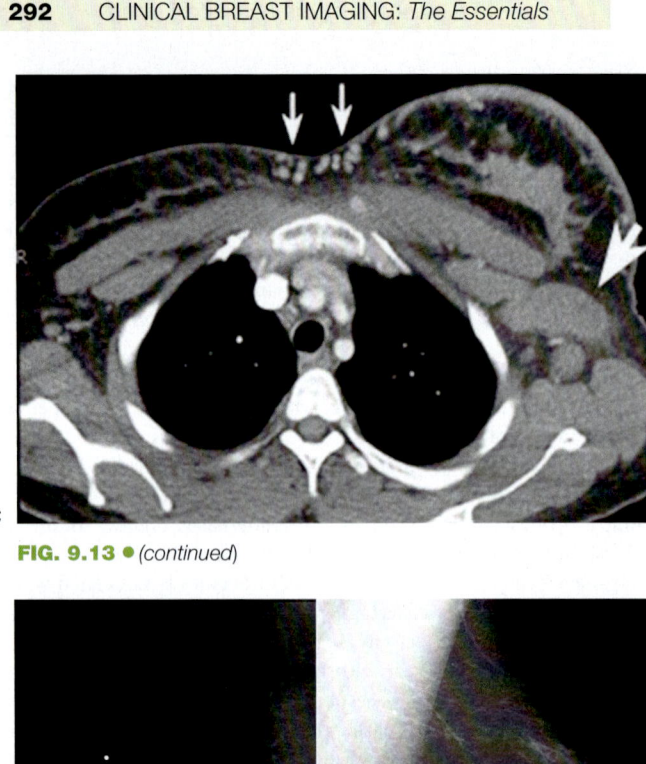

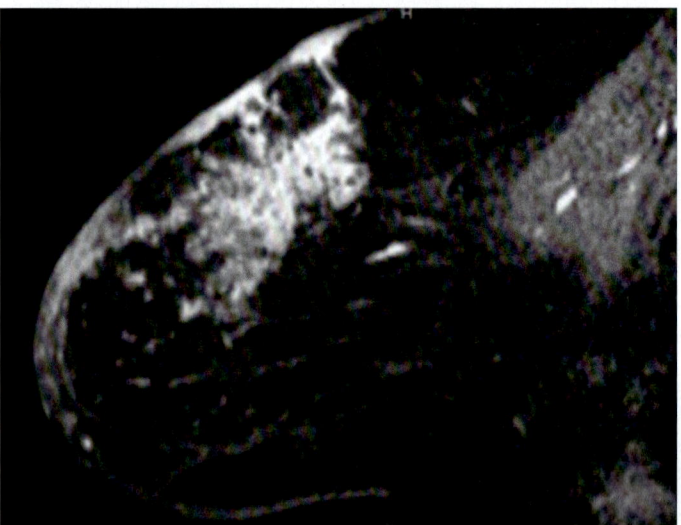

FIG. 9.14 • **Locally advanced invasive ductal carcinoma with skin involvement. A:** MLO views in a 76-year-old patient describing a "lump" in the right breast. Metallic BB denotes site of palpable finding. The right breast is smaller than the left with diffuse prominence of the trabecular markings and increased density localized to the superior aspect of the breast possibly corresponding to the palpable finding. **B:** Ultrasound image at site of "lump" demonstrates a hypoechoic mass in the dermal layer *(small arrows)* and an irregular mass *(long arrows)* with shadowing in the breast. Also note that normal soft tissue planes are not apparent, and the overall echogenicity of the tissue surrounding the mass is increased. This area is diffusely abnormal. **C:** MRI, sagittal T1-weighted reconstruction of the right breast post contrast. Non–mass-like regionally distributed heterogeneous enhancement is present superiorly associated with multiple sites of skin thickening and enhancement consistent with skin involvement; on sagittal T2-weighted fat-suppressed images (not shown), the skin masses are low in signal, and subcutaneous edema is present extending to the pectoral fascia. The patient is diagnosed with an invasive ductal carcinoma, high nuclear grade with multiple sites of skin involvement and 27 of 27 positive lymph nodes. The tumor is estrogen/progesterone receptor-negative, HER2/neu-positive.

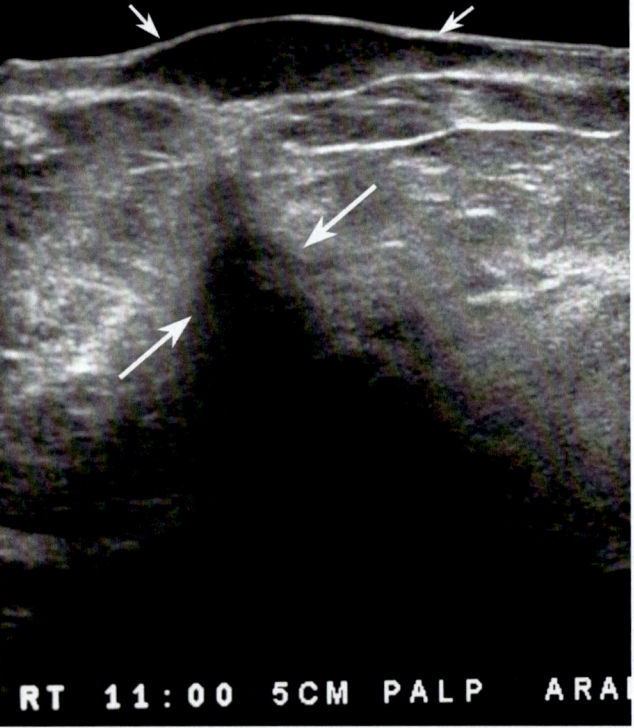

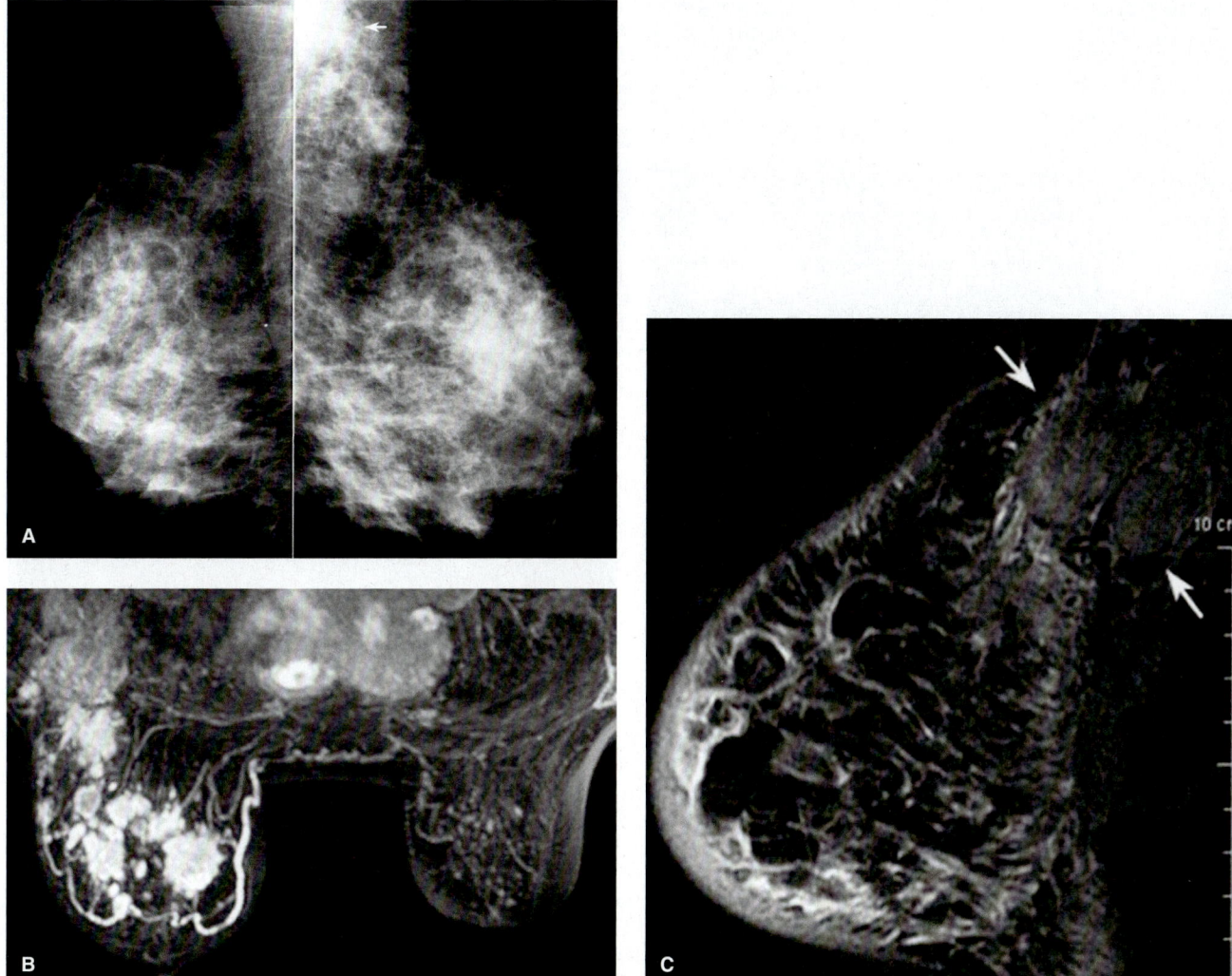

FIG. 9.15 • **Locally advanced invasive ductal carcinoma. A:** MLO views (technique used for right MLO: kVp = 25, mAs = 105, compression = 4.9 cm; technique used for left MLO: kVp = 32, mAs = 150, compression = 7.0 cm) in a 56-year-old patient. The left breast is larger and less compressible than the right. The overall density of the left breast is increased, and the contrast is decreased, a reflection of the higher kVp needed for exposure on the left compared with the right. On the MLO views, you can see increased density and prominence of the trabecular marking superimposed on the pectoral muscle as well as a mass (arrow) with indistinct margins in the axilla. Additionally, a possible mass with indistinct margins is noted in the upper inner quadrant of the left breast, zone B. Ultrasound images (not shown) confirm the presence of a round complex cystic and solid mass in the upper inner quadrant of the left breast and a macrolobulated mass with no identifiable fatty hilum in the left axilla. The patient is diagnosed with invasive ductal carcinoma with lobular features and metastatic disease to the axilla following ultrasound-guided core biopsies. The tumor is estrogen and progesterone receptor-negative, HER2/neu-positive. **B:** MRI, maximum intensity projection demonstrates multiple enhancing masses with spiculated margins in the left breast as well as abnormal and matted lymph nodes in the left axilla. Note asymmetrically increased vascular structures in the left breast. **C:** MRI, sagittal T2-weighted fat-suppressed image of the left breast. Skin thickening and diffuse edematous changes are noted, as are matted lymph nodes (arrows) with intermediate T2 signal in the left axilla. Following 4 months of neoadjuvant therapy, cPR and no metastatic disease to the axilla (0/5 LNs) are reported at the time of the mastectomy.

Recurrence After Breast-Conserving Therapy

Recurrences following breast-conserving therapy typically develop at the lumpectomy site. Rarely, patients can present with diffuse changes, including enlargement of the breast, skin thickening, increased density, and prominence of the trabecular markings (Fig. 9.17; also see Fig. 11.32). In some of these patients, the breast changes may be related to the development of axillary adenopathy and increased interstitial fluid in the breast.

Invasive Lobular Carcinoma

In addition to the more common localized presentations of invasive lobular carcinoma discussed in Chapter 8, patients may also have diffuse changes. The shrinking breast (Figs. 9.18 and 9.19), commonly reflecting invasive lobular carcinoma, is characterized by a progressive decrease in the size of the breast and an increasing prominence of the trabecular markings (21). On ultrasound, localized findings may be identified. This includes masses or an irregular, almost geometric

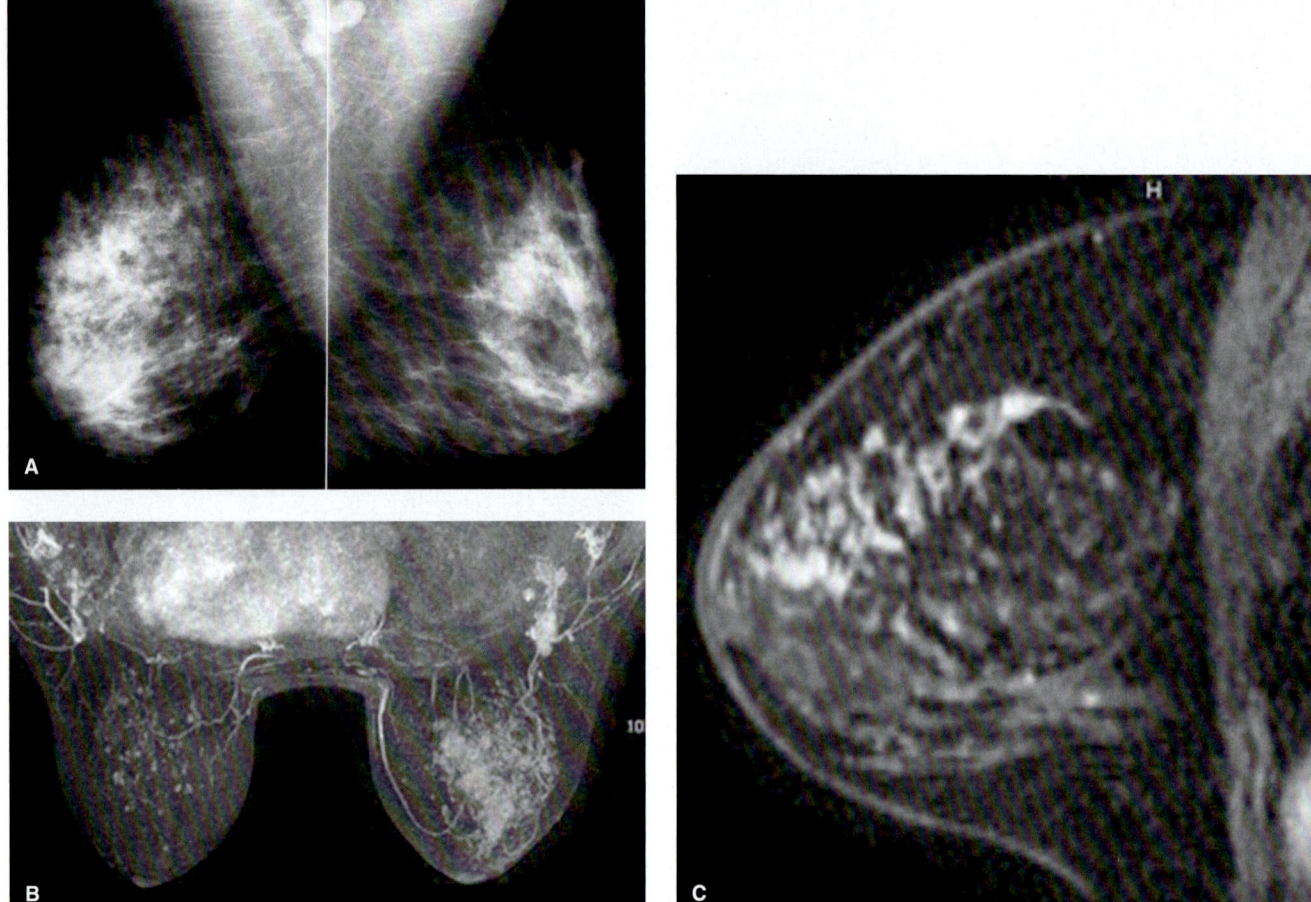

FIG. 9.16 • **Locally advanced invasive ductal carcinoma. A:** MLO views in a 47-year-old patient. The right breast is denser with a prominent diffuse "reticulonodular" pattern. If you are not actively thinking about diffuse changes, the finding may go undetected. An invasive ductal carcinoma high nuclear grade with metastatic disease to right axilla is diagnosed on ultrasound-guided cores biopsies (not shown). The tumor is estrogen and progesterone receptor-positive, HER2/neu-negative. **B:** MRI, maximum intensity projection demonstrating the extent of disease in the right breast. Foci of nonspecific enhancement are noted scattered in the left breast. **C:** MRI, T1-weighted sagittal reconstruction of the right breast image post contrast. Regionally distributed non–mass-like heterogeneous clumped and linear enhancement in the superior quadrants of the right breast. After neoadjuvant therapy, the MRI (not shown) demonstrates no focal abnormalities. A cPR with no metastatic disease to the axilla (0/12 LNs) is reported at the time of the mastectomy.

abrupt interface between thickened echogenic tissue and intense shadowing (Figs. 9.18C and 9.19C). Enlarged, morphologically abnormal lymph nodes may be imaged in the axilla mammographically and on ultrasound. Asymmetric breast size, thickened skin, edematous changes, one or multiple enhancing masses or non–mass-like enhancement are more readily identified on MRI (Fig. 9.19D). MRI is also useful in the detection of regional adenopathy (axillary, infra/supraclavicular, and internal mammary). Less commonly, the involved breast may be enlarged, less compressible, and characterized by diffuse increases in breast density indistinguishable from the classic presentation of patients with IBC.

Ductal Carcinoma In Situ

The overwhelming number of patients with ductal carcinoma in situ (DCIS) is diagnosed following the detection of calcifications on screening mammography. A mass (palpable or screen-detected), nipple discharge, Paget disease of the nipple, diffuse changes in the breast, localized or more diffuse distension of a ductal system, and areas of parenchymal asymmetry that may or may not be associated with calcifications are less common presentations of DCIS. An increasing number of patients are diagnosed following the detection of segmentally distributed clumped and linear enhancement or an enhancing mass on MRI with no other clinical or imaging findings (please see Table 6.6).

When DCIS presents as diffuse change, prominence of the trabecular markings may predominate (Fig. 9.20). Alternatively, asymmetry in the size and density of the involved breast with or without associated calcifications may be noted (Fig. 9.21; also see Fig. 5.38). On ultrasound, disruption of normal tissue architecture with irregular areas of hypoechogenicity, shadowing, calcifications (Fig. 9.21B), or dilated ducts (see Fig. 5.38) can be identified in some patients. An asymmetrically thickened breast with diffuse, non–mass-like enhancement (Fig. 9.21C) and edema may be seen on MRI; alternatively, segmentally distributed dilated ducts with surrounding enhancement on the post-contrast images may be noted (see Fig. 5.38). Although enlarged dense axillary lymph nodes may be found in these patients, these are reactive on core biopsy (e.g., metastatic disease in a patient with DCIS suggests unidentified invasive disease). In patients with diffuse changes, and

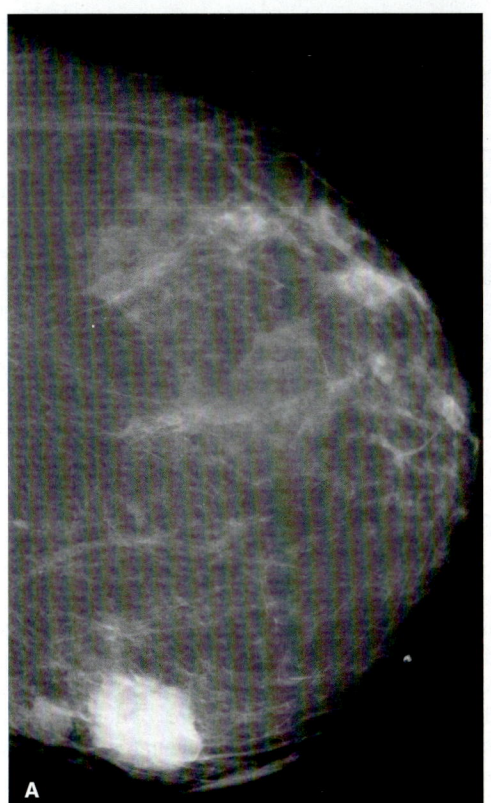
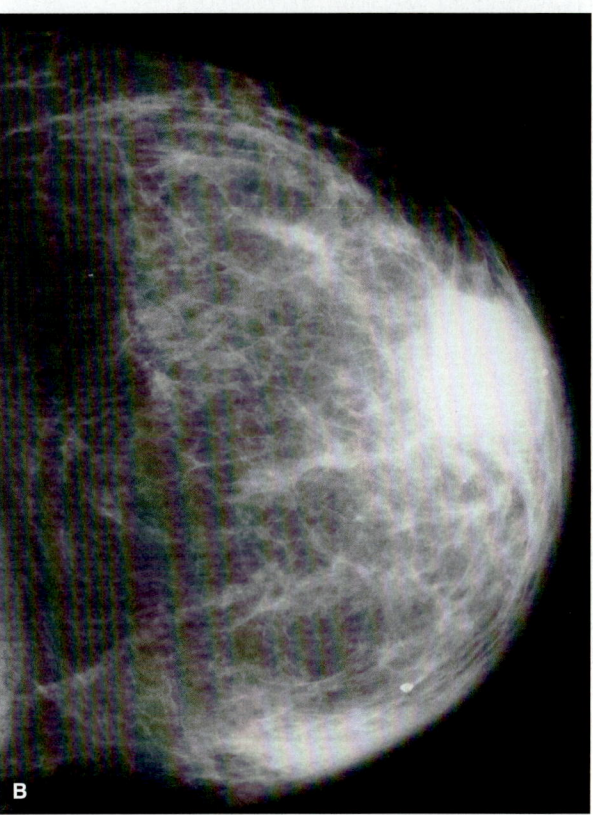

FIG. 9.17 • **Recurrent invasive ductal carcinoma. A:** Left CC view. Two round dense masses are imaged in the lower inner quadrant of the left posteriorly. Invasive ductal carcinoma is diagnosed and treated with lumpectomy and radiation therapy. **B:** Left CC view done 7 years after image shown in part **A**. The density of the left breast is significantly increased compared with prior studies done following treatment (not shown). Diffuse prominence of the trabecular markings is now apparent as well as a new round dense mass in the upper outer quadrant of the left breast anteriorly. Bilateral mastectomies are done at this time. A year later, the patient presented with metastatic disease to the brain.

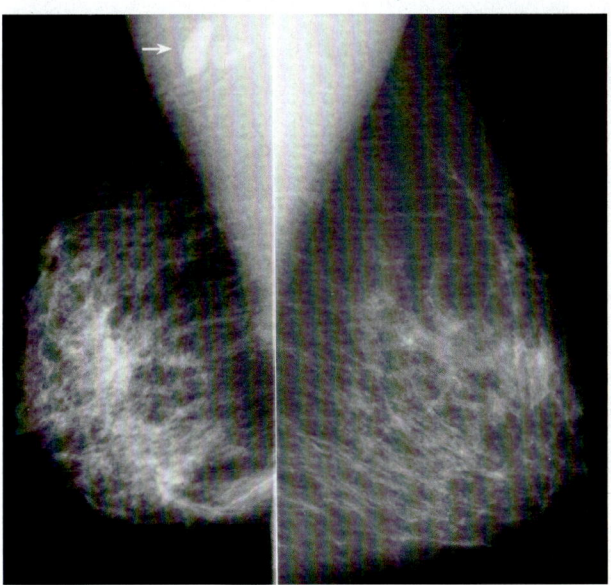
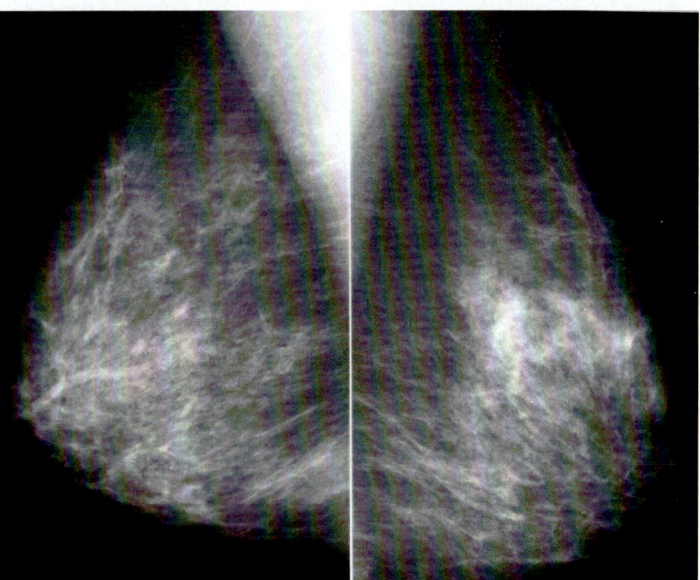

FIG. 9.18 • **Invasive lobular carcinoma.** Current MLO views in a 49-year-old patient **(A)** and MLO views for comparison, 3 years previously **(B)**. The right breast is now smaller (shrinking breast) than the left with diffuse prominence of the trabecular markings and an overall increase in the density of the parenchyma. A new oval dense mass (arrow in **A**) is seen superimposed on the right pectoral muscle. **C:** Ultrasound demonstrates an irregular mass with a thickened echogenic rim superficially, angular margins and intense shadowing distally in the upper inner quadrant of the right breast. Following ultrasound-guided core biopsies, the patient is diagnosed with invasive lobular carcinoma and metastatic disease to the axilla. Although she received neoadjuvant therapy, residual multifocal invasive lobular carcinoma (estrogen and progesterone receptor-positive, HER2/neu-negative) is found at the time of her mastectomy; sentinel lymph node biopsy (0/1 LN) is negative.

(continued)

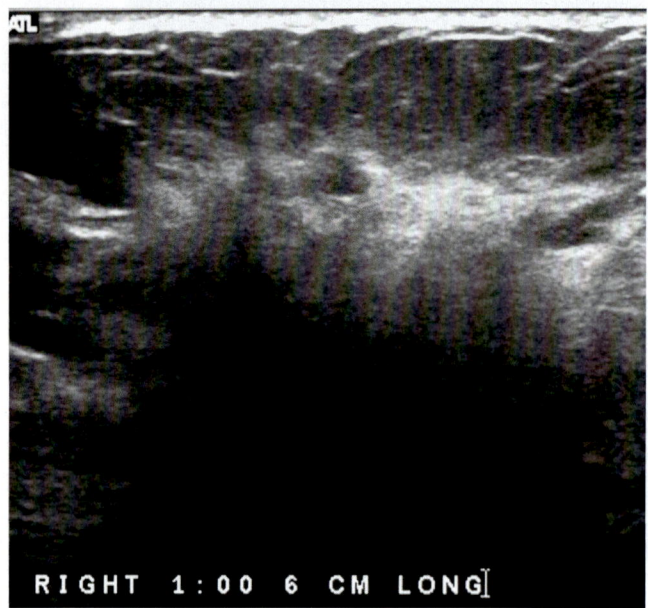

FIG. 9.18 • *(continued)*

a diagnosis of DCIS on core biopsies, an SLN biopsy should be considered at the time of the mastectomy. In the setting of diffuse DCIS, invasive disease may be identified in the mastectomy specimen, in which case the patient would need a full axillary dissection since SLN biopsy cannot be done after a mastectomy. It is also important to realize that invasive disease may be present but go undiagnosed since only representative sections from the mastectomy specimen are reviewed histologically.

Lymphoma

Lymphoma is primary to the breast when widespread or prior extramammary lymphoma is excluded (22). More commonly, lymphoma involves the breast secondarily. As discussed in Chapter 8, primary breast lymphoma may present with localized findings or with a more diffuse pattern of involvement (Fig. 9.22). Primary breast lymphomas are usually diffuse large B cell lymphomas (40% to 70%). Burkitt non-Hodkins lymphoma has been reported to involve the breasts of young, pregnant, or lactating women with an aggressive clinical behavior (7,8,22). Axillary and intramammary adenopathy are found in 30% to 40% of patients at the time of presentation (7,8).

PARENCHYMAL ASYMMETRY

In most women, breast tissue is symmetric. Rarely, women can have accessory tissue particularly in the axilla; this may be unilateral (Fig. 9.23A) or bilateral (Fig. 9.23B); this may be associated with accessory nipples. Although it may appear obvious, it is important to state at the onset that asymmetry cannot be established without the contralateral breast, and the term is used to describe "an area of fibroglandular-density tissue that is visible on only one projection, frequently representing superimposition of normal breast structures (summation artifact)." (23) Likewise, "developing parenchymal asymmetry" cannot be established in the absence of prior studies for comparison (Fig. 9.24). Parenchymal asymmetry may be characterized as "focal" when the island of tissue is localized, of similar size and density, and at approximately the same distance from the nipple in two or more projections (23,24). The tissue

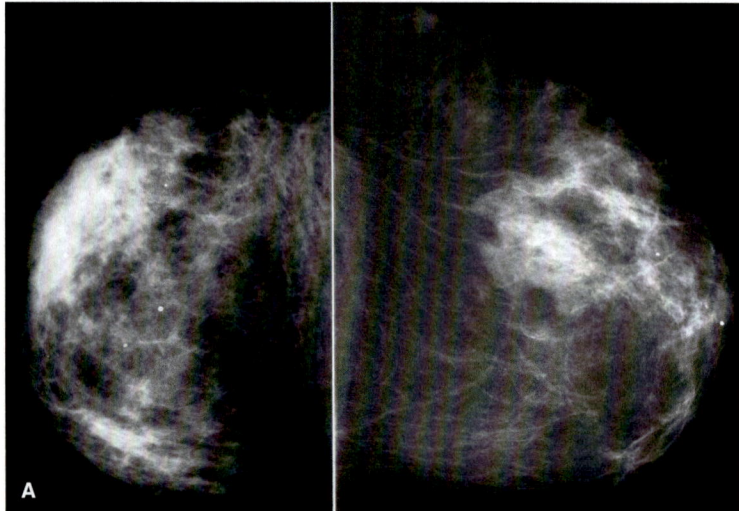

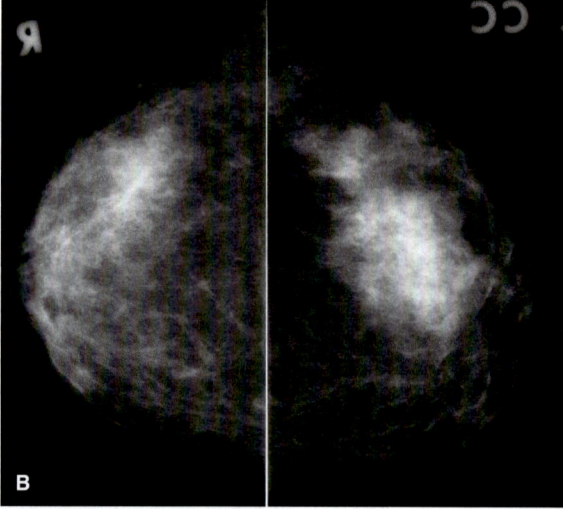

FIG. 9.19 • **Invasive lobular carcinoma. A:** Current CC views in a 65-year-old patient. **B:** CC views from 10 years before for comparison. The right breast is diffusely abnormal. It has decreased in size compared with the prior study and is smaller than the left breast. Diffuse prominence of the trabecular markings and an overall increase in the density of the breast is apparent. Also, incidentally noted is an increase in the amount of fat in the left breast with dispersal of the glandular tissue consistent with weight gain. **C:** Ultrasound. A vertically oriented mass with spiculated and angular margins as well as intense shadowing is imaged in the upper outer quadrant of the right breast. An invasive lobular carcinoma is diagnosed on core biopsy. The tumor is estrogen receptor-positive, progesterone receptor weakly positive and HER2/neu-negative. **D:** MRI, T1-weighted sagittal reconstruction of the right breast post contrast. Skin thickening is present. Although her known disease is in the upper outer quadrant of the right breast, multiple variably sized masses characterized by rapid wash in and wash out kinetic curves are identified predominantly, but not exclusively, in the lower quadrants of the right breast anteriorly. Skin thickening as well as subcutaneous and parenchymal edema extending to and along the pectoral fascia are apparent on T2-weighted fat-suppressed images (not shown).

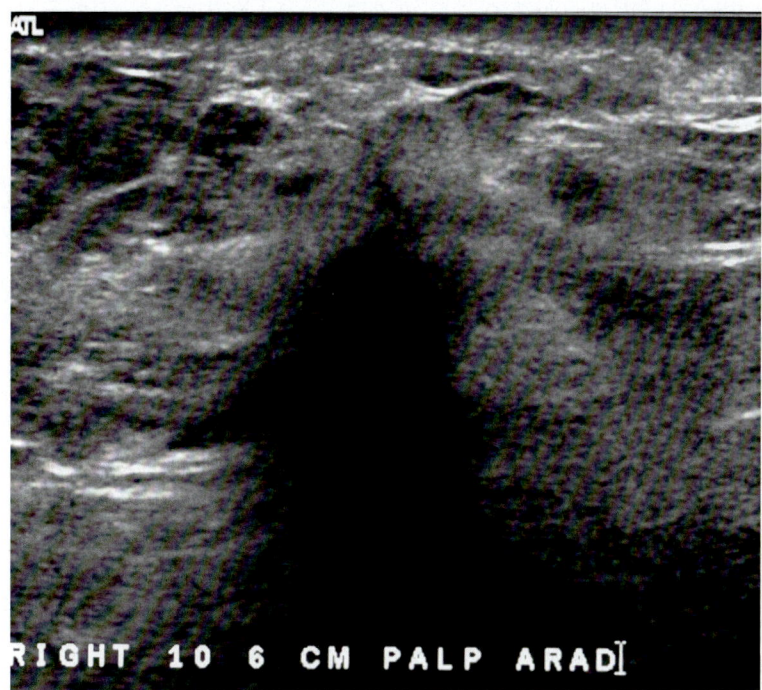
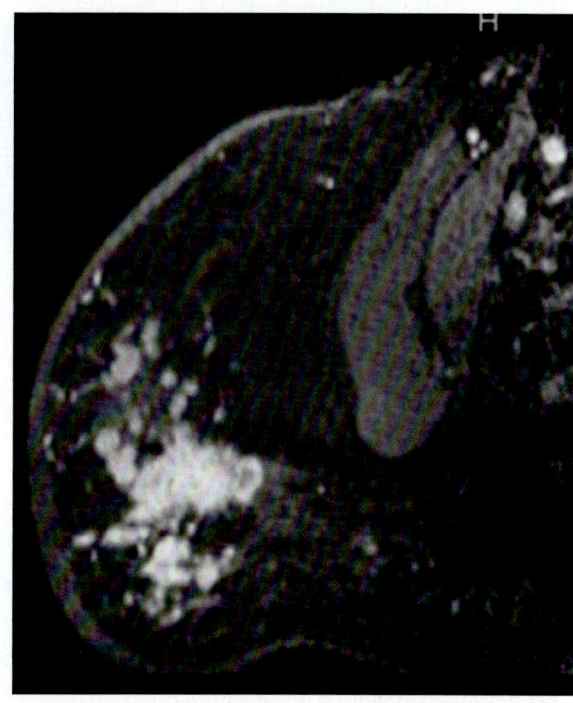

FIG. 9.19 • (continued)

demonstrates intermingled fat and a gradual transition into the surrounding fat. The abrupt interface characteristic of a mass is not seen (Fig. 9.24). Asymmetry is characterized as "global" when the asymmetry involves larger aspects or entire quadrants of the breast (Fig. 9.25) (23,24). The progressive development of parenchymal asymmetry may reflect a benign process (hormonal, pseudoangiomatous stromal hyperplasia [PASH], focal fibrosis); however, it is viewed with more concern, and patients should be evaluated with spot compression views, correlative physical examination, and ultrasound; if the ultrasound is negative but concerns persist following the physical examination or spot compression views, a stereotactically guided biopsy can be done.

Benign and malignant causes of parenchymal asymmetry are presented in Table 9.2. In many women, parenchymal asymmetry represents normal variation. It is also sometimes iatrogenic following excisional biopsy (see Fig. 11.4). Keep in mind, however, that on a single point in time, we have no way of knowing whether parenchymal asymmetry is stable or developing, and, as such, particularly in older women, evaluation is encouraged if there are no prior studies for comparison. Intervention is usually not warranted if there is no correlative physical finding and the ultrasound focused to the site of the asymmetry is normal. If the area of asymmetry is hard or indurated on physical examination, or if an abnormality is seen on ultrasound, biopsy may be indicated unless the history provides a good explanation for the findings. In addition to benign etiologies, malignant causes include invasive ductal (Fig. 9.26) and lobular carcinomas, DCIS (Fig. 9.27 and 9.28), in which case the parenchymal asymmetry may be associated with calcifications and lymphoma (Fig. 9.29).

PAGET DISEASE

Paget disease of the nipple represents 1% to 5% of all breast cancers with no reported age predilection (7,8). It is seen in less than 1% of

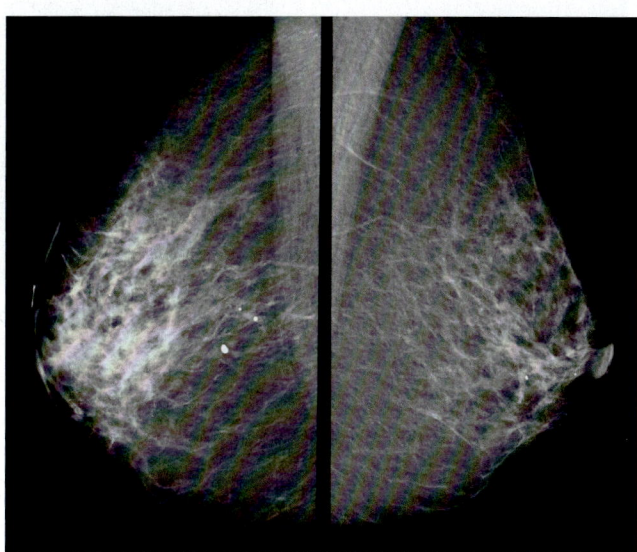

FIG. 9.20 • **DCIS.** MLO views in an 84-year-old patient. Diffuse prominence of trabecular markings is noted on the right. No malignant-type calcifications are identified. Multifocal DCIS, micropapillary, clinging and solid types are reported at the time of the mastectomy with no invasive disease identified.

men (7). Initial findings are limited to the nipple and include reddening with associated pruritus and pain. As the disease progresses, the nipple surface may be moist (oozing, gummy), there may be scaling, and eczematoid changes leading to ulceration, erosions (Fig. 9.30A), and crusting (Fig. 9.30B) of the nipple surface (25). It is usually a unilateral process associated with an underlying intraductal or invasive

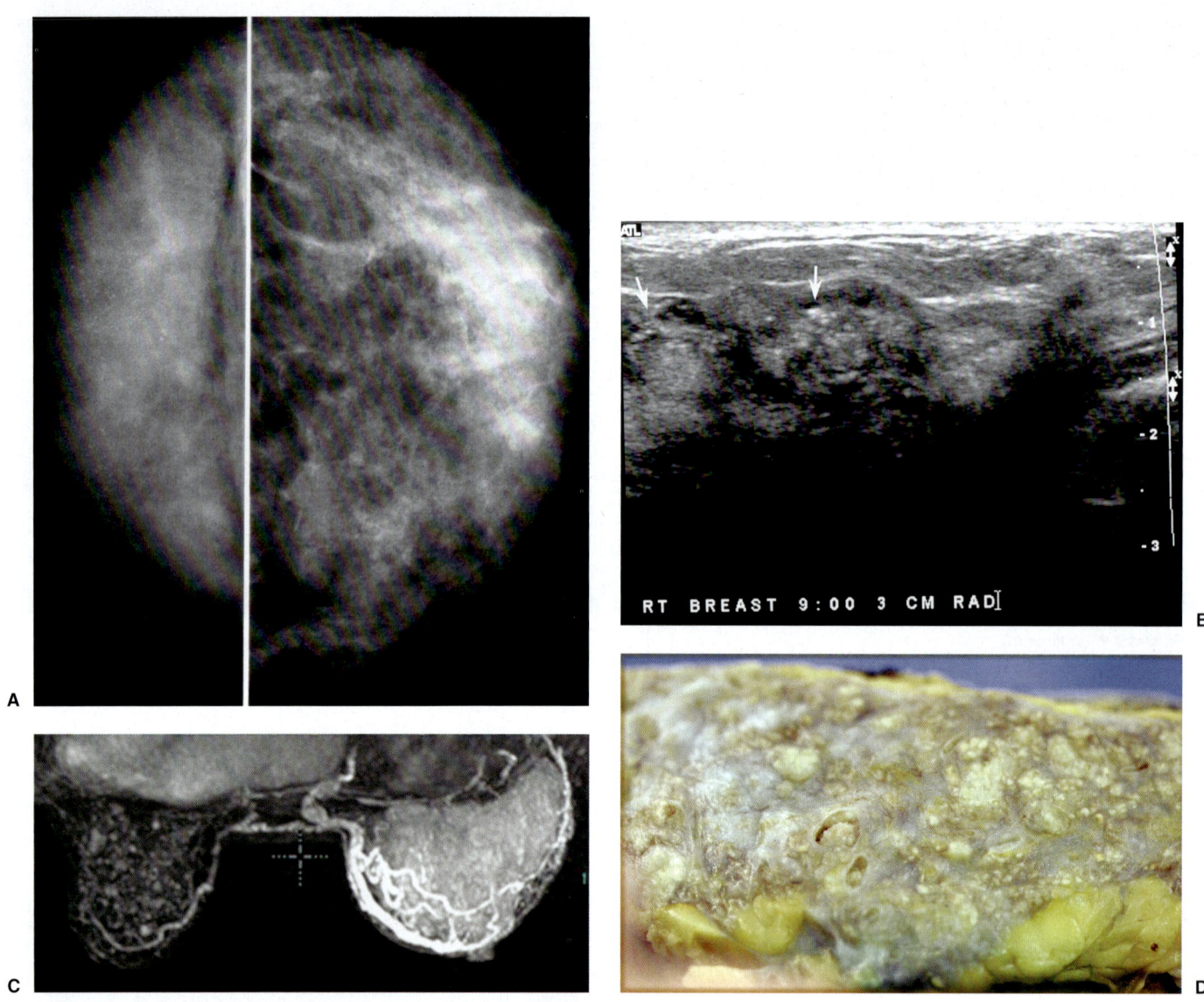

FIG. 9.21 • **DCIS. A:** CC views in a 45-year-old patient. The right breast is smaller. Fine pleomorphic calcifications are present diffusely scattered in asymmetrically dense breast parenchyma on the right. **B:** Representative ultrasound image demonstrates disruption of normal tissue architecture, distal shadowing, and rounded mass-like areas of tissue, some with numerous echogenic foci (*arrows*), reflecting the calcifications noted mammographically. **C:** MRI, maximum intensity projection. The right breast is thicker and on the MRI appears larger than the left. Diffuse enhancement and asymmetrically dilated venous structures are present. Foci of nonspecific enhancement are noted in the left breast. **D:** Gross image of the mastectomy specimen. Multiple variably sized ducts with intraluminal comedos are present. Diffuse, DCIS, high nuclear grade papillary and solid types with comedonecrosis and calcifications are described on the mastectomy specimen. Extensive sampling is done with no invasive disease identified. Sentinel lymph node biopsy (0/4 LNs) is negative.

ductal carcinoma in as many as 95% of patients. In addition to the nipple changes, patients can present with a concurrent palpable abnormality; invasive ductal carcinoma is diagnosed in 75% to 90% of patients presenting with a palpable finding. The nipple findings may be all that is apparent in 40% of women with an underlying invasive ductal carcinoma or in many of those with an underlying DCIS. Although the associated malignancy is commonly found in the central, subareolar aspect of the breast, it is peripheral in as many as 35% to 40% of patients. The associated DCIS is usually high grade with central necrosis, and the invasive lesions are typically poorly differentiated invasive ductal carcinomas (25–29).

In as many as 50% of patients, the mammogram is normal at the time of presentation. Alternatively, nipple retraction, nipple and areolar thickening, calcifications in the nipple and subareolar area, or a mass may be present (Fig. 9.30C). A mass or malignant-type calcifications as well as asymmetric tissue or distortion may be seen away from the subareolar area. Ultrasound may demonstrate an underlying hypoechoic mass; however, the findings may be nonspecific and include skin thickening, irregular areas of hypoechogenicity with disruption of normal tissue planes, and distended ducts that may demonstrate calcifications (26–29).

The high incidence of false-negative mammograms, in conjunction with the observation that even when there are mammographic

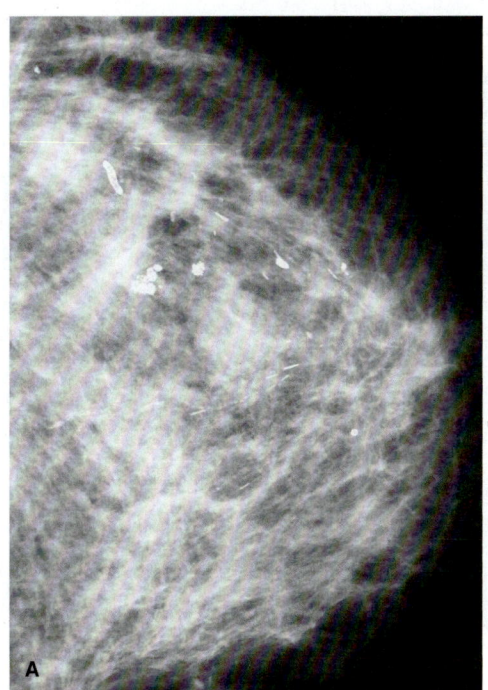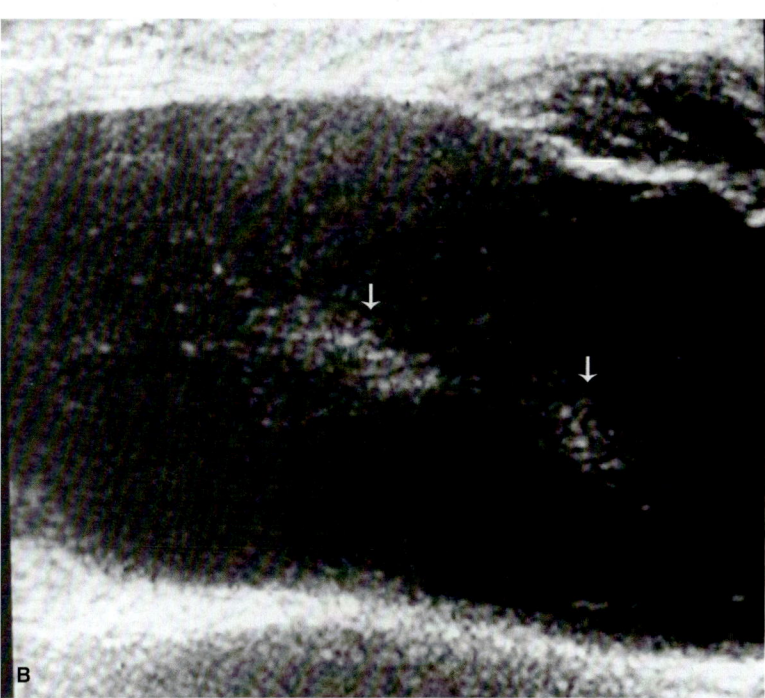

FIG. 9.22 • **Diffuse large B-cell lymphoma. A:** Left CC view. Increased density and diffuse prominence of the trabecular markings are noted involving the left breast. Dystrophic and rod-like calcifications are scattered in the parenchyma. **B:** Ultrasound, left axilla. Enlarged lymph nodes are noted. The cortex is markedly hypoechoic and thickened, with mass effect and attenuation *(arrows)* of the central hyperechoic hilum. Posterior acoustic enhancement is noted. (From Cardeñosa G. *Breast Imaging [The Core Curriculum Series]*. Philadelphia, PA: Lippincott Williams & Wilkins; 2003.)

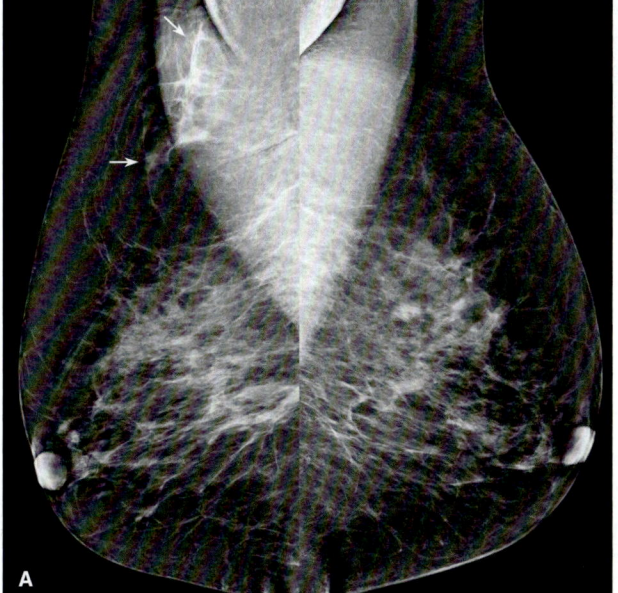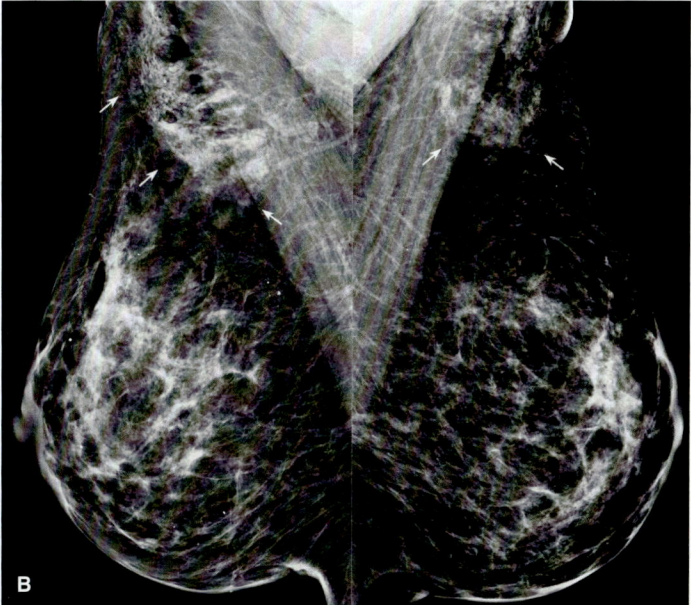

FIG. 9.23 • **Accessory glandular tissue in the axilla. A:** MLO views demonstrate asymmetric glandular tissue *(arrows)* superimposed on the right pectoral muscle, consistent with accessory glandular tissue in the axilla. Some women may have accessory nipples in the axillae or along the milk line extending bilaterally to the groin areas with variable amounts of associated glandular tissue. **B:** MLO views demonstrating accessory glandular tissue *(arrows)* bilaterally in the axilla, slightly more prominent on the right than the left. Some women with accessory glandular tissue in the axillae may present describing palpable findings with associated pain in the axillae that fluctuate with their cycles. On physical examination, prominent globular tissue is palpated, and normal tissue is imaged on ultrasound.

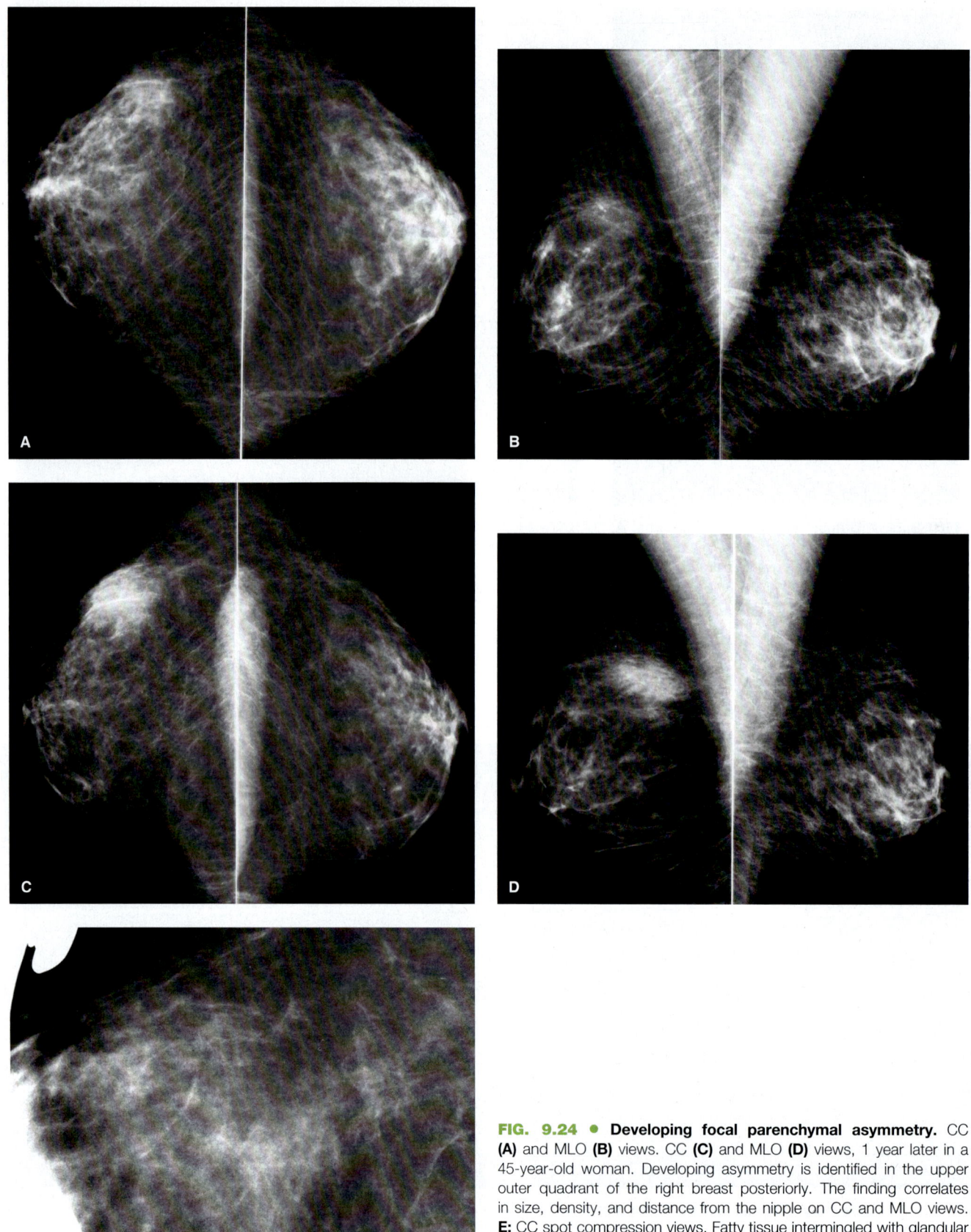

FIG. 9.24 • **Developing focal parenchymal asymmetry.** CC **(A)** and MLO **(B)** views. CC **(C)** and MLO **(D)** views, 1 year later in a 45-year-old woman. Developing asymmetry is identified in the upper outer quadrant of the right breast posteriorly. The finding correlates in size, density, and distance from the nipple on CC and MLO views. **E:** CC spot compression views. Fatty tissue intermingled with glandular tissue having a gradual transition into the surrounding tissue is seen on orthogonal spot compression views (only CC spot is shown). Normal tissue is palpated and imaged on ultrasound at the expected location of this finding. BI-RADS 2: Benign finding.

Miscellaneous Mammographic Findings 301

findings, the extent of the disease is underestimated in as many as 43% of patients, has led to reports describing the use of MRI in patients presenting with Paget disease (28,29). In these patients, MRI can demonstrate clinically and mammographically occult malignancy as well as the extent of the disease (e.g., multifocal and multicentric disease) in the breast. MRI findings, alone or in combination, include intense

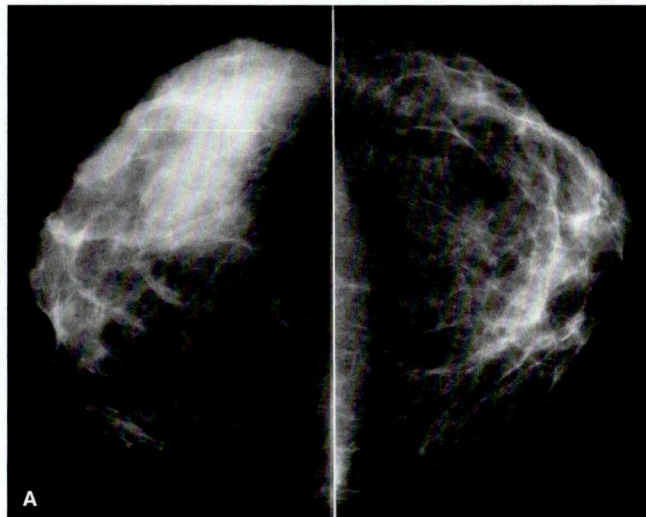
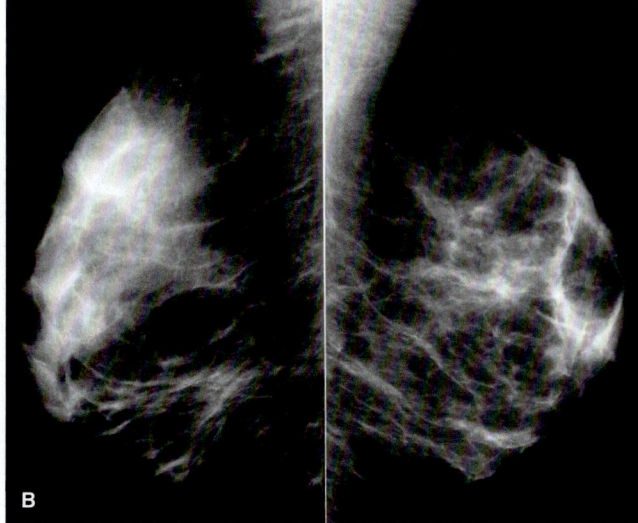

FIG. 9.25 • **Global parenchymal asymmetry.** CC **(A)** and MLO **(B)** views demonstrate asymmetric dense glandular tissue in the upper outer quadrant of the right breast. The tissue is scalloped, and a gradual transition is noted with the surrounding fatty tissue. BI-RADS 2: Benign finding.

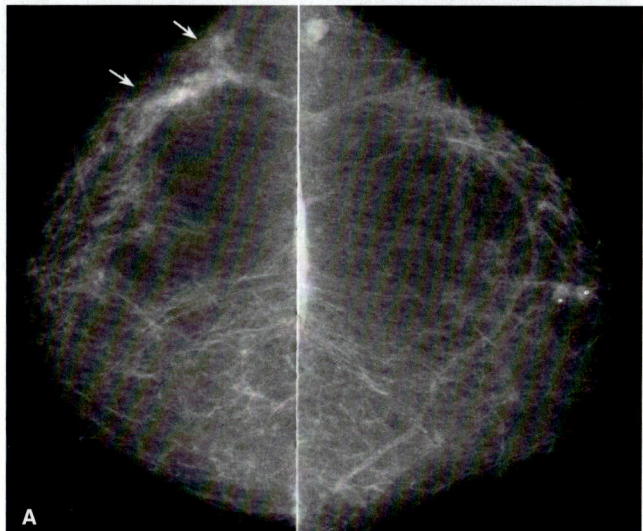
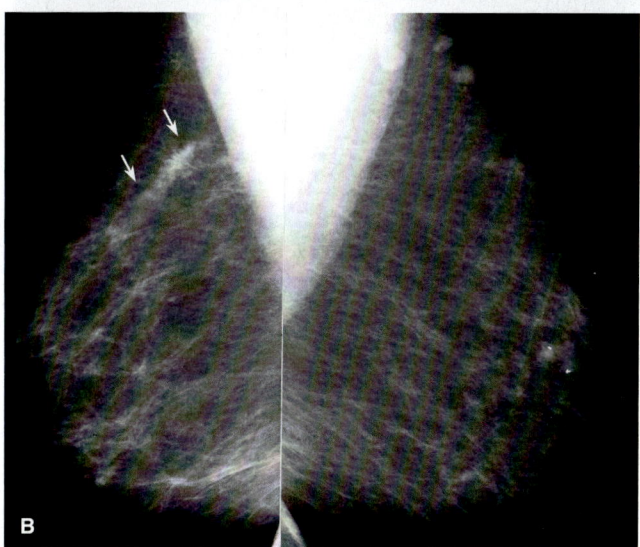

FIG. 9.26 • **Focal parenchymal asymmetry with calcifications, invasive ductal carcinoma and DCIS.** CC **(A)** and MLO **(B)** views in a 46-year-old patient. Focal parenchymal asymmetry *(arrows)* with associated fine pleomorphic calcifications is present in the upper outer quadrant of the right breast posteriorly. The tissue at this site is "rigid" in appearance. Incidentally noted are morphologically benign-appearing lymph nodes in the left axillary tail and axilla. **C:** Spot compression view, CC projection (MLO spot, not shown). The tissue persists, and the fine pleomorphic calcifications are limited to the site of the asymmetric tissue. **D:** MRI, axial T1-weighted axial image post contrast. Non–mass-like, segmentally distributed clumped and linear enhancement *(arrow)* is present in the upper outer quadrant of the right breast posteriorly correlating with the site of the mammographic findings. Homogeneously enhancing lymph nodes are noted in the axillae. Although DCIS nuclear grade 3 with a focus suspicious for invasion is described on the core biopsy, invasive ductal carcinoma grade 3 with DCIS is diagnosed at the time of the lumpectomy; SLN biopsy is negative (0/8 LNs). The tumor is triple-negative (estrogen and progesterone receptor- and HER2/neu-negative).

Table 9.2 DIFFERENTIAL: PARENCHYMAL ASYMMETRY

Normal variation
Accessory glandular tissue (axillary tail)
Prior surgery with removal of tissue in contralateral breast
Estrogen effect
Focal fibrosis
PASH
Trauma
Fat necrosis
Mastitis (granulomatous mastitis)
Invasive lobular carcinoma
Invasive ductal carcinoma
DCIS
Lymphoma

(continued)

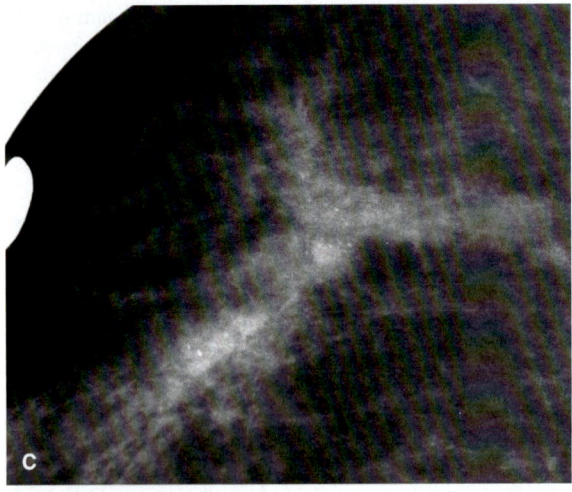
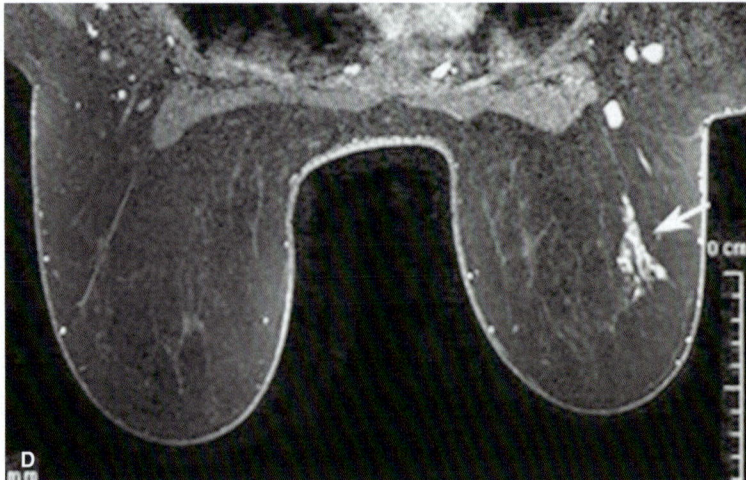

FIG. 9.26 • *(continued)*

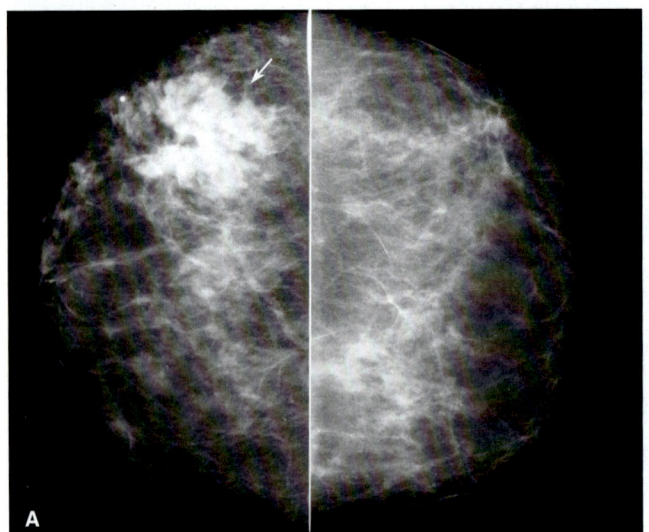
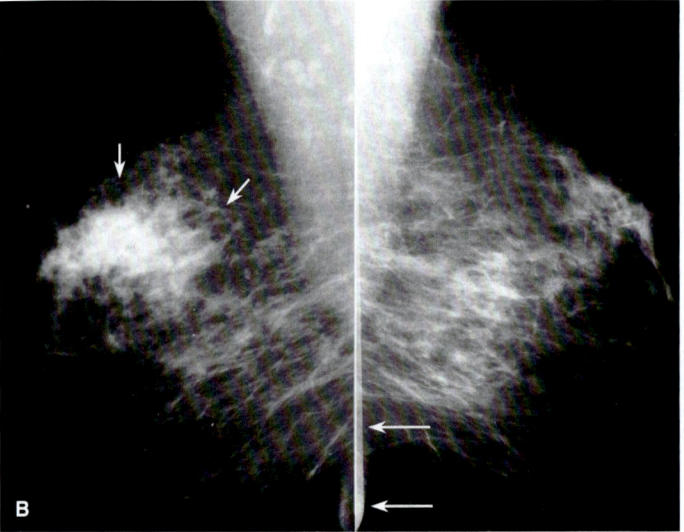

FIG. 9.27 • **Palpable focal parenchymal asymmetry, DCIS.** CC **(A)** and MLO **(B)** views in a 52-year-old patient who presents describing a "lump" in the right breast. Dense focal parenchymal asymmetry *(arrows)* is present in the upper outer quadrant of the right breast corresponding to the "lump" described by the patient. Metallic BB used to denote the palpable finding is seen on CC view, mostly "burned" out on the MLO. Also note artifact along the edge of the left MLO view *(long arrows)*. This results from film overlap as the films are fed in the processor (not an issue with digital systems). DCIS papillary type with no invasion is described on the lumpectomy specimen.

nipple enhancement, thickening, and enhancement of the nipple areolar complex, clumped and linear enhancement, or one or more enhancing masses (Fig. 9.30D, E). Including MRI in the diagnostic evaluation of patients with Paget disease is particularly appropriate when the mammogram is negative and the patient is considering conservative therapy (28–30).

The diagnosis of Paget disease can be made with a wedge biopsy, superficial "shave" biopsy of the epidermis, or punch biopsy of the nipple. The wedge biopsy is suggested as optimal for maximal evaluation of the epidermis and, often, a portion of the underlying lactiferous duct. Histologically, large cells with an abundant eosinophilic cytoplasm and large, pleomorphic nuclei with prominent nucleoli (Paget cells) infiltrate the epidermis of the nipple (26–29). It is also important to point out that some patients with a normal nipple are found to have Paget disease of the nipple microscopically following mastectomy for treatment of breast cancer.

Two theories of pathogenesis (31) are postulated in this disease: malignant cells from a pre-existing DCIS or invasive lesion migrate through the ducts along the basal membrane onto the nipple (epidermotropic). The coexistence of an underlying malignancy, as well as described similarities in the immunohistochemical staining of the Paget disease and that of the associated underlying carcinoma, are used to support the epidermotropic theory. The second theory suggests that the disease arises from malignant degeneration of existing cells in the epidermis of the nipple (intraepidermal transformation). Ultrastructural studies describing microvilli and desmosomal attachments between Paget cells and keratinocytes are used as evidence in support of the intraepidermal transformation theory.

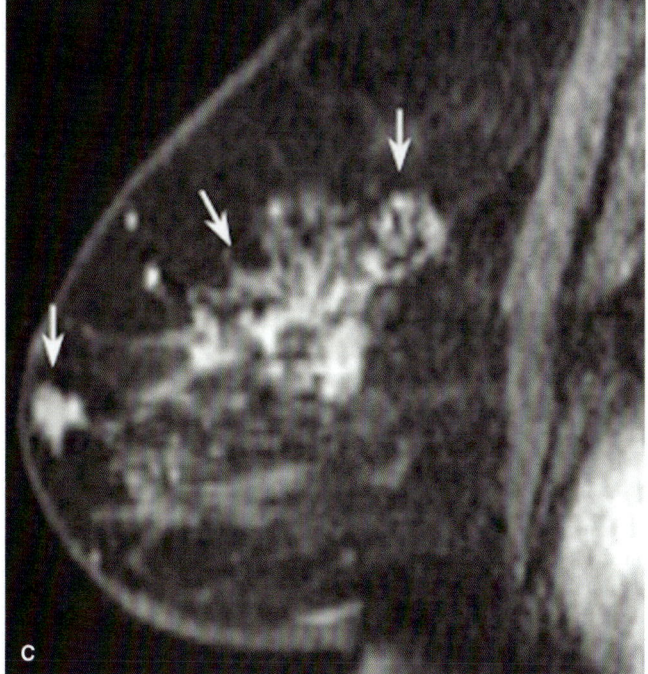

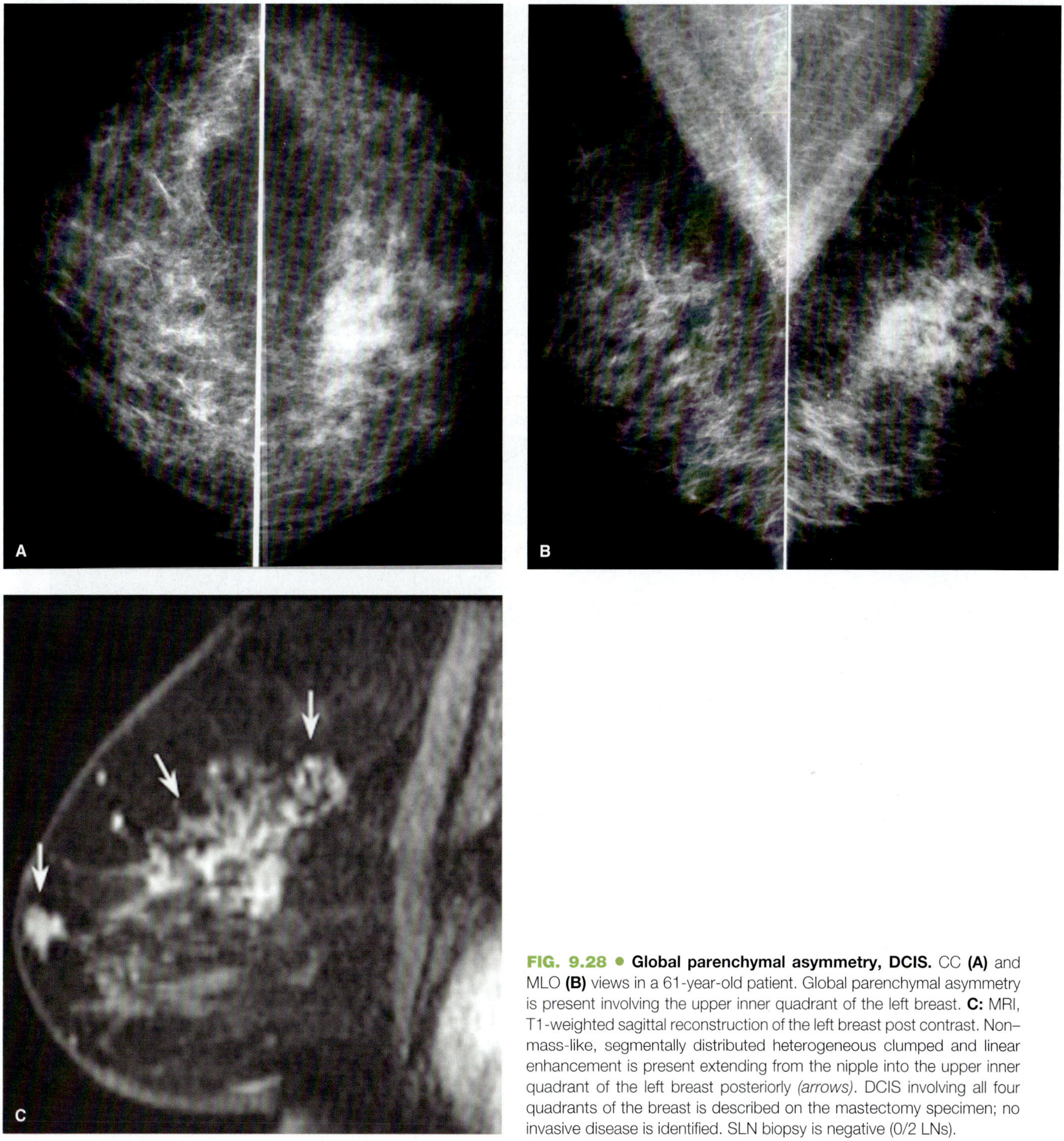

FIG. 9.28 • **Global parenchymal asymmetry, DCIS.** CC **(A)** and MLO **(B)** views in a 61-year-old patient. Global parenchymal asymmetry is present involving the upper inner quadrant of the left breast. **C:** MRI, T1-weighted sagittal reconstruction of the left breast post contrast. Non–mass-like, segmentally distributed heterogeneous clumped and linear enhancement is present extending from the nipple into the upper inner quadrant of the left breast posteriorly *(arrows)*. DCIS involving all four quadrants of the breast is described on the mastectomy specimen; no invasive disease is identified. SLN biopsy is negative (0/2 LNs).

Eczema, psoriasis, allergic contact dermatitis, lichen simplex chronicus, and squamous cell carcinoma in situ (Bowen disease) are diagnostic considerations at the time of presentation. Eczema is commonly characterized by a rapid time course, bilateral involvement, and sparing of the nipple (which is always involved in Paget disease). If there is nipple involvement, and symptoms persist or progress with topical steroid treatment, histological evaluation is indicated. Rarely, intraductal papillomas can protrude intermittently onto the nipple surface simulating Paget disease. Papillomas, however, can be reduced into the duct to demonstrate a normal nipple surface.

LOBULAR NEOPLASIA

The term lobular neoplasia (LN), introduced by Haagensen (25), was intended to move us away from the use of "carcinoma," and all of its implications, in lobular carcinoma in situ (LCIS). The use of "lobular neoplasia" has now been expanded to encompass a spectrum of proliferative processes, including lobular hyperplasia, atypical lobular hyperplasia (ALH), and LCIS; others have suggested using the term lobular intraepithelial neoplasia when referring to these lesions (32). Traditionally, LCIS has not been considered a premalignant lesion but

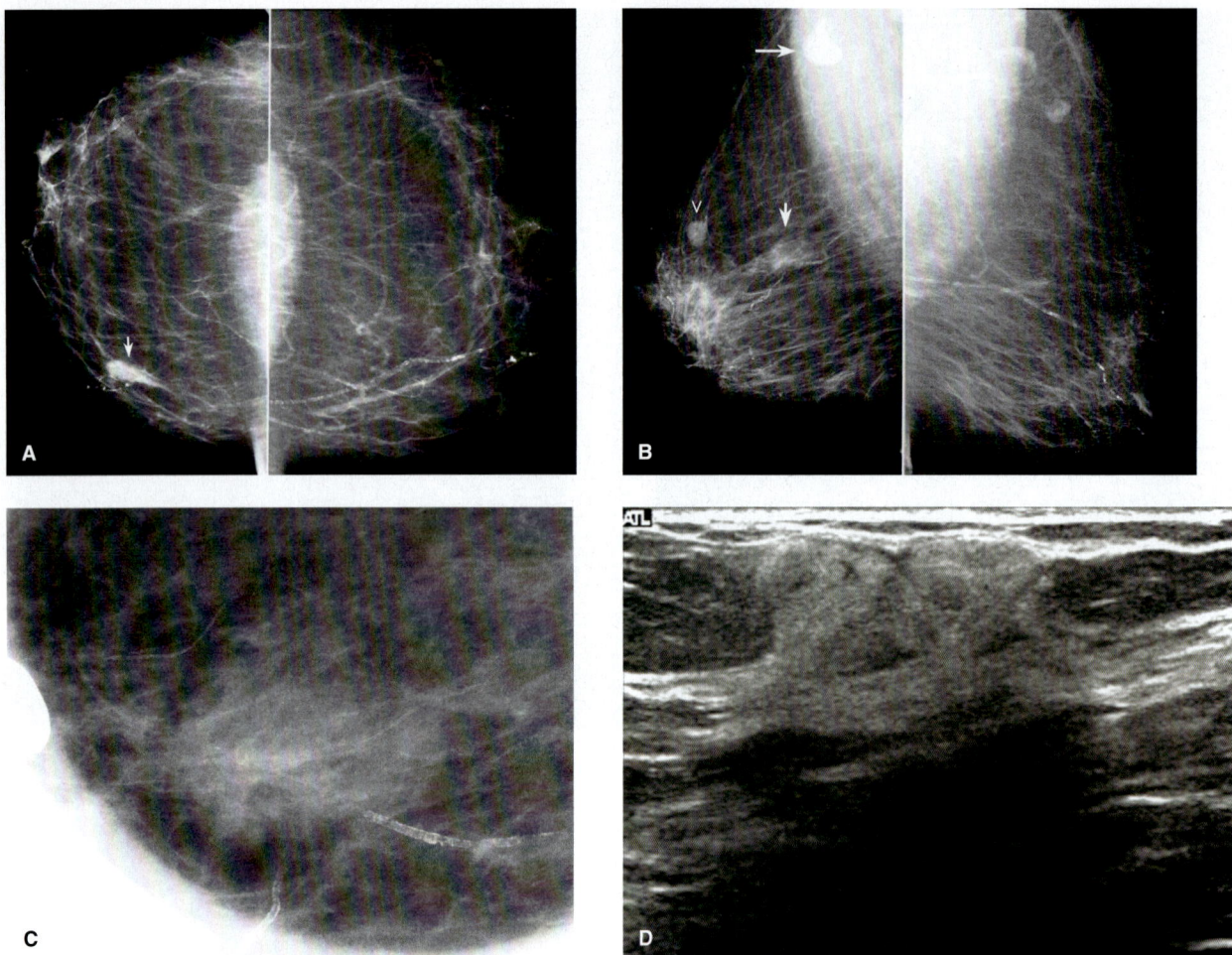

FIG. 9.29 • **Focal parenchymal asymmetry, lymphoma.** CC **(A)** and MLO **(B)** views in an 87-year-old patient. Focal parenchymal asymmetry *(short arrows)* is present in the upper inner quadrant of the right breast. It appears denser and more prominent on the CC view; low in density and harder to perceive on the MLO view. Also note intramammary *(arrowhead)* and dense lymph node *(long arrow)* in the right axilla. Morphologically normal appearing lymph nodes are present in the left axilla. Arterial calcification. **C:** Spot compression view, MLO view. Parenchymal asymmetry is confirmed on spot compression views (only one shown) with a gradual transition of the density, particularly involving the posterior aspect. **D:** Ultrasound. An irregular hyperechoic mass is imaged corresponding to the site of the asymmetry. Although hyperechogenicity is considered a benign feature, not all echogenic masses are benign. In this patient, the diagnosis is established following ultrasound-guided biopsy.

rather a marker lesion imparting one of the greatest lifetime risks (1%–2% increase per year; 30%–40% lifetime risk) for the subsequent development of breast cancer. Appropriately, these concepts are being challenged and are evolving rapidly such that in addition to being considered risk indicators, these lesions are now being discussed as possible nonobligate precursors of invasive cancer. Supporting this concept are the observations that LN is seen in the tissue surrounding invasive lobular carcinomas in as many as 90% of patients, and the similarities in the immunohistochemical profiles between the LN and associated invasive lobular carcinoma (loss of E-cadherin and β-catenin expressivity) (32–35).

Lobular neoplasia is an incidental finding on biopsies done for clinical findings, most commonly a palpable mass, or following biopsies done for mammographic findings, usually calcifications. Although there have been some reports of calcifications associated directly with LCIS (36), this is unusual. Unless the pathologist specifically states that calcifications are in areas of LN, we do not consider LN as a congruent histological finding for biopsies done for calcifications (see Chapter 12). Histologically, acini are expanded by monomorphic, discohesive cells in LCIS and only "partially" involved in ALH (7). Pleomorphic LCIS is a rare variant characterized by larger cells with abundant finely granular cytoplasm, apocrine differentiation, and atypical nuclei with prominent nucleoli (7). LN lesions are typically ER-, PR-positive, and do not express E-cadherin (E-cadherin is an adhesion molecule used to distinguish ductal from lobular proliferations; it is expressed in ductal processes but not in lobular proliferations) (7,37). Associated invasive disease has been reported in approximately 47% of women with LN with the likelihood of invasive ductal carcinoma equaling that of invasive lobular carcinoma. Interestingly, patients with ALH seem to be more likely to have associated invasive ductal carcinoma, while invasive lobular carcinoma is reportedly more common in patients with LCIS (86% vs. 23% for invasive lobular vs. invasive ductal carcinoma, respectively) (32,33).

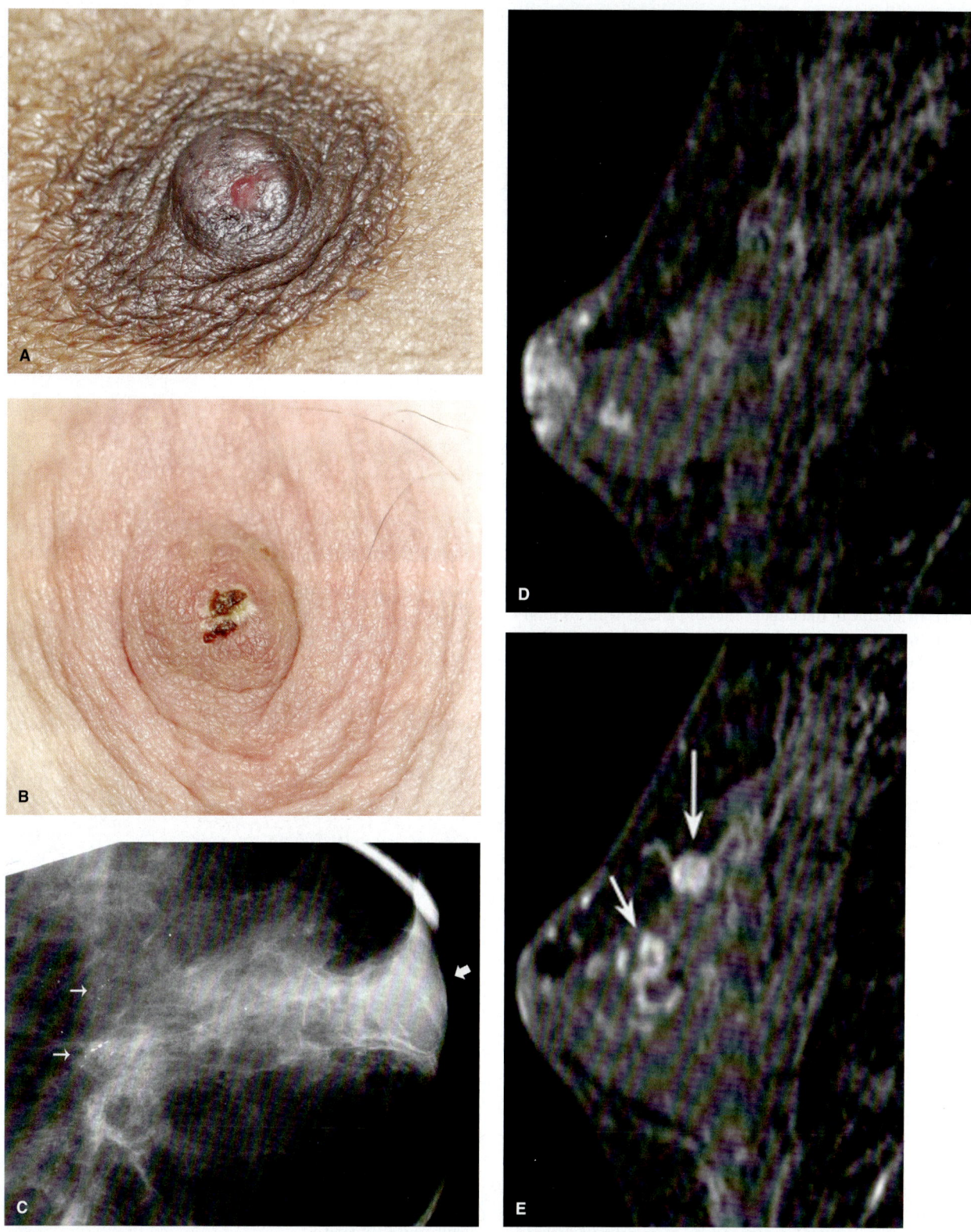

FIG. 9.30 • **Paget disease. A:** Erosion involving the surface of the nipple. Mammogram and ultrasound (not shown) are normal in this patient. **B:** Different patient. Crusting on nipple surface. The patient describes this as a "scab" that she picks at until it falls off, after which it forms again. **C:** Double spot compression magnification view of the left subareolar area demonstrates thickening and retraction of the nipple *(thick arrow)* with associated fine pleomorphic linear calcifications *(thin arrows)*. **D:** MRI, sagittal T1-weighted image of the left breast post contrast; different patient. Enhancement of the left nipple and subareolar area consistent with the patient's known diagnosis of Paget disease and DCIS. **E:** MRI, sagittal T1-weigthed image of the left breast postcontrast at a different location demonstrates additional areas of non–mass-like clumped and linear enhancement *(short arrow)* and one of several heterogeneously enhancing masses *(long arrow)* consistent with sites of invasive disease.

Lobular neoplasia is often a bilateral, multifocal process affecting premenopausal women. Although the traditional teaching has been that the risk of subsequent breast cancer development equally affects the breasts, recent publications suggest that the risk for subsequent breast cancer development is more likely to involve the breast and the site of the biopsied LN. As mentioned above, in women with isolated LCIS (no associated DCIS), the subsequent invasive lesion is almost always lobular. The management of patients with LN remains controversial, particularly as it relates to the diagnosis on core biopsy of an imaging-detected lesion (38–41). Some advocate excisional biopsy in all patients with LCIS on core biopsy citing upgrade to cancer in as many as 33% of patients on excisional biopsy (40). Others suggest excisional biopsy in patients who have another associated risk lesion (e.g., ADH); when there is clinical, imaging, and pathology discordance; if the pathologist experiences difficulty distinguishing LCIS from DCIS on the limited amount of tissue provided on a core; or when the pleomorphic variant of LCIS is diagnosed (7).

SOLITARY DILATED DUCT AND FOCALLY DILATED DUCT AWAY FROM SUBAREOLAR AREA

The solitary dilated duct is a rare finding on mammography. Sickles (42) described this as a probable benign lesion and recommended short interval follow-up to establish stability. More recently, Chang et al. (43) reported one of the larger series of patients with a solitary dilated duct, and suggested that the likelihood of malignancy in these patients may be greater than 2% such that a BI-RADS 4a assessment may be appropriate. In many women with one or two dilated ducts, no underlying etiology is identified (Figs. 9.31A and 9.32B). More commonly, the dilated duct is anechoic (Fig. 9.31B); however, in some patients internal echoes that are homogeneously isoechoic to slightly hyperechoic may be seen in the distended duct (Fig. 9.32B). Some patients with papillomas may present with a solitary dilated duct (Fig. 9.33). On physical examination, nipple discharge may be elicited. Dystrophic calcifications related to the papilloma can sometimes be seen in the dilated duct (Fig. 9.34), and in some, the calcifications have a distinct course, dense, curvilinear, hollowed out (what we refer to as the "hollow popcorns") appearance (Fig. 9.34C; also see Fig. 6.33B). When doing the ultrasound, technique is particularly important because, depending on the amount of pressure applied with the transducer, dilated ducts may collapse and refill as pressure is decreased. The identification of intraductal lesions is possible, particularly if the lesion is close to the nipple and provided the duct is dilated. The dilated duct can be followed for a variable distance away from the nipple, and often comes into and out of the scanning plane such that identification of lesions may be a challenge in some patients.

As discussed for patients with developing parenchymal asymmetry, the rapid or progressive development of an isolated dilated duct should be viewed with more concern since DCIS, commonly low nuclear grade, can present with the progressive or rapid development of distended ducts (Fig. 9.35). Our approach to these patients includes doing physical examination to determine whether there is nipple discharge followed by an ultrasound looking for an intraductal lesion. If discharge is found to be copious and arising from a single duct opening, we do a ductogram. In select patients with a developing solitary dilated duct, no nipple discharge on physical examination, or focal abnormality on ultrasound, MRI may prove helpful in identifying the underlying etiology (Fig. 9.36).

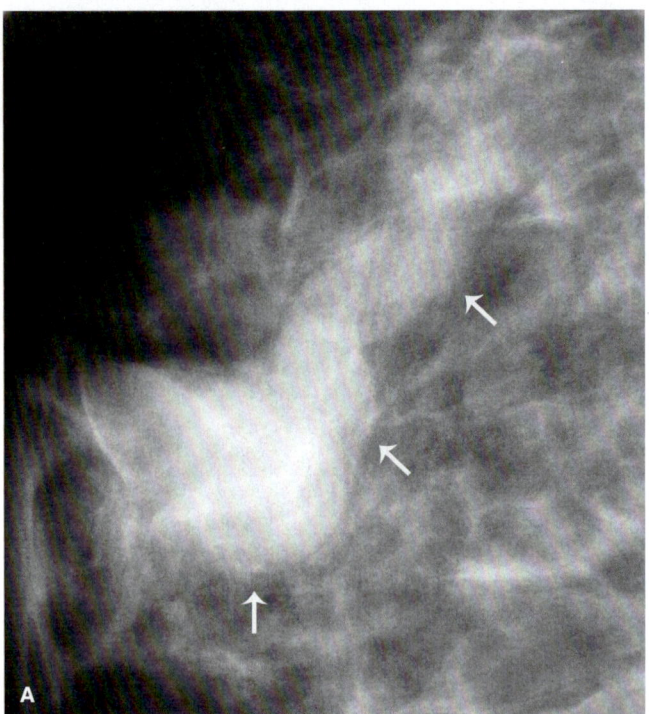

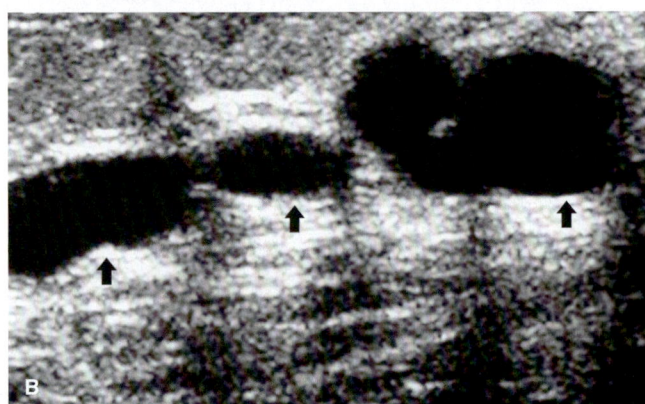

FIG. 9.31 • **Solitary dilated ducts. A:** Dilated duct *(arrows)*. This patient has a normal physical examination with no nipple discharge. **B:** Dilated anechoic duct *(arrows)* with no intraductal lesion identified during real-time scanning. This finding has been stable for 4 years. (From Cardeñosa G. *Breast Imaging [The Core Curriculum Series]*. Philadelphia, PA: Lippincott Williams & Wilkins; 2003.)

Even less common than the solitary dilated duct we have been discussing are patients who have focally dilated ductal structures identified on mammography and ultrasound away from the subareolar area. An isolated oblong (tubular), beaded structure is seen on the mammogram. An anechoic tubular structure is confirmed on ultrasound (Fig. 9.37). If no intraductal lesion is identified, we manage these patients conservatively.

DILATED VASCULATURE

Dilated venous structures (Fig. 9.38) can sometimes be seen in patients with fluid overload or, in situations where collateral flow develops, such as discussed above, in patients with superior vena cava syndrome. In many patients, no underlying cause is identified. Dilated

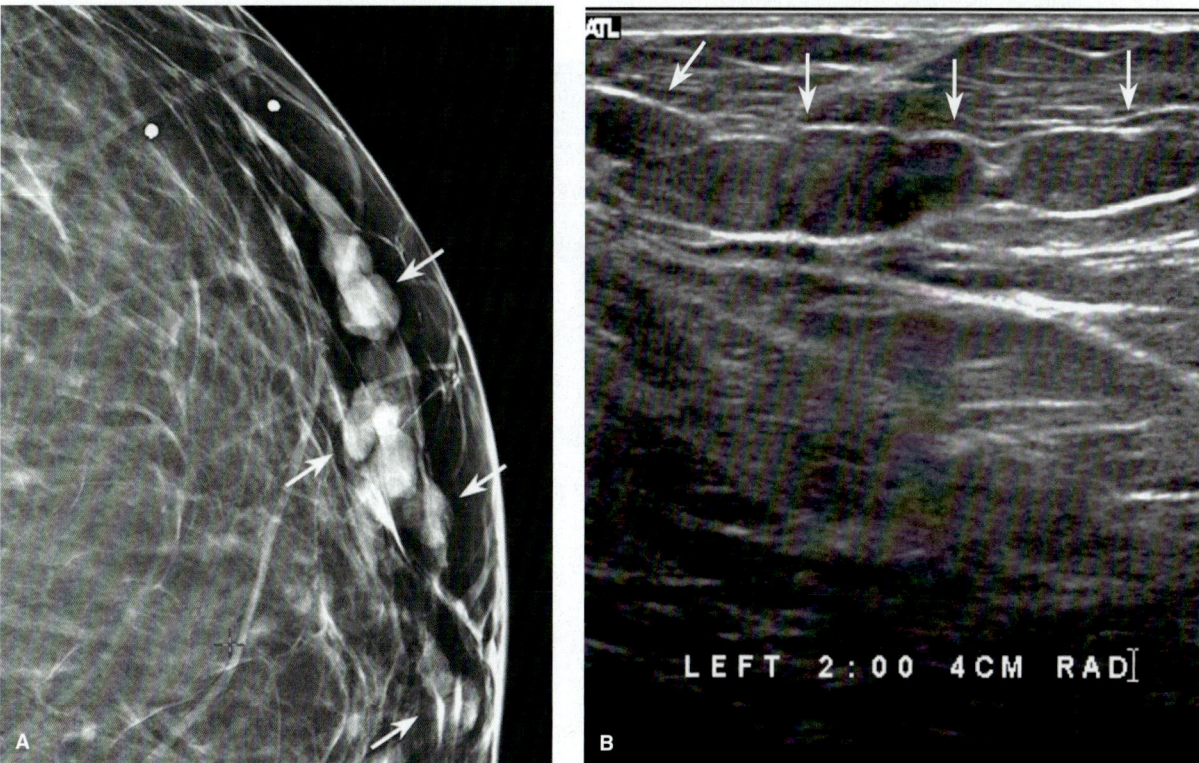

FIG. 9.32 • **Solitary dilated ducts. A:** Solitary dilated duct *(arrows)* extending from the nipple toward the lateral aspect of the left breast. **B:** Ultrasound. Dilated duct *(arrows)* with hyperechoic internal contents that can be seen "gurgling" during the study; no intraductal lesion is identified. Although most dilated ducts are anechoic, in some patients the contents are iso- to hyperechoic and demonstrate movement of the echoes when the transducer is held steady over the duct. On physical examination, no nipple discharge is elicited. This is a stable finding for 3 years.

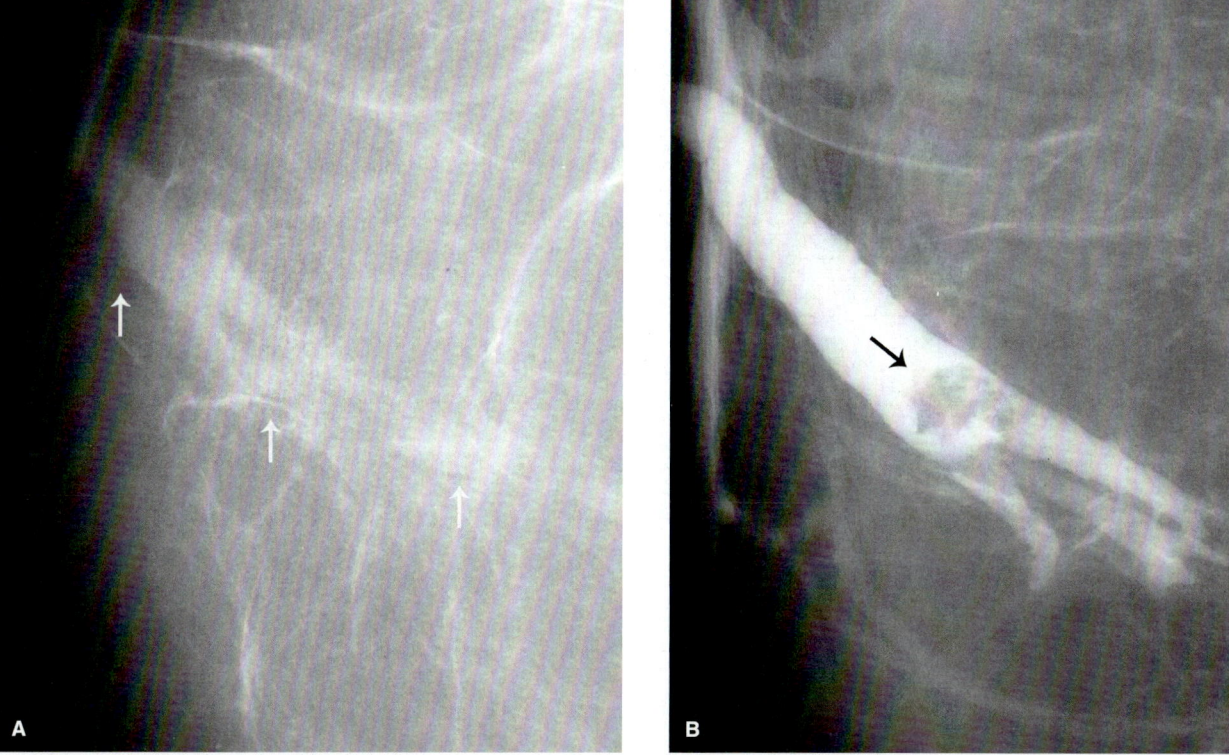

FIG. 9.33 • **Solitary dilated duct. Papilloma. A:** Solitary dilated duct *(white arrows)* is seen in the right breast. On physical examination, nipple discharge is elicited from a single duct. **B:** Ductogram demonstrates dilated duct with an intraductal lesion *(black arrow)*. An intraductal papilloma is diagnosed on excisional biopsy. (From Cardeñosa G. *Breast Imaging* [*The Core Curriculum Series*]. Philadelphia, PA: Lippincott Williams & Wilkins; 2003.)

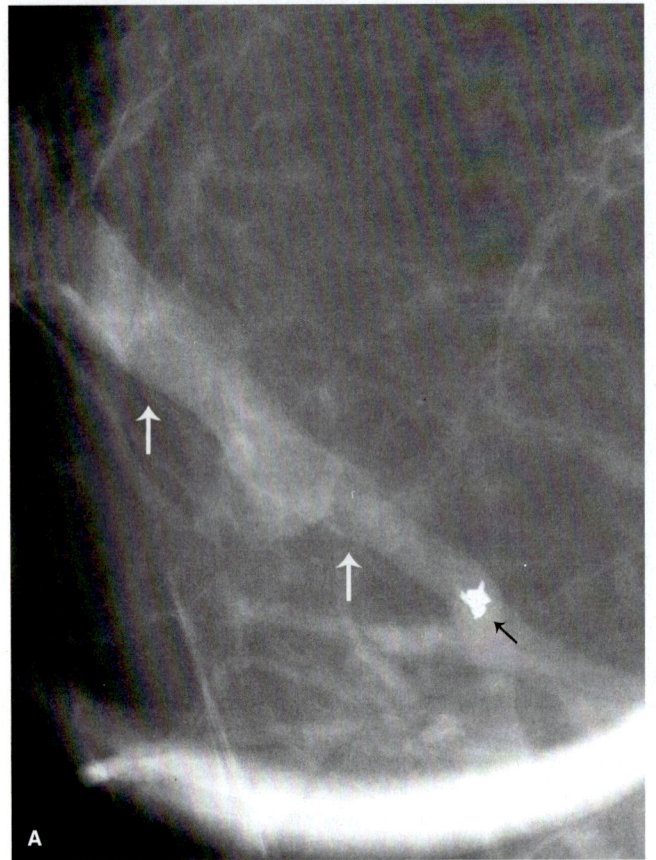
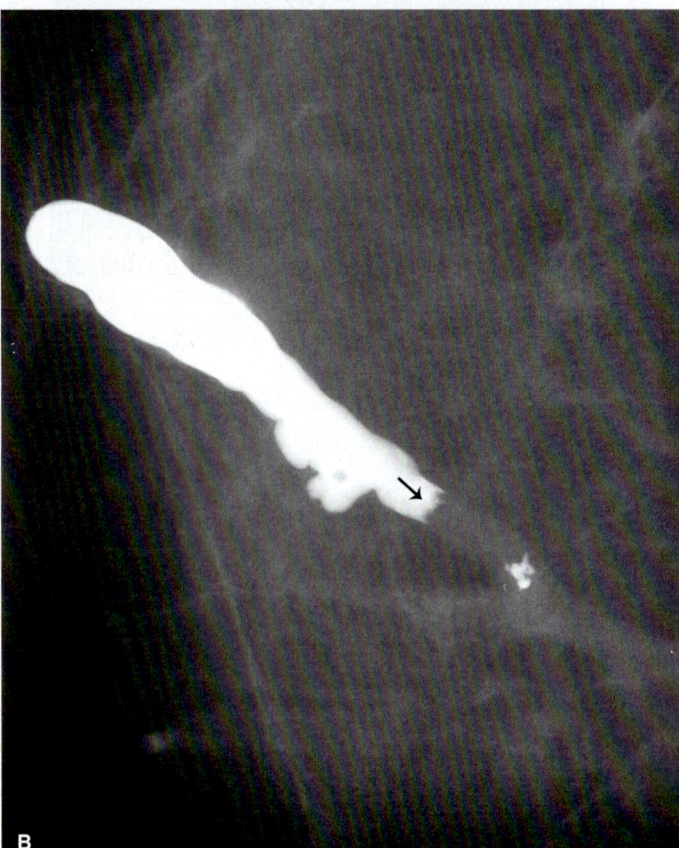
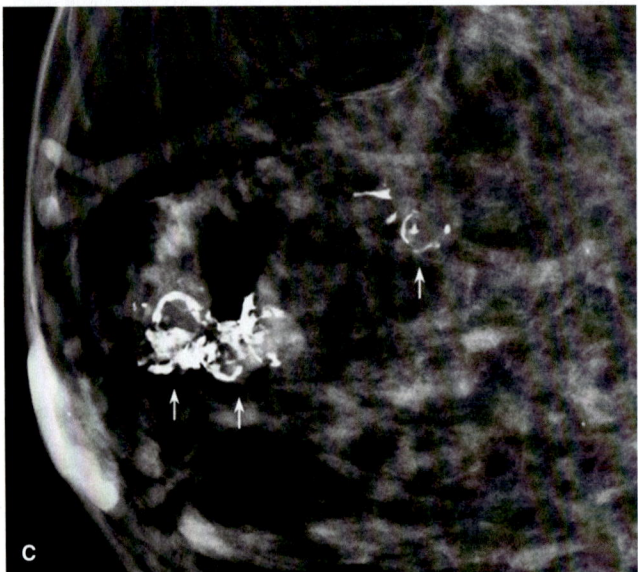

FIG. 9.34 • **Solitary dilated duct. Papilloma. A:** Solitary dilated duct *(white arrows)* with an associated intraluminal coarse dense dystrophic-type calcification *(black arrow)*. On physical examination, nipple discharge is elicited easily from a single duct opening. **B:** Ductogram demonstrates an intraductal lesion at the site of the calcifications *(black arrow)* with resulting duct obstruction. The suspected diagnosis of a papilloma is confirmed on an excisional biopsy. (From Cardeñosa G. *Breast Imaging [The Core Curriculum Series]*. Philadelphia, PA: Lippincott Williams & Wilkins; 2003.) **C:** Right CC view, photographically coned to the subareolar area in a different patient. Portions of a dilated duct with dense, coarse, and some curvilinear calcifications *(arrows)* are seen in the subareolar area; the calcifications are present at two separate sites. These "hollow popcorn" dystrophic-type calcifications typically develop in association with papillomas.

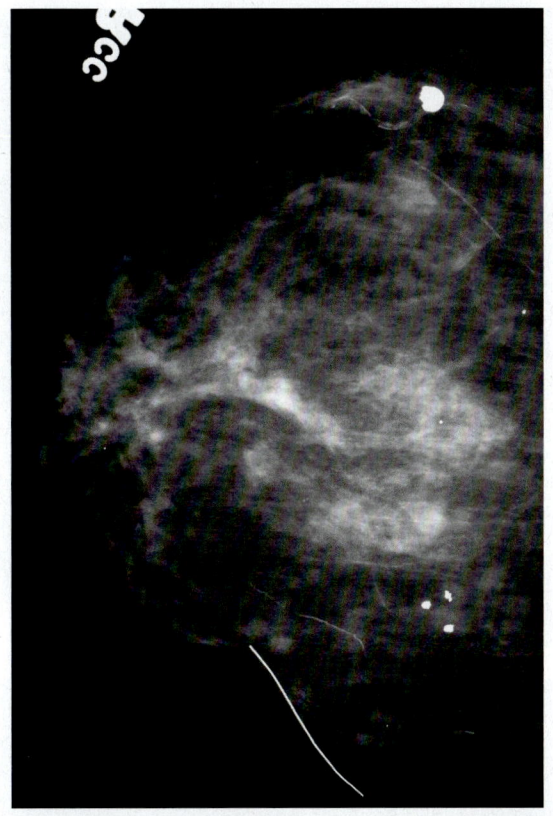
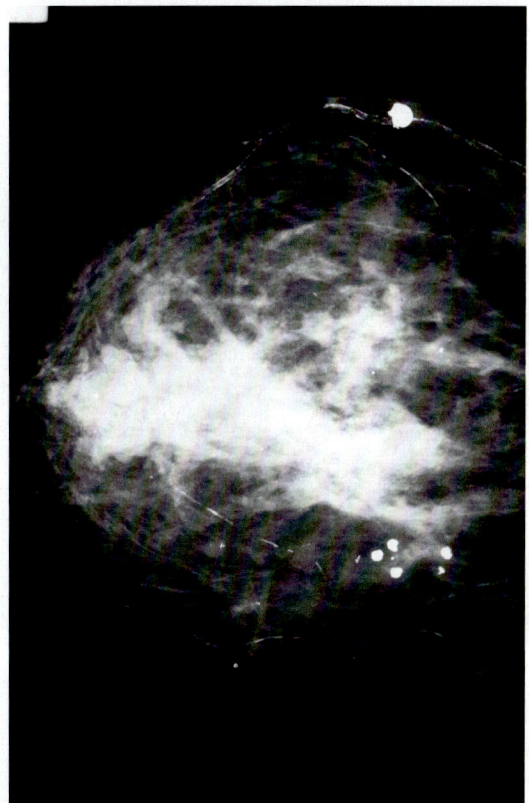
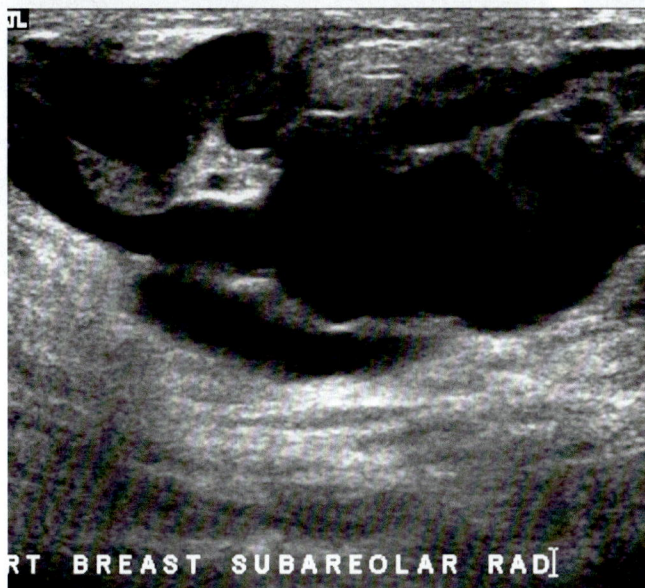

FIG. 9.35 • **Developing duct dilatation, extensive ductal carcinoma low nuclear grade. A:** Right CC view. **B:** Right CC view, 5 years later in a 64-year-old woman. The patient has developed dilatation of a duct extending from the nipple posteriorly in the lower central aspect of the right breast. On physical examination, copious discharge is elicited; however, the ductogram is not diagnostic because the injected contrast is diluted significantly by the amount of fluid in the duct. **C:** Ultrasound. Dilated anechoic fluid-filled ducts can be identified in the subareolar area and traced posteriorly for variable distances from the nipple. With the ducts coming into and out of the scanning field, identification of an intraductal lesion can be difficult; in this patient, no intraductal lesion could be found, and yet extensive DCIS low nuclear grade is diagnosed following excisional biopsy.

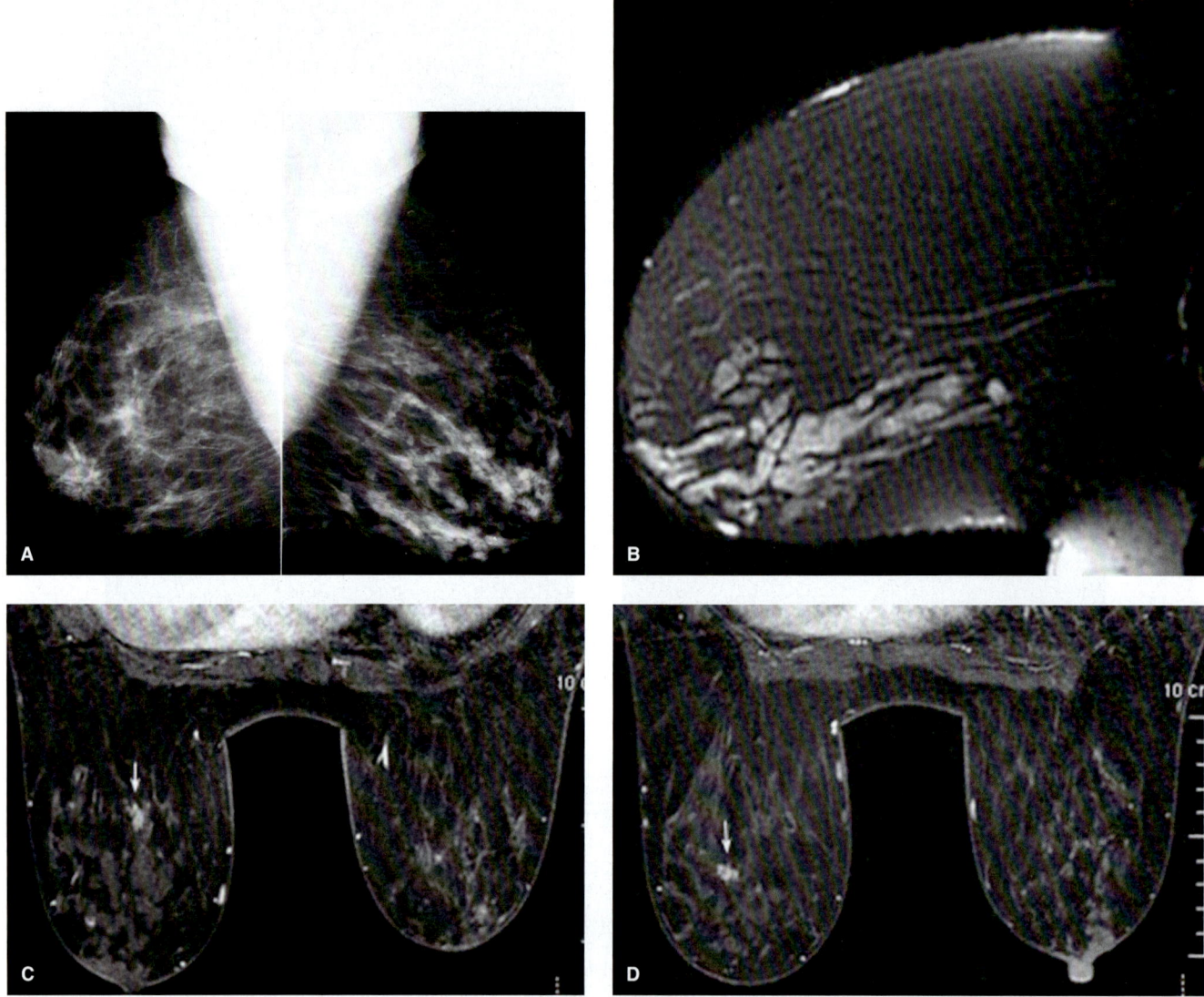

FIG. 9.36 • **Developing dilated ducts, DCIS and atypical ductal hyperplasia, atypical papilloma. A:** MLO views in a 53-year-old woman. Dilated, ectatic, tortuous ducts are present extending from the nipple posteriorly into the inferior quadrants of the left breast. These are new compared with the study done 1 year ago. On ultrasound, dilated ducts are identified; however, no intraductal lesion is seen. No discharge is elicited on physical examination. **B:** MRI, sagittal T2-weighted fat-suppressed image of the left breast. Dilated, fluid-filled (high T2-signal) ducts are imaged inferiorly in the left breast. **C:** MRI, axial T1-weighted image post contrast. An irregular mass with heterogeneous enhancement and spiculated margins *(arrow)* is imaged in one of the branches of the dilated ductal structure. **D:** MRI, axial T1-weighted image post contrast at a different scan plane. A second irregular mass heterogeneous enhancement and spiculated margins *(arrow)* is identified in another portion of the dilated duct. DCIS is diagnosed from the first site, and atypical ductal hyperplasia and an atypical papilloma are diagnosed from the second site on MRI-guided biopsies. The diagnoses are confirmed at the time of excision.

Miscellaneous Mammographic Findings   311

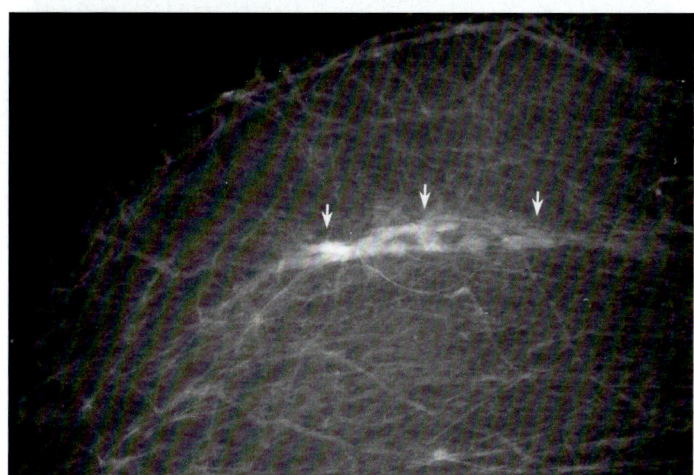
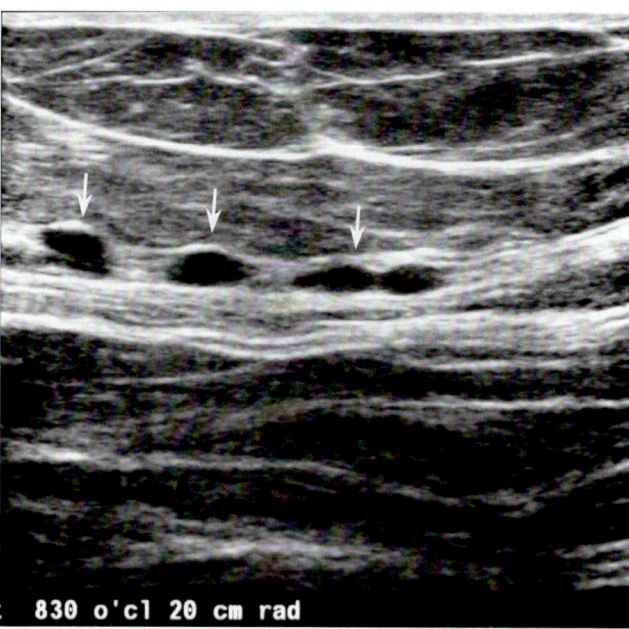

FIG. 9.37 • **Focal duct ectasia. A:** Right CC view, photographically coned to the lateral aspect of the breast. Isolated, focally dilated duct is noted in the upper outer quadrant of the right breast *(arrows)*. **B:** Ultrasound. Dilated duct is imaged coming into and out of the scanning plane *(arrows)*. No intraductal lesion is identified. Finding has been stable for 2 years. This type of isolated duct ectasia is rare, and the underlying etiology is not usually identified. We manage these patients conservatively unless there are indications (e.g., progression, localized finding on ultrasound, etc.) requiring a more aggressive approach.

venous structures can be seen on the anterior chest wall extending into the breasts bilaterally and may be imaged on the mammogram. In women with a diagnosis of breast cancer, dilated venous structures are not usually seen mammographically but can sometimes be particularly prominent in the affected breast on MRI (Figs. 9.15B and 9.21C; also see Figs. 5.26B and 5.28A). Han et al. (44) have suggested that increased ipsilateral whole breast vascularity as well as the presence of one or more vessels adjacent to breast cancers on MRI may serve as predictors of a poor prognosis. Their data suggest that increased whole breast vascularity may be a significant predictor of larger tumor size, metastatic disease, as well as nuclear and histologic grade (44).

MONDOR DISEASE

Mondor disease is an uncommon, self-limited thrombophlebitis involving a superficial vein of the breast. The thoracoepigastric vein, coursing obliquely over the lateral quadrants of the breasts from the epigastrium to the anterior axillary line, is the most commonly affected; the lateral thoracic vein coursing along the lateral margin of the pectoralis major muscle is involved less frequently. Patients present describing a cord of tenderness corresponding to the course of the vein. Linear dimpling can be seen in some patients particularly when they raise their arm (Fig. 9.39A). In some women, superficial, linear, serpiginous nodularity (e.g., simulating the appearance of varicose veins in the leg) can be seen corresponding to the thrombosed vein. This condition

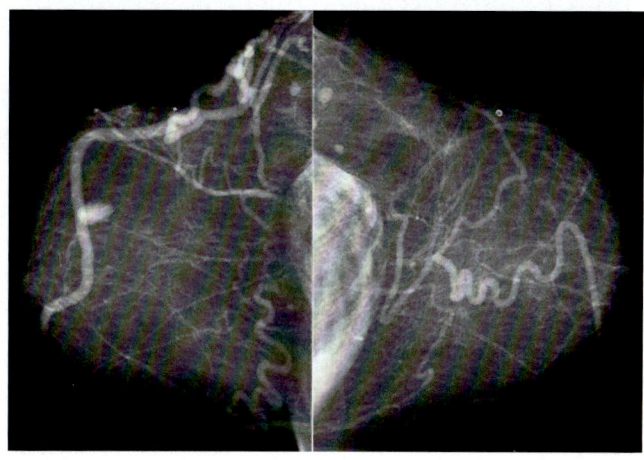

FIG. 9.38 • **Dilated veins.** CC views. Dilated venous structures are noted bilaterally. No known etiology.

usually resolves spontaneously and requires no aggressive intervention. Patients need to be reassured of the likely benign etiology of this condition and supported with nonsteroidal anti-inflammatory agents as needed for symptomatic relief. A cause for Mondor disease is not identified in most patients; however, a list of some reported causes is provided in Table 9.3.

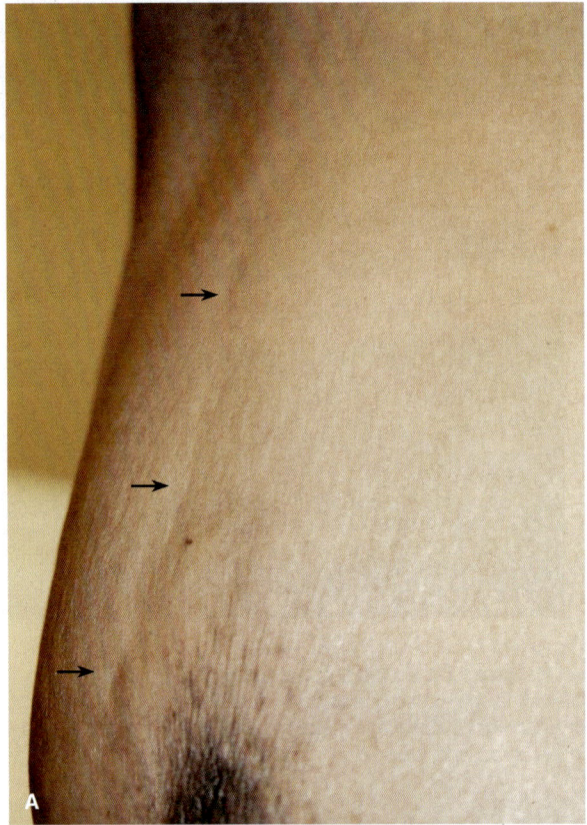
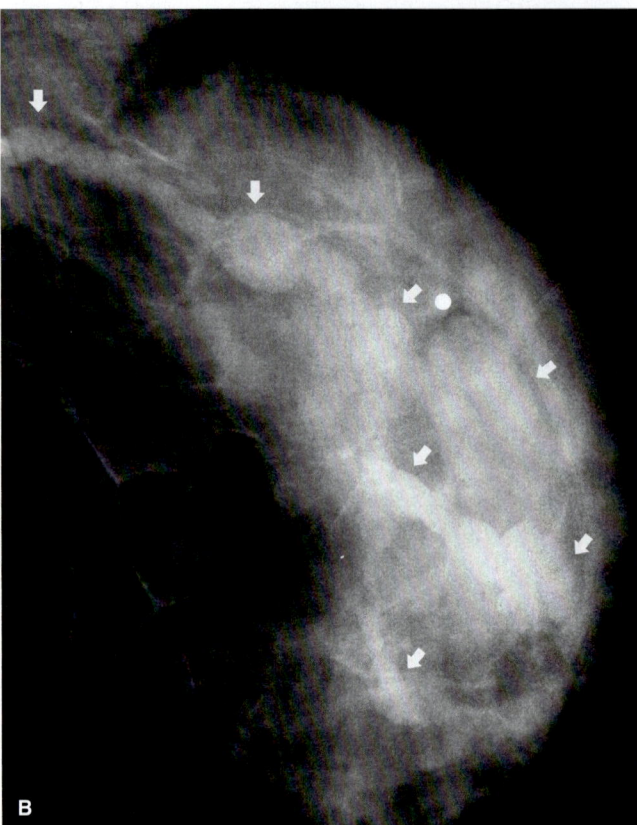
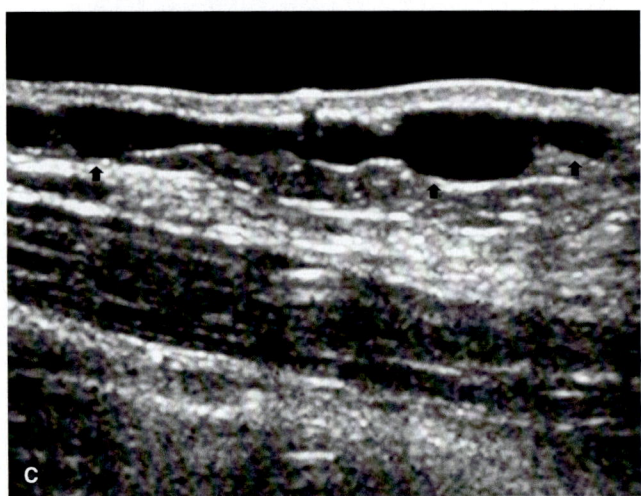

FIG. 9.39 • **Mondor disease. A:** Linear dimpling *(arrows)* elicited when the ipsilateral arm is raised; this correlates with a painful cord described by the patient following vigorous exercise. **B:** Different patient. A serpiginous, tubular structure with a beaded appearance *(arrows)* is imaged coursing from the axilla into the breast anteriorly. **C:** On physical examination, subtle protuberant nodularity is seen on the surface of the breast. A standoff pad is used to evaluate the skin and subcutaneous tissue. A serpiginous, anechoic tubular structure *(arrows)* is imaged on ultrasound subcutaneously. No flow is seen in this structure with Doppler. Skin thickness is normal. Symptoms and findings resolved completely 8 weeks following presentation. (From Cardeñosa G. *Breast Imaging [The Core Curriculum Series]*. Philadelphia, PA: Lippincott Williams & Wilkins; 2003.)

Mammographically, a vein or rope-like density is imaged corresponding to the area of dimpling; this may be associated with subcutaneous thickening (10). In women with nodularity, the vein may have a bead-like appearance (Fig. 9.39B). The dilated venous structures may be striking (Fig. 9.40A). On ultrasound, a superficial serpiginous, tubular structure (46) can be imaged corresponding to the area of dimpling in some patients (Figs. 9.30C and 9.40B). Internal echoes may be seen in the dilated venous structures (Fig. 9.40B, C) with no flow acutely; however, increased flow may be seen in the surrounding tissue. In some patients, the ultrasound is normal. On follow-up studies 6 to 8 weeks after presentation, the imaged venous structure may not be apparent mammographically or sonographically. Rarely, the thrombosed vein may calcify (47).

Table 9.3 **CAUSES OF MONDOR DISEASE**

Idiopathic
Breast trauma
Breast surgery
Breast cancer
Extensive physical activity
Dehydration
Cellulitis
Core needle biopsy (45)

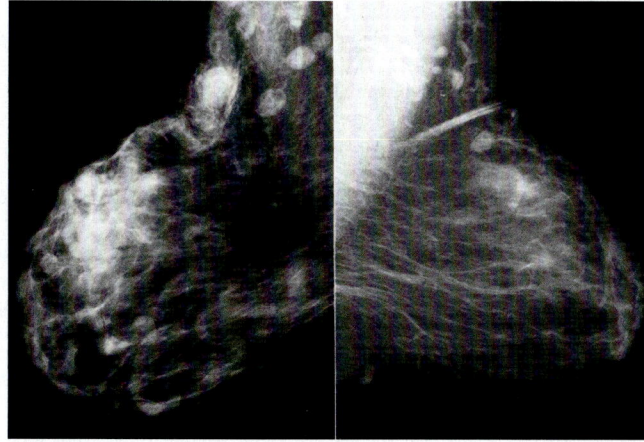
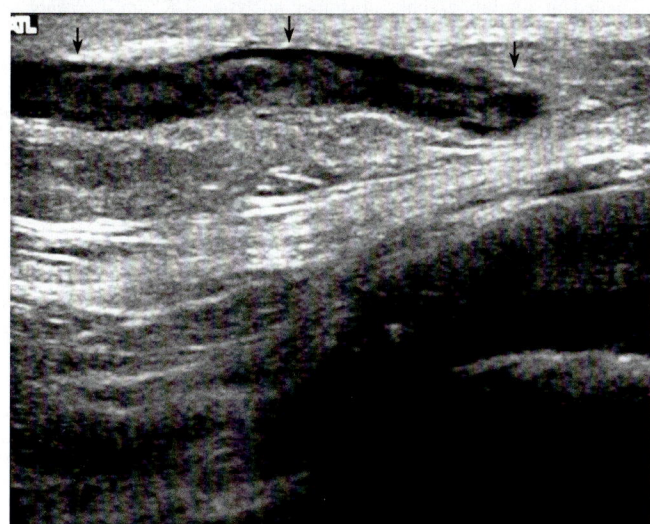
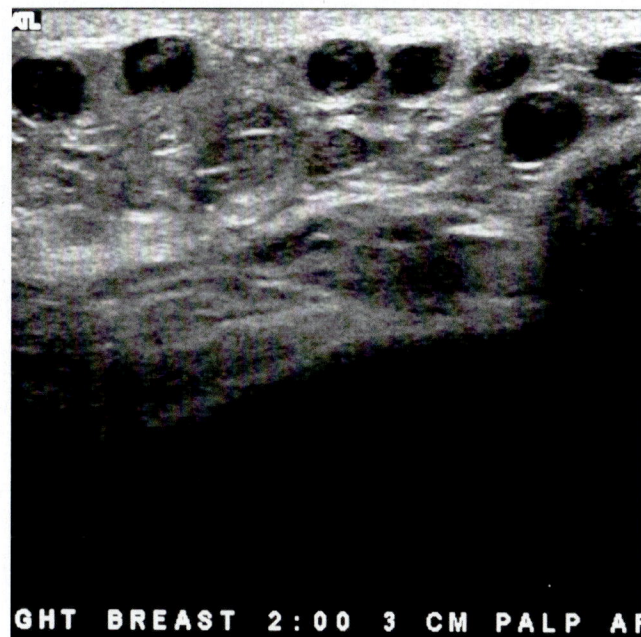

FIG. 9.40 • **Mondor disease. A:** MLO views. An asymmetrically dilated, tortuous venous structure is present in the right breast and right axilla. **B:** Ultrasound (radial) upper inner quadrant right breast. A dilated tubular structure *(arrows)* is imaged notable for the presence of internal echoes and no flow on Doppler. **C:** Ultrasound image (antiradial). Multiple rounded dilated venous structures with internal echoes are seen in cross section coming into and out of the scan plane; these can be followed from the upper inner quadrant of the right breast to the right axilla.

References

1. Cao MM, Hoyt AC, Bassett LW. Mammographic signs of systemic disease. *Radiographics*. 2011;31:1085–1100.
2. Dilaveri CA, Mac Bride MB, Sandhu NP, et al. Breast manifestations of systemic disease. *Int J Womens Health*. 2012;4:35–43.
3. An YY, Kim SH, Cha ES, et al. Diffuse infiltrative lesion of the breast: clinical and radiologic features. *Korean J Radiol*. 2011;12:113–121.
4. Mendelson EB. Imaging the postoperative breast. *Radiol Clin North Am*. 1992;30:107–138.
5. Dershaw DD. Evaluation of the breast undergoing lumpectomy and radiation therapy. *Radiol Clin North Am*. 1995;33:1147–1160.
6. Chansakul T, Lai KC, Slanetz PJ. The postconservation breast, part I: expected imaging findings. *AJR Am J Roentgenol*. 2012;198:321–330.
7. Rosen PP. *Rosen's Breast Pathology*. 3rd ed. Philadelphia, PA: Lippincott Williams & Wilkins; 2008.
8. Tavassoli FA. *Pathology of the Breast*. 2nd ed. New York, NY: McGraw Hill; 1999.
9. Vinayagam R, Cox J, Webb L. Granulomatous mastitis: a spectrum of disease. *Breast Care (Basel)*. 2009;4:251–254.
10. Ruiter AM, Vegting IL, Nanayakkara WB. Idiopathic granulomatous mastitis: a great imitator? *BMJ Case Rep*. 2010. doi:10.1136/bcr.03.2010.2844.
11. Han BK, Choe YH, Park JM, et al. Granulomatous mastitis: mammographic and sonographic appearances. *AJR Am J Roentgenol*. 1999;173:317–320.
12. Ozturk M, Mavili E, Kahriman G, et al. Granulomatous mastitis: radiological findings. *Acta Radiol*. 2007;48:150–155.
13. Gurleyik G, Aktekin A, Aker F, et al. Medical and surgical treatment of idiopathic granulomatous lobular mastitis: a benign inflammatory disease mimicking invasive carcinoma. *J Breast Cancer*. 2012;15:119–123.
14. Dawood S, Merajver SD, Viens P, et al. International expert panel on inflammatory breast cancer: consensus statement for standardized diagnosis and treatment. *Ann Oncol*. 2011;22:515–523.
15. Kim T, Lau J, Erban J. Lack of uniform diagnostic criteria for inflammatory breast cancer limits interpretation of treatment outcomes: a systematic review. *Clin Breast Cancer*. 2006;7:386–395.
16. Anderson WF, Schairer C, Chen BE, et al. Epidemiology of inflammatory breast cancer. *Breast Dis*. 2005;22:9–23.
17. Yang WT, Le-Petros HT, Macapinlac H, et al. Inflammatory breast cancer: PET/CT, MRI, mammography and sonography findings. *Breast Cancer Res Treat*. 2008;109:417–426.
18. Kushwaha AC, Whitman GJ, Stelling CB, et al. Primary inflammatory carcinoma of the breast: retrospective review of the mammographic findings. *AJR Am J Roentgenol*. 2000;174:535–538.
19. Günhan-Bilgen I, Ustün EE, Memiş A. Inflammatory breast carcinoma: mammographic, ultrasonographic, clinical and pathological findings in 142 cases. *Radiology*. 2002;223:829–838.
20. Gianni L, Eiermann W, Semiglazov V, et al. Neoadjuvant chemotherapy with trastuzumab followed by adjuvant trastuzumab versus neoadjuvant chemotherapy alone in patients with Her2-positive locally advanced breast cancer (the NOAH trial): a randomized controlled superiority trial with a parallel Her2-negative cohort. *Lancet*. 2010;375:377–384.
21. Harvey JA, Fechner RE, Moore MM. Apparent ipsilateral decrease in breast size at mammography: a sign of infiltrating lobular carcinoma. *Radiology*. 2000;214:883–889.
22. Brogi E, Harris NL. Lymphomas of the breast: pathology and clinical behavior. *Semin Oncol*. 1999;26:357–364.

23. Sickles, EA, D'Orsi CJ, Bassett LW, et al. ACR BI-RADS® Mammography. In: ACR BI-RADS® Atlas, Breast Imaging Reporting and Data System. Reston, VA, American College of Radiology; 2013.
24. Sickles EA. The spectrum of breast asymmetries: imaging features, work-up, management. *Radiol Clin North Am.* 2007;45:765–771.
25. Haagensen CD. *Diseases of the Breast.* 3rd ed. Philadelphia, PA: WB Saunders; 1986.
26. Burke ET, Braeuning MP, McLelland R, et al. Paget disease of the breast: a pictorial essay. *Radiographics.* 1998;18:1459–1464.
27. Ikeda DM, Helvie MA, Frank TS, et al. Paget disease of the nipple: radiologic-pathologic correlation. *Radiology.* 1993;189:89–94.
28. Lim HS, Jeong SF, Lee JS, et al. Paget disease of the breast: mammographic, US and MR imaging findings with pathologic correlation. *Radiographics.* 2011;31:1973–1987.
29. Morrogh M, Morris EA, Liberman L, et al. MRI identified otherwise occult disease in select patients with Paget disease of the nipple. *J Am Coll Surg.* 2008;206:316–321.
30. Corsi F, Sartani A, Galli D, et al. Usefulness of preoperative diagnosis with magnetic resonance imaging for conservative surgery in Paget's disease of the breast. *Breast Care (Basel).* 2010;5:26–28.
31. Karakas C. Paget's disease of the breast. *J Carcinog.* 2011;10:31.
32. Bratthauer GL, Tavassoli FA. Lobular intraepithelial neoplasia: previously unexplored aspects assessed in 775 cases and their clinical implications. *Virchows Arch.* 2002;440:134–138.
33. Gomes DS, Balabram D, Porto SS, et al. Lobular neoplasia: frequency and association with other breast lesions. *Diagn Pathol.* 2011;6:74.
34. Reis-Filho JR, Pinder SE. Non-operative breast pathology: lobular neoplasia. *J Clin Pathol.* 2007;12:1321–1327.
35. Buerger H, Simon R, Schafer KL, et al. Genetic relation of lobular carcinoma in situ, ductal carcinoma in situ and associated invasive carcinoma of the breast. *Mol Pathol.* 2000;53:118–121.
36. Georgian-Smith D, Lawton TJ. Calcifications of lobular carcinoma in situ of the breast: radiologic-pathologic correlation. *AJR Am J Roentgenol.* 2001;176:1255–1259.
37. Singhai R, Patil VW, Jaiswal SR, et al. E-Cadherin as a diagnostic biomarker in breast cancer. *N Am J Med Sci.* 2011;3:227–233.
38. Nagi CS, O'Donnell JE, Tismenetsky M, et al. Lobular neoplasia on core needle biopsy does not require excision. *Cancer.* 2008;112:2152–2158.
39. Sohn VY, Arthurs ZM, Kim FS, et al. Lobular neoplasia: is surgical excision warranted. *Am Surg.* 2008;74:172–177.
40. Arpino G, Allred DC, Mohsin SK, et al. Lobular neoplasia on core needle biopsy-clinical significance. *Cancer.* 2004;101:242–250.
41. Destounis SV, Murphy PF, Seifert PJ, et al. Management of patients diagnosed with lobular carcinoma in situ at needle core biopsy at a community-based outpatient facility. *AJR Am J Roentgenol.* 2012;198:281–287.
42. Sickles EA. Management of probably benign breast lesions. *Radiol Clin North Am.* 1995;33:1123–1130.
43. Chang CB, Lvoff NM, Leung JW, et al. Solitary dilated cut identified at mammography: outcomes analysis. *AJR Am J Roentgenol.* 2010;194:378–382.
44. Han M, Kim TH, Kang DK, et al. Prognostic role of MRI enhancement features in patients with breast cancer: value of adjacent vessel sign and increased ipsilateral whole-breast vascularity. *AJR Am J Roentgenol.* 2012;199:921–928.
45. Jaberi M, Willey SC, Brem RF. Stereotactic vacuum-assisted breast biopsy: an unusual cause of Mondor's disease. *AJR Am J Roentgenol.* 2002;179:185–186.
46. Conant EF, Wilkes AN, Mendelson EB, et al. Superficial thrombophlebitis of the breast (Mondor's disease): mammographic findings. *AJR Am J Roentgenol.* 1993;160:1201–1203.
47. Bassett LW, Jackson VP, Jahan R, et al. *Diagnosis of Disease of the Breast.* Philadelphia, PA: WB Saunders; 1997.

CHAPTER SELF-ASSESSMENT QUESTIONS

1. Screening images (left and right). No prior studies are available. With respect to the focal parenchymal asymmetry in the left breast what is indicated:

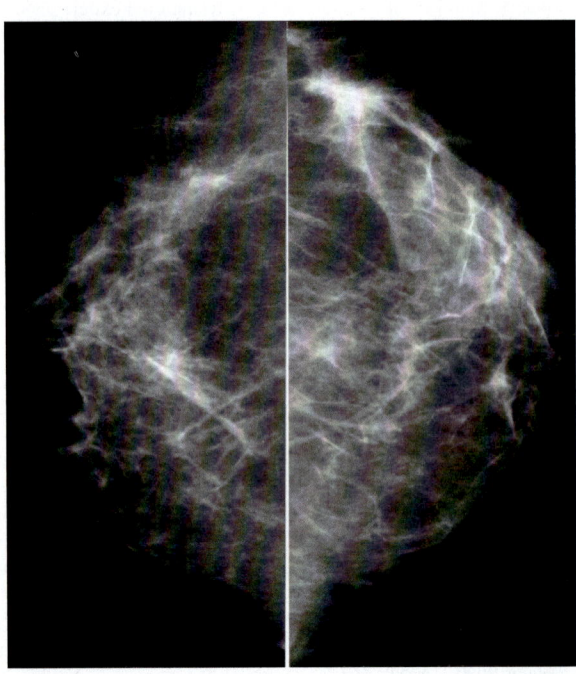
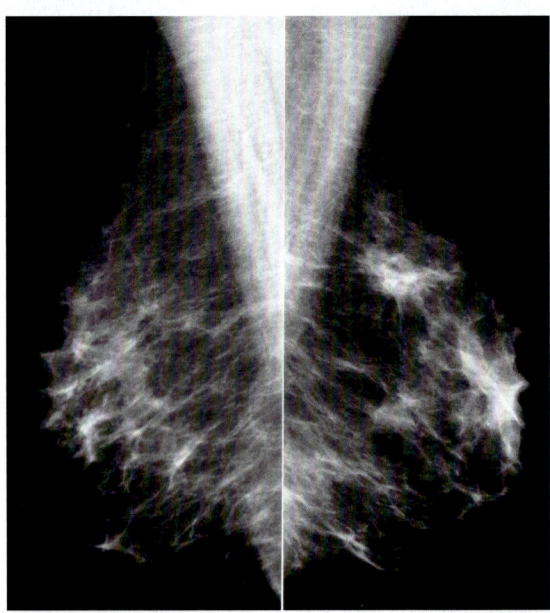

A. Correlative physical examination
B. Six-month follow-up to adequately establish a baseline
C. Magnetic resonance imaging
D. Nothing other than an annual screening mammogram; this is a normal variant

2. The pathology report on a needle biopsy of these calcifications reads: "Lobular carcinoma in situ (LCIS), pleomorphic variant." What additional information do you want from the pathologist?

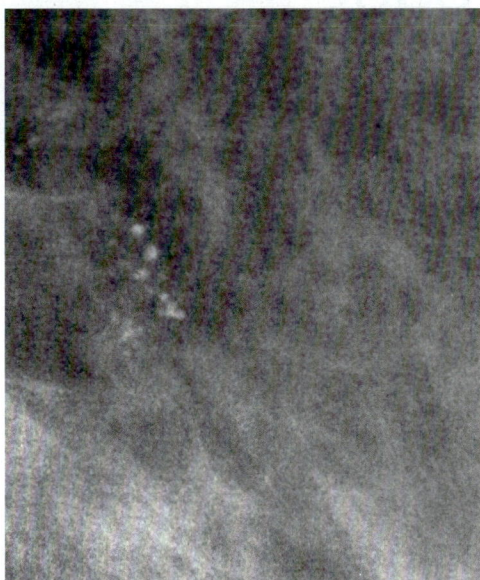

A. Does the LCIS extent to the margins of the cores?
B. Is the lesion estrogen and progesterone receptor positive?
C. How extensive is the LCIS on the cores?
D. Where are the calcifications?

Answers to Chapter Self-Assessment Questions

1. A If no prior films are available, spot compression views and correlative physical examination are indicated in patients with focal parenchymal asymmetry. Short-term follow-up and the probably benign category should not be used without additional evaluation (e.g., spots, physical examination, and possibly ultrasound). This finding alone is not an indication for magnetic resonance imaging. Lastly, remember: Make no assumptions; although this may represent normal variation, we do not make this assumption at the screening setting but rather fully evaluate the patient as describe.

2. D Lobular carcinoma in situ (LCIS), including the pleomorphic variant, is usually an incidental finding for biopsies done for calcifications, less commonly a mass detected mammographically or clinically. In this patient, it is imperative that the pathologist tell you where in the tissue the calcifications are located since a ductal carcinoma in situ may also be present. The extent of LCIS or margin involvement on core samples is not assessed or relevant in the management of these patients. Most LCIS is positive for estrogen and progesterone receptors; however, this is also not a factor in the management of patients with this diagnosis on core biopsies. In this patient, the LCIS is an incidental finding; the calcifications are localized to areas of proliferative fibrocystic changes.

The Male Breast 10

LEARNING OBJECTIVES

1. Presentation, imaging findings, and potential causes of gynecomastia
2. Risk factors for breast cancer in men
3. Imaging findings in men with breast cancer
4. Metastatic disease to the breast in men

Our approach to men presenting with breast-related symptoms includes marking the area of concern with a metallic BB and obtaining craniocaudal and mediolateral oblique views of the symptomatic side. Following review of these images, we may obtain views of the contralateral breast for comparison. If benign changes are diagnosed, no further evaluation is undertaken. Spot compression and spot compression magnification views are obtained as needed for evaluation of findings suggestive of an underlying cancer.

Mammographically, the normal male breast is predominantly fatty with prominent pectoral muscles and a small nipple. Rarely, the sternalis muscle (1,2) may be imaged in men (Fig. 10.1). When present, breast tissue in men is primarily composed of subareolar ducts with no significant branching and sparse surrounding stroma. Lobular units are rare. Consequently, lesions arising in the lobules such as cysts, fibroadenomas, sclerosing adenosis, lobular neoplasia, and invasive lobular carcinoma are rare in men who are not taking exogenous estrogen (e.g., for prostate cancer treatment). All of the breast lesions discussed for women can occur in men, however, with a significantly lower incidence (particularly, as already mentioned, the lobular-derived lesions).

The principles for positioning the male breast are the same as those described for women. The compression paddle used routinely for screening studies can make it difficult for the technologist to hold the male breast in place. Specifically, as compression is applied, the technologist may find it difficult to slide her hand out from under the paddle without scraping her knuckles or letting go of the breast prematurely. Some equipment manufacturers provide a paddle that is half the width (see Fig. 2.2A) of the standard compression paddle for imaging male patients (these paddles are also useful in women who have small breasts or those with implants for the implant-displaced views).

Breast imaging studies in men are scheduled as diagnostics since the patients present with breast-related symptoms. Cooper and associates (3) suggest that mammography is not necessary in men under the age of 50 whom present with diffuse breast enlargement or a palpable non-indurated central subareolar mass unless there are other strong clinical indications such as skin changes or bloody nipple discharge. In their series, none of 43 male patients under age 50 were found to have breast cancer (3). Although there is no significant data supporting screening mammography in men, it may be something to consider in those who have a personal history of breast cancer or in families with male breast cancer and the *BRCA2* gene. It is also unknown if screening should be done routinely in transgender (male to female) patients.

GYNECOMASTIA

Gynecomastia is common, reportedly occurring in 57% of men over the age of 44 (4). Gynecomastia is the enlargement of the male breast with secondary branching of the subareolar ducts and proliferation of surrounding stroma. Patients present describing a "lump" behind the nipple; some men describe pain with the lump. Gynecomastia may be uni- or bilateral, symmetric (Fig. 10.2) or asymmetric (Fig. 10.3). Cooper et al. (3) described unilateral involvement in 33% of their patients with gynecomastia and in 33% it was asymmetric. Appelbaum et al. (4) reported 61 patients with gynecomastia, 55 of which had bilateral mammograms: in 84% of the patients the gynecomastia was asymmetric, in 2% it was symmetrical, and in 14% it was unilateral. Increases in serum estradiol levels, combined with decreases in testosterone levels, are thought to be the etiologic factors governing the development of gynecomastia. At this time, there is no known association between gynecomastia and breast cancer in men. Some of the causes of gynecomastia are listed in Table 10.1.

Three patterns have been described for gynecomastia mammographically (3–7). The *nodular* pattern is characterized by focally increased tissue in the subareolar area (Fig. 10.4) that may fan out symmetrically from the nipple. It has been suggested that this represents the early phase of gynecomastia and corresponds to florid gynecomastia histologically. The epithelial lining of the ducts is hyperplastic and the surrounding stroma is edematous, loose, and cellular. The *fibrous* or *dendritic* pattern appears as retroglandular tissue with prominent fibrous extensions that radiate out into the fatty tissue. Histologically, this is fibrous gynecomastia and reflects long-standing changes; there is ductal proliferation with dense fibrotic stroma. *Diffuse* glandular gynecomastia is the third pattern; it simulates the heterogeneously dense breast in women (Fig. 10.5). Appelbaum et al. (4) describe 61

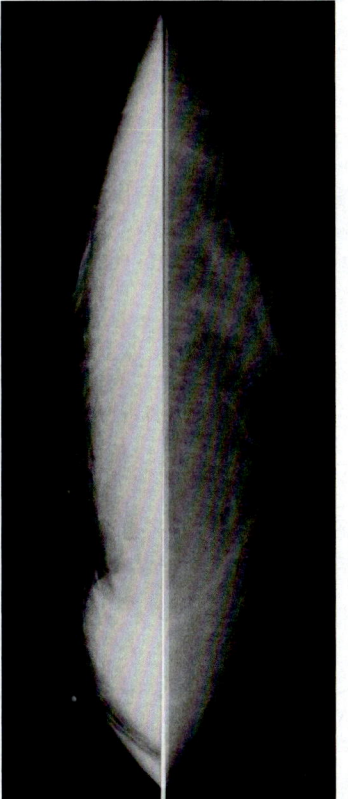
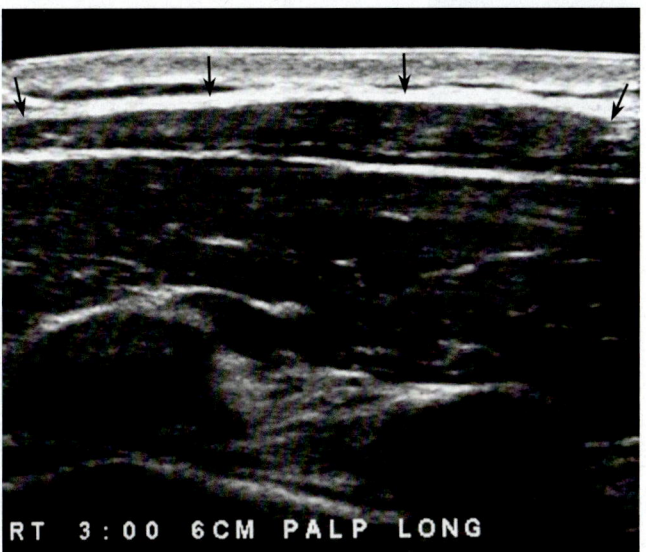
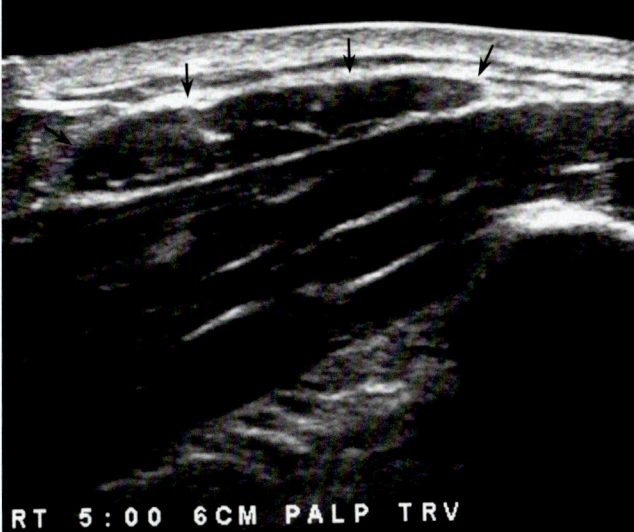
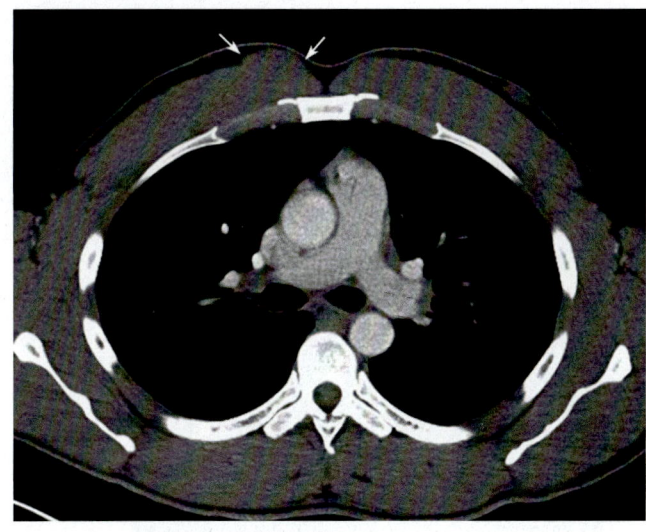

FIG. 10.1 • Sternalis muscle. A: Craniocaudal views in a 33-year-old weightlifter describing a "lump" in the lower inner aspect of the right breast. Metallic BB is used to denote the palpable finding. **B:** Ultrasound, sagittal plane. On physical examination, the "lump" described by the patient is hard and can be followed in a longitudinal course medially in the right breast close to the sternum. A hypoechoic tubular structure *(arrows)* is seen in the subcutaneous tissue overlying the deep pectoral fascia. **C:** Ultrasound, transverse plane. In cross-section, an oblong mass-like structure *(arrows)* with internal striations is imaged corresponding to the palpable finding described by the patient. A miniscule amount of subcutaneous fat is present interposed between the skin and the palpable finding. Also, note the thickness of the pectoral muscle in this athletic patient. **D:** CT scan. In cross-section, an oval mass *(arrows)* is noted superimposed on the right pectoral muscle. This is actually a tubular structure coursing along the anteromedial edge of the pectoral muscle consistent with a sternalis muscle.

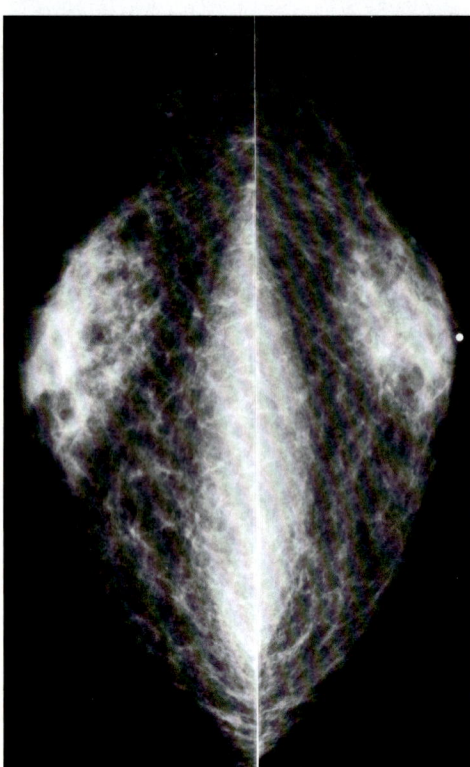

FIG. 10.2 • **Gynecomastia, symmetric.** Craniocaudal views in a 49-year-old man. Glandular tissue is noted centered on the nipples and fanning out into the surrounding fatty tissue. Metallic BBs (not readily apparent on the right) used to denote palpable finding. BI-RADS 2: Benign finding.

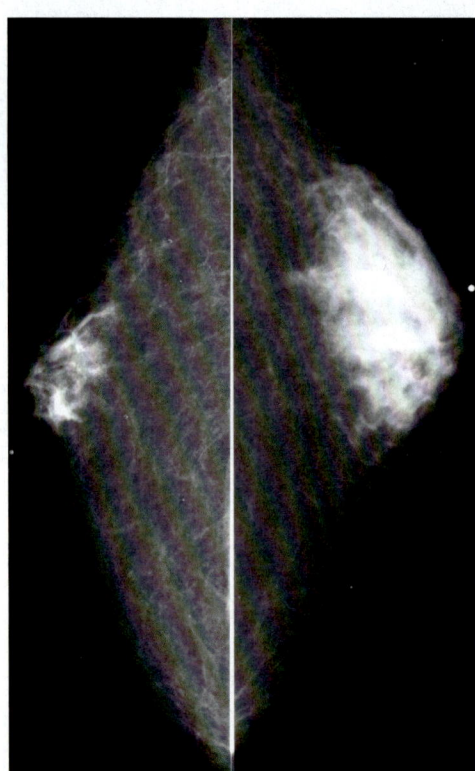

FIG. 10.3 • **Gynecomastia, asymmetric.** Craniocaudal views in a 61-year-old man. Glandular tissue is present bilaterally; however, it is asymmetric with more tissue seen in the left breast compared with the right. Metallic BBs denoting palpable findings. BI-RADS 2: Benign finding.

Table 10.1 CAUSES OF GYNECOMASTIA

Idiopathic
Physiologic
  Neonate (placental estrogens)
  Puberty (imbalance in androgen–estrogen ratio)
  Elderly (decreases in plasma testosterone levels)
Diseases with estrogen excess
  Testicular tumors (Leydig cell, Sertoli cell, testicular germ cell)
  Non-testicular tumors (lung, liver, renal, adrenocortical, hepatocellular)
  Cirrhosis
  Endocrine abnormalities (hypo- or hyperthyroidism)
  Nutritional deprivation
Androgen deficiency
  Aging
  1° hypogonadism; Klinefelter syndrome (XXY)
  2° hypogonadism (trauma, orchitis, cryptorchidism, irradiation, hydrocele)
  Renal failure (and hemodialysis)
Drugs
  Estrogenic activity (anabolic steroids, exogenous estrogen—diethylstilbestrol for prostate CA, digitalis, heroin, marijuana, alcohol)
  Inhibition of testosterone action or synthesis (cimetidine, diazepam, phenytoin, spironolactone, vincristine, methotrexate)
  Idiopathic mechanism (furosemide, isoniazid, methyldopa, nifedipine, reserpine, theophylline, verapamil)
Systemic disorders (unknown mechanism)
  Non-neoplastic diseases of the lung
  Chest wall trauma
  HIV

patients with histologically proven gynecomastia: 77% had nodular, 20% dendritic, and 3% diffuse patterns mammographically. In some men presenting with breast enlargement and tenderness, fatty tissue alone is imaged on the mammogram (Fig. 10.6).

On ultrasound, the findings seen with gynecomastia are nonspecific. In some patients, normal appearing tissue is imaged corresponding to the palpable abnormality fanning out from under the nipple. In others, the tissue may have an irregular appearance with long hypoechoic spicules possibly leading to confusion regarding the diagnosis (Fig. 10.4B). We do not routinely ultrasound patients in whom the mammographic findings are diagnostic of gynecomastia. Ultrasound is done if the diagnosis of gynecomastia remains in doubt after the mammogram, if there are findings not centered in the subareolar area or a mass is identified mammographically.

The management of gynecomastia is variable. In patients with drug-related gynecomastia, attempts can be made to eliminate the causative agent or, if this is not possible, another drug can be tried. No intervention is indicated unless the symptoms are severe or if the patient is bothered by the changes in the breast. Patients with significant symptoms may undergo surgical excision of the tissue. Unless there is a significant change in the physical findings, no imaging follow-up is recommended. Once it has developed, gynecomastia does not usually resolve particularly if the underlying cause is not identified (e.g., idiopathic).

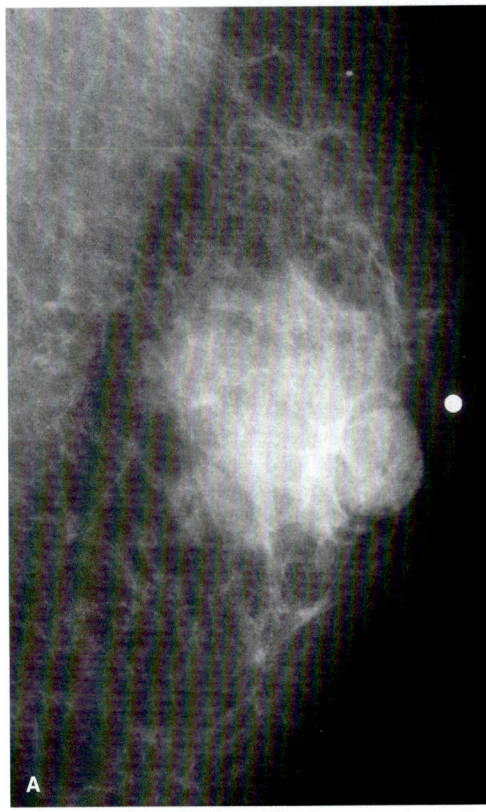
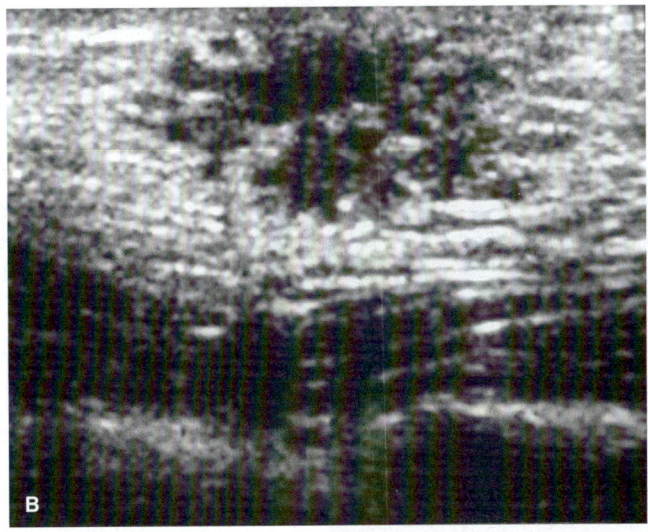

FIG. 10.4 • **Gynecomastia, nodular pattern. A:** Mediolateral oblique view in a 94-year-old man presenting with a "lump" in the left breast. Metallic BB denotes palpable finding. Round glandular tissue is imaged corresponding to the mass. Scalloping of the density is noted, consistent with tissue. **B:** Ultrasound. Irregular mass-like area of mixed echogenicity with internal hypoechoic serpiginous tubular-like structures (likely ducts) radiating out symmetrically from the nipple. The irregular spiculated-like appearance of this tissue should not be confused with a mass having spiculated margins. BI-RADS 2: Benign finding. (From Cardeñosa G. Breast Imaging [The Core Curriculum Series]. Philadelphia, PA: Lippincott Williams & Wilkins; 2003.)

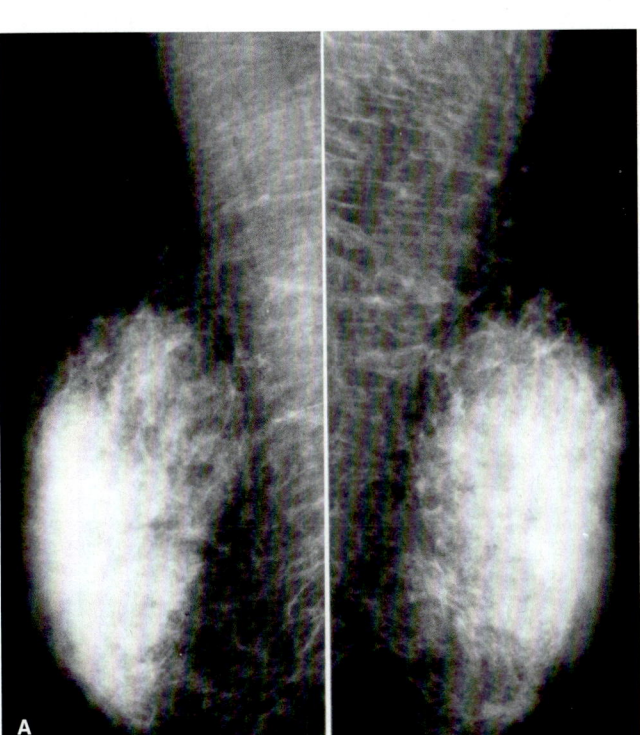
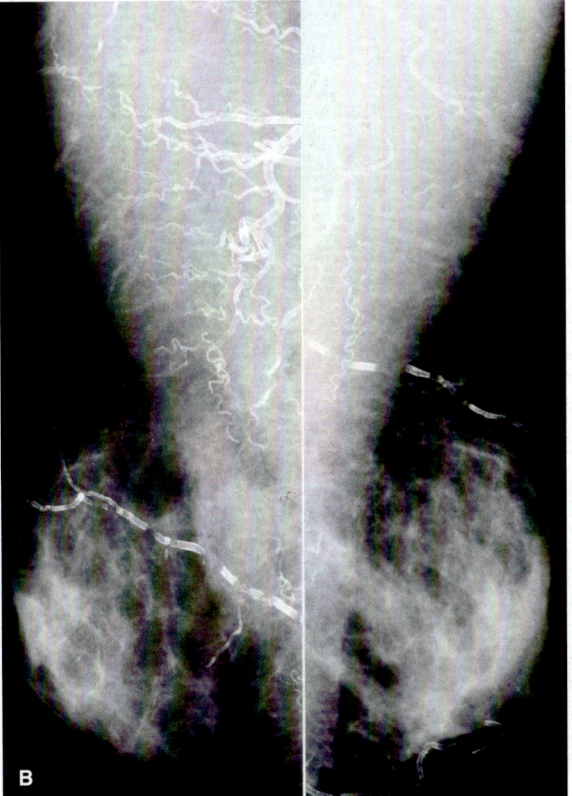

FIG. 10.5 • **Gynecomastia, diffuse pattern. A:** Mediolateral oblique views in a 35-year-old man. Bilateral symmetrically dense glandular tissue is present. In the absence of an explanation for this amount of gynecomastia in a 35-year-old patient, hormonal and testicular evaluation is indicated. **B:** Mediolateral oblique views in a 56-year-old man. Bilateral symmetrically dense glandular tissue is present. Extensive calcification of the arteries is noted in a patient with end-stage renal disease and hyperparathyroidism. Also, note prominence of the pectoral muscles.

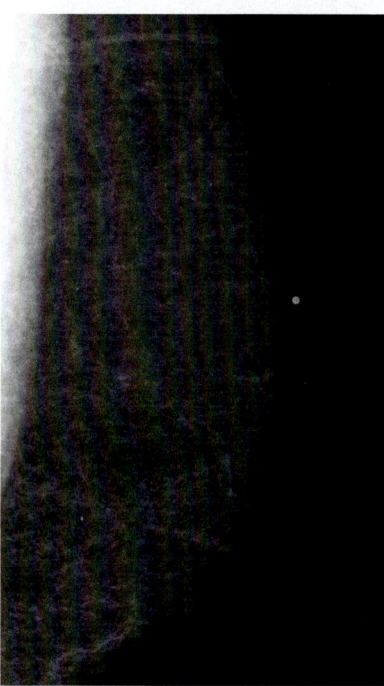

FIG. 10.6 • **Fatty tissue.** Left mediolateral oblique view. When fatty tissue is imaged corresponding to a palpable finding, it is sometimes called pseudo-gynecomastia. (From Cardeñosa G. *Breast Imaging [The Core Curriculum Series]*. Philadelphia, PA: Lippincott Williams & Wilkins; 2003.)

BENIGN LESIONS

Fat-containing masses in men are benign and have appearances similar to those described for women. These include lipomas, lymph nodes (Fig. 10.7), hematomas, and fat necrosis (Fig. 10.8). Water density masses seen in men include epidermal inclusion cysts, abscesses (Fig. 10.9), papillomas, pseudoangiomatous stromal hyperplasia (Fig. 10.10), and focal fibrosis (diabetic mastopathy). As mentioned previously, cysts and fibroadenomas as lobular derivatives are not usually seen in men.

BREAST CANCER

Breast cancer in men represents approximately 1% of all breast cancers and 0.2% of all cancers diagnosed in men; breast cancer in men is thought to be unrelated to gynecomastia. It is estimated that 2,360 men will be diagnosed with breast cancer in 2014 and that 430 men will die of breast cancer–related complications (in contrast 232,670 women and 40,000 breast cancer–related deaths among women are expected in 2014) (8). Risk factors for breast cancer in men are listed in Table 10.2.

Clinically, some reports suggest that male patients present at an older age (median age of 67) than female patients with a painless, hard mass most commonly in the subareolar area or, second in frequency, the upper outer quadrant of the breast; they can, however, occur anywhere in the breast. Skin or nipple retraction may be present and, some patients, present with spontaneous nipple discharge. Axillary

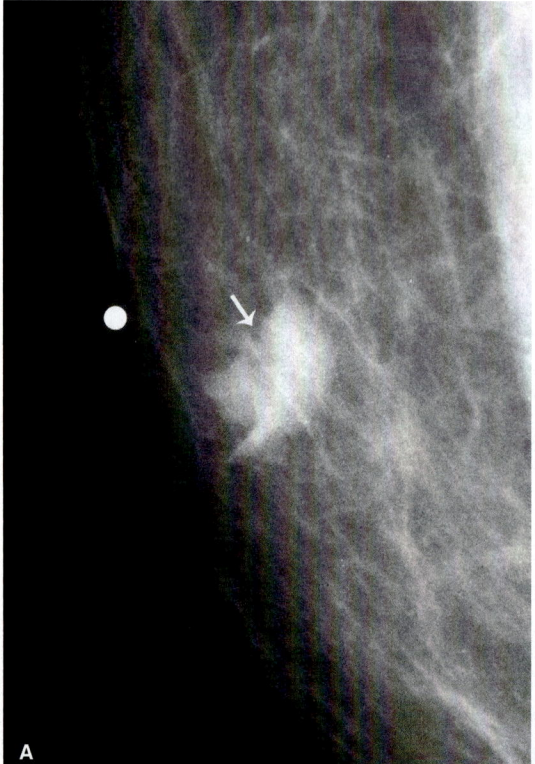

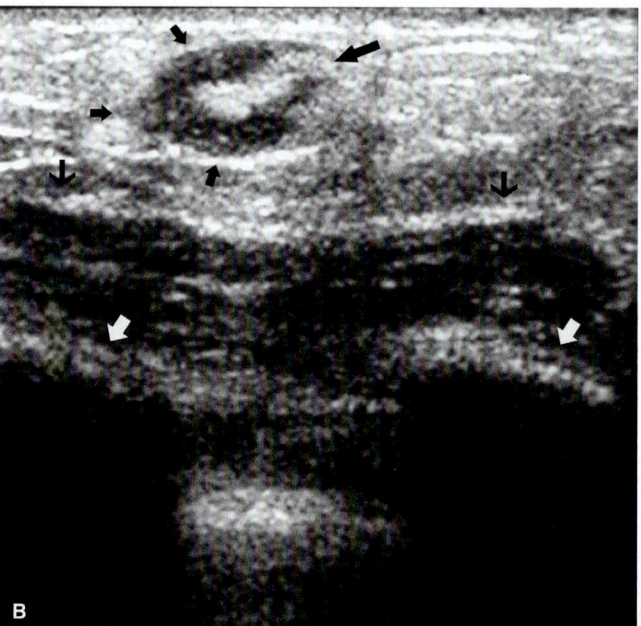

FIG. 10.7 • **Intramammary lymph node, medial. A:** Spot compression view in a 37-year-old man presenting with a "lump" *(arrow)*. Metallic BB used to denote palpable finding. Mass *(arrow)* with indistinct margins and the suggestion of a fatty notch is imaged on the spot view. **B:** Ultrasound. Oval hypoechoic mass *(small thick black arrows)* with a hyperechoic fatty hilar region *(large black arrow)* is imaged corresponding to the palpable mass. The ultrasound features are consistent with an intramammary lymph node. Deep pectoral fascia *(thin black arrows)*; ribs *(white arrows)* with associated shadowing. (From Cardeñosa G. Breast Imaging [The Core Curriculum Series]. Philadelphia, PA: Lippincott Williams & Wilkins; 2003.)

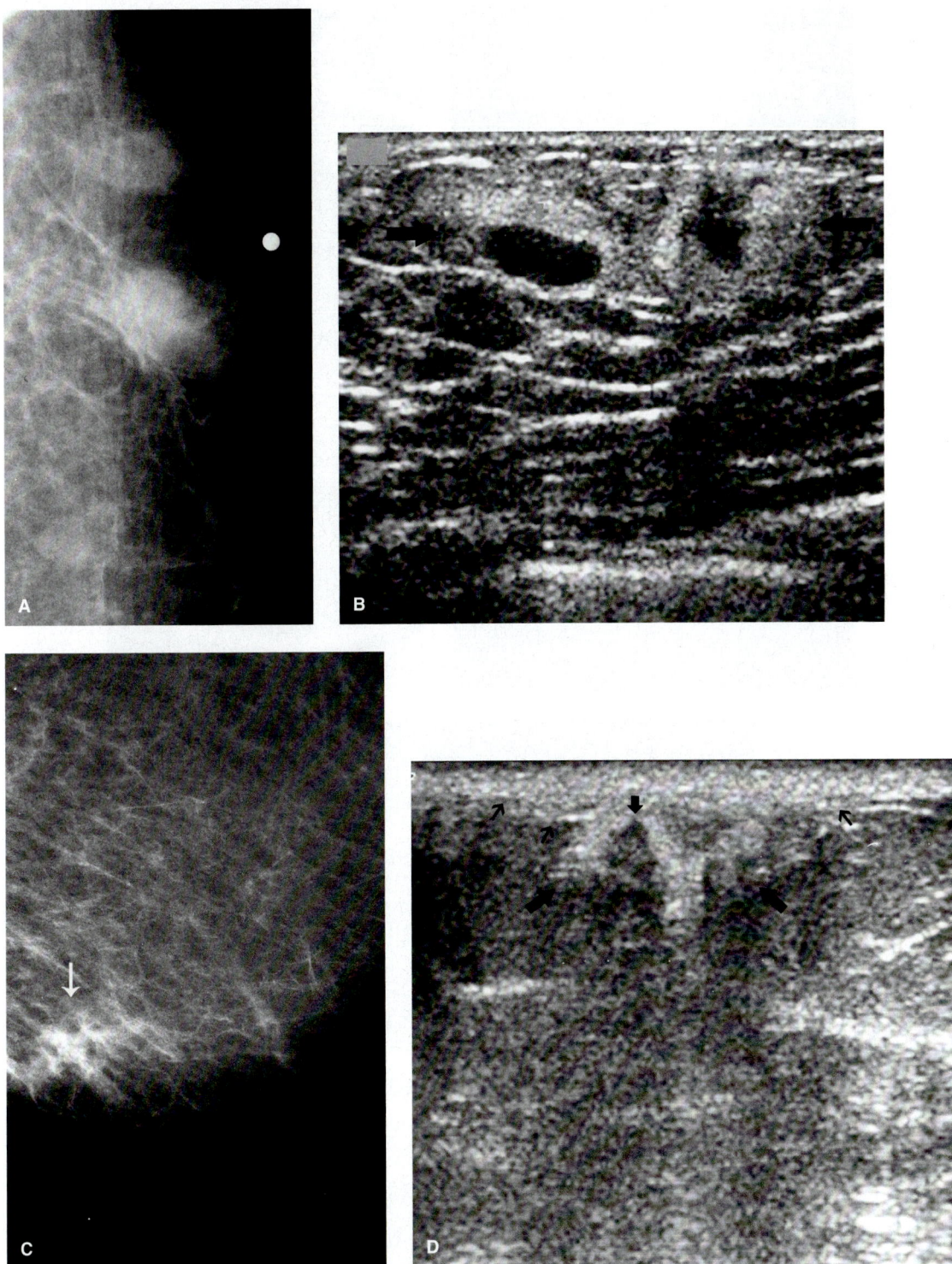

FIG. 10.8 • **Fat necrosis. A:** Left craniocaudal view. Two adjacent iso- to low-density masses with indistinct margins are imaged corresponding to a "lump" described by a 74-year-old man. Metallic BB used to denote palpable finding. **B:** Ultrasound. Two adjacent hyperechoic masses *(arrows)* with central hypoechoic areas are imaged corresponding to the palpable finding. The ultrasound features of these lesions are consistent with fat necrosis. Follow-up ultrasound 6 weeks later (not shown) demonstrates near complete resolution of the findings. **C:** Left mediolateral oblique view in a different patient presenting with a "lump." Architectural distortion is imaged at site of clinical concern *(arrow)*. **D:** Ill-defined area of hyperechogenicity *(thick long arrows)* with heterogeneity as well as an area of hypoechogenicity *(thick short arrow)* and some shadowing corresponding to the site of the palpable finding. The ultrasound features are consistent with fat necrosis. Associated skin thickening is noted *(thin arrows)*. The patient has a history of trauma to this site with complete resolution of the imaging findings on follow-up studies (not shown). (From Cardeñosa G. Breast Imaging [The Core Curriculum Series]. Philadelphia, PA: Lippincott Williams & Wilkins; 2003.)

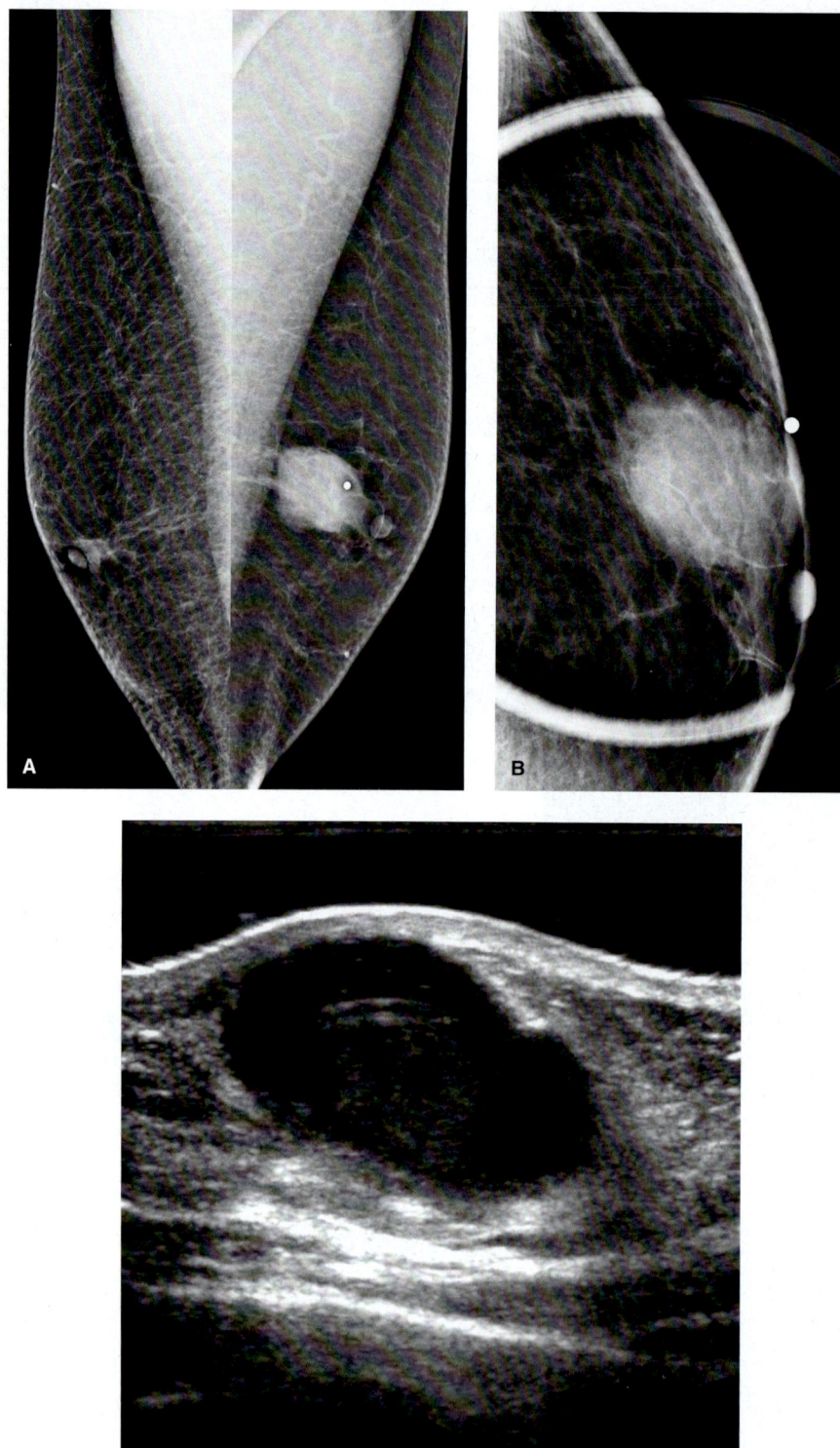

FIG. 10.9 • **Abscess. A:** Mediolateral oblique views in a 64-year-old man presenting with a "lump" in the left breast. Metallic BB used to denote site of "lump." Note small nipples typical of male patients. **B:** Spot tangential view demonstrates a round isodense mass with indistinct margins as well as focal skin thickening. Metallic BB denotes the palpable finding. **C:** Ultrasound. On physical examination, a 3 cm round area of erythema is noted at the left periareolar margin at the 3 o'clock position. No significant tenderness is elicited at this site. A complex cystic and solid mass with posterior acoustic enhancement is imaged abutting the skin correlating to the clinical and mammographic findings. An aspiration with possible core biopsy to follow is discussed with the patient. Approximately, 2 mL of thick purulent fluid is aspirated.

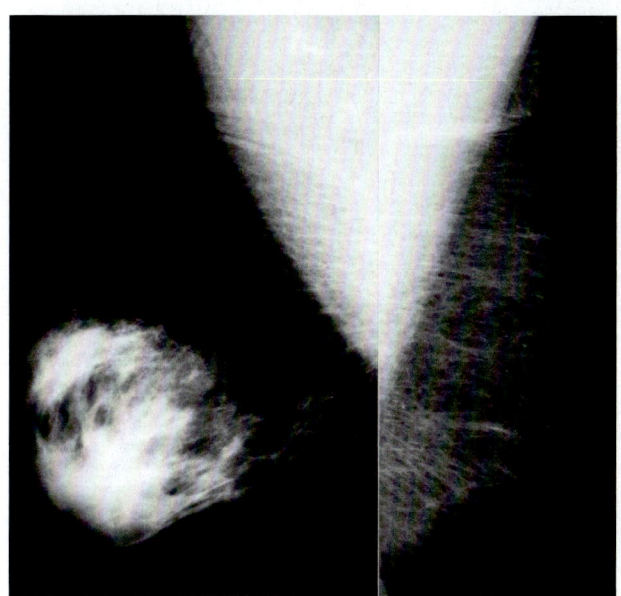 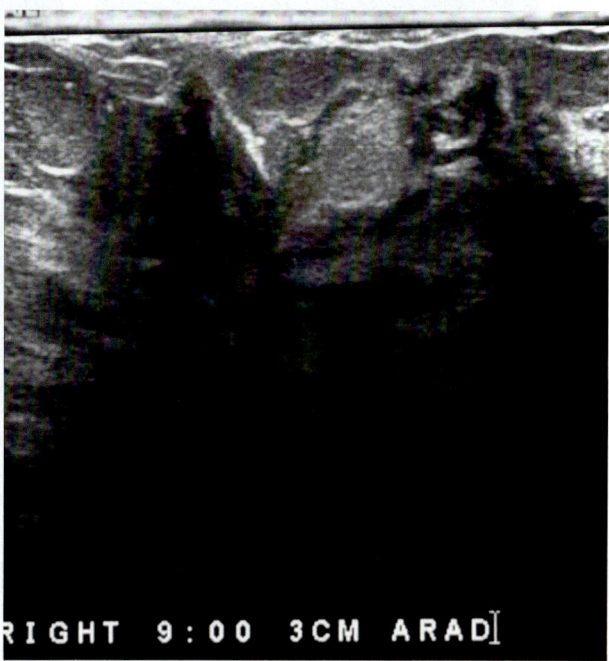

FIG. 10.10 • **Unilateral dense gynecomastia and pseudoangiomatous stromal hyperplasia (PASH). A:** Mediolateral oblique views in a 53-year-old man who presents describing rapid enlargement of the right breast with a more focal site of nodularity laterally. The right breast is larger than the left and further characterized by the presence of dense glandular tissue. Fatty tissue is imaged in the left breast. **B:** Ultrasound. Irregular masses with disruption of normal tissue planes and shadowing are imaged at the site of nodularity described by the patient laterally in the right breast. With rotation of the transducer, these areas become less prominent. Gynecomastia and PASH are diagnosed on an ultrasound guided core biopsy through this tissue. Although PASH typically presents with a mass, rapid breast enlargement has been described as an unusual presentation (see Chapter 7) for PASH.

Table 10.2	RISK FACTORS FOR MALE BREAST CANCER
Advanced age	
History of chest radiation (ionizing)	
Occupational exposure (electromagnetic field radiation)	
Cryptorchism	
Testicular injury	
Mumps (after age 20)	
Klinefelter syndrome	
Liver dysfunction (cirrhosis, schistosomiasis, malnutrition)	
Family history of breast cancer (*BRCA2*)	
Men of Jewish descent	
Exogenous estrogen use	

adenopathy is identified in approximately 50% of patients at the time of presentation. As with breast cancer in women, prognosis depends on the status of the axillary lymph nodes and the size of the tumor at the time of diagnosis. Unfortunately, many men delay seeking medical attention for breast cancer–related signs and symptoms.

Invasive ductal carcinomas represent 85% of all the cancers diagnosed in male patients. Associated ductal carcinoma in situ (DCIS) is found in 35% to 50% of patients (9–12). DCIS, in the absence of an infiltrative component, is much less common, representing approximately 5% of all breast cancers in male patients. Papillary carcinoma is the most common subtype diagnosed in male patients (9) with mucinous carcinomas also reported. The tumors are commonly estrogen and progesterone receptor positive.

A non-calcified, round or oval mass with circumscribed to indistinct margins eccentrically localized in the subareolar area is the most common mammographic finding in men with breast cancer (Fig. 10.11A, B). A mass with spiculated margins (Fig. 10.12A) that may be associated with skin or nipple retraction may also be seen (Fig. 10.12C) (12). Calcifications reflecting DCIS (Fig. 10.13) may be present associated with a mass or possibly extending beyond a mass. When present, the calcifications have been described as coarser, fewer in number, less commonly linear, and more scattered than those seen with breast cancers in women.

On ultrasound, the findings in male breast cancer are similar to those described for cancers occurring in women. This includes a hypoechoic mass with a heterogeneous echotexture (Fig. 10.11D, E), a vertically oriented mass with spiculated and angular margins,

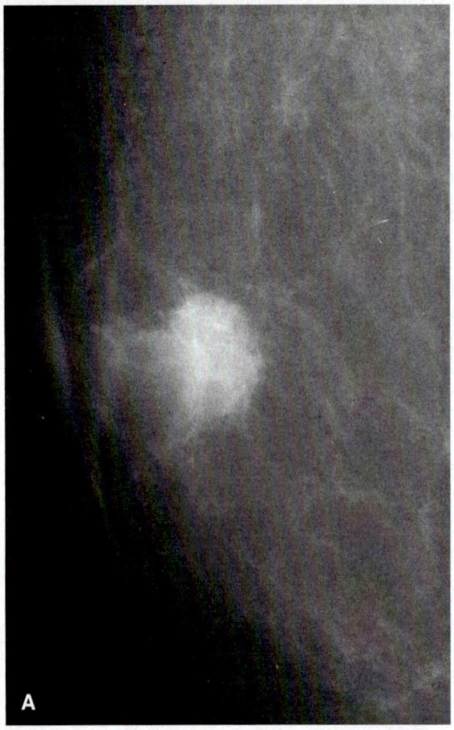

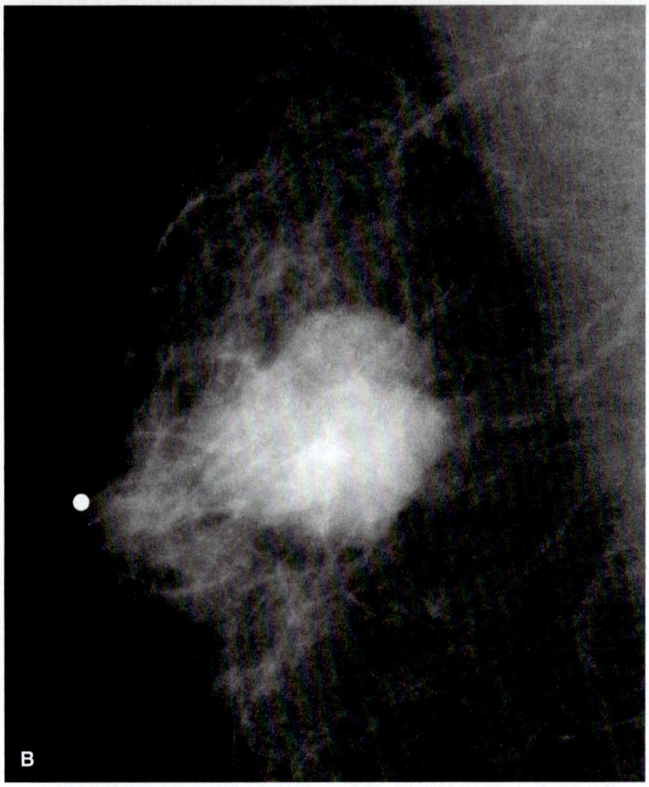

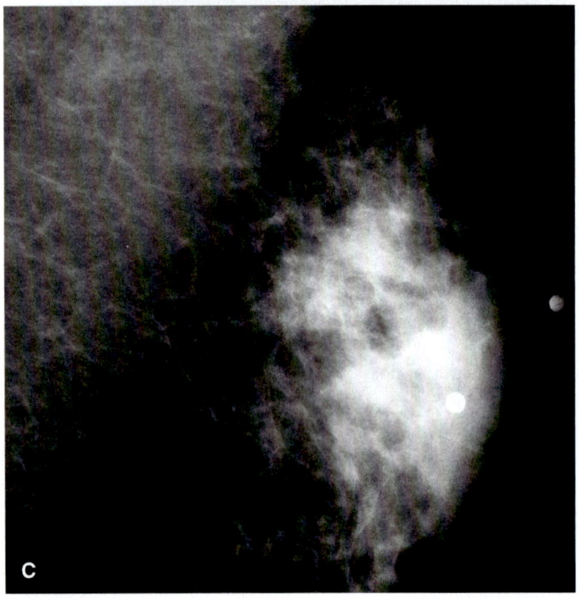

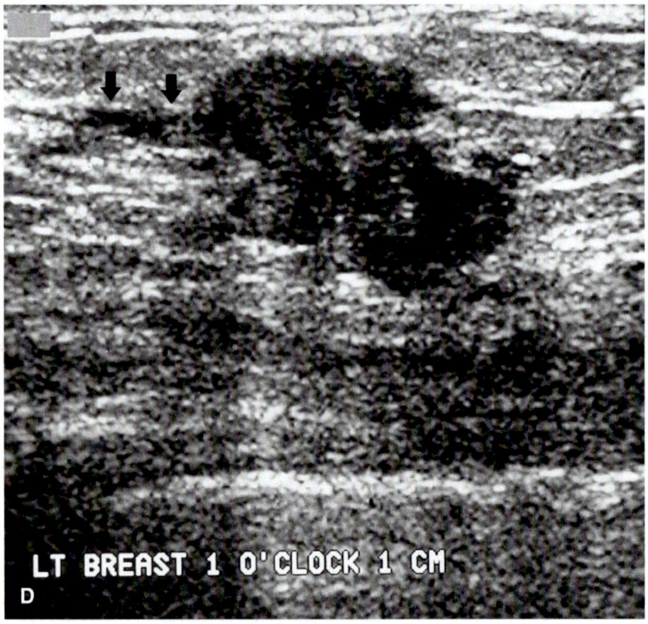

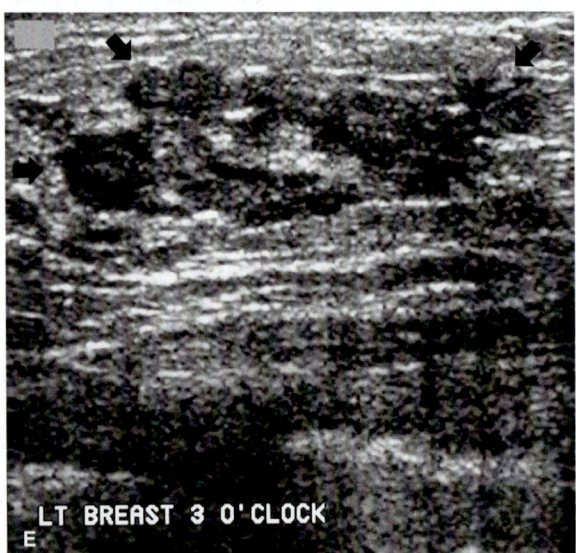

FIG. 10.11 • **Invasive ductal carcinomas, not otherwise specified. A:** Craniocaudal view, right breast. A round isodense mass with ill-defined and circumscribed margins is identified eccentrically positioned in the right subareolar area. **B:** Mediolateral oblique view, right breast different patient. A 57-year-old man on dialysis for chronic renal failure presents describing a "lump" in the right breast. A round dense mass with indistinct margins is imaged corresponding to the palpable finding. Metallic BB denotes site of palpable finding. **C:** Mediolateral oblique view of the left breast 2 years later in the patient shown in part **B** who now presents with two "lumps" in the left breast. Dense glandular tissue is imaged corresponding to the sites of the palpable findings (metallic BBs denote areas). **D:** Horizontally oriented, mass with a heterogeneous echotexture, indistinct, angular margins, and duct extension *(arrows)* is identified on ultrasound at 1 o'clock, 1 cm from the left nipple corresponding to one of the two palpable findings. **E:** A horizontally oriented mass *(arrows)* with heterogeneous echotexture, indistinct margins and microlobulation is imaged at the 3 o'clock position *(arrows)* corresponding to the second palpable finding. Multifocal breast cancer (metachronous) is confirmed on biopsies. (From Cardeñosa G. Breast Imaging [The Core Curriculum Series]. Philadelphia, PA: Lippincott Williams & Wilkins; 2003.)

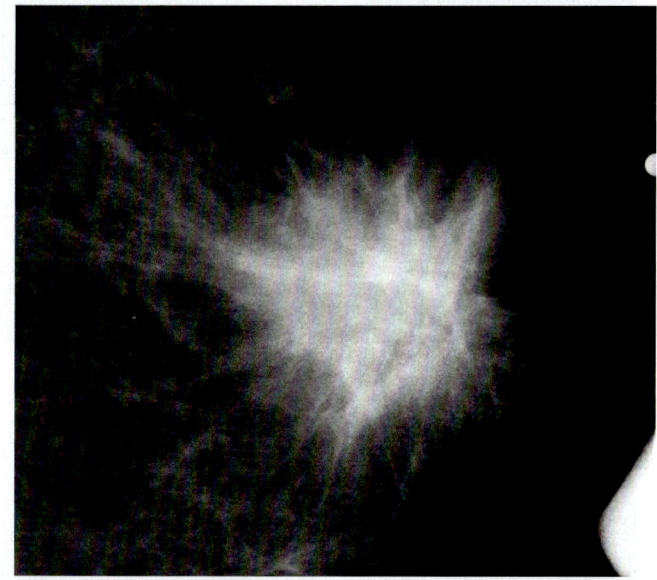
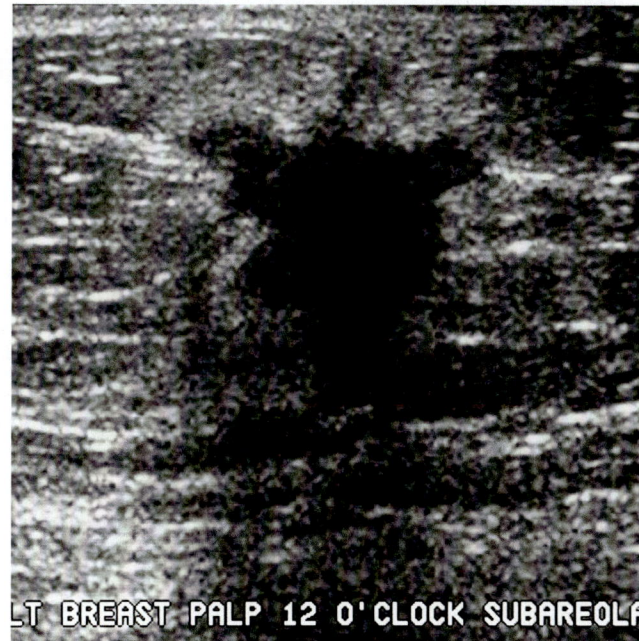
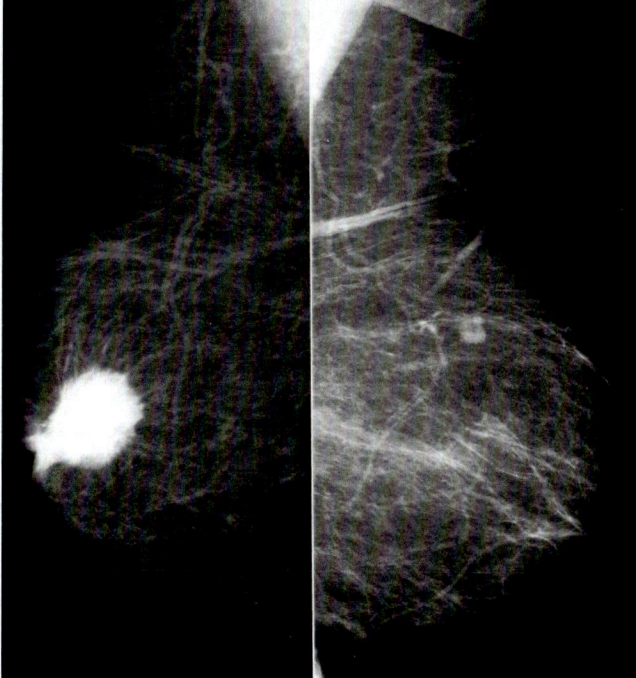

**FIG. 10.12 • Invasive ductal carcinoma, not otherwise specified.
A:** Spot compression view, left subareolar area in a 75-year-old man who presents describing a "lump" in the left breast. Metallic BB used to denote palpable finding. A dense mass with spiculated margins is imaged in the left subareolar area. **B:** Ultrasound. A vertically oriented, hypoechoic mass with angular margins, an echogenic rim, and shadowing are imaged corresponding to the clinically and mammographically apparent mass. (From Cardeñosa G. Breast Imaging [The Core Curriculum Series]. Philadelphia, PA: Lippincott Williams & Wilkins; 2003. **C:** Mediolateral oblique views in a 53-year-old man describing a "lump" in the right breast. The right breast is smaller than the left. An oval dense mass with spiculated margins is imaged in the right subareolar area with associated skin thickening and nipple retraction.

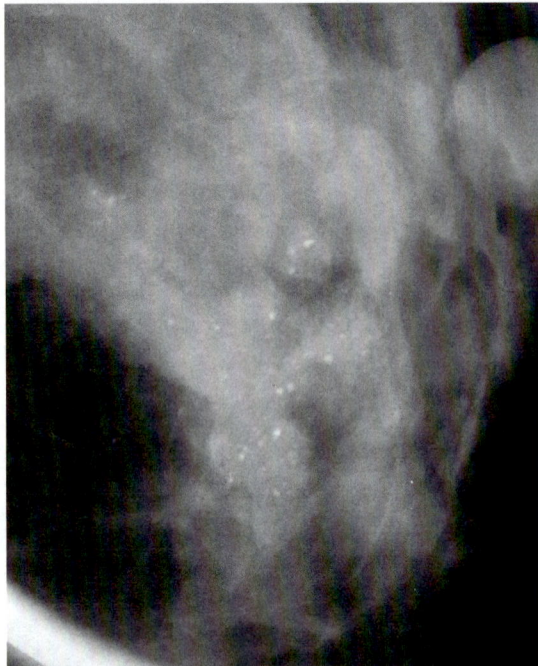

FIG. 10.13 • **Invasive ductal carcinoma, not otherwise specified with associated ductal carcinoma in situ.** Spot compression magnification view demonstrates an irregular mass with indistinct, macrolobulated margins and associated coarse heterogeneous calcifications. (From Cardeñosa G. *Breast Imaging [The Core Curriculum Series]*. Philadelphia, PA: Lippincott Williams & Wilkins; 2003.)

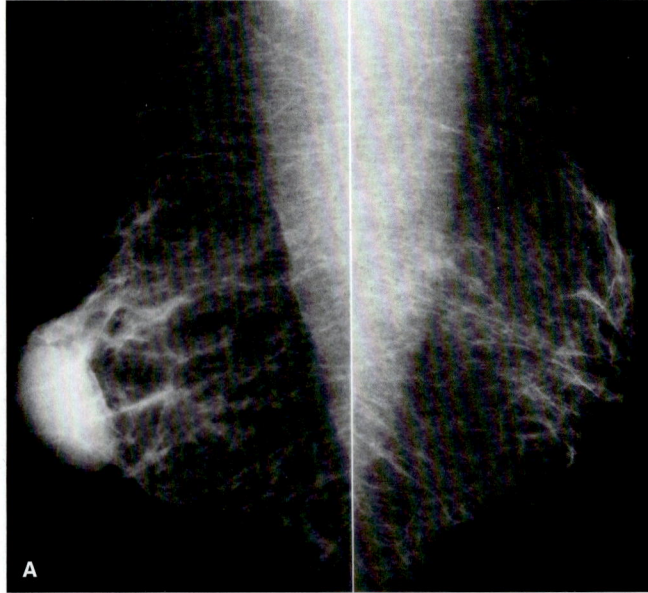

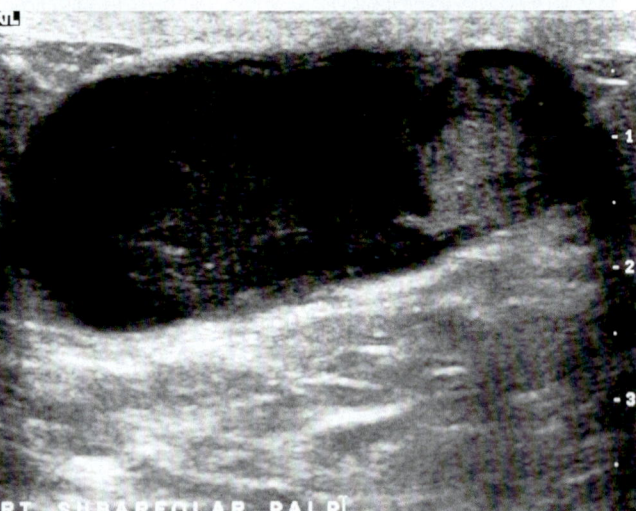

FIG. 10.14 • **Encapsulated papillary carcinoma, intermediate to high grade. A:** Mediolateral oblique views. A dense mass with circumscribed margins is imaged in the right subareolar area corresponding to a "lump" described by this 65-year-old man. **B:** Ultrasound. Complex cystic and solid mass that is predominantly cystic with a solid component. Please remember that in patients with complex cystic and solid masses, the diagnosis is not established in over 50% patients with an aspirate alone. This patient had three separate fine needle aspirations (palpation guided) all of which yielded benign results. It was only after an ultrasound-guided aspiration of the fluid and core biopsy of the remaining solid component that an accurate diagnosis was obtained on the core samples. Please see Figure 12.17 for aspiration and core biopsy images.

an echogenic rim and shadowing (Fig. 10.12B) or a complex cystic and solid mass. Associated features may include a ductal extension or a branch pattern. Complex cystic and solid masses (Fig. 10.14) are seen commonly in patients with papillary lesions (9). The MRI features of cancers developing in men are similar to those seen in women (Fig. 10.15).

Breast cancer in men is usually treated with mastectomy and either sentinel lymph node biopsy or axillary dissection. Radiation therapy may be given to the chest wall for larger lesions and chemotherapy may be added based on the status of the axillary lymph nodes. Although there is no data in the literature to support the use of screening mammography on the contralateral breast, we recommend this for men in our practice with a history of breast cancer.

METASTATIC DISEASE

Metastatic carcinoma to the breast in men is rare. Prostate cancer is the most commonly reported (10,11); hematopoietic (Fig. 10.16), lymphoreticular, melanoma and lung (Fig. 10.17) cancers occur less frequently. Mammographically, a round mass with circumscribed to indistinct margins is the most common finding. On ultrasound, a mass with circumscribed to indistinct margins and a homogeneous (Fig. 10.18) or a heterogeneous hypoechoic echotexture may be seen. A complex cystic and solid mass is seen when there is associated tumor necrosis. Posterior acoustic enhancement may be seen with some of the more rapidly growing lesions.

The Male Breast

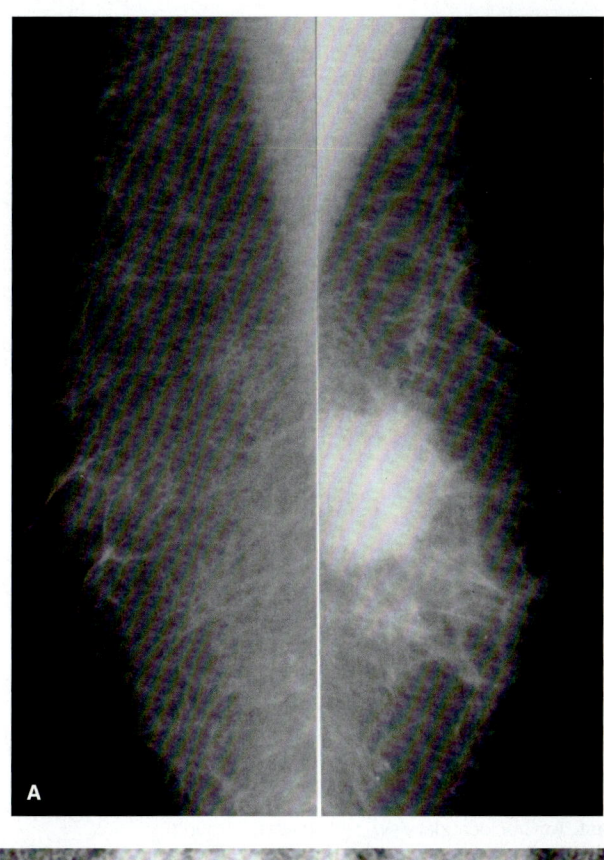
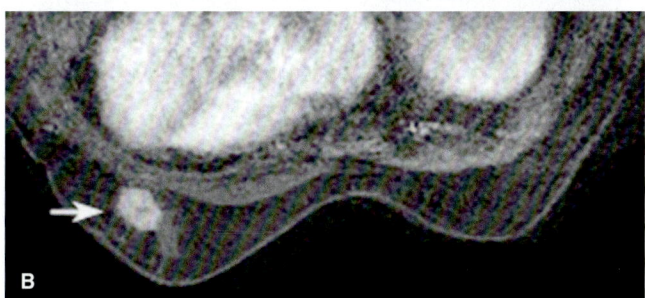
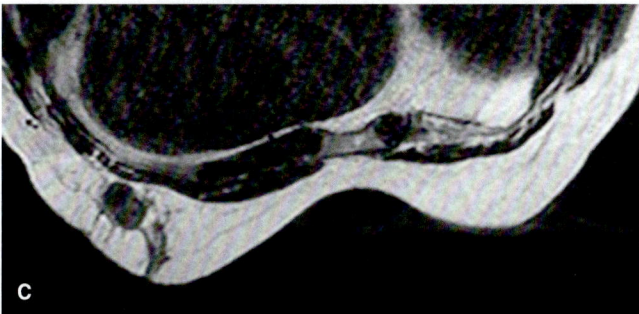

FIG. 10.15 • **Invasive ductal carcinoma. A:** Mediolateral oblique views in a 57-year-old man. Although positioning is not optimal, a high-density mass with indistinct margins is partially imaged in the left breast posteriorly. **B:** Magnetic resonance imaging, axial T1-weighted image, post contrast. An oval mass *(arrow)* with heterogeneous enhancement and spiculated margins is imaged in the left breast posterolaterally. This mass demonstrates rapid wash in and a mixture of wash out and plateau-type–delayed kinetic curves. **C:** Magnetic resonance imaging, axial T2-weighted image. An oval mass with low T2 signal is imaged in the left breast correlating to the known site of malignancy.

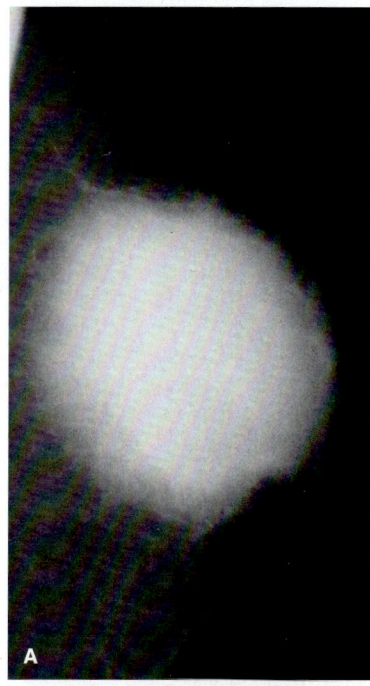
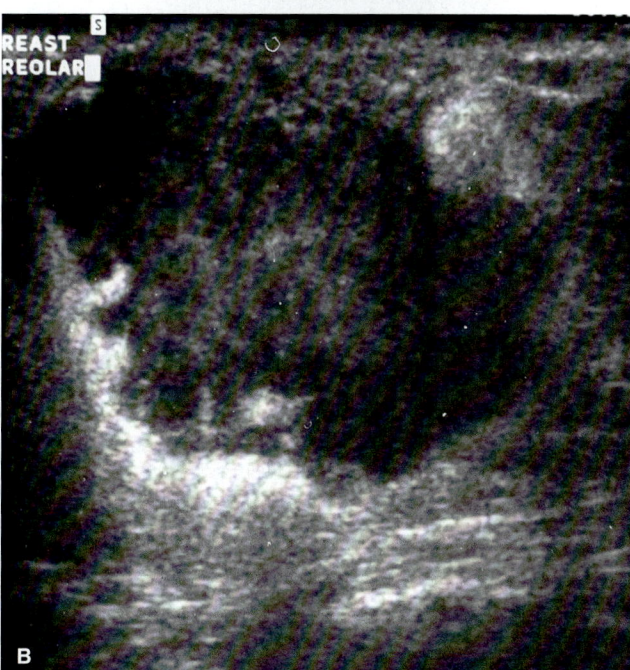

FIG. 10.16 • **Metastatic leukemia. A:** Craniocaudal view, left breast. A dense mass with indistinct margins is imaged in left subareolar area in a 21-year-old male patient with a history of leukemia. **B:** Ultrasound. Irregular, vertically oriented, heterogeneously hypoechoic mass with angular margins, an echogenic rim, and some posterior enhancement corresponding to the palpable mass in the subareolar area of the left breast. (From Cardeñosa G. *Breast Imaging [The Core Curriculum Series]*. Philadelphia, PA: Lippincott Williams & Wilkins; 2003.)

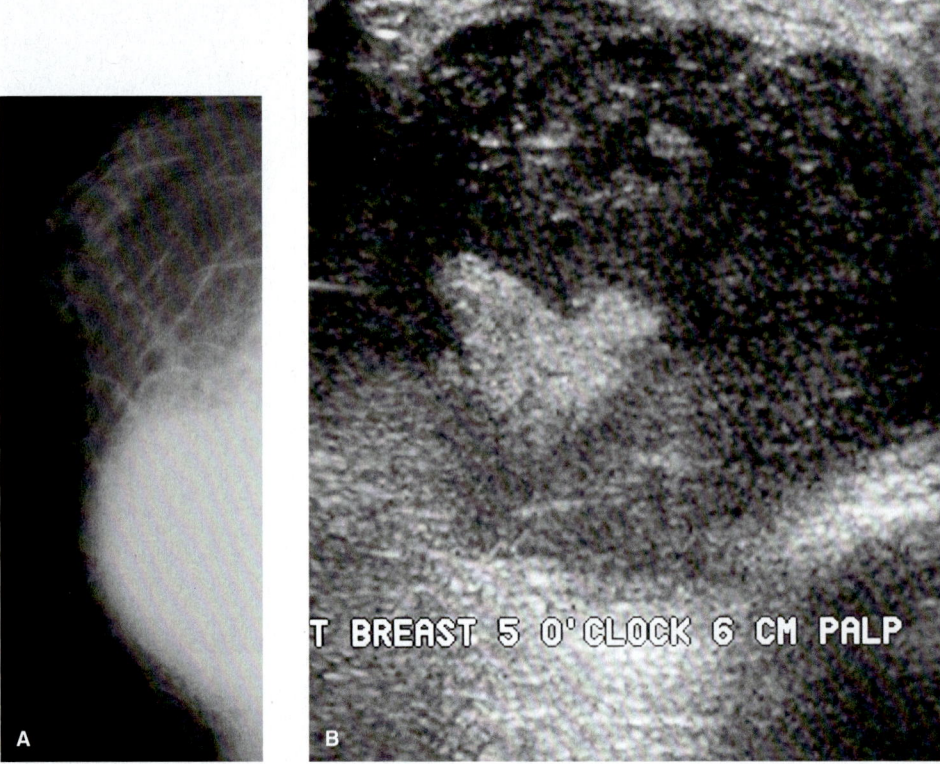

FIG. 10.17 • **Metastatic lung carcinoma to the breast. A:** Craniocaudal view, right breast. A round high-density mass with indistinct margins is partially imaged posteromedially in the right breast, in a 77-year-old male patient with a history of lung cancer. **B:** Ultrasound. Round mass with a heterogeneous echotexture and posterior acoustic enhancement. (From Cardeñosa G. *Breast Imaging [The Core Curriculum Series]*. Philadelphia, PA: Lippincott Williams & Wilkins; 2003.)

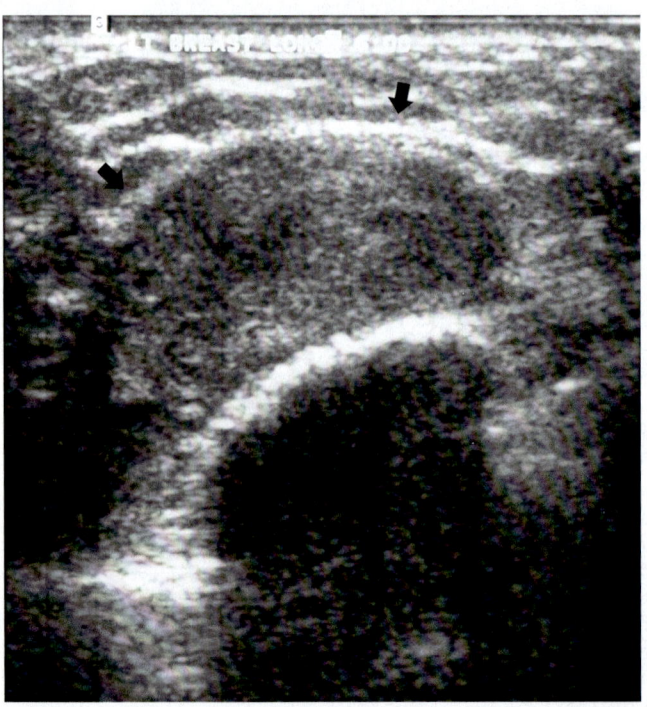

FIG. 10.18 • **Pleomorphic liposarcoma.** An 86-year-old patient presents describing a "lump" in the left breast. The palpable finding could not be imaged mammographically. An oval, homogeneously hypoechoic mass with circumscribed margins is imaged readily on ultrasound corresponding to the palpable finding *(arrows)*. Rib with associated shadowing is imaged deep to the mass. As illustrated in this patient, and previously discussed, ultrasound is helpful in evaluating areas that may be difficult to image with mammography. (From Cardeñosa G. *Breast Imaging [The Core Curriculum Series]*. Philadelphia, PA: Lippincott Williams & Wilkins; 2003.)

References

1. Bradley FM, Hoover HC, Hulka CA, et al. The sternalis muscle: an unusual normal finding seen on mammography. *AJR Am J Roentgenol.* 1996;166:33–36.
2. Raikos A, Paraskevas GK, Tzika M, et al. Sternalis muscle: an underestimated anterior chest wall anatomical variant. *J Cardiothorac Surg.* 2011;6:73.
3. Cooper RA, Gunter BA, Ramamurthy L. Mammography in men. *Radiology.* 1994;191:651–656.
4. Appelbaum AH, Evans GFF, Levy KR, et al. Mammographic appearances of male breast disease. *Radiographics.* 1999;19:559–568.
5. Dershaw D. Male mammography. *AJR Am J Roentgenol.* 1986;146:127–131.
6. Chantra PK, So GJ, Wollman JS, et al. Mammography of the male breast. *AJR Am J Roentgenol.* 1995;164:853–858.
7. Hendrix TM, Tobin CE, Resnikoff LB, et al. Breast imaging case of the day. *Radiographics.* 1996;16:452–455.
8. Siegel R, Ma J, Zou Z, Jemal A. Cancer Statistics, 2014. *CA Cancer J Clin.* 2014;64:9–29.
9. Yang WT, Whitman GJ, Yuen EHY, et al. Sonographic features of primary breast cancer in men. *AJR Am J Roentgenol.* 2001;176:413–416.
10. Rosen PP. *Rosen's Breast Pathology.* 3rd ed. Philadelphia, PA: Lippincott Williams & Wilkins; 2008.
11. Tavassoli FA. *Pathology of the Breast.* 2nd ed. New York, NY: McGraw Hill; 1999.
12. Matthew J, Perkins GH, Stephens T, et al. Primary breast cancer in men: clinical, imaging and pathologic findings in 57 patients. *AJR Am J Roentgenol.* 2008;191:1631–1639.

CHAPTER SELF-ASSESSMENT QUESTIONS

1. Craniocaudal and mediolateral oblique views (left and center) as well as a spot tangential view (right) of the right breast in 47-year-old man presenting with a "lump." What is the most likely diagnosis?

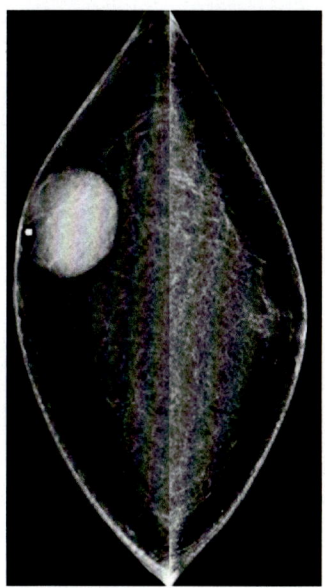
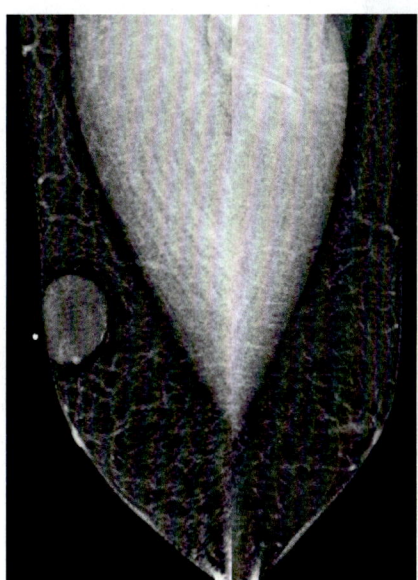
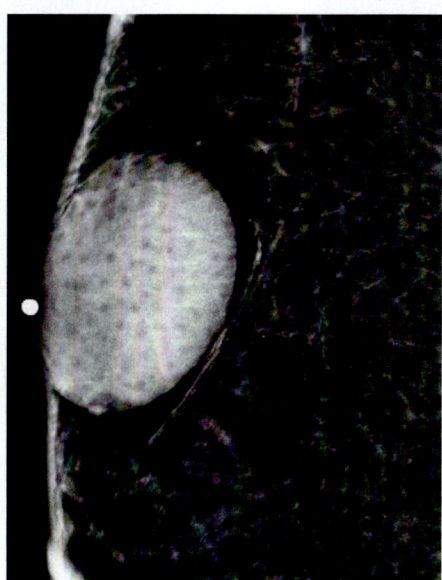

A. Cyst
B. Fibroadenoma
C. Sebaceous cyst
D. Invasive lobular carcinoma

2. Craniocaudal and mediolateral oblique views (top and bottom) in 39-year-old man presenting with "lumps" bilaterally. What would you recommend?

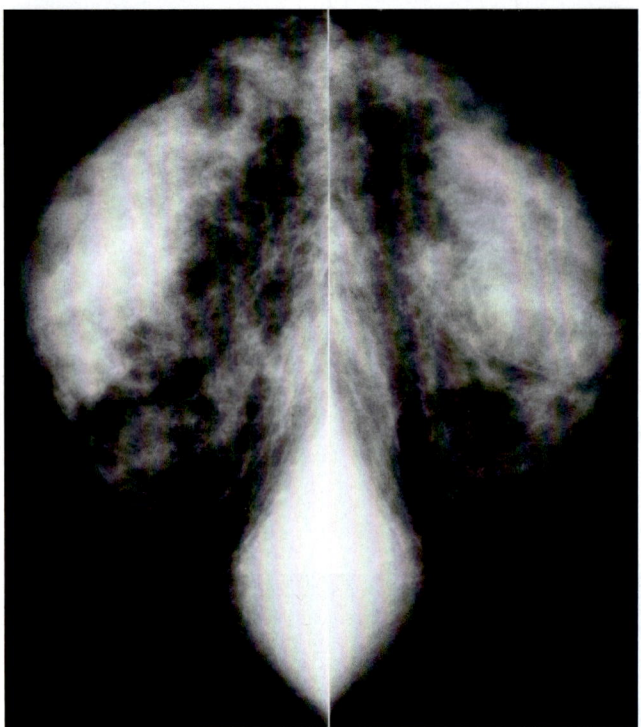

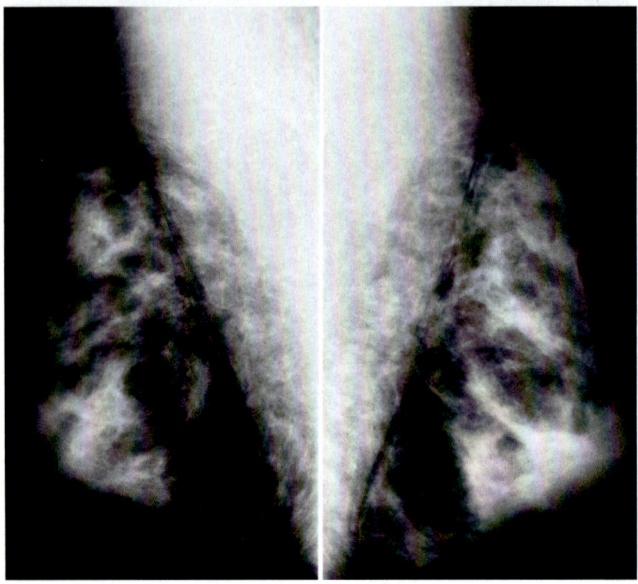

A. Annual mammography for increased breast cancer risk
B. Bilateral whole breast ultrasound
C. Six-month follow-up mammogram
D. Detailed drug history, hormone levels and a testicular examination

Answers to Chapter Self-Assessment Questions

1. C The images demonstrate an isodense mass with circumscribed margins. A lucency (best seen on the MLO view) outlines the borders of the mass suggesting a skin location; the relationship of this lesion to the skin is confirmed on the spot tangential view. Cysts, fibroadenomas and invasive lobular carcinomas are all lobular derivatives; lobules and lobular-derived pathology are not typically seen in normal men (e.g., men with no exposure to exogenous estrogen).

2. D Gynecomastia is present bilaterally. Note prominence of the pectoral muscles medially, commonly seen in men. Gynecomastia requires no additional follow-up and is not associated with increased risk of breast cancer; consequently annual studies are not appropriate. Gynecomastia may be seen in newborns, during puberty and in elderly men; however, in a 39-year-old patient, the main concern should center on why he has developed this degree of gynecomastia. A detailed drug history should be the starting point. If not drug related, hormone levels and a careful testicular exam may be appropriate to exclude an estrogen-secreting tumor.

The Altered Breast

11

LEARNING OBJECTIVES

1. Imaging findings and evolution of biopsy-related changes
2. Imaging findings of trauma-related changes in the breast
3. Imaging findings and evolution of changes expected following lumpectomy and radiation therapy
4. Medical complications related to breast hypertrophy
5. Imaging findings associated to reduction mammoplasty
6. Imaging women with implants
7. Imaging implant-related complications

EXCISIONAL BIOPSY CHANGES

Accurate pre-operative wire localization methods facilitate minimal volume biopsies and an increasing number of minimally invasive imaging-guided needle biopsies have reduced the need for excisional biopsies. Consequently, the likelihood of an excisional biopsy creating a permanent change that affects subsequent mammographic interpretations has decreased significantly. When post-operative changes occur, they often resolve in the first several months after the procedure. Unless a mammogram is done in the first 6 months following a biopsy, annual mammograms are normal in over 50% of these women (1–3) and, in those women in whom a change is seen, it is often recognizable as related to a biopsy particularly when correlated with history to the site of the biopsy.

The technologists take a careful history, inspect the breast, and document the site of any scars on the patient's history sheet. This allows the interpreting radiologist to correlate any findings on the mammogram with prior biopsy sites. Although we do not routinely mark biopsy scars at the time screening studies are done, thin wires or metallic BBs can be used (2). Given the expense associated with these markers, in conjunction with the high number of women who have had at least one breast biopsy, we reserve the use of markers for the few patients a year in whom there is a question about an area of mammographic concern correlating with a biopsy site. Most importantly, when reviewing images, we want to minimize distractions that may interfere with our ability to identify early-stage breast cancers; metallic makers (e.g., for nipples) and wires are a distraction that, in most patients, provide no useful diagnostic information (Fig. 11.1).

Changes that may be seen on a mammogram correlating with excisional biopsy sites include skin thickening and retraction, distortion (Fig. 11.2) that is often seen best in one of the standard views and subtle or not apparent in the other view, and a round, oval, or irregular mass possibly fat-containing with spiculated or indistinct margins (Fig. 11.3) (4). Depending on the amount of tissue excised, generalized

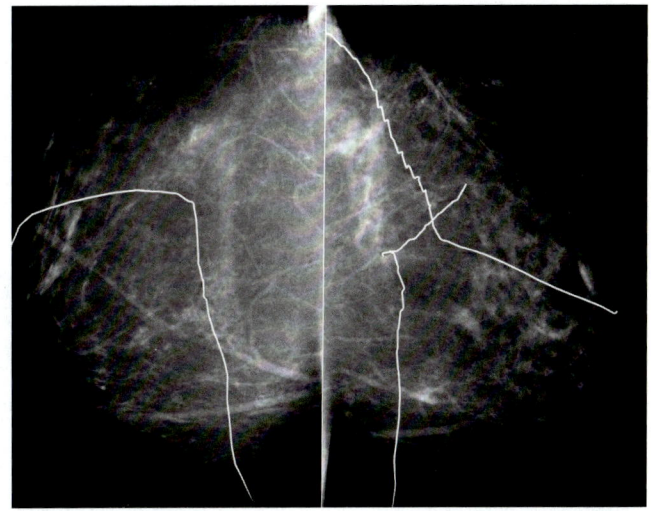

FIG. 11.1 • **Biopsy markers.** CC views. Wires used to mark prior incisions for a reduction mammoplasty. The first things you notice are the wires distracting you from the task at hand. Given the potential for distraction, lack of changes related to prior biopsies in more than 50% of patients, and the cost of the markers, we do not routinely mark prior biopsy sites. Even in patients with post-biopsy changes, the findings are distinctive enough that, in combination with the history, a confident diagnosis is made without the use of markers. For similar reasons, we do not use nipple markers. (From Cardeñosa G. *Breast Imaging [The Core Curriculum Series]*. Philadelphia, PA: Lippincott Williams & Wilkins; 2003.)

observations may include asymmetry in the size of the breasts with the operated breast being smaller and parenchymal asymmetry such that less tissue is present at the surgery site compared with remaining tissue at the corresponding site in the contralateral breast (Fig. 11.4). Except for the asymmetric breast size and resulting parenchymal asymmetry

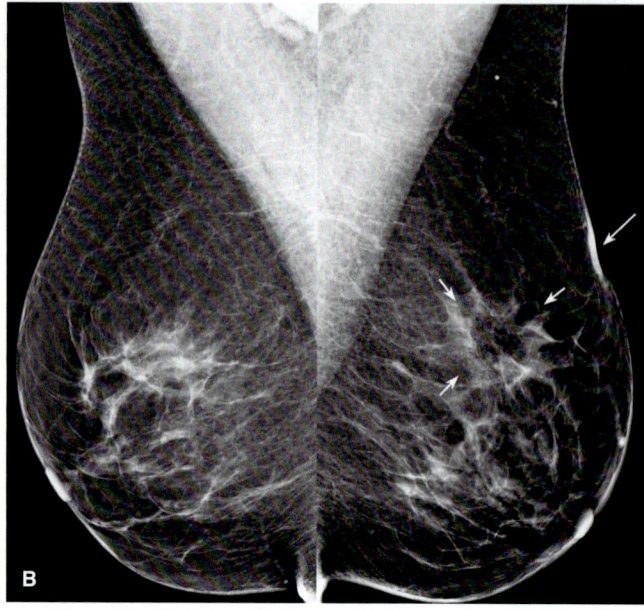

FIG. 11.2 • **Biopsy-related changes, left breast.** CC **(A)** and MLO **(B)** views in a 48-year-old woman 3 years after an excisional biopsy of the left breast. Distortion *(arrow)* is apparent laterally in the left breast on the CC projection. Focal skin thickening *(long arrow)* and distortion *(short arrows)* on the MLO view, the overall configuration and fat content of which, is different from the appearance of this area on the CC view. When distortion is seen more prominently in one of the two standard projections, review the patient's history for prior breast surgery. Reviewing the mammograms of women who have had prior excisional biopsies is a good way to teach yourself how to detect subtle areas of distortion.

seen in some patients, focal changes usually resolve completely on serial mammograms, remain stable after the first year or slowly evolve with time (Fig. 11.5). Increasing amounts of fat centrally in a mass, dispersion of the density, oil cyst formation, and the development of dystrophic calcifications are changes that can be seen on follow up (1–4). Occasionally, retained fragments of the localization wire (Fig. 11.6A), needle tips, or foreign bodies (Fig. 11.6B) may be seen at prior surgical sites.

When biopsy changes are noted mammographically and correlated to a biopsy site, evaluation with ultrasound or magnetic resonance imaging (MRI) is not usually indicated. Ultrasound and MRI findings, however, will vary significantly depending on the timing of

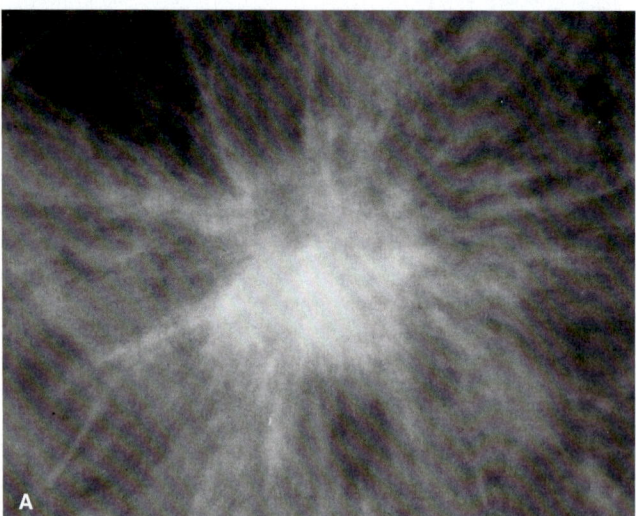
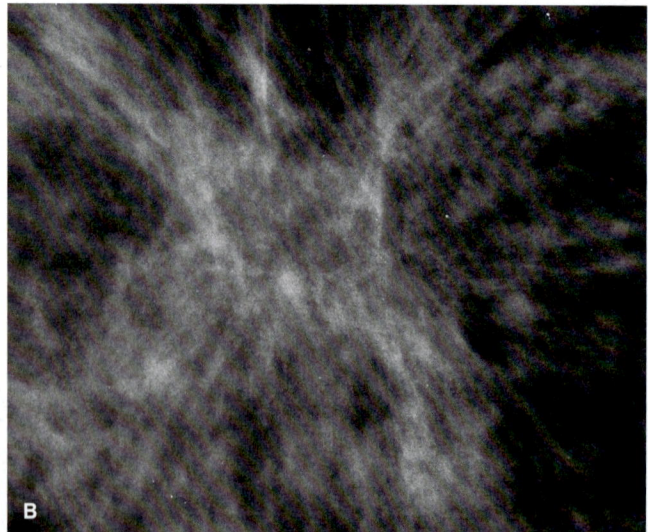

FIG. 11.3 • **Biopsy-related fat necrosis. A:** An isodense round mass with spiculated margins is imaged corresponding to a prior biopsy site. **B:** On a follow-up study, the previously noted central density (mass) has been replaced with fat and the remaining finding is best described as distortion. This may stabilize, or if the soft tissue component continues to resolve, an oil cyst and dystrophic calcifications may develop. You should use biopsy changes such as these to test your ability to detect subtle areas of distortion and spiculation. If you can detect these findings in patients who have had a biopsy, you will probably detect small, subtle breast cancers presenting with distortion on screening studies. (From Cardeñosa G. *Breast Imaging [The Core Curriculum Series]*. Philadelphia, PA: Lippincott Williams & Wilkins; 2003.)

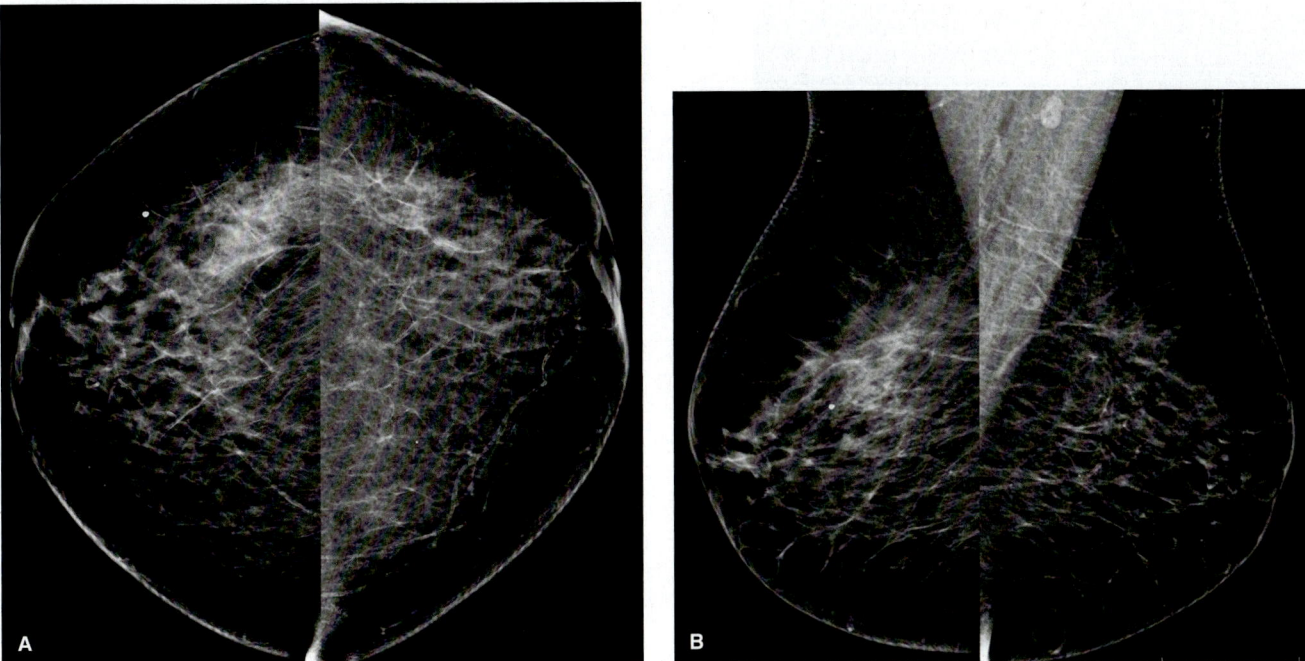

FIG. 11.4 ● **Biopsy changes, left breast.** CC **(A)** and MLO **(B)** views in a 68-year-old woman many years following an excisional biopsy of the left breast. Parenchymal asymmetry is evident with less tissue noted in the upper outer quadrant of the left breast. Subtle skin changes are noted laterally in the left CC and distortion is noted superiorly in the left oblique view.

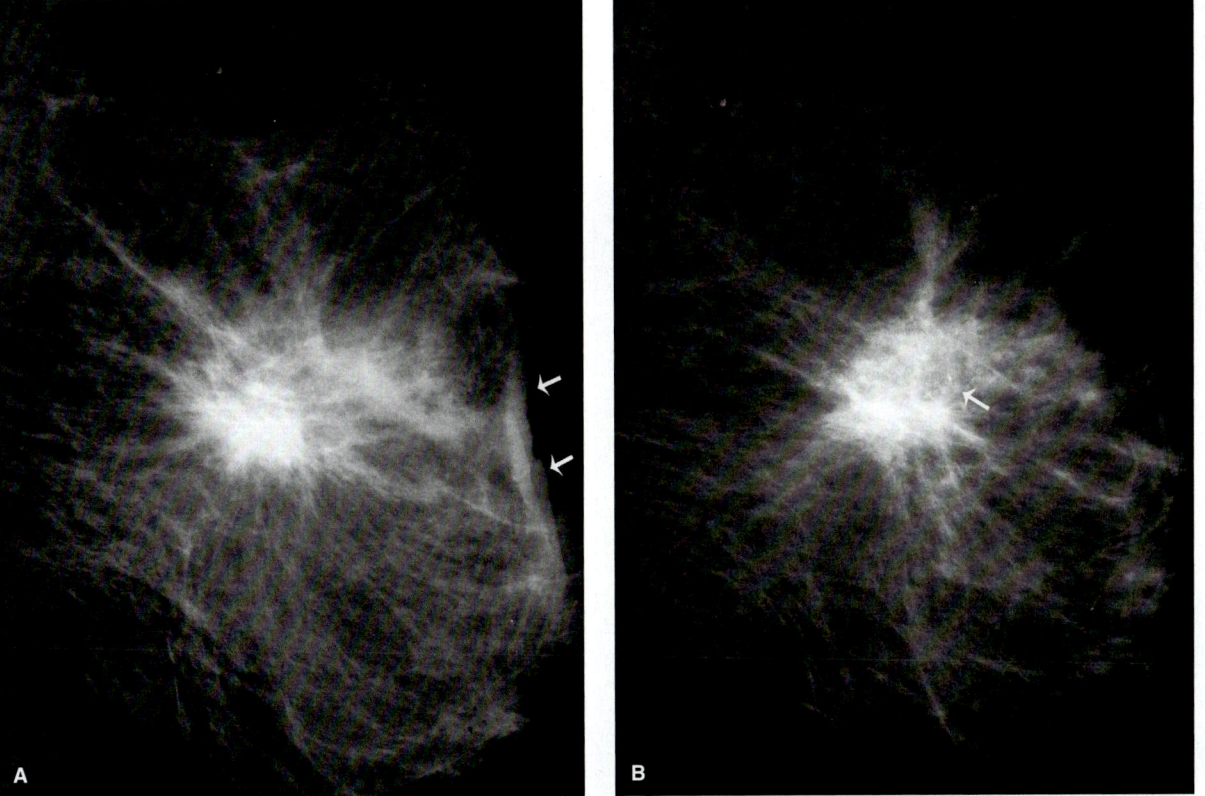

FIG. 11.5 ● **Evolution of biopsy changes. A:** MLO view photographically coned to the anterior aspect of the left breast obtained 2 months following an excisional biopsy. A mass with spiculated margins and associated distortion is noted correlating to the excisional biopsy site. Skin changes including thickening, distortion, and retraction are present *(arrows)*. **B:** Six months following the image in part **A**, 8 months following the biopsy. The mass persists, however, is smaller and less dense. A lucent area is developing in the center *(arrow)* associated with some punctate calcifications. Skin changes are less prominent. **C:** One year following the biopsy. The overall size and shape of the remaining density is changed compared with the mass seen in **A** and **B**. Distortion persists and dense, coarse calcifications are now present centrally. (From Cardeñosa G. *Breast Imaging [The Core Curriculum Series]*. Philadelphia, PA: Lippincott Williams & Wilkins; 2003.)

(continued)

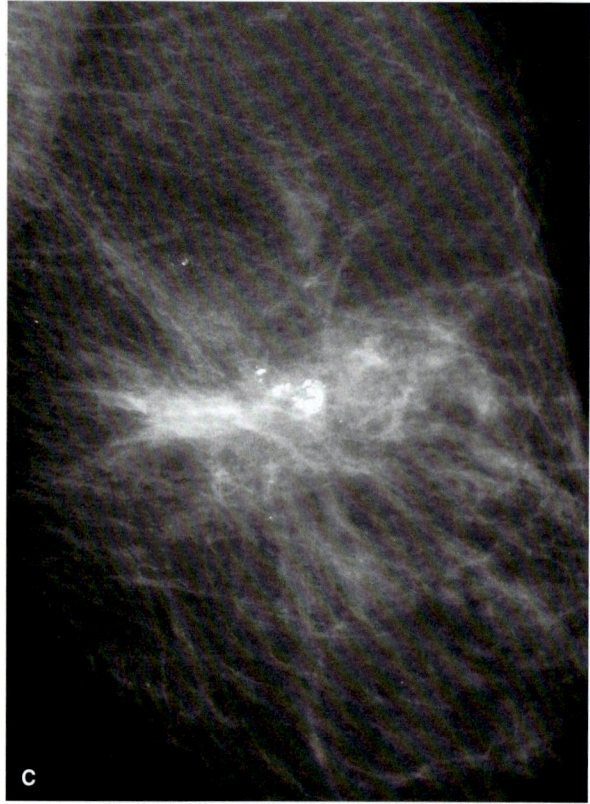

these studies to the biopsy. Acutely, biopsy changes on ultrasound may be characterized by increases in the echogenicity of the tissue, loss of normal soft tissue planes, fluid collections (Fig. 11.7A) that may be complex and skin thickening. Distortion and shadowing (5) that may be seen best in one plane and become less apparent as the transducer is rotated 90-degrees are common findings at long-standing biopsy sites.

On MRI, an irregular mass with mural or internal areas of high T1 and T2 signal and minimal or no enhancement is a common finding for acute hematomas (Fig. 11.7B–D; also see Fig. 5.9); if enhancement is present, it is often thin and peripheral in location. Subacute and chronic post-operative fluid collections may demonstrate a heterogeneously high T2 signal with intermediate to low T1 signal and internal non-enhancing nodules. Minimal enhancement may be noted involving the wall of the collection. Following re-absorption of post-operative fluid collections, increased non-enhancing soft tissue with distortion, an associated fat signal and skin changes (retraction, focal thickening) may be apparent.

Post-operative changes are characterized by progressive resolution or stability needs to be established on annual studies. This is particularly important in patients with a high-risk lesion (e.g., atypical ductal hyperplasia, lobular neoplasia, and multiple peripheral papillomas) diagnosed on excisional biopsy, or those with a personal or significant family history of breast cancer. In these patients, a mammogram 6 months after the biopsy is helpful in establishing the presence of any biopsy change (e.g., a new baseline for the patient). Changes seen 6 months after a biopsy are unlikely to represent recurrent or interval cancer. On subsequent studies, however, we expect the changes to

FIG. 11.5 • (continued)

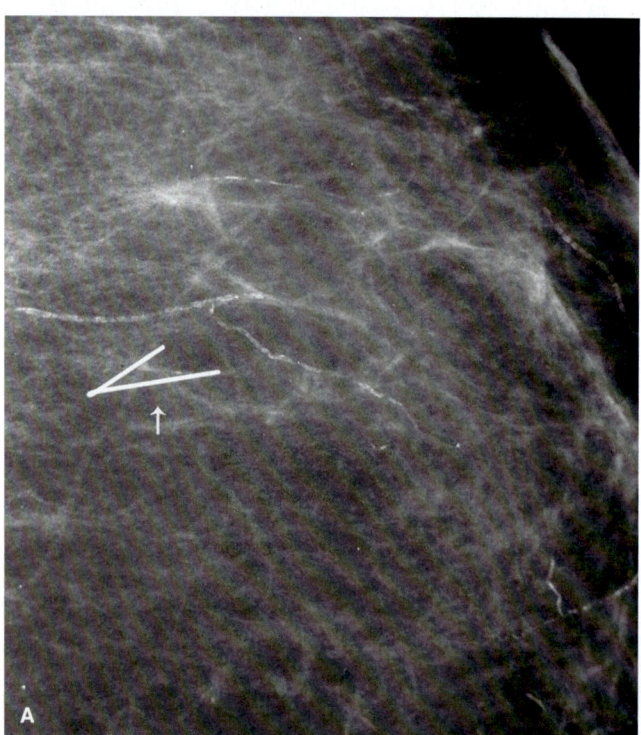
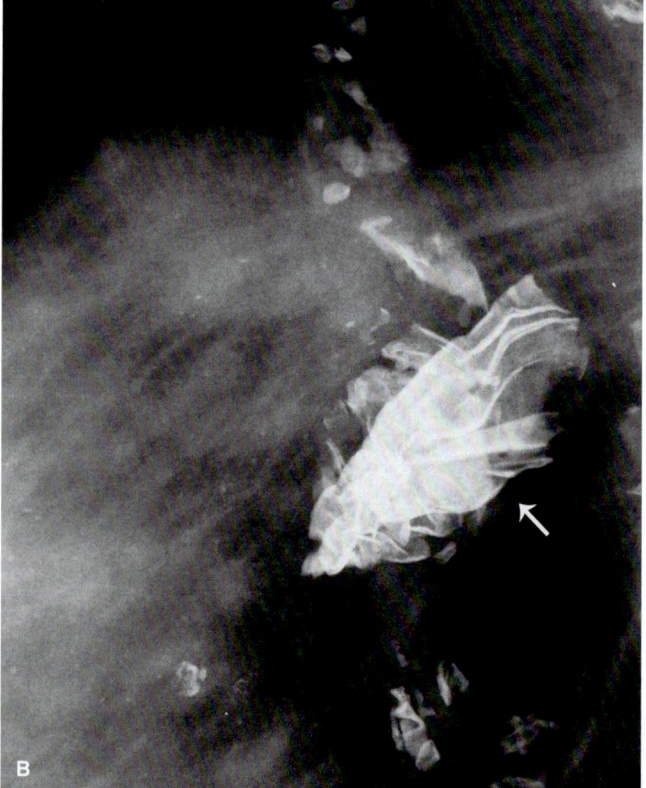

FIG. 11.6 • **Retained localization wire fragment and foreign body. A:** Intraoperative transection of the localization wire can result in retained wire fragments in the breast (arrow). Vascular calcification is present. **B:** Different patient. Radiopaque foreign body (arrow) is noted corresponding to a prior biopsy site. (From Cardeñosa G. *Breast Imaging [The Core Curriculum Series]*. Philadelphia, PA: Lippincott Williams & Wilkins; 2003.)

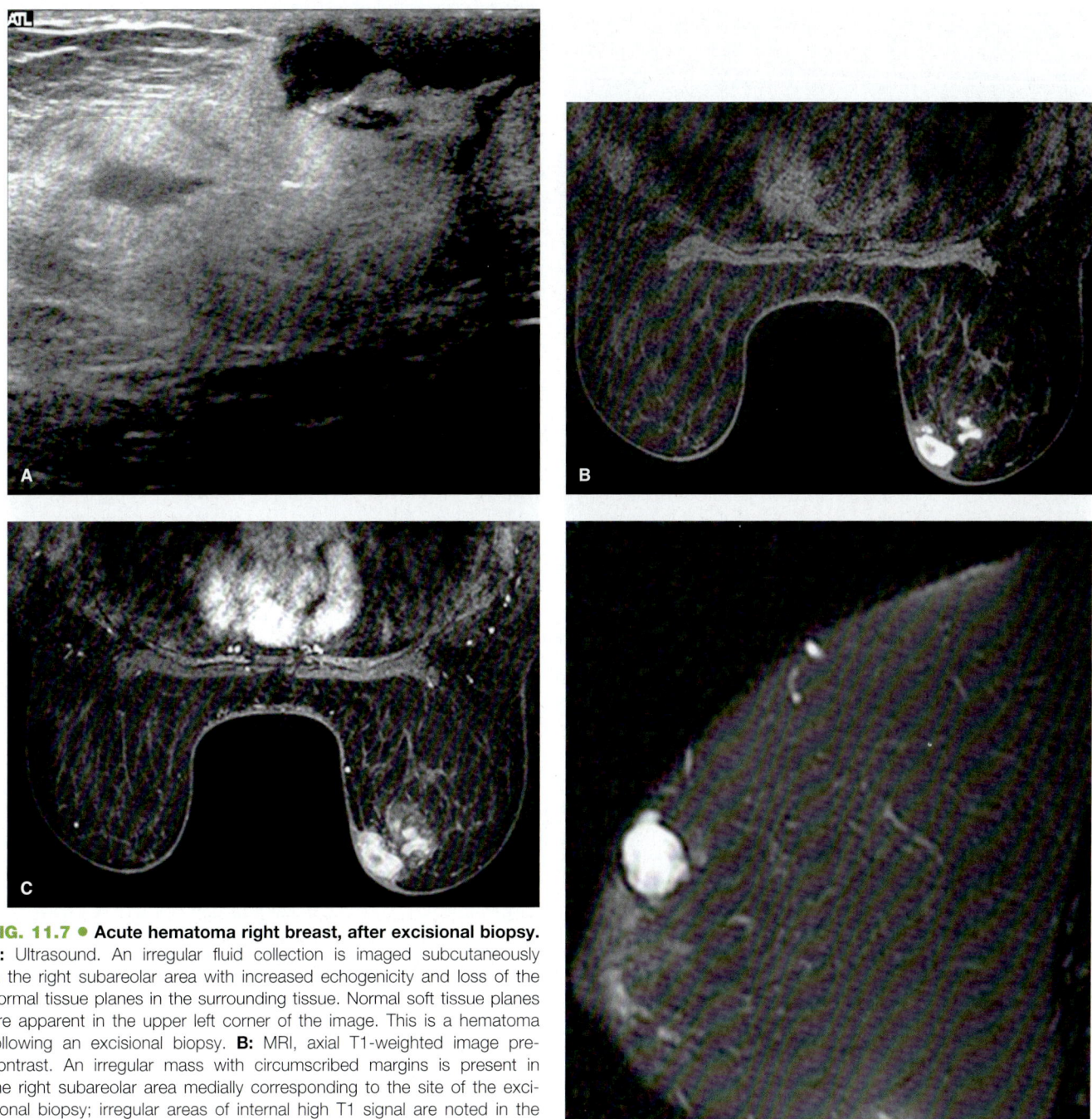

FIG. 11.7 • Acute hematoma right breast, after excisional biopsy. A: Ultrasound. An irregular fluid collection is imaged subcutaneously in the right subareolar area with increased echogenicity and loss of the normal tissue planes in the surrounding tissue. Normal soft tissue planes are apparent in the upper left corner of the image. This is a hematoma following an excisional biopsy. **B:** MRI, axial T1-weighted image precontrast. An irregular mass with circumscribed margins is present in the right subareolar area medially corresponding to the site of the excisional biopsy; irregular areas of internal high T1 signal are noted in the mass. **C:** MRI, T1-weighted image post contrast. No enhancement is noted in the mass. **D:** MRI T2-weighted sagittal fat-suppressed image of the right breast. Heterogeneously high T2 signal is noted in the right subareolar mass corresponding to areas of high T1 signal shown in part **B** consistent with an acute hematoma.

stabilize or, more commonly, evolve, becoming less prominent with time. Increases in distortion or density at a biopsy site after the initial 6-month post-operative study warrant a biopsy recommendation and a review of the original pathology (Fig. 11.8). As yearly studies accrue on a patient, comparison is made to the earliest post-operative study available. Subtle progressive changes may not be readily apparent from year to year, but can be quite obvious, if comparison is made to the earliest available post-operative study (Fig. 11.9).

VACUUM-ASSISTED IMAGING-GUIDED BIOPSY

Vacuum-assisted, imaging-guided breast biopsies with an 11G (less commonly 14G) needle can result in complete removal of small lesions. In these patients, a radiopaque marker (often a titanium clip) is deployed to mark the site of the lesion. In patients having biopsies for MRI detected, mammographically occult lesions, the clip marks the

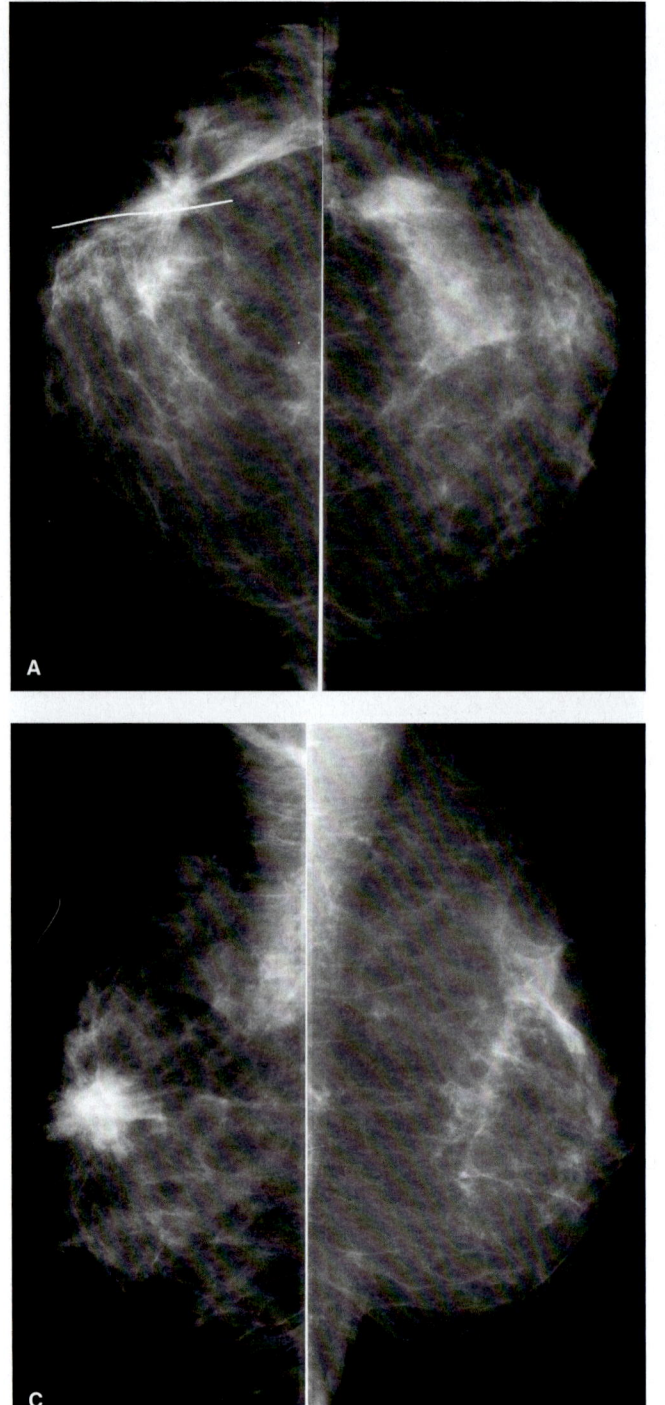

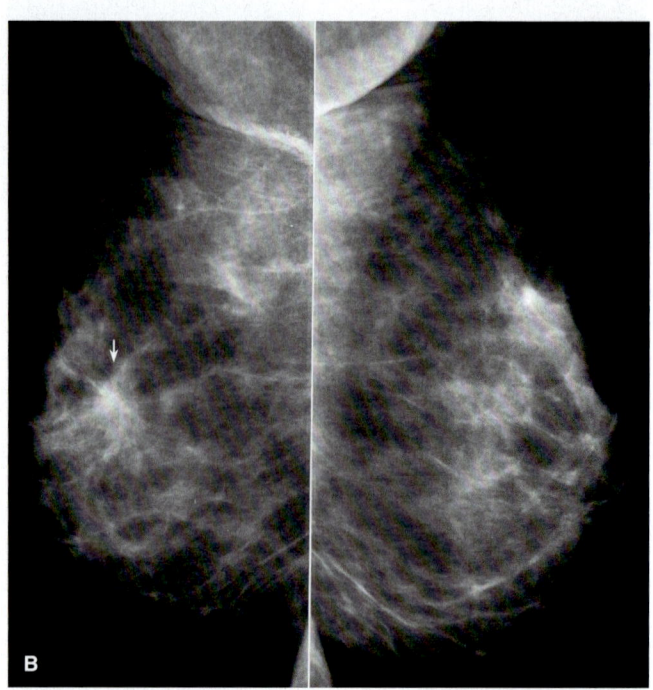

FIG. 11.8 • Invasive ductal carcinoma, not otherwise specified (NOS) occurring at prior biopsy site. CC **(A)** and MLO **(B)** views. A mass with spiculated margins and associated distortion is noted at a biopsy site *(metallic wire)* in the upper *(arrow* on MLO) outer quadrant of the right breast. Findings are attributed to the biopsy. Notice that at this point, the mass is more apparent on the CC projection. **C:** MLO views one year later. An irregular dense mass with spiculated margins and associated distortion is now apparent. The mass has increased in size and density compared with the prior study. Imaging-guided biopsy is done to establish the diagnosis of invasive ductal carcinoma. Apparent increases in density and distortion at a prior biopsy site warrant comparison with the earliest and all subsequent post-operative studies available. If the change is significant as in this patient, it may be appreciated from one year to the next; however, in many patients, the progression evolves slowly and may not be apparent from one year to the next.

site of the MRI detected abnormality for future reference. If a high-risk lesion or malignancy is diagnosed, the radiopaque marker is localized pre-operatively so that the high-risk lesion can be more completely characterized or wide excision of a malignancy can be accomplished. The clip usually remains at, or close to the biopsy site; however, migration of the clip can occur (6,7). If the patient does not undergo surgery, the radiopaque marker is seen on follow-up studies.

If a clip is deployed during an imaging-guided biopsy, orthogonal images are done to document the accuracy of clip placement immediately after the biopsy procedure; we also comment if the original lesion is removed in its entirety. In addition to the radiopaque marker, an air locule or locules (Fig. 11.10) increased density in a tubular configuration (Fig. 11.11) in one of the images and more mass-like on the orthogonal view (e.g., denoting the needle track), and increased soft tissue stranding or a mass may be seen at the biopsy site (Fig. 11.12). If present, imaging-guided biopsy changes usually resolve within the first several days following the biopsy and do not produce long-term sequelae. If an MRI is done following an imaging-guided biopsy, fluid collections will usually have a high T2 signal, and the T1 signal will vary depending on the timing of the MRI with respect to the biopsy (in the acute setting they may have a high T1 signal that decreases with time); these are sometimes noted along the distribution of the needle track (Fig. 11.13).

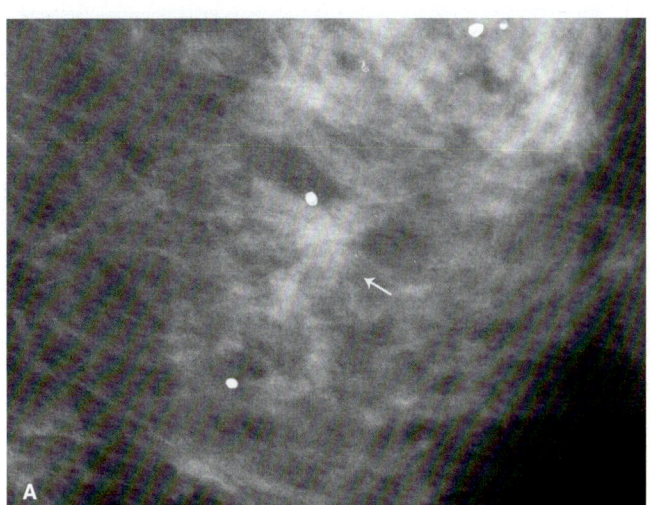
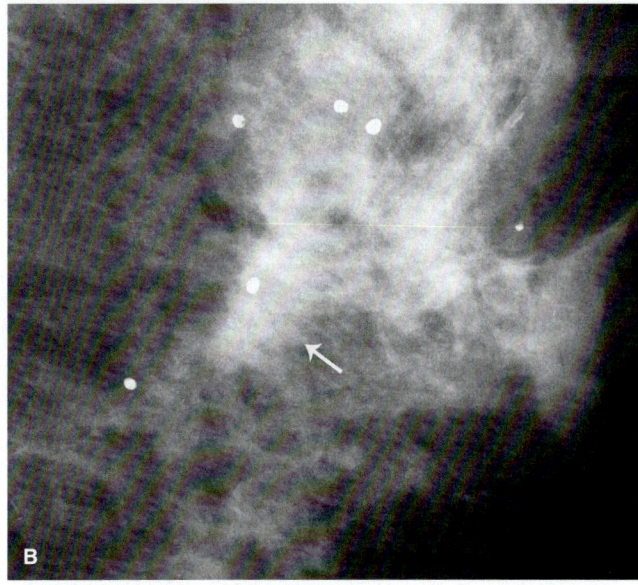

FIG. 11.9 • **Invasive ductal carcinoma, not otherwise specified, at prior biopsy site. A:** Minor distortion is noted at a prior biopsy site *(arrow)*. **B:** Three years following the image in part **A**. An irregular mass *(arrow)* with indistinct margins is apparent at the prior biopsy site. When comparison is made to the earliest study following the biopsy (image shown in part **A**), changes are easier to detect. Imaging-guided biopsy is done in this patient to establish the diagnosis. When evaluating distortion and densities associated with prior biopsy sites, be sure to look at the earliest post-operative study available, since slowly evolving changes may not be readily apparent from one year to the next. Benign coarse calcifications are seen in the adjacent tissue. (From Cardeñosa G. *Breast Imaging [The Core Curriculum Series]*. Philadelphia, PA: Lippincott Williams & Wilkins; 2003.)

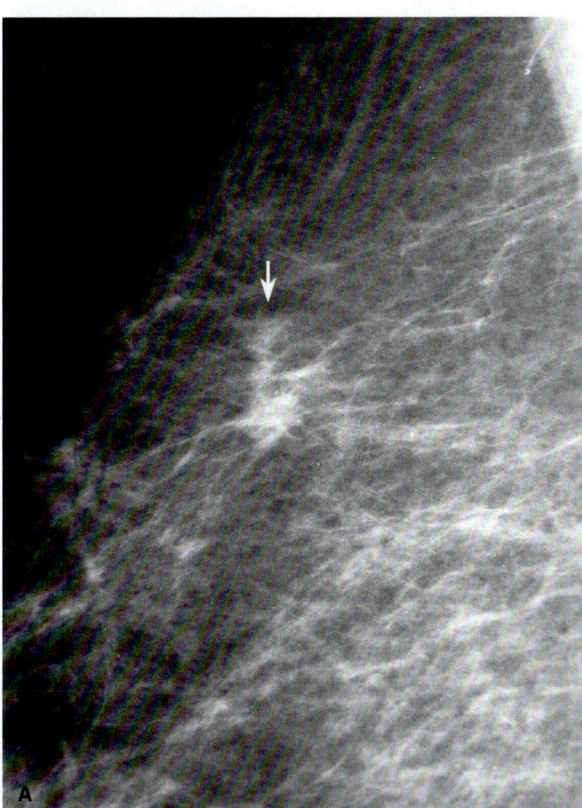
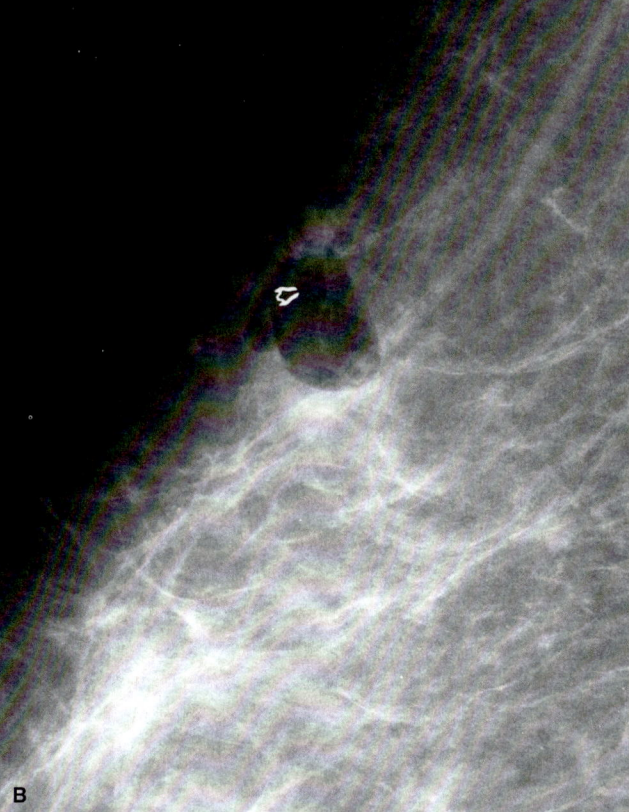

FIG. 11.10 • **Invasive ductal carcinoma, NOS, clip post–vacuum-assisted breast biopsy. A:** MLO view of the right breast photographically coned to the upper aspect of the breast. An irregular mass *(arrow)* with spiculated margins is identified superiorly in the right breast. **B:** Ninety-degree lateral (LM) view done after an 11G vacuum-assisted biopsy. The clip and an air locule are seen on orthogonal views (only one view is shown) at the biopsy site. A biopsy marker (in this patient a titanium micromark clip) is deployed to denote the location of the lesion and follow-up orthogonal images are done immediately after the biopsy to verify clip placement. As in this patient, with vacuum-assisted biopsies, small lesions or cluster of calcifications may be completed removed with the biopsy procedure. If cancer, or a high-risk lesion is diagnosed, and more tissue needs to be excised, the clip is localized and excised with the surrounding tissue on the day of the patient's definite surgical procedure. (From Cardeñosa G. *Breast Imaging [The Core Curriculum Series]*. Philadelphia, PA: Lippincott Williams & Wilkins; 2003.)

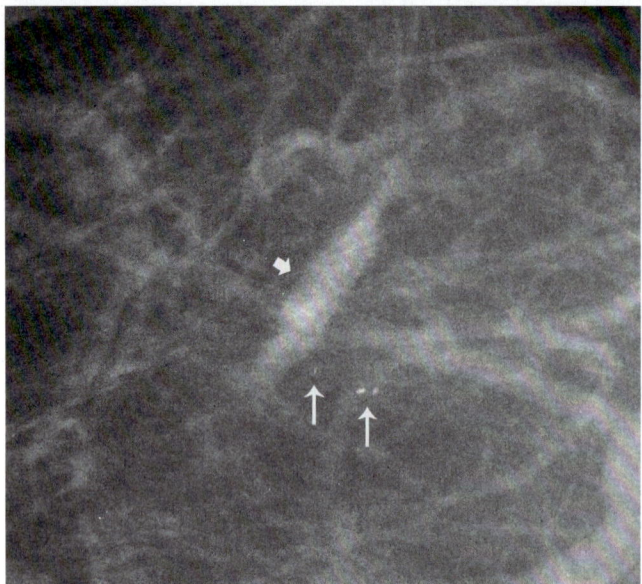

FIG. 11.11 • **Hematoma, post–vacuum-assisted breast biopsy.** Tubular area of increased density *(thick arrow)* is seen along the course of the 11G needle track. In the orthogonal view (not shown), this simulates a round mass. A clip is not deployed because calcifications *(thin arrows)* remain at the biopsy site following the procedure. DCIS is diagnosed on the core biopsy and confirmed on the lumpectomy specimen. (From Cardeñosa G. *Breast Imaging [The Core Curriculum Series]*. Philadelphia, PA: Lippincott Williams & Wilkins; 2003.)

TRAUMA

Following trauma to the breast, patients may present acutely with an ecchymosis at the site of the trauma. Irregular areas of increased density, a mass reflecting the presence of a hematoma (Fig. 11.14A; also see Fig. 7.55), parenchymal asymmetry, or focal prominence of the trabecular markings (Fig. 11.15; also see Fig. 9.7) may be seen mammographically. On ultrasound, a hyperechoic or complex cystic and solid mass (Fig. 11.14B; also see Fig. 7.55B) may be seen alternatively; mass-like areas of hyperechogenicity with internal hypo- to anechoic areas are common sonographically. Clinically, the ecchymosis resolves. Mammographic and sonographic findings also usually resolve; however, some patients develop a hard palpable mass on physical exam that is often a fat-containing mass mammographically (Figs. 11.14D, 11.16A, and 11.17A). Alternatively, an oil cyst and dystrophic calcifications may develop at the site of trauma (Fig. 11.16B). Many patients do not present acutely following the trauma but rather months after the incident. Consequently, if a fat-containing mass is seen mammographically with hyperechogenicity and internal hypoechogenicity on ultrasound (Fig. 11.17B), specifically ask the patient about trauma. Also, before assuming a mammographic finding is related to trauma, consider the location of the lesion; trauma is typically going to involve the upper quadrants of the breasts, and it is unlikely to involve the lower central aspects of the breasts posteriorly. In some patients on anti-coagulants, hematomas may develop with the patient having no recollection of significant trauma (Fig. 11.17).

Following a seat belt injury, patients may present with a band-like area of increased density corresponding to the course of the seat belt. The findings are localized to the upper inner or central quadrants of the left breast or the lower inner quadrant of the right breast when the patient is the driver. Findings in the upper inner quadrant of the right breast (Fig. 11.18) or lower inner quadrant of the left breast may be identified when the patient is the front seat passenger (8).

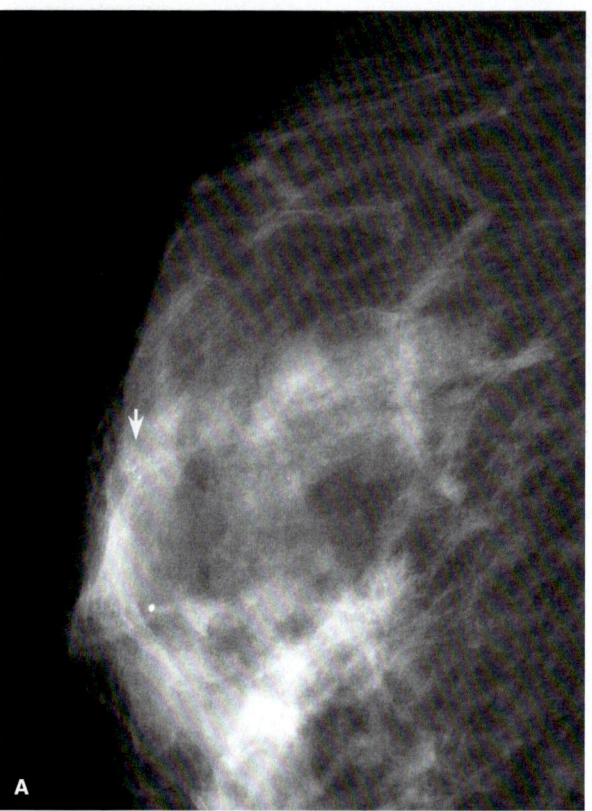

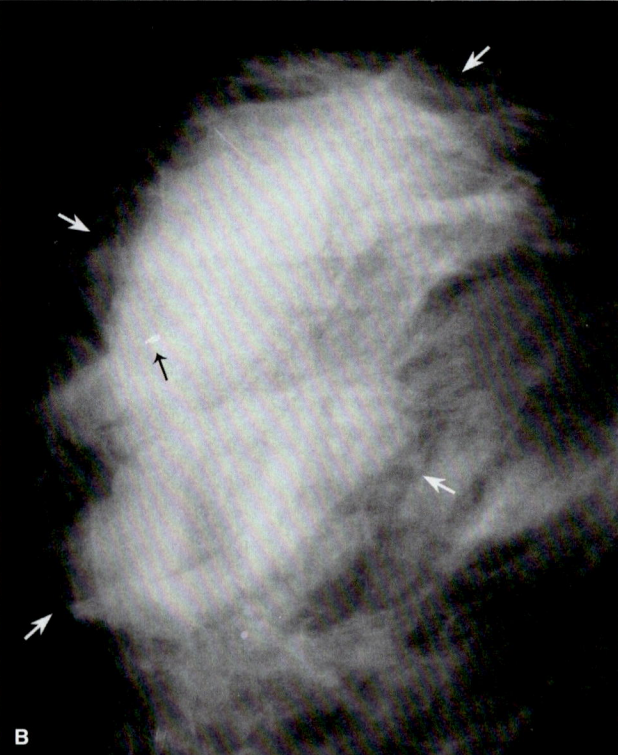

FIG. 11.12 • **Hematoma, post–vacuum-assisted breast biopsy. A:** MLO view, right breast pre-biopsy. Grouped fine pleomorphic calcifications *(arrow)*. **B:** Micromark clip is deployed *(black arrow)* at the site of the vacuum-assisted biopsy (11G) for calcifications (benign changes described histologically). Increased density *(white arrows)* is noted related to the presence of a hematoma. Although not common, hematomas can occur following imaging-guided breast biopsies. These typically resolve spontaneously. Rarely, surgical evacuation is needed. (From Cardeñosa G. *Breast Imaging [The Core Curriculum Series]*. Philadelphia, PA: Lippincott Williams & Wilkins; 2003.)

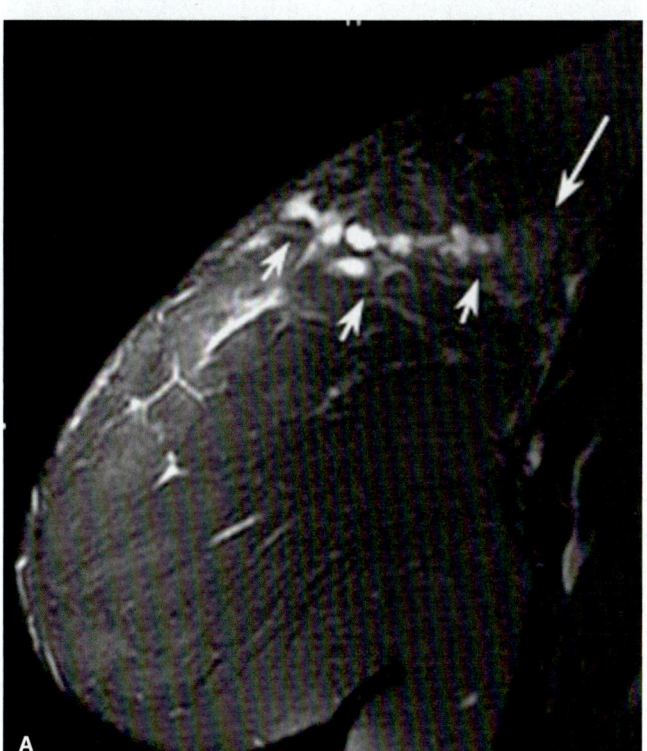
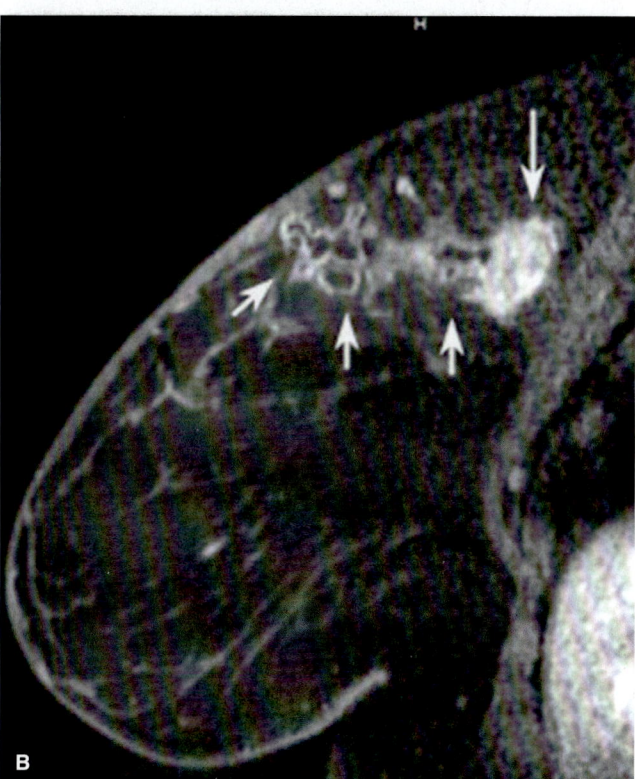

FIG. 11.13 • **Invasive ductal carcinoma, NOS, needle track post-biopsy. A:** MRI, sagittal T2-weighted fat-suppressed image of the right breast. A mass *(long arrow)* with a low T2 signal is imaged upper aspect of the right breast posteriorly. Multiple smaller masses *(short arrows)* characterized by a high T2 signal extend linearly from the skin to mass denoting the needle track formed during an ultrasound-guided 14G biopsy of the mass. Edematous changes (high T2 signal) are noted in the surrounding tissue. **B:** MRI, sagittal T1-weighted reconstruction of the right, post contrast. Oval mass *(long arrow)* with heterogeneous enhancement and irregular margins is noted correlating to the mass seen on the T2 image shown in part **A** and the site of the patient's known malignancy. Non-enhancing soft tissue stranding is noted along the needle track *(short arrows)*; the masses with high T2 signal noted in part **A** have a low T1 signal and demonstrate minimal peripheral enhancement. Note skin thickening and enhancement corresponding to the skin entry site for the biopsy.

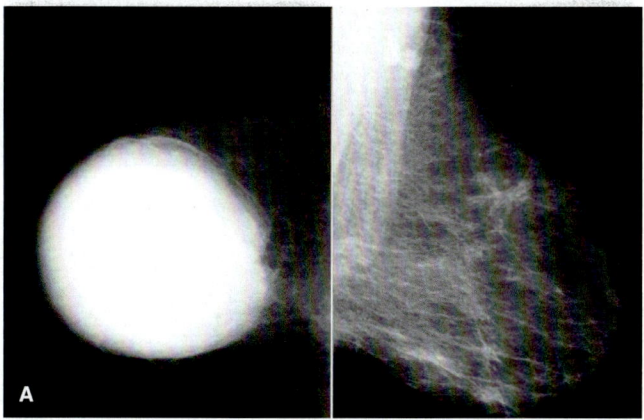
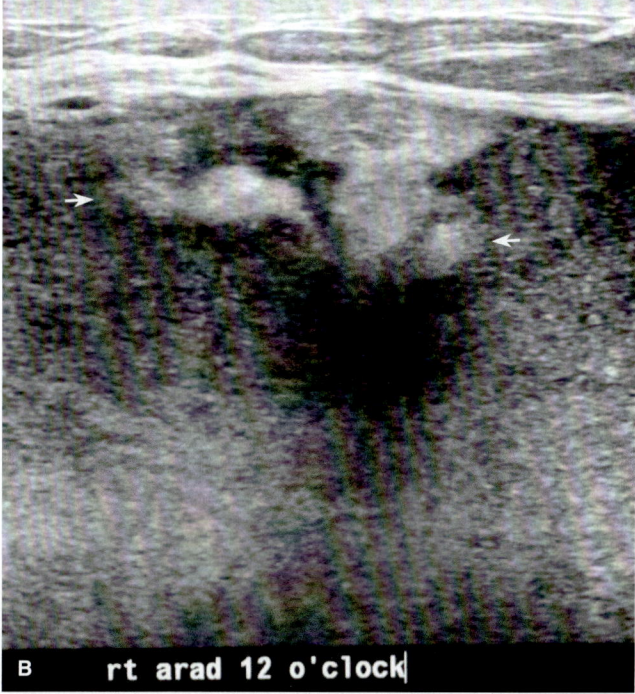

FIG. 11.14 • **Hematoma, evolution. A:** MLO views. Acutely following trauma, a round dense mass with circumscribed margins is present almost completely involving the right breast. In an attempt to penetrate through the mass, the remainder of the breast tissue is "burned" out. Technical factors for the exposure of the right breast: compression = 9.9 cm, kVp = 35, mAs = 400. **B:** Ultrasound. Given the size of this mass, it is imaged in parts. This image is a fair representation of the lesion with cystic areas and hyperechoic mural nodules *(arrows)*. **C:** MLO views. A round dense mass with circumscribed margins persists 2 years after the accident; however, it has decreased in size. **D:** MLO views 5 years after the accident. Multiple low-density and fat-containing masses with circumscribed margins are now seen at the site of the original hematoma.

(continued)

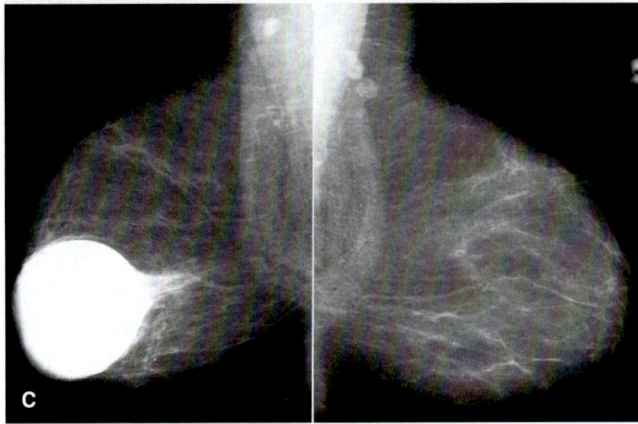
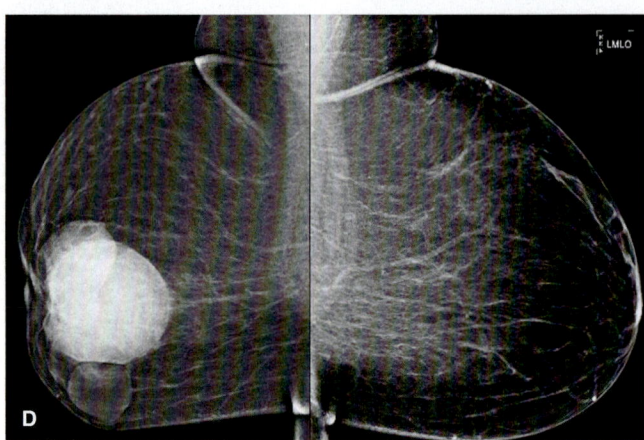

FIG. 11.14 • *(continued)*

CONSERVATIVE BREAST CANCER TREATMENT

The primary aim of breast conserving treatment is adequate local control of breast cancer. Wide surgical margins are desired in minimizing local recurrences. The cosmetic results, however, are an important secondary consideration. If a substantial amount of tissue needs to be removed to obtain clear margins in a patient with a small breast, cosmesis may not be acceptable. Radiation therapy is used to control any residual occult breast cancer. It is begun 2 to 5 weeks after the lumpectomy. Treatment is given 5 days a week for a total of 5 weeks and delivers 45 to 50 Gy to the affected breast. A boost to the lumpectomy site may be given using an electron beam or iridium implant, increasing the total dose delivered to 60 to 66 Gy (2). Although not all patients with breast cancer are good candidates, high doses of radiation therapy delivered over a 5-day period to the site of the tumor (brachytherapy) are being used with early results comparable to those of whole breast radiation. The other alternative being used with increasing frequency is neoadjuvant therapy as the initial treatment. This approach has been traditionally reserved for patients with inflammatory carcinoma; however, it is now being extended to include two other groups of patients: (i) those with known metastatic disease to the axilla in whom systemic disease is a concern and (ii) those with larger primary lesions in whom conservative therapy is not a good option at the time of presentation but for whom it can become an option if the tumor shrinks (see Chapter 5 for additional discussion regarding imaging in these patients).

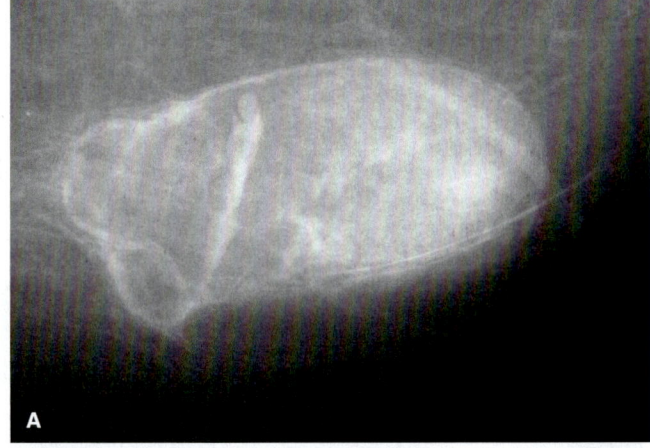
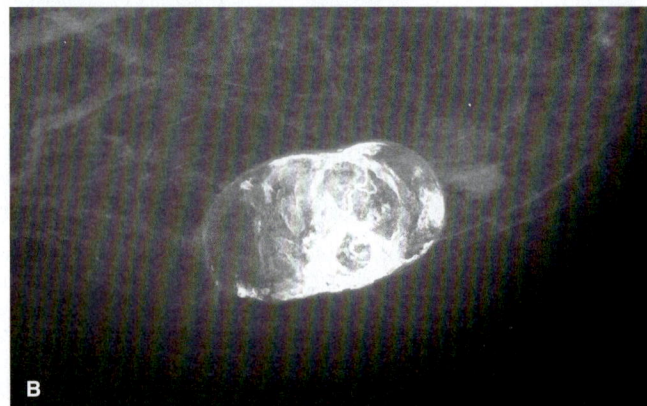
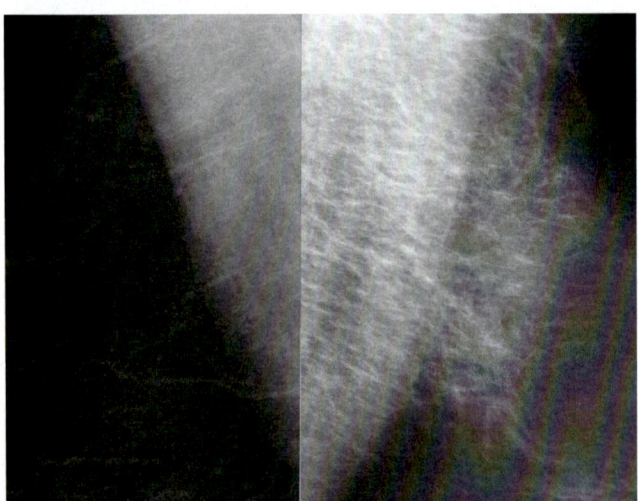

FIG. 11.15 • **Hematoma.** MLO views photographically coned to the upper portion of the images. Thickening and increased density of the trabecular markings is seen corresponding to the site of an ecchymosis in the upper portion of left breast following trauma to the breast. (From Cardeñosa G. *Breast Imaging [The Core Curriculum Series]*. Philadelphia, PA: Lippincott Williams & Wilkins; 2003.)

FIG. 11.16 • **Hematoma, evolution. A:** Oval fat-containing mass is imaged corresponding to a site of trauma in the left breast. **B:** Seven years later, the mass is smaller with dense dystrophic mural calcifications (From Cardeñosa G. *Breast Imaging [The Core Curriculum Series]*. Philadelphia, PA: Lippincott Williams & Wilkins; 2003.).

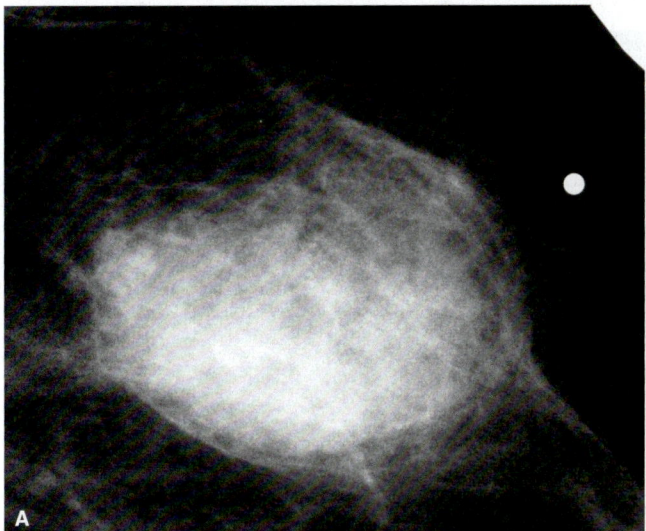

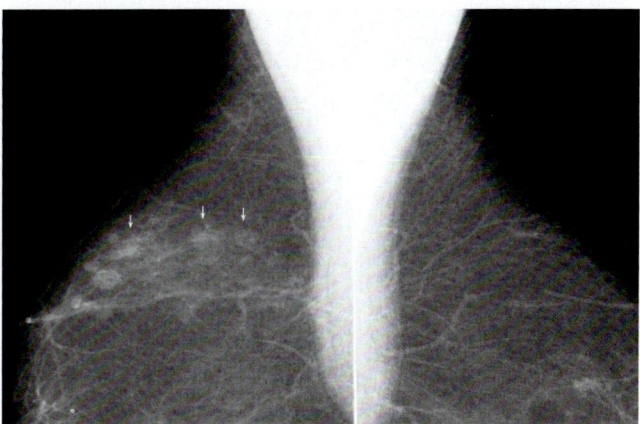

FIG. 11.18 ● **Seat belt injury, oil cysts.** MLO views. Linearly distributed oil cysts in a patient following a car accident several years previously.

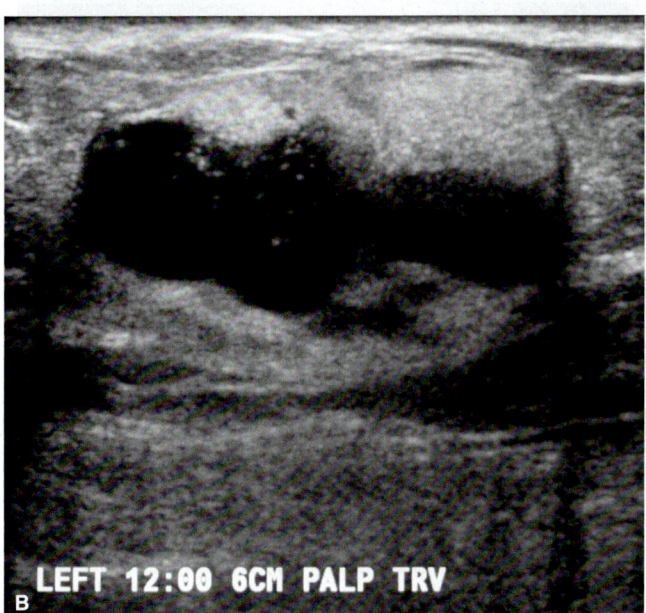

FIG. 11.17 ● **Hematoma. A:** Spot tangential view done at the site of "lump" described by the patient (metallic BB denotes palpable finding). Fat-containing (e.g. mixed density) mass with indistinct margins and internal halo is imaged at the site of the palpable finding. **B:** Ultrasound, transverse (TRV) plane. On physical examination a healing ecchymotic area is apparent on the skin overlying the palpable finding. The patient states she is on Coumadin and bruises easily. An oval mass with hyperechoic and anechoic components (heterogeneous echotexture) is imaged corresponding to the palpable and mammographic finding in the left breast. BI-RADS 2: Benign finding.

Mammographic changes related to whole breast radiation therapy involve the breast diffusely and are primarily related to edema. These include skin and trabecular thickening resulting in increases in parenchymal density and reduced breast compressibility. The changes usually resolve within the first 2 years following treatment (Fig. 11.19; also see Fig. 9.1). Technical factors for adequate exposure of the remaining breast tissue may need to be adjusted accordingly. In the acute setting, skin thickening, dilated lymphatics, and increased tissue echogenicity may be seen on ultrasound following radiation therapy. Residual skin thickening is seen in approximately 20% of women 2 years after radiation therapy (2). Rarely, patients develop fairly extensive fat necrosis

that involves the breast diffusely (e.g., not localized to the lumpectomy site) with progressive fibrosis, contracture, and patient discomfort (Fig. 11.20). It is unclear if this process is related solely to the radiation or if it reflects a combination of radiation therapy and surgical effect. Long-term complications of radiation therapy are now also being seen with increasing frequency in part a function of an increase in the number of follow-up years in women who have had whole breast radiation therapy for breast cancer. Patients may present with pulmonary fibrosis, pleural effusions, rib fractures (osteonecrosis), and secondary malignancies often sarcomatous in nature involving the skin (e.g., cutaneous angiosarcomas), breast parenchyma (Fig. 11.21), or soft tissues of the chest and upper abdominal wall (Fig. 11.22) included in, or surrounding, the radiation field (9,10).

The findings seen mammographically following lumpectomy are variable, usually evolve with time and are localized to the surgical site (Fig. 11.19). These include irregular increases in density, distortion, a mass with spiculated margins (fat necrosis), and a mass at the lumpectomy site reflecting a post-operative fluid collection as well as localized skin thickening and retraction. On MRI, non-enhancing distortion and a non-enhancing mass with spiculated margins are the most common findings noted at prior lumpectomy sites; associated skin thickening and retraction are also seen and, in some patients, depending on the location of the original tumor, tenting of the pectoral muscle.

Fat necrosis developing at the lumpectomy site is variably sized and characterized by an irregular mass with indistinct, or more commonly spiculated margins, or distortion alone (Fig. 11.19C, D). As the acute inflammatory changes associated with fat necrosis resolve, the mass or area of distortion decreases in size and density, and oil cysts or dystrophic calcifications (Fig. 11.23) can be seen developing at the lumpectomy site (2,4,11–17). On ultrasound, fat necrosis often results in disruption of normal soft tissue planes as well as distortion and intense shadowing at the surgical site sometimes associated with an irregular mass (5).

Fluid collections are seen in as many as 50% of patients within the first 4 weeks after the lumpectomy (2). An oval or round (Figs. 11.19A, B and 11.24A) mass with circumscribed to indistinct or spiculated margins (Fig. 11.24C) is identified at the lumpectomy site. These are variable in density; however, some are relatively low in density particularly when considering their size. They may have lucent locules or fluid–fluid levels. An internal halo may be present partially outlining the inner margin of the mass (Fig. 11.25). On ultrasound, complex cystic and solid masses with septations (Fig. 11.26A; also see

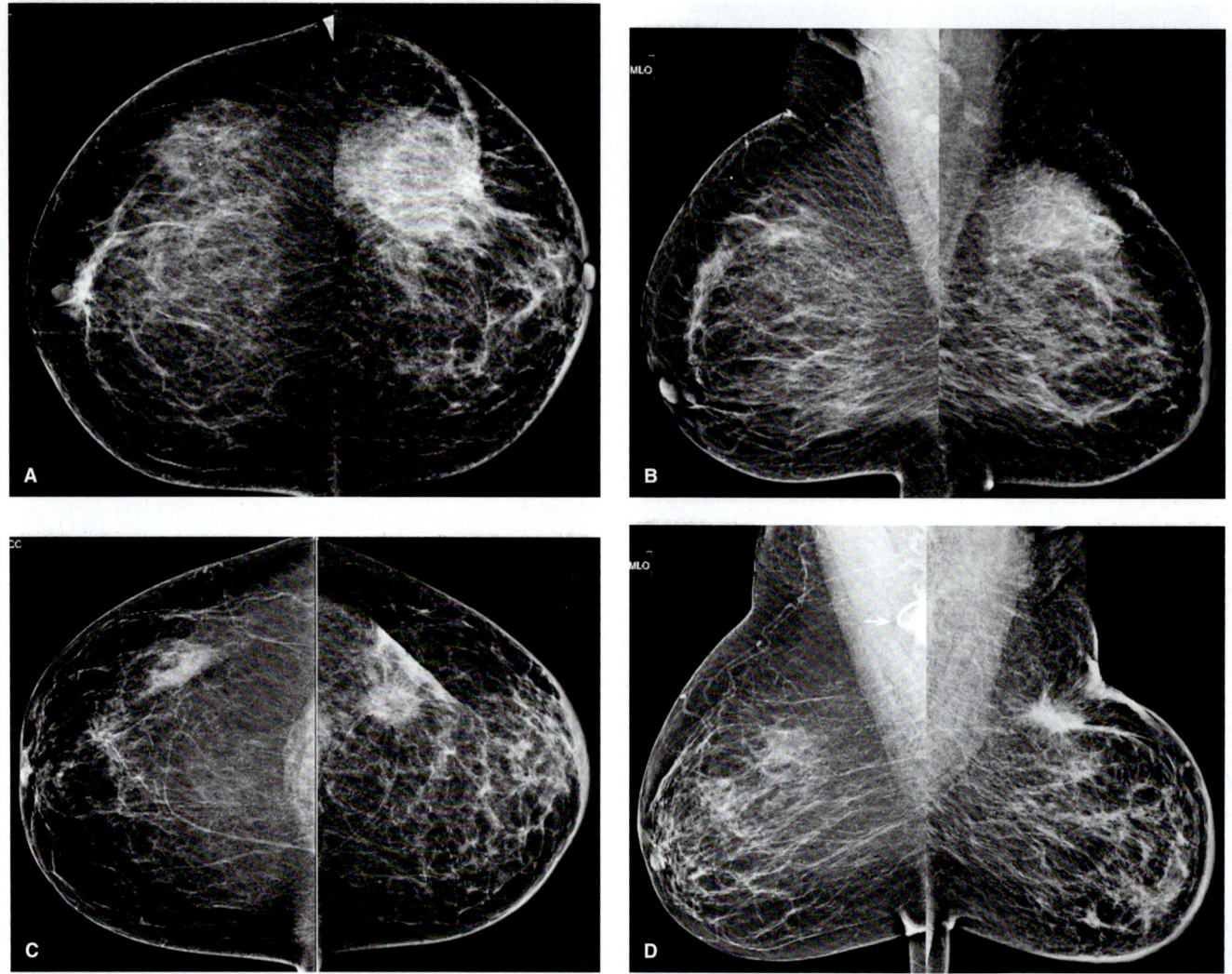

FIG. 11.19 • **Lumpectomy and radiation therapy changes.** CC **(A)** and MLO **(B)** views done in a 55-year-old patient. First study post lumpectomy and radiation therapy for DCIS in the left breast. The left breast is smaller than the right. Diffuse skin thickening as well as increased and thickened trabecular markings reflecting edematous changes related to the radiation therapy are noted involving the left breast. A round low-density mass with indistinct margins is imaged in the upper outer quadrant of the left breast consistent with a fluid collection at the lumpectomy site. Thickening and retraction of the skin are noted localized to the lumpectomy site. Compare the technical factors used for exposure on the right CC view: compression = 55 mm, kVp = 25, mAs = 165 with those used for the left CC: compression = 66 mm, kVp = 27, mAs = 236; the difference in compression reflect decreased compressibility of the radiated breast and the needed increase in kVp and mAs are related primarily to skin thickening. CC **(C)** and MLO **(D)** views in a 65-year-old patient. First study post lumpectomy and radiation therapy for a high-grade invasive ductal carcinoma in the left breast. The left breast is smaller than the right. Diffuse skin thickening as well as increased and thickened trabecular markings reflecting edematous changes related to the radiation therapy are noted involving the left breast. A mass with spiculated margins is imaged in the upper outer quadrant of the left breast associated with localized skin thickening and retraction. Note the appearance (shape and density) of the mass between the MLO and the CC views. One of the imaging features of fat necrosis at lumpectomy sites is a differential appearance between the routine views: it is often more apparent in one projection (in this patient the MLO) compared with the other (CC). Compare the technical factors used for exposure on the right CC view: compression = 49 mm, kVp = 24, mAs = 165 with those used for exposure on the left CC: compression = 58 mm, kVp = 26, mAs = 185. A round density and a tube *(arrow)* are partially imaged in the right axilla related to the presence of a central venous access catheter.

Fig. 4.29B), thickened walls, or echogenic nodules (Fig. 11.26B; also see Fig. 4.29A) are imaged corresponding to the masses seen mammographically. Less commonly a complex cystic and solid mass that is predominantly solid with cystic spaces (Fig. 11.24B and 11.26C) or a nearly anechoic mass is seen. Most fluid collections resolve within the first 2 years after the lumpectomy; however, some may persist for years. If the patient is asymptomatic, aspiration is not indicated and should be avoided because, in many patients, the fluid re-accumulates rapidly after percutaneous drainage, the re-accumulated fluid collection may be larger than the starting point and chronic draining sinuses can develop (Fig. 11.27; also see Fig. 4.30). Draining sinuses can be hard to manage and affect the patient's quality of life significantly.

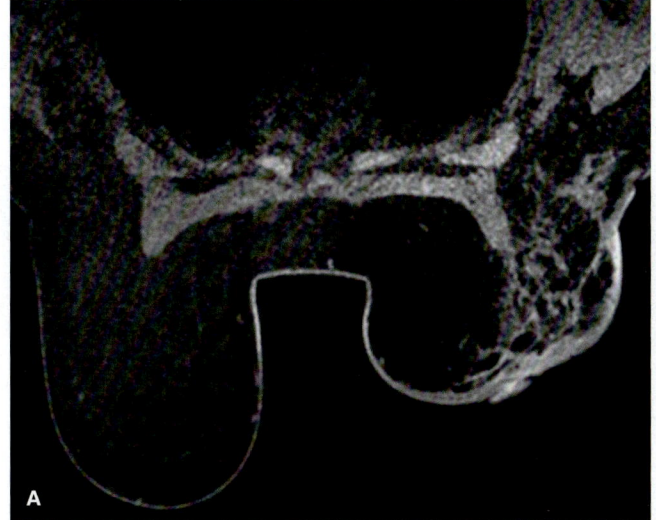

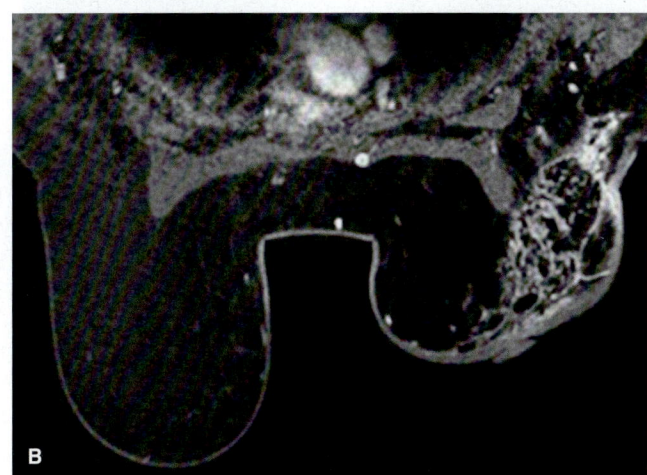

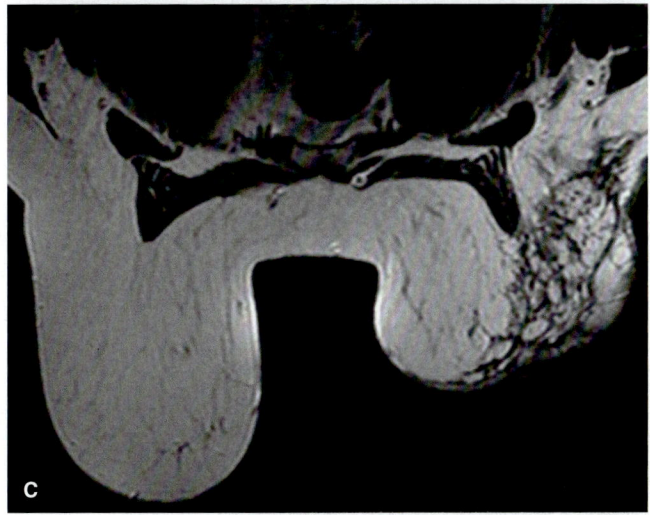

FIG. 11.20 • **Fat necrosis.** MRI, axial T1-weighted image pre contrast **(A)**, MRI axial T1-weighted image, post contrast **(B)** and MRI, axial T2-weighted image **(C)** all at the same scan position, in a 57-year-old patient 2 years following lumpectomy and radiation therapy who presents describing a hard mass in the right breast with significant associated pain and discomfort (unable to tolerate a mammogram). The right breast is smaller and deformed compared with the left. An irregular mass with a thin rim and internal septations that enhance, irregular margins and internal fat is imaged encompassing the lateral quadrants of the right breast. The findings are consistent with fat necrosis following lumpectomy and radiation therapy.

The signal characteristics of post-operative fluid collections on MRI are variable depending on the age of the collection. Acutely, they may demonstrate high T1 and T2 signal with minimal rim enhancement. As the collection ages, it decreases in size, the margins become better defined and the T1 signal usually decreases. Fluid–fluid levels may be apparent (Fig. 11.28).

Currently, there is no consensus on an appropriate follow-up protocol for patients following lumpectomy. If the patient is asymptomatic following conservative breast cancer therapy, the American College of Radiology practice guidelines on screening and diagnostic mammography (18) leaves the decision on how to schedule (e.g., as screening or diagnostic studies) these patients at the discretion of the imaging facility. Some facilities recommend 6-month follow ups of the treated breast for 3, 5, or 7 years and annual imaging of the contralateral, presumably normal breast (2). In our practice, we obtain a pre-radiation mammogram on patients who presented with an extensive area of calcifications. Rarely, we identify patients with residual calcifications at the lumpectomy site (14) who may benefit from re-excision before radiation therapy is started. Following completion of radiation therapy, we schedule patients for diagnostic studies annually for 7 years after which we return them to screening. We are not routinely obtaining 6-month follow ups of the treated breast following conservative therapy since there is nothing to suggest that recurrences grow any faster than primary lesions. In addition to routine views (CC and MLO), we obtain a spot compression magnification view of the lumpectomy site in tangent to the x-ray beam.

When evaluating these patients, it is helpful to have information on those features of the initial tumor that may influence the likelihood of recurrence including tumor size and grade, proximity of tumor to margins, presence of an extensive intraductal component, lymphovascular space involvement, and lymph node status. Additionally, it is helpful to know if the patient had radiation, chemotherapy, and if she is being treated with tamoxifen. Ideally, the patient's imaging evaluation at the time of diagnosis is available for review since recurrences often resemble the appearance of the primary. The likelihood of recurrence is low in the first 2 years following treatment; it may be that some of the lesions identified within this time period reflect residual (inadequately treated) disease and not necessarily a recurrence. In the first 7 years following treatment, recurrences are likely to arise at or close to the lumpectomy site (Figs. 11.29 and 11.30); after this, recurrences or second primaries develop with an equal frequency anywhere in the breast (Fig. 11.30) (19–21). Fine pleomorphic calcifications with linear forms or demonstrating linear distribution, developing at prior lumpectomy sites should be biopsied (Fig. 11.29). Developing masses (Fig. 11.31) or increases in the size and density of architectural distortion at the lumpectomy site may also indicate recurrence. Rarely, recurrences will

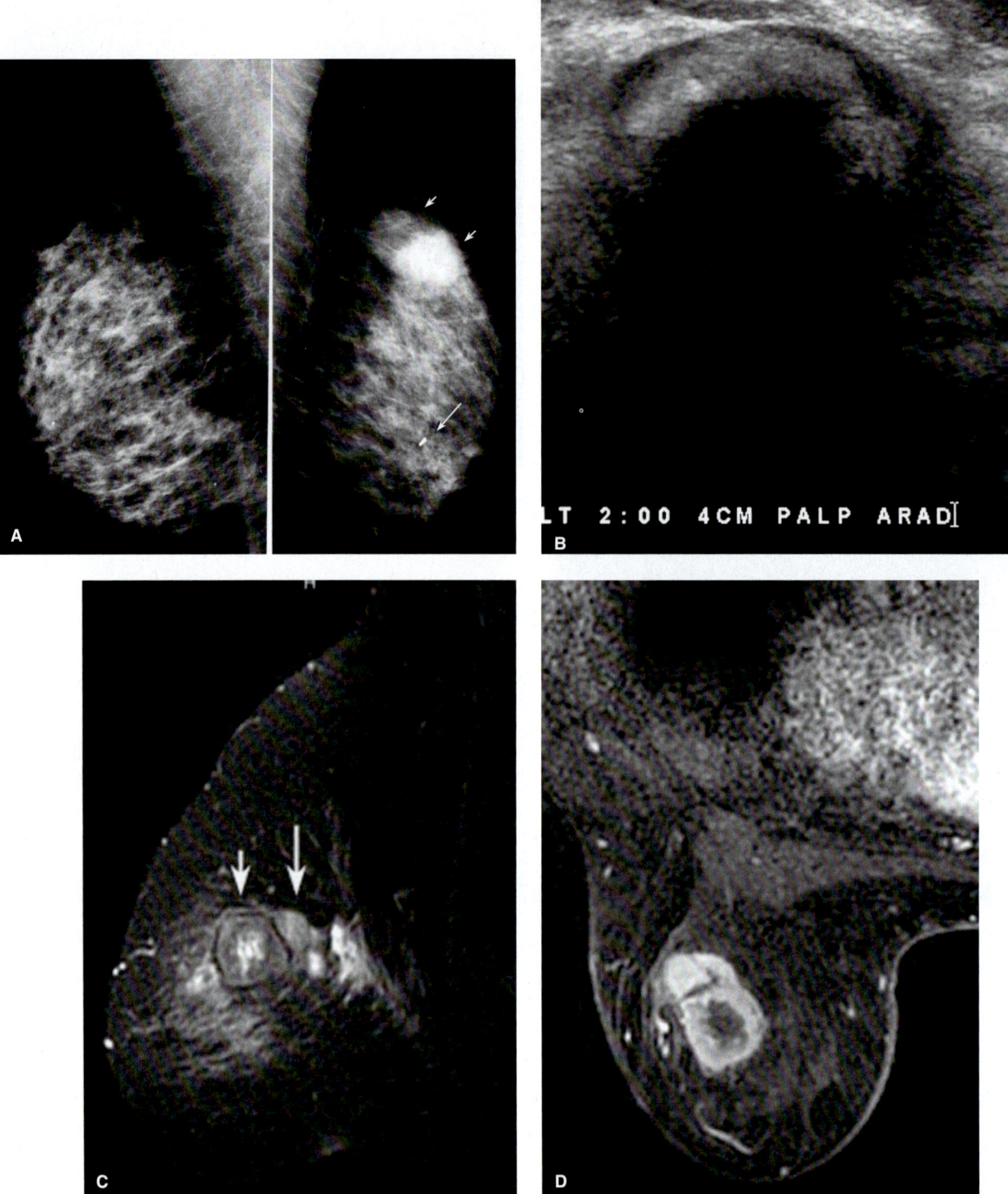

FIG. 11.21 • **Radiation induced osteosarcoma. A:** MLO views in a 64-year-old woman 8 years following lumpectomy and radiation therapy for invasive ductal carcinoma in the left breast. The left breast is smaller. An oval mass *(short arrows)* with two components, one dense (anteriorly) and the other isodense is identified in the upper outer quadrant of the left breast; this is new compared with the prior study. A metallic clip *(long arrow)* with surrounding distortion is seen inferiorly denoting the prior lumpectomy site. **B:** Ultrasound. A mass with a thickened echogenic curvilinear component and intense shadowing as well as circumscribed margins superficially and indistinct margins laterally is imaged corresponding to the dense portion of the mass. A giant cell neoplasm (metaplastic or giant cell) is reported on the ultrasound-guided core specimens. **C:** MRI sagittal T2-weighted image of the left breast, fat suppressed. A mass with internal high T2 signal and intermediate T2 signal peripherally is imaged corresponding to the mammographic and ultrasound finding. Also note the sharp demarcation between the round *(short arrow)* component anteriorly (dense mammographically) and the more posterior portion *(long arrow)* of the mass. Edematous changes are noted as "wispy" high T2 signal in the surrounding tissue extending to the pectoral fascia. **D:** MRI, T1-weighted axial image of the left breast, post contrast. Bilobed mass, the anterior portion of which demonstrates thickened irregular rim enhancement with rapid wash-in and wash-out delayed kinetics. Low internal T1 signal correlates to the high T2 signal seen in the mass, part **D** consistent with internal necrosis. An osteosarcoma, presumably radiation induced, is diagnosed following a left mastectomy.

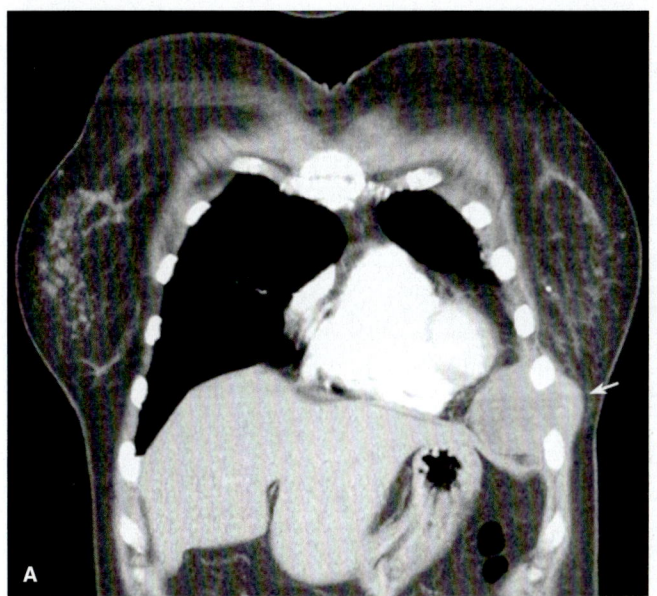
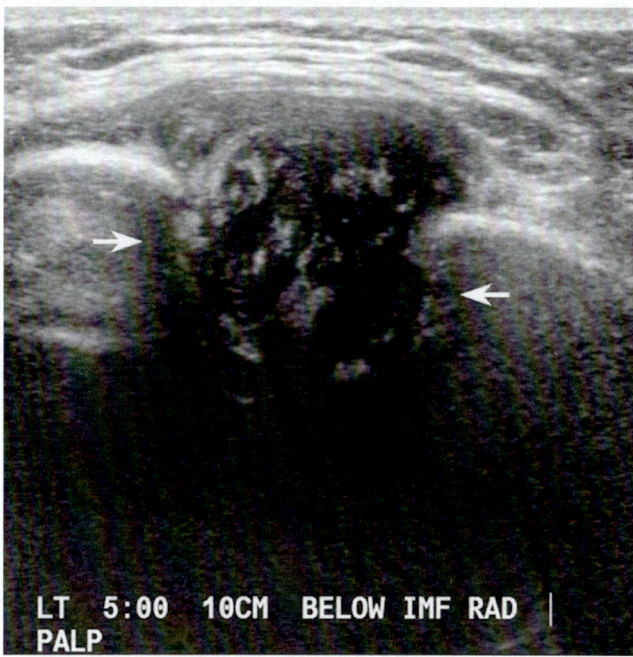

FIG. 11.22 • **Radiation induced chest wall sarcoma. A:** Coronal reconstruction of a chest CT scan in a 63-year-old patient who had bilateral lumpectomies and radiation therapy 12 and 8 years previously. A mass *(arrows)* is present anteriorly involving the soft tissues of the lower chest wall and upper abdominal wall on the left extending through and displacing the ribs; one of the ribs is eroded. **B:** Ultrasound image demonstrating the portion of the mass *(arrows)* extending though the ribs. Initial diagnosis is established on an ultrasound-guided biopsy. A radiation induced high-grade spindle cell sarcoma is diagnosed on the en-bloc chest wall resection. Also described is invasion of the seventh through ninth ribs; however, no involvement of the pleura is seen.

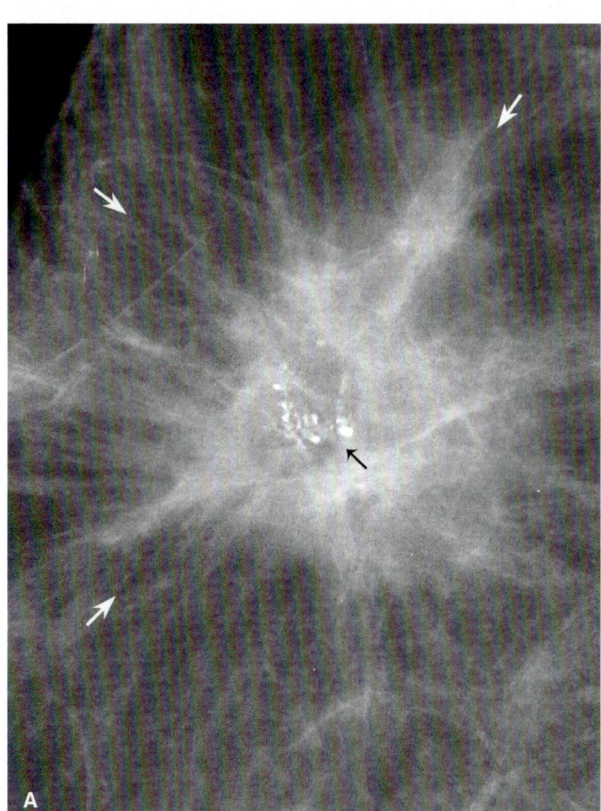
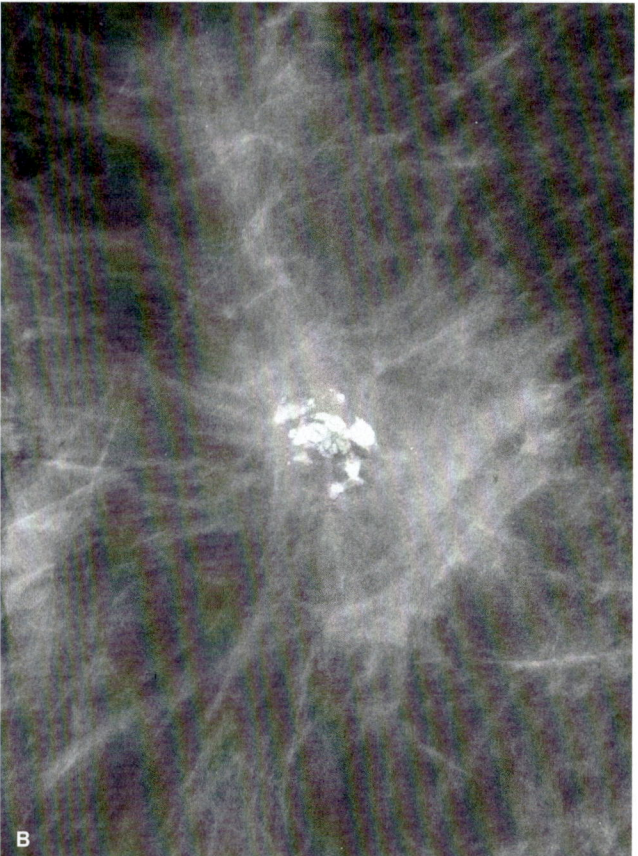

FIG. 11.23 • **Evolving fat necrosis, post lumpectomy and radiation therapy. A:** Irregular fat-containing mass with spiculated margins *(white arrows)* consistent with fat necrosis and oil cyst at a lumpectomy site. Coarse calcifications are developing in the oil cyst *(black arrow)*. **B:** One year later, the mass and associated distortion have decreased in size and density, while the dystrophic calcifications continue to develop. (From Cardeñosa G. *Breast Imaging [The Core Curriculum Series]*. Philadelphia, PA: Lippincott Williams & Wilkins; 2003.)

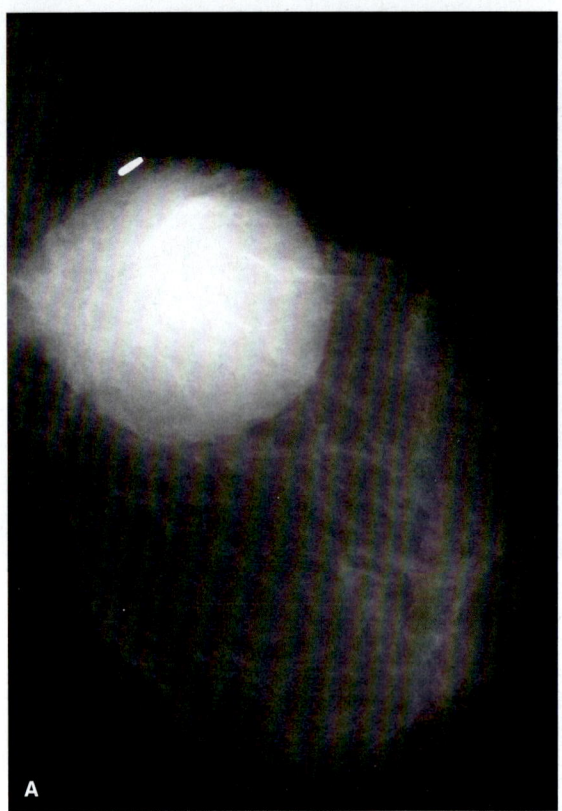
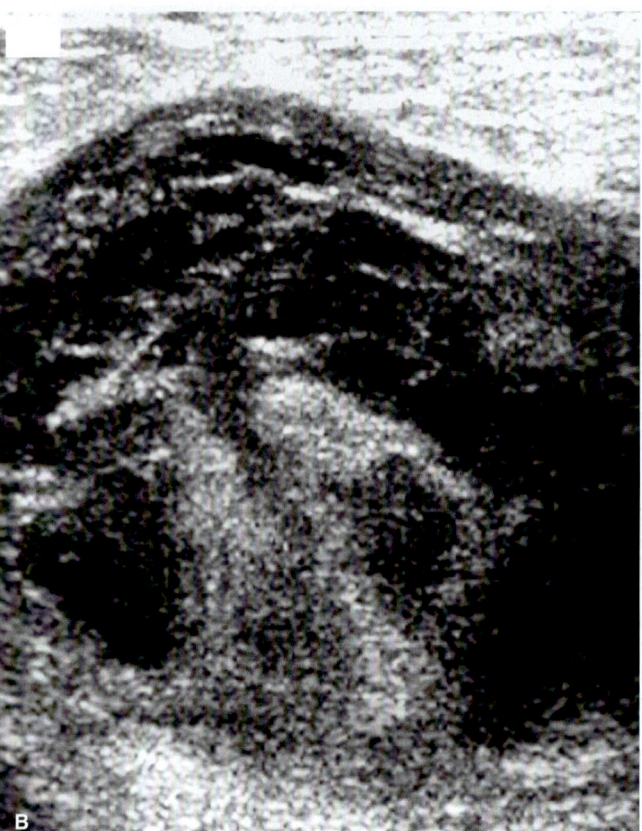
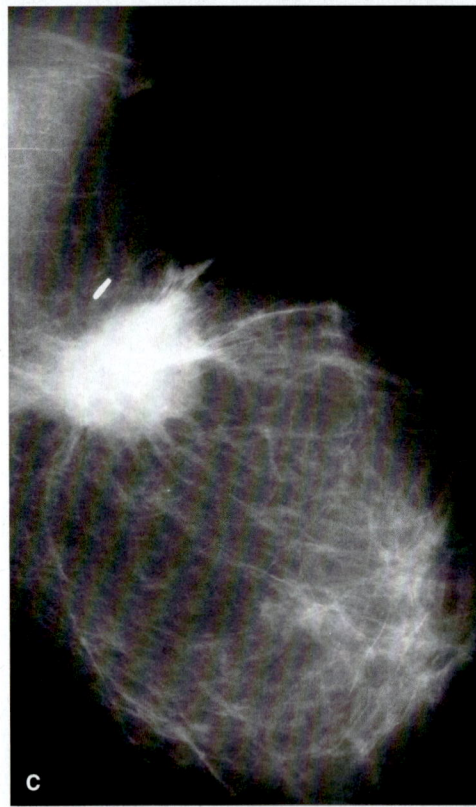

FIG. 11.24 • **Post-lumpectomy fluid collection. A:** Left MLO view. A round dense mass with circumscribed margins is imaged at a lumpectomy site in the left breast. A surgical clip is note at the superior edge of the mass. **B:** Ultrasound. A complex cystic and solid mass is imaged corresponding to the mass seen mammographically. No intervention is warranted unless superimposed infection is suspected. When rapidly decompressed (e.g., aspirated), these may recur quickly and sometimes attain a size greater than that of the original collection. **C:** Follow-up left MLO view. The mass is smaller and the margins are now spiculated. (From Cardeñosa G. *Breast Imaging [The Core Curriculum Series]*. Philadelphia, PA: Lippincott Williams & Wilkins; 2003.)

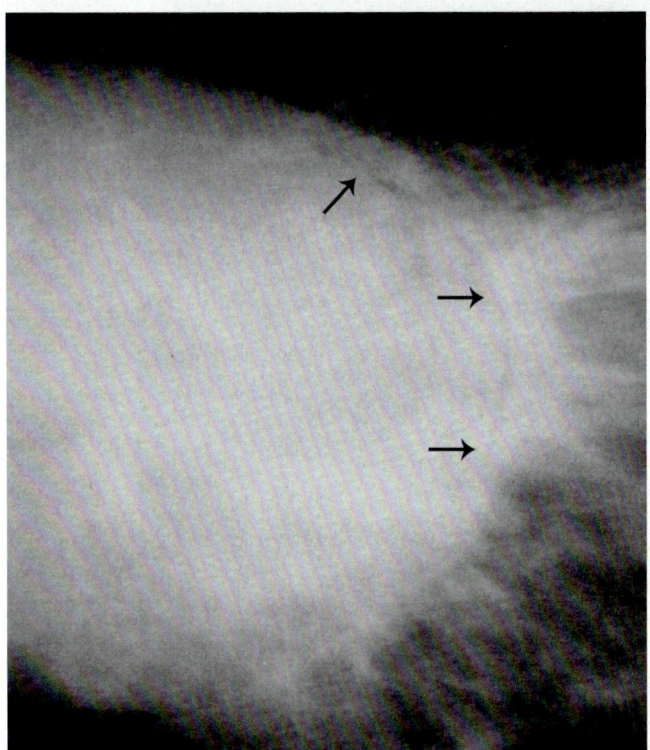

FIG. 11.25 • **Post-lumpectomy fluid collection, internal halo.** An oval mass with circumscribed and spiculated margins is partially imaged at the lumpectomy site. An "internal halo" is present *(arrows)* along the anterior edge of the mass. Interior halos at typically seen in post-operative or traumatic fluid collections. (From Cardeñosa G. *Breast Imaging [The Core Curriculum Series]*. Philadelphia, PA: Lippincott Williams & Wilkins; 2003.)

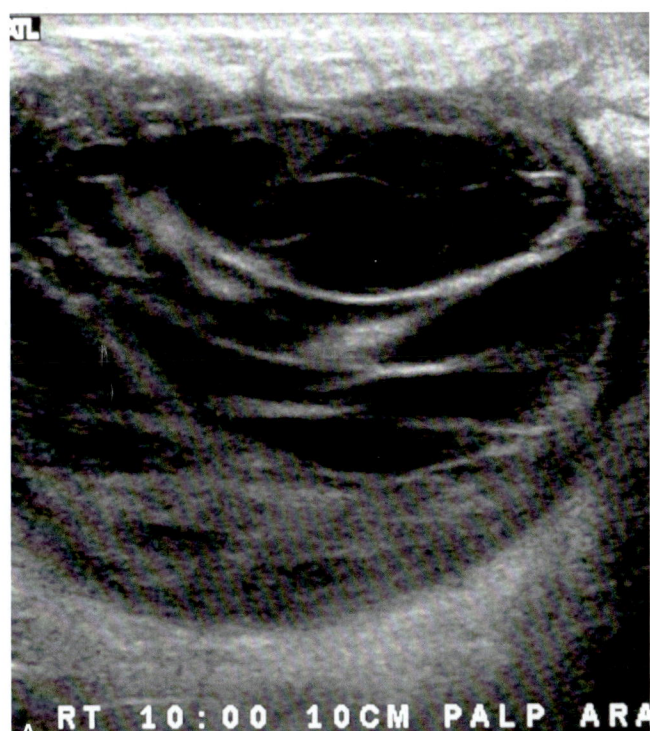

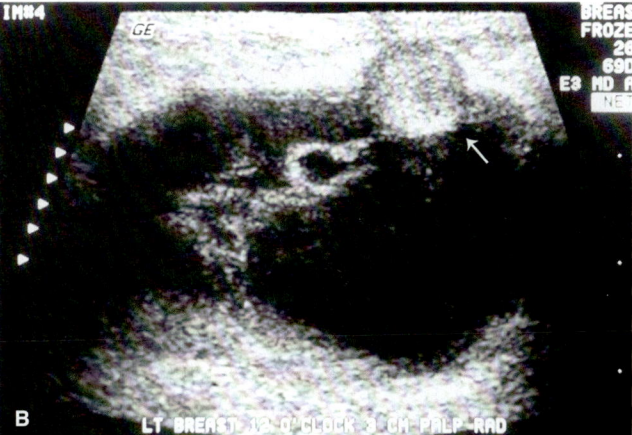

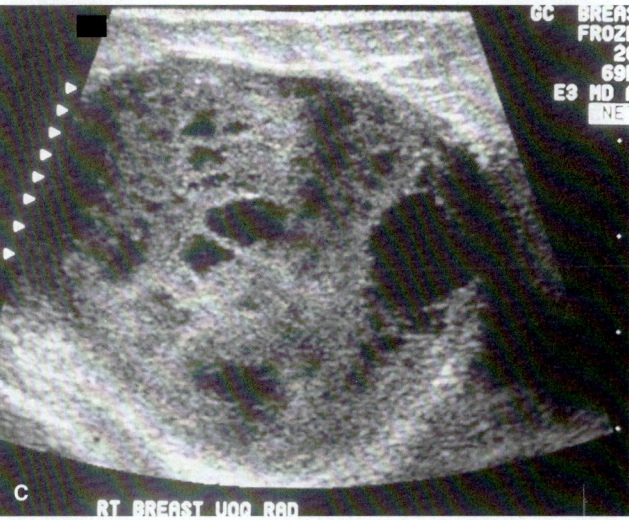

FIG. 11.26 • **Post-lumpectomy fluid collections. A:** A complex cystic and solid mass with internal septations and posterior acoustic enhancement is imaged corresponding to the lumpectomy site in the right breast. Note increased echogenicity of the tissue interposed between the collection and the skin. **B:** Complex cystic and solid mass with posterior acoustic enhancement is imaged corresponding to a lumpectomy site in the left breast. The echogenic mass *(arrow)* corresponds to an oil cyst associated with the fluid collection on the patient's mammogram (not shown). **C:** Complex cystic and solid mass that appears predominantly solid with cystic spaces corresponding to a known lumpectomy site. Unless superimposed infection is suspected, no intervention is warranted in these patients. These collections commonly resolve spontaneously. (**B** and **C:** (From Cardeñosa G. *Breast Imaging [The Core Curriculum Series]*. Philadelphia, PA: Lippincott Williams & Wilkins; 2003.)

FIG. 11.27 • **Draining sinuses developing following aspirations of post-lumpectomy fluid collections.** Oval air locule *(arrow)* is present associated with an area of distortion at the lumpectomy site. Draining sinus developing after repeated aspirations of a post-operative fluid collection (also see Fig. 4.30). (From Cardeñosa G. *Breast Imaging [The Core Curriculum Series]*. Philadelphia, PA: Lippincott Williams & Wilkins; 2003.)

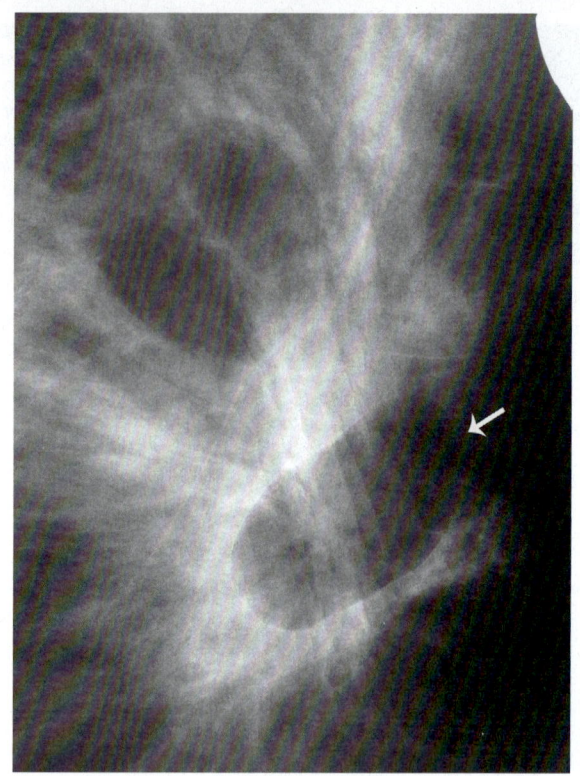

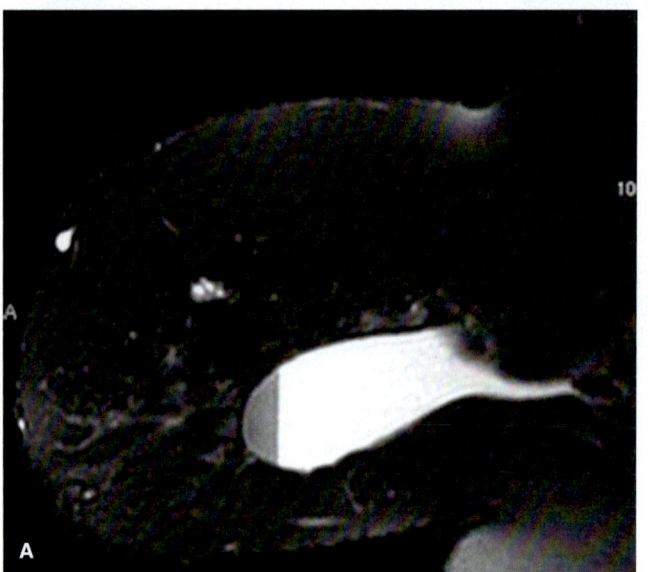

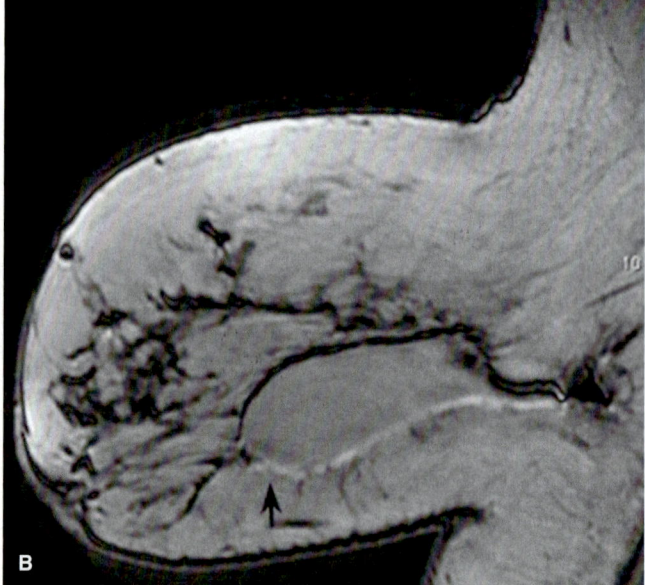

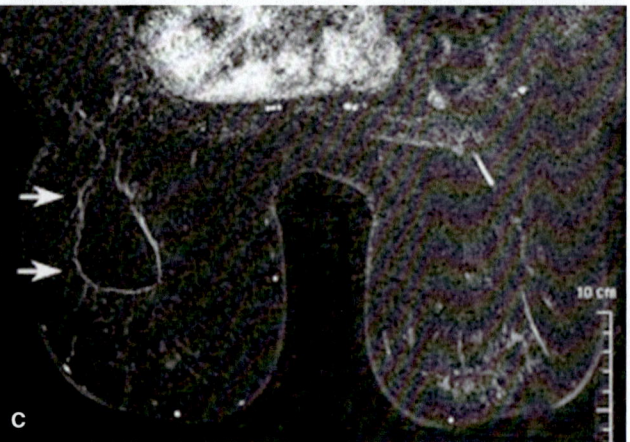

FIG. 11.28 • **Fluid collection, acute post-lumpectomy. A:** MRI, sagittal T2-weighted, fat-suppressed image of the left breast. An oval mass with circumscribed margins and a predominantly high T2 signal and a fluid–fluid level anteriorly (patient is prone) 14 days following the lumpectomy. **B:** MRI, sagittal T1-weighted image left breast. The oval mass *(arrow)* demonstrates an intermediate to high T1 signal, consistent with a resolving hematoma. The fluid–fluid level is not as apparent on this sequence. **C:** MRI, axial T1-weighted subtraction image. A thin enhancing wall but no internal enhancement characterizes the post-op fluid collection *(arrows)*.

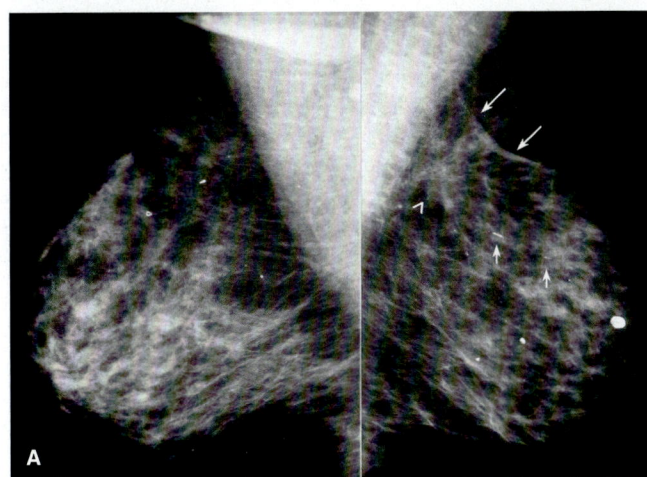
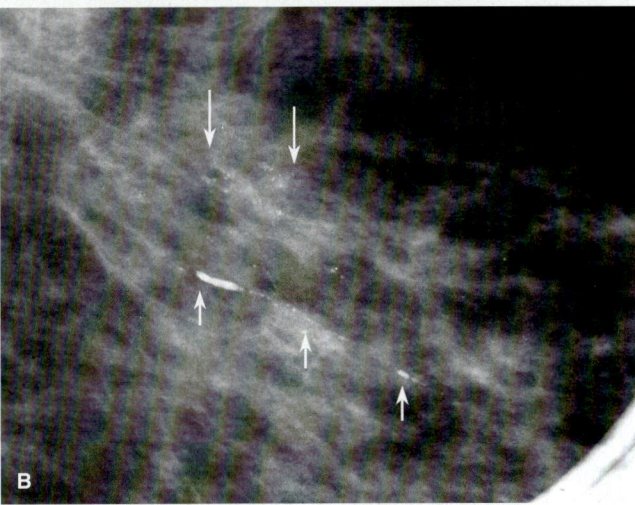

FIG. 11.29 • **DCIS, recurrent. A:** MLO views in a 72-year-old patient following lumpectomy and radiation therapy for DCIS in the upper outer quadrant of the left breast posteriorly. The left breast is smaller than the right. Distortion *(arrowhead)* is present in the upper outer quadrant of the left breast posteriorly associated with focal skin thickening and retraction *(long arrows)*. As compared with prior studies (not shown), calcifications *(short arrows)* including round, punctate and linear forms some in a linear orientation are noted at the anterior edge of the lumpectomy site. **B:** Spot compression magnification view, MLO projection. Linear and punctate calcifications *(short arrows)* in a linear distribution as well as clusters of fine pleomorphic calcifications *(long arrows)* are seen extending anteriorly from the lumpectomy site. Severe atypical ductal hyperplasia is reported on the core biopsy. DCIS intermediate-grade solid type with comedonecrosis is diagnosed on the excision biopsy.

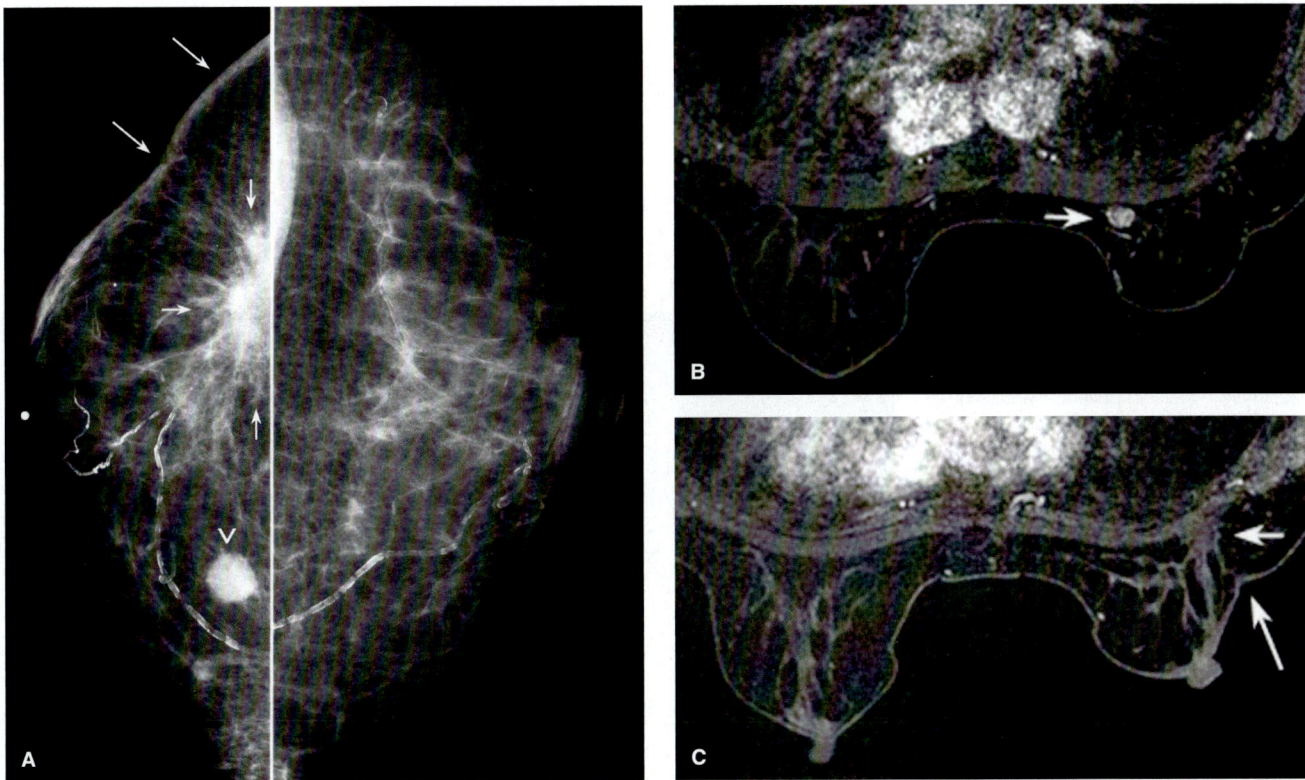

FIG. 11.30 • **Invasive ductal carcinoma, NOS new primary in a patient post-lumpectomy and whole breast radiation. A:** CC views in a 72-year-old patient presenting with a "lump" in the right breast. The right breast is smaller and deformed with nipple deviation, skin thickening *(long arrows)* laterally as well as distortion and spiculation *(short arrows)* posteriorly corresponding to the lumpectomy site (8 years previously); these findings are stable in appearance. A dense round mass *(arrowhead)* is present posteromedially in the right breast corresponding to the "lump" described by the patient. Vascular calcifications are incidentally noted bilaterally. A round mass with angular margins is imaged on ultrasound (not shown) corresponding to the palpable mass. Diagnosis is established on an ultrasound-guided core biopsy. **B:** MRI, axial T1-weighted image post contrast demonstrates a mass *(arrow)* with circumscribed margins and heterogeneous enhancement corresponding to the patient's new primary. **C:** MRI, axial T1-weighted image post contrast lower scan position. Skin retraction *(long arrow)* and slight thickening, lateral deviation of the right nipple, and non-enhancing distortion *(short arrow)* that extends to the pectoral fascia is imaged corresponding to the patient's right lumpectomy site.

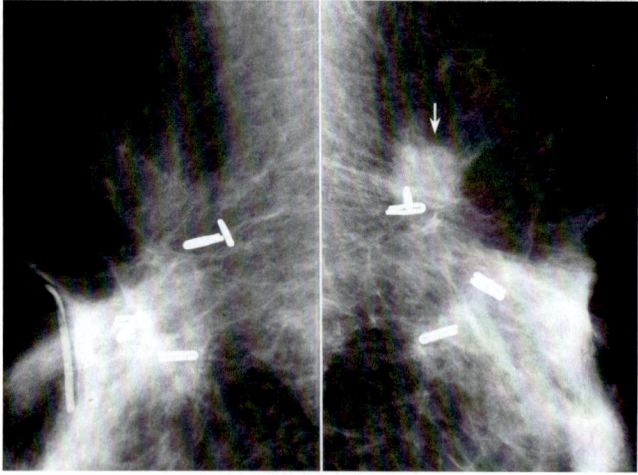

FIG. 11.31 • **Invasive ductal carcinoma not otherwise specified, recurrent.** MLO views of the left breast 3 years apart shown back to back (e.g., current MLO on the right half of the image; MLO from 3 years ago, flipped and on the left half of the image). The patient is 6 years post-lumpectomy and radiation therapy. An area of distortion with associated surgical clips is noted superiorly in the left breast corresponding to the prior lumpectomy site. On the current study, a round mass *(arrow)* with spiculated margins is noted at the site of the superior most clip; confirmed on spot compression views (not shown). A vertically oriented mass with angular margins and shadowing is seen on ultrasound (not shown) corresponding to the mass seen mammographically. Ultrasound-guided biopsy is done to confirm the diagnosis of recurrent invasive ductal carcinoma.

present with diffuse changes (Fig. 11.32; also see Fig. 9.17). In addition to meticulously evaluating the treated breast, carefully evaluate the contralateral side, since patients with a personal history of breast cancer are at increased risk for the development of breast cancer in the contralateral side (Fig. 11.33; also see Figs. 2.47 and 8.18). Aggressively pursue developing changes with spot compression or spot compresson magnification views, correlative physical examination and ultrasound.

MASTECTOMY SITE

After the breast is removed palpation of the chest wall is easier. Only a small amount of tissue is interposed between the examining fingers and the chest wall. Consequently, in patients following mastectomy, recurrences developing at the mastectomy site are usually palpable on a thorough physical examination. Imaging of the mastectomy site probably adds little to the care and management of these patients (2,22). However, some investigators advocate a single mediolateral oblique (MLO) view of the mastectomy side view because some recurrences (e.g., ductal carcinoma in situ) may be imaged before they become clinically detectable (Fig. 11.34) (L. Tabar, personal communication). Unless the patient has a large pannus at the mastectomy site, we are not routinely imaging the mastectomy site. Rarely, patients develop reactive fluid collections at the mastectomy site (Fig. 11.35), surrounding tissue expanders (Fig. 11.36) or following explanation of a reconstruction implant (Fig. 11.37), and we are asked to evaluate the patients for an associated infection or recurrence.

RECONSTRUCTION FOLLOWING MASTECTOMY

Reconstruction after mastectomy can be done at the time of the mastectomy (immediate) or it can be delayed. Implants or autologous tissue transplantation are used for reconstruction. When an implant is used for the reconstruction, posterior tissue along the pectoral fascia

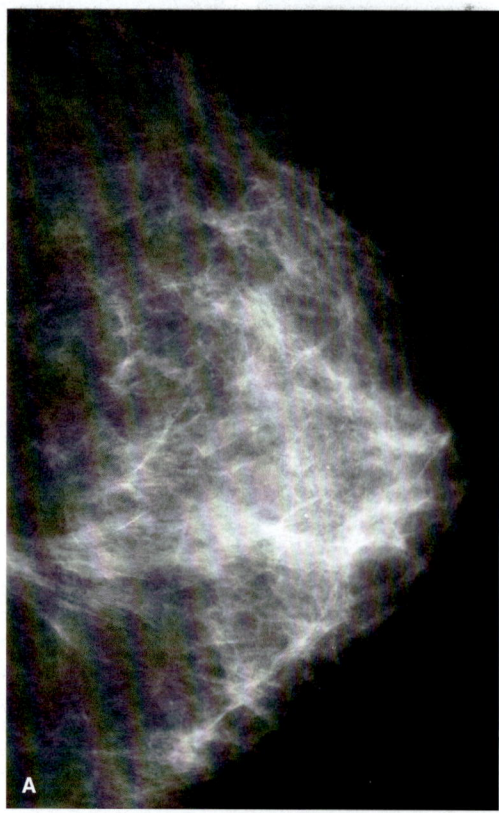
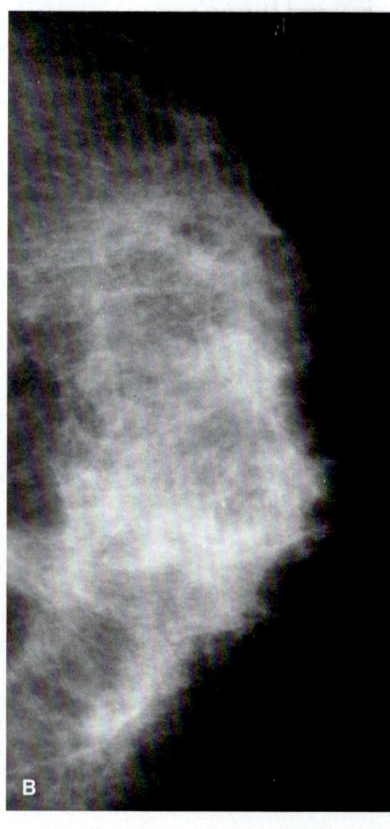

FIG. 11.32 • **Invasive ductal carcinoma, NOS, recurrence with diffuse changes and distant metastases. A:** CC view, left breast in a 54-year-old patient 2 years following lumpectomy, radiation therapy, and chemotherapy for an invasive ductal carcinoma in the left breast. No obvious abnormality is apparent. **B:** CC view left breast, 1 year after image in part **A** and 3 years following original treatment. The left breast is smaller (shrinking) than previously with a diffuse increase in the overall density of the parenchyma. **C:** Bone scan done at this time demonstrates diffuse uptake in the left breast *(thick arrows)* as well as increased uptake by the inferior portion of the sternum *(thin arrow)*. **D:** Chest CT scan image demonstrates skin thickening *(thin arrow)* medially on the left and thickening and irregularity of the pectoral muscle *(thick arrows)*. Although not shown, a lytic lesion could be seen with bone windows involving the inferior most portion of the sternum. Diffuse involvement of the breast is diagnosed on excisional biopsy. (From Cardeñosa G. *Breast Imaging [The Core Curriculum Series]*. Philadelphia, PA: Lippincott Williams & Wilkins; 2003.)

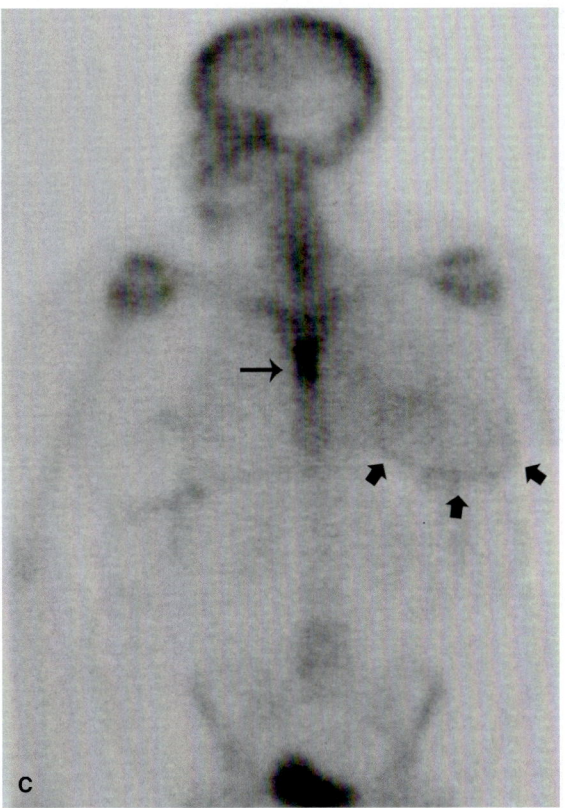
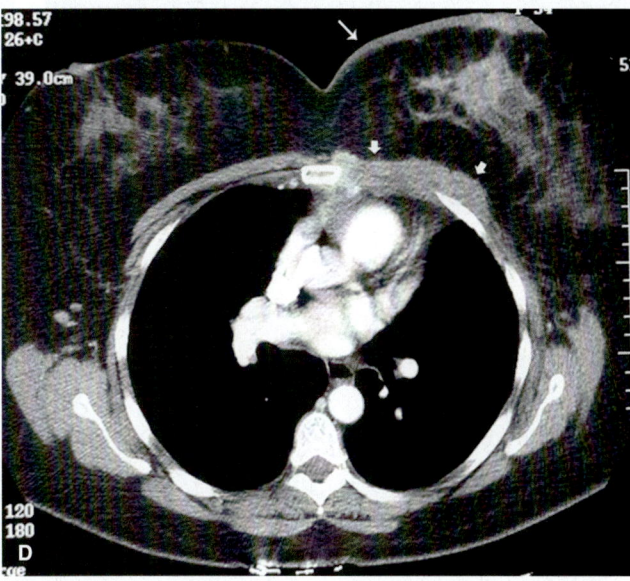

FIG. 11.32 • *(continued)*

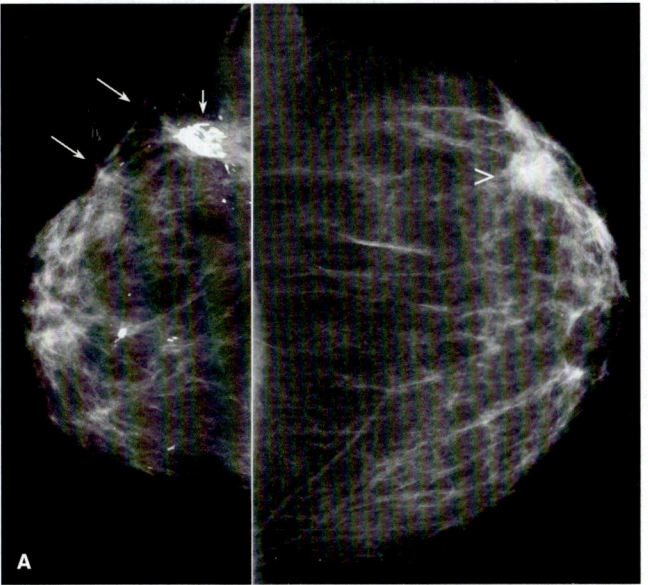
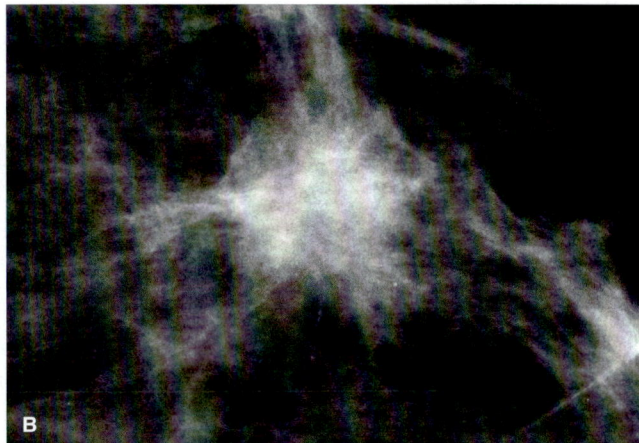

FIG. 11.33 • **Metachronous invasive ductal carcinoma, not otherwise specified in a patient with prior contralateral malignancy. A:** CC views in a 62-year-old patient with a history of right breast cancer treated with lumpectomy and radiation therapy 11 years previously. The right breast is smaller with distortion and a dense dystrophic calcification *(short arrow)* noted at the prior lumpectomy site in the upper outer quadrant of the breast posteriorly. Localized skin thickening and retraction *(long arrows)* is also noted at the lumpectomy site. A new mass is identified in the upper outer quadrant of the left breast zone B. **B:** Spot compression views (only one is shown) confirm the presence of a dense, round mass with spiculated margins as well as some associated calcifications. Invasive ductal carcinoma, high nuclear grade is diagnosed on an ultrasound-guided core biopsy. **C:** MRI axial T1-weighted image post contrast. A rim-enhancing mass *(arrow)* with spiculated margins is imaged at the site of the patient's new malignancy. Also note the right breast is smaller with focal skin thickening laterally. **D:** MRI axial T1-weighted image post contrast at the level of the lumpectomy site in the right breast. Skin thickening and retraction *(long arrow)* is seen associated with increased, irregular, non-enhancing soft tissue *(short arrow)* extending from the skin posteriorly with tenting of the pectoral muscle.

(continued)

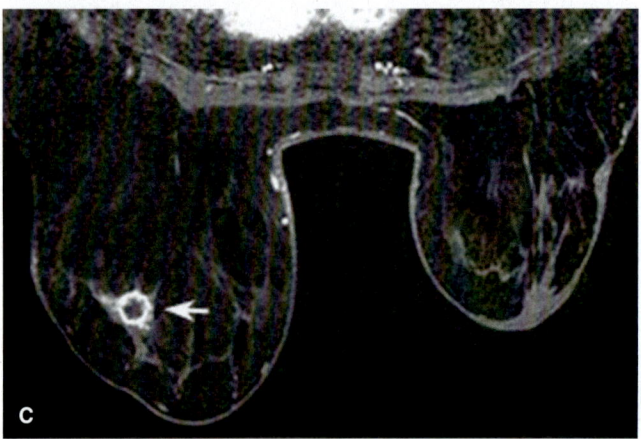
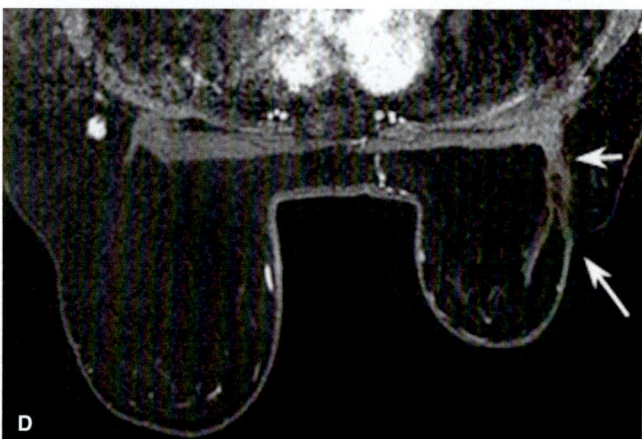

FIG. 11.33 • *(continued)*

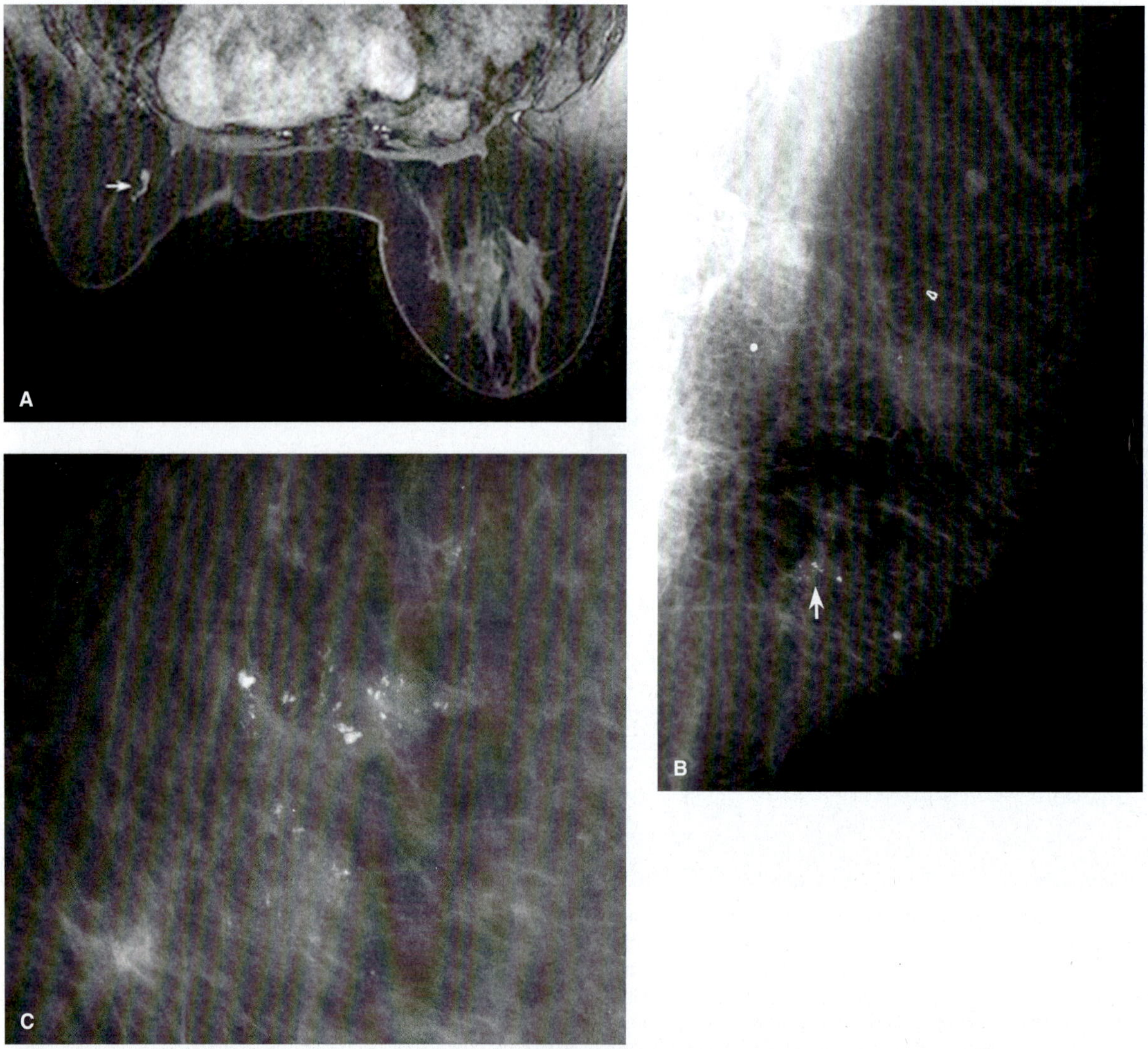

FIG. 11.34 • **DCIS left mastectomy site. A:** MRI axial T1-weighted image post contrast in a patient who had a left mastectomy for breast cancer 9 years previously. Non–mass-like clumped and linear enhancement *(arrow)* is noted medially at the mastectomy site. **B:** MLO view of the left mastectomy site. A cluster of calcifications *(arrow)* is imaged corresponding to the area of enhancement seen on the MRI. **C:** Spot compression magnification view. Cluster of coarse heterogeneous calcifications correlating to the non–mass-like enhancement seen on MRI. DCIS high-grade solid type with comedonecrosis is reported histologically.

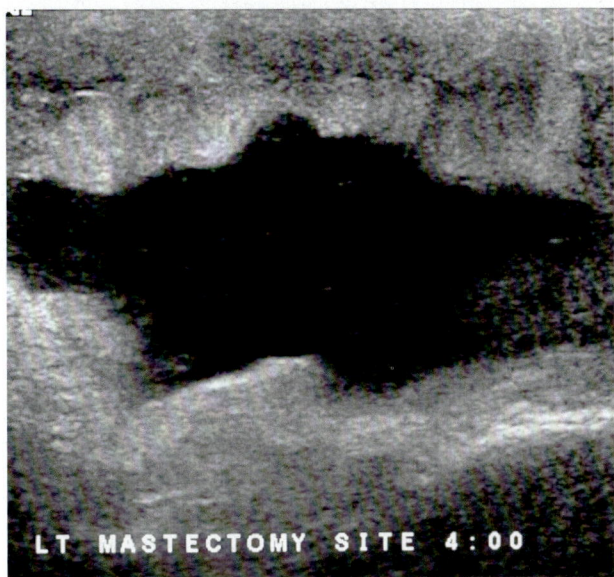

FIG. 11.35 • **Reactive fluid collection, left mastectomy site.** Ultrasound. An irregular fluid collection is imaged in the lower outer aspect of the left mastectomy site in a 51-year-old patient 8 days following the mastectomy. Skin thickening and diffuse echogenicity in the surrounding tissue reflect operative changes. Given the recent surgery and the lack of complexity in the collection it was considered reactive, however, because of tenderness and overlying erythema 12 mL of serous fluid is obtained on aspiration. Gram stain and cultures are negative.

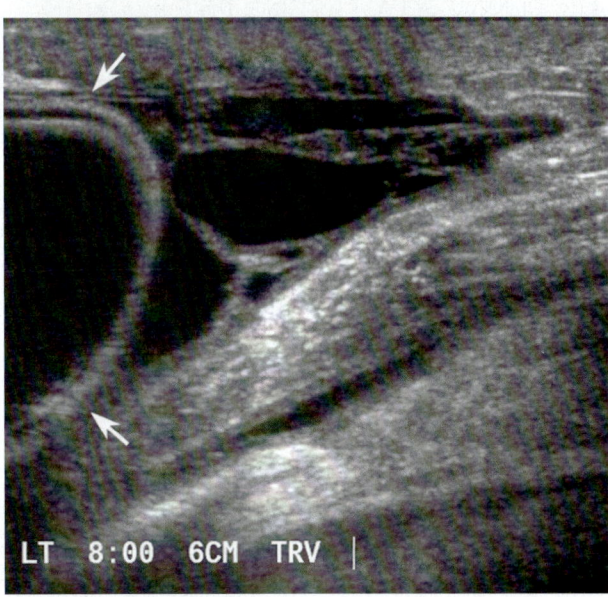

FIG. 11.36 • **Reactive fluid collection around an expander, left mastectomy site.** Ultrasound. A fluid collection with septations is imaged in the lower inner aspect of the left mastectomy site surrounding a partially filled expander *(arrows)*. Erythematous changes are noted at the time of the ultrasound; however, relatively little tenderness is elicited. Based on the clinical and imaging findings, the impression is that of reactive fluid; however, an aspiration is done. Serosanguineous fluid is aspirated. Gram stain and cultures are negative.

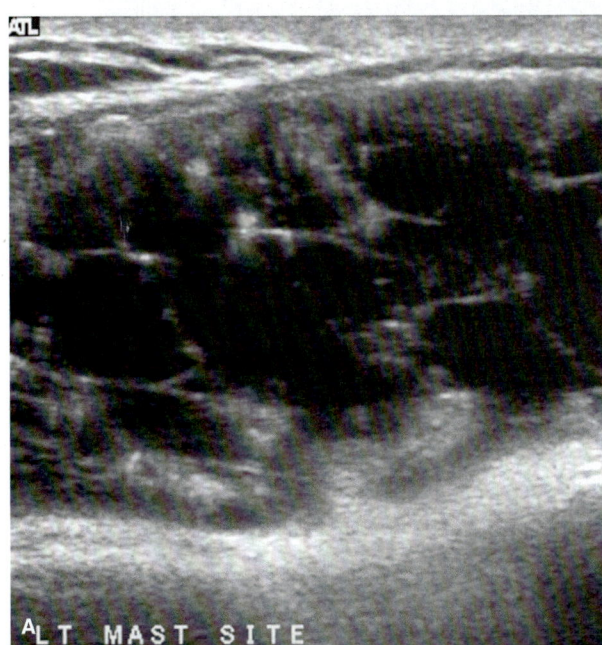

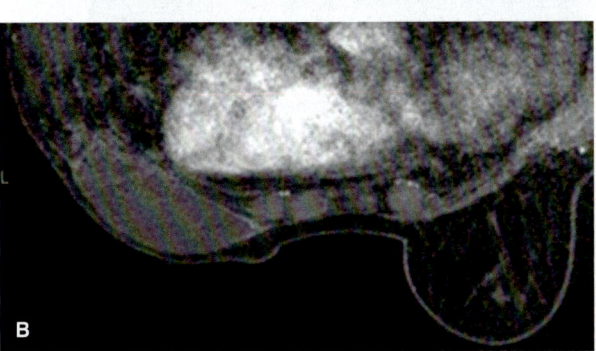

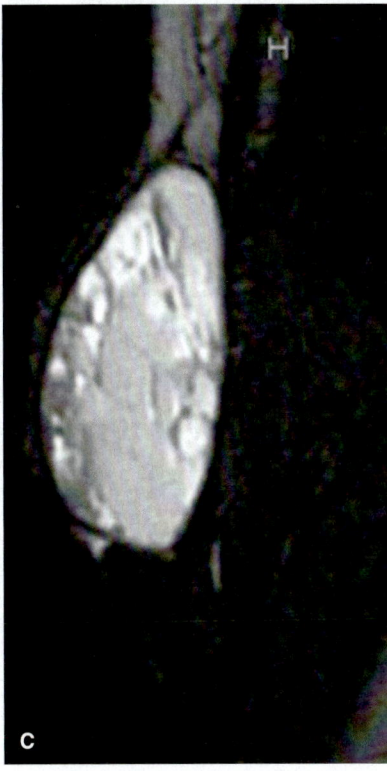

FIG. 11.37 • **Fluid collection at implant explanation site, right mastectomy. A:** Ultrasound. Complex fluid collection is imaged at the left mastectomy site in a 62-year-old patient who had a mastectomy with immediate implant reconstruction 22 years ago. The implant was removed 17 years ago. She now presents describing swelling at the mastectomy site; she has no associated pain or redness. **B:** MRI, axial T1-weighted image post contrast. Intermediate T1 signal is noted at the mastectomy site, the contour and shape of which is consistent with a fluid collection developing in the capsular pocket previously occupied by the implant. No associated enhancement or enhancing masses to suggest a recurrence are identified at the left mastectomy site or in the axilla. The right breast is normal. **C:** MRI, sagittal T2-weighted image of the left mastectomy site. Heterogeneously high T2 signal imaged the contour and shape of which suggest the development of a fluid collection at the site previously occupied by the implant (e.g., within the preexisting capsule).

cannot be imaged mammographically and as such we do not image the affected side. However, if patients with an implant reconstruction present with a palpable finding, ultrasound is helpful in evaluating the area of concern. Rarely, recurrences or second primaries can be imaged in these patients with ultrasound (Fig. 11.38A). MRI can also be helpful in establishing and evaluating the presence of recurrences after mastectomy with implant reconstruction; the multiplanar capabilities of MRI are particularly helpful in demonstrating the relationship of the recurrence to chest wall structures (Fig. 11.38B–D).

If autologous tissue transplantation is done, we do a single MLO view of the reconstruction. The goal is to identify recurrences occurring at the chest wall, deep to the reconstruction (23). Patients with autologous tissue transplantation have tissue interposed between the examining fingers and the chest wall limiting physical examination. This is particularly

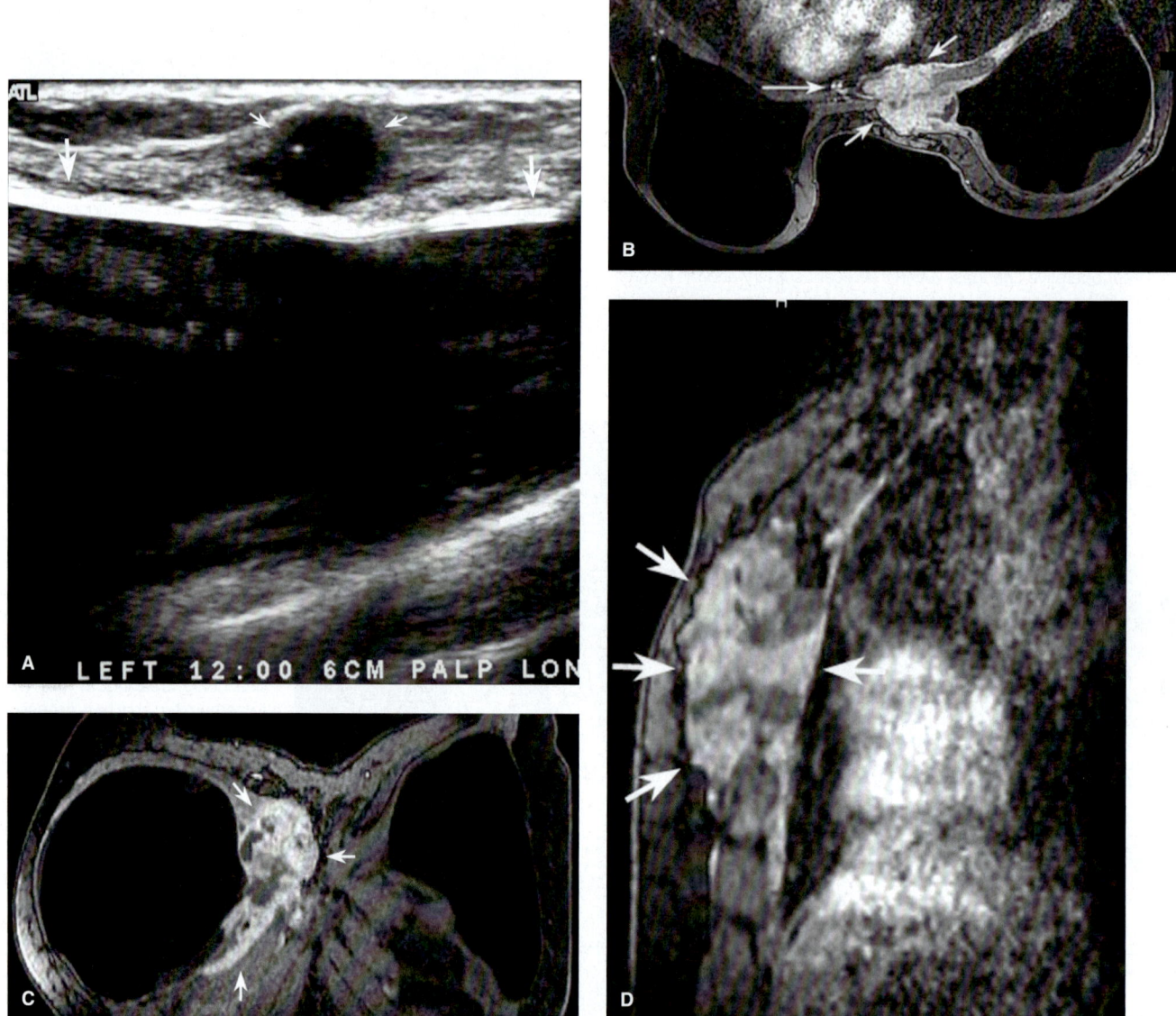

FIG. 11.38 • **Recurrent invasive ductal carcinoma high nuclear grade after mastectomy and implant reconstruction. A:** Ultrasound. A round markedly hypoechoic mass *(thin arrows)* with spiculated margins is imaged in the subcutaneous tissue interposed between the implant *(thick arrows)* and the skin. This corresponds to a "lump" described by the patient 3 years following her mastectomy and immediate reconstruction. Diagnosis is established following an ultrasound-guided core biopsy. **B:** MRI axial T1-weighted image post contrast in a 62-year-old patient who presents describing a mass in along the upper inner edge of her right implant. She had mastectomies with implant reconstructions for breast cancer on the right 3 years ago. A mass *(short arrows)* with heterogeneous enhancement and circumscribed margins is imaged along the upper inner aspect of the right implant posteriorly extending to the chest wall and surrounding one of the upper costochondral junctions. Although the internal mammary vessels are apparent on the left *(long arrow)*, they cannot be identified on the right. MRI, coronal **(C)** and sagittal **(D)** reconstructions post contrast. The multiplanar capability provided by MRI is helpful in delineating the tumor *(arrows)* and its relationship the chest wall structures. On the sagittal reconstructions, it is established that this tumor extends through two of the intercostal spaces.

applicable to those patients in whom fat necrosis hardens the tissue further limited physical examination. Autologous tissue reconstructions are done most commonly done using a transverse rectus abdominis myocutaneous (TRAM) flap. The latissimus dorsi muscle is sometimes used; however, the relatively small amount of tissue and the resulting size of the reconstruction are such that these are sometimes combined with implants. The appearance of the latissimus dorsi flap is distinctive in that the muscle with associated striations is seen superimposed on the upper portion of the pectoral muscle on the mammogram with fatty tissue anteriorly making up the "breast" mound. On cross-sectional imaging (CT, MRI), the slip of muscle is seen extending from the back anteriorly to overlie the pectoral muscle (Fig. 11.39).

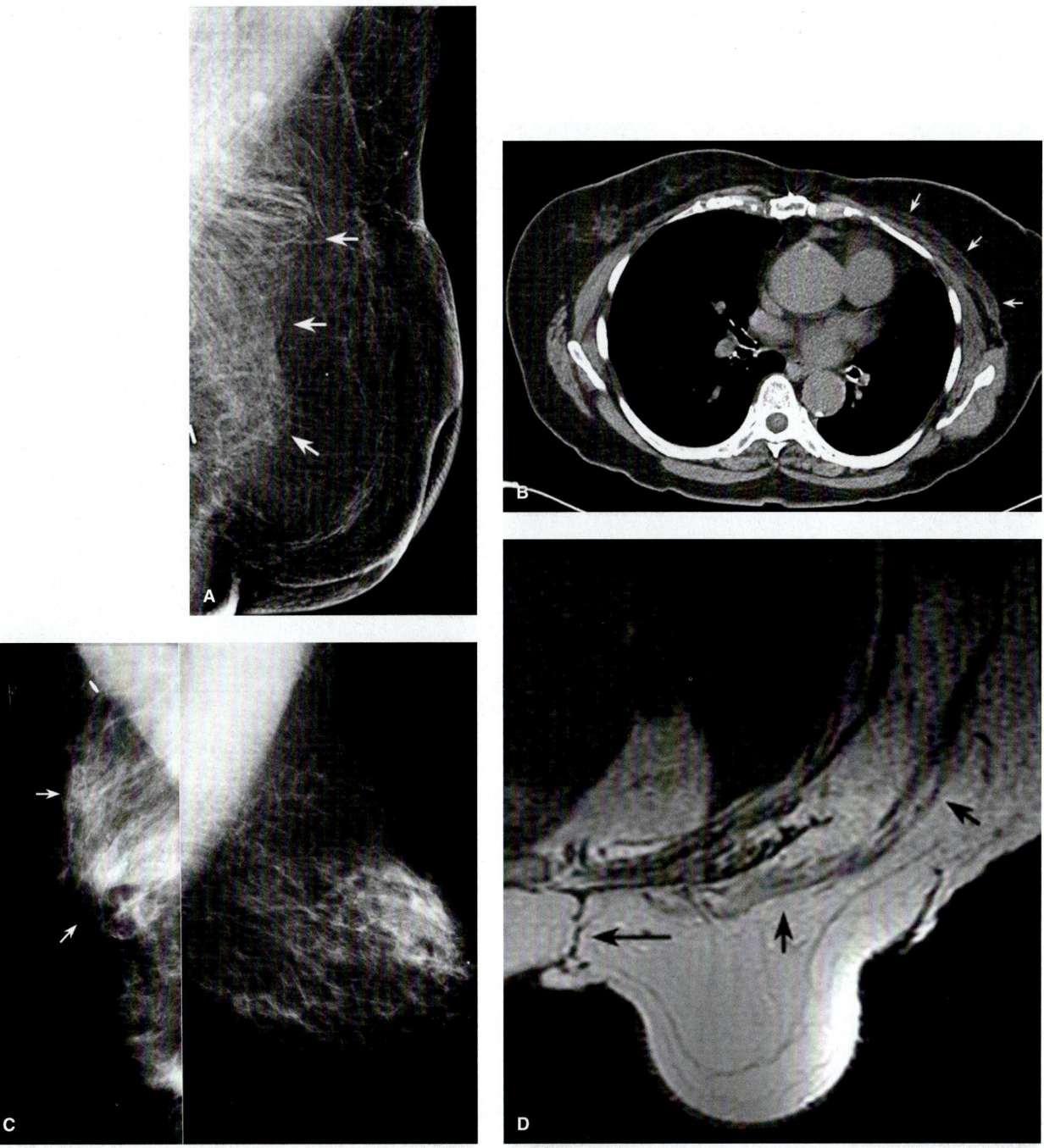

FIG. 11.39 • **Latissimus dorsi flap reconstructions. A:** Left MLO view. Curvilinear density *(arrows)* with striations (e.g., latissimus dorsi muscle) is noted partially overlying the pectoral muscle. **B:** CT scan image demonstrating the transplanted muscle *(arrows)* extending from the back towards the lateral aspect of the left mastectomy. Some fatty replacement of the muscle is apparent. Fatty tissue is noted making up the "breast" mound. **C:** MLO views. Transplanted muscle *(arrows)* is apparent partially overlying the right pectoral muscle superiorly. Note size asymmetry between the reconstruction on the right and the left breast. In some patients, the latissimus dorsi reconstruction is combined with an implant or, in other patients a reduction of the contralateral breast is done to better match the size of the reconstruction and remaining breast. **D:** MRI, axial T2-weighted image. The transplanted muscle *(short arrows)* is noted extending from the back anteriorly to overlie the pectoral muscle. Fatty tissue is noted making up the "breast" mound. An additional suture line is noted centrally *(long arrow)*.

The appearance of TRAM flaps is also distinctive on imaging. Irregular areas of increased density reflecting fat necrosis may develop at the superior (Fig. 11.40A, B) and less commonly inferior (Fig. 11.40C) aspects of the reconstruction. The rectus muscle is usually seen as a round- or triangular-shaped density posteriorly (24) abutting the inferior aspect of the pectoral muscle; with time, fatty replacement and atrophy of the transplanted muscle is apparent (Fig. 11.40). On follow-up studies, the superior and inferior areas of increased density decrease in size and many develop oil cysts or more commonly dystrophic calcifications. These calcifications may be curvilinear, coarse, "bubbly" or "lace-like." As illustrated in Chapter 6 (see Figs. 6.43A, and 6.46C, D) rarely, when calcifications begin to develop in areas of fat necrosis, they may be linear and resemble some of the calcifications that develop in association with ductal carcinoma in situ (DCIS) having central necrosis. Correlating the patient's history, with the location of the calcifications and their association with a lucent-centered mass is such that a biopsy or short interval follow up may be appropriate. On MRI, the rectus muscle is seen closely associated with the inferior aspect of the pectoral muscle. Variable amounts of fatty tissue are imaged anterior to the muscle. Bloom artifact from surgical clips

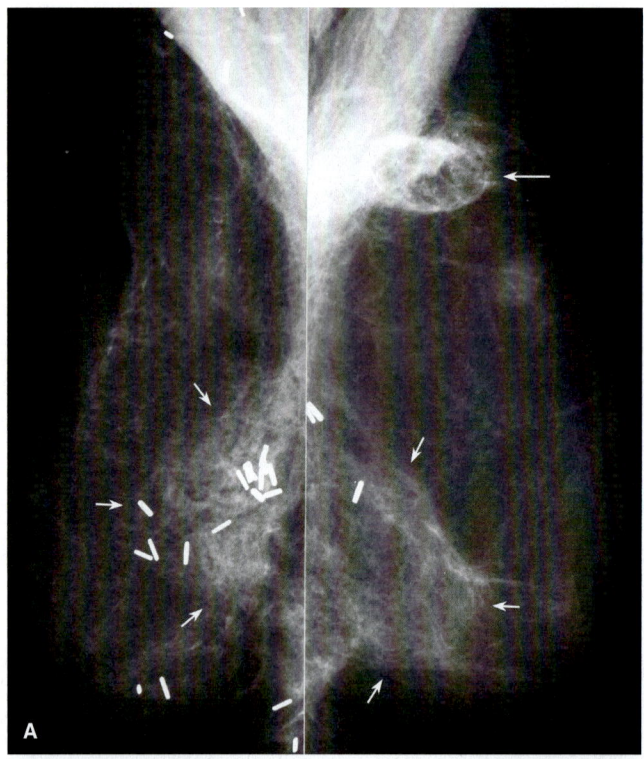

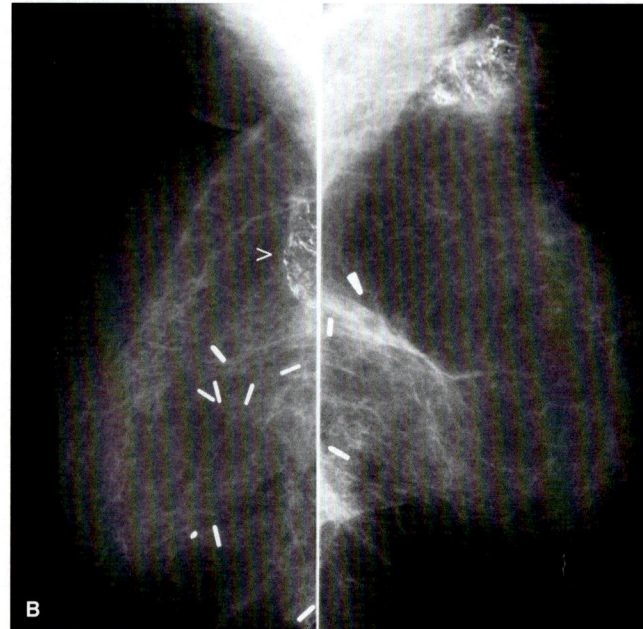

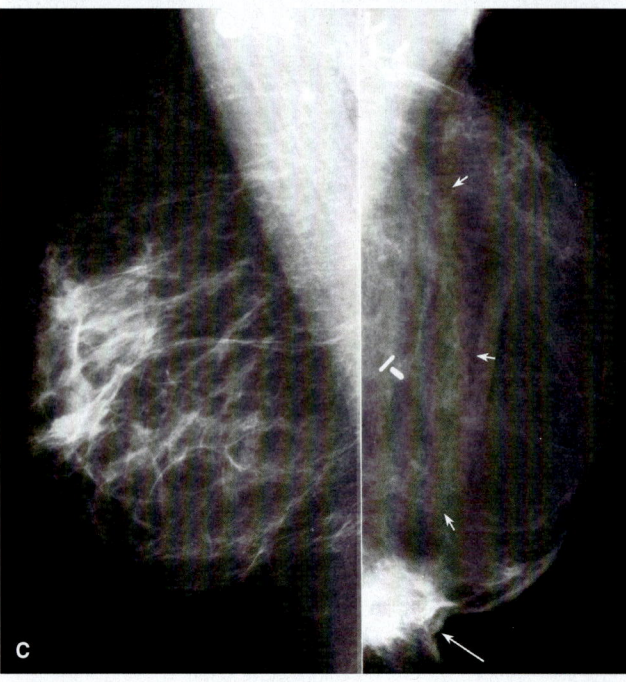

FIG. 11.40 • Transverse rectus abdominis myocutaneous (TRAM) reconstruction post mastectomy. A: MLO views. The patient had mastectomies with TRAM flap reconstructions. The rectus muscles *(short arrows)* are seen as variably sized triangular densities posteriorly at the inferior edge of the pectoral muscles with fatty tissue seen anterior to the rectus muscles. Surgical clips are noted associated with the muscles bilaterally (more on the right than the left); clips are also noted in the right axilla. A fat-containing mass *(long arrow)* is imaged superiorly on the left; this is a common site for fat necrosis following TRAM flap reconstructions. **B:** MLO views 2 years following the image in part **A**. The overall density of the rectus muscle on the left is decreased; on the right, the muscle is not included on the image. The fat-containing mass in the superior aspect of the left reconstruction has gotten smaller, and as expected for fat necrosis, is developing dystrophic-type calcifications (coarse curvilinear). An additional area of fat necrosis with associated dystrophic calcifications now also noted at the edge of the film on right just inferior to the pectoral muscle. **C:** MLO views in a different patient with a TRAM flap reconstruction on the left. A dense round mass *(long arrow)* with indistinct margins is image inferiorly in the TRAM, the second most common place for fat necrosis to develop following TRAM flap reconstructions. The rectus muscle *(short arrows)* is atrophic and almost completely fatty replaced. Surgical clips are situated in the posterior aspect of the rectus muscle.

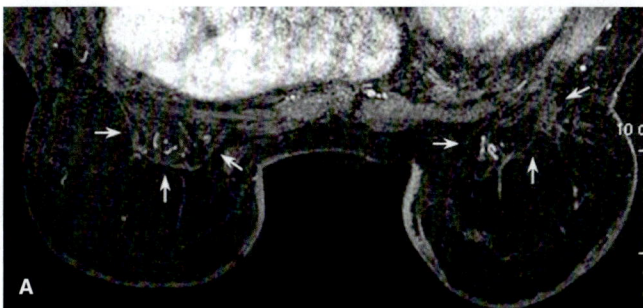
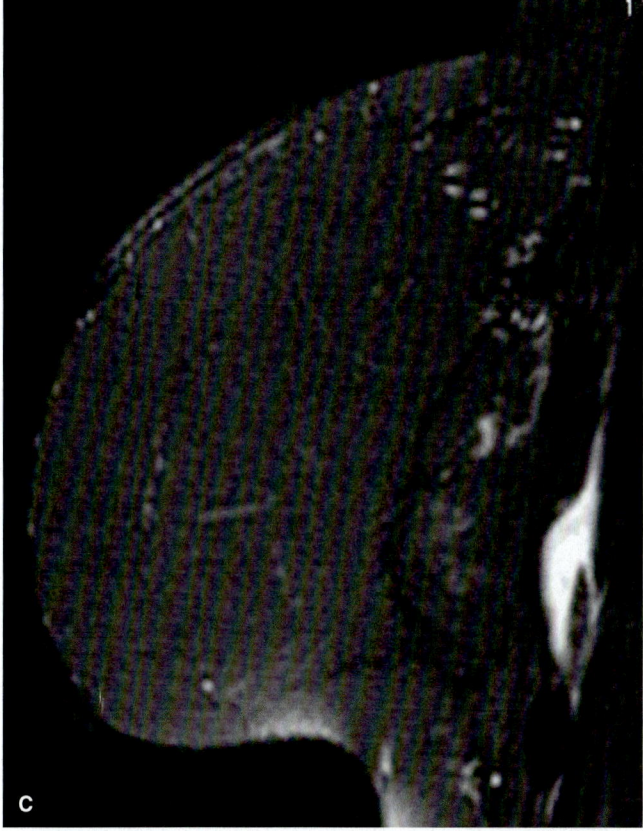
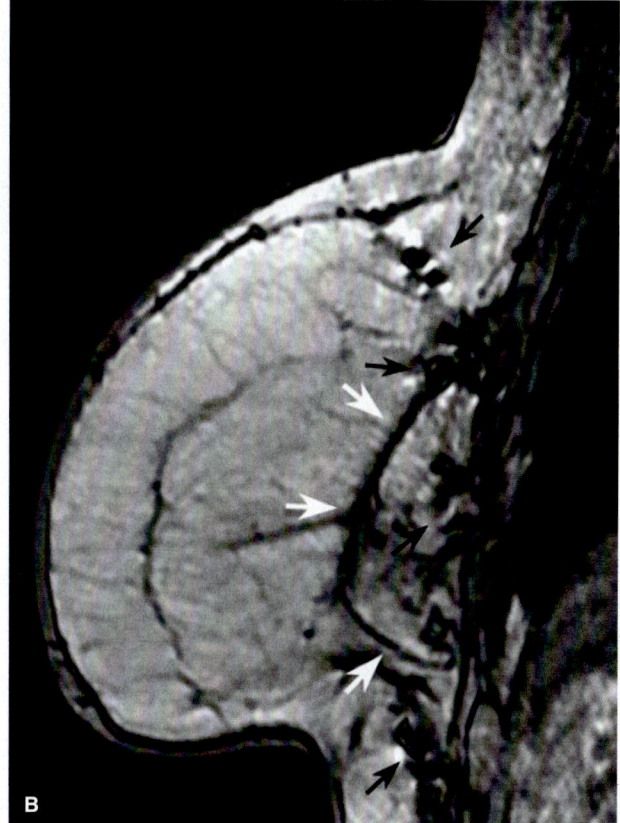

FIG. 11.41 • **Transverse rectus abdominis myocutaneous (TRAM) reconstruction post mastectomy, bilateral. A:** MRI axial T1-weighted post contrast image. The rectus muscles *(arrows)* almost completely fatty replaced can be seen abutting the pectoral muscles centrally. Also noted is the vascular pedicle needed for the viability of the flap. **B:** MRI, sagittal T1-weighted image of the right breast with no fat suppression. Demonstrating the position of the rectus *(white arrows)* as well as bloom artifact *(black arrows)* at several sites along the chest wall. **C:** MRI, sagittal T2-weighted, fat-suppressed image of the right breast. A predominantly fatty rectus muscle is seen posteriorly in the reconstruction with clips in the superior and inferior aspect of the reconstruction, posteriorly. A small amount of pleural fluid is also noted incidentally.

is often seen posteriorly above and below the rectus as well as in the rectus muscle (Fig. 11.41).

Although these procedures tend to be lengthy and recovery time is greater than for patient undergoing implant reconstruction long term, patients with flaps encounter less complications and the flaps reflect body weight changes something that does not occur in patients with implants. A prior caesarian section is a contraindication for the standard TRAM flaps. Additionally, the resulting abdominal wall weakness and possibility of ventral hernia development following TRAM flaps, have led to the development of microsurgical techniques for breast reconstruction using skin and subcutaneous tissue but with the preservation of the rectus muscle (e.g., the DIEP flap = deep inferior epigastric perforator flap), a procedure that may minimize the likelihood of these complications.

REDUCTION MAMMOPLASTY

Breast hypertrophy can lead to significant medical issues for affected women. These include respiratory compromise secondary to increases in chest wall weight, alterations in posture, back, thoracic and breast pain, shoulder grooving, intertrigal infections at the inframammary fold, and psychosocial issues. If the hypertrophy is asymmetric, unilateral reduction is indicated to achieve symmetry.

Several surgical procedures are now available for breast reduction. These usually involve the creation of lateral and medial flaps, and a flap for the nipple-areolar complex. A periareolar incision alone or in combination with a vertical scar to the inframammary fold and a horizontal scar along the inframammary fold is used to either reposition breast tissue or excise tissue and reposition the breast on the chest wall (25).

Potential complications of reduction mammoplasty include nipple necrosis and loss in up to 5% of patients (25). Patients who are smokers or have diabetes or hypertension and are obese have an increased incidence of this complication. Flap necrosis usually involving the lateral flap may occur. Some patients experience periareolar sensory deficits; these may resolve with time. Hypertrophic scarring, post-operative fluid collections, fat necrosis with subsequent oil cyst formation, loss of lactation, cosmetic disappointments (nipple position, asymmetry, breast shape, under or over reduction), re-growth, or recurrent hypertrophy are also potential complications (25).

Mammographic findings following reduction mammoplasty are variable but distinctive (26) and include non-anatomic distribution of glandular tissue (Fig. 11.42), swirling pattern of tissue inferiorly on MLO views (Fig. 11.43), upward tilting of the nipple which may become more prominent with time ("bottoming out") (Fig. 11.44), fibrotic bands in the subareolar area, and curvilinear along the lateral and medial edges on CC views (Figs. 11.45 and 11.46), distortion (Fig. 11.44), oil cysts (Fig. 11.45), skin calcifications distributed linearly along the healed scars, and dystrophic calcifications typically developing at sites of fat necrosis (Fig. 11.46) or oil cysts, both processes that are commonly seen following reduction mammoplasty. As mentioned previously, fat necrosis, oil cysts, and calcifications often evolve and become less prominent on follow-up studies (Fig. 11.46). Rarely, if skin is "entrapped" in the breast following these procedures, or any

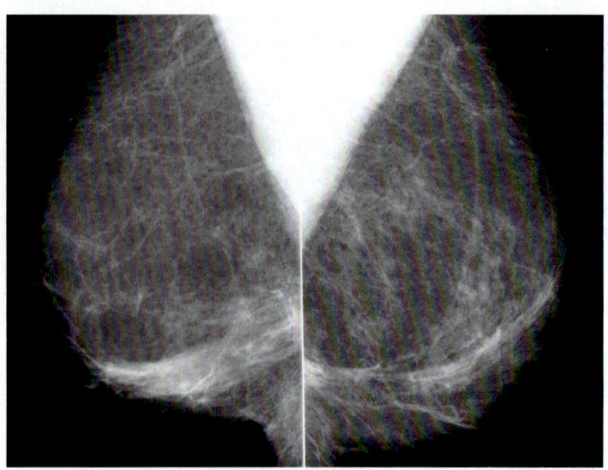

FIG. 11.43 • **Reduction mammoplasty.** MLO views in a woman following reduction mammoplasty, demonstrate inferiorly displaced tissue in a "swirling" pattern. Usually, tissue is more common in the upper outer quadrants of the breasts. Following reduction mammoplasty, however, the tissue often drops inferiorly and acquires this curvilinear appearance. The nipples on these patients commonly point superiorly secondary to reposition of the nipple-areolar complex. (From Cardeñosa G. *Breast Imaging [The Core Curriculum Series]*. Philadelphia, PA: Lippincott Williams & Wilkins; 2003.)

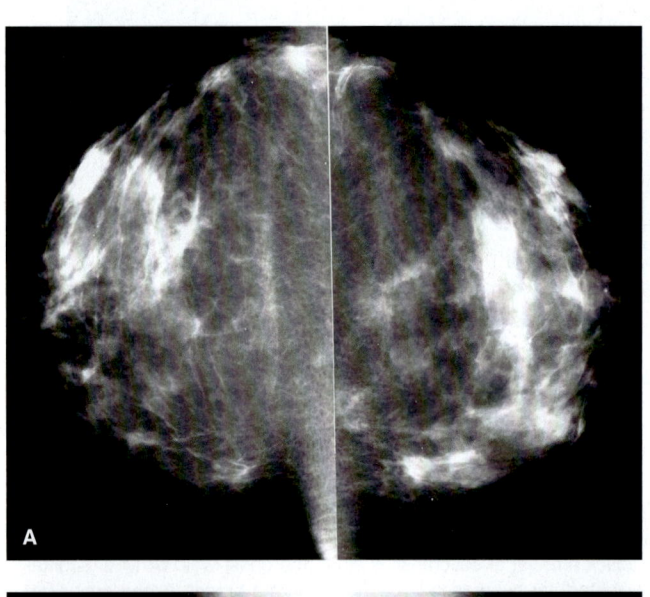

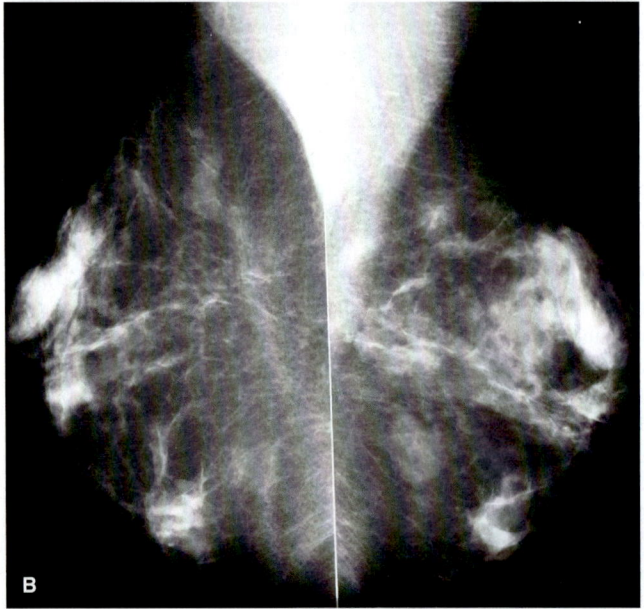

FIG. 11.42 • **Reduction mammoplasty.** CC **(A)** and MLO **(B)** views. Non-anatomically distributed islands of breast tissue following a reduction mammoplasty. (From Cardeñosa G. *Breast Imaging [The Core Curriculum Series]*. Philadelphia, PA: Lippincott Williams & Wilkins; 2003.)

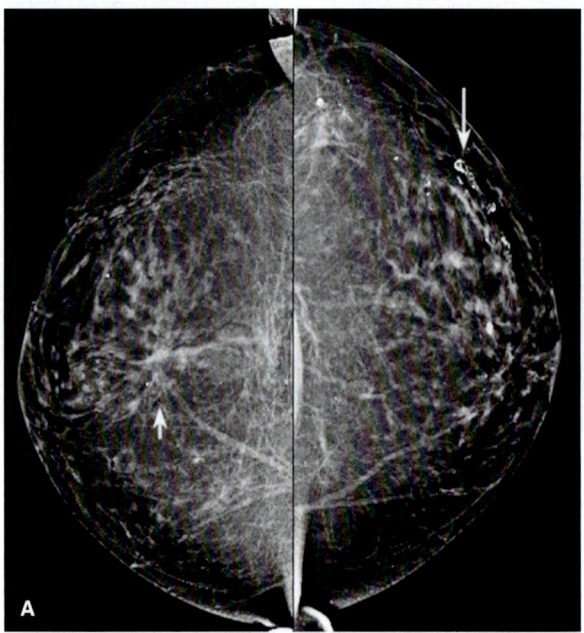

FIG. 11.44 • **Reduction mammoplasty.** CC **(A)** and MLO **(B)** views in a woman after a reduction mammoplasty. Distortion *(short arrows)* is noted in the lower central aspect of the right breast, zone B more apparent in the CC projection than on the MLO. Fat necrosis with dystrophic calcifications *(long arrows)* is present in the upper outer quadrant of the left breast anteriorly. Skin thickening and irregularity is noted primarily on the MLO views. Note upward tilt of the nipples. **C:** MRI axial T2-weighted image. Distortion *(arrows)* is noted centrally in the right breast. No enhancement is noted in this area on the post contrast sequences (not shown). **D:** MRI, sagittal projection T1-weighted non–fat-suppressed image of the right breast demonstrating the site of non-enhancing distortion *(arrow)* seen on the mammogram and corresponding to the area shown on the axial image in part **C**. **E:** MRI, sagittal projection T2-weighted fat-suppressed image of the left breast. Area of fat necrosis *(arrow)* is noted in the left breast correlating to the site of the dystrophic calcifications identified on the mammogram. On the sagittal projections, the breast are "tilting" upward.

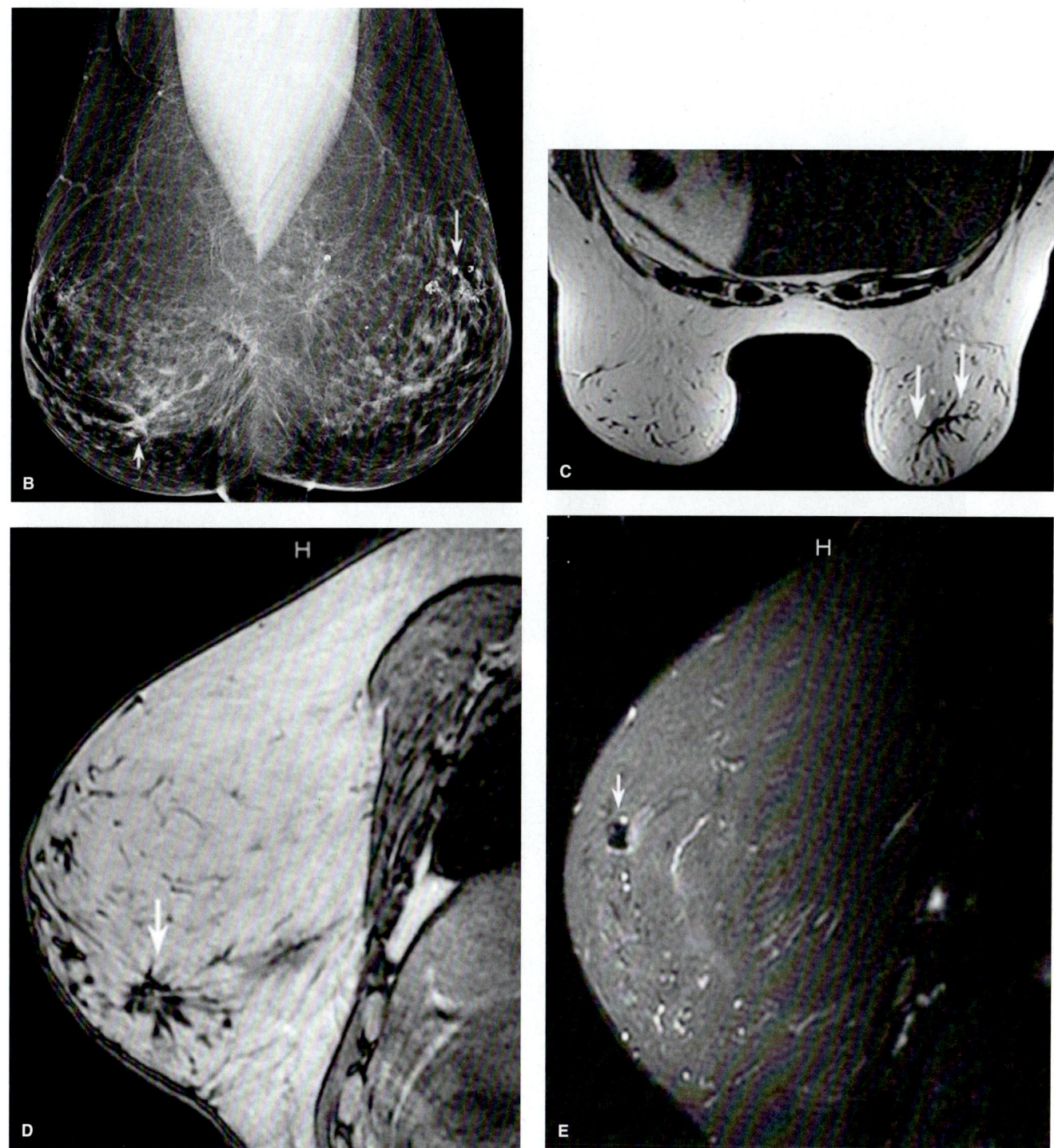

FIG. 11.44 • *(continued)*

other surgical procedure or trauma, epidermoid inclusion cysts may be seen presenting as a developing mass usually with circumscribed margins (Fig. 11.47) (27).

AUGMENTATION

As an attempt to improve on nature, breast augmentation has been beset with controversy from its earliest days when, in some instances, women themselves used injections of paraffin or after it became available, silicone. Many of these women encountered complications including the development of hard breast masses, draining sinuses, inflammatory reactions, tissue necrosis as well as pulmonary and cerebral emboli. Although paraffin and silicone injections have never been approved in the United States, we see women in whom the long-term sequelae of these procedures in the breast hamper our ability to detect early, potentially curable breast cancer (Fig. 11.48; also see Fig. 6.27). In the 1950s, polyvinyl alcohol sponges (Ivalon) were introduced and used for augmentation with good results, initially. With time, however, contracture, distortion, and hardness of the breasts developed in many patients. High rates of infection and extrusion

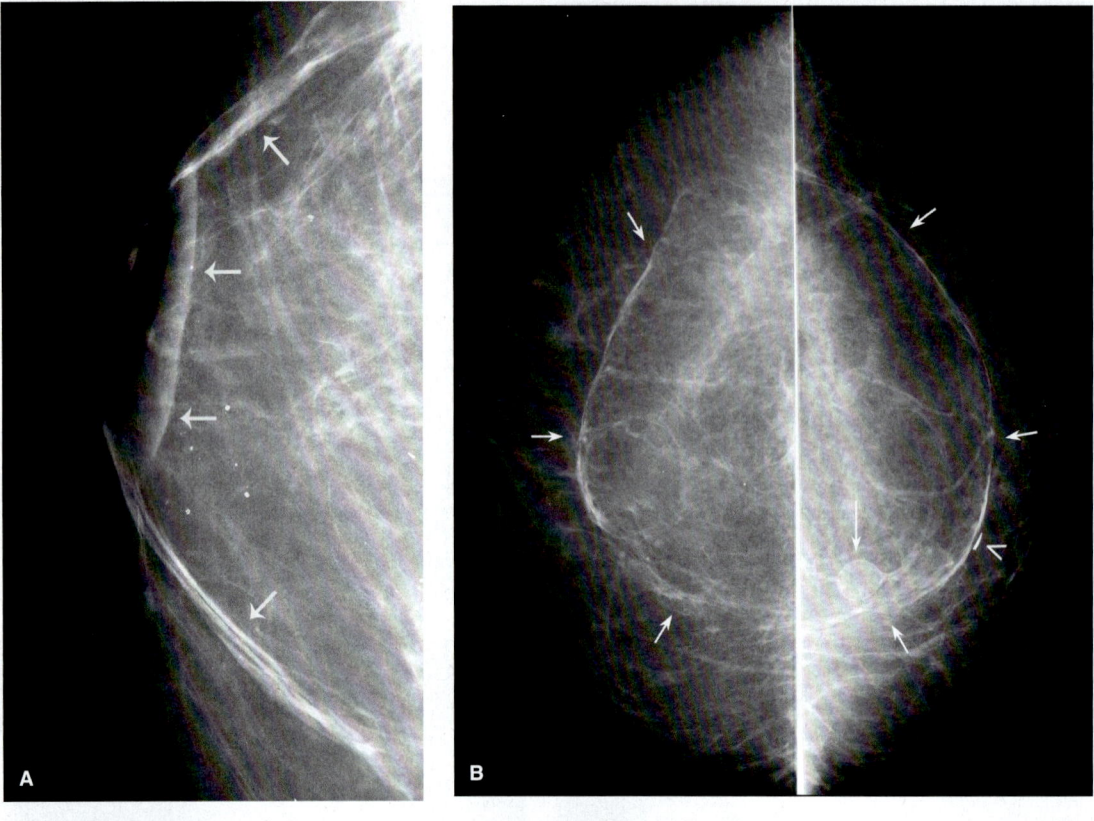
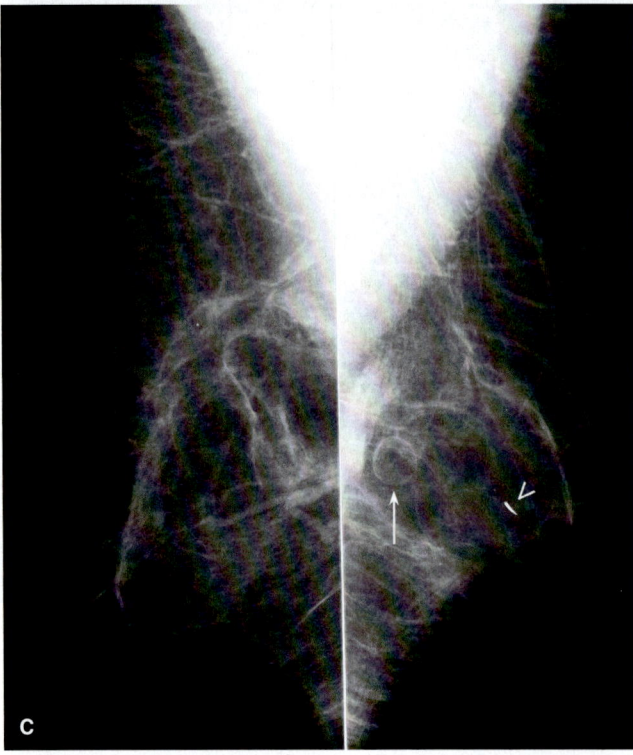

FIG. 11.45 • **Reduction mammoplasty and retained needle fragment. A:** CC view demonstrating fibrotic bands *(arrows)* seen in some patients following reduction. (From Cardeñosa G. *Breast Imaging [The Core Curriculum Series]*. Philadelphia, PA: Lippincott Williams & Wilkins; 2003.) CC **(B)** and MLO **(C)** views in a different patient after a reduction. Thin curvilinear densities *(short arrows)* are seen in the CC views in a non-anatomic distribution and gross distortion of normal tissue architecture and distribution is noted on the MLO views. An oil cyst *(long arrow)* is present posteromedially and centrally in the left breast. Also note a curvilinear high-density structure *(arrowhead)* in the left breast consistent with a retained needle fragment.

The Altered Breast 361

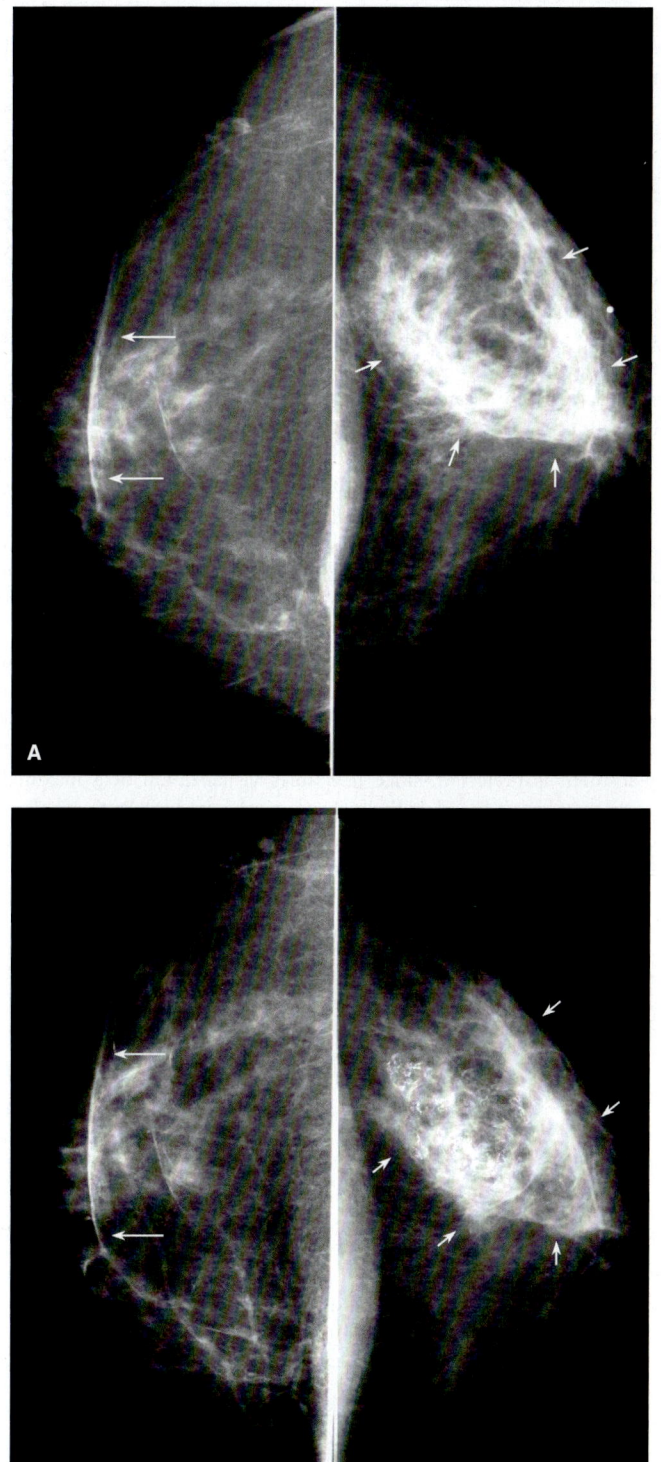

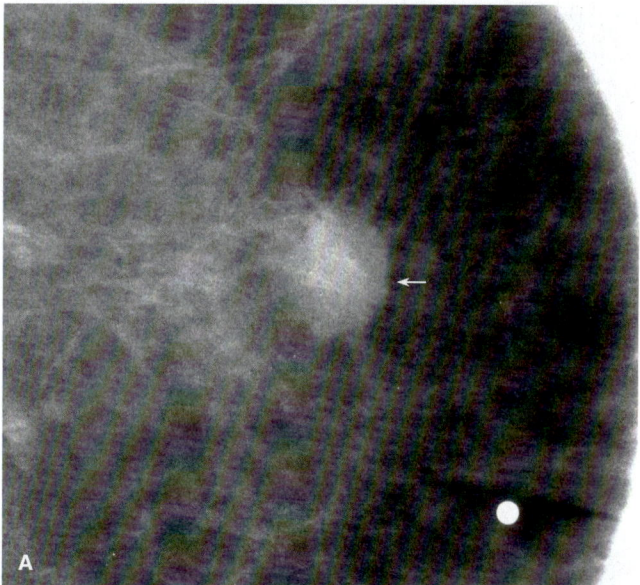

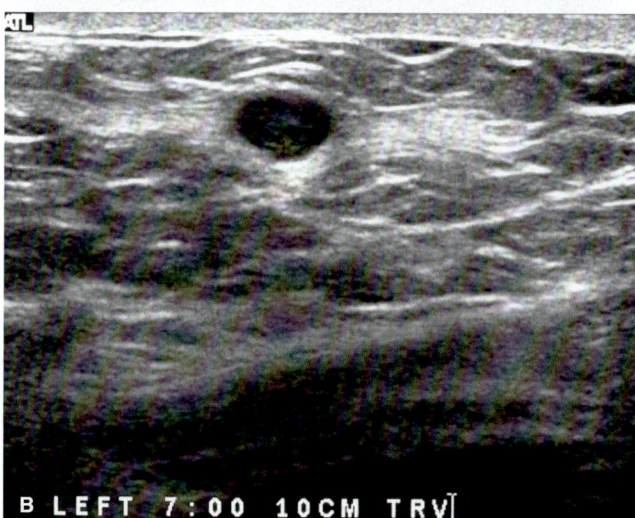

FIG. 11.47 • **Epidermoid inclusion cyst following reduction mammoplasty. A:** Spot compression view demonstrates an isodense mass *(arrow)* with circumscribed margins imaged in the left breast parenchyma at the site of a palpable finding. Metallic BB denotes site of palpable finding. **B:** Ultrasound. An oval mass with circumscribed margins and posterior acoustic enhancement is imaged in the breast parenchyma not associated with the skin and correlating to the mass shown in part **A**. An epidermoid inclusion cyst is described on core biopsy. Epidermoid inclusion cysts typically develop in the skin and are seen in association with the dermis on spot tangential views and ultrasound. However, following reduction mammoplasty portions of skin may be entrapped in the breast resulting in the development of this lesion in the parenchyma.

FIG. 11.46 • **Reduction mammoplasty. A:** CC views done 1 year following a reduction. **B:** CC views 2 years following the image in part **A**. A complex fat-containing (e.g. mixed density) mass *(short arrows)* with indistinct margins is noted occupying the lateral aspect of the left breast. On follow up, the mass has decreased in size and density with dense, coarse and "bubbly" calcifications now apparent; these findings are consistent with evolving fat necrosis. Also note band like area of increased density *(long arrows)* in the right subareolar area and the non-anatomic and disrupted appearance of the tissue in the right breast.

were reported when other sponges (Etheron, Polystan, polyurethane, and Teflon) were used.

When Cronin and Gerow reported on their use of a silicone gel prosthesis in 1963, a revolution took place that came to a grinding halt in April of 1992. After this date, the Food and Drug Administration (FDA) imposed a moratorium on the use of silicone prosthesis for the purposes of aesthetic augmentation; however, they could still be used for reconstructive purposes, in women with congenital abnormalities forthcoming to establish a cause-and-effect relationship. In 1999, the Institute of Medicine published a review on the safety of silicone breast implants concluding that local concerns were the primary safety issue with no existing evidence that implants had systemic health effects including cancer or autoimmune disorders.

In November of 2006, the FDA approved silicone breast prostheses made by two manufactures (Allergen and Mentor) for breast augmentation with requirements for the manufactures to undertake further studies to evaluate safety and effectiveness. It is suggested that patients with silicone breast implants be imaged with MRI 3 years following the initial surgery and every 2 years after that to evaluate patients for rupture that is not clinically apparent (reportedly "silent" rupture occurs in approximately 11% of patients). More recently, in January of 2011, the FDA issued a safety communication stating that patients with breast implants may have a small but increased risk of developing anaplastic large cell lymphoma in the capsule surrounding the implants.

Inframammary, periareolar, and transaxillary surgical approaches are used to place implants in a subglandular (retroglandular) or subpectoral (retropectoral) location. The subglandular position (see Fig. 2.29) is more commonly used reported in 77% to 87% of patients with implants (29). Subpectoral placement (see Fig. 2.30) of the implants may be associated with a lower incidence of capsular contraction possibly related to the movement of the pectoral muscle partially overlying the implant. Projection of the breast, however, may be limited when the implants are in a subpectoral in location. From the standpoint of screening women with implants for breast cancer, subpectoral implant placement is preferred, since it enables visualization of a maximal amount of breast tissue on the mammographic images. With subglandular implant placement, variable amounts of tissue are excluded and this may increase as capsular contraction develops (Fig. 11.49).

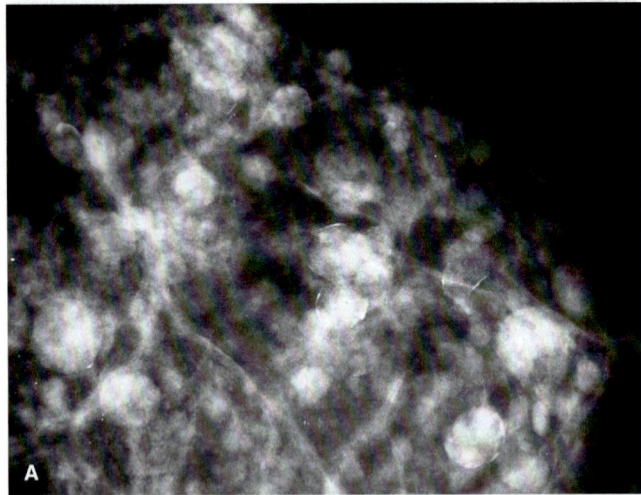

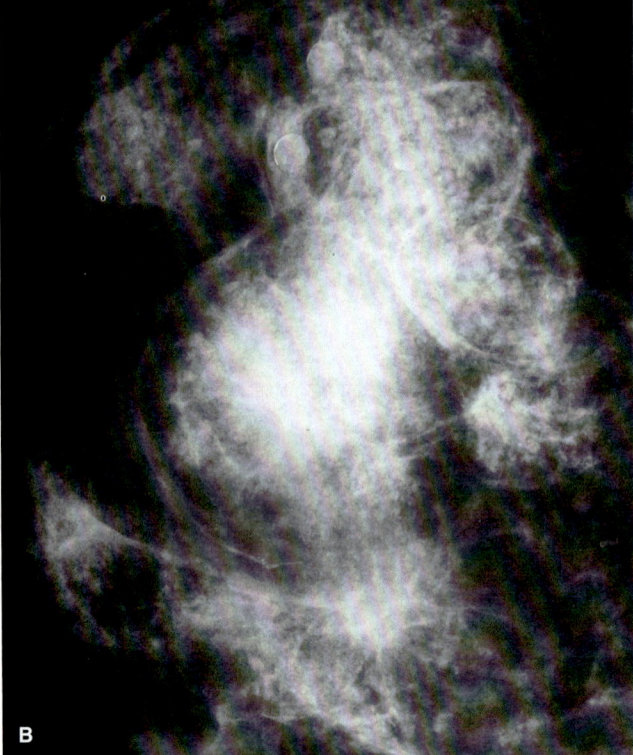

FIG. 11.48 • **Augmentation, subcutaneous silicone injections.**
A: A myriad of variably sized, round, dense masses are seen some with curvilinear (mural) calcifications consistent with silicone granulomas. **B:** Different patient with a slightly different pattern for subcutaneous silicone injections. Irregular high-density masses with associated distortion. Our ability to detect early breast cancer in these patients is significantly limited. It is unclear if MRI will be helpful. (From Cardeñosa G. *Breast Imaging [The Core Curriculum Series]*. Philadelphia, PA: Lippincott Williams & Wilkins; 2003.)

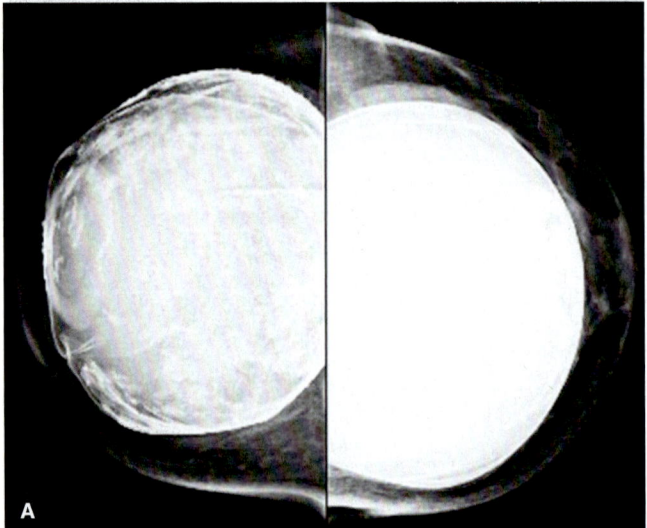

FIG. 11.49 • **Retroglandular implant placement with dense capsular calcification and encapsulation.** CC **(A)** and MLO **(B)** views with saline implants in the field of view. On the oblique views, the pectoral muscles are noted "diving" down posterior to the implants consistent a retroglandular location for the implants. Dense capsular calcification is present bilaterally (more apparent on the right) such that capsular contraction may limit the ability to displace the implants. Also note the round shape of the implant on the right best seen on the oblique view consistent with encapsulation. CC **(C)** and MLO **(D)** implant displaced (ID) views. Glandular tissue is excluded from the images when implants are subglandular in location particularly if the capsule is calcified and the implants are retroglandular. On the right, tissue visualization is significantly limited and the pectoral muscle is not imaged on the ID MLO view; a little more tissue is imaged on the left.

or those requiring replacement of their silicone implants. Like with other augmentation methods, as experience with silicone implants accrued, complications were reported including capsular contracture, gel bleed, rupture, pain, deformity, additional surgical procedures, and the potential association with autoimmune disorders (28). Although the FDA used reports of a potential link between silicone implants and autoimmune disorders to withdraw silicone implants from the market in 1992, this remains controversial. No definitive proof was

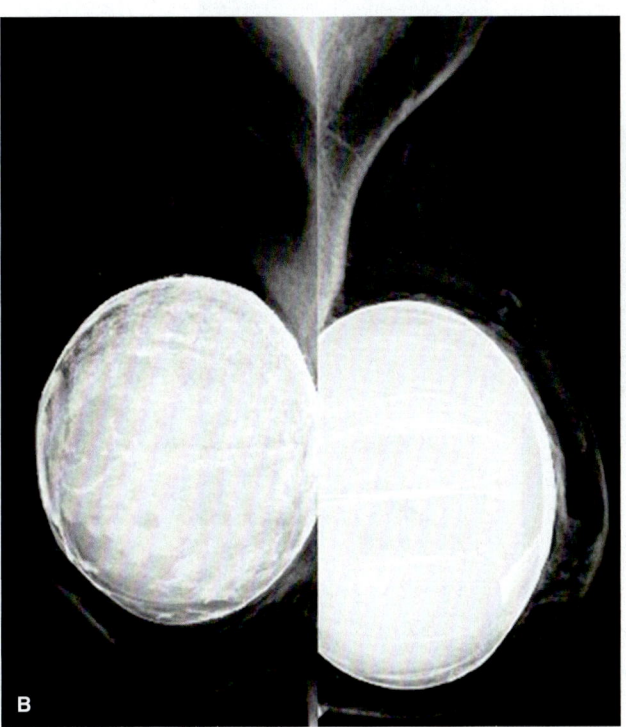
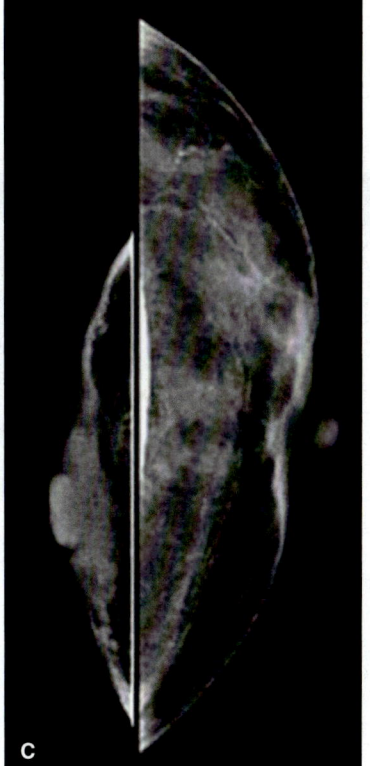
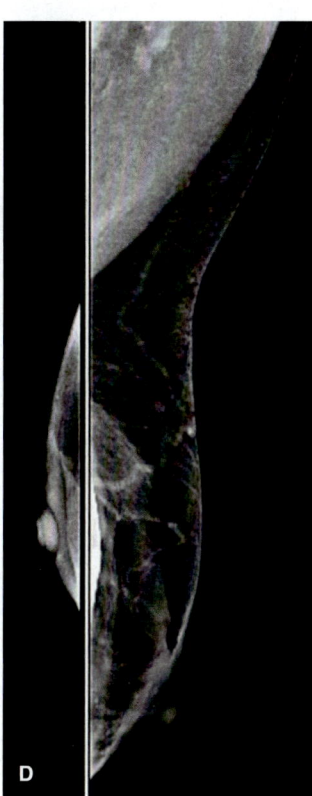

FIG. 11.49 • (continued)

The subglandular or subpectoral location of the implants and the type (silicone, saline, textured, or double lumen) can usually be determined mammographically. With subglandular placement, the pectoral muscle is seen acutely angling posterior to the implant (Fig. 11.49B; also see Fig. 2.29). With subpectoral placement, a strip of muscle of varying thickness can be seen covering the upper portion of the implant on the MLO views and may be seen overlying a portion of the implants anteriorly (sometimes medially) on CC views (see Fig. 2.30). Silicone implants are high in density such that wrinkles are not identifiable and tissue cannot be seen through them. Saline implants are less radiopaque than silicone so that wrinkles, folds, and valves are usually visible, and tissue is often faintly seen through them. Rarely, calcifications can develop on the valve of the saline implants. These calcifications may be fine pleomorphic (round, punctate) simulating the type of calcifications seen in DCIS (Fig. 11.50A). As different projections are obtained these calcifications are always associated with the valve of the implant (Fig. 11.50B, C). In other patients, the valvular calcifications are dense and coarse (Fig. 11.50B, C). Saline implants can collapse such that the implant shell is folded up on itself resulting in variably shaped dense structures posteriorly in the breast (Fig. 11.51). The textured polyurethane–coated implants are no longer used; however, they can be recognized on close inspection by subtle undulations of the implant surface in those patients who still have them in place. The textured implants reportedly had one of the lower rates of contracture but were removed from the market after reports emerged of an association between polyurethane and liver cancer in mice (30). In women with double lumen implants, different densities comprising the different components (saline and silicone) of the implants are apparent (Fig. 11.52). Contour deformities, contracture, surface undulations, wrinkles (Fig. 11.53A), bulges or herniations (Fig. 11.53B), capsular calcifications (Fig. 11.49), and extracapsular silicone may be seen mammographically. Gel bleed and intracapsular rupture are not seen mammographically but may be seen on MR imaging (31–33).

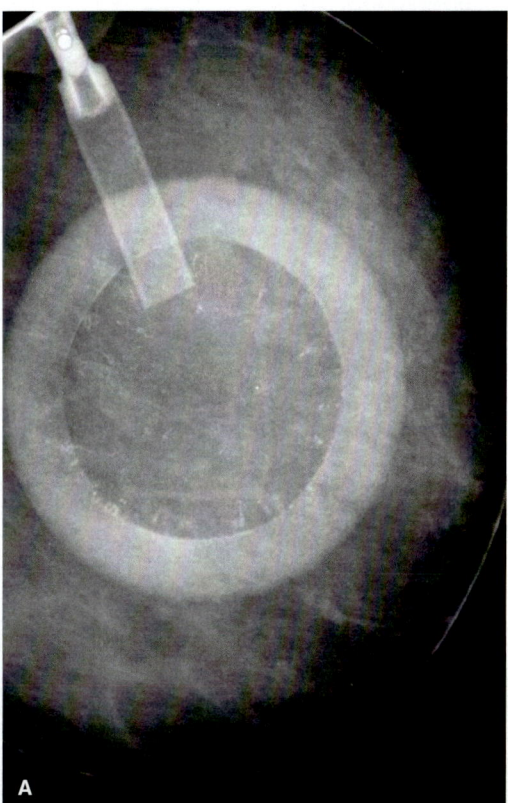

FIG. 11.50 • **Calcifications associated with saline implant valve. A:** Fine pleomorphic calcifications including some linear forms are present involving the valve of the saline implant. In all projections obtained these are associated with the valve of the implant. Right **(B)** and left **(C)** MLO views, different patient. Dense, coarse calcifications are noted associated with the valve of this type of saline implant.

(continued)

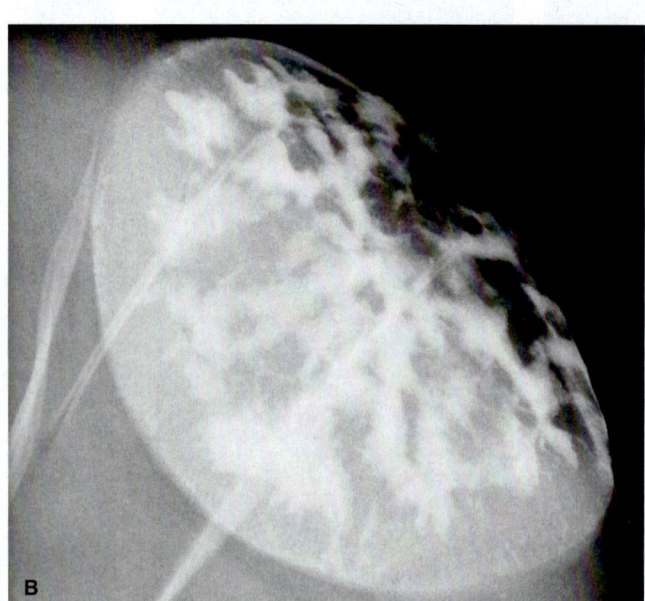
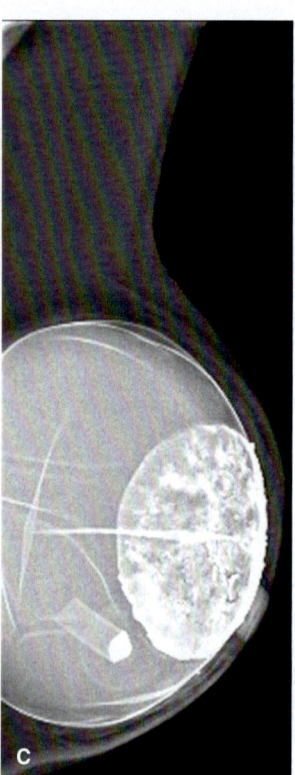

FIG. 11.50 • *(continued)*

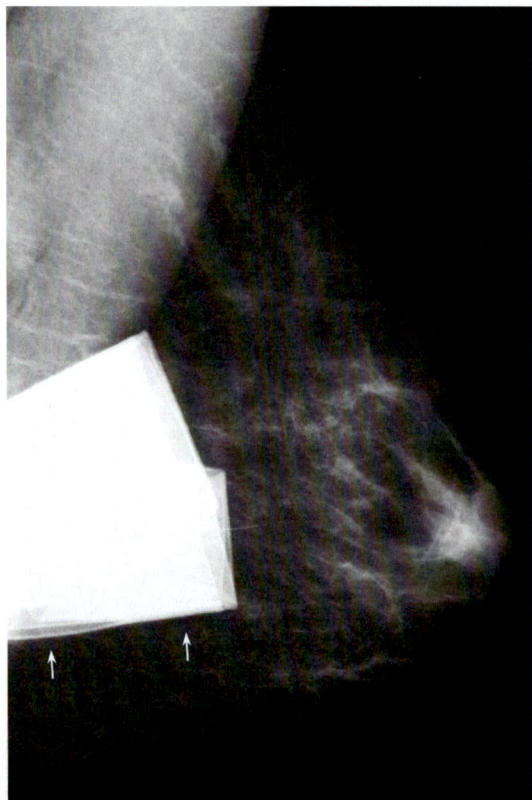

FIG. 11.51 • **Collapsed saline implant.** MLO view of the left breast. A collapsed saline implant *(arrows)* in a subglandular location is partially imaged posteriorly in the left breast. Saline implants may progressively decrease in size with an increase in the size and number of wrinkles and eventually they can collapse completely as in this patient.

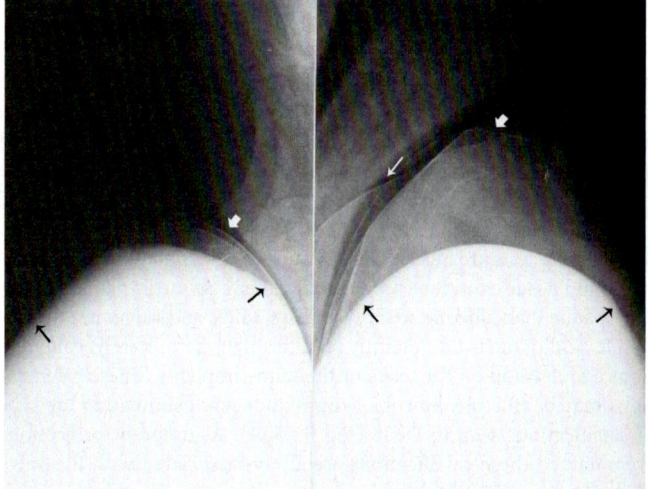

FIG. 11.52 • **Double lumen implants, subglandular in location.** Two different densities are seen associated with these implants. In this patient, the low-density saline component is on the outside *(thick white arrows)*. Silicone is the inner component *(black arrows)*. The pectoral muscle *(thin white arrow)* is seen posterior to the implants. (From Cardeñosa G. *Breast Imaging [The Core Curriculum Series]*. Philadelphia, PA: Lippincott Williams & Wilkins; 2003.)

As foreign bodies, all implants incite a reaction that is characterized by the deposition of an avascular and acellular matrix of continuous bands of fibrous tissue. These fibrous capsules can remain soft and pliable such that the augmented breast looks and feels natural. However, in many patients, the capsule contracts, "strangulating" the implant. This contracture results in a hard, palpable, visible, and relatively

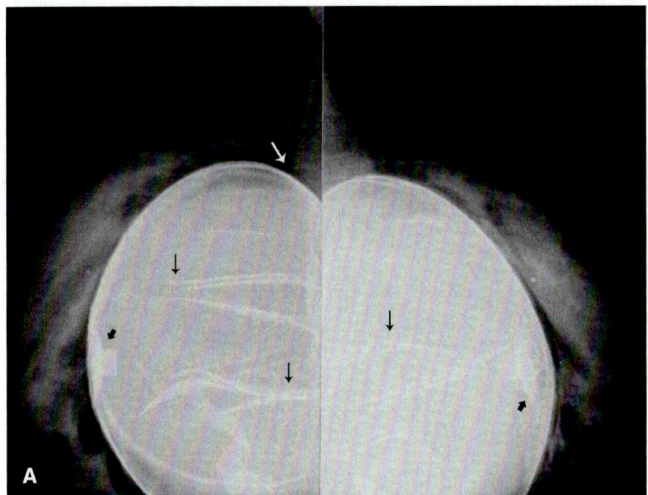
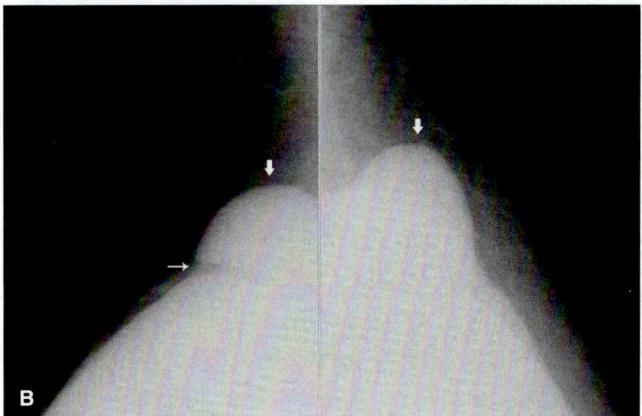

FIG. 11.53 • **Implant wrinkles; implant bulges. A:** The low density of the saline implants enables visualization of wrinkles involving the implants *(thin black arrows)* and the valves associated with some of the saline implants *(thick black arrows)*. The pectoral muscle is seen posterior to the implants *(white arrow)*. **B:** Silicone implants. In some patients, round or oval contour deformities *(thick arrows)* can be seen with areas of constriction noted *(thin arrow)*. The protrusions are well marginated likely representing a bulge or herniation of an intact implant through tears in the fibrous capsule. (From Cardeñosa G. *Breast Imaging [The Core Curriculum Series]*. Philadelphia, PA: Lippincott Williams & Wilkins; 2003.)

immobile, uncompressible implant. Usually, in a bilateral process, capsular contraction has been reported in as many as 74% of women with smooth-walled implants (29). In some patients, the capsule can calcify contributing to the hardness of the implant. Unless the capsule is calcified, it is not usually visible mammographically (Fig. 11.49; also see Fig. 6.17). Many causes for capsular contraction have been suggested including bleeding, subclinical infections, and inflammatory reactions; however, no definite etiologic factor has been identified.

Encapsulation can be treated with closed or open capsulotomies (25). A closed capsulotomy involves manual circumferential compression of the implant to "pop" the capsule. This releases and helps soften the feel of the implant. Potential complications associated with this procedure include bleeding, implant rupture, and an asymmetric capsular tear distorting the appearance of the breast. Gamekeeper's thumb resulting from an injury to the ulnar collateral ligament has been reported as a potential complication for the plastic surgeons doing closed capsulotomies. An open capsulotomy is the surgical alternative for releasing the implant from the capsule. The type of implant and placement (subglandular vs. subpectoral) can be changed at the time of an open capsulotomy in an attempt to minimize the likelihood of recurring capsular contraction.

During open capsulotomies silicone is often seen on the surface of intact implants and is found microscopically in the capsule around the implant. This reflects the slow egress of silicone fluid through the semipermeable implant shell; a process commonly referred to as "gel bleed." As pointed out by Middleton and McNamara (33), however, this phenomenon is more appropriately referred to as "silicone fluid bleed," since it is silicone fluid that egresses from the implant not the cross-linked silicone gel on the inside of the implant. All implants have an elastomer shell made of cross-linked silicone that creates a semipermeable barrier for the gel contents of the implant. The extent of the cross-linking on the shell is used to determine the rate of silicone fluid bleed as low or high. From the day implants are put in, silicone fluid bleeds out. The cross-linked silicone gel inside the implants escapes only following implant rupture and capsule tear. The silicone fluid bleed is not apparent mammographically or on ultrasound; however, it reportedly may account for silicone signal seen inside implant wrinkles (Figs. 11.54 and 11.55D) on MRI.

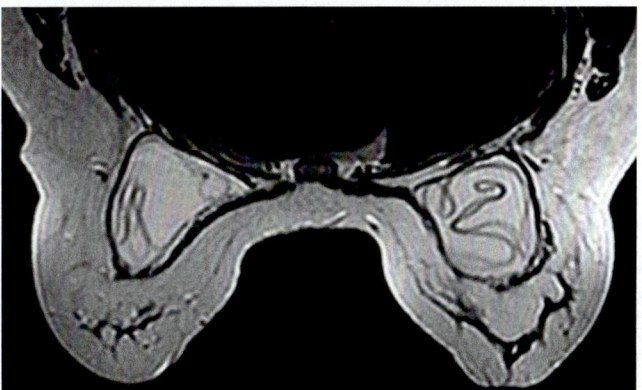

FIG. 11.54 • **Intracapsular implant rupture.** MRI, axial T2-weighted image. "Linguini sign." Implant shell is floating in the contents of the implant presumably contained by an intact capsule (fibrous tissue intended to wall off the implant). The capsule is seen as a signal void surrounding the implant. A "key hole" is seen in the right implant posteromedially. Note that silicone (bright signal) is seen in the "key hole." When this is seen in isolation (e.g., implant is otherwise intact), it is thought to possibly reflect silicone fluid bleed.

Implant rupture can be the result of direct trauma, closed capsulotomies, or aging of the implant with decomposition of the implant shell. Intracapsular rupture refers to the disruption of the implant shell with containment of the implant contents by the capsule formed by the patient. Reportedly, the implant shell is not identifiable in most women who have had silicone implants for more than 10 years. Intracapsular rupture cannot be diagnosed mammographically because the density of silicone precludes assessment of internal findings in the implant. The diagnosis of intracapsular rupture is best done with MRI (Figs. 11.54 and 11.55D), but can also be made with ultrasound (32,34–36). Fragments of the implant shell are imaged floating in the implant contained by an intact capsule. Extracapsular rupture results in the extrusion of implant contents outside of the capsule. When this is silicone, high-density amorphous material or high-density droplets can be seen surrounding the implant mammographically (Fig. 11.55A) (32,35). If long-standing,

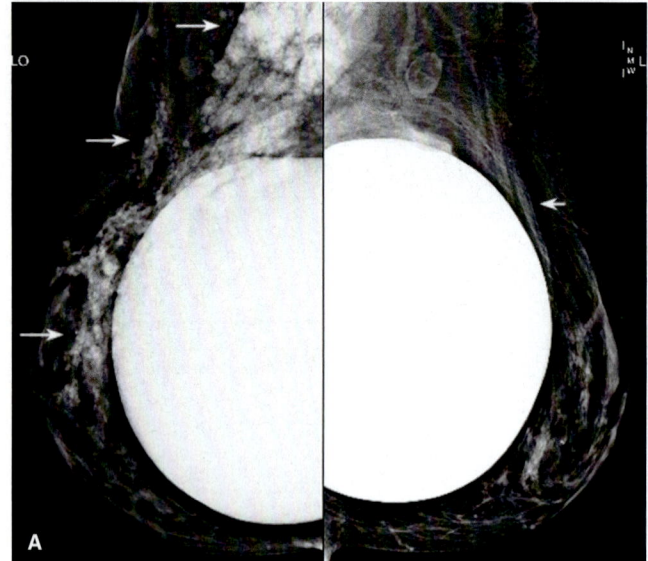
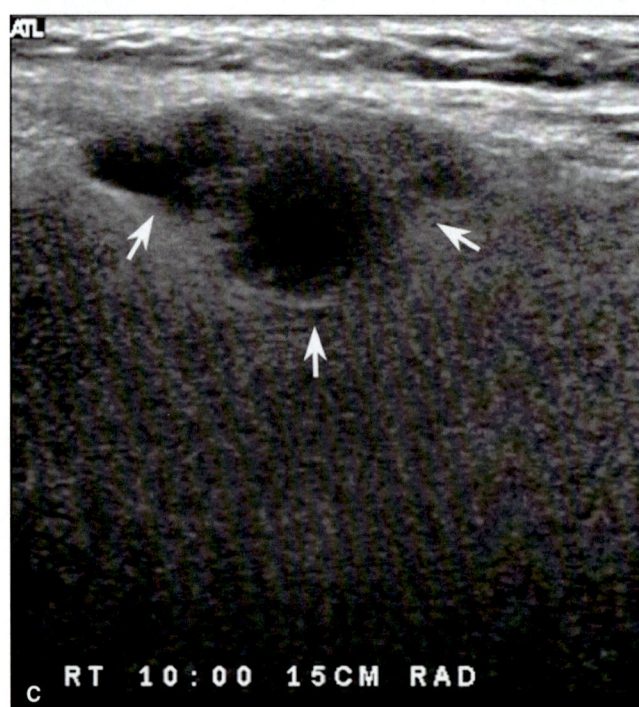
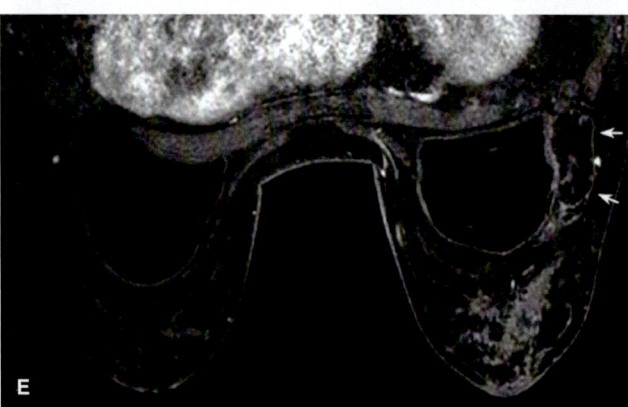
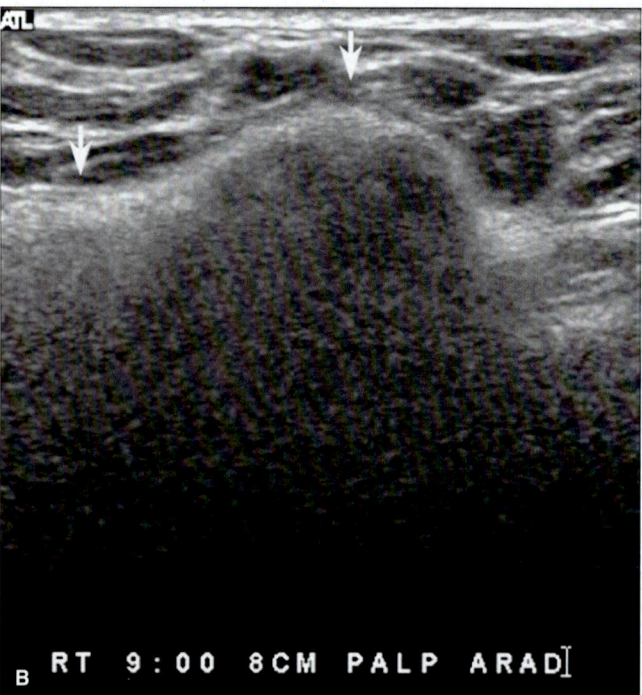
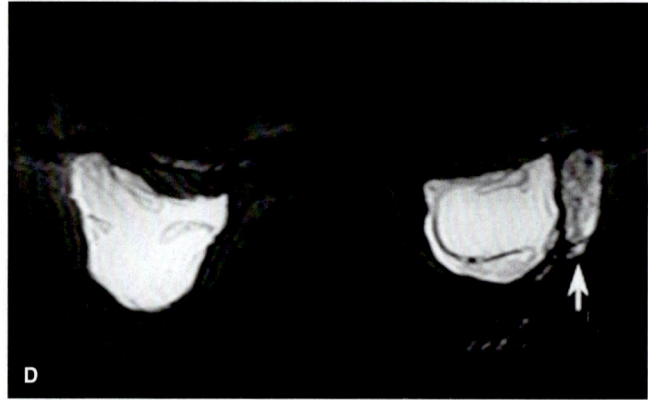

FIG. 11.55 • Extracapsular implant rupture. A: MLO views with silicone implants in the field of view. The implants are subpectoral in location (patient had previously had silicone implants in a subglandular location). A slip of pectoral muscle *(short arrow)* drapes the superior aspect of the implant on the left; however, it cannot be seen on the right secondary to high-density material *(long arrows)* noted extending from the lateral aspect of the breast in the CC view (not shown) into the axilla on the MLO view. The density of the material and its amorphous appearance is consistent with silicone. In some areas, it has a beaded appearance. A morphologically normal appearing lymph node is noted in the left axilla. **B:** Ultrasound. This is the described "snowstorm" appearance of extraluminal silicone on ultrasound. A mass-like protuberant, irregular echogenic line *(arrows)* is noted at this location below which high-specular echoes are seen. **C:** Ultrasound. A cluster of irregular hypoechoic masses *(arrows)* is imaged in the "snowstorm" consistent with silicone granulomas noted in this patient at a difference location in the right breast. These two appearances ("snowstorm" and hypoechoic masses) are the most common findings on ultrasound in patients with extravasated, extracapsular silicone. **D:** MRI, silicone sequence. Findings ("linguini") consistent with intracapsular rupture are noted bilaterally in the new implants. A collection of extracapsular silicone *(arrow)* is noted lateral to the right implant posteriorly; this correlates to the extracapsular silicone seen mammographically and the snowstorm on ultrasound. **E:** MRI, T1-weighted image, post contrast. The extracapsular silicone *(arrows)* collection is identified with no associated enhancement.

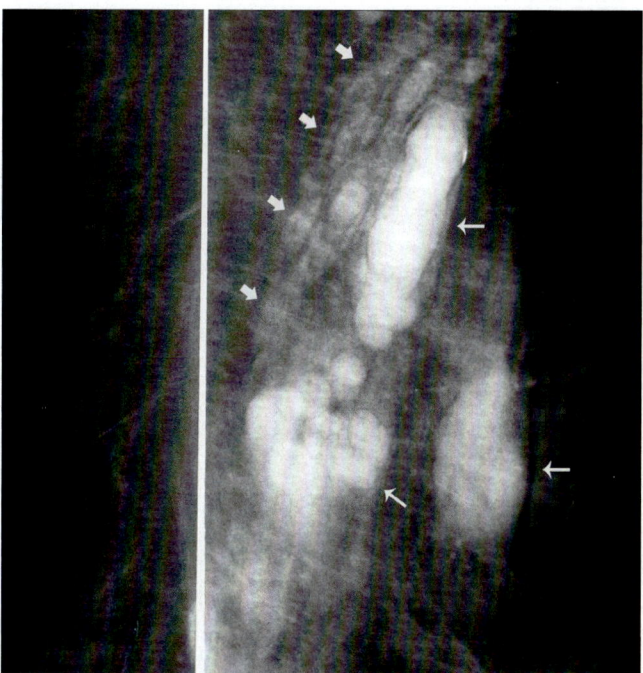

FIG. 11.56 • **Extracapsular implant rupture with silicone extending to axillary lymph nodes.** High-density material is seen increasing the density of several axillary lymph nodes *(thin arrows)*. Silicone is also seen in beaded, linear-like tracks *(thick arrows)*; this may represent silicone in lymphatic channels. This appearance is not seen acutely following extracapsular rupture; this represents a long-standing extracapsular rupture. (From Cardeñosa G. *Breast Imaging [The Core Curriculum Series]*. Philadelphia, PA: Lippincott Williams & Wilkins; 2003.)

silicone may be seen extending to the axilla and in association with axillary lymph nodes (Figs. 11.55A and 11.56). Sonographically, extravasated silicone and silicone granulomas may be seen as high-specular echoes deep to an echogenic line ("snowstorm") or as a hypoechoic masses (34–36), respectively (Fig. 11.55B, C). Extracapsular rupture is also evident on MRI with silicone noted outside of the implant capsule (Fig. 11.55D, E).

When implants are removed, uni- or bilateral fluid collections (Figs. 11.37 and 11.57A) may develop posteriorly in the breasts at the site occupied by the implants; these presumably form in the preexisting capsule. Alternatively, portions of the capsule may be seen as curvilinear densities (Fig. 11.57B) of variable thickness posteriorly. These may have, or develop, associated dystrophic calcifications (Fig. 11.57C). In some patients, distortion (Fig. 11.57D) or a mass with spiculated margins (fat necrosis) may be seen following explantation. On MRI, reactive fluid collections are rarely seen partially or completely surrounding otherwise intact implants in some patients.

ESTROGEN EFFECT

Natural and premature, surgically or chemically, induced menopause is associated with a variety of signs and symptoms some of which have significant health implications for the patient and others impact quality of life. Hormone replacement therapy (HRT) is used to treat some of the signs and symptoms associated with menopause. In women who have had a hysterectomy, estrogen replacement is given alone. For patients who have not had a hysterectomy, the risk of uterine cancer

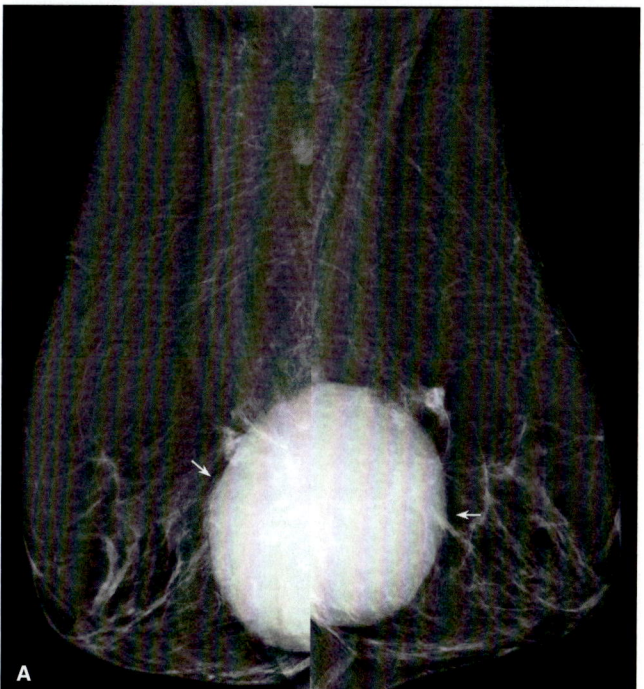

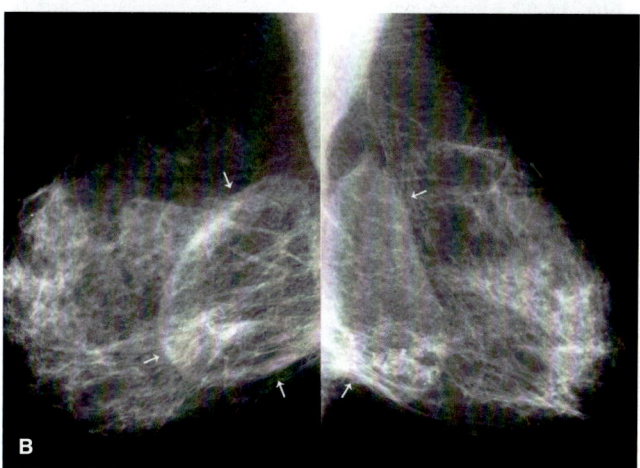

FIG. 11.57 • **Findings after implant removal. A:** MLO views. Round isodense masses *(arrows)* are partially imaged in the lower central aspect of the breasts posteriorly at sites previously occupied by implants. Seromas, presumably developing in the remaining capsules, are one of the findings that may be seen when implants are removed. These may evolve decreasing in size and sometimes developing dense dystrophic calcifications. **B:** MLO views, different patient. Curvilinear densities are seen posteriorly *(arrows)* in the breasts following removal of implants; dystrophic calcifications are noted developing in the inferior portion of the remaining capsule on the left. These densities represent remaining portions of the fibrous capsule. **C:** CC views, different patient. Circularly distributed dense, coarse calcifications *(long arrow)* are noted posteriorly in the retroareolar area on the right. These reflect remnants of a partially collapsed and calcified fibrous capsule. Non-anatomic symmetric curvilinear densities *(short arrows)* developing calcifications (along the medial portion) on the left can also be seen post-implant removal. **D:** MLO views, different patient. Bilateral irregular masses *(arrows)* with indistinct margins are noted at the inferior edges of the pectoral muscles likely reflecting fat necrosis from implant removal. Also note the distortion (straight lines) of the breast parenchyma bilaterally consistent with prior surgical procedures. Morphologically normal lymph nodes are noted in the right axilla.

(continued)

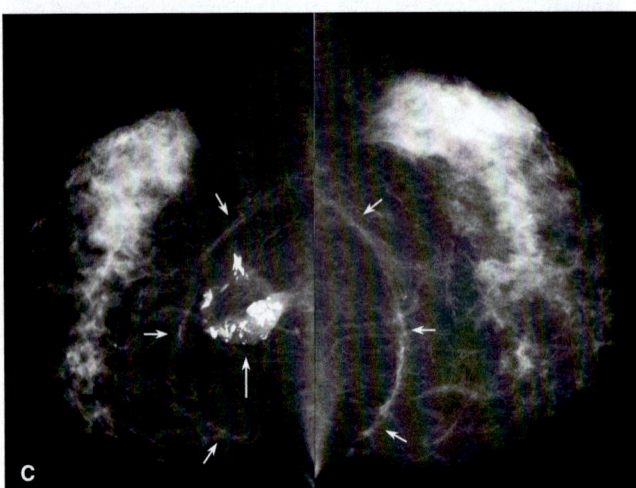
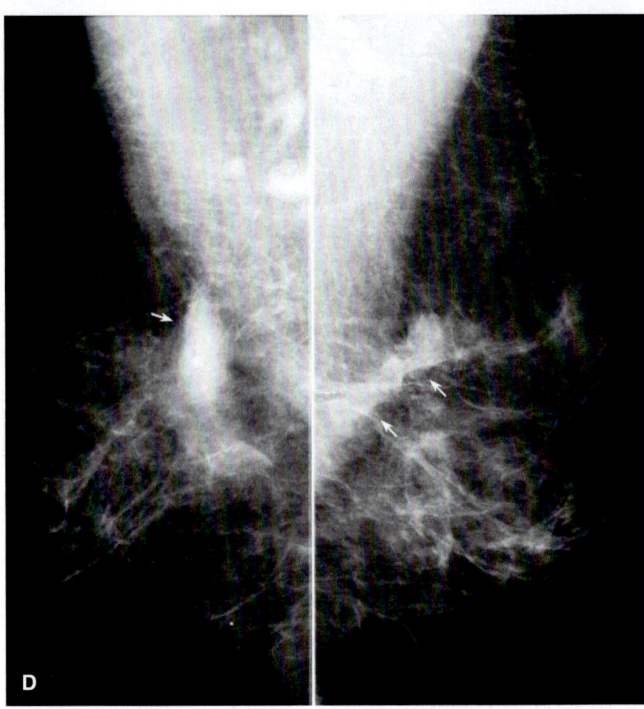

FIG. 11.57 • *(continued)*

is increased if estrogen is given continuously or unopposed; in these patients, estrogen needs to be stopped for a specified amount of time during the month or progesterone needs to be given.

Post-menopausal women burn fewer calories at rest, compared with pre-menopausal women such that, as estrogen levels decrease, women gain weight. Vasomotor symptoms including hot flashes and night sweats affect 85% of women undergoing natural menopause. These symptoms may be exacerbated in women undergoing premature, surgically or chemically induced menopause. These symptoms are significantly improved or relieved in a large number of women on HRT. Bone mineral density decreases rapidly during the first 5 years following menopause leading to osteoporosis and the increased risk of hip or wrist fractures. HRT is effective in preventing the decreases in bone mineral density seen post-menopausally and, in some women, it actually leads to increases in bone mineral density (37).

The issue of coronary artery disease and the potential preventive effect of HRT are controversial. Early studies suggest a protective effect for women on replacement therapy, while more recent studies suggest there may be no protective benefit. The potential role of HRT in breast cancer development also remains unclear. It would appear that at least for the first 10 years of therapy, there might be no significant increase of breast cancer among the women on HRT. Additional studies are needed to elucidate the nature of the relationship, if any, between HRT and the development or stimulation of breast cancers. It is a particularly difficult and controversial issue to address in young women with surgically or chemically induced menopausal symptoms who have a personal history of breast cancer (37). The concerns regarding breast cancer in patients on HRT have increased substantially in the last several years such that patients are either not being placed on HRT or are placed on lower doses.

Mammographically, no change is seen in the appearance of the breast parenchyma is 63% of patients on HRT. Diffuse density increases (Fig. 11.58) or cyst formation is reported in up to 24% of women receiving HRT. In approximately 12% of patients, breast density decreases slightly after therapy is instituted (37–39).

Tamoxifen is an anti-estrogenic medication currently used in the treatment and "prevention" of breast cancer. Decreases in the density of the breast parenchyma can be seen mammographically in a small number of women on tamoxifen (40). Conversely, increases in the density of the parenchyma can be seen when tamoxifen therapy is stopped (see Fig. 5.11). This "rebound" in the tissue and possibly associated cystic changes should not be mistaken for a recurrence presenting with diffuse findings.

MISCELLANEOUS
Weight Changes

Alterations in breast size, differences in the glandular-to-fatty tissue ratio, centimeters of compression, and technical factors needed to obtain an optimal image can be noted following significant changes in body weight. Weight loss can result in perceptible decreases in breast size and compression required to obtain an optimal image. Tissue density seemingly increases, as the amount of fatty tissue is reduced and glandular tissue aggregates becoming denser in some women (Fig. 11.59). Conversely, significant increases in weight lead to increases in breast size and dispersal of glandular tissue by increasing amounts of fatty tissue.

Foreign Bodies

In some patients, foreign bodies may be localized in the breast. Most patients are not aware of their presence and rarely recall the traumatic event. These include but are not limited to lead pencil tips, retained wire fragments (Fig. 11.6A) needle or needle fragments (Fig. 11.45B, C), bullet(s), metallic BBs or shrapnel (see Fig. 6.48C). The shape and density of these foreign bodies are usually distinctive enough to be able to characterize them (Fig. 11.60). With shrapnel, high-density particles can be seen detailing the track followed by the bullet in the breast. In some women, nipple rings may be present (see Fig. 2.37D). Following pre-operative wire localizations, wire fragments (Fig. 11.6A) are rarely noted on follow-up mammograms indicating that the localization wire was inadvertently transected during the excisional biopsy; other foreign bodies can also be seen following surgery (Fig. 11.6B).

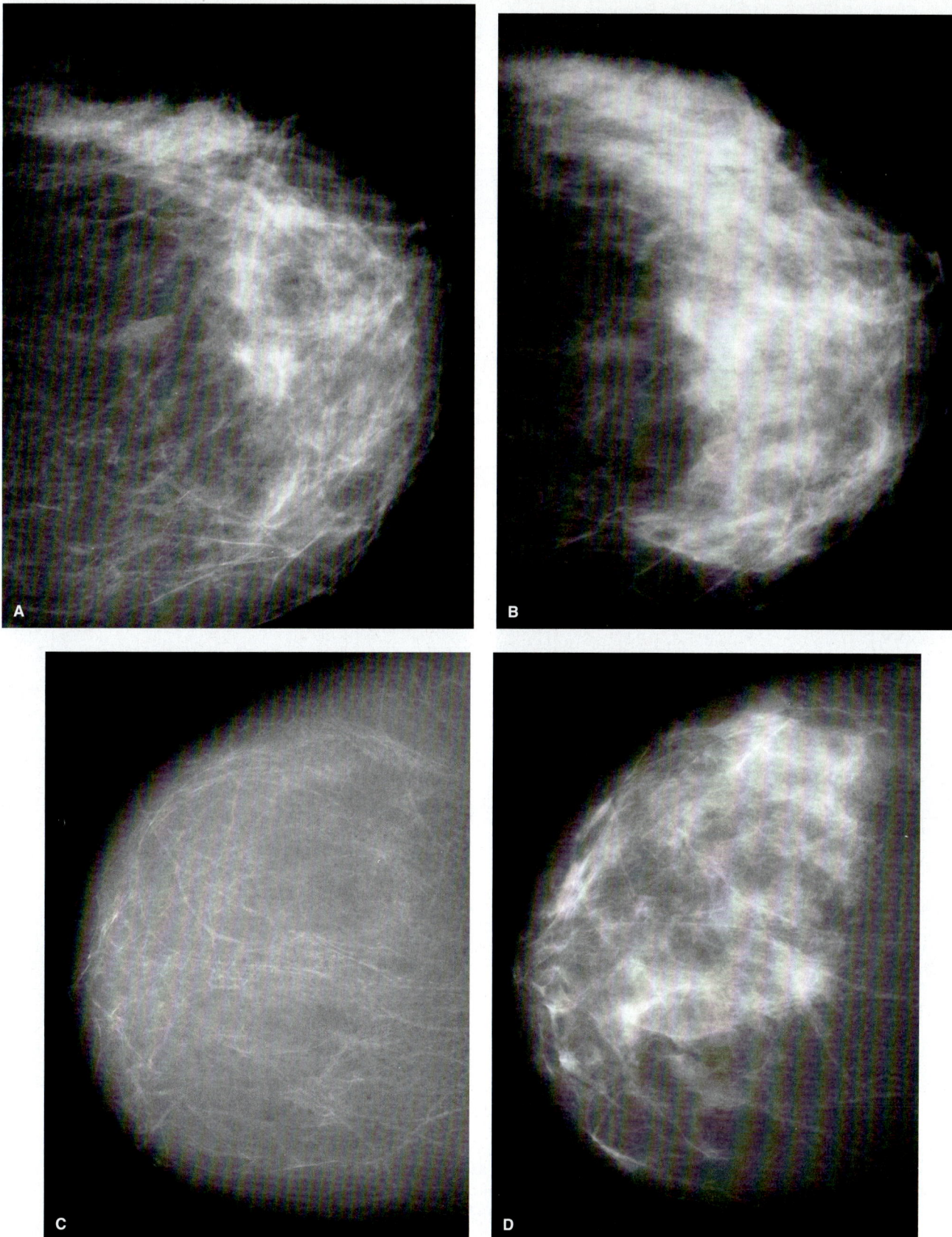

FIG. 11.58 • **Estrogen effect. A:** CC view of the left breast. Fibroglandular tissue is present. **B:** CC view of the left breast 1 year after image shown in part **A** and patient started on HRT. The increase in the amount and density of the breast tissue is related to HRT. **C:** CC view of the right breast in a different patient. Predominantly fatty tissue is imaged. **D:** CC view of the right breast 1 year after image shown in part **C** and patient started HRT. Glandular tissue is now present and likely related to HRT. These patients often describe associated breast engorgement and pain, which can be significant. Cysts also sometimes develop or enlarge after HRT is started. (From Cardeñosa G. *Breast Imaging [The Core Curriculum Series]*. Philadelphia, PA: Lippincott Williams & Wilkins; 2003.)

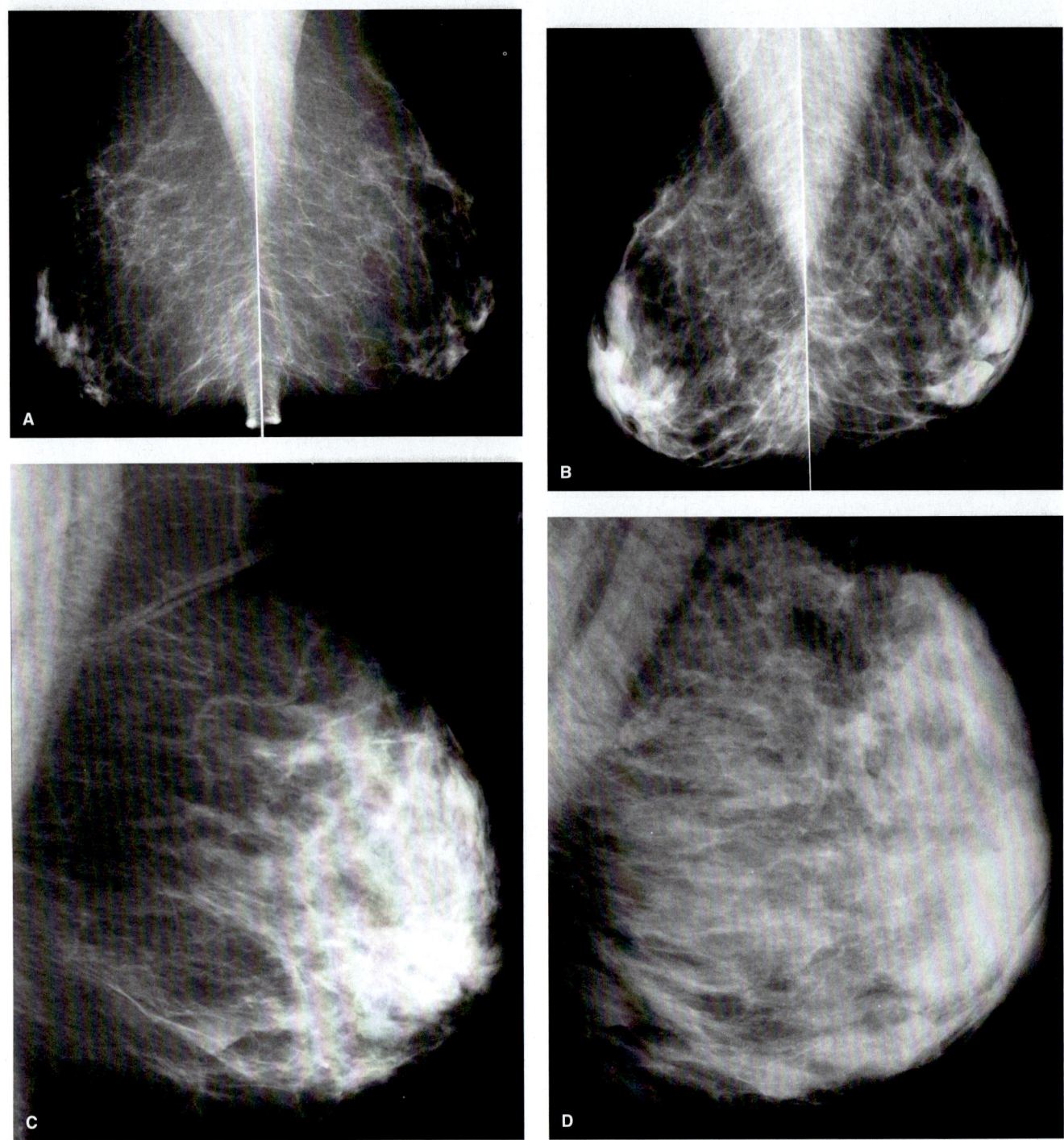

FIG. 11.59 • **Effect of weight changes. A:** MLO views. **B:** MLO views in the same patient shown in part **A** after a 60-lb weight loss. The amount of fatty tissue is reduced and glandular tissue has seemingly increased in amount and density. **C:** MLO view of the left breast in a different patient. **D:** MLO view in the same patient is shown in part **C** after a 150-lb weight loss. The amount of fatty tissue is reduced significantly and the glandular tissue appears increased in amount and density. The amount of compression applied and technical factors used for exposure were also adjusted. (From Cardeñosa G. *Breast Imaging [The Core Curriculum Series]*. Philadelphia, PA: Lippincott Williams & Wilkins; 2003.)

Dacron Central Line Cuff

A 4- to 6-inch subcutaneous tunnel in the medial aspect of the chest is made for Hickman catheter placement. A dacron cuff is used to anchor the catheter to the subcutaneous tissue midway between the skin and the venous entry points. These cuffs (rectangular objects with central lucency and peripheral linear density) may be palpable and are more commonly seen in the upper inner quadrant of the breast posteriorly. When the catheter is pulled out, the dacron cuff remains in place and may be seen on MLO views superimposed on the pectoral muscle and less commonly on the craniocaudal (CC) view (Fig. 11.61) (41).

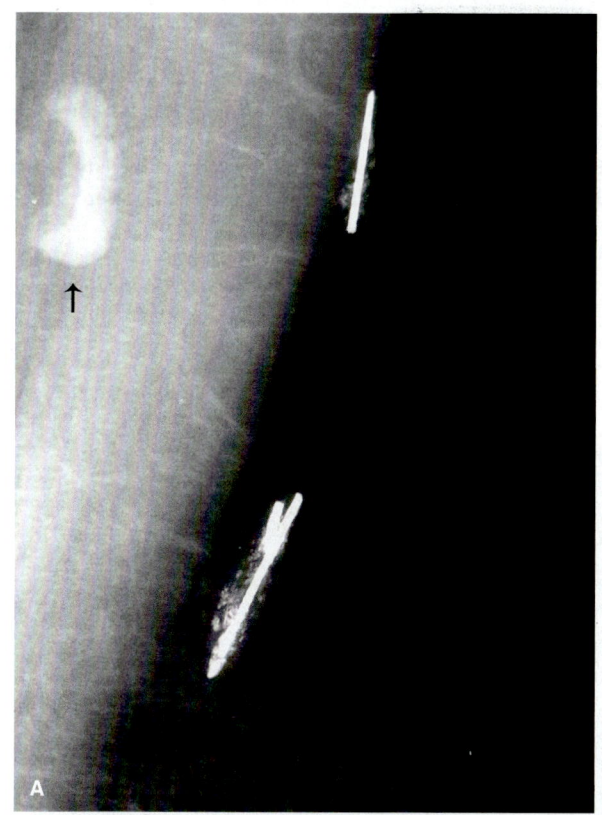
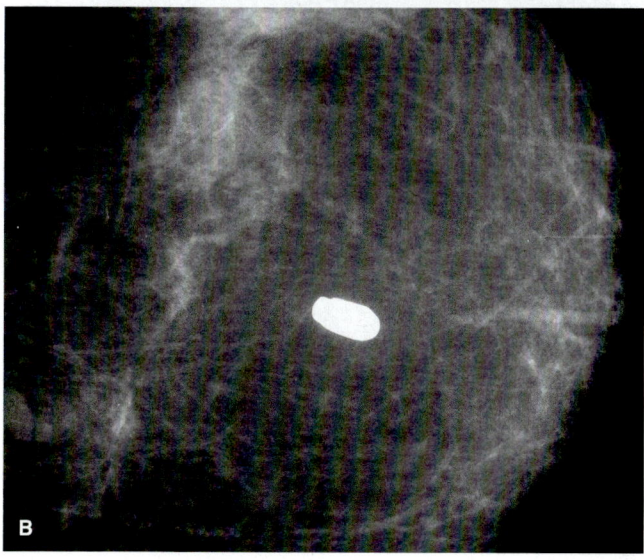

FIG. 11.60 • **Foreign bodies. A:** MLO view of the left breast photographically coned to the upper portion of the image. Needle fragments (2) with some surrounding dystrophic calcifications are noted at the anterior edge of the pectoral muscle. Incidentally noted is a morphologically normal appearing lymph node *(arrow)*. **B:** Photographically coned imaged of the left breast in a different patient. An oval high-density object is imaged in the breast consistent with a bullet. (From Cardeñosa G. *Breast Imaging [The Core Curriculum Series]*. Philadelphia, PA: Lippincott Williams & Wilkins; 2003.)

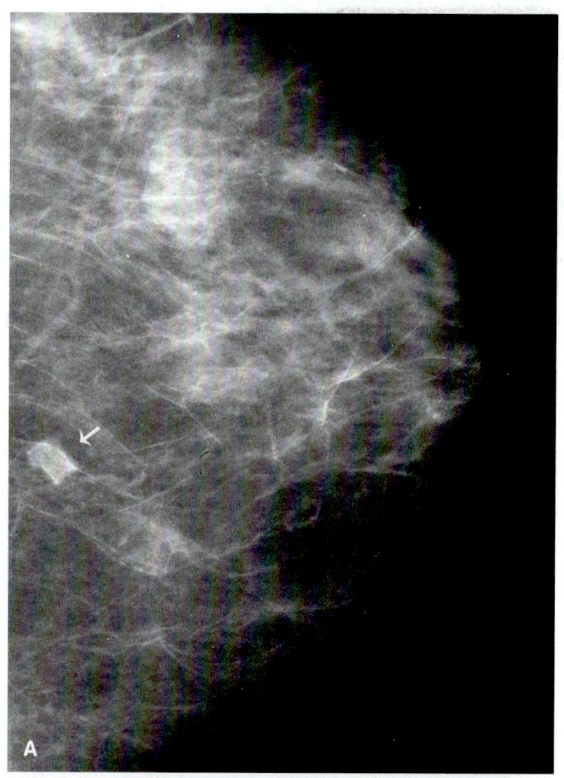
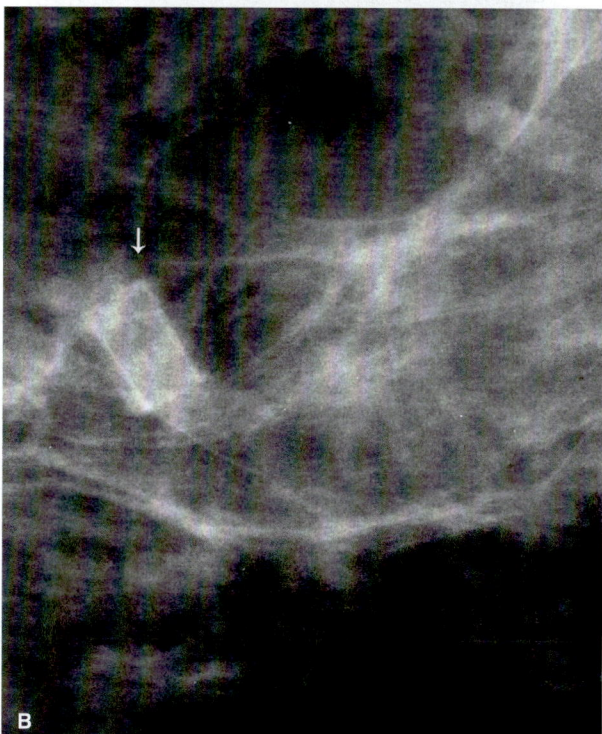

FIG. 11.61 • **Hickman catheter dacron cuff. A:** CC view. Rectangular object *(arrow)* with central lucency and peripheral density is imaged in the medial aspect of the left breast posteriorly. This represents a cuff used to anchor a central line. If this is included on the MLO view (not shown), it is usually seen superimposed on the pectoral muscle. **B:** Photographically coned image in a different patient. Close up of the cuff *(arrow)*. When present for a long time, the edges can become frayed and indistinct and some patients develop associated dystrophic calcifications. (From Cardeñosa G. *Breast Imaging [The Core Curriculum Series]*. Philadelphia, PA: Lippincott Williams & Wilkins; 2003.)

Abscess formation around the cuff has been reported and should be suspected when an irregular mass that may contain air is seen associated with the cuff (42).

Port-a-Catheters

Port-a-catheters are surgically placed on the chest wall of the upper inner quadrant of either breast posteriorly (when placed for breast cancer–related chemotherapy, they are usually placed on the side opposite that of the breast cancer). They provide convenient venous access for patients receiving chemotherapy. While in place, they can be seen as a round area of increased density on the MLO view often superimposed on the pectoral muscle (Fig. 11.19D) and less commonly medially on the CC view. In a small number of women, a mass reflecting a fluid collection (Figs. 11.62 and 11.63), area of spiculation (Fig. 11.63), or calcifications can be seen developing following removal of the catheter. These changes usually resolve on subsequent mammograms but initially, can simulate a malignancy. If the findings are directly correlated to the port-a-catheter site, a conservative approach is appropriate.

Pacemakers

Pacemakers may be partially or completely seen on mediolateral (see Fig. 2.37A) or lateromedial oblique (see Fig. 3.32) views superimposed

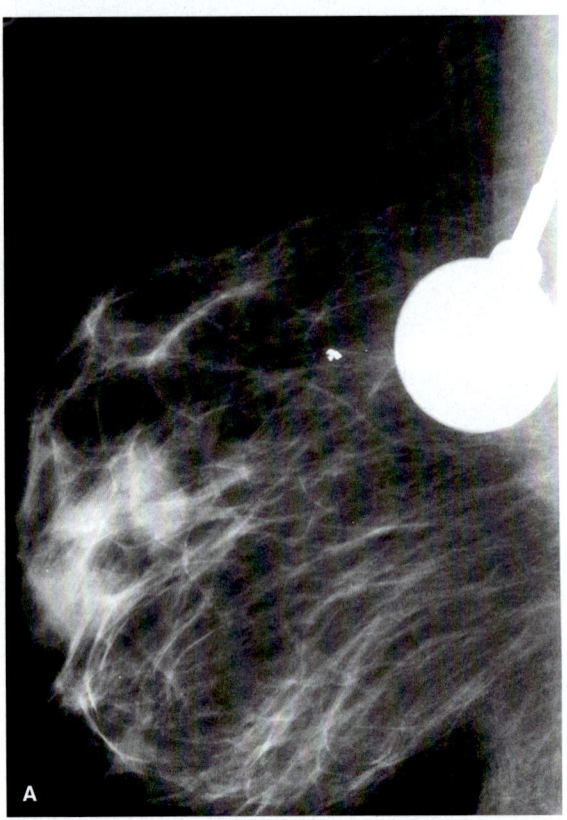

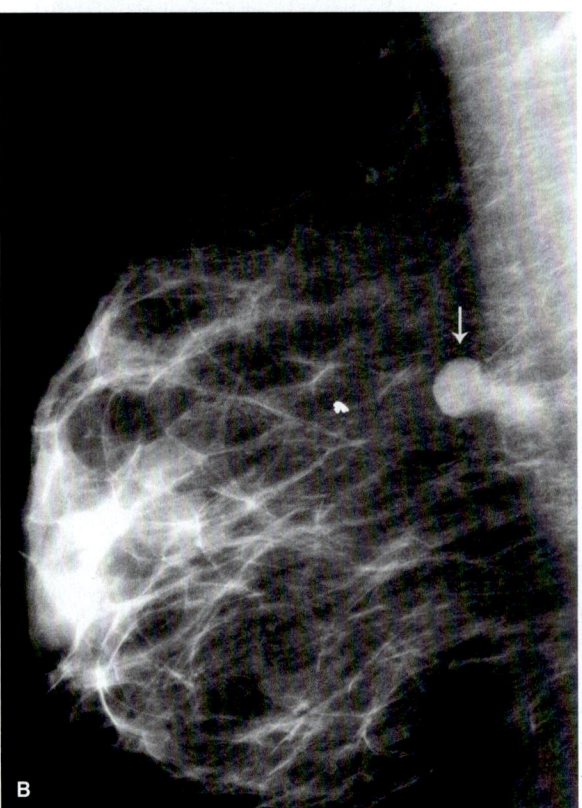

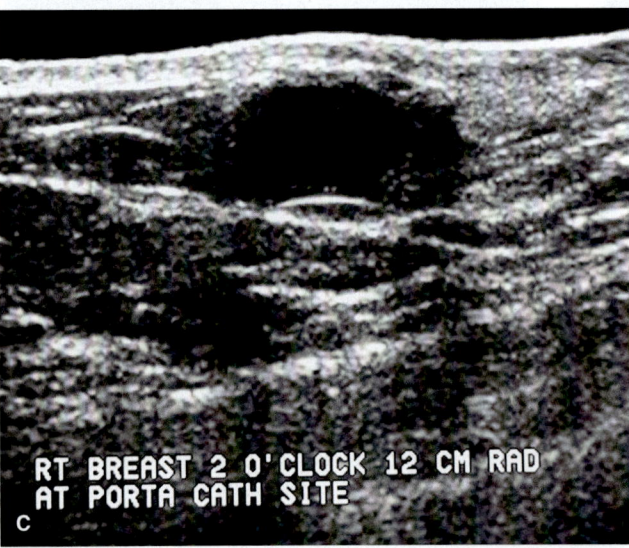

FIG. 11.62 • **Fluid collection at port-a-catheter site. A:** MLO view of the right breast in a patient with a port-a-catheter in place for chemotherapy. The catheter could also be seen in the medial aspect of the right breast posteriorly on the CC view (not shown). **B:** MLO view of the right breast done in the patient shown in part **A** after the removal of the port-a-cath. A mass *(arrow)* with circumscribed (anteriorly) and indistinct (posteriorly) margins anteriorly is seen corresponding to the site of the port-a-catheter on orthogonal views (CC view not shown). **C:** Ultrasound. A fluid collection is imaged corresponding to the mass seen mammographically in the upper inner quadrant of the right breast posteriorly. (From Cardeñosa G. *Breast Imaging [The Core Curriculum Series]*. Philadelphia, PA: Lippincott Williams & Wilkins; 2003.)

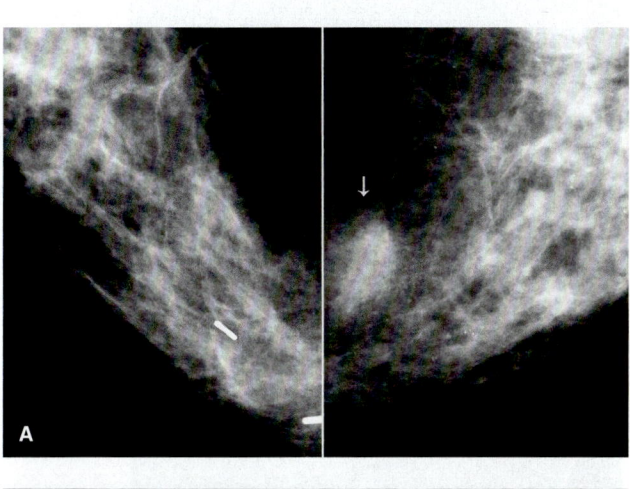
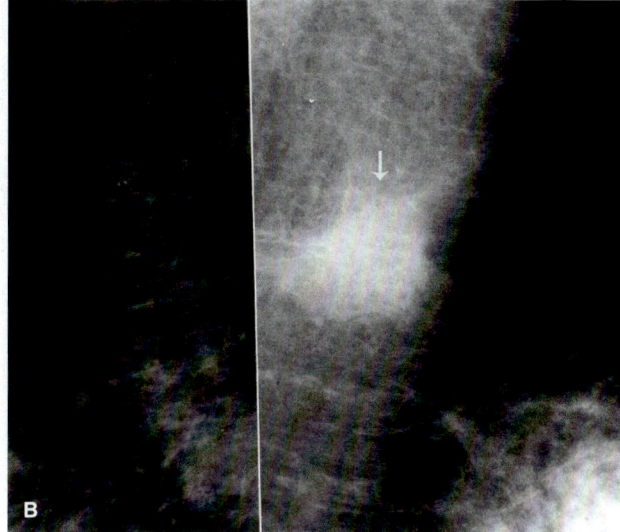
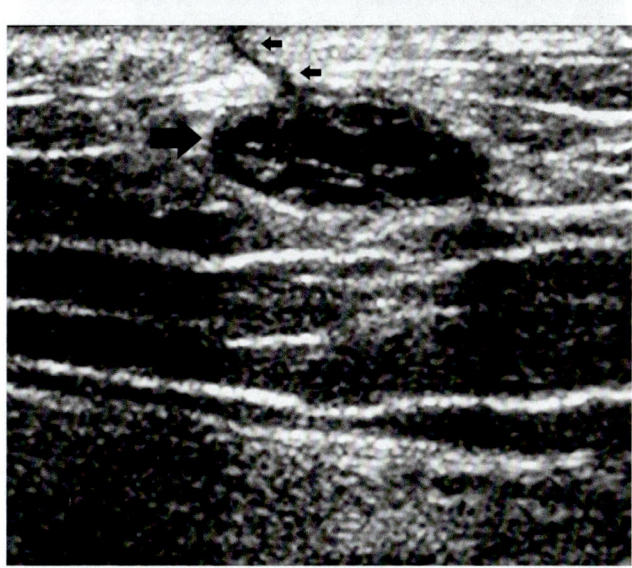

FIG. 11.63 • **Fluid collection at port-a-catheter site.** CC views photographically coned to the medial and posterior tissue **(A)** and MLO views photographically coned to the upper portion of the images **(B)**. An irregular mass with indistinct margins is noted in the upper inner quadrant of the left breast posteriorly in a patient following lumpectomy, radiation and chemotherapy for right breast cancer (clips seen on right CC view). **C:** Ultrasound. A complex cystic and solid mass *(large arrow)* with posterior acoustic enhancement and a track to skin *(small arrows)* is imaged in the upper inner quadrant of the left breast posterior correlating to the site occupied by the port-a-catheter used to administer chemotherapy. In our experience, findings at port-a-catheter sites following removal of the access cap are common and range from a round, oval, or irregular mass with indistinct to spiculated margins, distortion without an associated mass or less commonly dystrophic calcifications. These findings usually resolve on follow-up studies. (From Cardeñosa G. *Breast Imaging [The Core Curriculum Series]*. Philadelphia, PA: Lippincott Williams & Wilkins; 2003.)

on the pectoral muscle and less commonly on CC or from below (see Fig. 2.36) views. If the pacemaker is removed, pacemaker wires may remain and coarse calcifications or a fluid collection may develop in the cavity left by the pacemaker. Depending on the location and size of the pacemaker, positioning on the MLO view may be compromised and breast or axillary tissue may be excluded from view.

Hormonal/Aromatase Inhibitor as Primary Treatment for Breast Cancer

Rarely, in patients with significant co-morbidities precluding traditional surgical treatment, hormonal therapy may be tried to limit tumor growth, and in some, decrease the size of the lesion. If the tumor is estrogen receptor positive, patients can be placed on tamoxifen or an aromatase inhibitor. Although Femara (letrozole) is one of the more commonly known aromatase inhibitors, other includes Arimidex (anastrozole) or Aromasin (exemestane). These patients are followed clinically, and sometimes, mammographically to assess change. In some patients, the effects on the tumor can be quite dramatic (Fig. 11.64). If the tumor continues to increase in size, however, changing to another one of these drugs is appropriate. An aromatase inhibitor is also sometimes offered to patients who, after 5 years of tamoxifen, want to continue using a potentially preventive agent.

Transgender (Male to Female, MtF) Patients

An increasing number of patients at various stages in the male-to-female re-assignment process are being referred for screening. However, it is unknown if these patients have an increased risk of breast cancer and there is no data available to guide screening recommendations. The impetus for the referrals is use of high doses of estrogens partly for the purposes of stimulating breast development. In addition to estrogen, some of these patients undergo augmentation with implants or some present following the subcutaneous injection of silicone (Fig. 11.65).

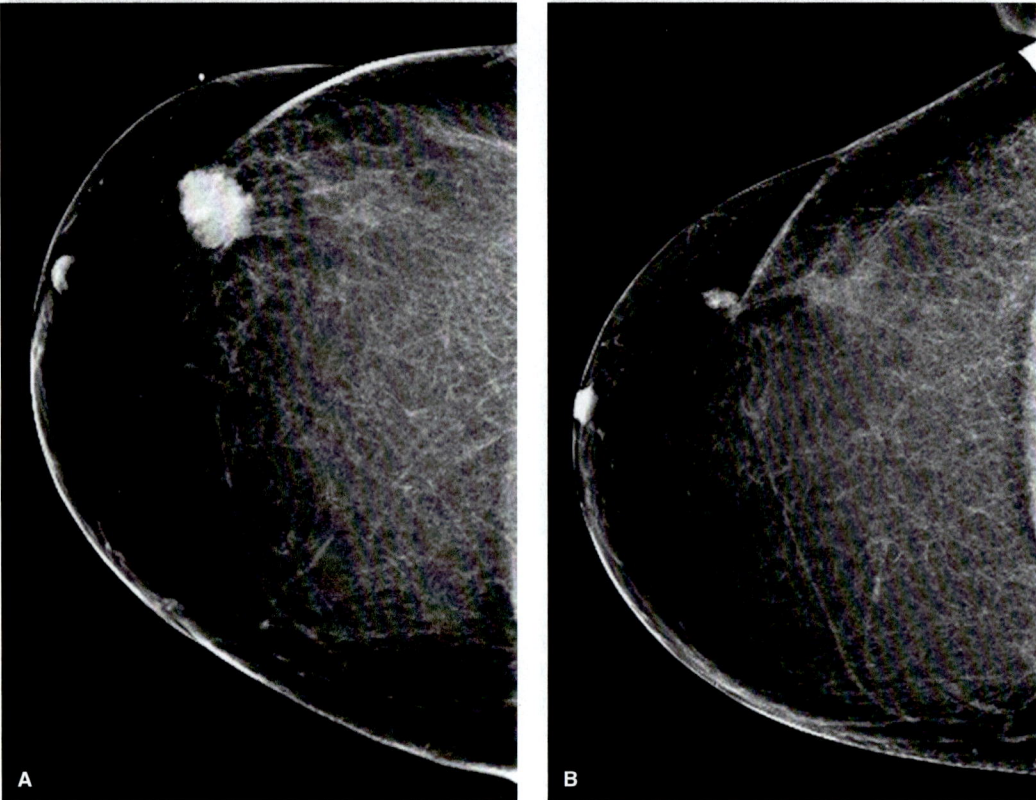

FIG. 11.64 • **Invasive ductal carcinoma, treatment with aromatase inhibitor. A:** CC view of the right breast in an 86-year-old patient presenting with a "lump." A dense round mass with microlobulated and indistinct margins and associated skin retraction is imaged in the lateral aspect of the right breast anteriorly corresponding to the palpable finding. An invasive ductal carcinoma grade 2 is reported on the ultrasound-guided core biopsy. The tumor is estrogen and progesterone receptor positive, HER2/neu-negative. Given other significant medical problems precluding surgery, and following lengthy discussions with the patient and her family, she was started on Femara with clinical response. **B:** CC view of the right breast 1 year after the image in part **A**. The mass is again noted, however, it is decreased in size.

FIG. 11.65 • **Transgender patients. A:** MLO views. In addition to the use of hormone therapy, this patient has had subcutaneous silicone injections. The kVp needed to obtain this exposure is high resulting in a "burn-out" of the pectoral muscles.

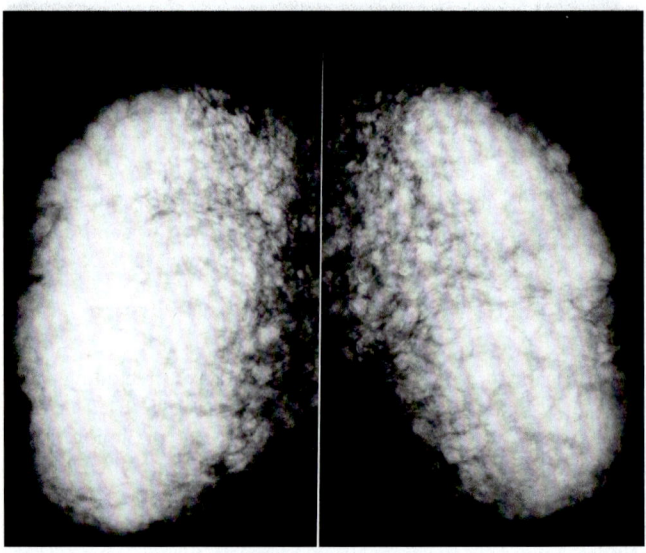

References

1. Sickles EA, Herzog KA. Mammography of the postsurgical breast. *AJR Am J Roentgenol*. 1981;136:585–588.
2. Mendelson EB. Evaluation of the postoperative breast. *Radiol Clin North Am*. 1992;30:107–138.
3. Stigers KB, King JG, Darvey DD, et al. Abnormalities of the breast caused by biopsy: spectrum of mammographic findings. *AJR Am J Roentgenol*. 1991;156:287–291.
4. Hogge JP, Robinson RE, Magnant CM, et al. The mammographic spectrum of fat necrosis in the breast. *Radiographics*. 1995;15:1347–1356.
5. Soo MS, Kornguth PJ, Hertzberg BS. Fat necrosis in the breast: sonographic features. *Radiology*. 1998;206:261–269.
6. Burbank F, Forcier N. Tissue marking clip for stereotactic breast biopsy: initial placement accuracy; long-term stability and usefulness as a guide for wire localization. *Radiology*. 1997;205:407–415.
7. Burnside ES, Sohlich RE, Sickles EA. Movement of a biopsy-site marker after completion of stereotactic directional vacuum-assisted breast biopsy: case report. *Radiology*. 2001;221:504–507.
8. DiPiro PJ, Meyer JE, Frenna TH, et al. Seat beat injuries of the breast: findings on mammography and sonography. *AJR Am J Roentgenol*. 1995;164:317–320.
9. Yi A, Kim HK, Shin HJ, et al. Radiation induced complications after breast cancer radiation therapy: a pictorial review of multimodality imaging findings. *Korean J Radiol*. 2009;10:496–507.
10. Noh JM, Huh SJ, Choi DH, et al. Two cases of post-radiation sarcoma after breast cancer treatment. *J Breast Cancer*. 2012;15:364–370.
11. Chansakul T, Lai KC, Slanetz PJ. The postconservation breast, part I: expected imaging findings. *AJR Am J Roentgenol*. 2012;198:321–330.
12. Harris KM, Costa-Greco MA, Baratz AB, et al. The mammographic features of the postlumpectomy, postirradiation breast. *Radiographics*. 1989;9:253–268.
13. Hassell PR, Olivotto IA, Mueller HA, et al. Early breast cancer: detection of recurrence after conservative surgery and radiation therapy. *Radiology*. 1990;176:731–735.
14. Bassett LW, Jackson VP, Jahan R, et al. *Diagnosis of Disease of the Breast*. Philadelphia, PA: WB Saunders; 1997.
15. Brenner RJ, Pfaff JM. Mammographic features after conservative therapy for malignant breast disease: serial findings standardized by regression analysis. *AJR Am J Roentgenol*. 1996;167:171–178.
16. Dershaw DD. Mammography in patients with breast cancer treated by breast conservation (lumpectomy with or without radiation). *AJR Am J Roentgenol*. 1995;164:309–316.
17. Krishnamurthy R, Whitman GJ, Stelling CB, et al. Mammographic findings after breast conservation therapy. *Radiographics*. 1999;19:S53–S62.
18. American College of Radiology. *ACR Practice Guideline for the Performance of Screening and Diagnostic Mammography*. Reston, VA: American College of Radiology; 2008:Resolution 24.
19. Liberman L, Van Zee KJ, Dershaw DD, et al. Mammographic features of local recurrence in women who have undergone breast-conserving therapy for ductal carcinoma in situ. *AJR Am J Roentgenol*. 1997;168:489–493.
20. Philpotts LE, Lee CH, Haffty BG, et al. Mammographic findings of recurrent breast cancer after lumpectomy and radiation therapy: comparison with primary tumor. *Radiology*. 1996;201:767–771.
21. Rissanen TJ, Makarainen HP, Mattila SI, et al. Breast cancer recurrence after mastectomy: diagnosis with mammography and US. *Radiology*. 1993;188:463–467.
22. Fajardo LL, Roberts CC, Hunt KR. Mammographic surveillance of breast cancer patients: should the mastectomy site be imaged? *AJR Am J Roentgenol*. 1993;161:953–955.
23. Helvie MA, Wilson TE, Roubidoux MA, et al. Mammographic appearance of recurrent breast carcinoma in six patients with TRAM flap breast reconstructions. *Radiology*. 1998;209:711–715.
24. Hogge JP, Zuurbier RA, de Paredes ES. Mammography of autologous myocutaneous flaps. *Radiographics*. 1999;19:S63–S72.
25. Georgiade NG, Georgiade GS, Riefkohl R. *Aesthetic Surgery of the Breast*. Philadelphia, PA: WB Saunders; 1990.
26. Miller CL, Feig SA, Fox JW. Mammographic changes after reduction mammoplasty. *AJR Am J Roentgenol*. 1987;149:35–38.
27. Fajardo LL, Bessen SC. Epidermal inclusion cysts after reduction mammoplasty. *Radiology*. 1993;186:103–106.
28. Bondurant S, Enster V, Herdman R, eds. *Safety of Silicone Breast Implants*. Washington, DC: National Academy Press; 1999.
29. Destouet JM, Monsees BS, Oser RF, et al. Screening mammography in 350 women with breast implants: prevalence and findings of implant complications. *AJR Am J Roentgenol*. 1992;159:973–978.
30. Hester TR. The polyurethane covered mammary prosthesis: facts and fiction. *Perspect Plast Surg*. 1988;2:135–169.
31. Mund DF, Farria DM, Gorczyca DP, et al. MR imaging of the breast in patients with silicone-gel implants: spectrum of findings. *AJR Am J Roentgenol*. 1993;161:773–778.
32. Everson LI, Parantainen H, Detlie T, et al. Diagnosis of breast implant rupture: imaging findings and relative efficacies of imaging techniques. *AJR Am J Roentgenol*. 1994;163:57–60.
33. Middleton MS, McNamara MP. *Breast Implant Imaging*. Philadelphia, PA: Lippincott Williams & Wilkins; 2003.
34. Harris KM, Ganott MA, Shestak KC, et al. Silicone implant rupture: detection with US. *Radiology*. 1993;187:761–768.
35. Ganott MA, Harris KM, Ilkanipour ZS, et al. Augmentation mammoplasty: normal and abnormal findings with mammography and US. *Radiographics*. 1992;12:281–295.
36. Rosculet KA, Ikeda DM, Forrest ME, et al. Ruptured gel-filled silicone breast implants: sonographic findings in 19 cases. *AJR Am J Roentgenol*. 1992;159:711–716.
37. Harris JR, Lippman ME, Morrow M, et al, eds. *Disease of the Breast*. 2nd ed. Philadelphia, PA: Lippincott Williams & Wilkins; 2000.
38. Stomper PC, Van Voorhis BJ, Ravnikar VA, et al. Mammographic changes associated with postmenopausal hormone replacement therapy: a longitudinal study. *Radiology*. 1990;174:487–490.
39. Berkowitz JE, Gatewood OMB, Goldblum LE, et al. Hormonal replacement therapy: mammographic manifestations. *Radiology*. 1990;174:199–201.
40. Cardenosa G, Eklund GW. Letter to the editor: Breast parenchymal change following treatment with tamoxifen. *Breast Dis*. 1992;5:55–58.
41. Beyer GA, Thorsen MK, Shaffer KA, et al. Mammographic appearance of the retained Dacron cuff of a Hickman catheter. *AJR Am J Roentgenol*. 1990;155:1204.
42. Ellis RL, Dempsey PJ, Rubin E, et al. Mammography of breasts in which catheter cuffs have been retained: normal, infected and postoperative appearances. *AJR Am J Roentgenol*. 1997;169:713–715.

CHAPTER SELF-ASSESSMENT QUESTIONS

1. Craniocaudal (CC) views (top-left and top-right), 1 year apart as well as CC (bottom-left) and mediolateral oblique compression (bottom-right) views in a patient who has had a lumpectomy and radiation therapy change for left breast cancer. What is indicated?

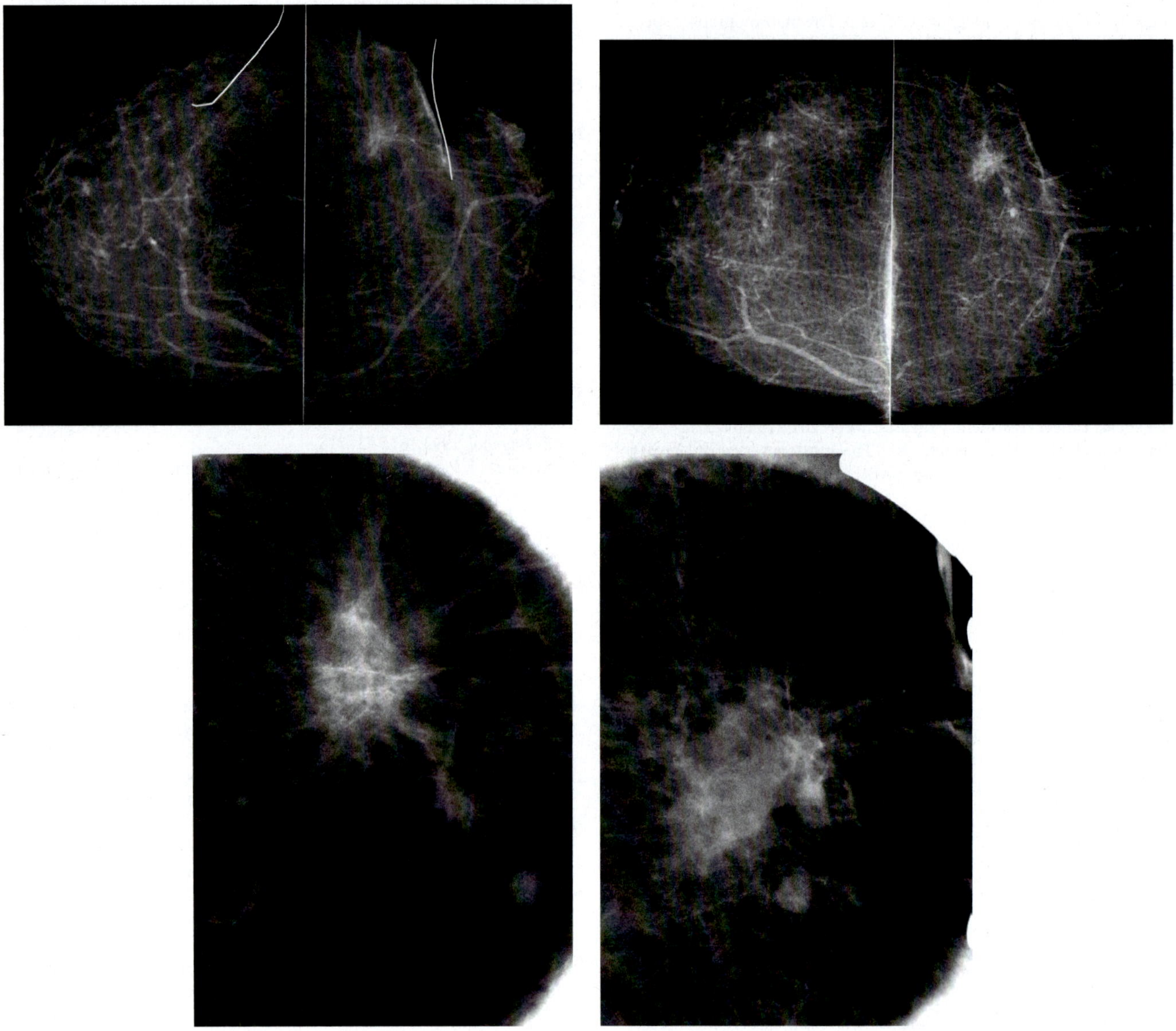

   A. Six-month follow-up
   B. Imaging guided biopsy
   C. Magnetic resonance imaging
   D. Mastectomy

2. MIP image from an MRI in a 52-year-old patient. What is most likely?

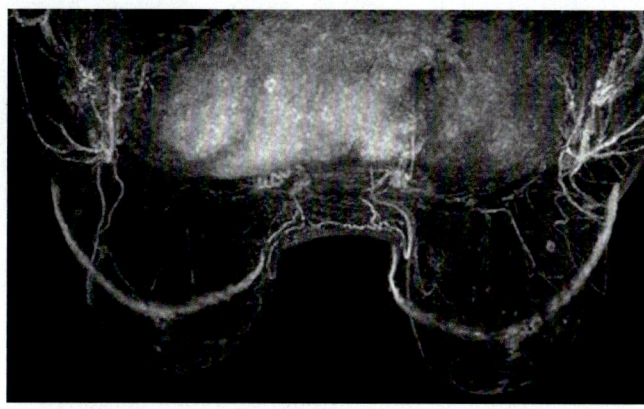

A. Explantation
B. TRAM flap reconstructions
C. Reduction mammoplasty
D. Artifact

Answers to Chapter Self-Assessment Questions

1. B On the current study, distortion associated with skin thickening and retraction is again noted laterally in the left breast. However, two new masses are confirmed on the spot compression views adjacent to the distortion. One is round with indistinct margins and the other is irregular with spiculated margins. With the interval development of these and their imaging features, biopsy of at least one of these is indicated. These masses are new and as such, if solid on ultrasound, 6-month follow-up is inappropriate. MRI is likely to be done following a diagnosis; however, it is not indicated before confirming the suspected diagnosis. In this patient, a second lumpectomy, or more commonly a mastectomy, is indicated only after histological confirmation is obtained. In this patient, an ultrasound-guided biopsy confirmed the suspected recurrence.

2. C This patient has had a recent reduction mammoplasty. The symmetric curvilinear bands of enhancement are related to post operative skin thickening and may resolve on subsequent studies.

Interventional Procedures 12

LEARNING OBJECTIVES

1. Ductography
   - Indications for procedure
   - How is the procedure done?
   - Findings and differential considerations
   - Diagnostic versus preoperative ductography
   - When should wire localization be used in conjunction with preoperative ductography?
2. Cyst aspiration and pneumocystography
   - Indications for cyst aspiration
   - Indications for pneumocystography
   - Procedures
   - Complex cystic masses: management
3. Needle biopsies
   - Indications for imaging-guided biopsies
   - Ultrasound, stereotactic, and MRI guidance
   - Clip placement
   - Post procedure patient management
   - Radiology–pathology concordance and patient management
4. Preoperative wire localizations
   - Indications
   - Approaches
5. Specimen evaluation
   - Radiography
   - Sonography
6. Paraffin block radiography
   - Indications
   - Orthogonal imaging

DUCTOGRAPHY

The evaluation and management of patients presenting with nipple discharge is variable among clinicians. Commonly, the prolactin level is checked and some of the discharge is submitted for cytological evaluation; if the results are normal, the patient usually undergoes no further workup unless the discharge is bloody. Patients with bloody nipple discharge are referred to a surgeon and may undergo a subareolar duct excision. The assumptions made with these approaches need to be challenged as outlined in Table 12.1.

Although ductography is not a perfect test, it can help address some of the issues raised by the assumptions presented in Table 12.1. The presence, location, and extent of lesions can be demonstrated in many

Table 12.1 **COMMON ASSUMPTIONS IN WOMEN WITH NIPPLE DISCHARGE**

Assumption	Fact
1. Negative cytology results reliably exclude pathology	Negative cytology does not reliably exclude significant pathology
2. Only bloody nipple discharge is significant	DCIS can present with serous or clear, heme occult negative nipple discharge[a]
3. The location and extent of a lesion in the duct can be reliably identified intra-operatively so that the dissection is extended as needed to include, but not transect, the lesion	Not all papillomas are close to the subareolar area, and when DCIS is present, it is often extensive and not subareolar in location
4. The pathologist can reliably identify the location of the lesion in the specimen submitted for histologic processing	Staining of the duct with methylene blue facilitates intra-operative identification of the duct for excision by the surgeon and during processing of the specimen by the pathologist

[a]How a patient notices the discharge is more important than the character of the discharge. Expressed nipple discharge is usually physiologic. Spontaneous nipple discharge needs to be evaluated regardless of its appearance.

patients with spontaneous nipple discharge. The location of the duct containing the lesion and its distribution in the breast can be established preoperatively. When findings consistent with duct ectasia or fibrocystic changes are diagnosed, surgery may be averted. Lastly, if preoperative ductography is done using a methylene blue:contrast (1:1) combination, the contrast allows us to verify that we cannulated the abnormal duct; the methylene blue stains the duct; so it is easy to identify by the surgeon intra-operatively and the pathologist at the time the specimen is processed. This helps assure that the lesion is localized, excised, and evaluated histologically.

Clinically, patients with intraductal lesions may present describing nipple discharge. When asked how they notice the discharge, patients invariably provide one (or all) of three histories. They notice dark spots on their bra cups or spots on their nightclothes, or after taking a hot bath or shower they notice their nipple is dripping. If the discharge is only expressed after vigorous manipulation of the breast and nipple, the likelihood of finding an intraductal lesion is low and ductography is not indicated. Patients should be discouraged from trying to express nipple discharge. As part of breast self-examination, they should be instructed to get into the habit of checking their bra cups for dark brown spots.

Ductography is a safe, easy, and simple contrast evaluation of a lactiferous duct (1–4). The only relative contraindication to ductography is the presence of mastitis and no significant complications have been described with the water-soluble contrast agents currently in use. Ductography is used to evaluate women presenting with spontaneous nipple discharge, regardless of the character of the discharge (Fig. 12.1). Adequate lighting and magnification of the nipple are helpful in identifying the secreting duct opening. Full-strength iodinated contrast material is drawn into a 3-mL Luer lock syringe. A 30G blunt-tip sialography needle with attached tubing is screwed onto the Luer lock syringe, making sure that the connection is tight so that air bubbles are not drawn into the syringe. Contrast material is run through the tubing until all air bubbles are removed from the system. Topical anesthesia and dilators are not needed for this procedure.

Although we place the patient in a supine position with the ipsilateral arm placed above her head, others do these procedures with the patient sitting up. The nipple is inspected for the presence of crusting or a minimally prominent, erythematous and patulous duct opening. After the visual inspection of the nipple, an alcohol wipe is used to swab the nipple and remove any keratin plugs that may obstruct the duct opening. Next, the breast is examined. A "trigger point" may be identified in some patients (5). When this "trigger point" is compressed, nipple discharge is obtained. As you move away from this point, the discharge stops. In patients with an intraductal lesion, the discharge is commonly copious and "projectile."

If you identify a trigger point, use it to elicit small amounts of discharge. Elicit just enough to moisten and glisten the duct opening. If a larger amount of discharge is obtained, other openings are flooded, precluding correct identification of the offending duct. With a clear idea of which opening the discharge is coming from, angle the cannula and place the tip in the duct opening. After the cannula is engaged in this manner, straighten it so that the cannula "falls" into the duct to the level of the hub. After cannulation, take a few seconds to observe the tubing. Since the tubing is now in a closed system with the cannulated duct, duct contents can sometimes be seen refluxing back into the tubing (Fig. 12.2A). If this does not happen, inject a small amount of the contrast and look at the nipple. As intraductal fluid is displaced by contrast, some of the fluid may come out to form a drop around the cannula (Fig. 12.2B). When either of these observations is made, you have some assurance that you cannulated the potentially abnormal duct.

A small amount of contrast (0.2–0.4 mL) is injected initially and the cannula is taped on the nipple. Injecting larger amounts of contrast at the onset may obscure small lesions (Fig. 12.3) or those that are close to the nipple. Full paddle magnification views in the craniocaudal (CC) and 90-degree lateromedial (LM) projections are obtained. After a review of these initial images, additional contrast can be injected, as needed to opacify the duct proximally (Fig. 12.3).

Little is known about the ductographic appearance of "normal" ducts. There seems to be considerable variation in length, amount of branching, distribution, and caliber (Fig. 12.4). Occasionally, a contained contrast blush is seen, the overall appearance of which suggests the possibility of lobular opacification (Fig. 12.3B, C). We use the sialography

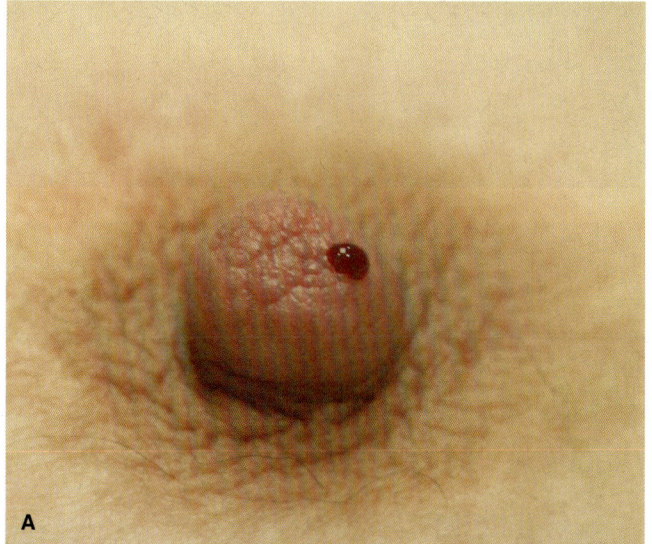
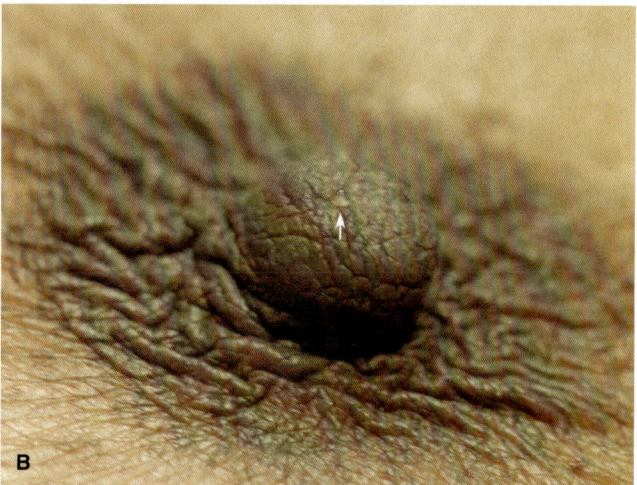

FIG. 12.1 • **Nipple discharge. A:** Bloody nipple discharge arising from a single duct opening. **B:** Clear nipple discharge *(arrow)* arising from a single duct opening. If the patient presents with nipple discharge, it is important to establish if it is expressed or spontaneous by asking the patient how she notices the discharge. If spontaneous, the character (bloody, clear, serous, etc.) of the discharge does not dissuade us from evaluating the patient with ductography. Breast cancers can present with clear or serous, heme occult negative discharge. (From Cardeñosa G. *Breast Imaging [The Core Curriculum Series]*. Philadelphia, PA: Lippincott Williams & Wilkins; 2003.)

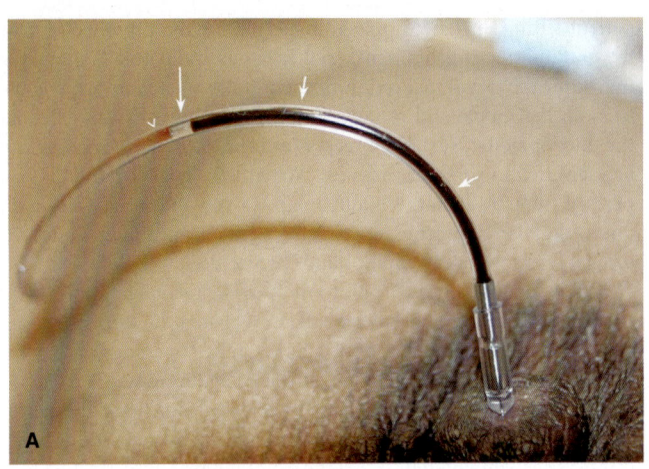
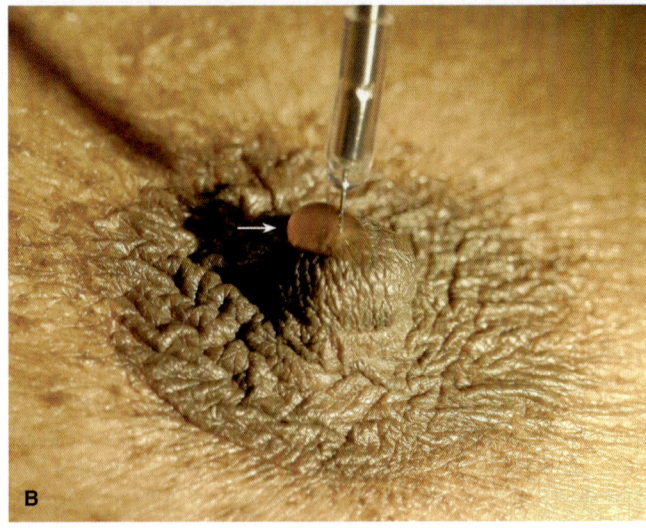

FIG. 12.2 • **Establishing accurate cannulation. A:** Cannula in the duct to the hub. Immediately after you cannulate the duct, look at the tubing for a few seconds before injecting contrast. The tubing is now in a closed system with the cannulated duct so duct contents can sometimes be seen refluxing into the tubing. If this is seen, it confirms cannulation of the duct producing the discharge. In this patient, the refluxing material is bloody *(short arrows)*. An air bubble *(long arrow)* is present in the tubing. Also note intermingling of bloody duct contents with the contrast *(arrow head)* in the tubing. When the discharge is clear or serous, mixing of the duct contents with the contrast can be seen occurring in the tubing. **B:** Duct contents forming a serosanguineous droplet around the cannula. If duct contents do not reflux into the tubing, duct contents can sometimes be seen forming a droplet *(arrow)* around the cannula as contrast is injected. The contrast displaces duct contents. When this is seen, it confirms cannulation of the duct producing the discharge. (From Cardeñosa G. *Breast Imaging [The Core Curriculum Series]*. Philadelphia, PA: Lippincott Williams & Wilkins; 2003.)

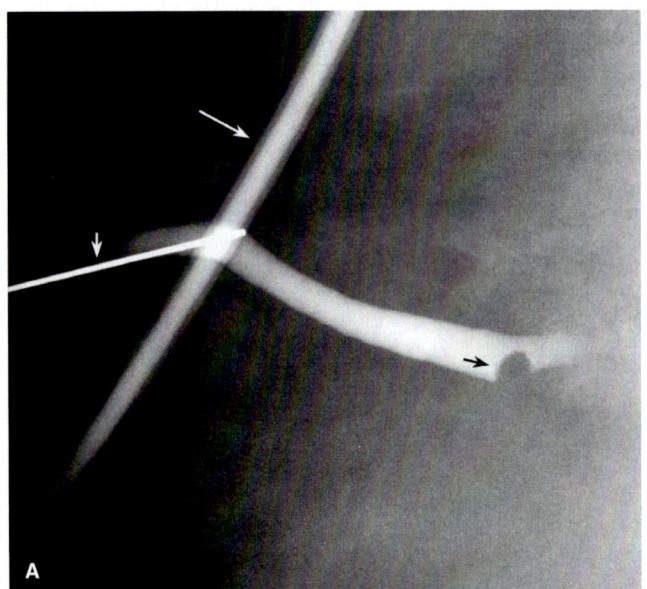
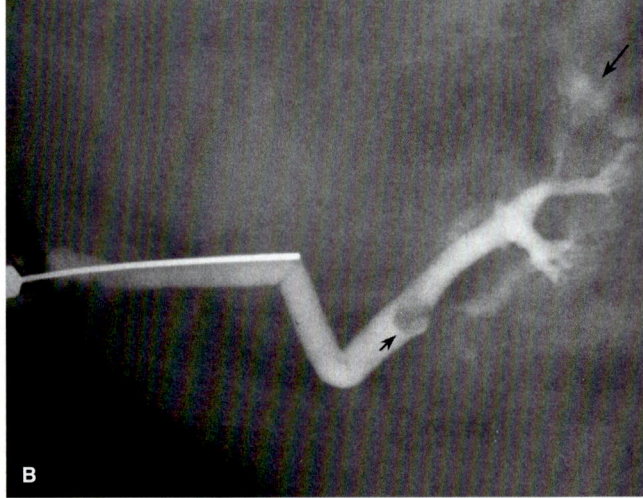
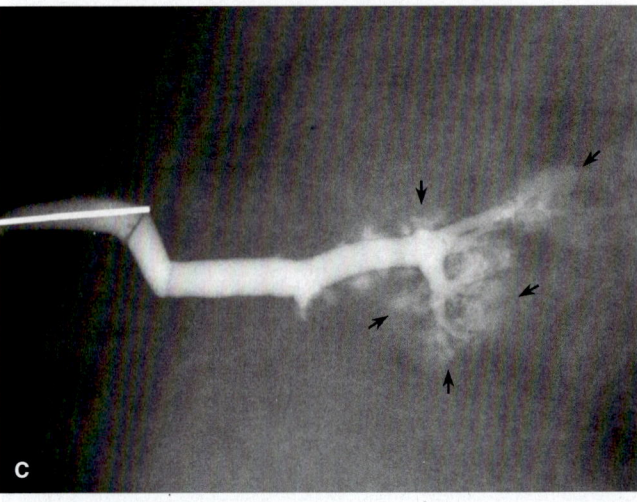

FIG. 12.3 • **Masking of lesion, "lobular blushing," papilloma. A:** Initial films following injection of 0.2 mL of contrast demonstrate a filling defect *(black arrow)* reflecting a papilloma. No proximal opacification of the duct is noted. Cannula *(short white arrow)* is noted in the duct. The tubing with contrast *(long white arrow)* should be moved out of the field of view by the technologist. **B:** Following the injection of an additional 0.2 mL of contrast, the filling defect *(short black arrow)* is still seen. Branches of the duct are now filling with contrast and there is some "blushing" *(long black arrow)* possibly reflecting contrast in lobular units. **C:** An additional 0.2 mL of contrast is injected. The lesion is no longer seen secondary to the amount of contrast injected. Contrast "blushing" is increasing *(arrows)*. Small lesions, and lesions that are close to the nipple, can be obscured if too much contrast is injected initially. A small amount is injected initially. If the cannula is left in place, it is easy to inject additional contrast as needed to evaluate the duct proximally. (From Cardeñosa G. *Breast Imaging [The Core Curriculum Series]*. Philadelphia, PA: Lippincott Williams & Wilkins; 2003.)

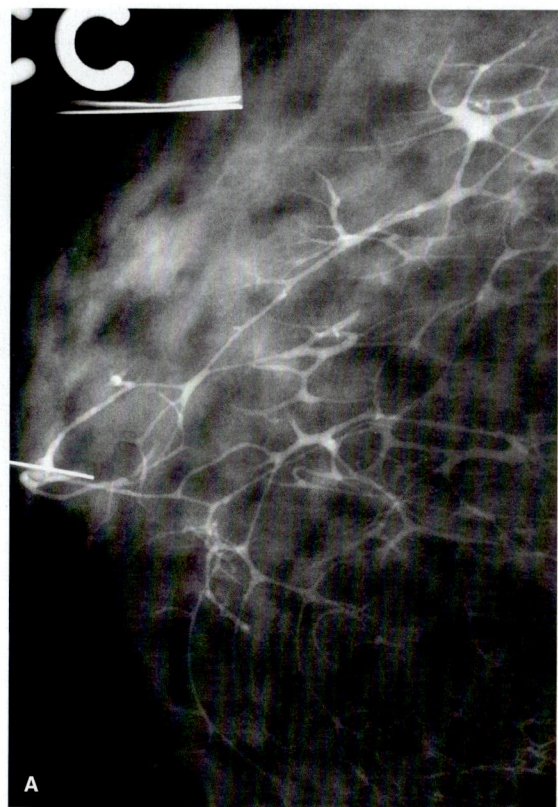

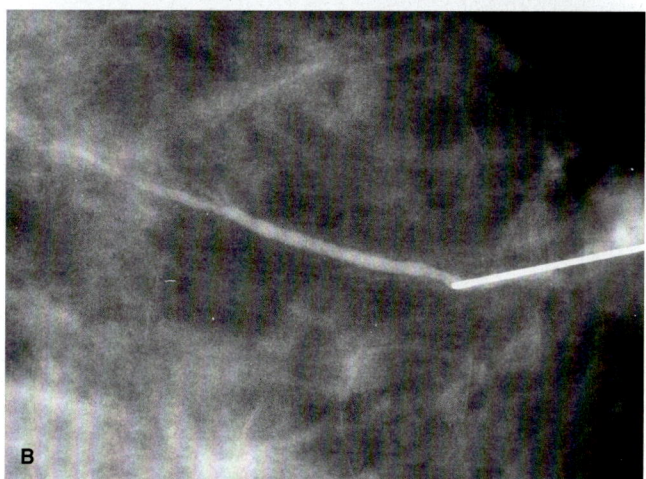

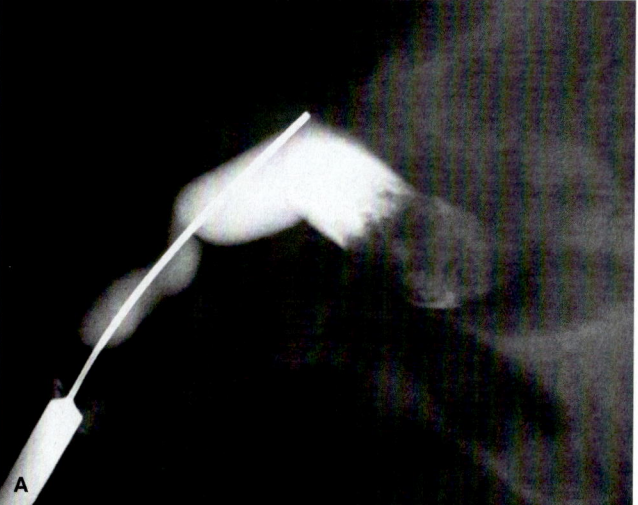

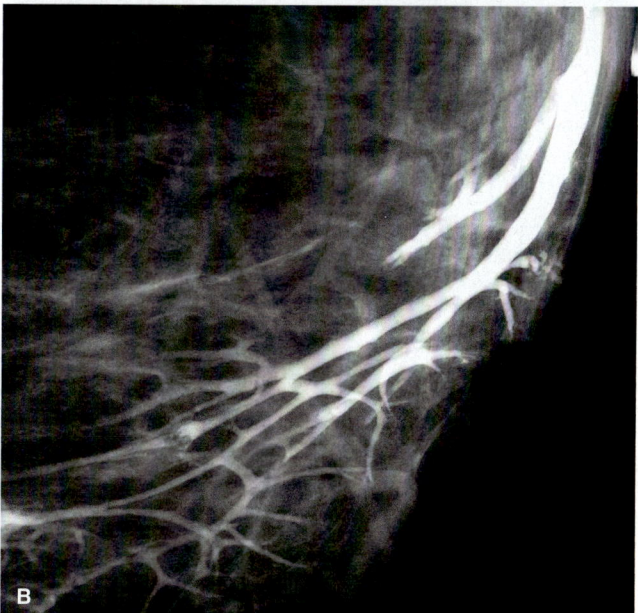

FIG. 12.4 • "Normal" ducts. **A:** If we use the cannula as an internal reference, this duct is normal in caliber. This duct demonstrates a wide area of drainage with a moderate amount of branching. No focal abnormality is apparent. **B:** Different patient. This duct has no detectable branch points and its distribution is limited in the breast. Normal caliber. As demonstrated in these two different patients, what we presume to be normal ducts are variable in length, branch pattern, and distribution in the tissue. (From Cardeñosa G. *Breast Imaging [The Core Curriculum Series]*. Philadelphia, PA: Lippincott Williams & Wilkins; 2003.)

cannula as an internal measure of duct caliber. Arbitrarily, we define normal duct caliber as up to three times the width of the cannula.

Solitary papillomas are diagnosed in approximately 50% of women presenting with spontaneous nipple discharge (1–7). Papillomas are most commonly found within dilated ducts in a subareolar location (see Figs. 9.33 and 9.34A, B). Although the entire duct may be dilated in these patients, the segment of duct between the lesion and the nipple is most commonly involved (Fig. 12.5A). Papillomas, however, can occur anywhere

FIG. 12.5 • Papillomas. **A:** A lesion is present obstructing the cannulated duct close to the nipple. The irregular interface at the obstructing site reflects contrast pooling in the interstices of the papilloma. The duct between the lesion and the nipple is dilated (compare to cannula). The subareolar location of this lesion in a distended duct is common with papillomas. **B:** Different patient. Opacified duct is moderately dilated. Do you see the lesion? In spite of the magnification technique, some of these lesions can be difficult to identify, and close evaluation of all branches is important. Imagine the limitations in evaluating ducts and detecting lesions without the use of magnification. **C:** Photographic coning to the area of the lesion demonstrates a filling defect (*arrows*) in the opacified duct shown in part **B**. The edges of the lesion are irregular consistent with contrast pooling in the interstices of the papilloma. Notice the distance from the nipple to the lesion. Although papillomas are often subareolar in location not all of them are. Without knowing the location of this lesion preoperatively, do you think the surgeon would extend his/her dissection to this point? Even if they did, can we be sure the pathologist would know where to look for the lesion? **D:** Different patient. The caliber of opacified duct is normal. An area of persistent narrowing and irregularity is noted involving a side branch of the duct (*arrows*). Although ductal carcinoma in situ is suspected in this patient, a papilloma is diagnosed after wire localization and excision. The findings of papillomas and ductal carcinoma in situ on ductography overlap therein the need for excisional biopsy. (From Cardeñosa G. *Breast Imaging [The Core Curriculum Series]*. Philadelphia, PA: Lippincott Williams & Wilkins; 2003.)

(continued)

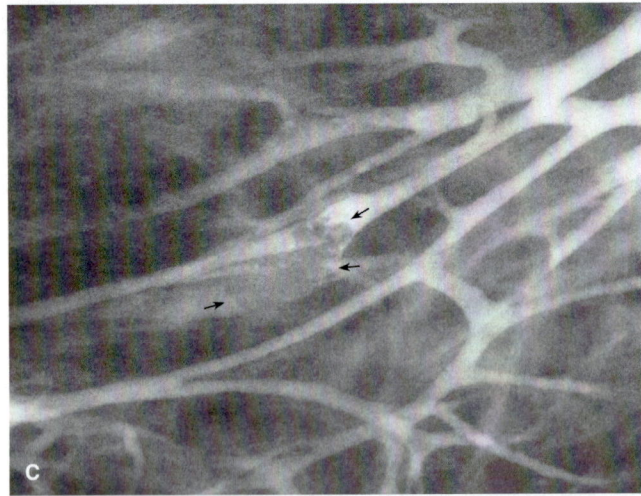

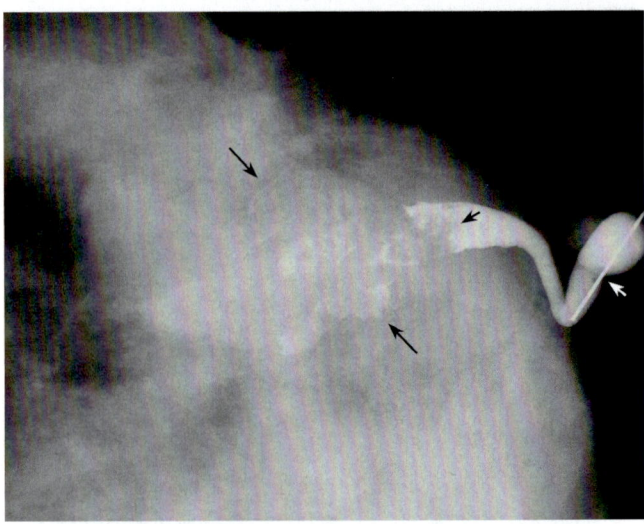

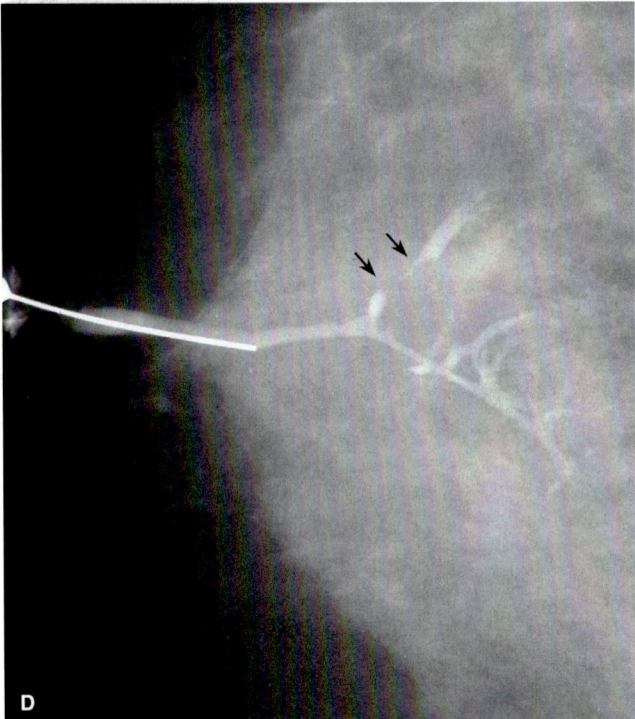

FIG. 12.5 • *(continued)*

FIG. 12.6 • **Papilloma, expanding and distorting the duct.** This lesion is obstructing the duct. Contrast is seen seemingly outside the confines of the duct *(black arrows)* but this is actually contrast in the interstices of the lesion and the duct itself is normal. If we use the cannula *(white arrow)* as an internal reference, this duct is dilated. (From Cardeñosa G. *Breast Imaging [The Core Curriculum Series]*. Philadelphia, PA: Lippincott Williams & Wilkins; 2003.)

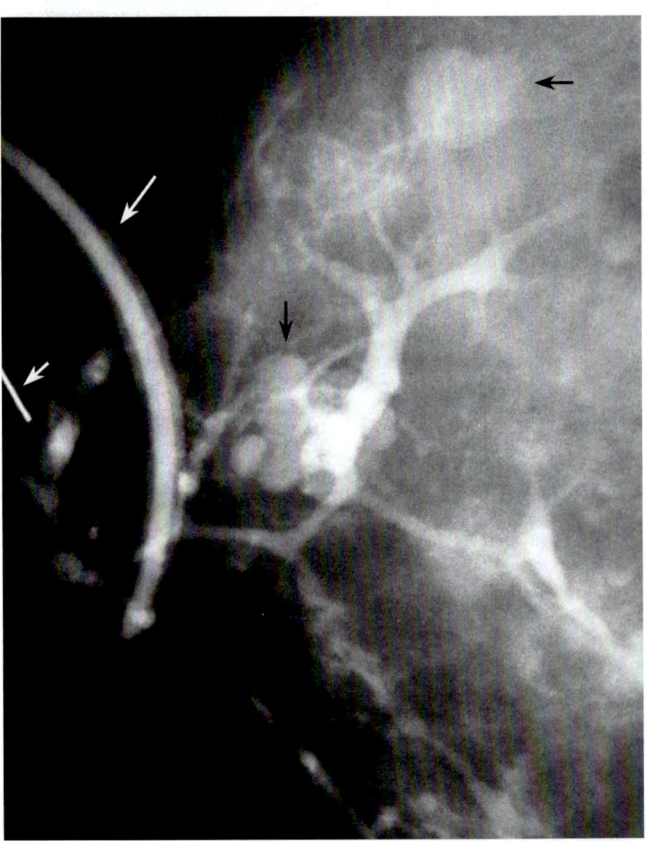

FIG. 12.7 • **Fibrocystic changes, connection to cysts.** Contrast is seen opacifying multiple cysts *(black arrows)*. A portion of the contrast containing tubing *(long white arrow)* used for the ductogram is seen superimposed on the breast. Ideally, the technologist moves the tubing away from the field of view. A small portion of the cannula *(short white arrow)* is seen at the edge of the image. (From Cardeñosa G. *Breast Imaging [The Core Curriculum Series]*. Philadelphia, PA: Lippincott Williams & Wilkins; 2003.)

in the duct, and duct dilatation is not always present. Filling defects (Fig. 12.5B, C; also see Fig. 9.33), obstruction of the main duct (Fig. 12.5A) or a branch, and, less commonly, wall irregularity (Fig. 12.5D) are ductographic findings in patients with papillomas. In some patients, contrast can be seen pooling irregularly in the interstices of the lesion. The lesions sometimes appear to expand and disrupt the integrity of the duct; however, when excised, the wall of these ducts is intact (Fig. 12.6). In patients with fibrocystic changes, the discharge is often green in color (7). Ductography findings include connection with one or several cysts (Fig. 12.7) or diffuse wall irregularities. Thick white pasty discharge (Fig. 12.8A) may be seen in patients with underlying duct ectasia as the cause of nipple discharge (7). These ducts are dilated in the subareolar region and often change abruptly in caliber as the duct courses proximally (Fig. 12.8B).

Lastly, breast cancer can present with spontaneous nipple discharge (1–7). In this group of patients, three subgroups should be considered: (i) patients with ductal carcinoma in situ (DCIS) arising in a papilloma; in this group the opacified duct is often dilated and one or multiple

Interventional Procedures **383**

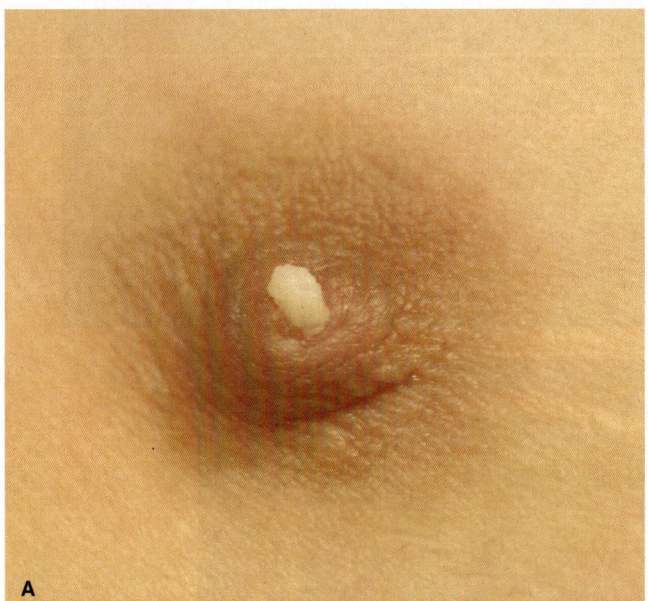

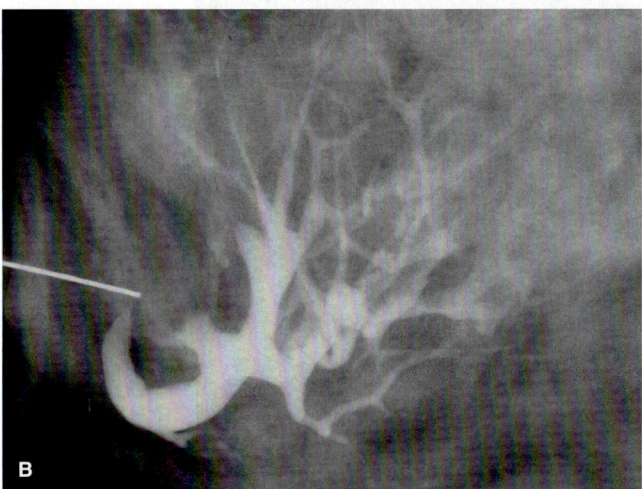

FIG. 12.8 • **Duct ectasia. A:** Thick white discharge (sometimes malodorous) is seen commonly in women with duct ectasia. **B:** Different patient. The duct is dilated in the subareolar area with an abrupt change in caliber. The more proximal branches of the duct assume a normal caliber. No focal finding is identified. (From Cardeñosa G. *Breast Imaging [The Core Curriculum Series]*. Philadelphia, PA: Lippincott Williams & Wilkins; 2003.)

intraductal lesions are identified (Fig. 12.9A); (ii) patients with DCIS in whom the duct is not usually dilated and the findings involve the opacified duct diffusely (Fig. 12.9B, C); and (iii) patients with invasive ductal carcinoma in whom a mass may be identified on the mammogram (Fig. 12.9D). Most of the patients with breast cancer who present with nipple discharge in groups (i) and (ii) have normal mammograms. Of all patients presenting with spontaneous nipple discharge, 5% to 8% will be diagnosed with breast cancer and it is commonly DCIS. A small number of patients presenting with spontaneous nipple discharge have a finding suggestive of cancer (e.g., malignant-type calcifications, mass with indistinct or spiculated margins) identified on the mammogram (Fig. 12.9D). In these patients, we do not assume that the nipple discharge is necessarily related to the mammographic finding. Until a relationship is established, these may represent synchronous yet unrelated processes (Fig. 12.9E–G). The findings on ductography in women with breast cancer overlap those described for papillomas. They include one or multiple filling defects, obstruction of the duct, and duct wall irregularity. Less common signs of cancer on ductography include contrast extravasation and displacement of the opacified duct (3).

Potential pitfalls include masking of small lesions, or those close to the nipple, if too much contrast is injected at the onset (Fig. 12.3). If masking of a lesion close to the nipple is suspected, a follow-up image can be done after the cannula is removed. Air bubbles may rarely be mistaken for a lesion. Air bubbles, however, are well defined, round, lucent, and change in position between images (Fig. 12.10). Rarely in some patients, an extensive amount of air outlines portions of the duct. This is probably not related to the contrast injection; however, the cause is not usually established. Duct perforation with contrast extravasation is uncommon. It is not easy to perforate a normal duct. It requires a certain amount of force, is painful and the patient describes a burning sensation as soon as

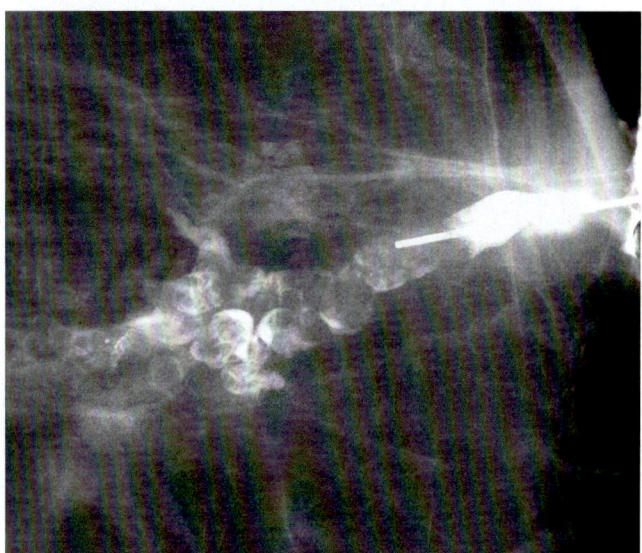

FIG. 12.9 • **Ductal carcinoma. A:** Intraductal lesion with interstices outlined by contrast. The duct is dilated between the lesion and the nipple. A papilloma with associated and adjacent ductal carcinoma in situ (low to intermediate nuclear grade with no central necrosis) is diagnosed histologically. **B:** Different patient. Magnified craniocaudal view of the anterior aspect of the left breast in a 42-year-old patient presenting with spontaneous nipple discharge. Her mammogram (not shown) is normal. A diffusely abnormal duct extends proximally into the upper central and lateral portions of the left breast. Multiple areas of narrowing and sacculation are identified, as are abrupt rounded terminations of the duct. Extensive ductal carcinoma in situ is described histologically. **C:** Different patient. The segment of the duct closest to the nipple *(arrows)* is normal. The remainder of the duct is diffusely abnormal with areas of sacculation and narrowing. Ductal carcinoma in situ is reported histologically. **D:** An irregular mass with spiculated margins is apparent on the mammogram. A side branch of the opacified duct is obstructed *(black arrow)* with a meniscus noted at the obstruction site. This corresponds to the site of the mass *(white arrows)* on orthogonal views (only one view is shown) consistent with an invasive ductal carcinoma in a patient with nipple discharge and a mass on her mammogram. **A–D** (From Cardeñosa G. *Breast Imaging [The Core Curriculum Series]*. Philadelphia, PA: Lippincott Williams & Wilkins; 2003.) **E:** Different patient with a mass in the left breast and nipple discharge. Spot compression view demonstrating a mass *(arrow)* in the left subareolar area laterally. **F:** Ultrasound. A complex cystic and solid mass is seen on ultrasound corresponding to the mass seen mammographically. **G:** Ductogram. An intraductal lesion obstructs the dilated duct *(long arrow)*. You cannot assume that the nipple discharge and mass detected mammographically are related. In this patient, the mass *(short arrow)* is an atypical papilloma and the intraductal filling defect identified on ductography is ductal carcinoma in situ, intermediate nuclear grade. In patients presenting with mammographic findings and nipple discharge, do not assume the two are related; separate processes may underlie the findings.

(continued)

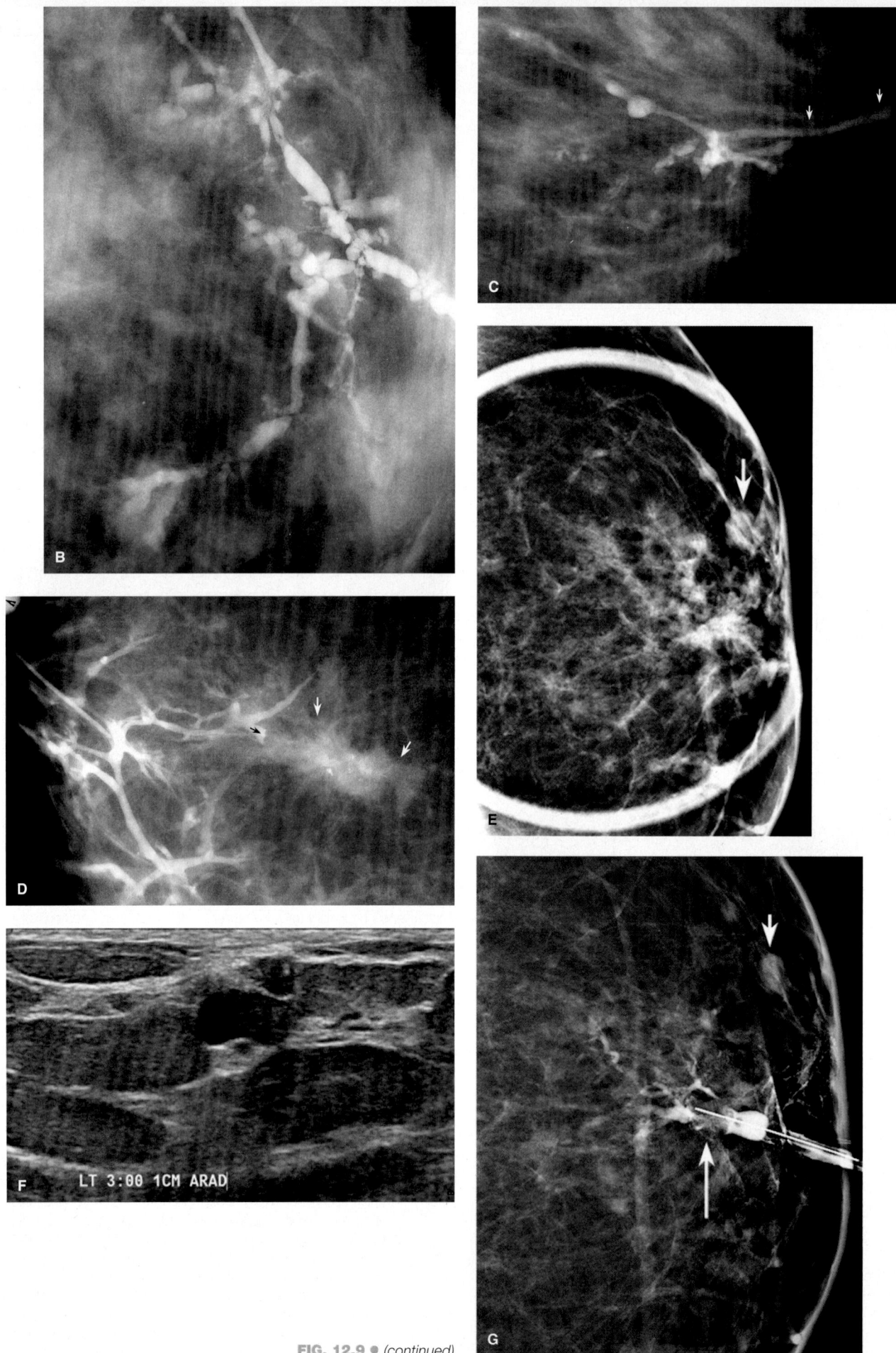

FIG. 12.9 • (continued)

Rarely, pseudolesions may be seen on ductography. Diffuse wall abnormalities may be seen on the initial ductogram; yet at the time of the preoperative ductography, the findings are not confirmed (Fig. 12.12). Nonspecific fibrocystic changes are diagnosed in these patients. It is unclear why this is seen; however, it may represent debris or clots in the lumen of the duct. Lastly, false negative ductography secondary to the cannulation of the wrong duct occurs in approximately 15% of patients. Duct openings are closely apposed on the surface of the nipple so identifying the one with the discharge can be a challenge. If a patient presents with a classic history (e.g., dark spots on the bra cup) and physical examination (focal crusting on the nipple, identifiable trigger point with copious discharge arising from a single duct opening) suggestive of an intraductal lesion, a normal ductogram is not accepted. The patient is asked to return for a repeat study or ultrasound can be used in an attempt to localize the lesion.

If an intraductal lesion is identified on ductography, excision is usually recommended. A preoperative ductography with a methylene blue:contrast combination (1:1) can be helpful to the surgeon intraoperatively and assures the pathologist will process and evaluate the lesion (Fig. 12.13A). Occasionally, in women with lesions that are a distance from the nipple, or proximal to multiple branch points in the duct, a wire localization of the lesion is done using the ductogram to guide the wire localization procedure (Fig. 12.13B, C). In these patients, the ductogram is done with undiluted contrast material (e.g., no methylene blue is injected).

After the study is completed, the cannula is removed and the nipple is covered with gauze or a nursing pad. This prevents contrast material from leaking out onto the patient's clothes. Many patients describe a significant reduction or complete cessation of the discharge for several

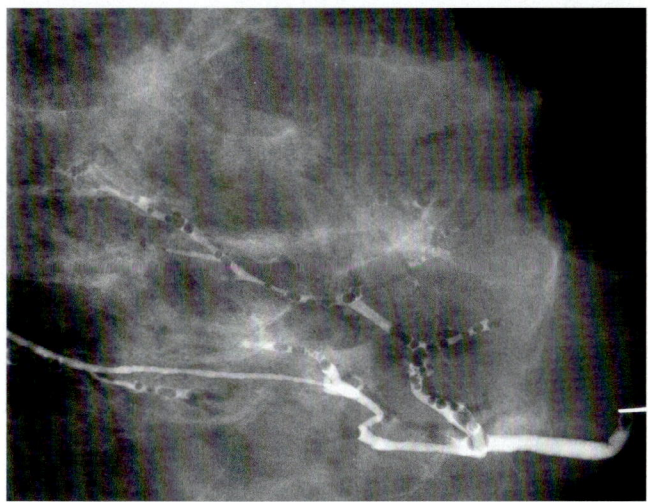

FIG. 12.10 • **Air bubbles.** Many circumscribed, round and oval lucent filling defects are noted throughout the opacified duct. Obtaining a second image will usually show that these change in position. (From Cardeñosa G. *Breast Imaging [The Core Curriculum Series]*. Philadelphia, PA: Lippincott Williams & Wilkins; 2003.)

you start injecting contrast. In attempting to distend small ducts, contrast extravasation proximally in side branches of the duct and opacification of lymphatic channels can sometimes be seen (Fig. 12.11). Patients with proximal extravasation tolerate the injection initially, but describe a burning sensation after a few drops of contrast have been injected.

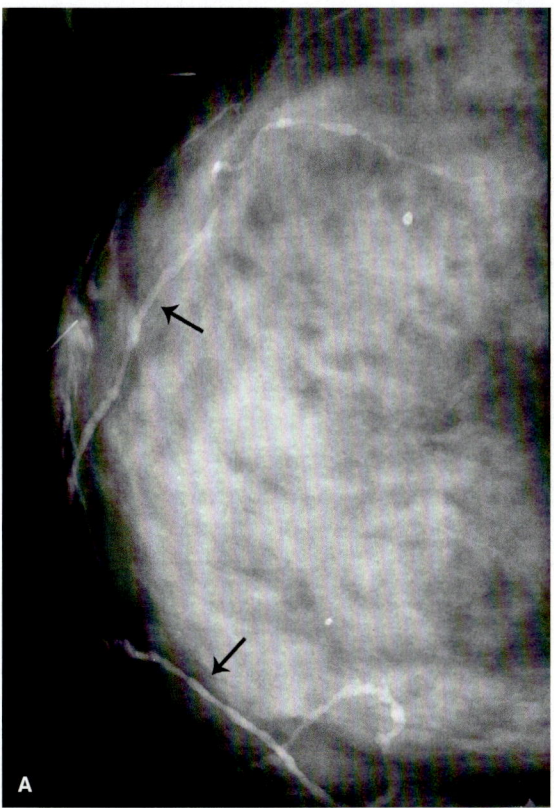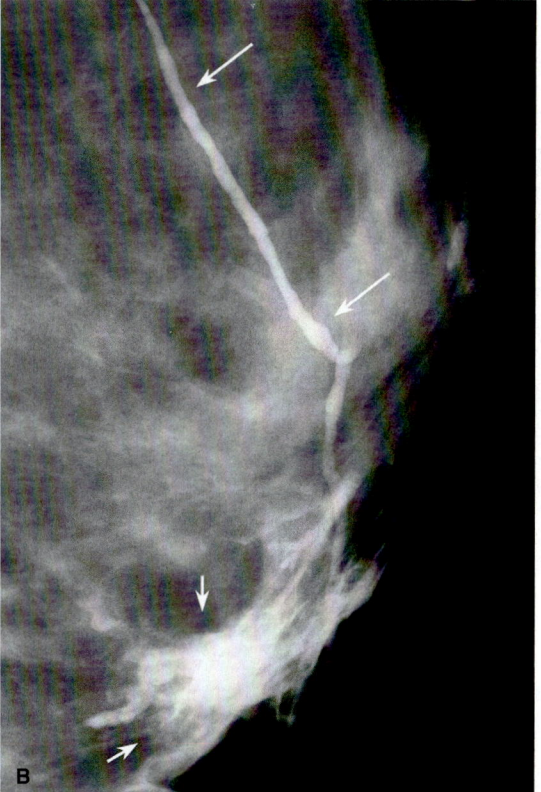

FIG. 12.11 • **Opacified lymphatic channels. A:** Tubular structures *(arrows)* are opacified with contrast. The random nonanatomic distribution of these structures (e.g., not ducts or vascular structures) is such that they are thought to represent lymphatic channels. **B:** Different patient. Proximal extravasation *(short arrows)* of contrast is noted resulting from an attempt to opacify additional branches in the cannulated duct. The patient describes burning as the extravasation occurs. A tubular structure *(long arrows)* in a nonanatomic distribution for a duct is opacified; this is thought to represent a lymphatic channel. (From Cardeñosa G. *Breast Imaging [The Core Curriculum Series]*. Philadelphia, PA: Lippincott Williams & Wilkins; 2003.)

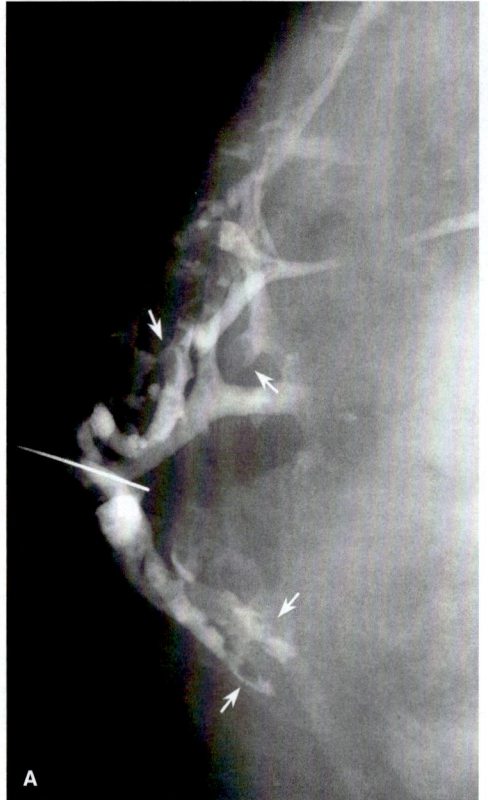
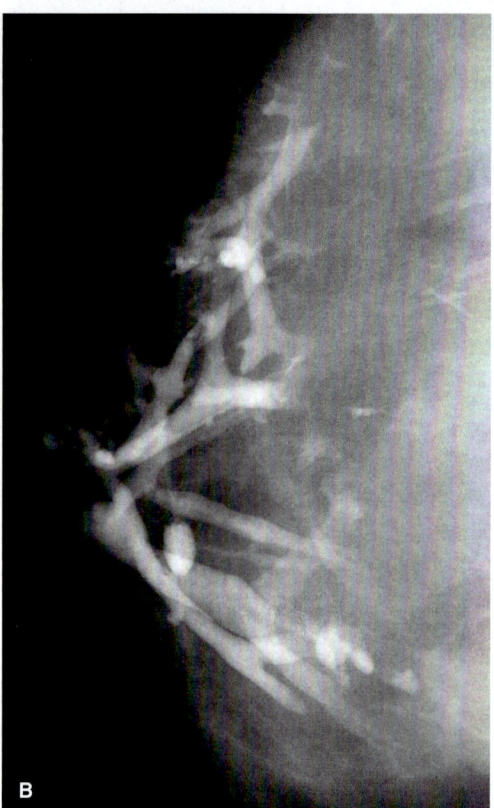
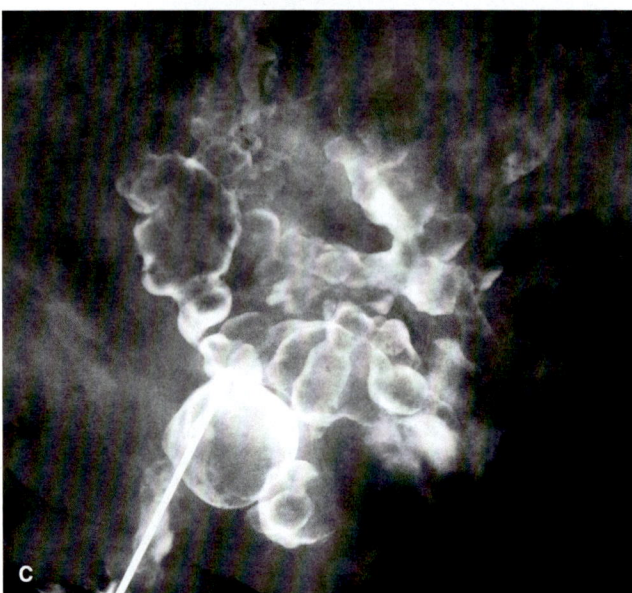

FIG. 12.12 • **Pseudo lesions. A:** Diagnostic ductogram demonstrates a diffusely irregular duct with filling defects and wall irregularities *(white arrows)*. Excision is recommended. **B:** Preoperative ductogram demonstrates a normal duct. Previously noted abnormalities are not reproduced. Nonspecific fibrocystic changes are reported histologically. **A, B** (From Cardeñosa G. *Breast Imaging [The Core Curriculum Series]*. Philadelphia, PA: Lippincott Williams & Wilkins; 2003.) **C:** Different patient. Apparent filling defects diffusely involving a duct with focally dilated segments. It is unclear if these represent duct contents.

weeks following the ductogram. It is unclear why this occurs but it is usually not a problem for the preoperative ductogram since discharge is still obtained when pressure is applied in the subareolar area.

CYST ASPIRATION AND PNEUMOCYSTOGRAPHY

Aspiration of cysts is undertaken in three situations: (i) when there are associated symptoms (e.g., tenderness, burning), (ii) if observations are made on ultrasound such that the diagnosis of a cyst is in question, or (iii) at the patient's request. As cysts enlarge and tension on the wall and surrounding tissue increases, patients may describe discomfort and tenderness. Some investigators have suggested that as cysts enlarge, some of the fluid escapes into the surrounding breast parenchyma eliciting an aseptic inflammatory response. Aspiration under these circumstances often relieves the symptoms (2,8,9).

We consider aspiration when the ultrasound findings are not diagnostic of a cyst and sometimes do pneumocystography in patients in whom we suspect an intracystic or mural abnormality (Fig. 12.14). Palpation, ultrasound, or mammography can be used to guide the aspiration. Even with palpable cysts, our preference is to aspirate them using ultrasound guidance. Direct observation with ultrasound expedites

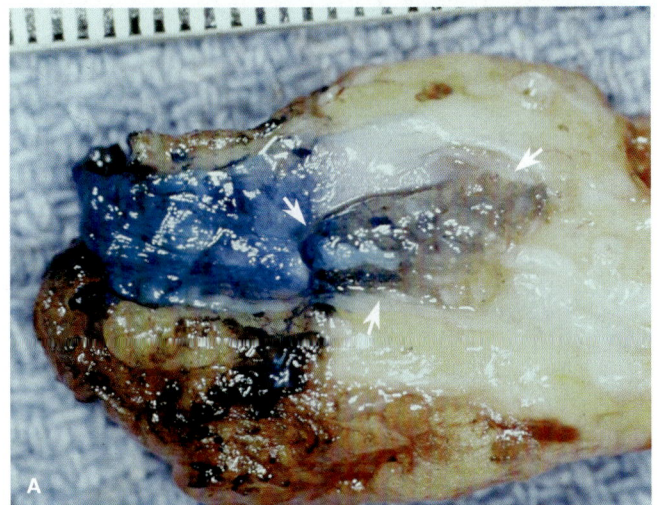
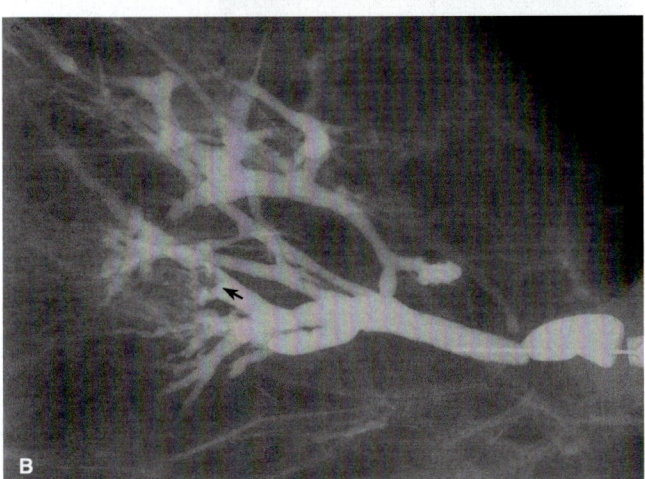
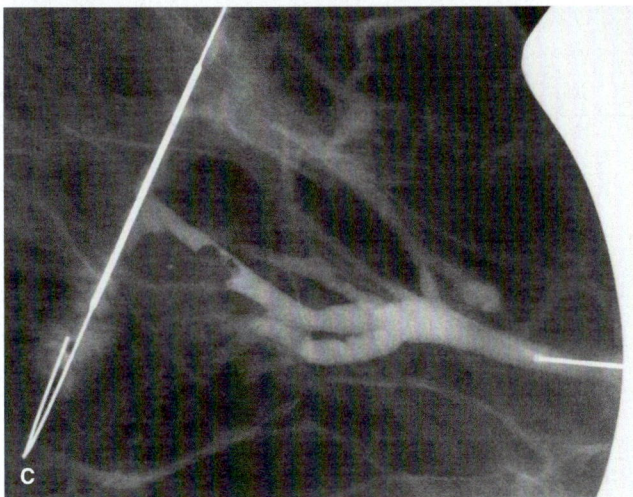

FIG. 12.13 • **Papillomas, preoperative ductogram with methylene blue or wire localization. A:** Methylene blue stained duct is opened and the lesion *(arrows)* is identified in the duct and evaluated histologically. Preoperative ductograms are done using a contrast:methylene blue (1:1) combination. The contrast enables the radiologist to confirm cannulation of the abnormal duct. The surgeon uses the methylene blue to identify the duct intra-operatively. The methylene blue also stains the duct and, as in this patient, the leading edge of the lesion, for the pathologist. **B:** Different patient. Diagnostic ductogram demonstrates a filling defect *(arrow)* in a side branch of an arborized duct. **C:** The day of surgery, the ductogram is repeated and used to guide wire localization. Mid-portion of reinforced wire segment is just posterior to the intraductal lesion. **B, C** (From Cardeñosa G. *Breast Imaging [The Core Curriculum Series]*. Philadelphia, PA: Lippincott Williams & Wilkins; 2003.)

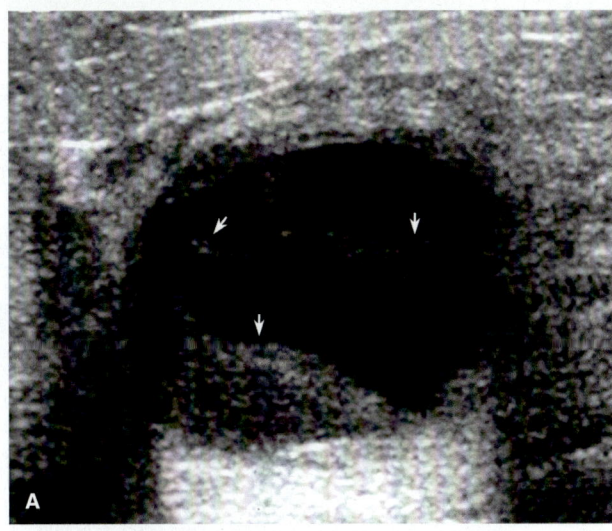
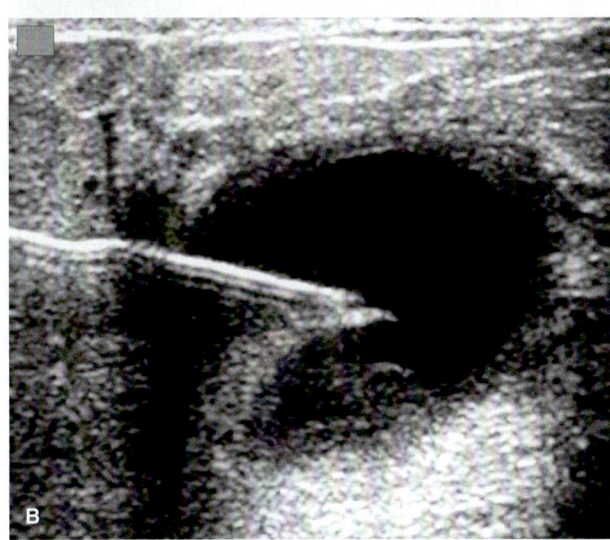

FIG. 12.14 • **Cyst aspiration and pneumocystography. A:** A seemingly complex cystic and solid mass with posterior acoustic enhancement is imaged corresponding to a lump described by the patient and a mass with obscured margins imaged on the mammogram. Internal echoes, apparent septations *(arrows),* and possible irregularity of the wall are noted. Aspiration and pneumocystography are done for diagnostic purposes. **B:** Needle with tip in the center of the mass. The aspiration is monitored during real time and the echoes are seen being aspirated into the needle. No residual abnormality is seen on ultrasound post aspiration. After the contents are aspirated, 50% of the volume of fluid aspirated is replaced with air. **C:** Ninety-degree lateral (LM) spot compression magnification view is done following the injection of air. A smooth-walled cyst cavity is seen with no intracystic or mural component. This is confirmed on orthogonal projections (craniocaudal spot compression view not shown). The findings are consistent with a cyst, possibly aseptically inflamed (given initial mural irregularities) warranting no further intervention or follow-up. **D:** Different patient. Two masses with circumscribed and indistinct margins are apparent mammographically in a 60-year-old patient presenting with a "lump." The metallic BB marks the site of the palpable finding. **E:** Ultrasound. A complex cystic and solid mass (predominantly solid with a solid component) is imaged correlating to the palpable finding. The other mass seen mammographically is a cyst (not shown). Aspiration and pneumocystography are done. The fluid is serous in appearance. "Findings consistent with cyst contents" are reported cytologically (the pathologist is aware that a papillary lesion is suspected). **F:** Pneumocystogram image demonstrates intracystic mass *(arrow)*. The remainder of the cavity has a smooth wall. Excisional biopsy following ultrasound-guided wire localization is done (see Fig. 12.41). In our experience, fluid reaccumulates (sometimes quickly) in patients with neoplastic (intracystic or mural) lesions - see Fig. 12.41 for the US on this patient on the day of the localization procedure and Fig. 12.18 for images on another patient. (From Cardeñosa G. *Breast Imaging [The Core Curriculum Series]*. Philadelphia, PA: Lippincott Williams & Wilkins; 2003.)

(continued)

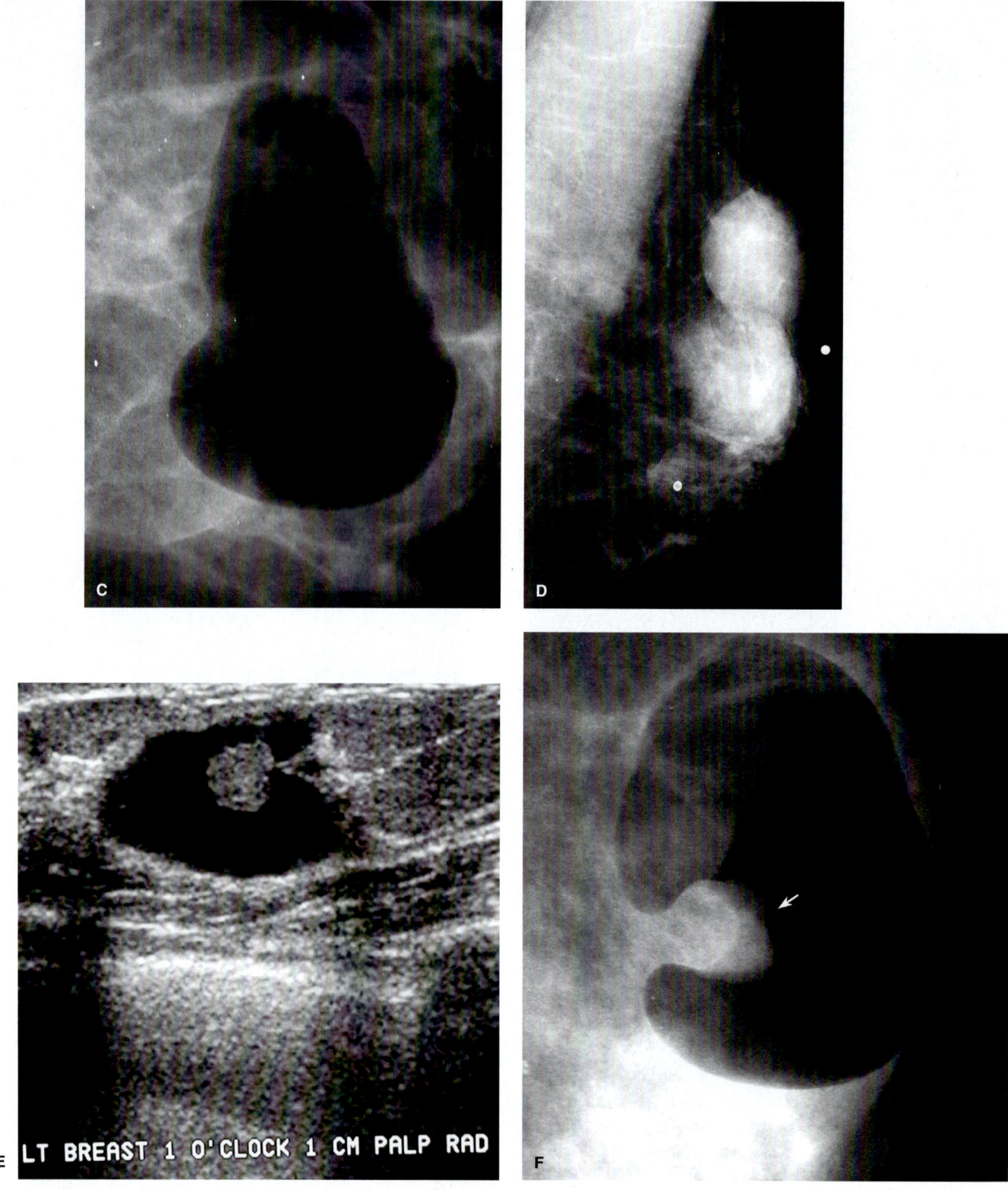

FIG. 12.14 • *(continued)*

needle movements and is helpful in determining the amount of pressure needed to puncture cyst walls that are sometimes thickened and inflamed. After the aspiration, no residual abnormality should be seen sonographically (Fig. 12.15). If a persistent abnormality is seen, a core biopsy is indicated. When pneumocystography is done, half the amount of aspirated fluid is replaced with air. Spot compression magnification views of the cyst are obtained in orthogonal projections (CC and 90-degree lateral views) to evaluate the cyst wall (Fig. 12.14C, F).

When using ultrasound guidance, we select an approach that enables us to introduce the needle parallel to the chest wall and transducer (see needle biopsy section for a more detailed description). The skin is cleaned with betadiene and alcohol. Lidocaine (1 or 2 mL of 1%) is

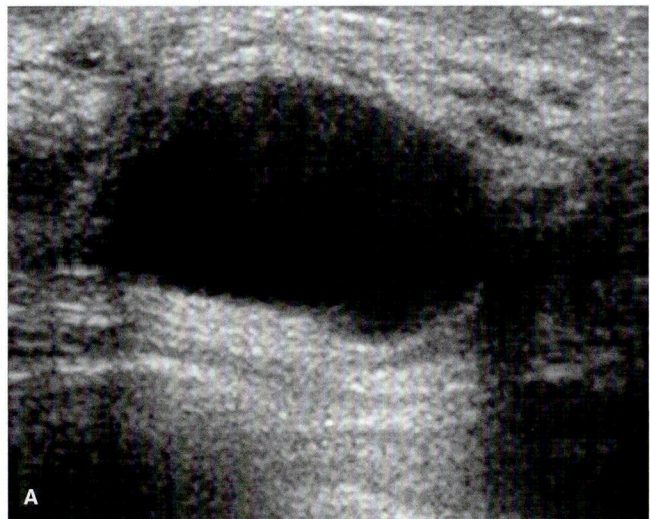

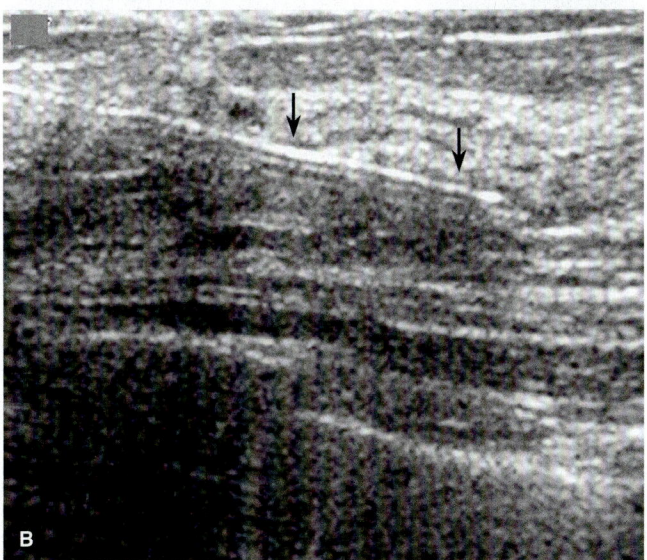

FIG. 12.15 • **Cyst aspiration. A:** Nearly anechoic cyst with posterior acoustic enhancement and internal echoes. The distribution of the echoes is such that they may not represent reverberation artifact. After local anesthesia is administered, a 20G needle is advanced into the lesion. An image to document needle positioning is done (not shown). **B:** The aspiration is monitored during real time and the echoes are seen being aspirated into the needle. No residual abnormality is seen post aspiration. This image done after the aspiration documents normal tissue surrounding the needle *(arrows)*. No additional intervention or follow-up is indicated in this patient. (From Cardeñosa G. *Breast Imaging [The Core Curriculum Series]*. Philadelphia, PA: Lippincott Williams & Wilkins; 2003.).

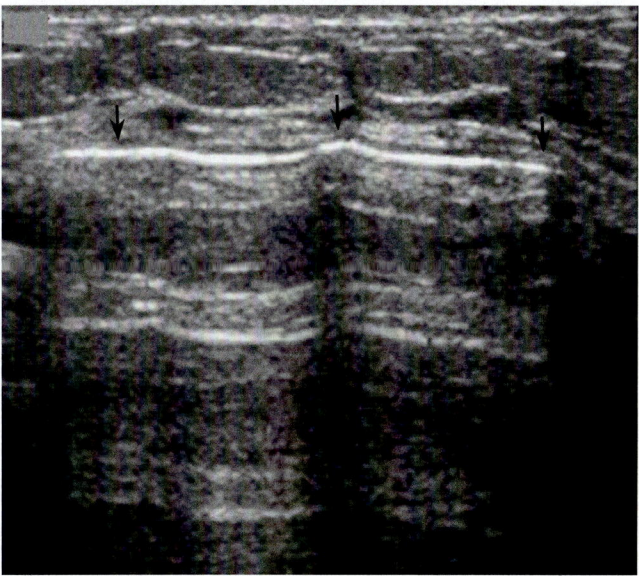

FIG. 12.16 • **Air.** An echogenic line *(arrows)* is seen following injection of air into a cyst cavity. Although not evident in this patient, shadowing may be seen in some patients deep to the injected air. In this patient, the air is injected in an attempt to reduce the likelihood of cyst recurrence. No mammographic images (e.g., pneumocystogram) are done post aspiration. (From Cardeñosa G. *Breast Imaging [The Core Curriculum Series]*. Philadelphia, PA: Lippincott Williams & Wilkins; 2003.).

used to slowly raise a skin wheal. Under ultrasound guidance, the anesthesia needle is advanced up to the cyst (but not into the cyst) and lidocaine is infiltrated along the expected course of the needle. A few minutes are allowed to elapse after the administration of the lidocaine. Using ultrasound guidance, a 20G spinal needle is used to puncture the cyst. When using real-time scanning, it is easy to appreciate how much pressure to apply in traversing the cyst wall. In some patients, the cyst wall indents significantly before it is pierced. With the tip of the needle in the center of the cyst (Fig. 12.14B), the inner stylet is removed and the needle is connected to a 10 mL syringe. Under direct ultrasound visualization, suction is applied until all of the contents are evacuated. There should be no residual abnormality following the aspiration. In patients with cysts having thick contents, an 18G spinal needle may be needed to completely evacuate the cyst. The aspirated fluid is not submitted for cytological evaluation unless the aspirate is bloody (or the patient requests it).

Air can be injected into the cyst cavity. Some investigators have suggested that injecting air may have a therapeutic benefit by reducing the likelihood of cyst recurrence (2,8,9). In these patients, no mammographic images are obtained after the air is injected. Alternatively, a pneumocystogram (2,8,9) can be done for diagnostic purposes to evaluate potential intracystic or mural lesions. After the cyst is drained, the needle is stabilized and the fluid-filled syringe is replaced with a syringe containing air. Fifty percent of the aspirated fluid is replaced with air. The needle and syringe are then removed. Sonographically, an irregular echogenic line is seen if air is injected (Fig. 12.16). For a pneumocystogram, spot compression magnification views of the cyst are done to evaluate the wall of the cyst and the appearance of the surrounding tissue (Fig. 12.14).

In women with small lesions, or when the lesion is deep in a larger breast or deep in the tissue, cyst aspirations can be done using mammographic guidance (see preoperative wire localization section). A fenestrated paddle is used to establish the coordinates for the lesion. With the patient still in compression, a 20G spinal needle is advanced slowly at the coordinates for the lesion as suction is applied. When fluid is obtained, the needle is stabilized until all of the fluid is aspirated. The needle is left in place and follow-up orthogonal images are obtained to document resolution of the lesion.

Management of Patients with a Complex Cystic and Solid Mass

If a large fluid component is present in patients with a complex cystic and solid mass, our approach is to aspirate the fluid and do core biopsies through the residual solid component (Fig. 12.17). Even when malignancy is present, fluid cytology alone is nondiagnostic (or misleading) in approximately 50% of patients; the diagnosis is made on core biopsies of the solid component (Fig. 12.17). If fluid cytology is often nondiagnostic, why not just core the solid component without first aspirating the fluid out? The fluid in some of these lesions can incite a significant aseptic inflammatory reaction if fluid is inadvertently

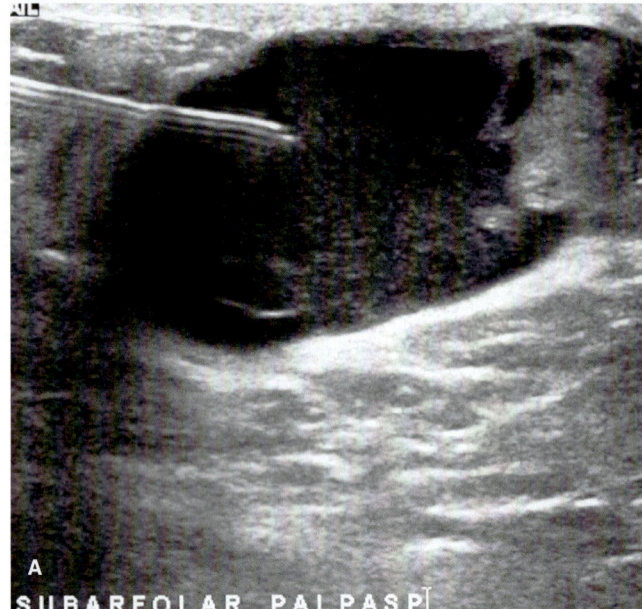

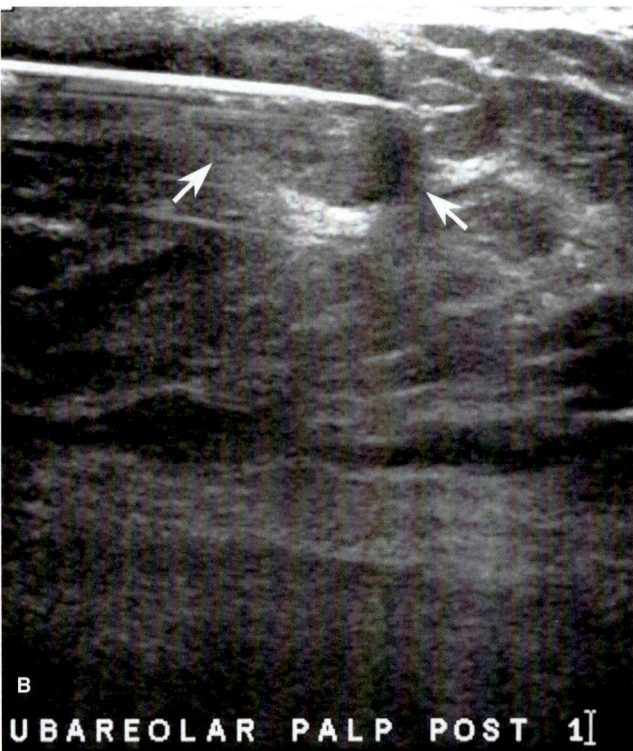

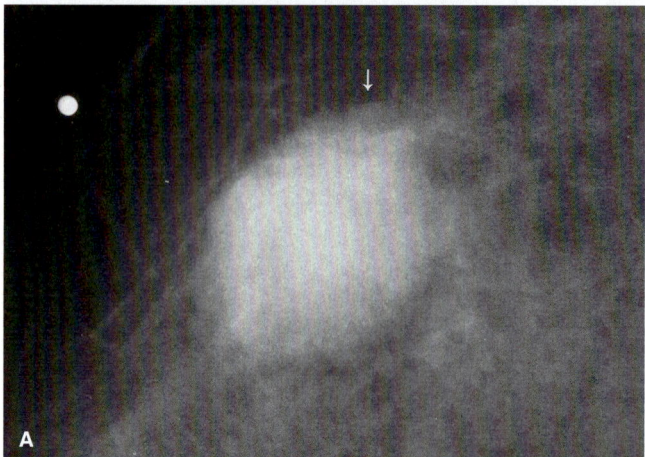

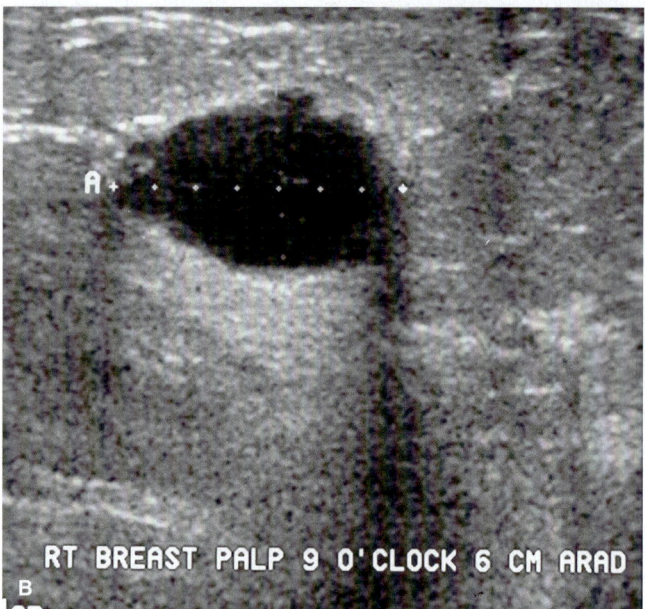

to weeks. We try hard to avoid precipitating these and in our experience, concerns regarding an inability to identify the solid component or localize the lesion at a later date if the fluid is first aspirated are not well founded. If a tumor is present and the source of the fluid, it will be apparent after aspiration and in most patients, the fluid reaccumulates within several days of the aspiration (Fig. 12.18).

FIG. 12.17 • **Encapsulated papillary carcinoma, intermediate to high grade. A:** Complex cystic and solid mass in a 65-year-old man. A 20G spinal needle is used to aspirate the fluid. In this patient, three prior fine-needle aspirations done using palpation guidance yielded nonspecific benign results. A solid mass remains after the aspiration. **B:** Post fire image demonstrating the core needle through the residual solid mass *(arrows)*. The diagnosis of a papillary carcinoma is made on the core biopsy and confirmed at the time of the mastectomy. Sentinel lymph node (LN) biopsy is negative (0/6 LNs). See Figure 10.14 for the diagnostic images on this patient.

FIG. 12.18 • **Invasive ductal carcinoma, not otherwise specified, poorly differentiated. A:** Spot tangential view in a 36-year-old patient who presents with a tender, "lump." Metallic BB marks the clinical finding. A round mass *(arrow)* with indistinct margins is imaged corresponding to the palpable finding. **B:** Ultrasound. A complex cystic and solid mass with lobulated margins and posterior acoustic enhancement is imaged correlating to the clinically and mammographically apparent mass. Closely evaluate the margins and note irregular microlobulations and spiculation. Aspiration is undertaken. **C:** Residual irregular abnormality is seen post aspiration; when abnormalities persist following aspiration, do a core biopsy. Fluid cytology is not diagnostic in approximately 50% of patients. In this patient, the fluid is submitted for cytology, and necrosis, inflammatory cells, and viable cells with atypia are reported. A course of antibiotics is prescribed and a follow-up ultrasound is scheduled. **D:** Ultrasound, 5 weeks after the aspiration. A round mass with a heterogeneous echotexture, angular margins, and posterior acoustic enhancement is imaged at the prior aspiration site. Ultrasound-guided core biopsy done to establish the diagnosis of an invasive ductal carcinoma, high grade. (From Cardeñosa G. *Breast Imaging [The Core Curriculum Series]*. Philadelphia, PA: Lippincott Williams & Wilkins; 2003.)

"spilled" into the surrounding tissue. When inadvertently induced, the inflammatory reaction simulates an acute mastitis with the patient describing significant tenderness, redness, and swelling of the breast. Since this is not bacterial, antibiotics are of no use. The patient is managed conservatively with symptoms subsiding slowly over several days

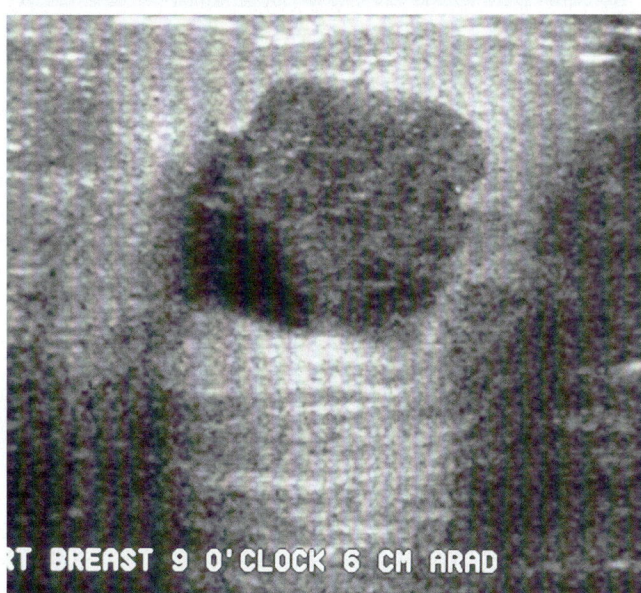

FIG. 12.18 • *(continued)*

FINE-NEEDLE ASPIRATION

Fine-needle aspiration (FNA) is a quick, reliable method of accurately establishing a diagnosis for breast and axillary masses; it is used successfully and advocated by many (10,11). Others contend that inadequate specimens (reported in as many as 47% of patients) and false negative rates (sensitivity range of 65%–99%; specificity of 64%–100% and accuracy of 81%–98%) are unacceptably high (10,11). FNA can be successfully used in evaluating patients with palpable and mammographically detected masses; it is of limited usefulness in evaluating clusters of calcifications. As with anything, however, good technique and experience are invaluable in maximizing the usefulness of the technique. Also, having a trained cytopathologist who is comfortable with breast aspirates is critical; the pathologist needs to be comfortable in making definitive statements regarding the adequacy of the sample and the presence of malignancy. However, keep in mind that if you provide an adequate amount of cellular material, the diagnosis can usually be made. Ideally, the cytopathologist is available while the aspiration is done so that the adequacy of the specimen can be determined immediately. If additional material is needed, more samples can be obtained.

For nonpalpable lesions, fenestrated paddles, stereotactic devices, or ultrasound can be used to accurately localize the lesion. At this time, we are almost exclusively doing ultrasound-guided FNAs primarily for lesions that may otherwise be difficult to approach with a core needle biopsy (Fig. 12.19). In some patients, with breast and axillary findings,

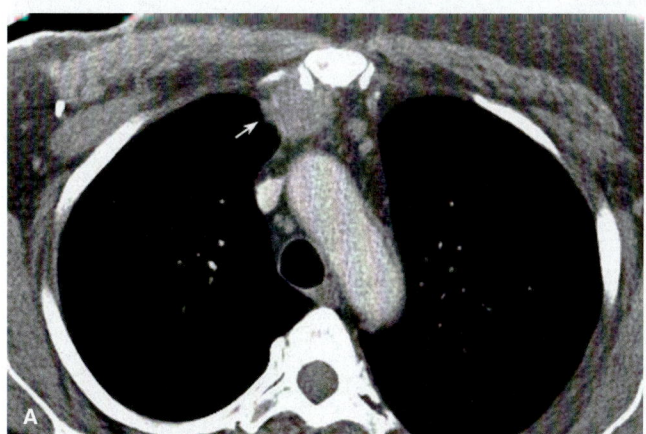

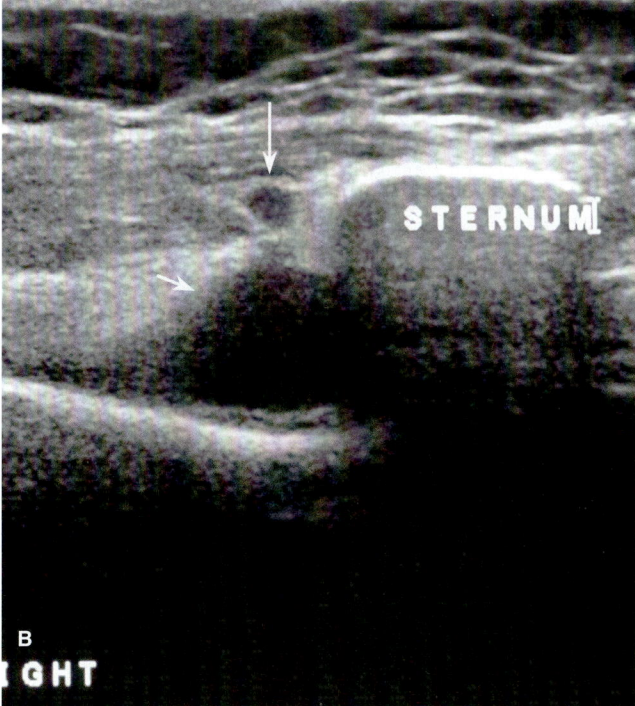

FIG. 12.19 • **Fine-needle aspiration, internal mammary lymph node. A:** Chest CT scan in a patient with a history of right breast cancer treated with mastectomy and axillary dissection. An abnormal internal mammary lymph node *(arrow)* is described. **B:** Ultrasound. A nearly anechoic mass *(short arrow)* is imaged adjacent to the sternum immediately deep to a pulsating vessel *(long arrow)*. **C:** Under ultrasound guidance, a 20G spinal needle *(short arrows)* is advanced into the mass. The pulsating vessel *(long arrow)* is monitored during the aspiration. With the needle in the mass, suction is applied and slow methodical incursions and excursions of the needle in the mass are monitored during real time making sure the needle does not go out of the mass at either end. Material is submitted on a slide for cytology and aspirates are also submitted in normal saline for cell block (hematoxylin & eosin, histology). **D:** Cell block material demonstrating malignant cells consistent with metastatic breast cancer. Notice the amount of cellular material available following fine-needle aspiration with the technique described.

(continued)

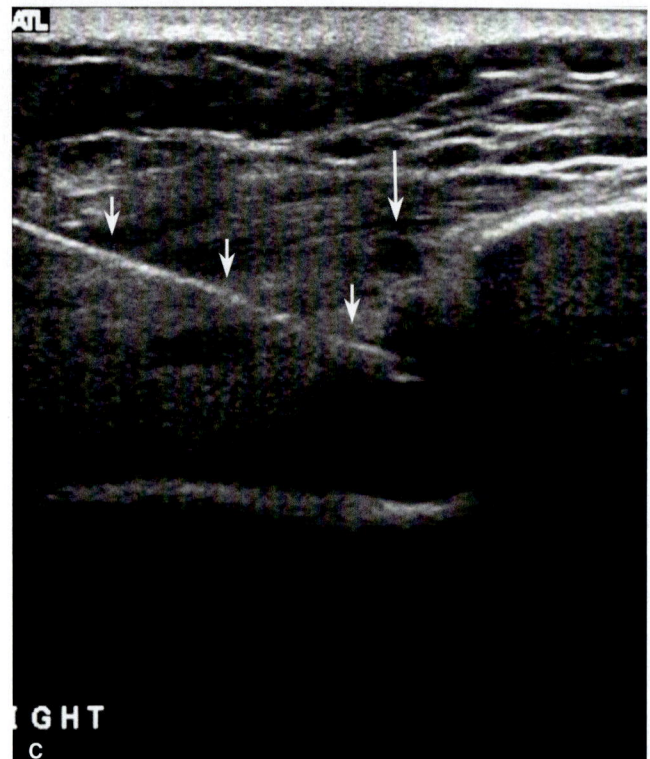

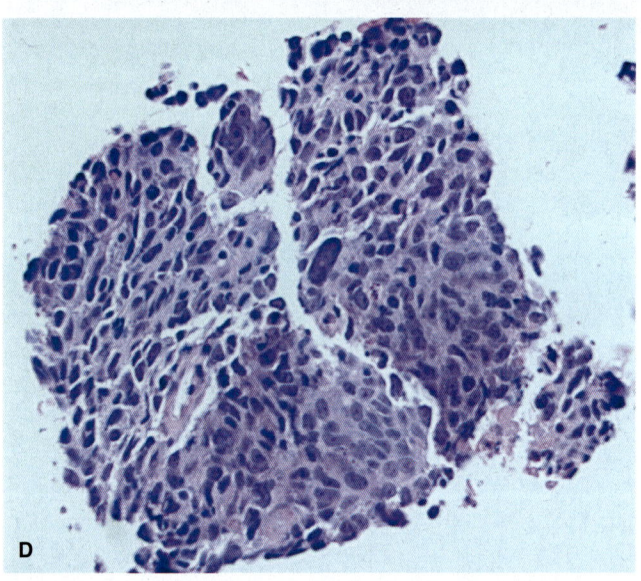

FIG. 12.19 • *(continued)*

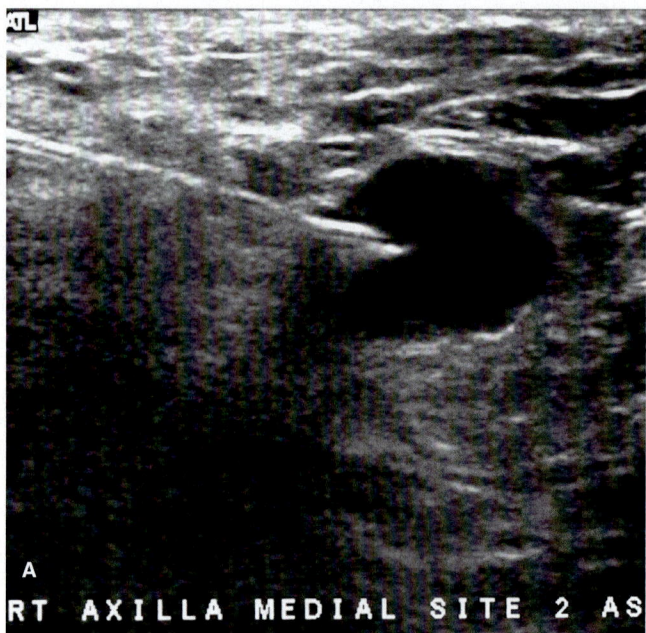

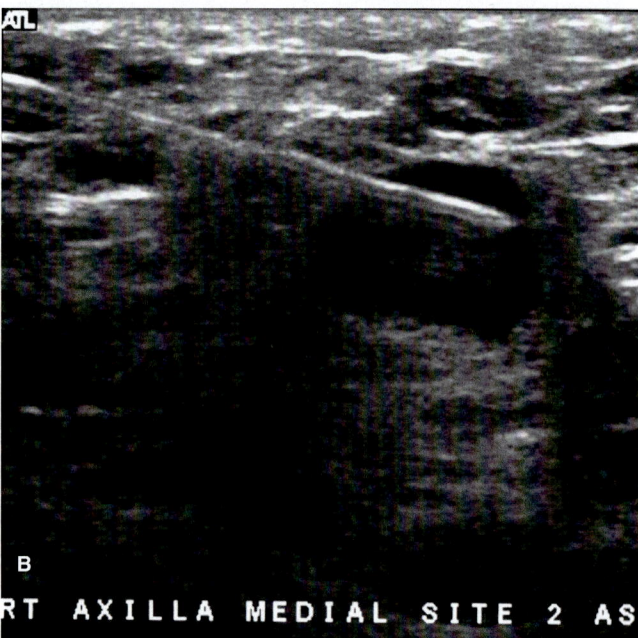

FIG. 12.20 • **Fine-needle aspiration, axillary lymph node. A:** Anechoic mass with some posterior acoustic enhancement in the right axilla likely representing metastatic disease to a lymph node in a patient with ipsilateral breast cancer (mammogram and ultrasound of breast mass not shown). Under ultrasound guidance, a 20G spinal needle is advanced to the superficial portion of the mass. Suction is applied. **B:** With suction being applied and under ultrasound guidance, the needle is slowly advanced through the mass but not beyond it. These two images illustrate the slow, repeated movements of the needle as suction is applied. With the needle tip just in the mass as shown in part **A**, suction is applied. Slow, methodical incursions and excursions of the needle from one end of the mass to the other are monitored with ultrasound. All of the movements of the needle when suction is being applied occur in the mass. After three or four movements (**A** to **B** to **A,** etc.) in the mass, suction is stopped and the needle is pulled out. Aspirates are submitted for cytology and histology (e.g., cell block). Metastatic breast cancer is reported with associated lymphoid elements.

we obtain cores of the breast mass so that enough material is available for receptor analysis (estrogen and progesterone receptors and HER2/neu) and do an FNA of the axillary finding for confirmation of suspected metastatic disease. The predetermined skin entry point is wiped with betadiene and alcohol; lidocaine (1%) is used to raise a skin wheal and is infiltrated along the expected course of the needle. For one-handed aspirations, the needle (22G or 25G) can be attached to a syringe in a pistol grip holder. Alternatively, with the tip of the needle in the center of the lesion, the needle can be attached directly to a syringe. As suction is applied and, under ultrasound guidance, the needle is slowly and methodically moved from one end of the lesion to the other making sure the needle does not come out of the lesion (Fig. 12.20). As incursions are made, the angle of the needle can be varied.

The suction is stopped before the needle is pulled out of the lesion. With the needle out of the breast, it is disconnected from the syringe and a syringe filled with air is attached and used to gently express the contents of the needle onto a glass slide. The material on the slide is smeared in one swift movement using another slide at a slight angle. Fixation is accomplished by allowing the material to air dry or placing the slide in 95% alcohol. In addition to the material smeared on slides for cytology, we also do one or two aspirates for cell block: the aspirated material is placed in normal saline and processed for cell block and hematoxylin and eosin staining (Fig. 12.19D). The methods used in handling the aspirates should be reviewed with the pathologist at your institution since there are variations.

NEEDLE BIOPSIES

At the onset of this discussion, it is important to point out that needles, guns, needle vacuum systems, and clips proliferate almost on a monthly basis. It is not my intention to discuss all available options exhaustively or even the pros and cons of each but rather to suggest that the tool selected is not nearly as important as the needed observations, evaluations, generation of appropriate differentials, and the critical thinking required to take care of patients. It is easy to biopsy every potential abnormality (including those that are obviously benign) with the largest and latest gadget, after which one or multiple clips are left behind. But is this really what is needed for optimal patient care? Why not approach each patient individually and, based on suspected histology (e.g., if invasive lobular is suspected, FNA of an axillary lymph node may not be the best tool to assess for metastatic disease), use the simplest approach that will provide an accurate diagnosis? In establishing the extent of disease, do we need to biopsy four or five sites or can we biopsy the extremes of a lesion or the two lesions that are furthest apart? Is vacuum assistance needed for every breast biopsy that is done? If vacuum is used, how many cores are needed: 5, 10, 20, or 50 and should the number of cores done be the same for all patients? If one or two cores with a 14G needle provide an accurate answer, why is this not done more often?

Some adamantly insist that clips need to be left in *all* patients after imaging-guided biopsies. Really? Is a clip really indicated in all patients following imaging-guided biopsies? Why not consider what is appropriate for the patient you are taking care of and tailor your approach accordingly? If the patient wants a mastectomy if diagnosed with breast cancer, why is a clip needed? If a patient with a 2- to 3-cm mass or one with segmentally distributed malignant-type calcifications wants a lumpectomy, are we suggesting that the percutaneous biopsy will leave no residual abnormality for the localization? For those who argue that the clip is useful in establishing concordance between a biopsied mass on ultrasound and the mammographic finding, I submit to you that this type of concordance needs to occur *before* any biopsy is done. There are simpler ways to establish mammographic–sonographic concordance than doing a vacuum-assisted biopsy, leaving a clip, and then finding out that you have not biopsied the area in question mammographically. Doing things because we can or haphazardly is not the answer. So, in this section I provide an overview of the basic principles and will discuss our approach and application of the basics. We strive to do what is needed to manage our patients appropriately. Optimal patient care is our compass, and critical, clinically-oriented thinking regarding what is best for our patients guides our approach. Accurate answers can often be obtained simply and expeditiously.

First described by Parker and associates, stereotactic-guided, and then ultrasound-guided, biopsies of breast lesions represent a significant advancement in patient care and management. These authors first described the use of a spring-loaded mechanism with a 14G needle and then a vacuum-assisted device that can be used with 14G, 12G, 11G, and 8G needles to increase the amount of tissue obtained (12–16). These techniques revolutionized the practice of breast imaging and are now well established with significant literature to support their routine use (12–22).

As already stated, the availability of these relatively simple techniques should not be used to replace or undermine complete clinical and imaging workups. If following a complete evaluation, a lesion is diagnosed as benign, the patient is asked to return for a screening mammogram in 1 year. If following evaluation a lesion fits the criteria for a probably benign lesion (see Chapter 13), we recommend a short-interval follow-up; typically this is a 6-month follow-up unless an inflammatory or post traumatic change is suspected, in which case a 3-month follow-up may be done rarely. However, findings, and all available options, including imaging-guided and excisional biopsies, are discussed with the patient. If the patient requests an imaging-guided biopsy, it is done. If a biopsy is indicated following complete clinical and imaging evaluations, it is important to consider what you will accept as a diagnosis and what you will do if the findings are discordant. At every step of the process, concordance is critical, and you as the radiologist must establish it. Are clinical and imaging findings concordant? Stated differently, is what the patient is feeling the same as what is seen on the images? Is what you are seeing on the mammogram concordant with the ultrasound finding? Is what is imaged on ultrasound concordant with an MRI finding? Are pathology results obtained for a clinical, mammographic, ultrasound, or MRI finding concordant with the finding? If discordant, what is the next step? Should repeating an imaging-guided biopsy be the next best step? What makes us think that using the same tool we will be any more successful 2 or 3 days from now if we weren't able to get a congruent result today?

At the time a biopsy recommendation is made, we should ask ourselves what are we willing to accept as a diagnosis for the finding and, given the diagnostic considerations, what will be our next step if we obtain different results. If the pathology results do not correlate with the imaging features of the lesion you need to be prepared to repeat the biopsy or refer the patient for an excisional biopsy (see Figs. 4.53, 5.37, and 8.21). If you decide to repeat the biopsy, please don't just repeat what you did before expecting different results but rather consider doing it with a different needle system, approach, or imaging modality.

Commonly used sampling methods include automated gun-needle combinations and directional vacuum-assisted biopsy probes (Fig. 12.21). The automated gun-needle combinations are spring loaded to move the two components making up the devices. The inner sampling needle has a 4- to 5-mm needle tip followed by a tissue trough that is either 10 to 15 mm (short throw) or 21 to 25 mm (long throw) in length. The larger throw needles are preferred since more tissue is obtained. The second component is an outer cutting cannula. When the "gun" is fired, the inner sampling needle moves forward followed almost instantaneously by the outer cutting cannula; this in effect cuts the tissue and secures a core of tissue in the trough (Fig. 12.22). If you are using a long throw needle, the mechanism advances 2.5 cm through the tissue and lesion being targeted. After each firing, the needle is pulled out so the tissue can be removed.

These "guns" have a cocking mechanism. The first position in the mechanism exposes the tissue trough; the second position, prepares the gun for another firing by withdrawing the sampling needle back into the outer cannula. The guns have a safety device to prevent premature firing during needle positioning and a trigger to set the needle mechanism in motion. Reusable and disposable guns are available; the reusable guns are more cost effective and seem to have more force in propelling the needle forward and cutting through dense fibrous tissue. Needle lengths available include a 10 cm long needle used primarily for ultrasound-guided biopsies, 13 cm and a 16 cm long needle used

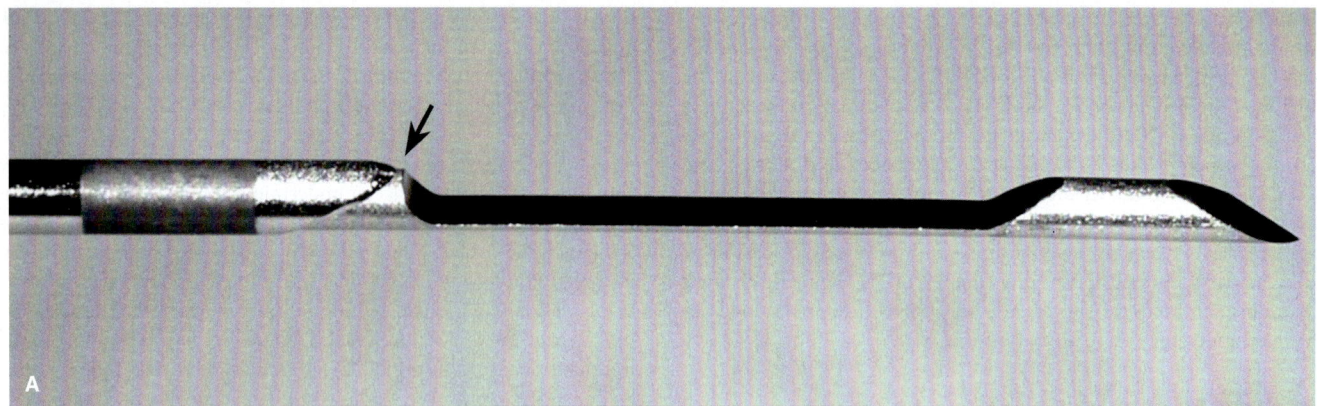

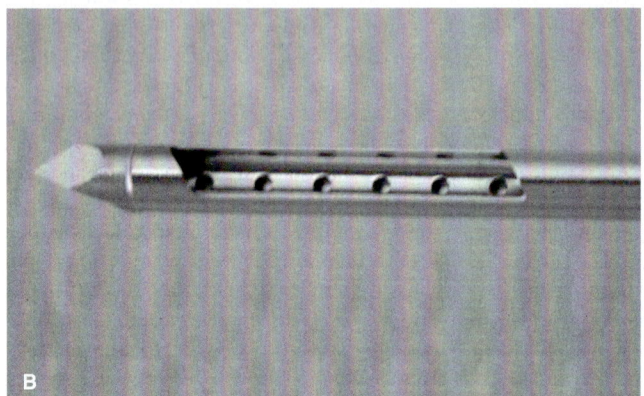
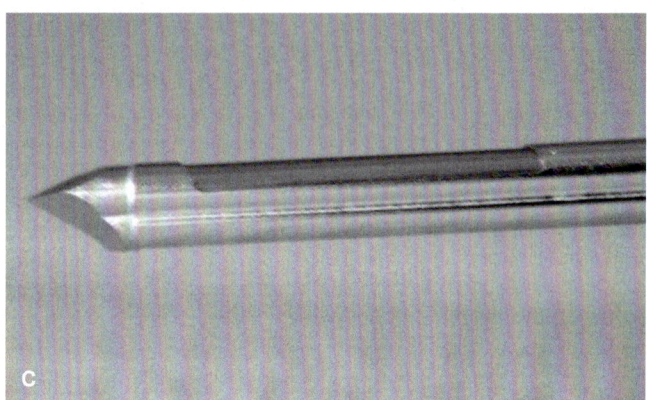

FIG. 12.21 • **Needles. A:** Close-up of a 14G needle with a 22 mm tissue trough used in spring-loaded systems. In addition to the tissue trough, the inner mechanism has a 5-mm-sharp cutting portion. When the gun is fired, the inner mechanism advances into the lesion and almost instantaneously the outer sheath *(arrow)* follows, effectively entrapping a piece of the tissue in the trough. **B:** Close-up of an 11G needle used with one of the directional vacuum-assisted biopsy probes. Note the small openings in the dependent portion of the tissue trough used to create the suction that helps entrap the tissue in the trough. As the trough is covered, the tissue is cut and sucked out into an external filtered tissue collection chamber. **C:** Same needle seen in **B** with the tissue trough closed. In this position, the needle can be turned slightly so as to obtain another sample.

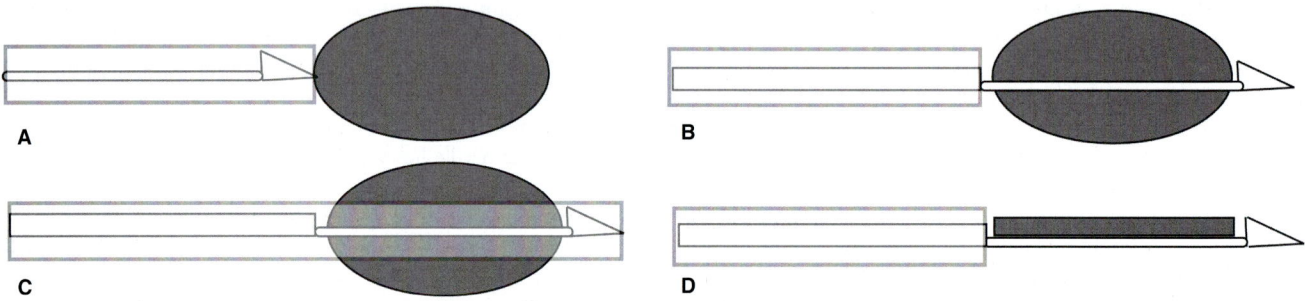

FIG. 12.22 • **Diagram illustrating needle movement with the spring-loaded systems. A:** Prefire needle position. The tip of the needle is positioned at the leading edge of the mass. **B** and **C:** When the "gun" is fired, the inner stylet moves through the tissue and lesion for either 1.5 or 2.2 cm depending on the throw of the needle. This is followed almost instantaneously by the outer sheath (cutting) of the needle. This cuts through the tissue, securing a small core of tissue in the trough. An image documenting the post fire position of the needle is done. For small lesions, we obtain an orthogonal image of the needle to demonstrate the relationship of the needle to the lesion; ideally, the lesion surrounds the barrel of the needle. **D:** At this point, images are done to document the relationship of the needle to the lesion after which the needle is pulled out and the specimen is teased off the trough and placed in 10% formalin for tissue fixation. See Figure 12.29 for ultrasound images of a biopsy using this technique.

for stereotactically guided procedures. It is helpful to have the patient hear the "pop" the gun makes when it is fired before starting the procedure so that during the procedure she is not startled by the sound.

Several gun-needle combinations are available that enable you to advance the needle in a post fire, prebiopsy position. While these systems can be used in the manner just described earlier, they also permit you to advance the inner mechanism with an exposed tissue trough into the lesion such that you control the final position of the needle tip (Fig. 12.23A–C). When the gun is fired in the breast to obtain the specimen, the tip of the needle does not move but rather the outer cutting sheath moves almost instantaneously over the exposed portion of the needle and trough to secure the specimen. These needles come

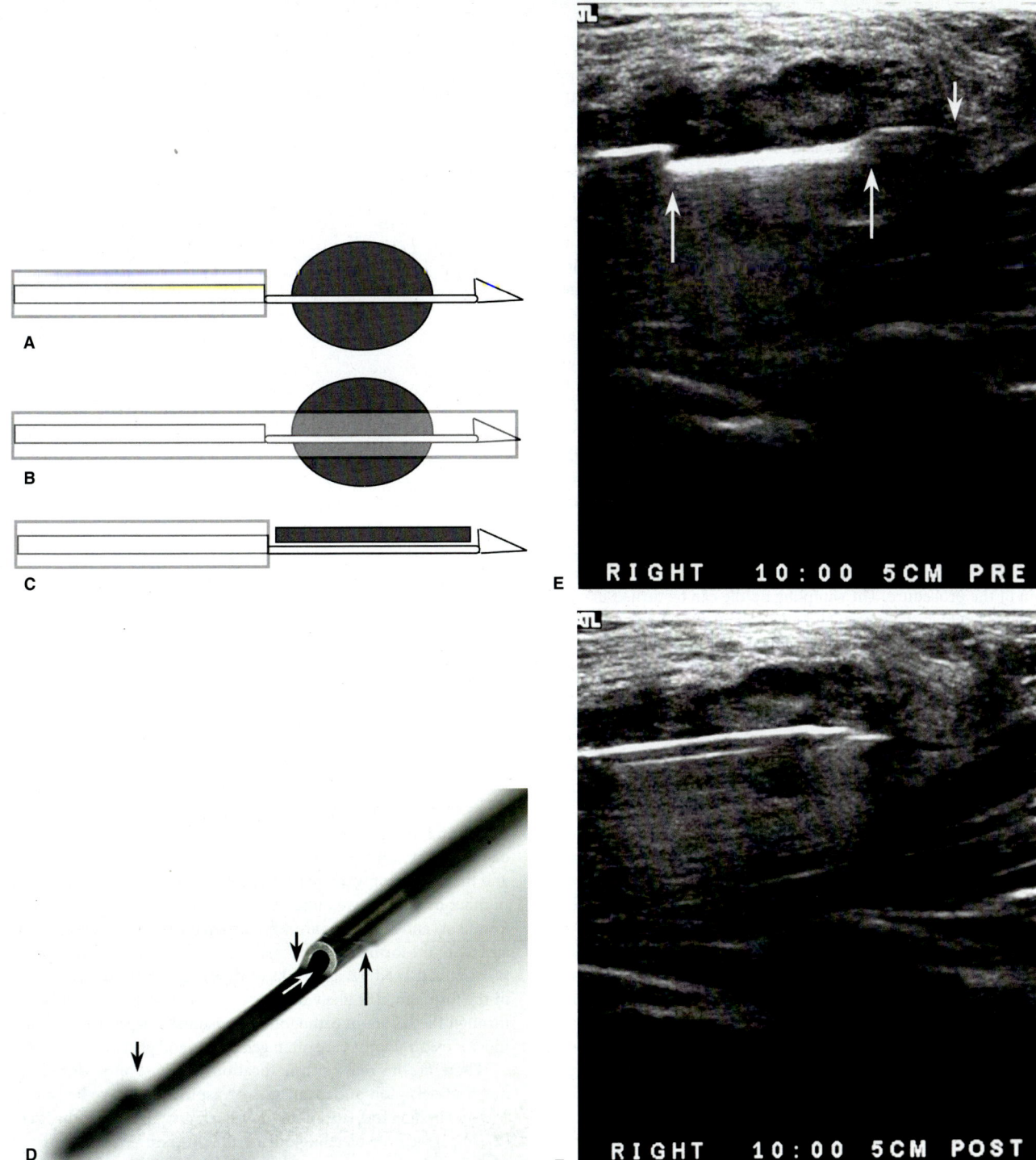

FIG. 12.23 • **Needle placement using the prefire, prebiopsy mode. A:** Before advancing the needle in the breast, the gun is cocked and fired once so that the inner mechanism and tissue trough are exposed. The needle is then advanced into the lesion under ultrasound guidance. If the needle is advanced parallel to the transducer, the tissue trough is readily recognized on ultrasound and can be positioned in the lesion being biopsied. You determine the final position of needle tip (e.g., the tip of the needle will not change in position after the gun is fired a second time to obtain the specimen). A prebiopsy image is done to document the relationship of the needle to the lesion. **B:** The gun is then fired a second time propelling the outer cutting sheath to move over the inner portion of the needle entrapping some of the tissue in the trough. At this point, we obtain post biopsy orthogonal ultrasound images to demonstrate the relationship of the needle to the lesion. **C:** The needle is pulled out of the breast and the specimen is teased off and placed in 10% formalin for fixation. **D:** Photographically coned image of the needle in the post fire, prebiopsy, position. The tissue trough is exposed *(short arrows)*. The tip of the needle is blurred in order to adequately demonstrate the hole *(white arrow)* in the needle that helps create some suction when the outer cutting cannula *(long arrow)* passes over the tissue trough in effect procuring the tissue sample. **E:** Post fire, prebiopsy image, demonstrating exposed tissue through *(long arrows)* in the lesion. The location of the tip of the needle *(short arrow)* is readily apparent and will not change when the biopsy is done. In this patient, two passes with a 14G needle yielded no tissue. **F:** Post biopsy image. The tissue trough is no longer apparent. The tip of the needle is unchanged in position. A core the length of the tissue trough is obtained on the first and only pass using this system.

in various gauges and some have minimal vacuum assistance through a hole in the central portion of the needle mechanism (Fig. 12.23D). Our use of these systems is limited primarily to two situations: (i) if after one or two tries we are unable to obtain tissue with the 14G gun-needle combination. This is not common but does occur when a lesion is particularly hard and densely fibrotic. The 14G needle recoils out of the lesion rather than going through it. Alternatively, the needle may move through the lesion, however, scant or no tissue is found in the trough or (ii) when the lesion we are trying to sample is in a precarious location (e.g., axilla, close to the chest wall, or an implant). This system allows for a controlled advance of the needle. Rather than the needle sharply and rapidly moving 2.5 cm in the breast or axilla after the gun is fired, you control the advance of the needle through the lesion under ultrasound guidance (Fig. 12.23E, F), and after positioning, when the gun is fired, the needle does not advance further into the tissue.

Different needle gauges (e.g., 14G, 11G) can be used with the directional vacuum-assisted biopsy probes. A needle with a tissue trough, a cutting mechanism, perforations that enable the creation of a vacuum, and suction when the tissue chamber is closed is advanced into, or in close proximity to, the lesion (Fig. 12.21B, C). As tissue samples are obtained, they are automatically sucked from the trough into a filtered tissue collection chamber outside of the breast for retrieval at the completion of the procedure. The sampling needle can be turned in small increments while in the breast, and after each turn is made, the tissue trough is exposed, the cutting mechanism moves over the sampling needle and suction is applied enabling retrieval of the core. Tissue can be sampled in small increments circumferentially (360 degrees) or in a 180-degree radius without having to take the needle out of the breast between samples; after each slight turn of the needle the tissue is suctioned out of the needle into collection chamber using vacuum assistance. Larger amounts of tissue are consistently obtained with these devices and as such are preferred for sampling calcifications that are more loosely clustered and similar in morphology: with these biopsy systems, targeting of the same calcification on the stereo pair is not as critical as it is when the procedure is done using the spring-loaded 14G mechanisms. The vacuum and suction used with these systems can make up for some imprecision in the targeting.

When using vacuum assistance, and depending on the number of cores obtained, small masses and tight clusters of calcifications can be removed piecemeal such that placement of a clip is indicated to mark the site of the lesion. If a cancer is diagnosed on the cores, the clip is used to localize the site of the tumor bed for wide excision and assessment of the margins. In patients in whom a clip is deployed, CC and 90-degree lateral views are done to document the location of the clip at the end of the procedure. The vacuum-assisted systems are also recommended when doing MRI-guided biopsies; for these procedures, clip deployment is also indicated, particularly since in most patients, the lesions are usually not apparent with mammography or ultrasound.

We continue to do most of our biopsies using ultrasound guidance and a spring-loaded 14G core biopsy needle. This includes some patients with calcifications. Our general rule is: if we can see the lesion with ultrasound, we prefer to do the biopsy using ultrasound guidance. In our practice, stereotactically guided biopsies are done in two groups of patients: (i) those in whom the lesion cannot be seen on ultrasound with enough confidence to do the biopsy (this is mostly patients with calcifications; however, it also includes a small number of patients who have predominantly fatty tissue and an isoechoic mass [e.g., no ultrasound correlate] or those with distortion) and (ii) patients with large breasts and a centrally or posteriorly located small lesion. In these patients, immobilization of the breast and lesion with compression may facilitate and expedite the biopsy procedure. Depending on the size and tightness of a calcification cluster, we will use a spring-loaded 14G system or for more loosely clustered calcifications, vacuum assistance.

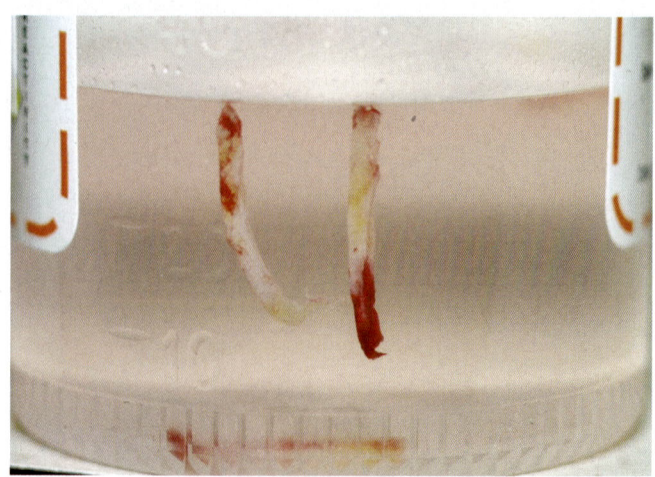

FIG. 12.24 • **Cores.** In conjunction with the imaging done during the procedure, stiff, white cores that "dip" or "sink" are suggestive of adequate sampling. When doing ultrasound-guided core biopsies, we routinely examine our core samples carefully to help determine the number of cores needed to establish a diagnosis. The appearance of the cores itself may be diagnostic helpful. (From Cardeñosa G. *Breast Imaging [The Core Curriculum Series]*. Philadelphia, PA: Lippincott Williams & Wilkins; 2003.)

The prone position and the turning of the head and neck required for stereotactic biopsies using dedicated tables are not well tolerated by some patients. Likewise with add-on stereotactic devices, positioning in some patients can be awkward (e.g., when using a medial approach). Ultrasound-guided biopsies are quick, easy on the patient, require no compression, and use no radiation. The ability to do orthogonal views of the needle and establish its relationship to the lesion during ultrasound-guided procedures is helpful in determining the accuracy of the biopsy. This, in conjunction with the appearance of the cores and their behavior when placed in the formalin, helps us determine the number of samples we obtain to establish a diagnosis. If a core is yellow, floats and fat locules are seen dispersing from its edges onto on the surface of the formalin, additional cores are obtained. If the core is stiff, predominantly white, and sinks or dips (Fig. 12.24) as soon as it is put in the formalin, it is likely diagnostic, particularly if the needle is seen through the lesion on orthogonal ultrasound images. Core samples of mucinous carcinomas are often gelatinous and glisten (see Fig. 8.31A).

There are no real contraindications to these procedures. We do not routinely stop anticoagulants or aspirin and have had no issues with hematoma formation; this approach is supported in the literature (23,24). If we note bleeding during the procedure, we take extra time to tamponade between passes and at the end of the procedure. In our experience, aspirin use, with its long-term effects on platelet function, is associated with a greater likelihood of bleeding than Coumadin.

Ultrasound Guidance

Prior to undertaking an ultrasound-guided biopsy of a mammographically detected lesion, it is important to review the mammogram and ultrasound images to make sure the lesion seen on ultrasound correlates with the mammographic finding (see triangulation discussion in Chapter 3). If there is ever a question about the correlation, confirmation is obtained before the biopsy is done. For these patients, all of the preliminary steps (e.g., povidone-iodine and alcohol cleaning of the skin, lidocaine 1% for local anesthesia) for an ultrasound-guided core biopsy are taken, except the skin nick is not made until correlation is established. The needle used to inject the lidocaine (or a 20G spinal needle) is advanced to the lesion and taped in place and a mammographic image is obtained. This helps to determine the relationship of

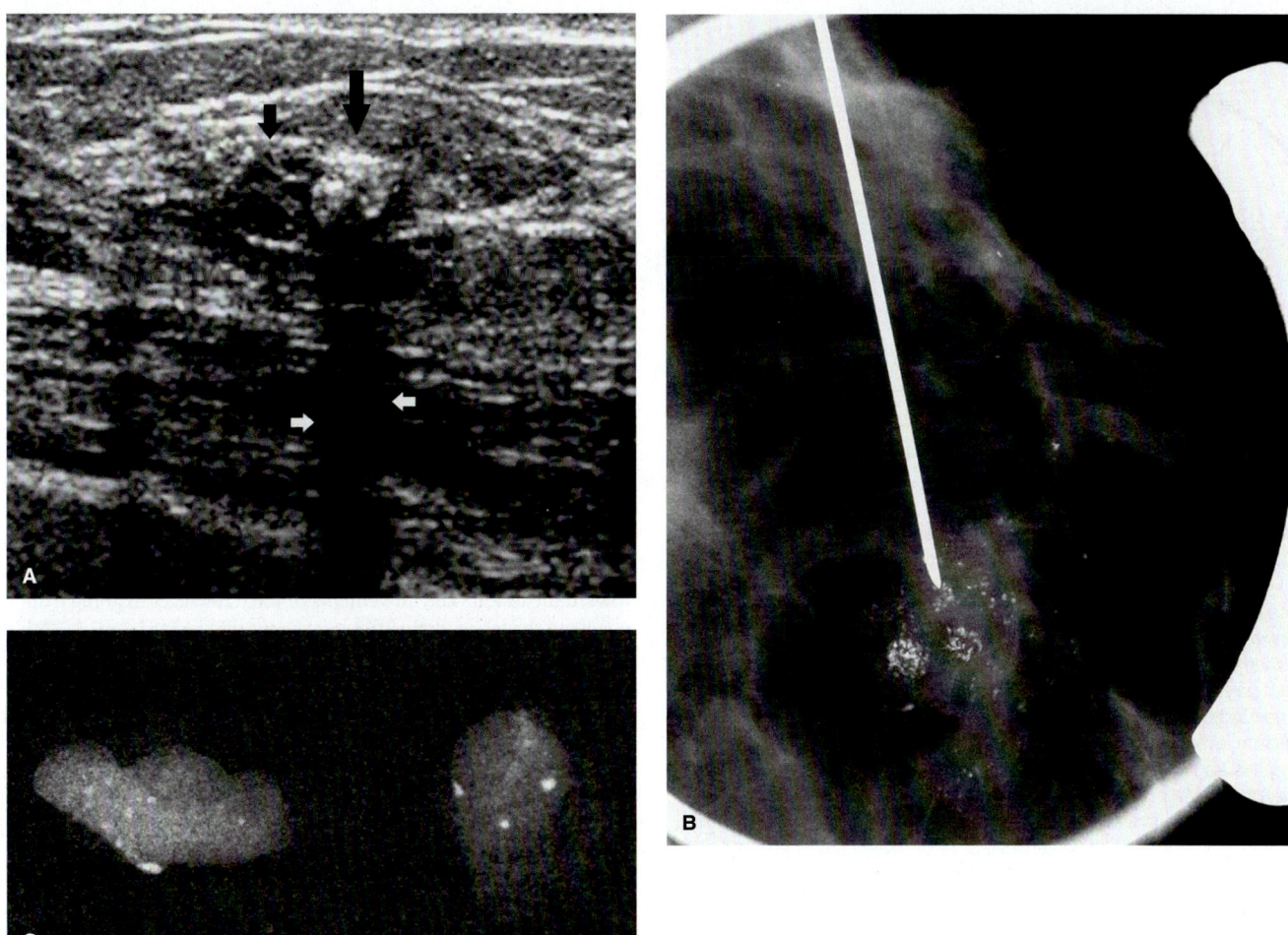

FIG. 12.25 • Correlating ultrasound and mammography findings: ductal carcinoma in situ, with central necrosis and areas of associated invasive ductal carcinoma. **A:** Ultrasound. An irregular area of hypoechogenicity *(short thick black arrow)* and focal hyperechogenicity *(long thick black arrow)* associated with shadowing *(white arrows)*. **B:** Spot compression view of the left breast demonstrates the needle used to inject lidocaine at the site of the calcifications and tissue we want to biopsy. When we are in doubt regarding correlation between mammogram and ultrasound findings, we advance the needle we use to administer the lidocaine, or a 20G spinal needle, to the suspected lesion under ultrasound guidance, tape it to the skin, and obtain a follow-up mammogram to document correlation. The biopsy is completed under ultrasound guidance using a 14G needle. **C:** A radiograph of the cores demonstrates calcifications associated with the two cores obtained to establish the diagnosis in this patient. (From Cardeñosa G. *Breast Imaging [The Core Curriculum Series]*. Philadelphia, PA: Lippincott Williams & Wilkins; 2003.)

the needle to the lesion seen mammographically (Fig. 12.25). If correlation between mammographic and ultrasound findings is established, the patient is returned to the ultrasound room and the biopsy is done. As experience increases with establishing ultrasound and mammographic correlation, the need for this extra step decreases significantly.

For ultrasound-guided procedures, the lesion is localized and an approach is selected. We select a skin entry point that allows us to approach the lesion with the needle parallel to the transducer and chest wall. When the needle is parallel to the transducer, it is easy to see it in its entirety. If the needle is angled, it becomes difficult to localize the tip of the needle (Fig. 12.26); given the rapid almost instantaneous movements of the needle after the gun is fired, knowing the location of the needle tip at all times is critical. The possibility of a pneumothorax is virtually eliminated if the needle is moved parallel to the chest wall and you are able to localize the tip easily. As a routine, we hold the gun upside down. If the gun is held upright, it is difficult in some situations to advance the needle without some angulation (Fig. 12.27). The skin entry site using this method is usually a distance from the transducer so that contamination of the biopsy site is minimized and the likelihood of getting blood on the transducer is reduced. Clean technique and lidocaine (1%) are used. With ultrasound, lidocaine (1%) rarely obscures the lesion and as such we use approximately 10 mL of lidocaine on the skin and along the expected track of the needle to the lesion. We infuse the lidocaine using ultrasound guidance to ensure that lidocaine is deposited up to the lesion but not in the lesion. This also provides an idea regarding the trajectory that needs to be taken and helps establish a plane through the tissue. A small skin nick is made with a no. 11 surgical blade.

Although some advocate having a technologist hold the transducer over the lesion as the radiologist advances the needle, this is probably more awkward and difficult (it has been likened to two people trying to drive a stick shift car: one manipulating the clutch and the other the stick shift). The movements of the transducer are useful in knowing how to make fine adjustments to the position of the needle. Consequently, at our facility, the radiologist doing the procedure manipulates the transducer with one hand (usually their nondominant hand) and the gun-needle combination with the other (dominant hand).

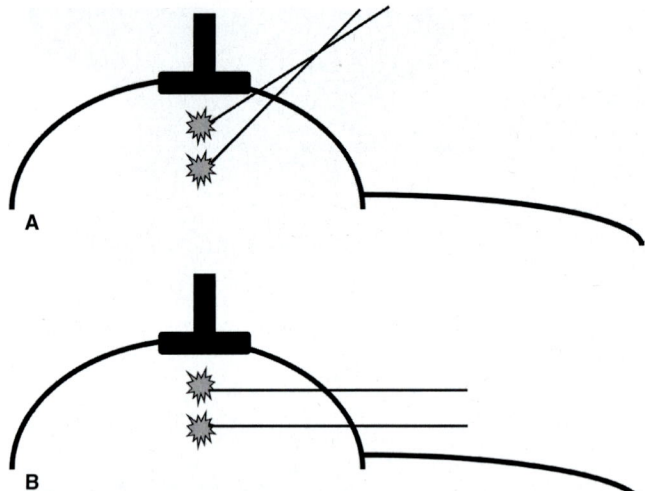

FIG. 12.26 • **Ultrasound, approach to lesion. A:** When the needle is introduced close to the transducer by necessity, it is angled downward making it difficult to see the needle in its entirety. Since the needle is going to advance in the breast almost instantaneously when the gun is fired, it is critical to know the relationship of the tip of the needle to the lesion and chest wall. **B:** When the skin entry point is a distance from the transducer and the needle is kept parallel to the transducer, movements can be imaged. The position of the needle tip and its relationship to the lesion is established easily. With this approach, even the thin localization wires are readily imaged (see Fig. 12.42). Using this approach, the needle is parallel to the chest wall. Consequently, the likelihood of a pneumothorax is almost completely eliminated. Also, since the skin entry site is a distance from the transducer, the likelihood that the needle or skin entry site is contaminated, or of getting blood on the transducer, is minimized. (From Cardeñosa G. *Breast Imaging [The Core Curriculum Series]*. Philadelphia, PA: Lippincott Williams & Wilkins; 2003.)

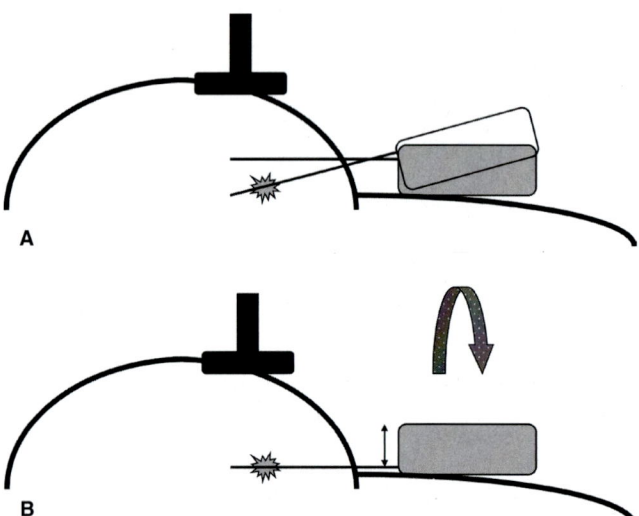

FIG. 12.27 • **Gun orientation for deep lesions. A:** When doing a biopsy of a lesion that is deep in the breast, or in a small-breasted patient or, in a patient with a protuberant abdomen, consider how you hold the "gun." Since the needle comes out of the gun barrel close to the top, there is some "dead space" between the needle and the bottom of the gun. This causes you to angle the needle down as you try to approach the lesion. **B:** With the gun flipped upside down, the needle is almost flush with the skin and can be advanced deep in the breast parallel to the chest wall. The tip of the needle can be identified without difficulty as the lesion is approached with the needle parallel to the chest wall. The likelihood of a pneumothorax is almost completely eliminated. (From Cardeñosa G. *Breast Imaging [The Core Curriculum Series]*. Philadelphia, PA: Lippincott Williams & Wilkins; 2003.)

With this approach, only one hand is moved at a time: if you are moving the transducer, don't move the needle; if you are moving the needle, keep the transducer still. When advancing the needle focus your attention on, and look at, the position of your hands rather than the ultrasound screen. So, at the onset, center the lesion on the ultrasound screen and use the transducer to apply firm pressure over the lesion to minimize its movement as the needle is advanced. Then look at your hands and advance the needle toward the transducer and the expected location of the lesion in one movement (e.g., move your dominant hand holding the needle toward your nondominant hand holding the transducer: your brain usually knows where your other hand is). After advancing the needle to the expected location of the lesion, look at the ultrasound screen again. The needle is often apparent in close proximity to the lesion being targeted. If the needle is not seen, the gun-needle combination is stabilized and the transducer is moved minimally from one side to the other looking for the needle (Fig. 12.28). When moving the transducer, keep it straight up and down and parallel to the floor; specifically, do not rock (angle) the transducer. If the needle is not found with these maneuvers, the skin entry point is approached with the transducer to localize the needle so that it can be followed back toward the lesion. The movements of the transducer in going from the needle to the lesion define the movement that has to be made with the needle. If the transducer is moved to the right in going from the needle to the lesion, the needle needs to be readjusted slightly toward the right. These are fine, delicate movements (the lesion is approached in small increments) until the needle is brought in line with the lesion. Also in doing these movements, the needle is not pulled back out and readvanced but rather it is a subtle sweeping motion of your arm from right to left or left to right. Prefire images are obtained to document the relationship of the needle to the lesion (Fig. 12.29A). The patient is warned she is going to hear a "pop" in the room before firing the gun. Post fire images are obtained demonstrating the relationship of the needle to the lesion on orthogonal images (Fig. 12.29B, C). Make sure that the needle is seen in its entirety. When only a portion of the needle is imaged, the transducer and needle are misaligned; so check your hands and make sure they are lined up (Fig. 12.29D, E). Usually minimal movements of the transducer are needed to enable visualization of the needle in its entirety (Fig. 12.29A, B). After documentation of needle positioning, the needle is taken out of the breast and the specimen is teased off the trough and placed in 10% formalin. If additional cores are obtained, air tracks may be seen in the lesion and should not be mistaken for the needle (Fig. 12.30). Air often has a beaded appearance, and if the transducer is held over the lesion for a few seconds, the bubbles will shift in position. Depending on the images and the appearance of the cores, the number of passes is individualized for each patient. Core radiography is obtained when calcifications are the target (Fig. 12.25C).

In a patient with a lesion deep in the breast, a couple of maneuvers can be used to facilitate approaching the lesion with the needle parallel to the chest wall (Fig. 12.31). The one we use most commonly involves "diving" the needle down in a controlled manner at the skin entry point to the expected depth of the lesion. The gun is then leveraged down so the needle can now be advanced in more horizontal plane. Alternatively, the tip of the needle can be wedged into the lesion and the gun is again leveraged down so that the needle and lesion are raised. The third approach available is to deposit and create a pool of saline deep to the lesion that helps raise the lesion. We have not found this method that helpful because after the first pass, the fluid collection generally dissipates, precluding a second pass without the injection of more saline. When using this last method, it is best to use saline and not lidocaine since you do not want to "numb" the pectoral fascia.

The beauty of using ultrasound guidance for biopsy procedures is the inherent flexibility that ultrasound provides. In some patients,

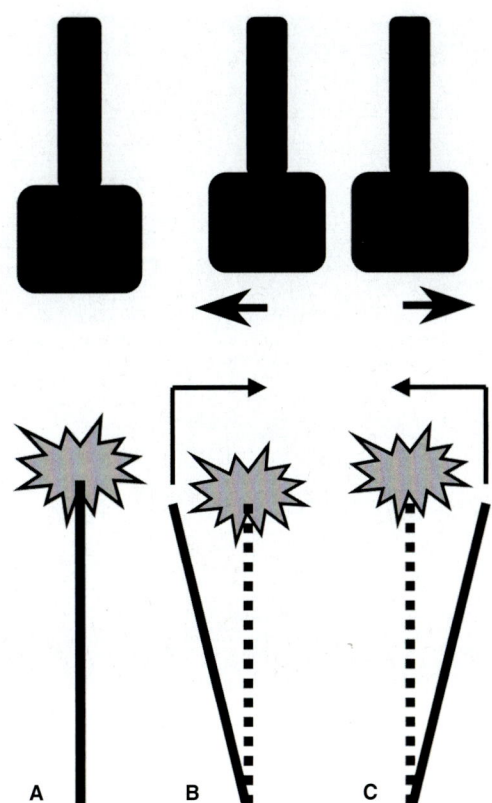

FIG. 12.28 • Using transducer movements to determine needed needle adjustments in approaching a lesion. A: With the transducer over the lesion, look at your hands and advance the needle toward the transducer and the location of the lesion in one movement. With experience, you will frequently see the needle coming into the field of view (it's amazing but your right hand usually knows where your left hand is!). Also focus on your hands, not the ultrasound image. **B:** If you advance the needle to the expected location of the lesion and you do not see it coming into the field of view (e.g., the lesion). STOP moving the needle. Move the transducer minimally to the left and right of the lesion to localize the needle. Do not rocket (angle) the transducer but rather move it slightly to the right of the lesion and then to the left. In this case, you find the needle to the left of the lesion. As you go from the needle back to the lesion, the movement of the transducer tells you what you need to do with the needle. This does not require you to pull the needle out and readvance, but rather you need to slightly sweep your arm holding the needle to the right. Using fine, delicate, slow sweeping movements of the needle and transducer, you "walk" the needle to the lesion. As you make the adjustments remember to only move one hand at a time. If you are moving the needle, keep the transducer over the lesion. If you are moving the transducer to find the needle, do not move the gun/needle mechanism. **C:** In this case, you find the needle to the right of the lesion. In going from the needle back to the lesion, the transducer is moved to the left. The needle and transducer are slightly swept to the left until the needle is seen lining up with the lesion. (From Cardeñosa G. *Breast Imaging [The Core Curriculum Series]*. Philadelphia, PA: Lippincott Williams & Wilkins; 2003.)

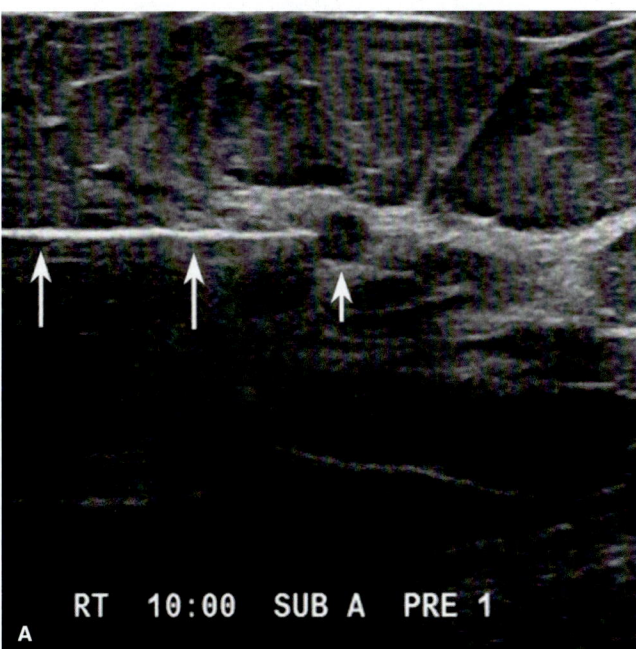
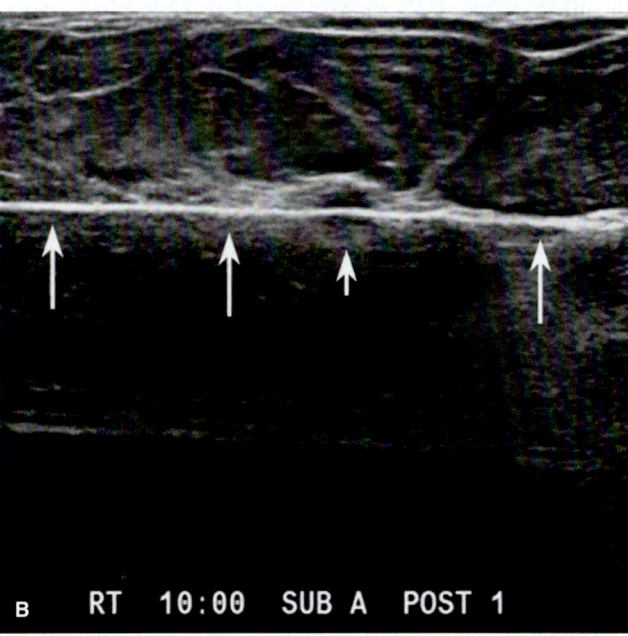

FIG. 12.29 • Ultrasound-guided procedures. A: Prefire image demonstrates needle *(long arrows)* tip at edge of a mass *(short arrow)*. The needle is parallel to the transducer and chest wall; it is seen in its entirety. The patient is warned that she will hear a pop and the gun is fired and the needle movement is watched on real time. **B:** Post fire image demonstrates that the needle *(long arrows)* is through the mass *(short arrow)*. **C:** Orthogonal view of the lesion and needle demonstrates that the needle *(black arrow)* is through the mass *(white arrow)*. The orthogonal image of the needle is particularly helpful when doing biopsies of small masses wherein averaging on the longitudinal image of the needle may be misleading; on the orthogonal view, the needle may be seen to be skimping the edge of the lesion and not actually through the mass. When the needle is seen surrounded by the mass and the core is stiff, you can be confident that the lesion has been biopsied. **D:** Different patient. Post fire image. The needle is only partially seen *(arrows)*. This reflects a needle transducer misalignment. When you see this, look at your hand and line the transducer up over the needle. **E:** Post fire image with a focus on the alignment of the transducer over the needle in the lesion. The needle *(arrows)* is now seen in its entirety through the lesion; the tip of the needle is easily identified beyond the lesion.

(continued)

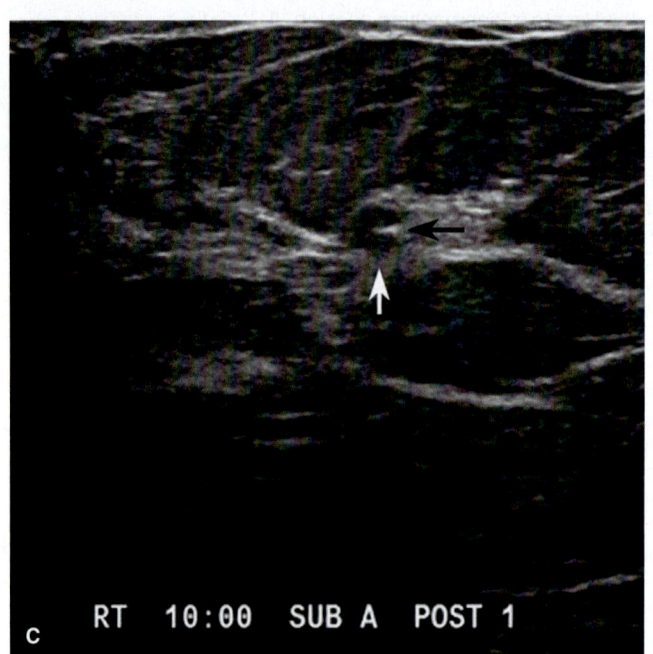
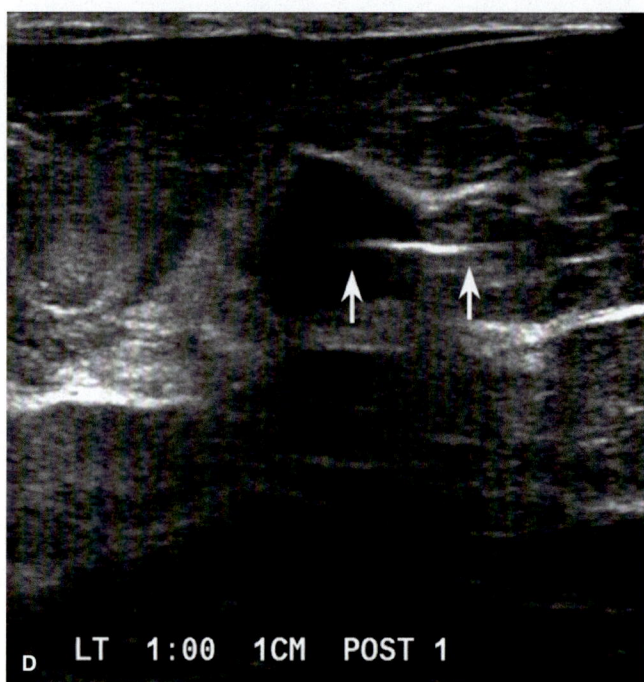
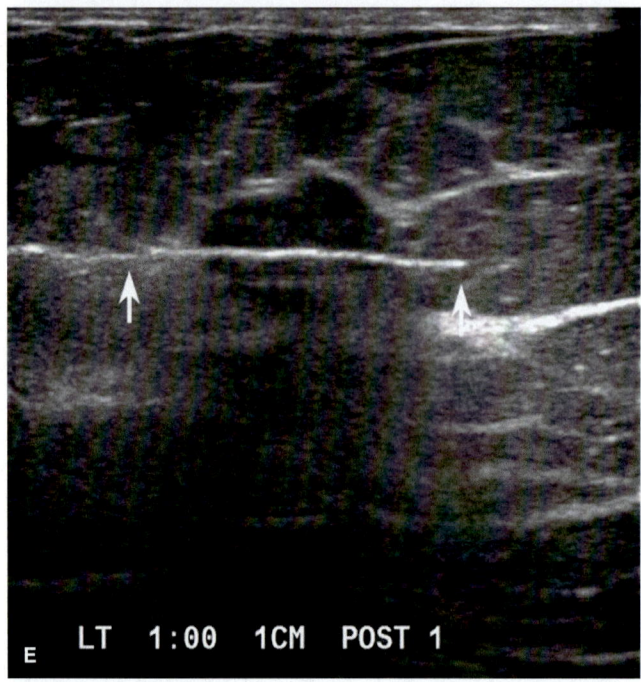

FIG. 12.29 • *(continued)*

depending on the location of the findings, different areas can be biopsied using one skin nick by altering the direction of the needle trajectory (Fig. 12.32). For example, if biopsies of a mass in the upper outer quadrant of the breast and a potentially abnormal lymph node in the ipsilateral axilla are indicated, these can often be approach through one skin nick. The position of the skin nick is established by scanning one lesion with the transducer in a transverse orientation while approaching the axillary finding in a more longitudinal orientation (Fig. 12.32). The orientation of the transducer dictates the trajectory to be used when advancing the needle.

Complications with these procedures are uncommon. As already mentioned, bleeding with hematoma formation is rare even in patients on Coumadin or aspirin (23,24). When bleeding occurs, it is often apparent during the procedure (Fig. 12.33), in which case we stop and tamponade the bleeding before proceeding. Cellulitis or, less commonly, mastitis is also rare. As already mentioned, aseptic inflammatory reactions may develop in patients with complex cystic and solid masses if the fluid is not aspirated before biopsies of the solid component are done or those in whom fluid-filled ducts are inadvertently transected. Lastly, pneumothoraces can occur; however, if needle movements are done parallel to the chest wall and monitored using ultrasound, this should not occur.

Stereotactic Guidance

Dedicated prone tabletops and add-on devices attached to mammography units are available. In determining the approach, the shortest

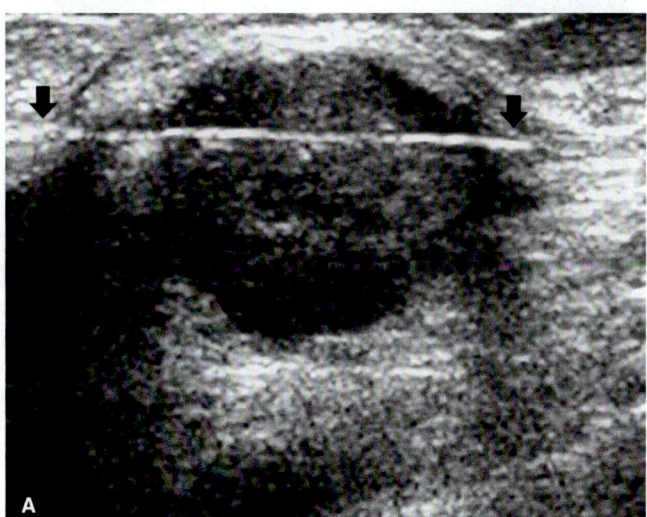 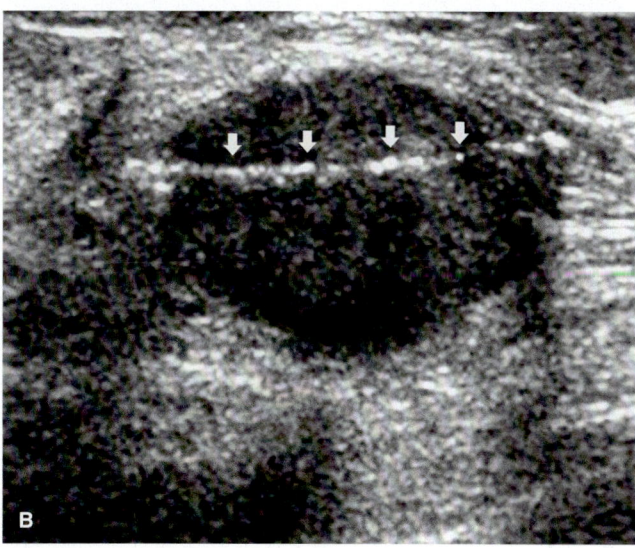

FIG. 12.30 • **Air in needle track, poorly differentiated, invasive ductal carcinoma, not otherwise specified. A:** Round mass with posterior acoustic enhancement in a 73-year-old patient. The needle (14G) is through the mass *(arrows)*. Note the needle is imaged in its entirety, reflecting transducer needle alignment. **B:** After the first pass, air *(arrows)* is seen moving back and forth along the needle track. Air has a beaded appearance, and when observed during real time, the bubbles shift in position as the mass is compressed. Be careful not to mistake this for your needle. (From Cardeñosa G. *Breast Imaging [The Core Curriculum Series]*. Philadelphia, PA: Lippincott Williams & Wilkins; 2003.)

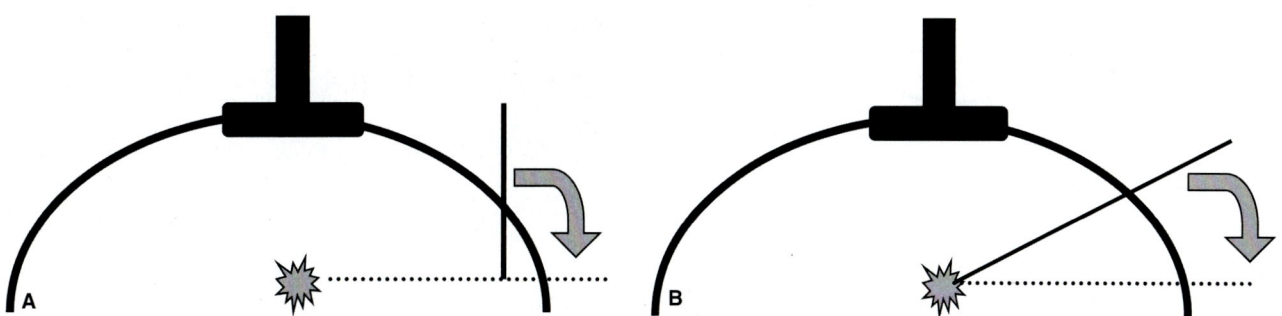

FIG. 12.31 • **Maneuvers to reach deep lesion and approach them parallel to the chest wall. A:** At the skin entry site, the needle is "dived" down carefully and in a controlled manner to the expected depth of the lesion. The gun/needle mechanism is levered down so the needle is now horizontal. **B:** Alternatively, the tip of the needle is wedged into the lesion and the gun/needle mechanism is levered down raising the needle and with it the lesion at the tip. (From Cardeñosa G. *Breast Imaging [The Core Curriculum Series]*. Philadelphia, PA: Lippincott Williams & Wilkins; 2003.)

distance from the skin to the lesion is desirable. This is established by reviewing CC and 90-degree lateral views (Fig. 12.34). If it is determined that the shortest distance to the lesion is by taking a mediolateral (ML) approach (e.g., the lesion is closest to the medial aspect of the breast on the CC view), the patient is positioned on the table so that compression with the fenestrated paddle is applied on the medial aspect of the breast in a 90-degree ML. A scout is taken to document that the lesion is imaged in the fenestrated portion of the paddle. If the lesion is seen, stereo-pair images are obtained by moving the x-ray tube 15 degrees to the right and then 15 degrees to the left. Multiple targets are selected on the stereo pair if the 14G gun-needle combination is being used or one point is selected in the center or at the inferior edge of the area of interest for the vacuum-assisted devices (Fig. 12.35). Using reference points on the images, the computer calculates horizontal (X), vertical (Y), and depth (Z) coordinates for the lesion. Lidocaine is used to raise a skin wheal; for stereotactic procedures with the 14G needle, care needs to be exercised in the amount of lidocaine used. Lidocaine can sometimes obscure the lesion or with calcifications it can spread the calcifications apart. A skin nick is made big enough to accommodate whichever needle you are using. The needle is advanced into the breast at the predetermined coordinates. For the automated gun-needle combinations, the 14G needle is advanced to within 5 mm of the Z value; for the directional vacuum-assisted biopsy probes, the 11G needle is advanced to within 2 mm of the Z value (verify this number with the manufacturer of the system you are using since it may vary) and prefire films are obtained (Fig. 12.35B). If the needle is lined up with respect to the lesion, the gun is fired and post fire images (prebiopsy with the vacuum-assisted systems) are obtained (Fig. 12.35C). If using the 14G gun-needle combination, the needle is taken out of the breast and the specimen is teased off the trough. When using a vacuum-assisted device, the needle is not taken out of the breast after each sample is obtained but rather samples are suctioned into a filtered tissue collection chamber. The needle is turned incrementally and additional samples can be obtained circumferentially or around a 90- or 180-degree radius depending on the relationship of the needle to the lesion being sampled. As mentioned previously, if there is a possibility that the entire lesion is removed with the biopsy, a metallic clip is deployed through the needle and stereo images can be taken (Fig 12.35D)

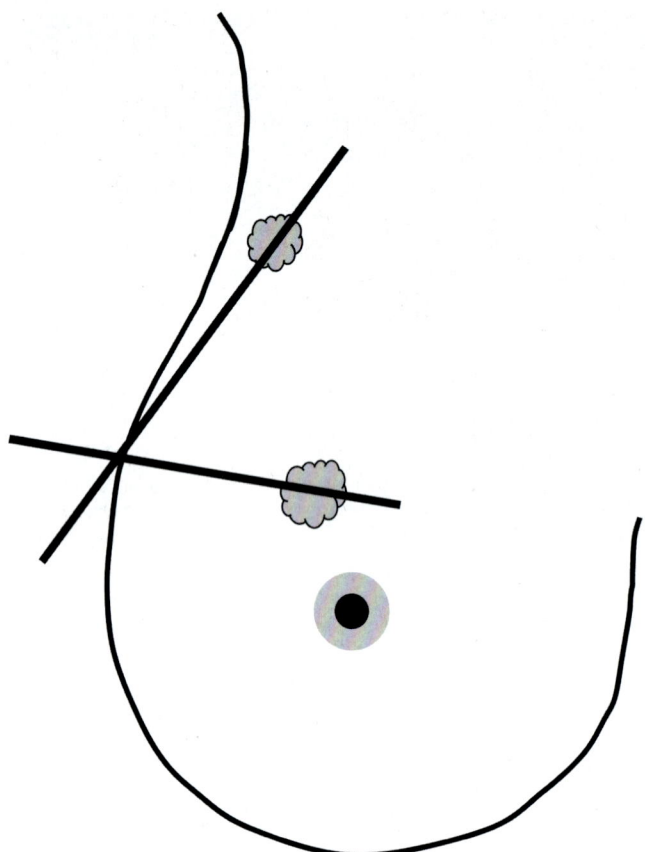

FIG. 12.32 • **Approaching two different lesions through one skin entry site.** For biopsies using ultrasound guidance, a line from the skin entry site to the lesion defines the needed trajectory of the needle. By changing the direction of the needle, two separate lesions may be amenable to biopsy through one skin nick. In this example, the needle is oriented almost horizontal (transducer is held transversely, radial) to biopsy the mass in the breast. To biopsy a morphologically abnormal lymph node in the axilla, the needle is directed more vertically (transducer in a more longitudinal or antiradial orientation) toward the axilla. If the distance to one of the two lesions is longer than that reachable by a 10-cm needle, the 14G needles are also available in lengths of 13 and 16 cm.

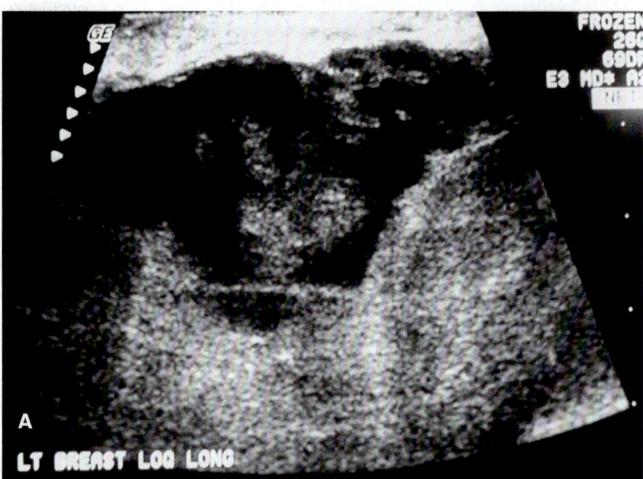

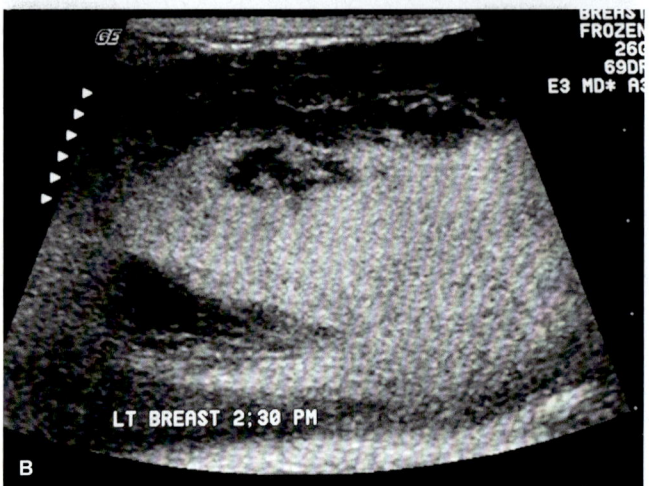

FIG. 12.33 • **Invasive ductal carcinoma, not otherwise specified. Acute bleed during imaging-guided biopsy. A:** Complex cystic and solid mass. Ultrasound-guided biopsy using 14G needle is done on a patient taking no medications. When the needle is removed from the breast after the first pass, blood actively squirted out through the skin nick. Pressure with ice packs kept on the area for 20 minutes until bleeding stopped. **B:** Ultrasound image approximately 40 minutes after first pass demonstrates hyperechogenic material in the mass consistent with blood. Immediately after the first pass, the echogenic material (blood) could be seen on real time, swirling in the mass and increasing in amount. (From Cardeñosa G. *Breast Imaging [The Core Curriculum Series]*. Philadelphia, PA: Lippincott Williams & Wilkins; 2003.)

to verify clip deployment before the needle is taken out of the breast. If a clip is deployed, follow-up orthogonal images are obtained mammographically to document clip placement. If the biopsy is being done for calcifications, core radiography is done to verify there are calcifications in the cores (Fig. 12.35E).

Rarely in several specific circumstances stereotactically guided procedures are not possible: (i) in patients with lesions that are close to the chest wall or far posterolaterally in the breast, it may not be possible to include the lesion in the fenestrated paddle precluding a stereotactically guided procedure; (ii) depending on the smallest needle throw permitted by the system you use, if the breast compresses to 1.5 cm or less ("pancake breast"), a stereotactically guided procedure may not be possible; and (iii) if the patient is unable to lie prone for 30 to 60 minutes, however, this may be overcome if you have the ability to do stereotactically guided biopsies on an upright unit.

Magnetic Resonance Guidance

When an enhancing mass or non-mass like enhancement is identified on breast MR only, or if concordance with mammographic and ultrasound findings is in question, the biopsy is done using MRI guidance.

The patient is prone, her breast is cleaned, and a compression paddle with multiple square fenestrations (Fig. 12.36A, B) is used to immobilize the breast. The breast needs to be taut, but care is taken not to apply too much compression; otherwise enhancement of lesions may be affected. Lesions are approached laterally, and with some systems, a medial approach can also be used. When using the lateral approach, both breasts are placed in the coil. For a medial approach, the contralateral breast is kept out of the coil by a plate placed over the upper portion of the coil. The resulting thickness of the excluded breast can, in effect, lift the patient up away from coil so that variable amounts of posterior tissue may be excluded from the coil (e.g., the breast does nor fall completely into the coil). Additionally, with some of the systems, the compression paddle used for a medial approach is shallower such that there is one less row of available squares (Fig. 12.36B). Consequently, depending on

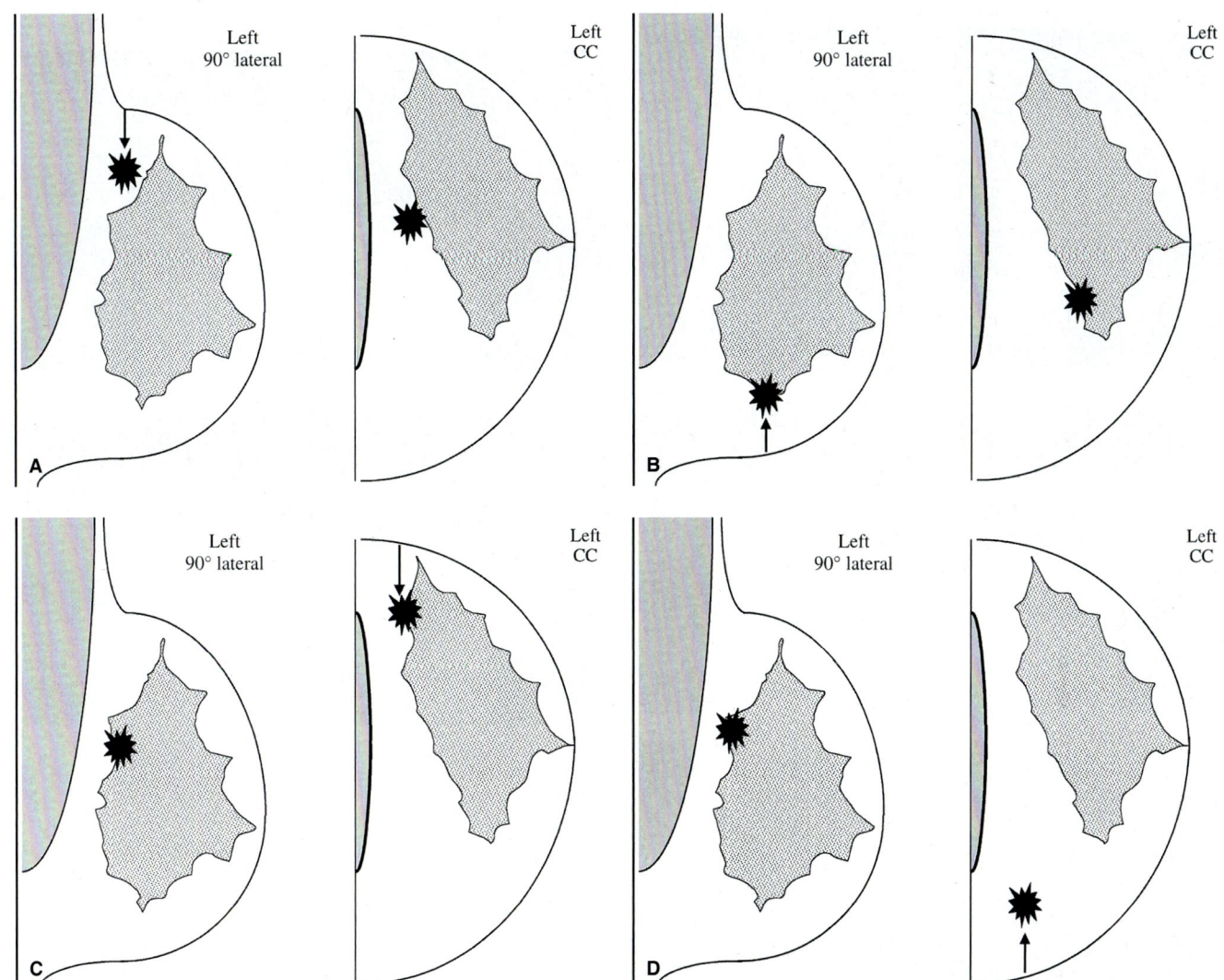

FIG. 12.34 • **Selection of approach for stereotactically guided biopsies and mammographically guided wire localizations. A:** Craniocaudal (CC) and 90-degree lateral views are reviewed. The shortest distance from the skin to the lesion determines the approach used. In this case, the lesion is closest to the superior skin surface on the 90-degree lateral view *(arrow)*. The patient is positioned in a CC projection for the biopsy or localization: the superior skin surface is compressed with the fenestrated compression paddle. **B:** In this example, the lesion is closest to the inferior surface of the breast on the 90-degree lateral view *(arrow)*. The patient is positioned using a from below (FB) projection for the biopsy or localization: the inferior skin surface is compressed using the fenestrated compression paddle. **C:** In this case, the lesion is closest to the lateral skin surface on the CC view *(arrow)*. The patient is positioned using a 90-degree lateromedial (LM) projection for the biopsy or localization: the lateral aspect of the breast is compressed using the fenestrated compression paddle. **D:** Here, the lesion is closest to the medial skin surface on the CC view *(arrow)*. The patient is positioned using a 90-degree mediolateral (ML) projection for the biopsy or localization. With this view, the medial aspect of the breast is compressed using the fenestrated compression paddle. (From Cardeñosa G. *Breast Imaging [The Core Curriculum Series]*. Philadelphia, PA: Lippincott Williams & Wilkins; 2003.)

the patient's body habitus, only lesions in the anterior two-thirds of the breast can be sampled consistently using a medial approach.

Imaging sequences used for MRI-guided biopsies varies among facilities. Our imaging sequence for these patients includes a sagittally acquired T1-weighted fat-suppressed sequence with 1-mm-thick slices through the potentially abnormal breast (or bilateral if bilateral biopsies are being done) and axially acquired T1-weighted images bilaterally (unless a medial approach is being used, which precludes bilateral scanning) precontrast. These images are used to confirm adequate positioning so that the expected site of the lesion is in the fenestrated portions of the paddle and that the fiducial marker is apparent (Fig. 12.37A). The same sequences are then repeated following a 20-mL bolus of contrast.

Using commercially available software, the breast (right vs. left) being biopsied, approach (lateral vs. medial) and needle system in use are inputted into the software. We scroll to the image best demonstrating the fiducial marker so that system detects its location (Fig. 12.37B). Then scroll to the image with the lesion and mark the location of the lesion using the cursor. The software calculates the depth (Z) of the lesion in the breast as well as the X and Y coordinates of the lesion and indicates which square fenestration in the compression paddle overlies the lesion. More specifically, the software marks which of the holes

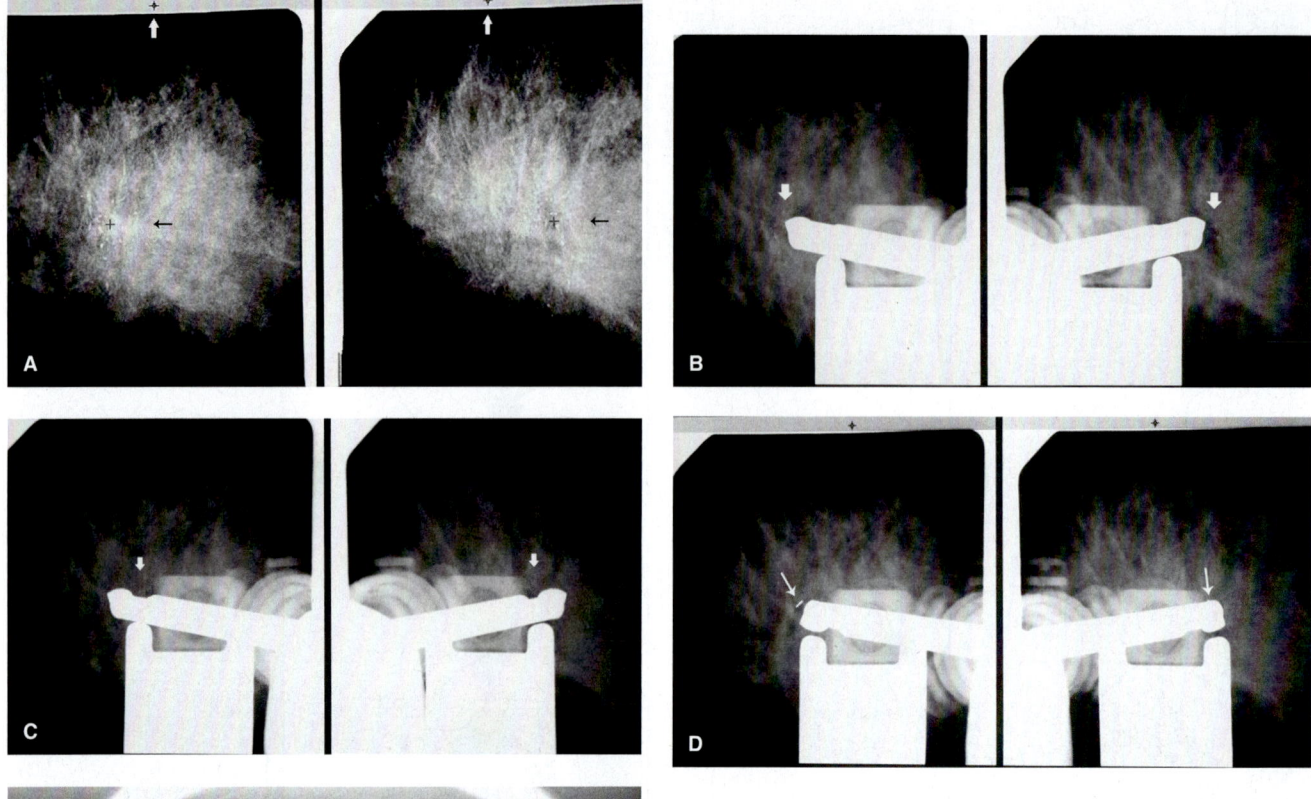

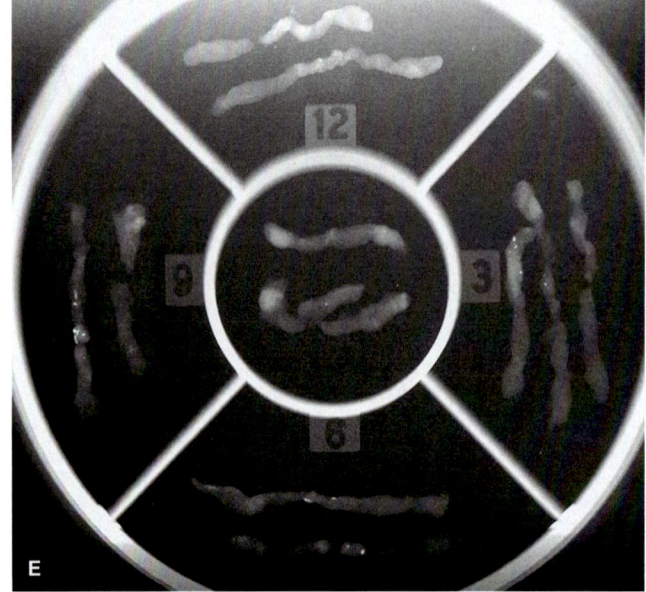

FIG. 12.35 • **Stereotactically guided breast biopsy. A:** Stereo scout images in a patient with a cluster of calcifications for directional vacuum-assisted biopsy with 11G needle. Cluster of calcifications is seen in both images *(black arrows)*. Reference cursors appropriately positioned *(white arrows)*. Point in calcification cluster selected *(black hatch mark)* for targeting. The unit calculates X, Y, and Z coordinates for the area of interest. Coordinates determined by the unit are dialed in and the needle is advanced to within 2 mm of the Z value. **B:** Prefire images. The calcifications are just beyond the tip of the needle *(arrows)*. The patient is warned that she will hear a "pop" when the gun in fired. **C:** Post fire, prebiopsy images. The calcifications now surround the needle notch *(arrows)*. Biopsies of the cluster are taken circumferentially (360 degrees). **D:** Stereo pair after deployment of the clip. The clip *(arrows)* is seen well in one of the two stereo pairs and only a small portion is seen on the right-hand image. Craniocaudal and 90-degree lateral views are obtained (not shown) to document clip positioning. **E:** Core radiograph. Calcifications are present in several of the cores. Ductal carcinoma in situ is diagnosed on the cores. (From Cardeñosa G. *Breast Imaging [The Core Curriculum Series]*. Philadelphia, PA: Lippincott Williams & Wilkins; 2003.)

in the nine-hole needle guide should be used to advance the needle. Lidocaine (10 mL of 1%) is used to raise a skin wheal and deposited along the expected track of the needle. The nine-hole needle guide is inserted in the square fenestration overlying the lesion (Fig. 12.37C). A rubber stopper on the introducer sheath is used such that the portion of the rubber stopper distal to the patient is placed at the calculated depth for the lesion (Fig. 12.37D). The introducer stylet is placed through the introducer sheath and this in turn is placed through the hole in the needle guide determined to be closest to the lesion. Using a rotating motion, the introducer stylet is advanced so that the rubber stopper on the introducer sheath (e.g., determined depth of the lesion) is up against the nine-hole needle guide. The stylet is replaced with the localizing obturator and the patient is scanned to establish the adequacy of targeting. If the obturator is imaged in association with the lesion (Fig. 12.37E–G), it is removed and replaced with the biopsy hand piece. As samples are obtained, 10 mL of lidocaine (1%) with epinephrine (1:100,000) is injected slowly. Depending on the position of the needle relative to the area of interest, tissue is sampled 360-degrees around the needle or in whatever radius maximizes sampling of the lesion. After the samples are obtained, the biopsy cavity is lavaged with normal saline after which we suction out the biopsy cavity as much as possible. The hand piece is removed and a clip is deployed through the introducer sheath. We have found that suctioning the biopsy cavity after the biopsy and saline lavage reduces the likelihood and extent of clip migration. Although we do not routinely scan patients after clip placement, some advocate that this be done to document the

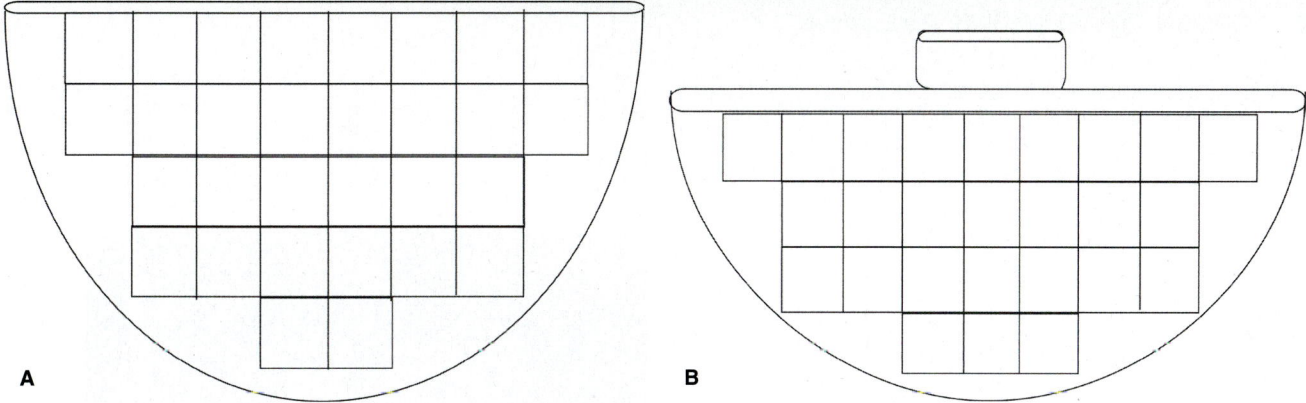

FIG. 12.36 • **Compression paddles used for magnetic resonance imaging-guided biopsies. A:** Lateral approach. Curved compression paddle with square fenestrations used with one of the available MRI systems to approach lesions from the lateral aspect of the breast. Vertically, five rows of squares are available. With other systems, the compression paddle is rectangular with eight rows of squares across and six down. **B:** Medial approach. Compression paddle used with one of the available MRI systems to approach lesions from the medial aspect of the breast. Vertically, four rows of squares are available with this paddle.

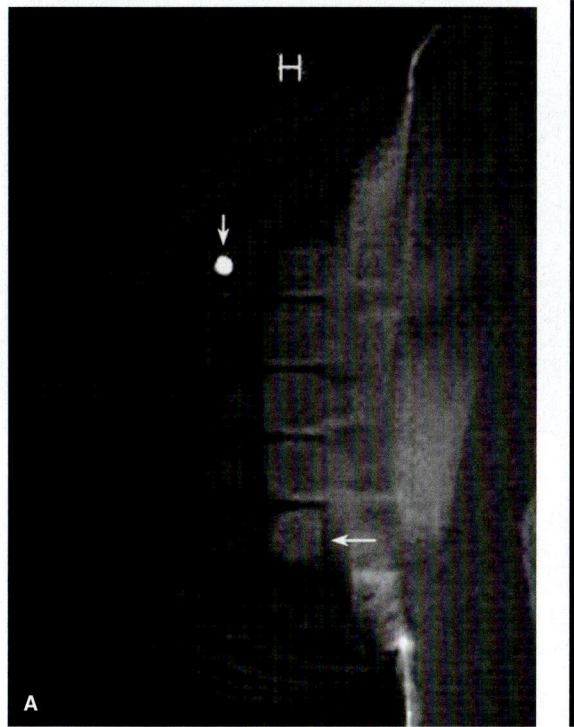
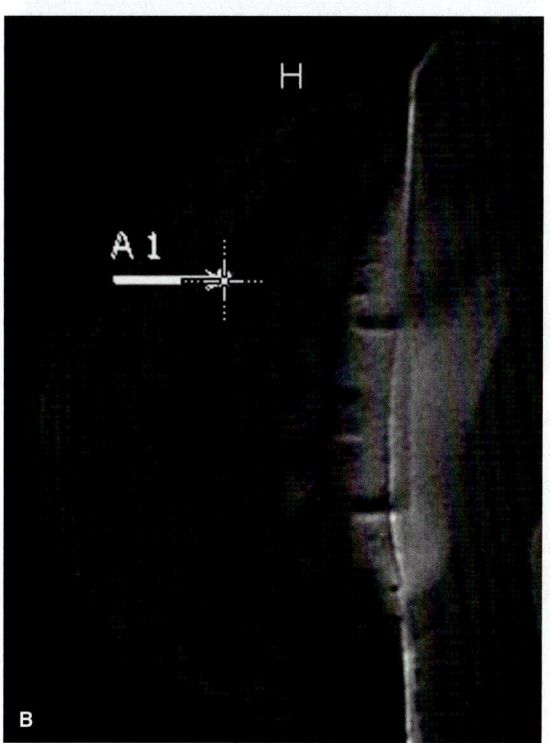

FIG. 12.37 • **Magnetic resonance imaging (MRI)-guided biopsies. A:** The fiducial marker *(short arrow)* and edge of paddle *(long arrow)* are identified. We place the cursor at the edge of the paddle so that as we scroll into the tissue we can establish the relationship of the anticipated location of the lesion to the edge of the paddle. This is particularly helpful when using a medial approach, since some posteromedial tissue is commonly excluded from under the paddle. **B:** The software recognizes the location of the fiducial and positions cursor at the fiducial marker. Scroll to the image best demonstrating the lesion and place the cursor at the lesion. The software uses the indicated location of the fiducial and lesion to calculate the X, Y, and Z for the lesion. **C:** Diagram of compression paddle with nine-hole needle guide placed in the square indicated by the system software as overlying the lesion. The software will also indicate which of the nine holes to use in advancing the stylet into the breast. **D:** Diagram of the introducer sheath with the rubber stopper placed at the calculated depth (30) for the lesion. In this example, the part of the rubber stopper distal to the patient is placed at 30. **E:** Sagittal T1-weighted image post contrast to assess the adequacy of targeting. A signal void with a round central high T1 signal *(short arrow)* is seen at the inferior and posterior aspects of the mass *(long arrow)* to be biopsied. With the needle system being used, the central high T1 signal denotes the positioning of the tissue notch when the obturator is replaced by the biopsy hand piece. Since the needle will be at the inferior and posterior edge of the lesion, theoretically the diagnosis can be established with samples taken from the 12 through the 9 o'clock positions; in actuality we took samples in a 180-degree radius above the needle (9 to 12 and through to 3 o'clock positions). **F:** Axial T1-weighted image demonstrates the central high T1 signal of the obturator and, in this patient, as you scroll image by image above the obturator, the lesion comes into the field of view within 1 to 2 mm of the obturator. The central high T1 signal *(arrows)* indicates where the tissue through will be when the biopsy hand piece is placed through the introducer sheath. See Figure 5.27 for the diagnostic MRI images on this patient. **G:** Different patient. A sagittal T1-weighted image is done following the contrast bolus to assess the adequacy of targeting. A signal void with a round central high T1 signal *(short arrow)* is seen at the inferior edge of the irregular heterogeneously enhancing mass *(long arrow)* to be biopsied. Since the localizing obturator (and eventually the tissue notch) is at the inferior edge of the lesion, samples are taken in a 180-degree radius above the needle (9 to 12 through 3 o'clock positions). See Figure 8.21 for diagnostic images on this patient.

(continued)

FIG. 12.37 • *(continued)*

relationship of the clip to the biopsy site on MRI. Once the patient is taken out of the magnet, she is asked to turn so that she is lying on her back and pressure is applied to the biopsy site for approximately 10 minutes after the procedure. Orthogonal mammographic images are done to document clip placement. The tissue collection chamber is unscrewed from the hand piece and the cores are removed by using the thin metal spatula in the filtered tissue collection chamber. They are placed in 10% formalin and submitted for histologic evaluation.

CLIP PLACEMENT TO MARK TUMOR LOCATION

As already discussed, clip placement after imaging-guided biopsy is considered mandatory by some; however, it is not indicated, and we do not do it, in all patients. Placement of a clip is indicated when: (i) based on the size of the lesion and the biopsy method used (e.g., 14G vs. vacuum), a lesion may be removed in its entirety with the needle biopsy procedure; (ii) patients are undergoing an MRI-guided biopsy; (iii) neo-adjuvant therapy is planned (25). In this last group of patients, the original tumor may resolve completely during the course of therapy (Fig. 12.38). If the patient elects to undergo conservative breast therapy, the clip marks the site of the original tumor and can be localized the day of the patient's lumpectomy. (iv) More recently, surgeons have been advocating placement of a clip after imaging-guided biopsies of axillary lymph nodes particularly if neo-adjuvant therapy is planned. If metastatic disease is diagnosed pre-therapy, the patient will undergo an axillary dissection at the time of definitive surgery. A specimen radiograph done at the time of the axillary dissection can be used to verify excision and histological evaluation of the lymph node with known disease pretherapy.

Patient Management after Imaging-Guided Biopsy Procedures and Radiologic–Pathologic Concordance

After an imaging-guided procedure, the needle track and biopsy site are compressed for at least 10 minutes. The patient is provided a small ice pack that fits in her bra to minimize any bruising or discomfort and is told that there are no restrictions following the biopsy. She is provided the radiologist's business card that includes a telephone number, a pager number, and an email address; some of us provide patients our cell numbers as well. The patient is instructed to contact the radiologist

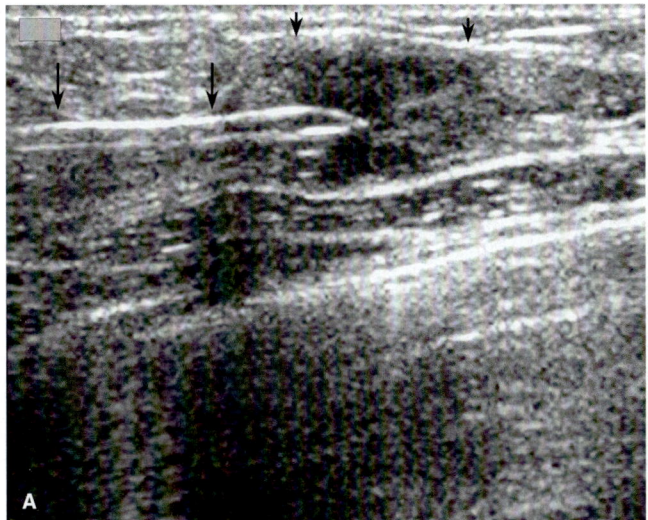

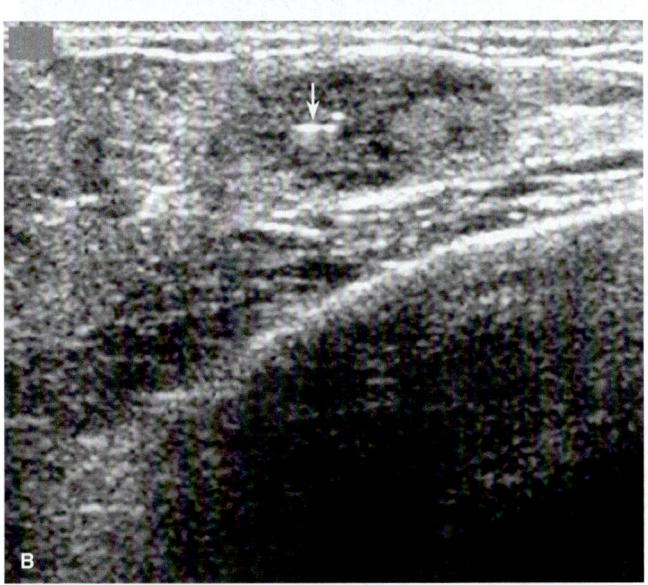

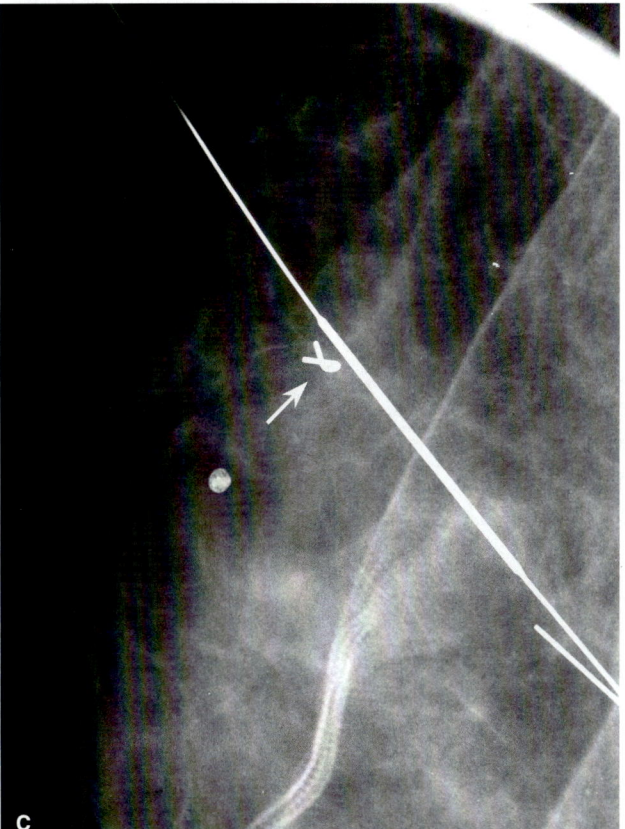

FIG. 12.38 • **Ultrasound-guided clip placement. A:** With the tip of the needle *(long arrows)* in the center of the mass *(small arrows)*, the clip is deployed to mark the site of the tumor. If the tumor completely regresses with neo-adjuvant therapy, the clip is used to preoperatively localize the site of the original tumor. The mass in this patient is a known, poorly differentiated, invasive ductal carcinoma, not otherwise specified with metastasis to at least one ipsilateral axillary lymph node in a 57-year-old patient undergoing neo-adjuvant therapy. **B:** The clip *(arrow)* is seen in the mass after the needle is removed. Craniocaudal and 90-degree lateral views (not shown) are done after the procedure to establish the adequacy of clip placement. **C:** After neo-adjuvant therapy, the clip is used to localize the site of the original tumor. The clip *(arrow)* is seen adjacent to the superficial portion of the reinforced wire segment. (From Cardeñosa G. *Breast Imaging [The Core Curriculum Series]*. Philadelphia, PA: Lippincott Williams & Wilkins; 2003.)

directly with questions or concerns. A follow-up appointment is scheduled for the patient usually the next business day after the biopsy.

Our pathologists have committed to a 24-hour turnaround time for patients undergoing imaging-guided breast biopsies during the week (results for biopsies done on Friday are available on Monday morning). First thing every week day morning, results are discussed directly with the pathologist at which time any issues regarding the imaging features of the lesion or the histology can be considered jointly. As stated repeatedly throughout the text, it is imperative that the breast imaging radiologist doing these procedures establishes concordance at every step of the process: from the clinical signs and symptoms to imaging findings, between the different imaging modalities, and lastly, to close the loop, between imaging findings and reported histology. When we recommend and do an imaging biopsy, we think about acceptable diagnostic considerations for the abnormality we sampled in the context of the relevant history as well as the clinical and imaging findings. We always try to think two and three steps ahead for our patients. Depending on the reported histology, what is indicated for the patient?

When the patient comes in for her appointment the day following the biopsy, the radiologist checks the biopsy site and discusses the results with the patient directly. When indicated based on the biopsy results, appointments for an MRI (the same day or within a day or two of the office visit) and consultation with one of our oncologic surgeons are made for the patient; if no additional appointments are needed, appropriate follow-up recommendations are discussed with the patient. Although the 24-hour turnaround time for biopsy results is in place because we think it is optimal patient care, in many ways we also benefit significantly. With the imaging features of the lesion (and procedure-related issues) fresh in our minds, we are given histologic results. Knowing the histology within a day of the biopsy is an incredible learning experience for the imagers, effectively leading to improvements in our prognostic abilities regarding likely histologic results for different imaging findings. It is through this process that we have learned much about which lesions need to be pursued aggressively even when the needle biopsy results describe benign findings and which do not. In addition to being appreciated by patients, it is an invaluable learning tool.

Patients with benign findings that are radio pathologically congruent (e.g., fibroadenoma) are returned to screening. Only rarely, is a 6-month follow-up recommended following a biopsy with congruent results. If the findings are not congruent, we usually refer the patient for an excisional biopsy. We are using MRI in some of these patients: if the lesion in question enhances on MRI (Fig. 12.39), an MRI-guided

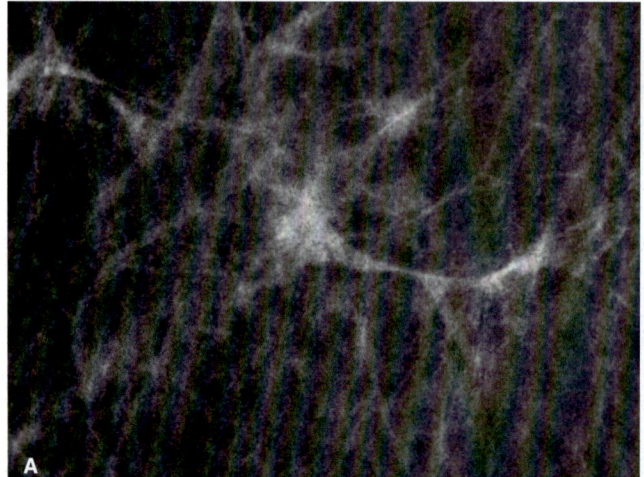
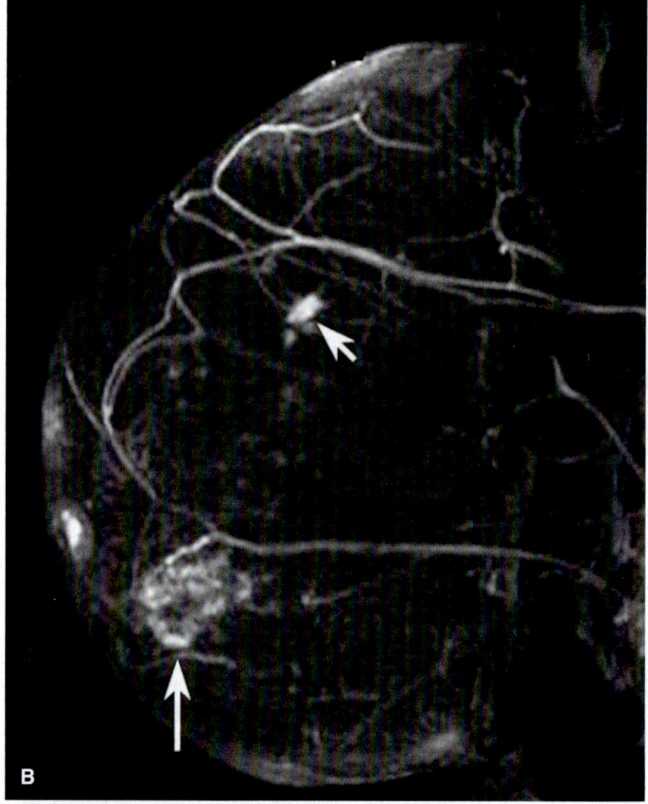

FIG. 12.39 • **Radiology–pathology correlation. A:** Spot compression view. A mass with spiculated margins is confirmed on orthogonal spot compression views (only CC projection shown). This represents a new finding in a 75-year-old patient (prior studies not shown). Benign breast tissue is reported on an ultrasound-guided core biopsy. This is not congruent with the imaging findings. An MRI is done confirming an irregular, heterogeneously enhancing mass with spiculated margins correlating to the mammographic finding. An MRI-guided biopsy is done. It is important to emphasize that given the mammographic features of this lesion, surgical consultation for excision is appropriate if no mass is identified on the MRI. **B:** Maximum intensity projection imaging from biopsy planning MRI. The irregular mass with heterogeneous enhancement is readily apparent *(short arrow)*. A hematoma with some peripheral enhancement is seen inferiorly *(long arrow)* related to the ultrasound-guided biopsy procedure. **C:** Sagittal T1-weighted image done following the contrast bolus to assess the adequacy of targeting. A signal void with a round central high T1 signal *(short arrow)* is seen at the lower anterior edge of the irregular heterogeneously enhancing mass to be biopsied. Since the localizing obturator, and eventually the tissue notch is at the anterior inferior edge of the lesion, six cores are done in a 180-degree radius to include the posterior tissue (12 through 3 to 6 o'clock positions); samples of tissue anterior to the needle are not done in this patient.

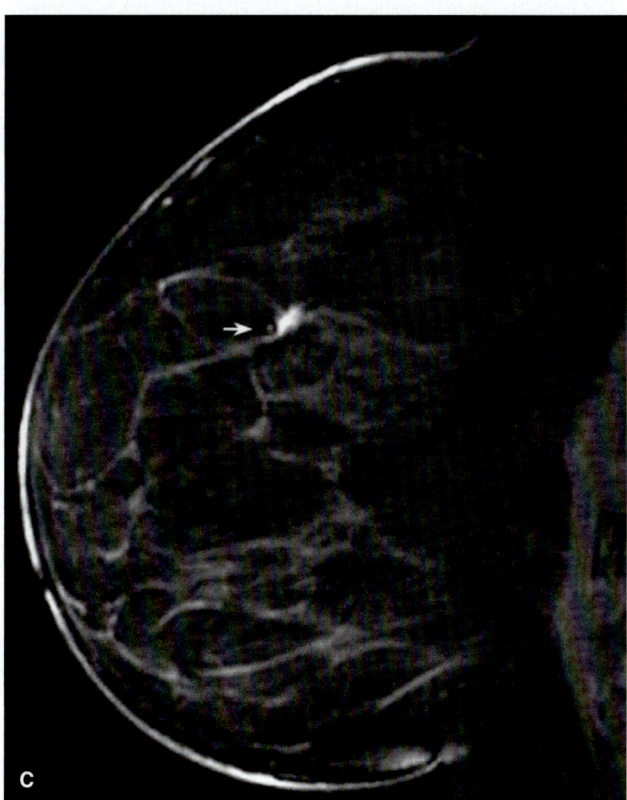

FIG. 12.39 • *(continued)*

biopsy can be done. If the lesion does not enhance, however, the patient is scheduled with one of the surgeons for excision.

With a diagnosis of atypical ductal hyperplasia (ADH), excision is always recommended; 20% to 56% and 0% to 38% of patients with ADH diagnosed with 14G automated systems or directed vacuum-assisted devices, respectively, are upstaged to malignancy (usually DCIS) on excision (26–29); patients with flat epithelial atypia (30,31), columnar cell change with atypia, atypical papillomas, and mucocele-like lesions are also referred for surgical biopsy. Excisional biopsy is also recommended if a fibroepithelial lesion is described and in some patients with "cellular" fibroadenomas if the pathologist is concerned the lesion could represent a phyllodes tumor.

Controversy surrounds the appropriate management of lobular neoplasia (e.g., atypical lobular hyperplasia and lobular carcinoma in situ) (32–44), papillary lesions (44–46), and complex sclerosing lesions (44) diagnosed on imaging-guided biopsies. In our practice, the decision to excise lobular neoplasia takes into consideration: (i) pertinent history and clinical, imaging, and histologic findings and (ii) follows a discussion with the pathologist regarding the extent of the process: is the process extensive in the cores? Does the lobular neoplasia account for the mammographic finding, or is it an incidental observation to the lesion precipitating the biopsy? In our experience, patients with incidentally noted foci of lobular neoplasia alone do not warrant an excisional biopsy. Although rare, if pleomorphic lobular carcinoma in situ is reported following a core biopsy, excision is always recommended.

In patients with screen-detected, otherwise asymptomatic papillary lesions, we are also not recommending excisional biopsy routinely. However, in symptomatic, older (>65) patients with larger papillary lesions in whom the likelihood of malignancy is higher and sampling bias may be an issue we recommend excisional biopsy. Lastly, for patients with complex sclerosing lesions, we recommend excision; as many as 33% of these patients may have an associated tubular carcinoma or DCIS (usually low nuclear grade).

PREOPERATIVE WIRE LOCALIZATIONS

As the number of imaging-guided breast biopsies increases, preoperative wire localizations decrease. At this time, we do preoperative wire localizations almost exclusively in patients who have already had an imaging-guided biopsy with a diagnosis of breast cancer or a lesion such as ADH that requires excisional biopsy. Rarely, in patients who, for technical reasons (e.g., cluster of calcifications in a breast compressing to 1.5 cm or less), cannot undergo imaging-guided biopsy, preoperative wire localization is done for diagnostic purposes. As with core biopsies, the number of localizations done with ultrasound guidance has increased in the last several years. When the area to be localized is not readily apparent on ultrasound (e.g., small metallic clips, calcification clusters, or, less commonly, isoechoic masses), or in a patient with a large breast and a small lesion posteriorly, mammographic guidance can be used and is described below.

Localizations have also been done using a free-hand, anteroposterior approach. Although some can do these easily, safely, and quickly, the approach requires skill and can be associated with an increased risk of pneumothorax (needle is advanced toward the chest wall). Based on CC and mediolateral oblique (MLO) (or 90-degree lateral) views, the location of the lesion is estimated. With the patient in a seated position, the needle is advanced toward the "estimated" location of the lesion "blindly" in an uncompressed breast (anterior to posterior). CC and 90-degree lateral views of the breast are done to establish the relationship of the needle to lesion. Depending on what is seen on these images, the needle may need to be repositioned once or several times before it is close enough to the lesion for the patient to go to the operating room. This approach is based on serial approximations and requires much skill on the part of the radiologist. It is often more time-consuming with possibly additional radiation exposures depending on how many sets of images have to be done and is inherently less accurate and safe when compared with the parallel to the chest wall mammographic approach, described in detail below. Similarly, the use of stereotactic or MRI guidance for preoperative wire localizations is not usually indicated and as such beyond the scope of this basic text.

Ultrasound Guidance

Basically, if we can see the lesion with ultrasound (and this includes some patients with calcifications), we do the localization using ultrasound guidance. Ultrasound-guided procedures are easier on patients since they are supine and no compression or radiation is used. Consequently, vasovagal reactions are almost completely eliminated. Ultrasound-guided localizations also facilitate the surgical approach. Unlike mammographically guided localizations during which the patient is sitting up with her breast pulled out and compressed, the patient is often supine for ultrasound-guided localizations simulating her position in the operating room. In conjunction with the use of a wire to skewer the lesion, an X is placed on the skin overlying the lesion and the surgeon is provided the distance from the skin to the lesion (and wire) to further facilitate the excision of the lesion. The incision can be made so as to intercept the wire rather than dissecting along the wire, as many surgeons do, after mammographically guided localizations.

A variety of needle-wire systems is available including spring hookwire (47), modified spring hookwire (48–50), "J" wire (51), and "barb" wire systems. These come in various lengths, including 3, 5, 7, 9, 11, and 15 cm. We use the modified spring hookwire; however, any of these systems accomplishes the goal of the localization procedures, which is to provide a guide or "road map" for the surgeon in removing the lesion in question while sparing as much of the surrounding normal tissue. The modified springhook wire has a hook at the end that helps anchor the wire in place and a 2-cm-long reinforced segment that is 1 cm from the tip of the hook. The reinforced segment adds stiffness to that portion of the wire minimizing the likelihood that the wire is inadvertently transected (cauterized). Additionally, it provides a reference point for describing the location of the lesion with respect to the wire for the surgeon. We aim to place the reinforced wire segment within or in close proximity to the lesion. Although the hook anchors the wire, it is important that the wire not be used as a retractor particularly in predominantly fatty breast tissue; otherwise, the wire can be dislodged accidentally.

If ultrasound guidance is used, the patient is supine or in a slight oblique position. As described for ultrasound-guided needle biopsies, a skin entry point is selected that will allow the needle to be advanced to and through the lesion parallel to the chest wall and transducer (Fig. 12.40). Lidocaine (1%) is used to raise a skin wheal and a small amount is used along the expected course of the needle from the skin to the lesion. A needle that is long enough to go beyond the lesion by at least 1 cm is selected. With the tip of the needle 1 cm beyond the lesion, the reinforced wire segment will be in close proximity to the lesion. The wire is removed from the needle and set aside to prevent premature deployment or contamination.

Under ultrasound guidance, the needle is advanced through the lesion and beyond it by 1 cm. If the lesion is small, an orthogonal view of the needle is done to document the relationship of the needle to the lesion (Fig. 12.41). The wire is passed through the needle so that the burnish mark on the wire is at the hub of the needle. The needle is pulled out of the breast making sure that the wire is not advanced into

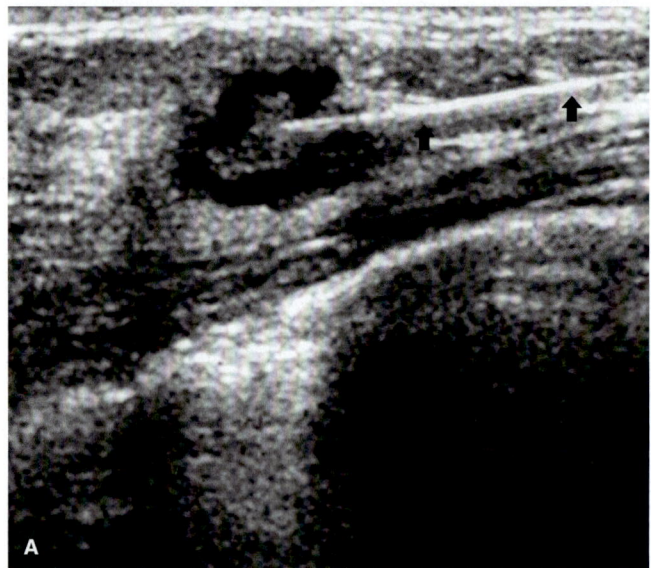

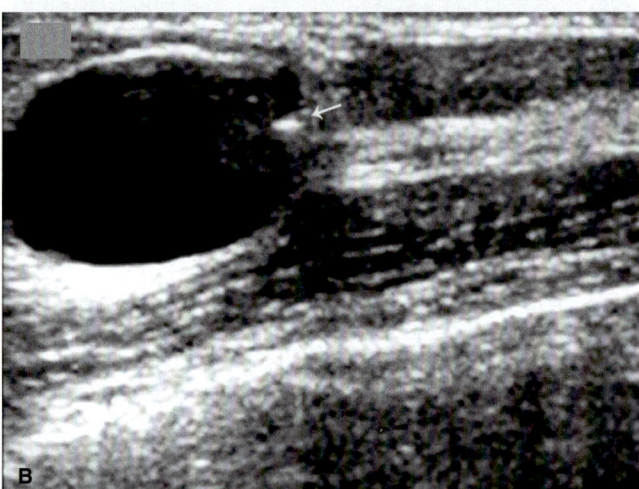

FIG. 12.41 • **Preoperative ultrasound-guided wire localization, papilloma. A:** Using ultrasound guidance, the needle *(arrows)* is placed through an intracystic mass. Note needle is parallel to deep pectoral fascia. Please see Figure 12.14D–F for diagnostic images on this patient. **B:** Orthogonal ultrasound image demonstrating the relationship of the localization needle to the intracystic mass. The needle is imaged in cross section *(arrow)* through the stalk of the intracystic lesion. **C:** A single mammogram image demonstrates the relationship of the localization wire to the mass *(arrow)*. As desired, the reinforced wire segment is through the posterior portion of the mass *(arrow)*. Only one mammographic image is obtained. Depending on the approach used to place the wire, a craniocaudal or 90-degree lateral view is done such that compression is applied parallel to the course of the wire; we do apply compression in a direction that would be perpendicular to the wire. **D:** Specimen. A "blue domed cyst" *(short arrow)* correlating to the localized mass is apparent when the specimen is inspected. The localization wire is seen extending beyond the specimen *(long arrow)*. **E:** The lesion is transected; fluid is released. Grossly, the papilloma *(long arrow)* is seen attached to the wall of the cyst. The remainder of the cyst wall *(short arrows)* is smooth as expected based on the ultrasound and pneumocystogram images shown in Figure 12.14E, F. The black on the surface of the specimen reflects the use of ink to establish the proximity of lesions to the margins of the specimen. Different colored inks (or suture material/knots) can be used to orient the specimen for the pathologist (e.g., anterior, posterior, lateral, and medial margins). (From Cardeñosa G. *Breast Imaging [The Core Curriculum Series]*. Philadelphia, PA: Lippincott Williams & Wilkins; 2003.)

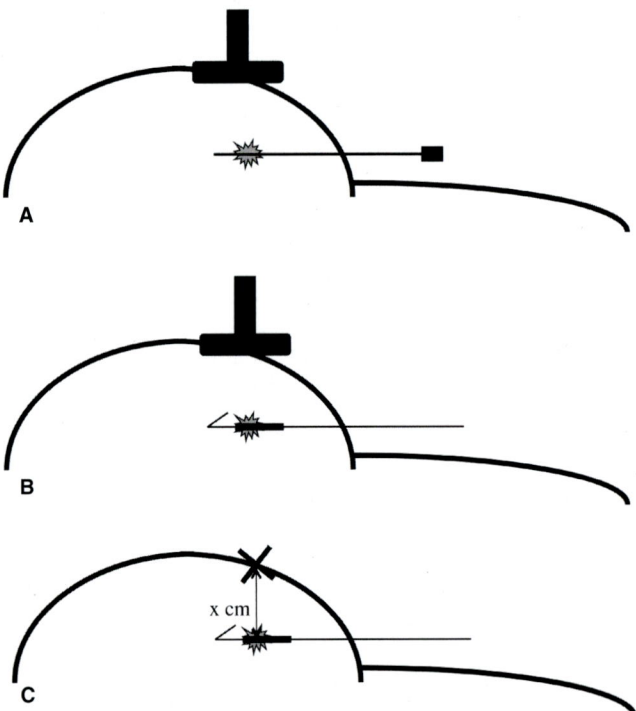

FIG. 12.40 • **Ultrasound-guided preoperative wire localization. A:** With the transducer over the lesion, the localization needle is advanced through the lesion. Orthogonal images of the needle are obtained when localizing small lesions. If the needle is through the lesion on the orthogonal ultrasound images, the wire is deployed and the needle is pulled out of the breast. **B:** As long as the thin localization wire is parallel to the transducer, it can be imaged in its entirety. Its position through the lesion is documented in orthogonal planes. **C:** The distance from the skin to the lesion and wire is measured and an *X* is placed on the skin directly over the lesion. This assists the surgeon in intersecting the wire rather than following it in from the skin entry point. (From Cardeñosa G. *Breast Imaging [The Core Curriculum Series]*. Philadelphia, PA: Lippincott Williams & Wilkins; 2003.)

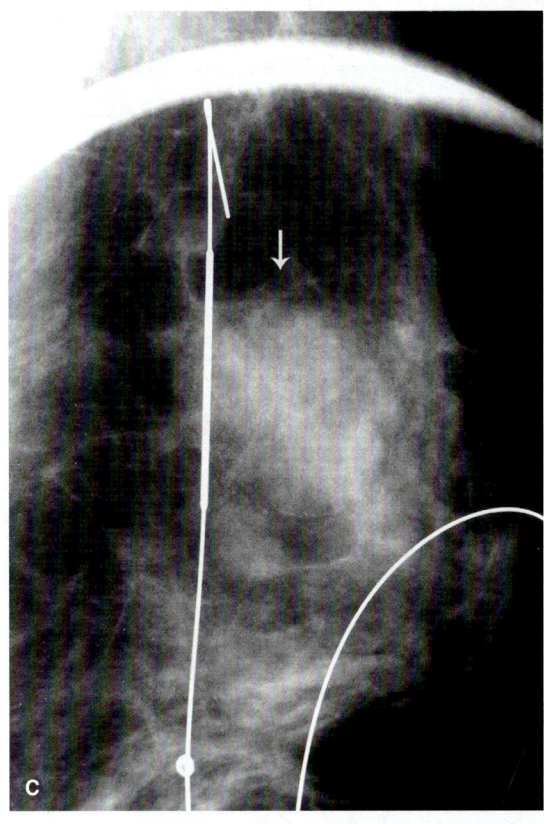
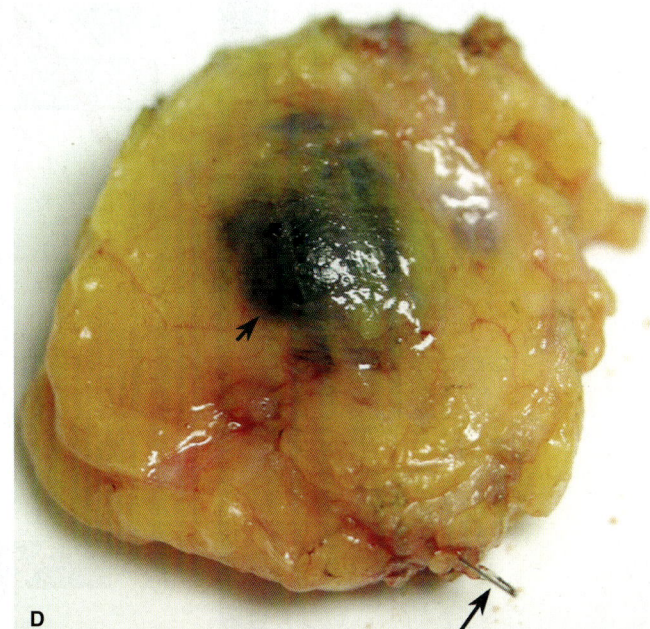
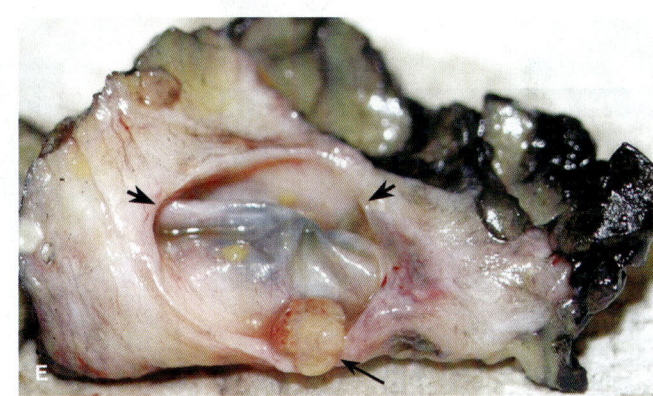

FIG. 12.41 • *(continued)*

the breast or pulled out with needle inadvertently. Ultrasound images of the wire and its relationship to the lesion are taken in orthogonal planes. The distance from the skin to the lesion is measured and, using an indelible marker, an *X* is marked on the skin directly over the lesion (Fig. 12.42). A single mammographic image is obtained with compression applied parallel to the course of the wire (Fig. 12.41C). After the hookwire is deployed, we do not compress the breast perpendicular to the wire; this can result in unwanted movements in the wire, including having the wire pull out from the lesion completely (accordion effect) (Fig. 12.43A–C). If the wire is pulled out of a lesion, a second wire needs to be placed (Fig. 12.43D).

Mammographic Guidance

Safe, precise localizations can also be accomplished by using mammographic guidance (47–55). CC and MLO views are reviewed to determine the shortest distance from the skin to the lesion; keep in mind that lateral lesions will move down and medial lesions will move up in going from an MLO to a 90-degree lateral view. If a question persists regarding the shortest distance to a lesion, a 90-degree lateral view can be done (Fig. 12.34). To determine what the length of the needle should be, measure the distance from the skin to the lesion and select a needle that is long enough to go beyond the lesion by at least 1 cm.

Several compression paddles are available for mammographically guided wire localization procedures. The most commonly used has a

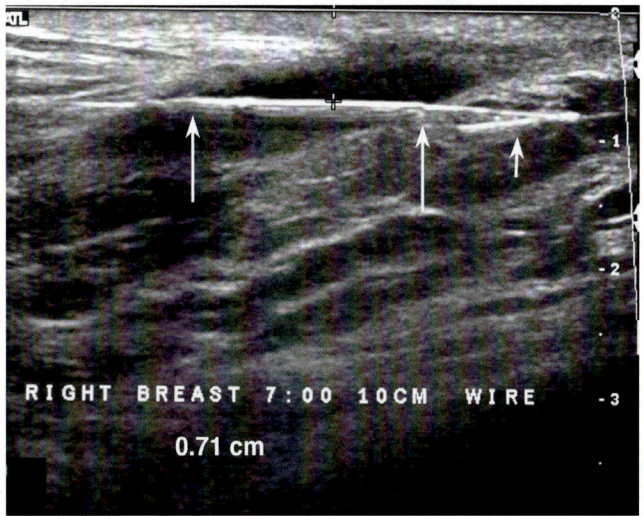

FIG. 12.42 • **Ultrasound image of localization wire.** If the wire is parallel to the transducer it can be seen in its entirety. The hook of wire *(short arrow)* is beyond the lesion being localized. The reinforced wire segment *(two long arrows)* is through the lesion. An *X* is placed on the skin overlying the lesions and wire. In this patient, the lesion and wire are 0.7 cm from the skin *(calipers)*. Rather than follow the wire from the skin entry site, the surgeon can intercept the wire at the site of the lesion.

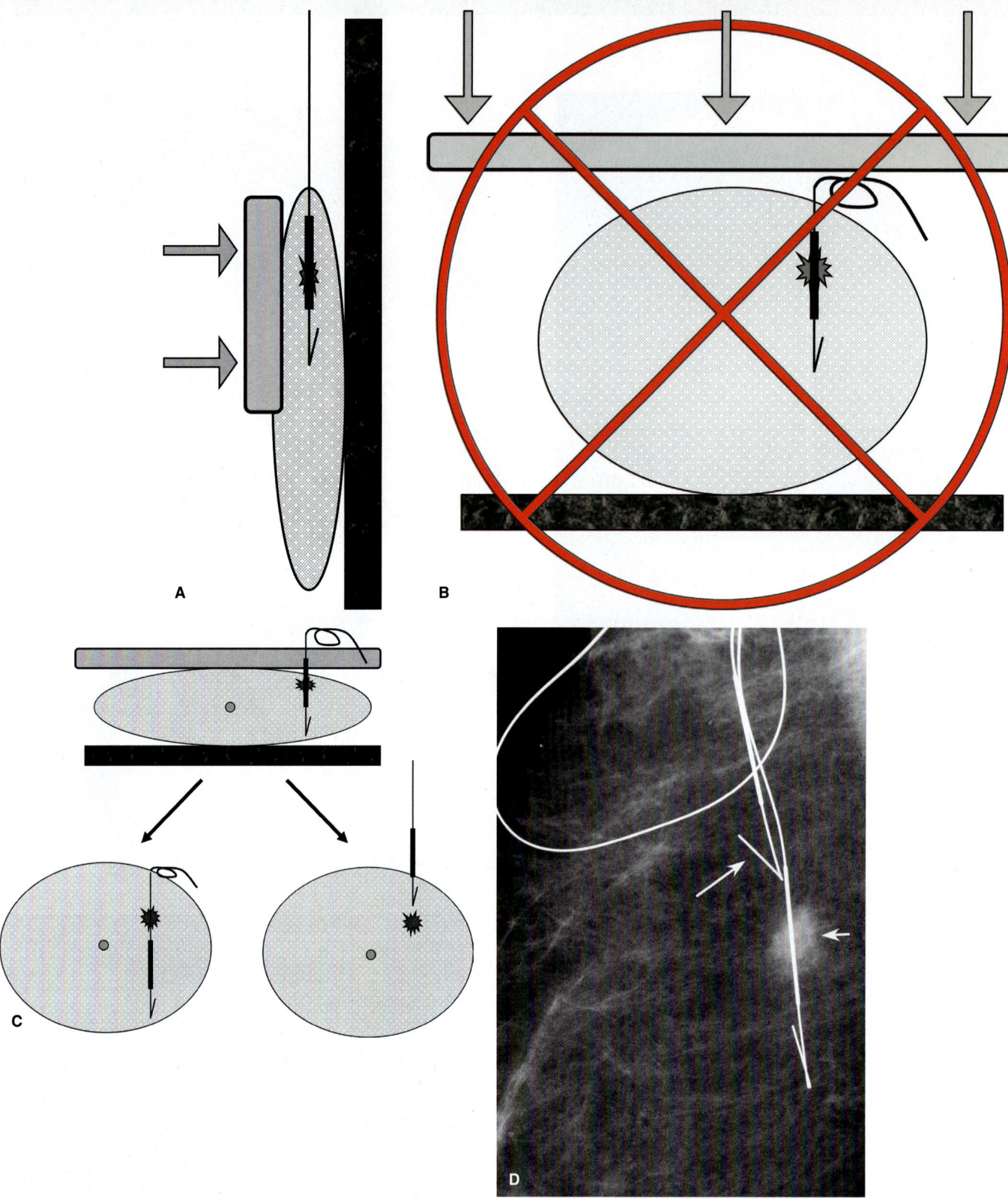

FIG. 12.43 • **Localization wires should be compressed parallel to their course, not perpendicular. A:** After the wire is in position following ultrasound-guided wire localizations, we compress the breast parallel to the wire without any hesitation. **B:** We do not, however, compress the breast perpendicular to the wire. **C:** If the breast is compressed perpendicular to the course of the wire, the wire can be advanced further into the breast or pulled out of the lesion. Having the wire advance beyond the lesion is not as big an issue as having the wire pull out of the lesion. If the wire is pulled out of the lesion, a second wire needs to be used to localize the lesion adequately. **D:** The first wire *(long arrow)* is short of the lesion. This is not an acceptable wire position; in effect, the lesion has not been localized. We do not remove the first wire percutaneously but rather use a second wire. As desired, the reinforced segment of the second wire *(short arrow)* is in the lesion and the hook of the wire is beyond the lesion. In addition to labeling the wires and the images that accompany the patient to the operating room, we communicate directly with the surgeon and explain the need for the second wire. Both wires are removed at the time of surgery. (From Cardeñosa G. *Breast Imaging [The Core Curriculum Series]*. Philadelphia, PA: Lippincott Williams & Wilkins; 2003.)

single fenestration with radiopaque markers along two sides for ease of coordinate mapping and needle placement. These types of paddles come in two sizes: as full compression paddles (the size of those used for routine screening views) or as smaller paddles (the size of a spot compression paddle). The small paddles are particularly useful in women with small breasts, or in patients with posterior, axillary or subareolar lesions (Fig. 12.44). In these situations, optimal compression and breast immobilization are difficult to accomplish with a full-sized compression paddle. The second type of localization paddle contains multiple perforations arranged at set intervals. With this type of paddle, the perforations need to be large enough to allow passage of the needle hub so the compression paddle can be released when the gantry is repositioned for the orthogonal view. A relatively minor disadvantage of these multiple perforation (hole) paddles is that repositioning of the breast may be required if the lesion does not project directly below one of the perforations (Fig. 12.45).

Let us consider a patient with DCIS diagnosed following a stereotactically guided biopsy of a cluster of calcifications in the left breast. She now presents for preoperative wire localization of the remaining calcifications (DCIS). The screening images (CC and MLO) views are reviewed to establish the shortest distance from the skin to the calcifications. If after reviewing the initial images a question persists

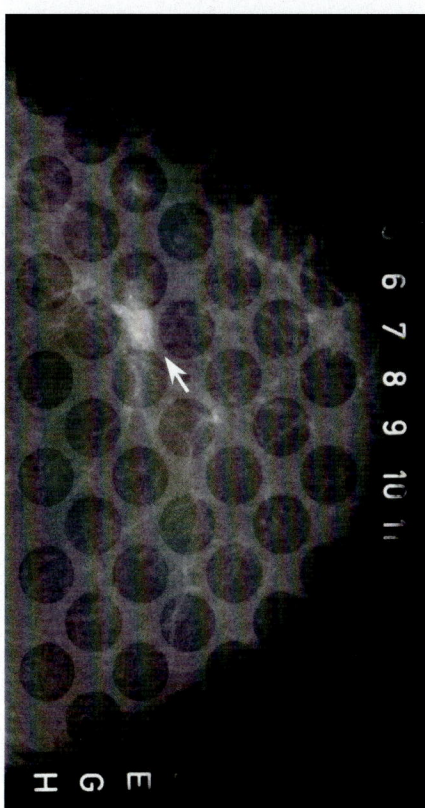

FIG. 12.45 ● **Multiple hole localization paddle.** In this patient, a multiple hole paddle is used for the localization procedure. The mass *(arrow)* is between two of the holes. Consequently, if you want to place the wire through the lesion, the patient needs to be repositioned so that lesion is under one of the perforations otherwise the wire will be in the adjacent tissue.

regarding the shortest distance, a 90-degree lateral view can be done. In this patient, calcifications are closest to the lateral aspect of the breast; the distance from the skin to the calcifications on the CC view is measured to determine the length of the needle to be used. The starting position for the patient is a 90-degree lateromedial (LM) view (Fig. 12.46A) using the fenestrated compression paddle. Firm compression is used to prevent inadvertent patient motion; the technologist marks the corners of the fenestration on the patient's skin so it is easy to determine if she moves after the initial image is done. The coordinates for the location of the lesion are established on this initial image. Using the centering light of the mammographic unit, a shadow of the coordinates for the lesion is cast onto the patient's compressed breast. The skin is cleaned with betadiene and alcohol. Lidocaine (1%) is used to raise a skin wheal. The wire is removed from the needle before starting and set aside; this prevents premature deployment or contamination of the wire. Using a 45-degree angle, the tip of the needle is placed at the intersecting point of the coordinates after which, using the centering light of the mammographic unit, the needle is aligned so that the shadow of the needle hub projects onto the interesting point for the coordinates (if the hub of the needle is held with the thumb and index fingers, and the rest of fingers are splayed away, the radiologist's hand will not interfere with the ability to see the shadow of the coordinates and needle hub). The needle is advanced as far as possible in one motion perpendicular to the skin and parallel to the chest wall and a repeat 90-degree lateral view is done to establish the relationship of the needle to the calcifications in this projection (Fig. 12.46B). On this image, the hub and tip of the needle should be superimposed on

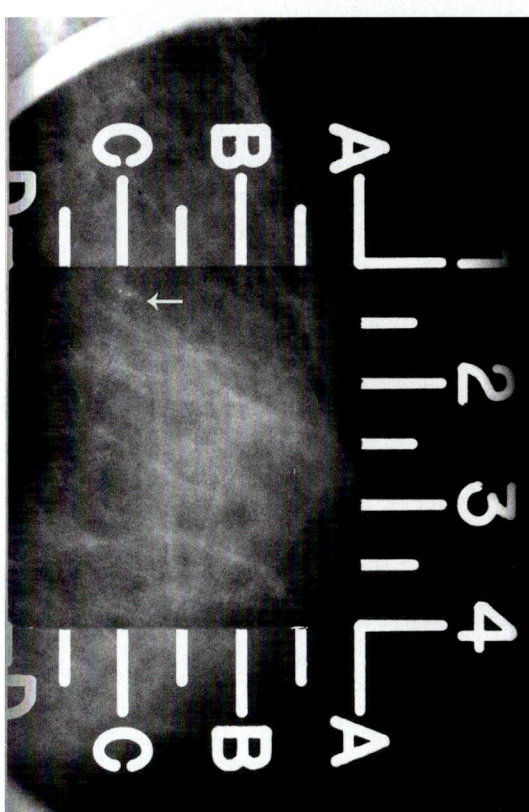

FIG. 12.44 ● **Spot localization paddle.** In this patient, a fenestrated spot compression paddle is used to localize a cluster of calcifications *(arrow)* in the axillary tail of the left breast. The posterolateral location of the calcifications and a thin breast *(compression = 1.5 cm)* preclude stereotactically guided biopsy. This fenestrated spot compression paddle with an alphanumeric grid is particularly helpful in patients with a small breast or in localizing lesions that are located posteriorly, high in the axilla or in the subareolar area. These areas are hard to access and compress adequately with the standard-sized fenestrated compression paddle. (From Cardeñosa G. *Breast Imaging [The Core Curriculum Series]*. Philadelphia, PA: Lippincott Williams & Wilkins; 2003.)

the lesion such that if a long enough needle was selected, the lesion is skewered. Also, since the wire is placed through the needle, this image serves to describe the eventual relationship of the lesion to the wire in this plane (e.g., this projection need not, and should not, be repeated after the wire is deployed; it would require that compression be applied perpendicular to the wire). Compression is released slowly allowing breast tissue to reexpand around the needle so that the hub is flush with the skin surface. At this point the patient, who has remained stationary, is encouraged to sit back and relax while the x-ray tube is rotated 90 degrees.

The patient's breast is repositioned with the needle now parallel to the detector; in this patient it is a CC view. Compression for this orthogonal image is best done with the spot compression paddle. Use of the spot paddle at this point allows us to determine the position of the tip of needle and its relationship to the lesion while permitting easy access to the hub of the needle for adjustments in needle positioning. If a larger paddle is used, the space between the detector and the compression paddle may limit access for needle repositioning and deployment of the wire (Fig. 12.47). The CC spot compression view in this patient (Fig. 12.43C) establishes the relationship of the needle to the lesion in the orthogonal plane. If the tip of the needle is beyond the lesion by more than 1 cm it can be pulled out as much as needed before the wire is deployed.

On the third image (in this patient a CC view), the location of the lesion along the course of the needle is determined. If the needle is more than 1 cm beyond the lesion, it is pulled out enough so that the tip is approximately 1 cm beyond the lesion. With this needle positioning, the reinforced wire segment will be in close proximity to the lesion. If the needle is in satisfactory position, the wire is advanced through the needle until the burnish mark on the wire is at the hub of the needle. The wire is then held in place as the needle is pulled out (similar to what is done during a catheter exchange). Care is needed to make sure

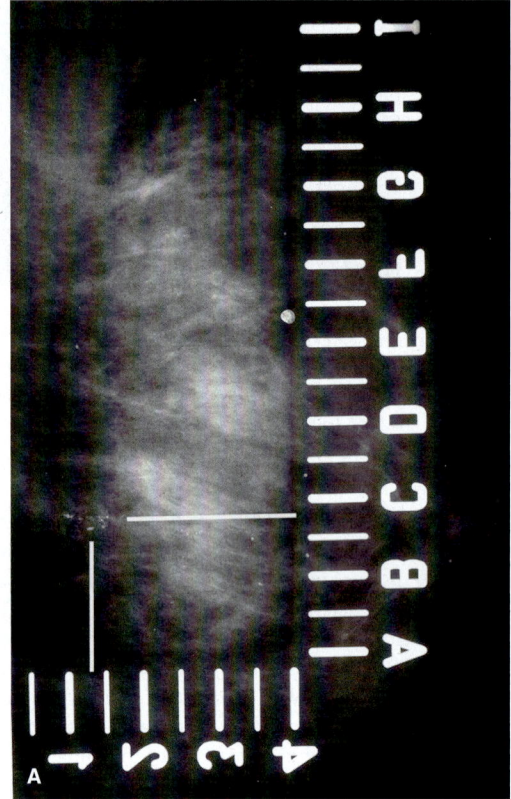 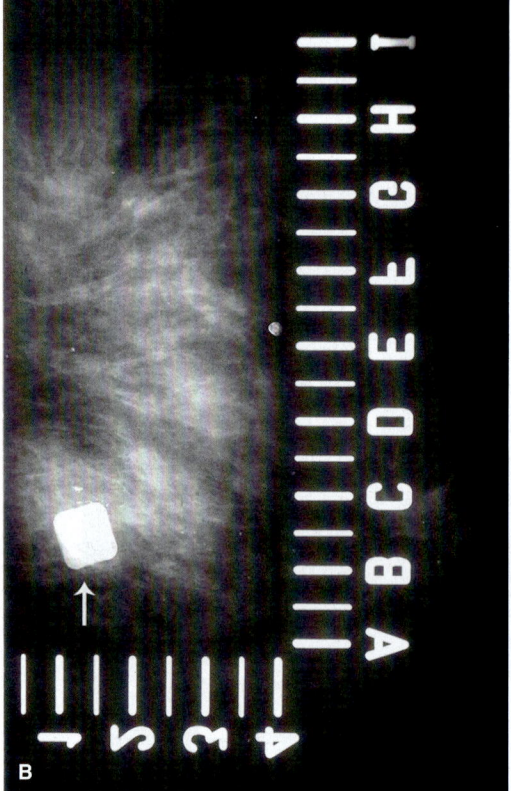

FIG. 12.46 • **Mammographically guided preoperative wire localization. A:** Ninety-degree lateromedial (LM) view in a patient with a cluster of calcifications closest to the lateral skin surface on the craniocaudal (CC) view. A 90-degree LM view is the starting point using the standard-sized fenestrated compression paddle. The coordinates for the cluster of calcifications are determined *(white lines)*. Collimator cross hairs are positioned so that a shadow is cast on the woman's breast at these coordinates. The needle is advanced in one movement to the hub and a repeat 90-degree LM is obtained. **B:** 90-degree LM. Hub of needle *(arrow)* is superimposed on calcification cluster. If a long enough needle has been selected the calcifications will be found along the course of the needle. This view defines the positioning of the wire (wire is passed through needle) so this view does not need to be repeated after the wire is deployed. Compression is released and a craniocaudal (CC) view is obtained to determine the location of the calcifications along the course of the needle. **C:** CC view using the spot compression paddle. Patient remains in compression after this view is done until after the wire is deployed. Needle is through the posterior edge of the calcification cluster. The wire is deployed. **D:** Repeat CC view. Superficial portion of reinforced wire segment is at the posterior edge of the calcification cluster. **E:** Specimen radiograph. Localized calcifications have been excised. Wire with hook has been excised. Proximity to one of the margins *(arrow)* is discussed with the surgeon. Although the specimen radiograph is a two-dimensional representation of a three-dimensional structure, proximity to the margins can sometimes be suggested based on the image. Coordinates for the three areas of calcifications *(thick arrows)* are indicated for the pathologist. (From Cardeñosa G. *Breast Imaging [The Core Curriculum Series].* Philadelphia, PA: Lippincott Williams & Wilkins; 2003.)

Interventional Procedures

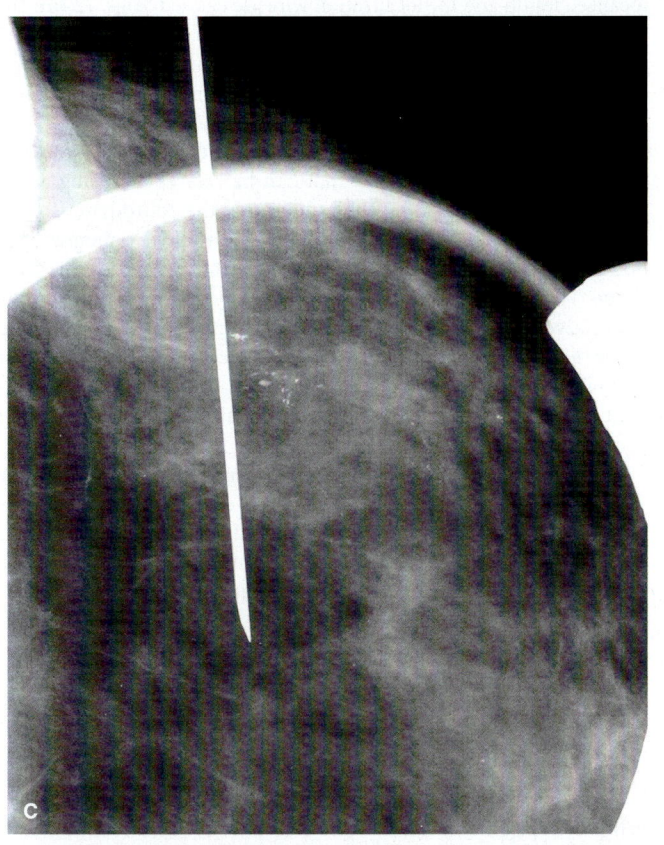
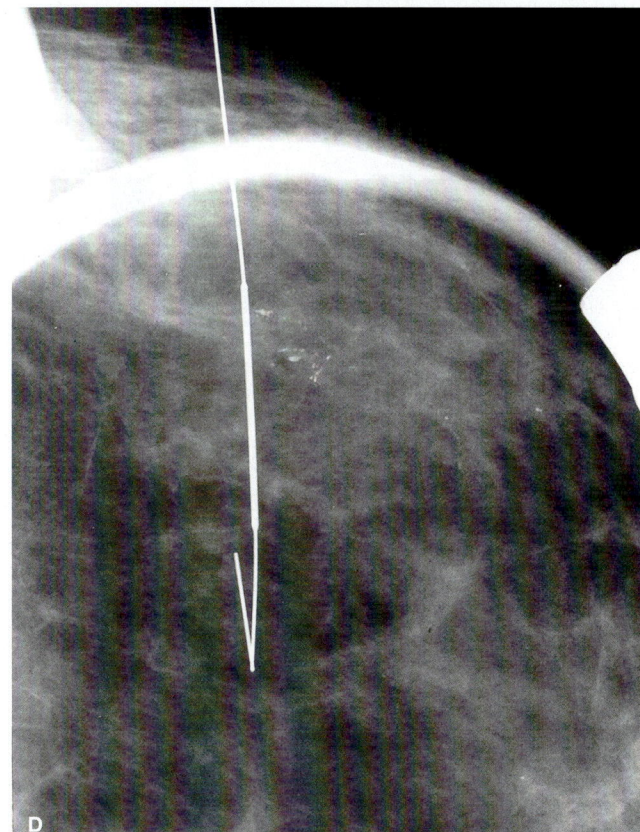
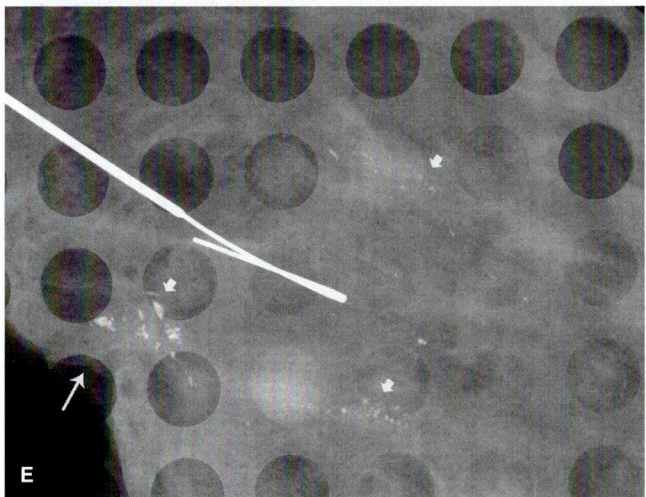

FIG. 12.46 • *(continued)*

the wire is not advanced into the breast as the needle is pulled out or that the wire is not pulled out with the needle (Fig. 12.48). After the needle is pulled out, a hemostat flush to the skin is used to bend the wire 90 degrees; this prevents the wire from advancing into the breast inadvertently and it helps the surgeon recognize if the wire pulls out of the breast slightly when the patient is mobilized (e.g., relationship of bend in the wire to the skin). A repeat CC view (Fig. 12.46D) is obtained to document the position of the wire and its relationship to the localized lesion. Compression is released and the external portion of the wire is secured to the skin. A theoretical localization using a CC approach and an actual localization using a 90-degree ML approach are presented for review (Figs. 12.49 and 12.50). In patients with multiple lesions or an extensive area of calcifications not undergoing mastectomy, multiple wires are used to localize each mass or to bracket an area of calcifications (Fig. 12.51).

SPECIMEN RADIOGRAPHY

Following imaging-guided wire localization, surgical specimens are radiographed (56,57), or when the lesion is not readily identified on a radiograph, an ultrasound of the specimen can be done. Imaging the specimen serves several purposes, including documentation that the

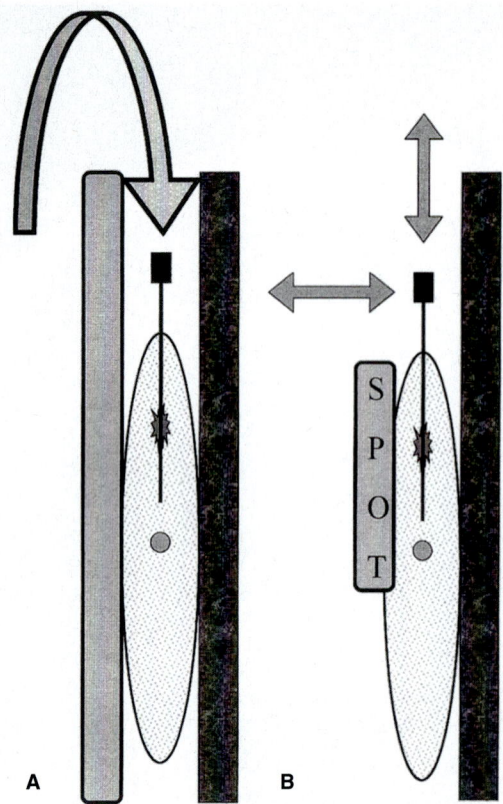

FIG. 12.47 • Use of spot compression paddle during mammographically guided wire localization. **A:** When obtaining the orthogonal view to document the relationship of the needle to the lesion, access to the hub of the needle may be limited if the large compression paddle is used. **B:** If the spot compression paddle is used, however, there is easy access to the hub of the needle. The needle can be pulled out slightly and in a controlled manner if the tip is beyond the lesion by more than 1 cm. It is also easy to stabilize the wire so there is no inadvertent motion of the wire as the needle is pulled out. (From Cardeñosa G. *Breast Imaging [The Core Curriculum Series]*. Philadelphia, PA: Lippincott Williams & Wilkins; 2003.)

localized lesion and the localization wire are excised (Figs. 12.46E and 12.50E). The specimen radiograph is also used to orient the pathologist to the location of the lesion in the specimen and the proximity of the lesion to the margins can sometimes be determined. Rarely, unsuspected lesions are identified in the specimen.

The specimen is placed in a container and compressed with an insert that has multiple holes that can be referenced using an alphanumeric grid. Based on the radiograph, the coordinates for the lesion are indicated for the pathologist. Specimen radiography is done with compression of the specimen and magnification technique. The radiograph can be obtained on a mammography unit or, alternatively, dedicated specimen radiography units are available. After the radiograph is obtained and verification of lesion removal is established the surgeon is notified with the results; if there are concerns about proximity to a margin, this is discussed with the surgeon.

With lesions that are not apparent mammographically and localized with ultrasound, an ultrasound of the specimen is done. A protective sheath is put on the transducer and a small amount of gel is applied to the specimen. The transducer is manipulated over the specimen in a systematic manner to determine the location of the lesion (Fig. 12.52). When the lesion is identified, a pin or needle can be put through it to mark the area for the pathologist; the individuals processing the specimen in pathology are alerted to the presence of a needle in the specimen.

PARAFFIN BLOCK RADIOGRAPHY

When a biopsy is done for calcifications and the calcifications are not apparent on the microscopic slides, we can assist the pathologist by doing a radiograph of the paraffin blocks (58,59). Magnified images of the blocks are obtained using the lowest possible kVp with an mAs of 5 to 6. The block or blocks with calcifications is identified and an orthogonal view of this block is obtained to establish the depth of the calcifications in the block (Fig. 12.53).

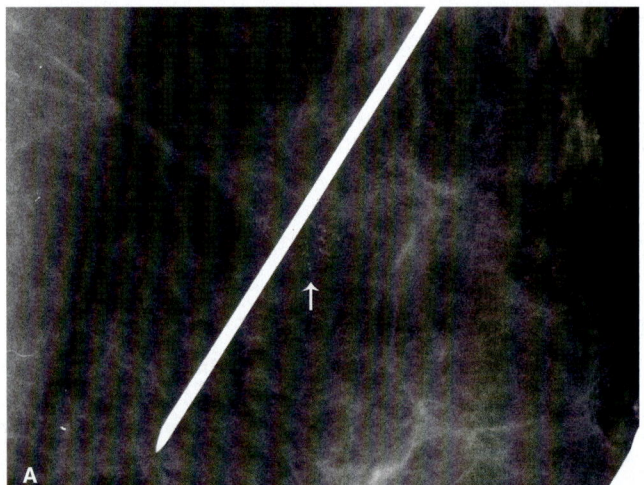
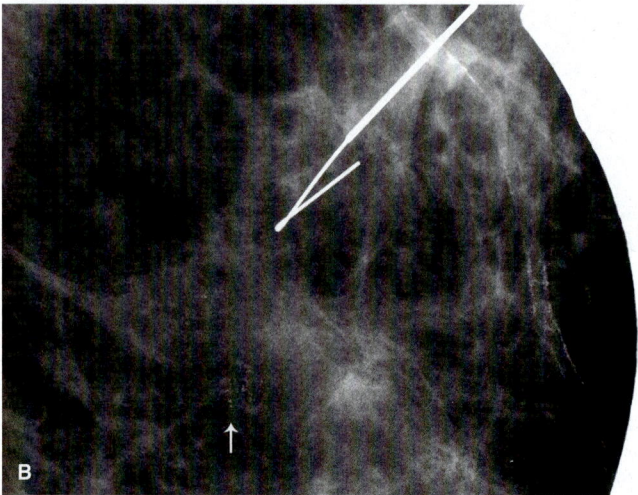

FIG. 12.48 • Inadvertent withdrawal of wire. **A:** Cluster of calcifications *(arrow)* is seen along the course of the needle. The wire is deployed. As the needle is pulled out, the wire needs to be stabilized (much as is done with a catheter exchange). Care must be exercised to not advance the wire as the needle is pulled out or to withdraw the wire with the needle. **B:** On the final image taken to document the relationship of the wire to the calcifications, it is clear that the wire was partially and inadvertently pulled out with the needle. The hook and reinforced segment of the wire are short of the cluster of calcifications *(arrow)*. When the wire is short of the lesion as in this patient, a second wire needs to be deployed; otherwise it becomes difficult for the surgeon to excise the area of concern. (From Cardeñosa G. *Breast Imaging [The Core Curriculum Series]*. Philadelphia, PA: Lippincott Williams & Wilkins; 2003.)

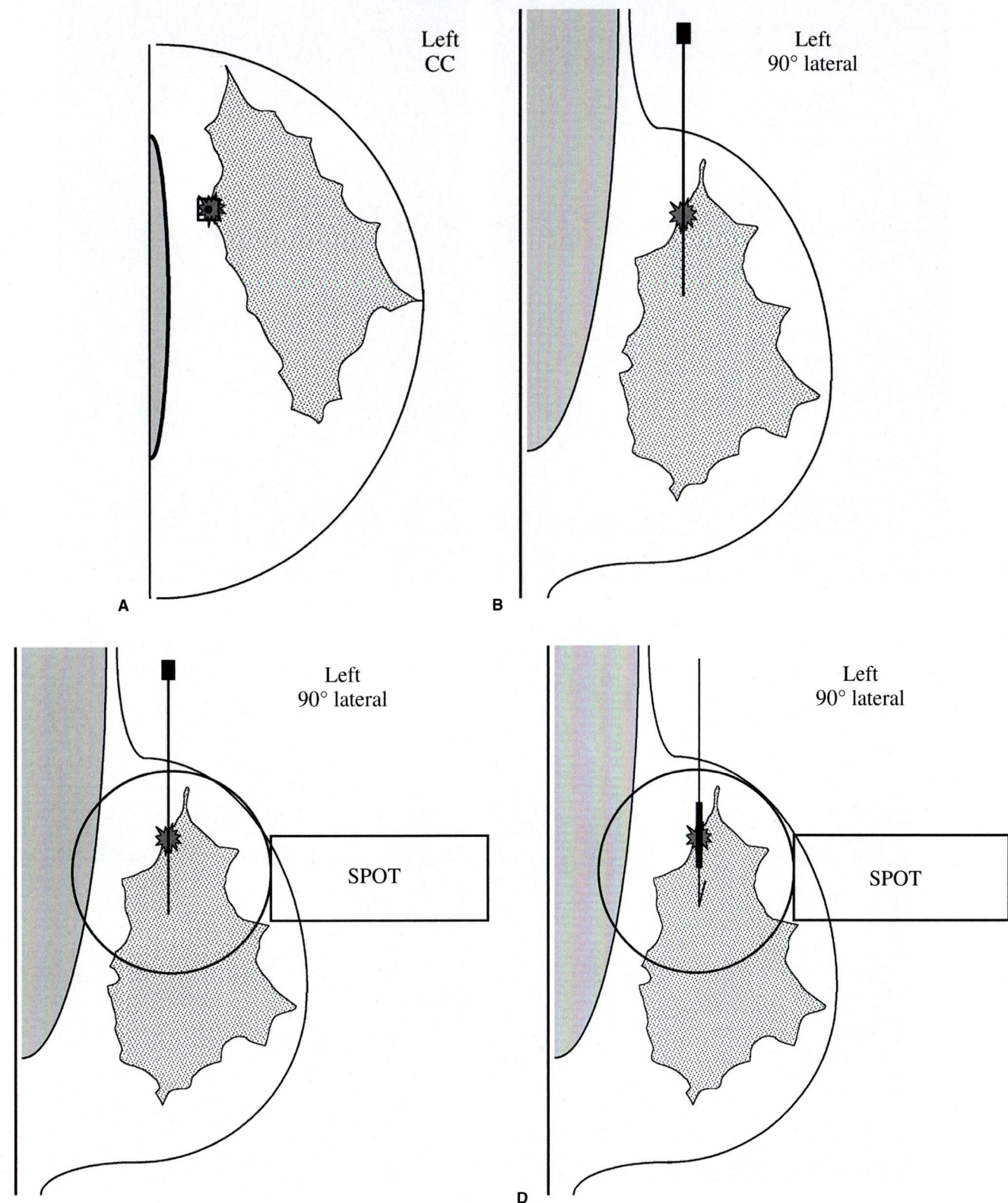

FIG. 12.49 • **Diagram of preoperative wire localization for a lesion closest to the superior skin surface. A:** With the patient in a craniocaudal position, the needle is advanced in the breast all the way to the hub. This image should show the hub of the needle and the needle superimposed on the lesion. Compression is released. **B:** The orthogonal view (in this example a 90-degree lateral view) is obtained to document the relationship of the needle to the lesion and the location of the tip. The tip of the needle should be approximately 1 cm beyond the lesion. **C:** The 90-degree lateral view is done using a spot compression paddle so there is easy access to the hub of the needle. The patient is kept in compression after this view is done. **D:** The wire is deployed and a second 90-degree lateral view is obtained to document final wire positioning. This image and that shown in A describe the relationship of the wire to the lesion and are sent to surgeon for use during the excision.(From Cardeñosa G. *Breast Imaging [The Core Curriculum Series]*. Philadelphia, PA: Lippincott Williams & Wilkins; 2003.)

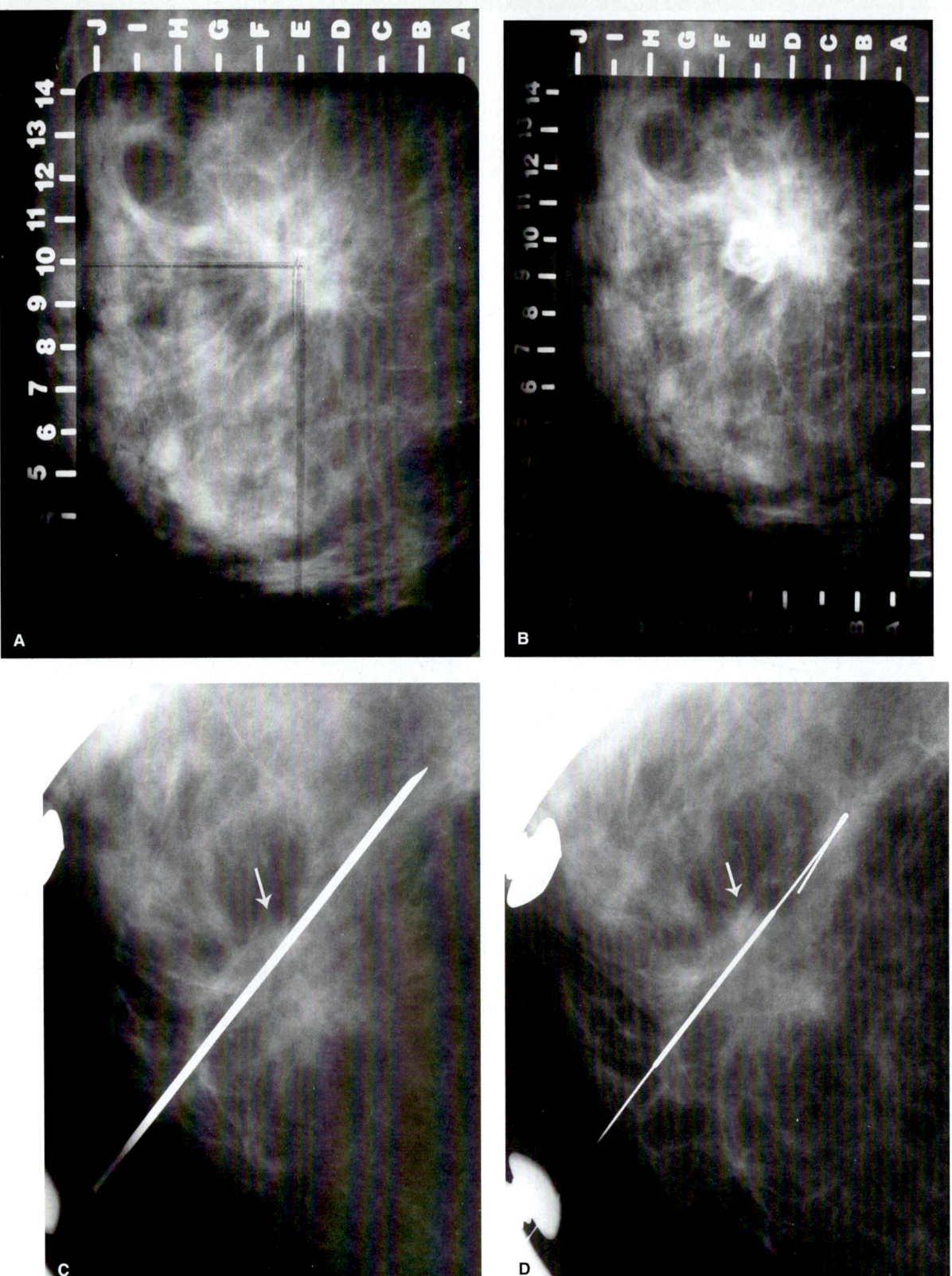

FIG. 12.50 • **Mammographically guided wire localization, 90-degree mediolateral approach. A:** Ninety-degree mediolateral (ML) view with fenestrated compression paddle. Coordinates for the spiculated mass are determined *(dark lines)*. The needle tip is placed at the intersection of the coordinates and advanced to the hub. **B:** Ninety-degree ML view after needle placement. The hub of the needle is superimposed on the anterior edge of the mass. If a long enough needle was selected the lesion is skewered. At this point, compression is released and the orthogonal view is obtained; in this patient, it is a craniocaudal (CC) view. **C:** CC view done using a spot compression paddle. This view demonstrates where the mass *(arrow)* is located along the course of the needle. If the tip of the needle is more than 1 cm beyond the lesion, the needle can be pulled out as much as needed. The wire is deployed and the needle is taken out making sure the wire is not moved as the needle is manipulated. **D:** Final image taken in the CC projection demonstrates reinforced wire segment through the spiculated mass *(arrow)*. **E:** Specimen radiograph confirms excision of the mass and wire. (From Cardeñosa G. *Breast Imaging [The Core Curriculum Series]*. Philadelphia, PA: Lippincott Williams & Wilkins; 2003.)

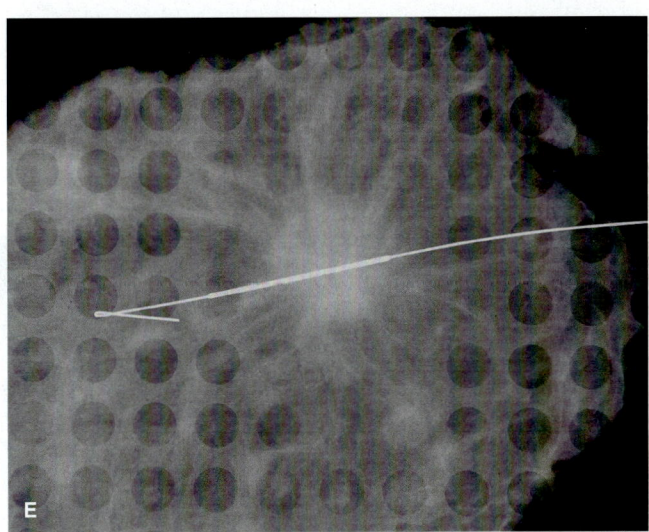

FIG. 12.50 • *(continued)*

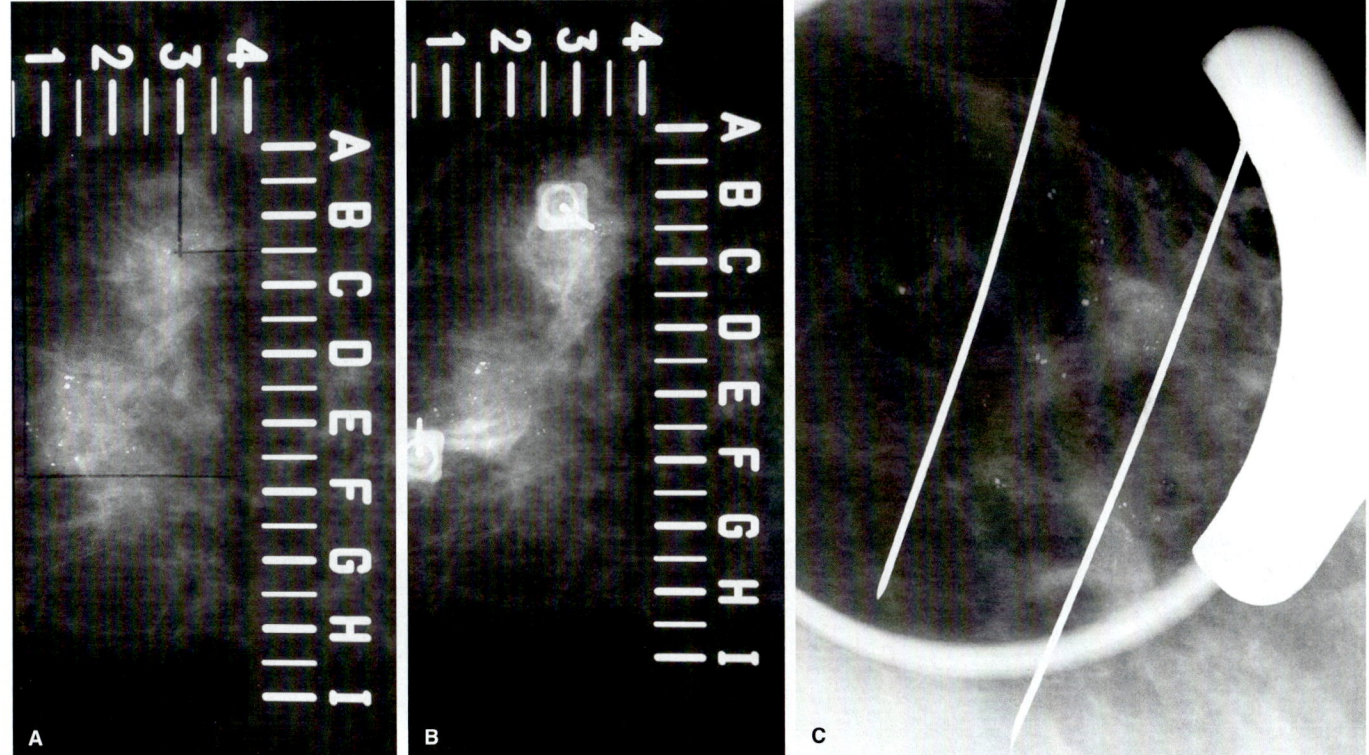

FIG. 12.51 • **Bracketing. A:** Ninety-degree lateral (LM) view. Fenestrated compression paddle with alphanumeric grid used to compress the lateral aspect of the breast. Coordinates for the calcification clusters *(dark lines)* are determined as shown. Needles are advanced at the two sets of coordinates. **B:** Ninety-degree LM view. After needles are placed, a repeat LM view is done to document the relationship of the needles to the calcification clusters in this plane. Compression is released making sure the needle hubs are secured so they are not inadvertently pulled out as the compression paddle is released. **C:** Craniocaudal (CC) view done using spot compression paddle. Calcifications are seen surrounding both needles. The patient stays in compression as the wires are deployed. **D:** Repeat CC view. Although the patient has moved slightly, the relationship of the wires to the calcifications can be determined. **E:** Specimen radiograph demonstrates wide area of calcifications in the specimen bracketed by the wires. Ductal carcinoma in situ is diagnosed. In patients with extensive areas of calcifications or multiple masses, multiple wires are used to bracket the area of concern for the surgeon. (From Cardeñosa G. *Breast Imaging [The Core Curriculum Series]*. Philadelphia, PA: Lippincott Williams & Wilkins; 2003.)

(continued)

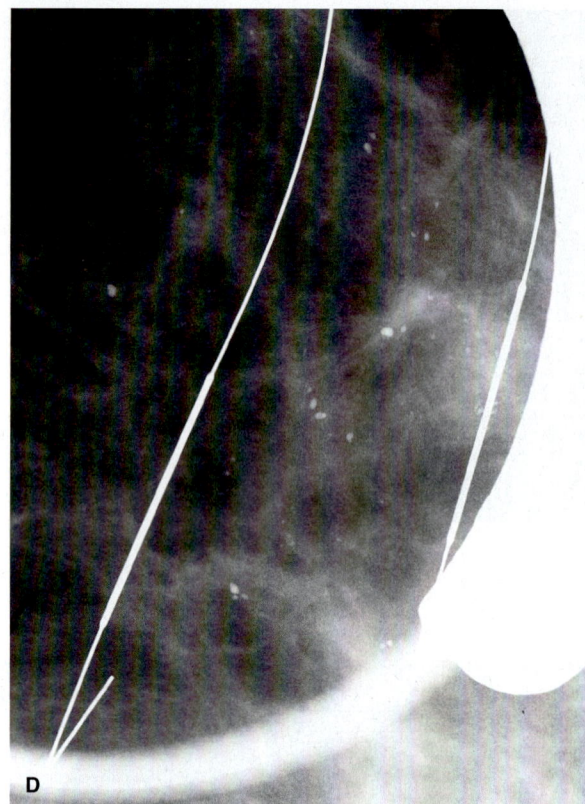
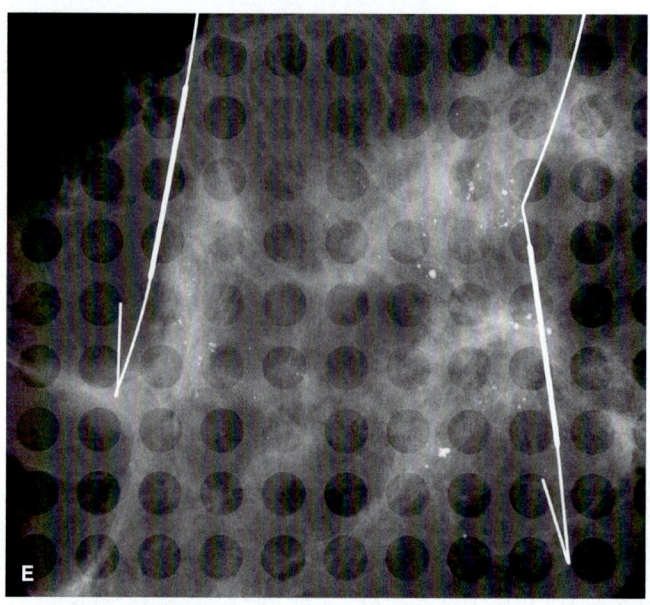

FIG. 12.51 • *(continued)*

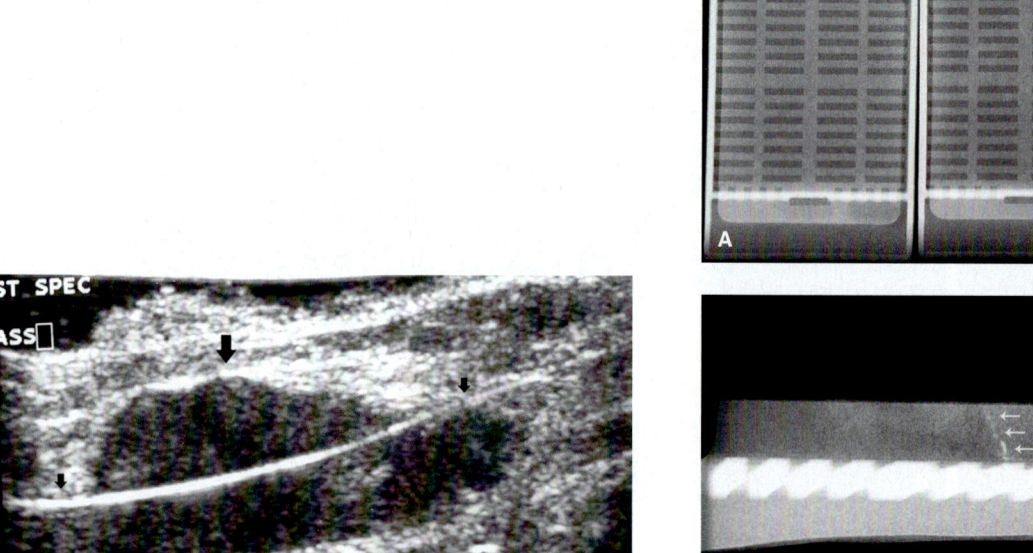

FIG. 12.52 • **Specimen sonogram.** If the lesion is not seen mammographically, ultrasound can be used to document excision of the lesion. Mass *(large arrow)* is readily seen in the specimen with the wire through it *(small arrows)*. (From Cardeñosa G. *Breast Imaging [The Core Curriculum Series]*. Philadelphia, PA: Lippincott Williams & Wilkins; 2003.)

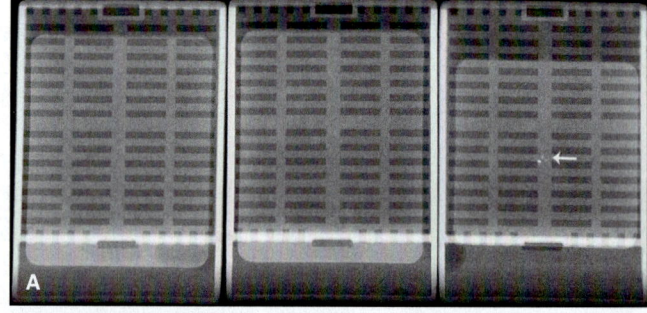
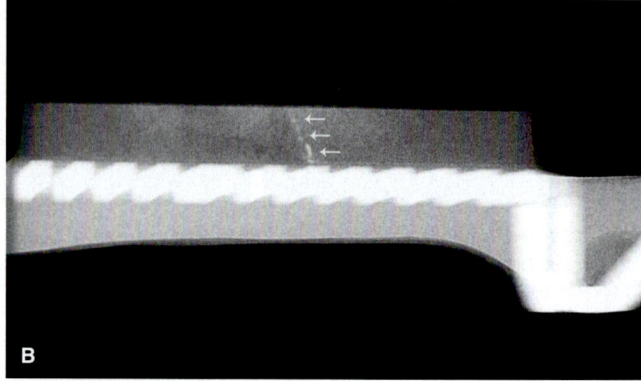

FIG. 12.53 • **Paraffin block radiography. A:** If the pathologist is unable to identify calcifications on the slides, the paraffin blocks can be radiographed (likewise, if there is any un-sectioned tissue, this can also be radiographed). The block containing the calcifications *(arrow)* is identified. **B:** Orthogonal view of the block. This is obtained to determine the depth of the calcifications *(arrows)* in the block. (From Cardeñosa G. *Breast Imaging [The Core Curriculum Series]*. Philadelphia, PA: Lippincott Williams & Wilkins; 2003.)

References

1. Cardenosa G, Doudna C, Eklund GW. Ductography of the breast: technique and findings. *AJR Am J Roentgenol.* 1994;162:1081–1087.
2. Fajardo LL, Jackson VP, Hunter TB. Interventional procedures in diseases of the breast: needle biopsy, pneumocystography and galactography. *AJR Am J Roentgenol.* 1992;158:1231–1238.
3. Leborgne R. *Estudio radiologico del sistema canalicular de la glandula mamaria normal y patologica.* Montevideo, Uruguay: Impresora Uruguaya S.A., Juncal 1511; 1943.
4. Tabar L, Dean PB, Zoltan P. Galactography: the diagnostic procedure of choice for nipple discharge. *Radiology.* 1983;149:31–38.
5. Haagensen CD. *Diseases of the Breast.* 3rd ed. Philadelphia, PA: WB Saunders; 1986.
6. Woods ER, Helvie MA, Ikeda DM, et al. Solitary breast papilloma: comparison of mammographic, galactographic and pathologic findings. *AJR Am J Roentgenol.* 1992;159:487–491.
7. Leis HP, Cammarata A, LaRaja RD. Nipple discharge: significance and treatment. *Breast.* 1985;11:6–12.
8. Tabar L, Pentek Z, Dean PB. The diagnostic and therapeutic value of breast cyst puncture and pneumocystography. *Radiology.* 1981;141:659–663.
9. Ikeda DM, Helvie MA, Adler DD, et al. The role of fine-needle aspiration and pneumocystography in the treatment of impalpable breast cysts. *AJR Am J Roentgenol.* 1992;158:1239–1241.
10. Azavedo E, Svane G, Auer G. Stereotactic fine needle biopsy in 2594 mammographically detected non-palpable lesions. *Lancet.* 1989;1:1033–1035.
11. Jackson VP. The status of mammograhically guided fine needle aspiration biopsy of nonpalpable breast lesions. *Radiol Clin North Am.* 1992;30:155–166.
12. Parker SH, Lovin JD, Jobe WE, et al. Stereotactic breast biopsy with a biopsy gun. *Radiology.* 1990;176:741–747.
13. Parker SH, Lovin JD, Jobe WE, et al. Nonpalpable breast lesions: stereotactic automated large-core biopsies. *Radiology.* 1991;180:403–407.
14. Parker SH, Jobe WE, eds. *Percutaneous Breast Biopsy.* New York, NY: Raven Press; 1993.
15. Parker SH, Burbank F, Jackman RJ, et al. Percutaneous large-core breast biopsy: a multi-institutional study. *Radiology.* 1994;193:359–364.
16. Parker SH, Klaus AJ, McWey PJ, et al. Sonographically guided directional vacuum-assisted breast biopsy using a handheld device. *AJR Am J Roentgenol.* 2001;177:405–408.
17. Liberman L. Percutaneous imaging-guided core breast biopsy: state of the art at the millennium. *AJR Am J Roentgenol.* 2000;174:1191–1199.
18. Liberman L, Fahs MC, Dershaw DD, et al. Impact of stereotaxic core biopsy on cost of diagnosis. *Radiology.* 1995;195:633–637.
19. Liberman L, Feng TL, Dershaw DD, et al. US-guided core breast biopsy: use and cost effectiveness. *Radiology.* 1998;208:717–723.
20. Meyer JE. Value of large-core biopsy of occult breast lesions. *AJR Am J Roentgenol.* 1992;158:991–992.
21. Perez-Fuentes JA, Longobardi IR, Acosta VF, et al. Sonographically guided directional vacuum assisted breast biopsy: preliminary experience in Venezuela. *AJR Am J Roentgenol.* 2001;177:1459–1463.
22. Fornage BD, Coan JD, David CL. Ultrasound-guided needle biopsy of the breast and other interventional procedures. *Radiol Clin North Am.* 1992;30:167–185.
23. Melotti MK, Berg WA. Core needle breast biopsy in patients undergoing anticoagulation therapy: preliminary results. *AJR Am J Roentgenol.* 2000;174:245–249.
24. Sommerville P, Seifert PJ, Destounis SV, et al. Anticoagulation and bleeding risk after core needle biopsy. *AJR Am J Roentgenol.* 2008;191:1194–1197.
25. Edeiken BS, Fornage BD, Bedi DG, et al. US-guided implantation of metallic markers for permanent localization of the tumor bed in patients with breast cancer who undergo preoperative chemotherapy. *Radiology.* 1999;213:895–900.
26. Liberman L, Cohen MA, Dershaw DD, et al. Atypical ductal hyperplasia diagnosed at stereotaxic core biopsy of breast lesions: an indication for surgical biopsy. *AJR Am J Roentgenol.* 1995;164:1111–1113.
27. Jackman RJ, Birdwell RL, Ikeda DM. Atypical ductal hyperplasia: can some lesions be defined as probably benign after stereotactic 11-gauge vacuum assisted biopsy, eliminating the recommendations for surgical excision? *Radiology.* 2002;224:548–554.
28. Philpotts LE, Shaheen NA, Jain KS, et al. Uncommon high-risk lesions of the breast diagnosed at stereotactic core needle biopsy: clinical importance. *Radiology.* 2000;216:831–837.
29. Reynolds HE. Core needle biopsy of challenging benign breast conditions: a comprehensive literature review. *AJR Am J Roentgenol.* 2000;174:1245–1250.
30. Khoumais NA, Scaranelo AM, Hoshonov H, et al. Incidence of breast cancer in patients with pure flat epithelial atypia diagnosed at core-needle biopsy of the breast. *Ann Surg Oncol.* 2013;20:133–138.
31. Lavoué V, Roger CM, Poilblanc M, et al. Pure flat epithelial atypia (DIN 1a) on core needle biopsy: study of 60 biopsies with follow-up surgical excision. *Breast Cancer Res Treat.* 2011;125:121.
32. Liberman L, Sama M, Susnik B, et al. Lobular carcinoma in situ at percutaneous breast biopsy: surgical biopsy findings. *AJR Am J Roentgenol.* 1999;173:291–299.
33. Berg WA, Mrose HE, Ioffe OB. Atypical lobular hyperplasia or lobular carcinoma in situ at core needle breast biopsy. *Radiology.* 2001;218:503–509.
34. Foster MC, Helvie MA, Gregory NE, et al. Lobular carcinoma in situ or atypical lobular hyperplasia at core-needle biopsy: is excisional biopsy necessary? *Radiology.* 2004;231:813–819.
35. Mahoney MC, Robinson-Smith TM, Shaughnessy EA. Lobular neoplasia at 11-gauge vacuum-assisted stereotactic biopsy: correlation with surgical excisional biopsy and mammographic follow-up. *AJR Am J Roentgenol.* 2006;187:949–954.
36. Karabakhtsian RG, Johnson R, Sumkin J, et al. The clinical significance of lobular neoplasia on breast core biopsy. *Am J Surg Pathol.* 2007;31:717–723.
37. Elsheikh TM, Silverman JF. Follow-up surgical excision is indicated when breast core needle biopsies show atypical lobular hyperplasia or lobular carcinoma in situ: a correlative study of 33 patients with review of the literature. *Am J Surg Pathol.* 2005;29:534–543.
38. Lewis JL, Lee DY, Tartter PI. The significance of lobular carcinoma in situ and atypical lobular hyperplasia of the breast. *Ann Surg Oncol.* 2012;19:4124–4128.
39. Esserman LE, Lamea L, Tanev S, et al. Should the extent of lobular neoplasia on core biopsy influence the decision for excision? *Breast J.* 2007;13:55–61.
40. Nagi CS, O'Donnell JE, Tismenetsky M, et al. Lobular neoplasia on core needle biopsy does not require excision. *Cancer.* 2008;112:2152–2158.
41. Destounis SV, Murphy PF, Seifert PJ, et al. Management of patients diagnosed with lobular carcinoma in situ at needle core biopsy at a community based outpatient facility. *AJR Am J Roentgenol.* 2012;198:281–287.
42. Atkins KA, Cohen MA, Nicholson B, et al. Atypical lobular hyperplasia and lobular carcinoma in situ at core breast biopsy: use of careful radiologic-pathologic correlation to recommend excision or observation. *Radiology.* 2013;269:340–347.
43. Brem RF, Lechner MC, Jackman RJ, et al. Lobular neoplasia at percutaneous breast biopsy: variables associated with carcinoma at surgical excision. *AJR Am J Roentgenol.* 2008;190:637–641.
44. Krishnamurthy S, Bevers T, Kuerer H, et al. Multidisciplinary considerations in the management of high-risk breast lesions. *AJR Am J Roentgenol.* 2012;198:W132–W140.
45. Rosen EL, Bentley RC, Baker JA, et al. Imaging-guided core needle biopsy of papillary lesions of the breast. *AJR Am J Roentgenol.* 2002;179:1185–1192.
46. Shin HJ, Kim HH, Kim SM, et al. Papillary lesions of the breast diagnosed at percutaneous sonographically guided biopsy: comparison of sonographic features and biopsy methods. *AJR Am J Roentgenol.* 2008;190:630–636.
47. Kopans DB, Meyer J. Versatile spring hookwire breast lesion localizer. *AJR Am J Roentgenol.* 1982;138:586–587.

48. Kopans DB, Deluca S. A modified needle-hookwire breast lesion localizer. *AJR Am J Roentgenol.* 1982;138:586–587.
49. Kopans DB, Lindfors K, McCarthy KA, et al. Spring hookwire breast lesion localizer: use of rigid-compression mammographic systems. *Radiology.* 1985;157:537–538.
50. Kopans DB, Swann CA. Preoperative imaging-guided needle placement and localization of clinically occult breast lesions. *AJR Am J Roentgenol.* 1989;152:1–9.
51. Homer MJ. Nonpalpable breast lesion localization using a curved-end retractable wire. *Radiology.* 1985;157:259–260.
52. Gisvold JJ, Martin JK. Prebiopsy localization of nonpalpable breast lesions. *AJR Am J Roentgenol.* 1984;143:477–481.
53. Hall FM, Frank HA. Preoperative localization of nonpalpable breast lesions. *AJR Am J Roentgenol.* 1979;132:101–105.
54. Meyer JE, Kopans DB, Stomper PC, et al. Occult breast abnormalities: percutaneous preoperative needle localization. *Radiology.* 1984;150:335–337.
55. Kalisher L. An improved needle for localization of nonpalpable breast lesions. *Radiology.* 1978;128:815–817.
56. Holland R. The role of specimen x-ray in the diagnosis of breast cancer. *Diagn Imaging Clin Med.* 1985;54:178–185.
57. Rebner M, Pennes DR, Baker DE, et al. Two view specimen radiography in surgical biopsy of nonpalpable breast masses. *AJR Am J Roentgenol.* 1987;149:283–285.
58. Cardenosa G, Eklund GW. Paraffin block radiography following breast biopsies: use of orthogonal views. *Radiology.* 1991;180:873–874.
59. Rebner M, Helvie MA, Pennes DR, et al. Paraffin tissue block radiography: adjunct to breast specimen radiography. *Radiology.* 1989;173:695–696.

CHAPTER SELF-ASSESSMENT QUESTIONS

1. Given this ductogram image, what do you think is indicated?

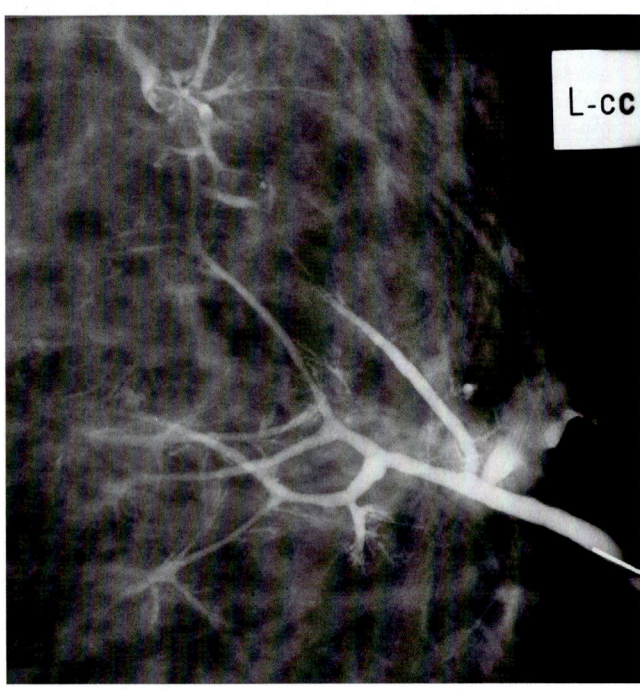

  A. Repeat ductogram
  B. Preoperative ductography and wire localization
  C. Magnetic resonance imaging
  D. Ultrasound

2. Patient with saline implants. Implant in the field of view (top-left and top-right), implant displaced (bottom-left and bottom-right), and photographically coned images of the left breast (left and right, respectively, in the following page). Arrows indicate location of relevant findings (seen best on the photographically coned images in the following page) on the displaced views. How would you approach this patient for preoperative wire localization?

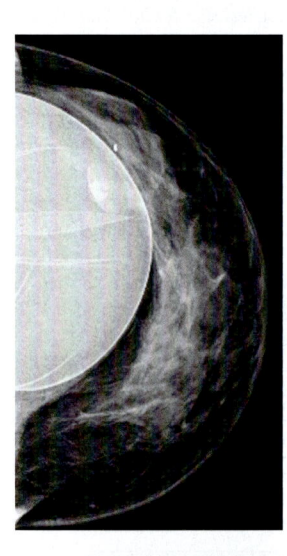
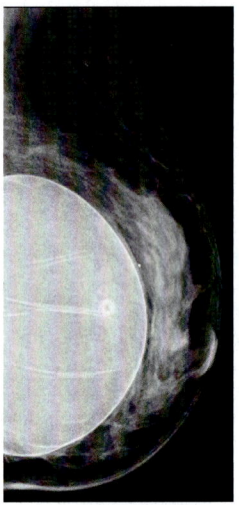
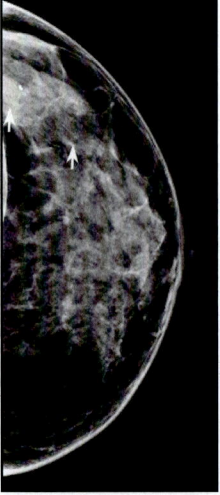
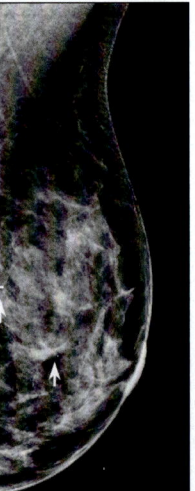

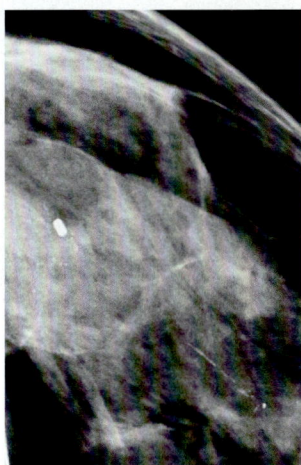
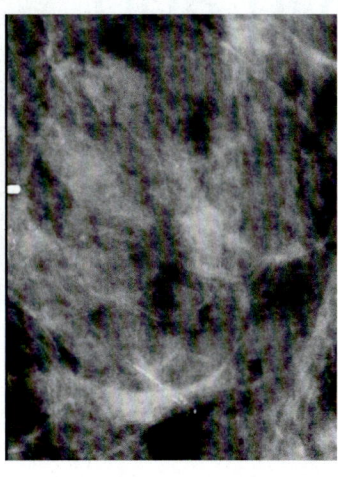

A. Given the implant, preoperative wire localization of the posterior most area (clip with surrounding calcifications) is not possible.
B. Given the implant, the patient is best managed with a mastectomy.
C. Use one wire to localize the clip and surrounding calcifications, and ask the surgeon to extend the dissection anteriorly and inferiorly to the second cluster.
D. Displace the implant for an LM projection and use two wires to localize the two clusters of calcifications.

Answers to Chapter Self-Assessment Questions

1. B An intraductal lesion is present (upper aspect of the image at the level of the LT CC marker). The lesion is several centimeters from the nipple in a nondilated side branch of the opacified duct. The likelihood that this will be identified reliably with ultrasound or intraoperatively by the surgeon is low. Magnetic resonance imaging is not indicated in this patient. Although a papilloma is suspected, an excisional biopsy is indicated (DCIS is in the differential and the patient is symptomatic). To localize the lesion accurately for the surgeon and pathologist on the day of surgery, a ductogram is done and used to guide a wire localization of the lesion.

2. D This patient has two lesions: a biopsy-proven invasive ductal carcinoma at the site of (biopsy clip) with surrounding malignant-type calcifications and a second separate cluster of fine linear branching calcifications that is approximately 2 cm inferior and medial to the site of the known malignancy. Implants are not a contraindication for needle biopsy, preoperative wire localization, or lumpectomy. Appropriate management of this patient requires localization of the two lesions to ensure adequate excision and pathologic evaluation. The lesions are closest to the lateral aspect of the breast, and as such a 90-degree lateral (LM) view with implant displacement is the starting point for the wire localization.

Communication and Accountability in Breast Imaging

13

LEARNING OBJECTIVES

1. Communication
2. The mammography report
   - Required components for reports—report organization
   - Assessment categories—BI-RADS
3. The probably benign concept
   - Definition of concept
   - Appropriate uses of this designation
   - Imaging algorithm for patients with a probably benign lesion
   - Likelihood of malignancy for different lesion types
4. Patient notification letters
5. Medical audit
   - Raw data needed
   - Derived data
   - Benchmarks

Communication in breast imaging is critical and takes many forms. Direct verbal communication with patients, family members, surgeons, pathologists, radiation and medical oncologists, plastic surgeons, and referring physicians is needed and helpful in optimizing patient care. Start by thinking of patients who present for breast imaging as "your patients." You are their doctor with respect to breast diseases. This simple acknowledgment brings with it incredible responsibilities. Consider the trust a patient places in you when she presents for screening or diagnostic mammography. I would suggest that this trust is one of the greatest honors anyone of us can be accorded. How do you handle this? Do you hide behind useless disclaimers in reports that say nothing? Do you have others speak for you? Do you see yourself as "just the radiologist"? After you have done a biopsy on a patient because you think she might have breast cancer, when and who discusses the results with her? Does she languish for days or a week or more waiting for the phone to ring? If we abdicate our responsibility to communicate biopsy results directly with patients, who establishes concordance between imaging and histological findings and who determines what the next step should be? Based on the imaging findings, are you involved and advocating for appropriate management of your patients?

The anxiety, concerns, and multiplicity of questions patients bring with them need to be recognized, accepted, and effectively addressed. I encourage direct communication with patients at every step of the process. Educate your patients and involve them in the decision-making process. I encourage residents and fellows to develop what is undoubtedly an art: how to approach patients, make them feel comfortable, and present them with options, recommendations, and results. We need to learn how to recognize when patients are ready to hear what we have to tell them and when it is appropriate to hold back.

In our practice, breast-imaging radiologists see all of our diagnostic patients. We see it as an opportunity to obtain a complete history from the patient with pertinent negatives, examine the patient, and do an ultrasound study if needed. Depending on the mammographic findings, an ultrasound, ductogram, or imaging-guided biopsies may be done. At each step, the radiologist communicates directly with the patient and involves her in the decision-making process. When discussing the need for a biopsy with a patient, I do not specifically mention the likelihood of cancer. I encourage questions and use them to guide me with respect to how in-depth the discussion needs to go. After the biopsy is done, I provide patients my card, which includes my office number, pager number, and email address, should any issues arise before I see them for their follow-up visit. I give them my cell number if I know I will be out of pager range. Immediately before I leave the room, I walk over to the patient, look her in the eye, and ask her if she has any questions for me. Most patients tell me they have no more questions for me. Some will, at that point, specifically ask me if I think what we biopsied is likely to be breast cancer. If it is, I tell them that I am concerned it could be but that we will have definitive results the next day. I take the question as an indication that they are ready to hear the answer. Honesty and direct answers have repeatedly served me well.

Following imaging-guided biopsies, we see most of our patients back the next business day. During the follow-up visit, we examine the biopsy site and, most importantly, discuss the results of the biopsy with her directly. When discussing results with a patient, particularly with a cancer diagnosis, I sit down, try to relax, and look them in the eyes. After giving them the results, I stop for a few minutes and give them time to process the information after which I let their questions again guide my discussion. I will sometimes gently extend a hand and touch their arm or shoulder. A box of tissues is always nearby so, if needed, I do not have to leave the room. In approaching these discussions, I keep in mind the one question I think most patients are considering even if they don't ask: "Am I going to die?" For many patients, this is immediately followed by another question that they often do not want to ask: "will I lose my breast?" So, I listen carefully for what the patient asks as well as what she does not ask to help guide me in how much information she is prepared to hear. I do not push information unless I think the patient is prepared to hear it. If the patient asks no questions, I refrain from saying anything regarding treatment options. I remind her that she has my card and I am available should she have any questions or if I can help in any way moving forward.

If the patient asks about treatment options, I provide an overview and make it clear that the surgeon will go into specifics and provide more details. I discuss appropriate options applicable to a given patient's situation. If, for an individual patient, I think one option is medically better suited than others, I provide the patient with my specific recommendation. I view it as my job and responsibility to not only give patients options but to specifically tell them what I think is best given their specific circumstance. Yet, I support and help them regardless of the decision they make. For the patients diagnosed with breast cancer, we make appointments for them for a breast MRI and to see one of our surgical oncologists. These patients leave our center knowing what to expect next, all needed appointments scheduled, and the assurance that we are available to help them through the process. If the biopsy results are benign and congruent with the imaging finding, we return the patient to annual screening.

Unfortunately, over the years, we have tried hard to insulate ourselves from patients by talking about "cases" and using words with implied negative connotations like "complain," "refuse," and "deny." We think of *patients* who present "*describing*" or "*reporting*" a symptom, or "*stating*" that they have no symptoms related to their breasts and who may "*decline*" a study or procedure we recommend. I think it is critical not to judge patients and recognize that they are often anxious and scared. Some are angry. It is not for me to judge someone if they have chosen to delay seeking care, but rather to help them once they have come to me for help. If a patient elects to forgo a procedure, I do not slam the door closed because she has chosen not to follow my recommendation, but rather, I leave the door wide open so she can walk back through it when she is ready. They usually come or call back seeking my help.

As clinical breast imagers, we are in a unique position to transition patients through a breast cancer diagnosis. Stop for a moment and consider the path many take: they have a screening mammogram and are otherwise feeling fine. They are called back for further evaluation, undergo a biopsy, and a couple of days later are being told they have breast cancer. Now what? How we handle the communications and help our patients through what can be an overwhelming process is critical. We can make a difference beyond having found an early potentially curable cancer and we should be focused on facilitating the process and advocating for optimal patient management.

THE MAMMOGRAPHY REPORT

As a critical form of communication, the mammographic report needs to be concise, accurate, and directive. It should be *clinically relevant*. For screening exams, a report with pertinent negatives is used for normal studies and a report stating there is a possible mass or a mass, distortion, or calcifications requiring further evaluation is issued for potentially abnormal studies. Description and characterization of findings is relegated to the diagnostic setting. Time and time again we find that the information available to us on the screening study is limited and may actually be misleading. In our opinion, trying to make definitive statements on a screening study is not optimal. As discussed in Chapter 2, the only assessment categories we use for screening studies are "1" (negative), "2" (benign), and "0" (need additional imaging evaluation or need prior studies for comparison).

In women who are called back for evaluation of a potential lesion on their screening mammogram, we need to first establish whether the lesion is real and, if it is, characterize it and make a decision about the next appropriate step. For a diagnostic exam in a patient presenting with a sign or symptom that may be related to a breast cancer, we need to correlate imaging findings (if any) to the area of clinical concern. This may require one or two mammographic images or an ultrasound and in some patients an imaging-guided needle biopsy. The bottom line: is there a finding that may represent breast cancer? What is the next step? Return to screen? Short-interval follow-up because you can justify that the lesion is probably benign? Or biopsy? On diagnostic studies all assessment categories are used although category "0" is rarely used (when prior studies have not reached our facility ahead of a diagnostic appointment). Our diagnostic reports are succinct in terms of characterizing the finding, describing the location and size, and providing specific recommendations or doing what we think is indicated for the patient.

Before dictating a report, ask yourself: what is clinically relevant? Review films with comparisons (if available) and make a decision as to what you think is going on; provide an appropriate recommendation and direction. Focus immediately on the relevant observations. Do not use the report to make up your mind, as you are describing every inconsequential "ditzel" and benign finding. If you do not have enough information to make up your mind, then do whatever you need to do to get the information. On clinically occult lesions, the radiologist interpreting the mammogram needs to provide guidance and a final recommendation.

Read your reports. Do they make sense? Are they logical and do they follow a logical progression? Or do you jump from one finding to the next or from one breast or axilla to the other? Make every effort to issue reports that are clinically relevant and helpful to the clinician. Eliminate excessive verbiage that is often confusing and can be misleading. Be precise; instead of saying a mass is small or large give a measurement in three planes. The description of a finding goes in the body of the report. The description of the findings needs to support and justify your impression and final recommendation. The impression should be succinct and a repetition of the findings is not appropriate. (Please see Appendix A for tables with ACR BI-RADS® lexicons for mammography, ultrasound and MRI findings).

In organizing your mammography reports provide the information listed in Table 13.1 (1–3). Examples of some of the templates we use for our screening and diagnostic reports are provided in Tables 13.2 and 13.3.

THE PROBABLY BENIGN CONCEPT

In order to demonstrate the viability of this concept, several issues need to be considered: (i) the imaging features of the lesions had to be defined so that lesions could be classified easily; (ii) the lesions placed

Table 13.1 **MAMMOGRAPHY REPORT OUTLINE**

Type of study (screening, diagnostic, ultrasound, etc.)
Reason for study
Comparison studies
Tissue type
Description of findings with pertinent negatives when appropriate
Location of lesion
Impression
Recommendation
Assessment category (required under the Mammography Quality Standards Act for all mammographic studies)
• BI-RADS 1: negative
• BI-RADS 2: benign
• BI-RADS 3: probably benign finding
• BI-RADS 4: suspicious abnormality, biopsy is indicated
    BI-RADS 4A (low suspicion)
    BI-RADS 4B (moderate suspicion)
    BI-RADS 4C (high suspicion)
• BI-RADS 5: highly suggestive of malignancy; biopsy is indicated
• BI-RADS 6: known biopsy-proven malignancy
• BI-RADS 0: incomplete, need additional imaging evaluation (or prior studies for comparison)

Table 13.2 **SAMPLE SCREENING REPORT TEMPLATES**
NORMAL There is a fibroglandular pattern. No masses or malignant-type calcifications are identified. Compared with prior studies. **IMPRESSION** No specific mammographic evidence of malignancy. Next screening mammogram is recommended in 1 year. BI-RADS 1: Negative. **POSSIBLE MASS** There is a fibrofatty pattern. A possible mass is noted in the right breast. Spot compression views and possible sonography are indicated for further evaluation. No masses or malignant-type calcifications are identified in the left breast. Compared with prior studies. **IMPRESSION** Possible mass, right breast. Additional evaluation is indicated. The patient will be contacted for this and a supplementary report will follow. No specific mammographic evidence of malignancy, left breast. BI-RADS 0: Need additional imaging evaluation. **MASS (SEEN IN TWO PROJECTIONS)** There is a dense fibroglandular pattern. A mass is noted in the right breast. Spot compression views and possible sonography are indicated for further evaluation. No masses or malignant-type calcifications are identified in the left breast. Compared with prior studies. **IMPRESSION** Mass, right breast. Additional evaluation is indicated. The patient will be contacted for this and a supplementary report will follow. No specific mammographic evidence of malignancy, left breast. BI-RADS 0: Need additional imaging evaluation. **CALCIFICATIONS** There is a fibroglandular pattern. A cluster of calcifications is noted in the left breast. Spot compression magnification views are indicated for further evaluation. No masses or malignant-type calcifications are identified in the right breast. Compared with prior studies. **IMPRESSION** Calcifications, left breast. Additional evaluation is indicated. The patient will be contacted for this and a supplementary report will follow. No specific mammographic evidence of malignancy, right breast. **NEED FOR PRIOR STUDIES** There is a fibrofatty pattern. A possible mass is noted in the right breast. Prior films are requested for comparison. No masses or malignant-type calcifications are identified in the left breast. **IMPRESSION** Possible mass, right breast. Awaiting prior films for comparison. A supplementary report with recommendation will follow when these become available. No specific mammographic evidence of malignancy, left breast. BI-RADS 0: Awaiting prior films for comparison.

in this category had to be shown to have low inherent malignant potential; (iii) changes needed to be detectable on follow-up studies; and (iv) it had to be proven that tumors were not upstaged when changes became apparent.

Localized findings defined as probably benign include: (i) clusters of small round or oval calcifications; (ii) *nonpalpable, noncalcified,* round or oval masses with predominantly circumscribed margins regardless of the size of the mass or the age of the patient; (iii) nonpalpable focal asymmetry with concave margins and interspersed fat; and (iv) asymptomatic, single dilated duct. Generalized findings described as probably benign include multiple (three or more) similar, randomly distributed findings bilaterally, including (i) multiple masses with circumscribed margins, (ii) small round or oval calcifications in tight clusters, or (iii) scattered individually throughout the breasts.

The probably benign BI-RADS 3 designation is used in the diagnostic setting only. We do not use this BI-RADS on screening studies since characterization of the lesion is required to justify the designation (1,4–11). Calcifications that appear benign on screening images may represent the "tip of the iceberg" with additional unsuspected calcifications and pleomorphic features on magnification views and sometimes those that appear linear and of concern are identified as benign with additional evaluation. Masses that appear to have circumscribed margins on the screening images may have small spiculations and indistinct margins on spot compression and spot compression magnification views. Ultrasound is undertaken because if the mass is a cyst, short-interval follow-up is not appropriate. Lastly, some of the lesions are characterized as benign after additional mammographic images or ultrasound, and short-interval follow-up is not indicated.

This designation is also only appropriate in women who have no prior studies. If the lesion is present on prior studies with no interval change or a decrease in size, a short-interval follow-up adds no

Table 13.3 SAMPLE DIAGNOSTIC REPORTS

Patient called back for evaluation of a MASS—biopsy needed
Spot compression views confirm the presence of a high-density mass with indistinct margins in the upper inner quadrant of the right breast, posteriorly.
On physical examination, I palpate normal tissue in the upper inner quadrant of the right breast. On ultrasound, a vertically-oriented mass with indistinct margins and shadowing is imaged at 1 o'clock, 7 cm from the right nipple, correlating to the finding described on the mammogram. This mass measures $1.4 \times 1 \times 0.8$ cm. Biopsy is indicated. Morphologically normal-appearing lymph nodes are imaged in the right axilla.

IMPRESSION
Mass, right breast. Biopsy is done and reported separately.
BI-RADS 4: Suspicious abnormality, biopsy is indicated.

Patient called back for evaluation of a MASS—benign
Spot compression views confirm the presence of a low-density mass with circumscribed margins in the upper outer quadrant of the right breast, anteriorly.
On physical examination, I palpate normal tissue in the upper outer quadrant of the right breast. On ultrasound, a cyst measuring $1.2 \times 1.1 \times 0.8$ cm is imaged at 10 o'clock, 2 cm from the right nipple correlating to the finding described on the mammogram. Since the patient is otherwise asymptomatic, no further intervention or short-interval follow-up is indicated.

IMPRESSION
Cyst, right breast. Next screening mammogram is recommended in 1 year.
BI-RADS 2: Benign finding.

Patient called back for evaluation of CALCIFICATIONS—biopsy is needed
Spot compression magnification views confirm a cluster of fine pleomorphic calcifications that includes linear forms in a linear orientation in the upper outer quadrant of the left breast, zone B. These encompass approximately $2 \times 1.5 \times 1$ cm of tissue. Biopsy is indicated.

IMPRESSION
Calcifications, left breast. Biopsy is done and reported separately.
BI-RADS 4: Suspicious abnormality, biopsy is indicated.

SYMPTOMATIC PATIENT
There is a dense fibroglandular pattern. No masses or malignant-type calcifications are identified in the left breast. A high-density lobulated mass with partially indistinct and obscured margins is imaged on a spot tangential view done at the site of a "lump" described by the patient in the upper outer quadrant of the right breast anteriorly.
On physical examination, I palpate a hard fixed mass at 11 o'clock, 2 cm from the right nipple. On ultrasound, a mass with indistinct margins and posterior acoustic enhancement is imaged correlating to the palpable and mammographic findings. This mass measures $2 \times 2.5 \times 1$ cm. Biopsy is indicated. Morphologically normal-appearing lymph nodes are imaged in the right axilla.

IMPRESSION
Mass, right breast. Biopsy is done and reported separately. No specific mammographic evidence of malignancy, left breast.
BI-RADS 4: Suspicious abnormality, biopsy is indicated.

ADDENDUM to reports requesting prior films—no new finding
Prior images from digital studies done at the Breast Center in Richmond, Virginia, on December 2, 2010, and December 2, 2011, are now available for comparison. Nodular asymmetry in the right breast can be seen previously. At this time, no new masses or malignant-type calcifications are identified.

IMPRESSION
No specific mammographic evidence of malignancy. Next screening mammogram is recommended in 1 year.
BI-RADS 1: Negative.

ADDENDUM to reports requesting prior films—call back
Prior images from digital studies done at the Breast Center in Richmond, Virginia, on December 2, 2010, and December 2, 2011, are now available for comparison. Spot compression views and possibly sonography are indicated for further evaluation of a mass in the right breast.

IMPRESSION
Mass, right breast. Additional evaluation is indicated. The patient will be contacted for this and a supplementary report will follow.
BI-RADS 0: Need additional imaging evaluation.

ADDENDUM to reports requesting prior films—no prior studies found
We have been unable to locate prior studies. Spot compression views and correlative physical examination are indicated for further evaluation of a possible mass in the right breast.

IMPRESSION
Possible mass, right breast. The patient will be contacted for this and a supplementary report will follow.
BI-RADS 0: Need additional imaging evaluation.

additional information. If the lesion has developed or increased in size compared with prior studies, and it is solid on ultrasound, a biopsy is indicated (not short-interval follow-up). Tracking the use of this category as part of the medical audit is useful information and may minimize its abuse.

The proposed imaging algorithm for patients with findings fulfilling the criteria for probably benign lesions calls for one extra study of the breast 6 months following the initial study. This is followed by a bilateral diagnostic study 6 months after the unilateral study is done (e.g., 1 year after initial study). Additional annual diagnostic studies are done 24 and 36 months following the initial study. Probably benign lesions and the data in support of follow-up are defined for mammographic findings. No comparable studies have been done to define what constitutes a probably benign lesion on ultrasound or MRI and there is no longitudinal data in support of follow-up (4–9).

As reported by Sickles, the likelihood of malignancy for probably benign lesions is 1.4% for solid masses with circumscribed margins, 0.6% for focal asymmetric densities, 0.4% for localized microcalcifications, 0.3% for multiple solid masses with circumscribed margins, and 0.2% for generalized microcalcifications (6,8). Seventeen cancers were diagnosed among the 3,184 lesions classified as probably benign, with 2 of the 17 cancers identified on the 6-month follow-up study (8). Although these data are used to advocate for 6-month follow-up studies on patients with probably benign lesions, one can argue that since only 2 of the 17 cancers were identified at 6 months, patients with appropriately classified probably benign lesions can be followed at annual intervals.

As already discussed, this category should not be used to circumvent complete mammographic workups or decision-making, nor should it be used for obviously benign lesions. Careful evaluation of lesions is required and strict adherence to the defined morphologic features of lesions is essential. Rosen et al. (10) in 2002, reported on 51 malignancies among 178 lesions assigned to the probably benign category. They found that none of the 51 lesions fulfilled the published criteria for the probably benign finding since 92% of the lesions had already demonstrated progression. These authors emphasize, "placing a lesion into this category is a poor substitute for incomplete or suboptimal evaluation" (10). Motion-blur degrading magnification views, inaccurate or incomplete localization of lesions, and failure to assess interval progression are cited as the most common failures encountered by these authors in reviewing the diagnostic evaluations of patients (10). Similarly, Lehman and colleagues (11) report that at least 80% of lesions designated as probably benign in a community mammography practice did not meet the morphologic criteria for this designation (see below). They describe finding amorphous, pleomorphic, branching and fine linear calcifications as well as masses with indistinct and spiculated margins among the lesions placed into the probably benign category (11). Many of their patients also had prior films available for comparison negating the appropriateness of the probably benign designation. These authors appropriately emphasize that even when strict criteria are applied with respect to the morphologic features of a lesion, it is essential to consider any patient history and clinical information that may increase the risk of malignancy (11).

Following appropriate workup, the findings and low likelihood of malignancy are discussed with the patient. Although a recommendation for short-interval follow-up (e.g., for masses) or annual follow-up (e.g., for calcifications) is made, options of imaging-guided and excisional biopsies are also discussed with the patient. A biopsy may be undertaken if the patient is particularly anxious, unlikely to return for follow-up, or is pregnant or planning a pregnancy.

PATIENT NOTIFICATION LETTERS

As regulated by MQSA, the results of mammographic studies and appropriate recommendations must be communicated directly to patients in writing using lay language. Forms with check-off boxes can be used, and if the studies are interpreted while the patient is still in your department, the notification can be given directly to the patient. If screening studies are batch interpreted, the letters have to be mailed within 30 days of the study. In an increasing number of states, patients with dense tissue must be notified that they have or may have dense tissue; the language to be used in the letters is usually specified by the statutes. In some states, statements regarding associated increased risk for breast cancer are also required.

MEDICAL AUDIT

One of the main purposes of the medical audit is to evaluate the accuracy of mammography and mammographic interpretation (1,12–15). As discussed in Chapter 1, the goal of mammography is the detection of early, potentially curable breast cancer, ideally under 1 cm in size. The medical audit aims to determine whether this goal is being accomplished and how much is being done to accomplish it (e.g., recalls, biopsies, 6-month follow-ups, etc.). It is also an incredibly wonderful teaching and learning tool. With review and feedback from our own follow-ups and biopsies we can improve so, the numbers should not be viewed statically but over a period of time.

For the medical audit, raw data that need to be tracked and collected are listed in Table 13.4 and derived data are listed in Table 13.5 (1,12–15). Please note that there is more than one definition for several of the items evaluated; so be precise when discussing these issues. Desirable goals are detailed in Table 13.6 (1,12–15).

Table 13.4 RAW DATA NEEDED FOR MEDICAL AUDIT

- Patient demographics
  - Age
  - Personal breast cancer history
  - Hormone replacement therapy
  - High-risk lesion on a previous biopsy (atypical ductal hyperplasia, lobular neoplasia)
- Audit periods
- Number of screening studies (asymptomatic women)
- Number of diagnostic studies (abnormal screening mammogram and symptomatic women)
- Number of first-time screens and number of repeat mammograms
- Number of women recalled for additional studies (assessment category "0")
- Number of women with biopsy recommendations (assessment categories "4" and "5")
- Number of short-interval follow-up recommendations (assessment category "3")
- Number of benign and malignant biopsies tracking needle biopsy separate from fine-needle aspiration
- Pathology tumor staging
  - Tumor size, histologic type, and grade
  - Nodal status

Table 13.5 DERIVED DATA FOR MEDICAL AUDIT

True positives (TP)	Breast cancer diagnosed within 1 year after a biopsy
True negative (TN)	No known breast cancer diagnosis within 1 year of a normal mammogram
False negative (FN)	Breast cancer diagnosed within 1 year of a normal mammogram
False positive (FP)	1. No breast cancer diagnosis within 1 year of an abnormal screening (categories "0," "4," and "5") 2. No breast cancer diagnosis within 1 year of an abnormal mammogram 3. Biopsy with benign findings within 1 year of a biopsy recommendation for an abnormal mammogram (categories "4" and "5")
Sensitivity	Probability of detecting cancer when cancer is present TP/(TP + FN)
Specificity	Probability of a normal mammogram when no cancer is present TN/(FP + TN); varies depending on FP definition used
Positive predictive value (PPV)	1. PPV of abnormal findings at screening: percent of screening studies with abnormal findings that result in breast cancer diagnosis TP/(TP + FP1) 2. PPV of biopsy recommendations: percent of patients with a biopsy recommendation with breast cancer diagnosis TP/(TP + FP2) 3. PPV of biopsies done: percent of all known biopsies done that resulted in breast cancer diagnosis TP/(TP + FP3)
Cancer detection rate	Number of cancers detected per 1,000 patients examined with mammography
Minimal breast cancers	Invasive carcinomas sized 1 cm or less or DCIS
Interval breast cancers	Breast cancers that become clinically apparent after a negative mammogram but before next screening mammogram is due

Table 13.6 DESIRED GOALS FOR SCREENING MAMMOGRAPHY

Sensitivity	>75%
Specificity	>90%
PPV	PPV1 = 5%–10%; PPV2 = 25%–40%
Tumor size	>50% stage 0 or 1 (screen detected) >30% are minimal (screen detected)
Node positive breast cancers	<25% of screen-detected cancers should be LN+
Cancer detection rate	6 to 10/1,000 among first screens (prevalent) 2 to 4/1,000 among repeat screeners (incident)
Recall rate	5% to 12% ideally individual improves with experience

References

1. D'Orsi CJ, Sickles EA, Mendelson EB, Morris EA et al. ACR BI-RADS® Atlas, *Breast Imaging Reporting and Data System*. Reston, VA, American College of Radiology; 2013.
2. D'Orsi CJ. *Use of the American College of Radiology Breast Imaging and Data System. RSNA Categorical Course in Breast Imaging Syllabus.* Chicago, IL: RSNA; 1995:77–80.
3. D'Orsi CJ, Kopans DB. Mammographic feature analysis. *Semin Roentgenol.* 1993;28:204–230.
4. Sickles EA. Probably benign breast lesions: when should follow-up be recommended and what is the optimal follow-up protocol? *Radiology.* 1999;213:11–14.
5. Sickles EA. Management of probably benign breast lesions. *Radiol Clin North Am.* 1995;33:1123–1130.
6. Sickles EA. *Management of Probably Benign Lesions. RSNA Categorical Course in Breast Imaging Syllabus.* Chicago, IL: RSNA; 1995:133–138.
7. Sickles EA. Nonpalpable, circumscribed, noncalcified solid breast masses: likelihood of malignancy based on lesion size and age of patient. *Radiology.* 1994;192:439–442.
8. Sickles EA. Periodic mammographic follow-up of probably benign lesions: results in 3,184 consecutive cases. *Radiology.* 1991;179:463–468.
9. Varas X, Leborgne F, Leborgne JH. Nonpalpable, probably benign lesions: role of follow-up mammography. *Radiology.* 1992;184:409–414.
10. Rosen EL, Baker JA, Soo MS. Malignant lesions initially subjected to short-term mammographic follow-up. *Radiology.* 2002;223:221–228.
11. Lehman CD, Rutter CM, Eby PR, et al. Lesion and patient characteristics associated with malignancy after a probably benign finding on community practice mammography. *AJR Am J Roentgenol.* 2008;190:511–515.
12. Sickles EA. Quality assurance: how to audit your own mammography practice. *Radiol Clin North Am.* 1992;30:265–275.
13. Linver MN, Osuch JR, Brenner RJ, et al. The mammography audit: a primer for the Mammography Quality Standards Act (MQSA). *AJR Am J Roentgenol.* 1995;165:19–25.
14. Linver MN. Plaudits for audits: the whys, wherefores and therefores. *Breast Imaging Categorical Course Syllabus.* American Roentgen Ray Society (99th Annual meeting); May 9–14, 1999; New Orleans, LA.
15. Sickles EA. *Auditing Your Practice. RSNA Syllabus Categorical Course in Breast Imaging.* Chicago, IL: RSNA; 1995:81–91.

CHAPTER SELF-ASSESSMENT QUESTIONS

1. Diagnostic left craniocaudal (top-left) and mediolateral oblique (top-right) views 6 months after a normal screening mammogram; ultrasound image (bottom) of the left breast at the time of current mammogram is also provided. Screening study six months ago represents a:

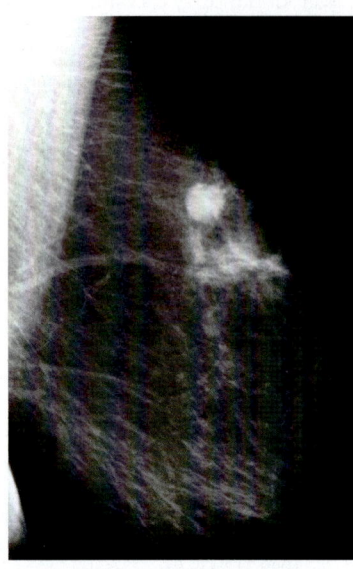
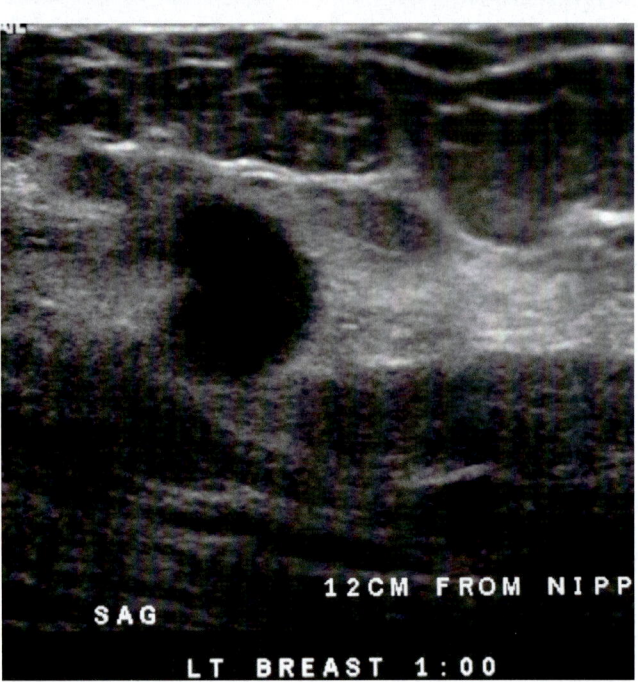

A. False-negative mammogram
B. False-positive mammogram
C. True-negative mammogram
D. True-positive mammogram

2. Spot tangential (left) and ultrasound image (right) of a palpable finding in a 40-year-old patient. Excisional biopsy confirms core biopsy diagnosis of malignant phyllodes. The diagnostic evaluation in this patient is considered:

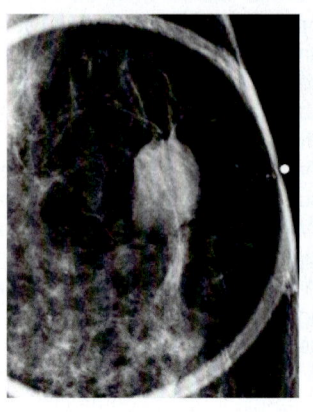
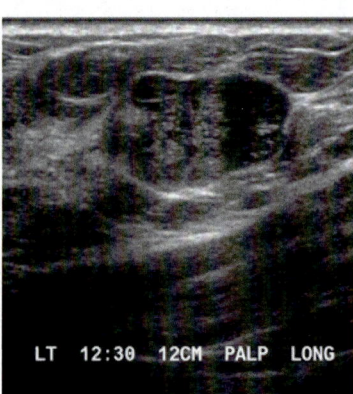

A. False-negative mammogram
B. False-positive mammogram
C. True-negative mammogram
D. True-positive mammogram

Answers to Chapter Self-Assessment Questions

1. A A false-negative screening study is defined as a tissue diagnosis of breast cancer within 1 year of the negative study (1). In the patient presented, the screening study was interpreted as negative. Six months later, she presents with a dense mass in the left breast and an ultrasound-guided biopsy confirms the suspected diagnosis of an invasive ductal carcinoma, high nuclear grade.

2. B False-positive studies may have three separate definitions (see Table 13.5). In this patient, a malignant phyllodes tumor is diagnosed on core biopsy; however, this is not breast cancer, and as such it is not a "true positive" but rather a false-positive study. The false-positive designation also applies to pathology-proven high-risk lesions (e.g., atypical ductal hyperplasia, atypical lobular hyperplasia, lobular carcinoma in situ, etc.) as well as breast sarcomas, lymphoma, metastases to the breast, and malignant phyllodes (1).

Self-Assessment Exam

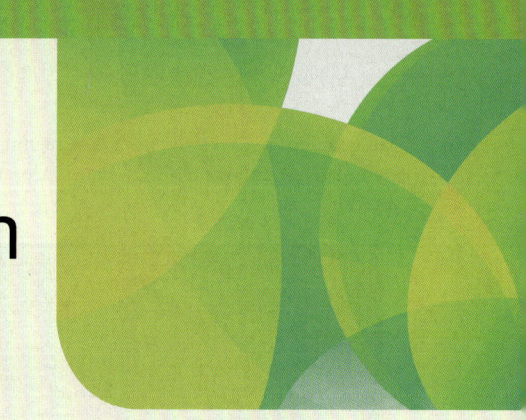

Self-Assessment Questions

1. What is the appropriate management for the patient with the lesion shown here?

   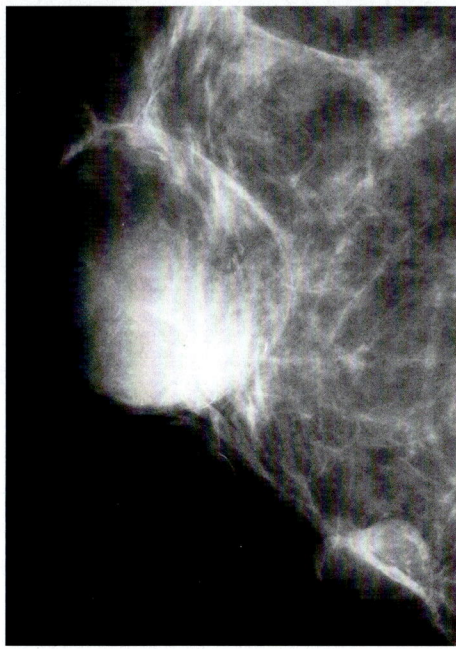

   A. Ultrasound
   B. Biopsy
   C. Annual screening mammography
   D. Short-interval follow-up

2. Sentinel lymph node biopsy is relatively contraindicated in
   A. Patients with multicentric disease
   B. Pregnancy
   C. Men with breast cancer
   D. Obese and older patients

3. Psammoma bodies in an axillary lymph node biopsy likely reflect metastatic disease from
   A. A necrotic invasive ductal carcinoma
   B. Ductal carcinoma in situ
   C. Endometrial carcinoma
   D. Papillary thyroid carcinoma

4. In this patient with a core biopsy-proven diagnosis of invasive ductal carcinoma, what would you recommend next?

   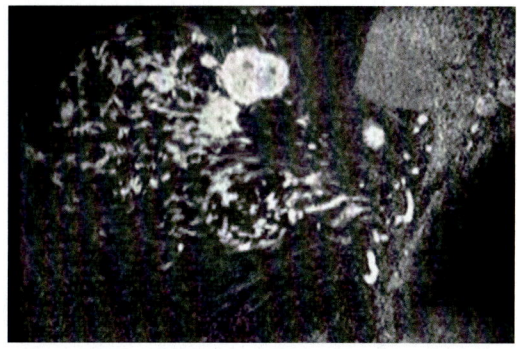

   A. "Second-look" ultrasound
   B. MRI-guided biopsy of non-mass like enhancement
   C. Mastectomy
   D. Lumpectomy with bracketing

5. In tumor staging, the "*yp*" designation defines pathology findings after
   A. Neo-adjuvant therapy
   B. Lumpectomy
   C. Sentinel lymph node biopsy
   D. Radiation therapy

6. The increased risk of breast cancer following high-dose radiation to the chest
   A. Peaks 20 to 25 years after the exposure occurs
   B. Preferentially affects the medial quadrants of the breasts
   C. Applies to men and women equally
   D. Applies to patients exposed between the ages of 10 and 30

7. Craniocaudal (CC) views from a screening mammogram. The mediolateral oblique (MLO) views are normal. What would you do?

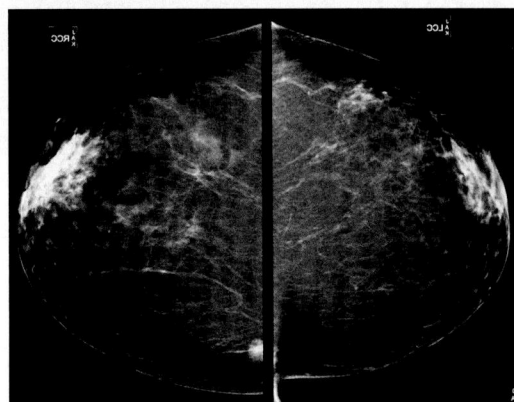

   A. Ask the technologist to check for a seborrheic keratosis
   B. Spot compression cleavage view and a 90-degree LM view
   C. Repeat the MLO view with attention to positioning
   D. Recommend 6-month follow-up for probably benign lesion

8. Criteria for lesion designation and longitudinal data in support of the probably benign concept are available for findings on
   A. Mammography
   B. Ultrasound
   C. Magnetic resonance imaging
   D. Physical examination

9. Which of the following is a common finding on ductography in patients with papillomas?
   A. Normal caliber but attenuated duct
   B. Narrowing of the duct
   C. Duct dilatation between the lesion and the nipple
   D. Contrast extravasation at the site of the lesion

10. What history most likely explains the findings in this patient?

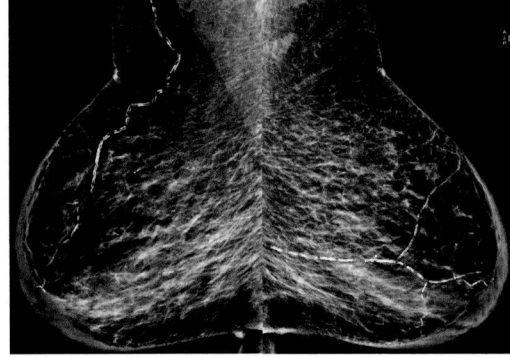

   A. Radiation therapy
   B. Adult-onset diabetes
   C. Hormone replacement therapy
   D. Renal failure

11. Which of the following is the likely stage in a patient presenting with Paget disease of the nipple and a 0.7-cm invasive lesion diagnosed following an MRI with normal-appearing regional lymph nodes:
    A. Stage 0
    B. Stage IA
    C. Stage IB
    D. Stage IIA

12. Breast cancer is most commonly diagnosed by
    A. Breast self-examination
    B. Clinical breast examination
    C. Screening mammography
    D. Screening breast ultrasound

13. Spot tangential view on a patient presenting with a new "lump." What is indicated?

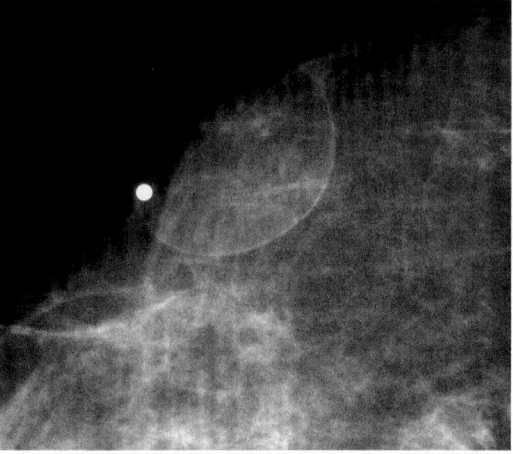

    A. A screening mammogram in 1 year
    B. Short-interval follow-up
    C. Correlative physical examination and ultrasound
    D. Fine-needle aspiration

14. The lesion associated with the highest lifetime risk for breast cancer is
    A. Atypical ductal hyperplasia
    B. Complex fibroadenomas
    C. Atypical lobular hyperplasia
    D. Lobular carcinoma in situ

15. Benchmark for screening mammography program
    A. Recall rates of 20% to 25%
    B. One cancer per 1,000 women screened
    C. Less than 25% of diagnosed breast cancers should be node positive
    D. Ductal carcinoma in at least 20% of patients

16. Under the Mammography Quality Standards Act (MQSA) mammography facilities must be
    A. Accredited every other year
    B. Inspected annually by Food and Drug Administration (FDA) or FDA designee
    C. Accredited by FDA
    D. Certified by ACR

17. What is appropriate a patient with a lesion having these imaging features?

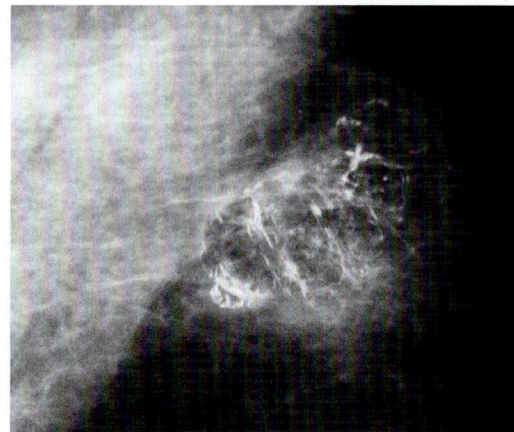

   A. Screening mammogram in 1 year
   B. Short-interval follow-up
   C. Spot compression magnification views
   D. Biopsy

18. Sentinel lymph node biopsies are usually done in patients
   A. With inflammatory carcinoma
   B. Undergoing mastectomy for DCIS
   C. With clinically abnormal lymph nodes
   D. With known metastatic disease to the liver

19. Stage of patients with a complete pathologic response (cPR) following neo-adjuvant therapy?
   A. Based on findings at the time of presentation
   B. Stage 0
   C. Based on the clinical findings after therapy
   D. Not provided

20. Given this mediolateral oblique view

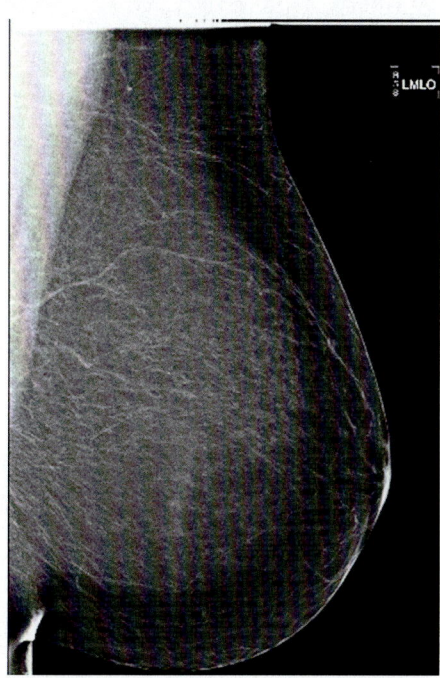

   A. An incorrect angle of obliquity was selected
   B. The service engineer needs to be contacted
   C. The grid was not plugged in
   D. Patient-related artifact

21. In patients with Zuska disease
   A. Ductal carcinoma in situ is diagnosed in as many as 50%
   B. No treatment is needed
   C. Periareolar fistula forms related to a subareolar abscess
   D. A punch biopsy of the skin is needed to establish the diagnosis

22. At this point in mammographically guided preoperative wire localizations, why is a spot compression paddle used?

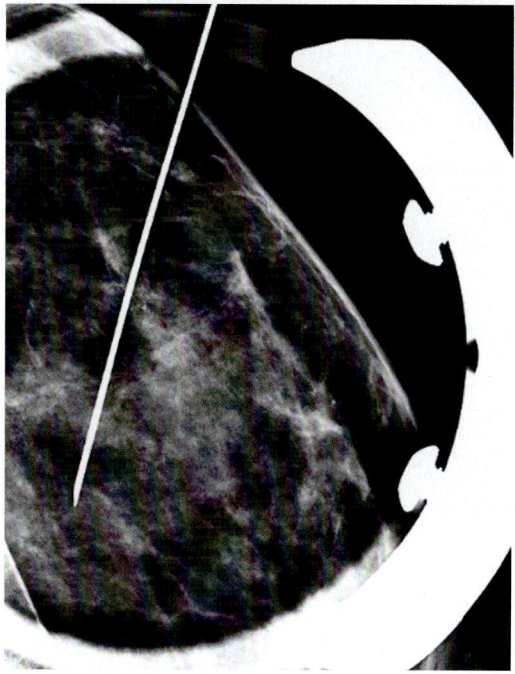

   A. To maximize immobilization of the patient
   B. To maximize visualization of the lesion
   C. Technologist preference
   D. Facilitates depth adjustment of needle

23. Rim calcifications are common in which of the following?
   A. Oil cysts
   B. Treated breast lymphoma
   C. Fibroadenomas
   D. Necrotic tumors

24. Which of the following is sometimes used to distinguish tubular carcinoma from sclerosing adenosis?
   A. E-cadherin
   B. Estrogen receptors
   C. p63
   D. Polarizing microscopy

25. On the basis of these images, what is indicated?

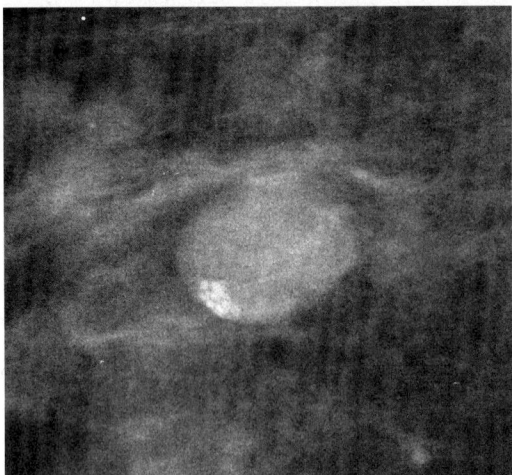
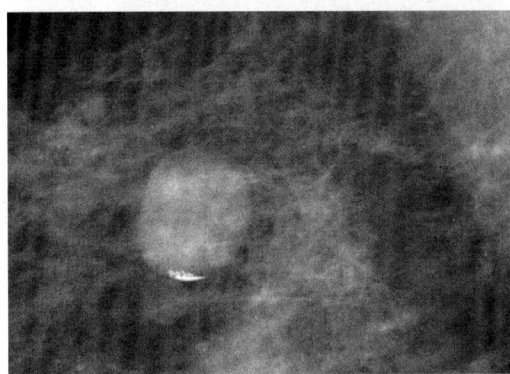

A. Annual screening mammography
B. Follow-up mammography in 6 months
C. Ultrasound
D. 90-Degree lateral view

26. Lesion measurements in breast imaging reports

A. Are best approximated with words such as small, medium, and large
B. Are not needed since size of tumors is best determined histologically
C. Should always be provided in three dimensions
D. Are not as accurate as those established clinically

27. On mammography, which of the following is the descriptor for the margins of a mass?

A. Stellate
B. Angular
C. Irregular
D. Obscured

28. Spot compression and ultrasound images. Which of the following is the likely diagnosis?

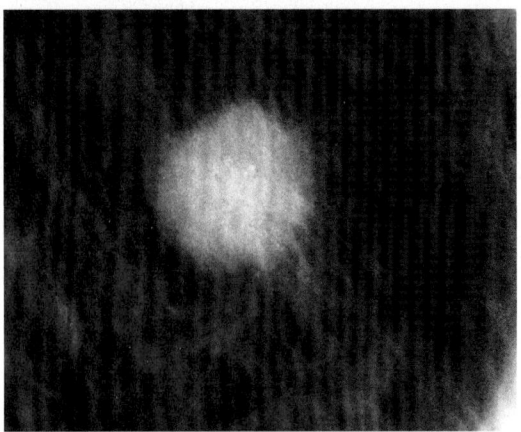
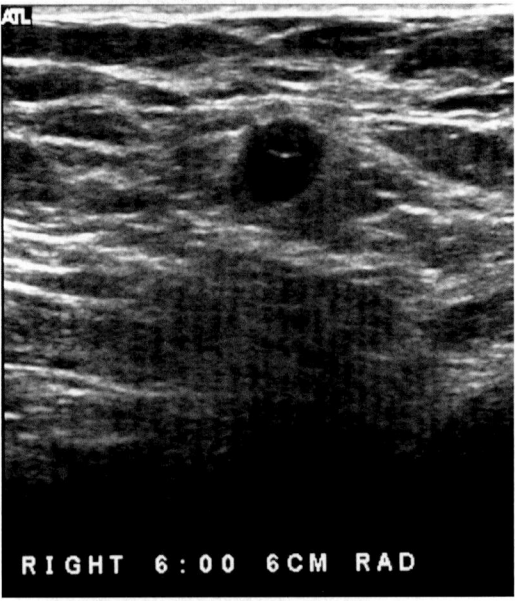

A. Cyst
B. Invasive ductal carcinoma, high grade
C. Invasive lobular carcinoma, low grade
D. Fibroadenoma

29. Which of the following is the most common cause of spontaneous nipple discharge?

A. Papilloma
B. Ductal carcinoma in situ
C. Duct ectasia
D. Fibrocystic changes

30. The diagnosis of inflammatory breast cancer requires

A. Identification of invasive lobular carcinoma histologically
B. Erythema, increased breast temperature, and peau d'orange changes
C. Presence of cancer cells in subdermal lymphatics
D. Diffuse changes mammographically

31. Gynecomastia is
    A. A risk factor for the subsequent development of breast cancer
    B. Almost always symmetrical
    C. Associated with reactive adenopathy
    D. Glandular tissue centered on the subareolar area

32. In this patient what is appropriate?

    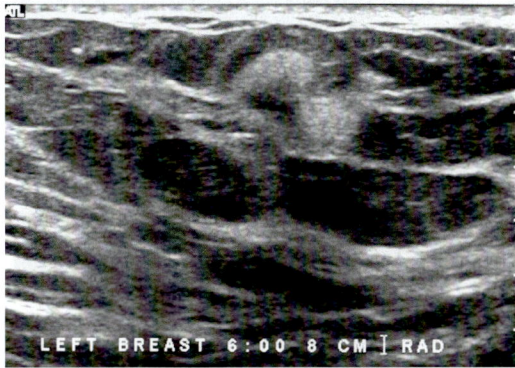

    A. Screening mammography
    B. Short-interval follow-up
    C. Core biopsy
    D. MRI

33. Under MQSA which of the following is required information on all mammography images?
    A. Name, city, state, and zip code for facility
    B. Initials of interpreting radiologist
    C. kV used for exposure
    D. Compression force

34. Which of the following is a precursor to invasive breast cancer in some patients?
    A. Multiple peripheral papillomas
    B. Lobular carcinoma in situ
    C. Atypical ductal hyperplasia
    D. Complex sclerosing lesions

35. Screening mammogram. What is your recommendation?

    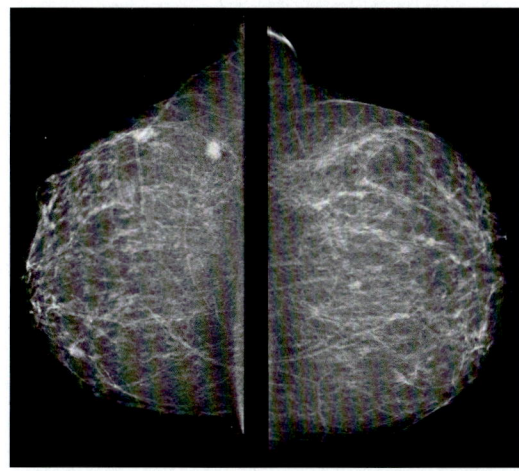

    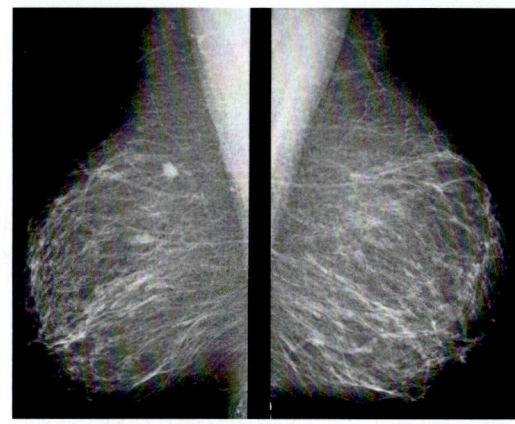

    A. Screening mammography in 1 year
    B. Biopsy
    C. Short-interval follow-up
    D. Additional imaging evaluation

36. A level I noncompliance violation following an FDA inspection of a mammography facility requires
    A. A written response to the FDA
    B. Immediate corrective action
    C. Corrective action before the next annual FDA inspection
    D. Corrective action within 30 days of the inspection

37. In reviewing this patient's history, what specifically are you looking for?

    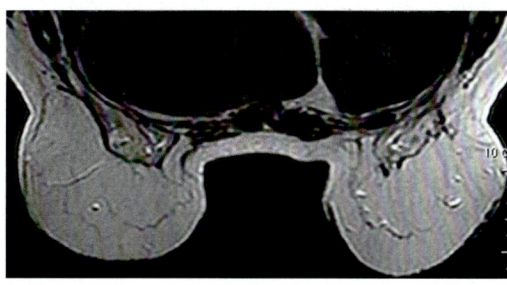

    A. TRAM flap reconstructions
    B. Prior trauma with air bag deployment
    C. Implant rupture
    D. Reduction mammoplasty

38. Low nuclear grade DCIS and LCIS are found associated with which of following invasive lesion in more than 50% of patients?
    A. Mucinous carcinoma
    B. Metaplastic carcinoma
    C. Medullary carcinoma
    D. Tubular carcinoma

39. Why was the MLO projection selected over the 90-degree lateral to be one of the screening views?
    A. Easier to position the patient
    B. Less painful
    C. Maximizes tissue inclusion
    D. Minimizes confusion between LM and ML

40. Which of the following lesions requires excisional biopsy when diagnosed on a core biopsy?
    A. Pseudoangiomatous stromal hyperplasia (PASH)
    B. Fibroepithelial lesion
    C. Complex fibroadenoma
    D. Apocrine metaplasia

41. Given the ultrasound features of this palpable mass in the left breast, what is the first thing you want to ask this patient about?

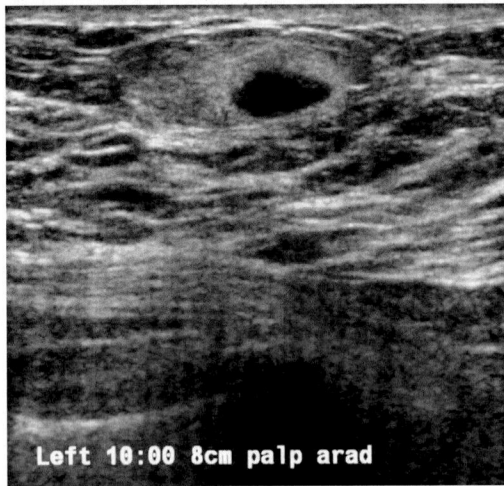

    A. Lactation
    B. Biopsy
    C. Mastitis
    D. Trauma

42. Which of the following describes the ultrasound appearance of many papillary carcinomas?
    A. Vertically oriented mass with intense shadowing
    B. Irregular mass with a thickened echogenic rim
    C. Complex cystic and solid mass
    D. Isoechoic and difficult to identify with ultrasound

43. Signal-to-noise ratios are calculated
    A. Using the phantom image
    B. By the radiologist at the workstation
    C. Semiannually using software in the digital unit
    D. On every patient

44. Small mass with spiculated margins
    A. Mucinous
    B. Medullary
    C. Papillary
    D. Tubular

45. What is the likely diagnosis in this patient?

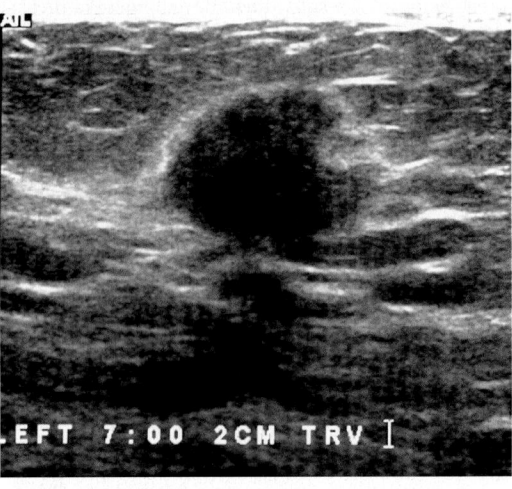

    A. Invasive ductal carcinoma, high grade
    B. Inflamed cyst
    C. Papillary lesion
    D. Reactive lymph node

46. Under MQSA, repeat analysis needs to be done
    A. Weekly
    B. Monthly
    C. Quarterly
    D. Semiannually

47. Which of the following is a common pathologic finding in patients with a subareolar abscess?
    A. Flat epithelial atypia
    B. Lobular carcinoma in situ
    C. Squamous metaplasia
    D. Columnar cell change

48. Ultrasound of "lump" described by the patient in the right breast. What is your recommendation?

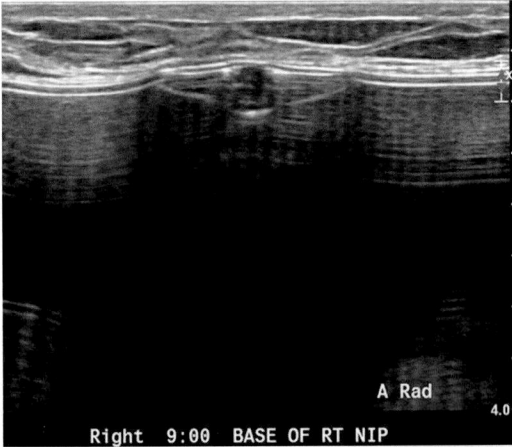

    A. Screening mammography in 1 year
    B. Referral to a plastic surgeon
    C. Short-interval follow-up
    D. US-guided fine-needle aspiration

49. Granular cell tumors reportedly arise from
    A. Epithelial cells
    B. Endothelial cells
    C. Fibroblasts
    D. Schwann cells

50. In women with silicone implants, mammography effectively demonstrates
    A. Capsule formation
    B. Intracapsular rupture
    C. Gel bleed
    D. Extracapsular rupture

51. MLO views from a screening mammogram. The CC views are normal. What would you do?

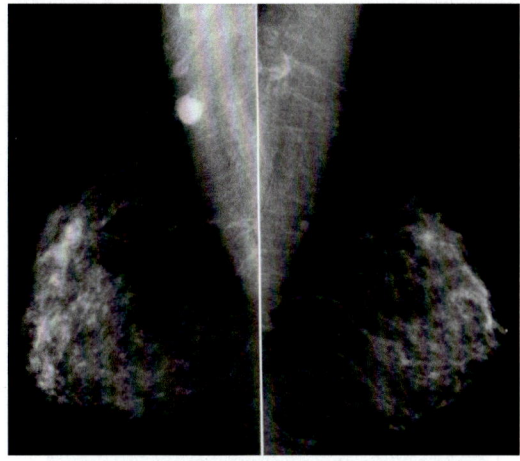

    A. Ultrasound lateral quadrants and the axillary tail of the right breast
    B. Spot in oblique projection and obtain a 90-degree lateral view
    C. Probable lymph node, recommend 6-month follow-up
    D. Benign finding, recommend screening mammography in 1 year

52. Screening MRI should be considered for a patient with
    A. An 18% lifetime risk for breast cancer
    B. A history of lymphoma and chest wall radiation at age 35
    C. Dense breast tissue and a personal history of breast cancer
    D. A first-degree relative with a known BRCA1 mutation

53. Given this specimen radiograph, what do you want to discuss with the surgeon?

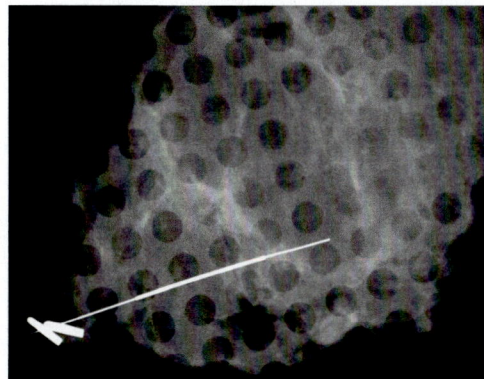

    A. Proximity of the lesion to one of the margins
    B. No obvious lesion is apparent
    C. Integrity of the wire
    D. Size of the specimen

54. Which of the following is a descriptor for calcifications suggestive of ductal carcinoma in situ?
    A. Grouped
    B. Segmental
    C. Regional
    D. Diffuse

55. Clinically, patients with subareolar abscesses commonly
    A. Have nipple rings
    B. Recur after surgical drainage
    C. Present during the third trimester of pregnancy
    D. Present after menopause

56. On this ultrasound image

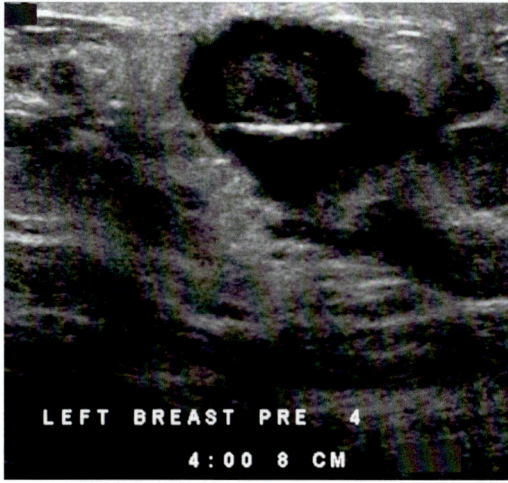

    A. Needle and transducer are misaligned
    B. Needle needs to be pulled back
    C. Needle is not imaged
    D. Needle placement is adequate for FNA

57. In patients with complex cystic and solid masses characterized by a significant fluid component
    A. Aspiration of the fluid and core biopsy of the solid component are indicated
    B. Cytology of fluid aspirate is effective in establishing an accurate diagnosis
    C. Short-interval follow-up is an acceptable recommendation
    D. A course of antibiotics is indicated prior to any intervention

58. Patients with diabetic mastopathy
    A. Have adult-onset type 2 diabetes
    B. Have ipsilateral axillary adenopathy
    C. Respond well to antibiotic therapy
    D. Are managed conservatively

59. Right CC (left) and MLO (right) views. What approach would you use for a mammographically guided preoperative wire localization?

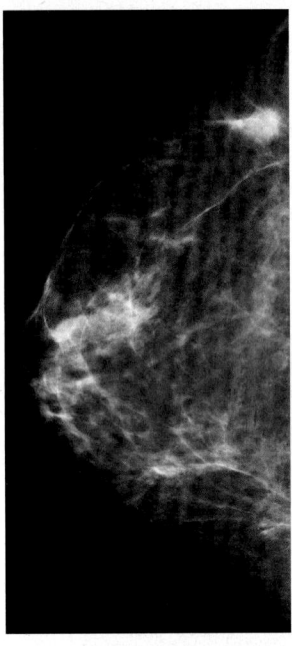
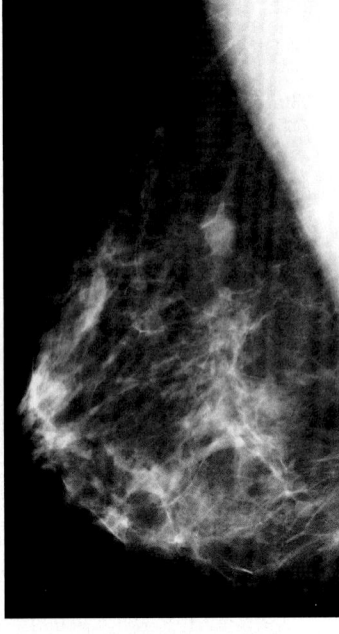

   A. Craniocaudal (CC)
   B. 90-Degree LM
   C. 90-Degree ML
   D. From below (FB)

60. In selecting an appropriate needle length for preoperative wire localizations, you need to be able to do which of the following?

   A. Go at least 1 cm beyond the lesion
   B. Go just beyond the lesion
   C. Reach the center of the lesion
   D. Reach the leading edge of the lesion

61. In women presenting with a breast "lump"

   A. Ultrasound is always indicated
   B. MRI is indicated if mammography and ultrasound are normal
   C. A spot tangential view can partially surround the lesion with fat
   D. Fine-needle aspiration is indicated

62. What BI-RADS® would you give these findings?

   A. 2: benign
   B. 3: probably benign
   C. 4A: suspicious
   D. 4C: suspicious

63. Which of the following is a common ultrasound appearance of mucinous carcinomas?

   A. Markedly hypoechoic
   B. Complex cystic and solid mass
   C. Isoechoic to slightly hyperechoic
   D. Intense shadowing

64. Under MQSA, phantom images need to be kept for

   A. Six months
   B. One year
   C. Two years
   D. Five years

65. Which of the following is recommended for management of patients with atypical ductal hyperplasia diagnosed by an imaging-guided biopsy:

   A. Diagnostic mammography in 1 year
   B. Short-interval follow-up
   C. Magnetic resonance imaging
   D. Excision

66. Nipple discharge is only significant if it is

   A. Noticed by the patient on her bra cup or night clothes
   B. Bloody
   C. Expressed after vigorous nipple compression
   D. Associated with abnormal cytology

67. Screening breast MRI in high-risk patient, postcontrast T1-weighted image. What would you recommend?

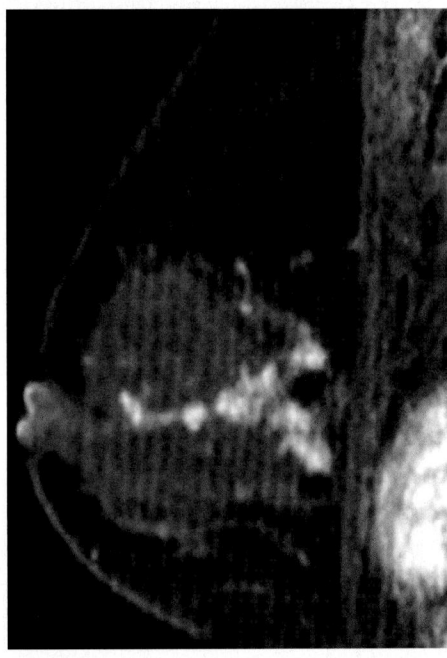

   A. Ultrasound
   B. MRI-guided biopsies
   C. MRI-guided clip placement for surgical excision
   D. Surgical referral for mastectomy

68. Multiple peripheral papillomas

   A. Are synonymous with "papillomatosis"
   B. Reflect a form of papillary epithelial hyperplasia
   C. Are characterized by a central fibrovascular core
   D. Are commonly present with nipple discharge

69. Metaplastic carcinomas are
    A. Rapidly growing lesions
    B. Commonly ER/PR positive
    C. HER2/neu positive
    D. Aggressive variants of invasive lobular carcinoma

70. In evaluating the ipsilateral lymph nodes with ultrasound in a patient with breast cancer
    A. Size (>1 cm) is most helpful in establishing the likelihood of metastatic disease
    B. Focal cortical hyperechogenicity warrants biopsy
    C. An anechoic mass reflects the presence of a cyst in accessory glandular tissue
    D. Cortical bulging is sampled with core biopsy or fine-needle aspiration

71. The "shrinking breast" is
    A. Seen in patients who have lost weight
    B. Typical in patients with inflammatory carcinoma
    C. Associated with invasive lobular carcinoma
    D. A therapy effect following lumpectomy and radiation therapy

72. Complex sclerosing lesions
    A. 1 cm or less in size
    B. Distortion
    C. Usually palpable
    D. Intense shadowing

73. Spot tangential view in a patient presenting with focal pain (BB marking site of pain). What is indicated?

    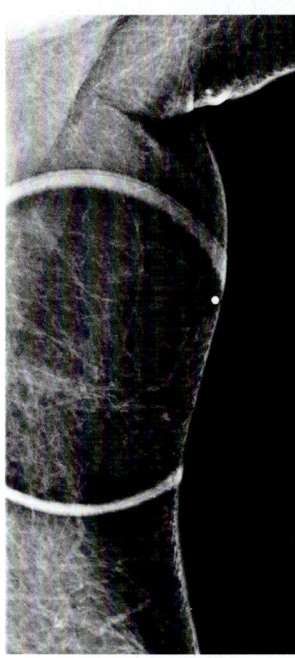

    A. Screening mammography in 1 year
    B. Follow-up in 6 months
    C. Physical examination and ultrasound
    D. Biopsy if clinically indicated

74. Focal parenchymal asymmetry
    A. Tissue seen in one projection
    B. Convex margins
    C. Homogeneously high in density
    D. Scalloping

75. Luminal A, luminal B, HER2, basal-like, and normal-like cancers are terms reflecting
    A. Molecular profiling of breast cancers
    B. Breast cancer growth patterns
    C. Variants of ductal carcinoma in situ
    D. Types of cancers seen in patients with BRCA1 mutations

76. This patient's breasts compress to 1 cm. What would you do?

    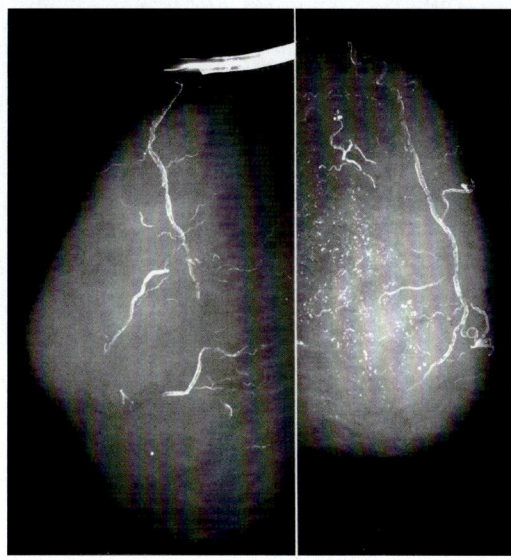

    A. Refer her to a surgeon for excisional biopsy
    B. Short-interval follow-up for renal disease-related calcinosis
    C. Ultrasound
    D. Annual screening mammography

77. False-negative assessment in the intraoperative evaluation of a sentinel lymph node is most commonly encountered with
    A. Invasive ductal carcinoma
    B. Invasive lobular carcinoma
    C. Metaplastic carcinoma
    D. Medullary carcinoma

78. In patients with malignant phyllodes tumors
    A. Lumpectomy followed by radiation therapy is the treatment of choice
    B. Sentinel lymph node biopsy is indicated
    C. Neo-adjuvant therapy may be needed with larger tumors
    D. Mastectomy is often required

79. In angiosarcomas,
    A. Immunohistochemical stains for endothelial cell markers may be indicated
    B. E-cadherin is used to confirm the diagnosis
    C. Cytokeratin profiling is needed
    D. p63 is used to distinguish low-grade lesions from high-grade lesions

80. Which of the following is the most likely explanation for these CC (left) and MLO (right) views?

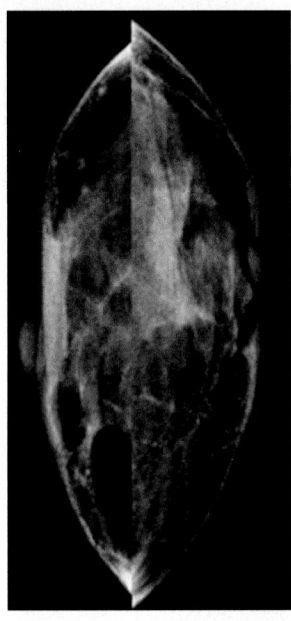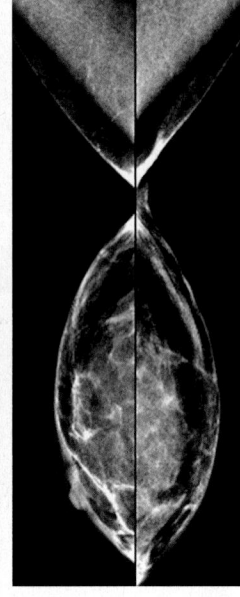

    A. Mammogram in male patient
    B. History of reduction mammoplasty
    C. Implant displaced views in patient with subglandular implants
    D. History of bilateral lumpectomies with radiation therapy

81. Displacement of epithelial cells following needle biopsy is reportedly more common with
    A. Invasive lobular carcinoma
    B. Papillary lesions
    C. Invasive ductal carcinoma
    D. DCIS

82. Human epidermal growth factor receptor 2 gene (HER2/neu)-amplified tumors
    A. Represent approximately 18% to 30% of breast cancers
    B. Are usually estrogen receptor positive
    C. Are characterized by low rates of recurrence
    D. Respond well to aromatase inhibitors

83. Based on this ultrasound image, what is the most likely diagnosis?

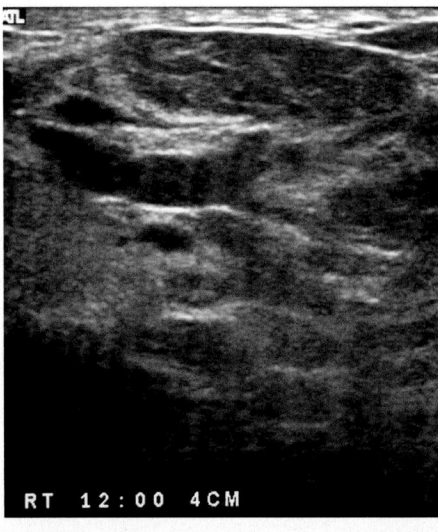

    A. Invasive ductal carcinoma
    B. Duct ectasia
    C. Fibroadenoma
    D. Papilloma

84. Wide surgical excision is the treatment of choice for
    A. Gynecomastia
    B. Complex fibroadenomas
    C. Fibromatosis
    D. Duct ectasia

85. For breast MRI
    A. Temporal resolution of 3 to 4 minutes is optimal
    B. GFR of 29 mL/min/1.73 m^2 contraindicates the study
    C. Hand injection of contrast is preferred
    D. Field strength of 0.5 T is ideal

86. What is the most likely diagnosis in this patient?

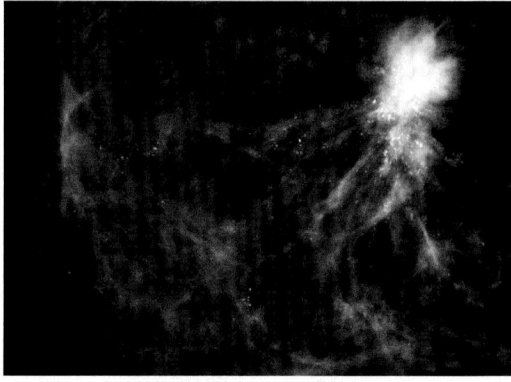

    A. Invasive ductal carcinoma with extensive ductal carcinoma in situ
    B. Invasive lobular carcinoma with associated lobular carcinoma in situ
    C. Postsurgical change and fat necrosis
    D. Locally advanced invasive ductal carcinoma

87. How would you manage the patient with the mammogram shown in question 86?
    A. Surgical excision with bracketing
    B. Core biopsies of mass and anterior most cluster of calcifications
    C. US-guided biopsy of mass
    D. MRI to determine what to biopsy

88. Which of the following is a common benign lesion with rapid wash-in and wash-out kinetics in a postmenopausal woman?
    A. Fibroadenoma
    B. Fibroadenolipoma
    C. Papilloma
    D. Lobular carcinoma in situ

89. Triple-negative tumors are
    A. Clinically detected with "negative" mammogram, ultrasound, and MRI
    B. Estrogen, progesterone, and HER2/neu negative
    C. p63, E-cadherin, and vimentin negative
    D. Metastatic in patients with normal physical examination, mammography, and ultrasound

90. Given the finding, what would you do?

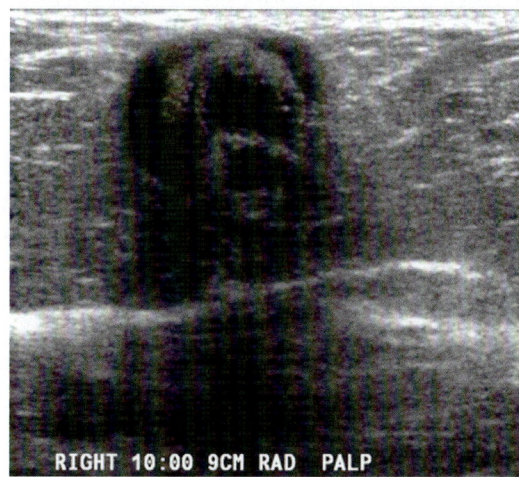

   A. Short-interval follow-up
   B. Aspiration
   C. Biopsy
   D. Correlation with mammogram

91. Injecting air into a cyst following aspiration
   A. Is associated with abscess formation
   B. Helps identify the aspirated cyst on subsequent mammograms
   C. May be therapeutic in some patients
   D. Is only indicated in patients with a possible intracystic lesion

92. What needs to be done at this point?

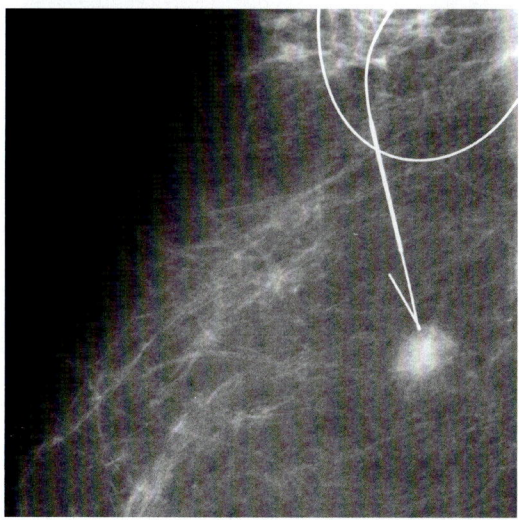

   A. Transfer patient to the operating room
   B. Place a second wire
   C. Advance the wire in further
   D. Pull this wire out and start all over

93. Which of the following is the contrast amount typically used for ductography?
   A. 0.2 to 0.4 mL
   B. 0.5 to 0.7 mL
   C. 0.8 to 1 mL
   D. 1.5 to 2 mL

94. Oncotype DX scores are used to
   A. Determine patients who might benefit from radiation therapy after mastectomy
   B. Determine patients who might benefit from screening with breast MRI
   C. Predict the likelihood of distant metastasis following trastuzumab treatment
   D. Estimate likelihood of recurrence in tamoxifen-treated patients with ER+, node negative disease

95. Given the findings, which of these would keep you from doing a biopsy on this patient?

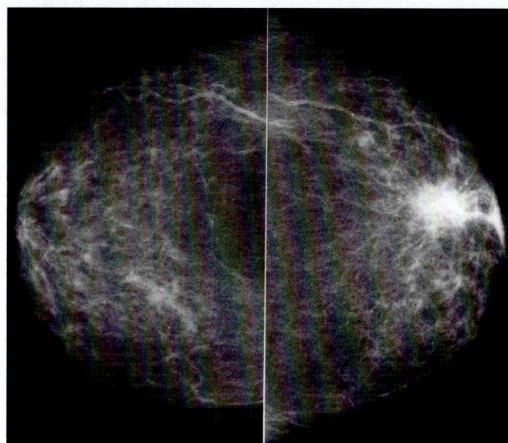

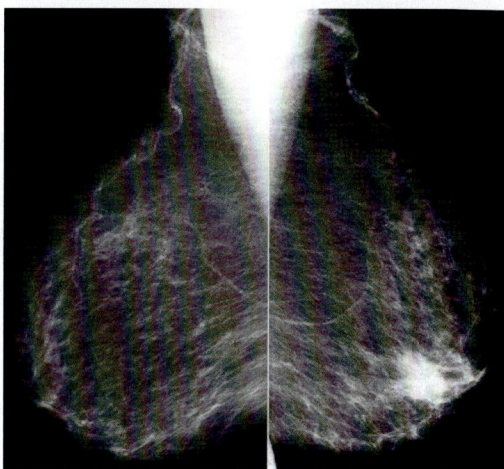

   A. 10-Year stability of the finding
   B. No associated enhancement on MRI at the site of the lesion
   C. Prior surgery correlated to the specific site of the lesion
   D. History of lactational mastitis 5 years ago

96. In women with intraductal lesions on ductography, wire localization should be considered
   A. In all patients
   B. With a lesion several branch points away from the nipple
   C. When requested by the surgeon
   D. When the duct is not dilated

97. Among your benign differential considerations for the findings, what is the most likely diagnosis?

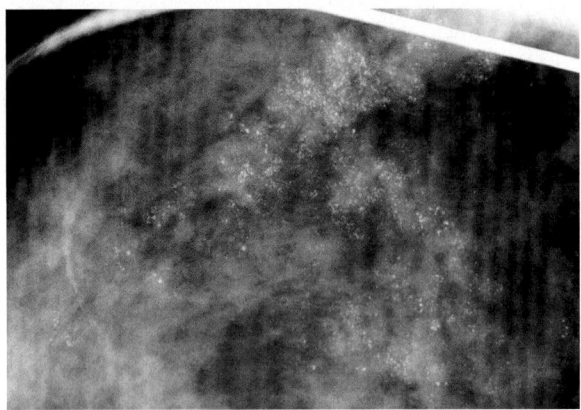

   A. Sclerosing adenosis
   B. Fibroadenoma
   C. Papillomas
   D. Fat necrosis

98. In educating patients regarding breast self-examination
   A. It should be done when breast pain is experienced only
   B. They should squeeze their nipples vigorously to detect discharge
   C. Instruct to start regularly after menopause
   D. Instruct them to check their bra cups periodically for dark brown spots

99. Based on this image, what is the "N" for this patient for the cTNM?

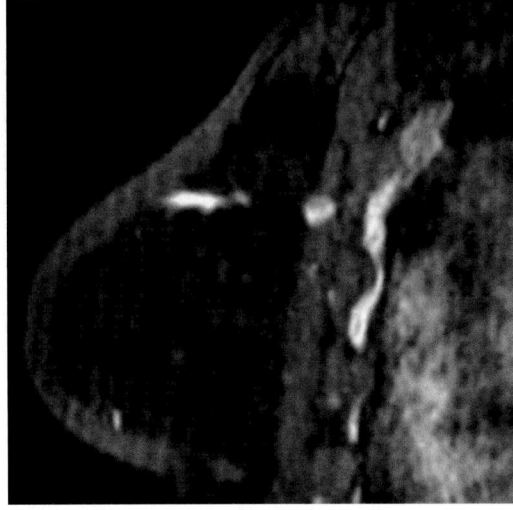

   A. N0
   B. N1
   C. N2
   D. N3

100. A false-negative mammogram is defined as a cancer:
   A. That is not apparent when a retrospective review of the prior study is done
   B. That is apparent on a retrospective review of the prior mammogram but not described on the mammogram
   C. Diagnosis within 1 year of a "normal" screening mammogram
   D. Diagnosis within 2 years of a "normal" screening mammogram

101. Which of the following is advised in the management of a 60-year-old woman with a new mass described as a cellular fibroadenoma on core biopsy
   A. Screening mammography
   B. Six-month follow-up
   C. MRI
   D. Excisional biopsy

102. Triple-negative cancers
   A. Are commonly interval cancers
   B. Are common in postmenopausal women
   C. Are less prevalent in African American women
   D. Represent close to 40% of all breast cancers

103. Based on this image, what is the most likely diagnosis?

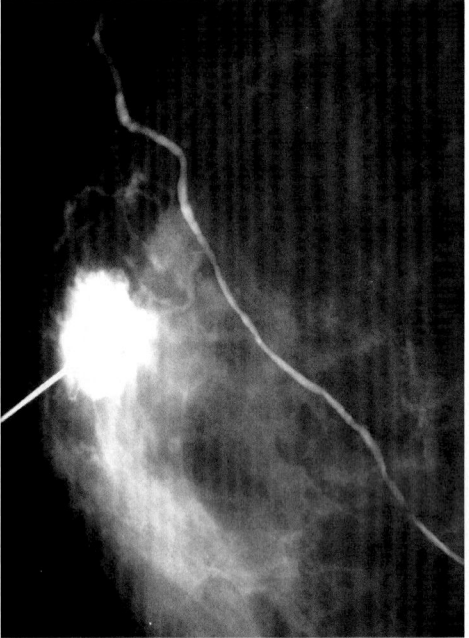

   A. Papilloma in a nondilated duct
   B. Extravasation with lymphatic opacification
   C. Ductal carcinoma in situ
   D. Invasive ductal carcinoma

104. The movement of a lesion between MLO and 90-degree lateral views is minimal when the lesion is
   A. In the axillary tail of the breast
   B. Close to the cleavage
   C. Anterior in the breast
   D. Retroareolar in location

105. The lesion shown is apparent on a mammogram from 4 years ago in a patient with a history of surgery in the contralateral breast

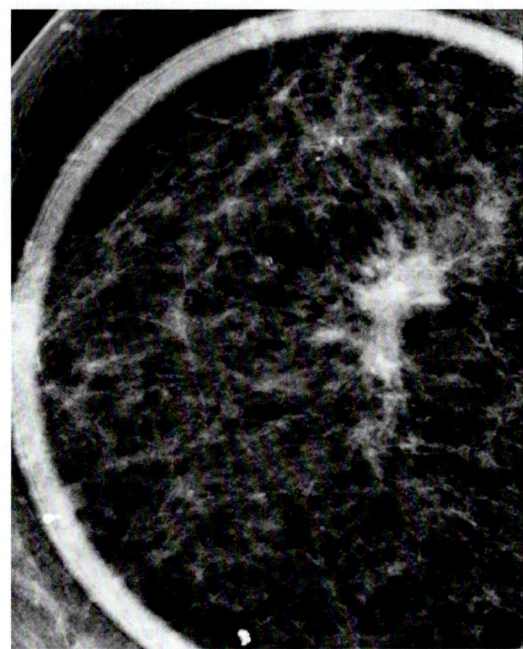

A. BI-RADS 4C
B. BI-RADS 4A
C. BI-RADS 3: probable benign finding, follow-up in 6 months
D. BI-RADS 2: benign finding, screening in a year

106. Mondor disease is characterized by
    A. Nipple involvement
    B. Fistula formation
    C. Thrombophlebitis
    D. Eczema on areola

107. Which of the following lesions can recur following excisional biopsy?
    A. Complex fibroadenomas
    B. Lactational adenomas
    C. Pseudoangiomatous stromal hyperplasia
    D. Fibroadenolipomas

108. What do you expect to see on this patient's mammogram?

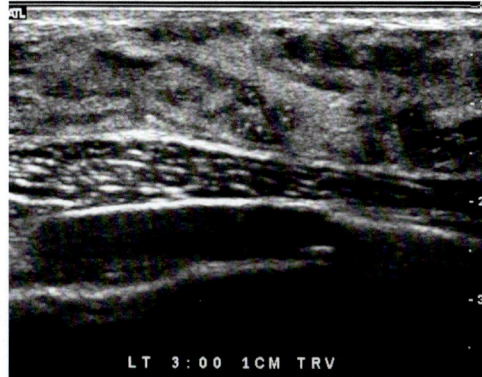

A. Dilated ducts
B. A mass with indistinct margins
C. Predominantly fatty tissue
D. Calcifications

109. Postsurgical changes
    A. Rarely resolve completely
    B. Are better seen on one of two orthogonal images
    C. Commonly develop calcifications
    D. Significantly affect mammography interpretations

110. Skin calcifications commonly develop
    A. Along the scars following reduction mammoplasty
    B. In skin folds in the axillary tail of the breast
    C. Predominantly in the periareolar area
    D. On thickened skin at lumpectomy sites

111. Spot compression (left) and US (right) image in a 45-year-old patient with new "lump" that is not tender. What is the leading consideration, and what would you recommend?

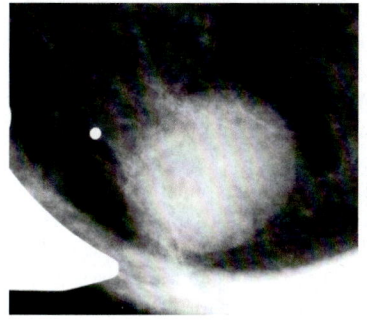 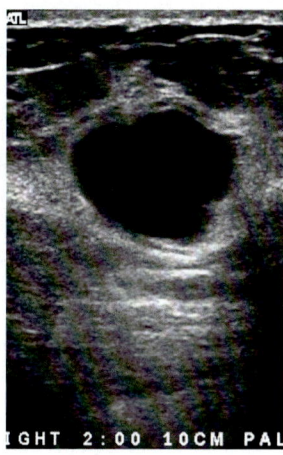

A. Abscess, aspirate
B. Cyst, screening mammography in 1 year
C. Necrotic invasive ductal carcinoma, core biopsy
D. Probable benign, follow-up in 6 months

112. Which of the following are (is) the gold standard in providing the evidence needed to support the use of screening to effectively decrease breast cancer mortality rates?
    A. Case-controlled studies
    B. Computer modeling
    C. Population-based trials
    D. Randomized controlled trials

113. Which of the following is a common cause of gynecomastia?
    A. Drugs
    B. Testicular tumor
    C. Chest wall trauma
    D. HIV

114. Metastatic pattern associated with invasive lobular carcinoma:
    A. Peritoneal seeding
    B. Lung
    C. Brain
    D. Liver

115. The MQSA covers
    A. Breast ultrasound
    B. Technologies for radiography of the breast
    C. Magnetic resonance imaging of the breast
    D. Breast-specific gamma imaging

Answers to Self-Assessment Questions

1. C A fat containing (mixed density) mass is imaged in the right subareolar area. Mixed-density masses are benign and require no additional evaluation or short-interval follow-up. In this patient, annual screening mammography is indicated. Differential considerations for mixed-density masses include lymph nodes, fibroadenolipomas, postoperative/traumatic fluid collections, galactocele, fat necrosis, and oil cysts.

2. B Sentinel lymph node (SNL) biopsies are relatively contraindicated in pregnant patients. If done on a pregnant patient, only sulfur colloid should be used. There are no data on the potential side effects of the vital blue dye on the fetus. SNLs are routinely done in obese and older patients as well as in men presenting with breast cancer. SNL biopsies are also done in patients with multifocal and multicentric disease.

3. D Psammoma bodies (see Fig. 8.56D) are distinctive round calcifications with an onion-like (laminar) appearance seen in patients with metastatic papillary thyroid carcinomas and ovarian papillary serous cystadenocarcinoma to the breast or axilla. Rarely, calcifications are seen in necrotic lymph nodes replaced with metastatic disease from breast primaries; however, they do not have the appearance of psammoma bodies histologically. The detection of calcifications on screening mammography is one of the more common presentations for ductal carcinoma in situ (DCIS); however, this disease is by definition an intraductal process and as such a metastatic disease, and, in particular, DCIS-related calcifications in lymph nodes are exceedingly rare. When metastatic disease is diagnosed in patients with DCIS, it is usually in patients with extensive DCIS and presumed to be related to undetected sites of invasion (e.g., false-negative pathology).

4. B In patients with known invasive breast cancer, preoperative MRI evaluation is indicated to establish the extent of the disease in the ipsilateral breast, assess regional lymph nodes (axilla, internal mammary) and evaluate the contralateral breast. In this patient diagnosed with invasive ductal carcinoma following an ultrasound-guided biopsy of a mass in the upper inner quadrant of the right breast, three heterogeneously enhancing masses are identified in the upper central to medial aspect of the right breast in zones B and C. Additionally, non-mass like clumped and linear enhancement is seen regionally distributed extending from the masses anteriorly and into the lateral quadrants of the right breast. The findings are consistent with multifocal disease and associated extensive ductal carcinoma in situ. In determining the appropriate management for this patient, if the non-mass like enhancement is confirmed to be DCIS, conservative therapy even following neo-adjuvant therapy is unlikely to be effective. Histologic confirmation of the suspected extent of the disease, however, should be obtained before doing a mastectomy. We would biopsy the furthest suspicious finding relative to the known site of malignancy. Second-look ultrasound is not helpful in patients with non-mass like enhancement. Unless the patient wants a mastectomy regardless of the findings, we do not do mastectomies without first obtaining histologic confirmation of the suspected extent of disease. Given the likely extent of disease, lumpectomy even with bracketing is likely to result in positive margins and unacceptable cosmetic results.

5. A The designation "yp" is used to describe the pathology stage in patients after neo-adjuvant therapy.

6. D The increased risk for breast cancer seen in patients following chest radiation manifests itself approximately 10 years after an exposure between the ages of 10 and 30. The risk is presumably related to scatter radiation and is not limited to the medial quadrants of the breasts. There are no data at this time regarding the risk of breast cancer in men who had chest radiation during adolescence.

7. B A mass is partially imaged posteromedially in the right breast. In patients with lesions that are seen in only one of the standard views, it is important to *make no assumptions*. Follow a stepwise, logical approach. Start by confirming and evaluating the lesion in the projection in which it is seen. In this patient, a spot compression cleavage view is used to confirm that there is a mass and use of the spot is likely to maximize the inclusion of posterior tissue so that the lesion can be seen in its entirety and margins can be evaluated. Once the lesion is confirmed in the CC projection, efforts are made to locate the lesion in the other image. In this patient, you can do rolled views to see if the lesion moves with superior or inferior tissue, or to maximize the inclusion of medial tissue, a 90-degree lateromedial (LM) view can be done. The 90-degree LM view places medial tissue against the imaging receptor, accomplishing two things: maximizing medial tissue inclusion and resolution (the lesion is placed closest to the detector). This mass does not have features to suggest a seborrheic keratosis (no interstices outlined by air). Although sebaceous cysts are common in the axilla and medial quadrants posteriorly, the margins and density of this lesion make this diagnosis unlikely. If positioning on the original MLO is acceptable, repeating the same projection is not usually helpful. Designation of a lesion into the probably benign category is not done on screening studies; it should be done only after complete evaluation with spot compression views, correlative physical examination, and an ultrasound study.

8. A The imaging features defining a lesion as probably benign, and the longitudinal data supporting periodic follow-up for these lesions, are available for findings on mammography only. Although in practice this designation is used for ultrasound and MRI findings, what constitutes a probably benign finding on ultrasound or MRI has not been defined, and the longitudinal data in support of short-interval follow-up are not available for these modalities. No definition or data exist regarding physical findings that may be associated with a low likelihood of malignancy.

9. C On ductography, papillomas often present as a filling defect(s), a mass obstructing the main duct or a branch, and, less commonly, a wall irregularity. The lesions sometimes appear to expand and disrupt the integrity of the duct; however, when excised, the wall of these ducts is intact. The lesion can occur anywhere in the duct; however, they are commonly subareolar in location. In many patients, ducts with papillomas are dilated, and it is the segment of the duct between the lesion and the nipple that is typically dilated. Why this portion of the duct is dilated is unclear; presumably, if the lesions actively secrete fluid/blood and the opening to the duct on the nipple is partially or completely blocked by keratin plugs, this portion of the duct can become distended over time. Traumatic perforation of a normal duct is exceedingly rare; it is painful, and the patients describe "burning" as soon as an effort is made to inject contrast. Rarely, contrast extravasation is a finding in patients with DCIS (described as "leaky" ducts); in these patients, the cannulation is not painful and the patient does not experience burning when the contrast is injected. In patients with DCIS and contrast extravasation on ductography, a follow up ductogram will replicate the finding.

10. D Diffuse skin thickening and prominence of the trabecular markings are present bilaterally. When diffuse changes are bilateral, fluid overload related to either cardiac or renal disease is one of the more common causes. When unilateral, acute radiation therapy change following lumpectomy is a common cause for skin thickening and diffuse prominence of the trabecular markings (see Table 9.1 for differential considerations in patients with diffuse changes). Parenchymal density increases, and the development of multiple masses may be seen in patients started on hormone replacement therapy; however, these changes are not usually associated with skin thickening or trabecular prominence. Adult-onset diabetes is not linked to any mammographic finding.

11. B Paget disease of the nipple alone is considered as an intraductal carcinoma and defined as Tis (Paget). When associated with an invasive lesion, the invasive lesion is used to define the tumor (T). Tumors that are less than or equal to 2 cm in size are designated as T1 lesions: (i) a T1mi is a tumor that is less than or equal to 0.1 cm in size; (ii) a T1a tumor is greater than 0.1 cm in size but less than or equal to 0.5 cm; (iii) T1b tumors are greater than 0.5 cm in size but less than or equal to 1.0 cm in size; and (iv) T1c tumors are greater than 1.0 cm but less than or equal to 2.0 cm in size. In this patient, the invasive lesion is described as 0.7 cm: it is a T1b tumor (greater than 0.5 cm in size but less than 1 cm). If the lymph nodes are confirmed normal on the sentinel lymph node biopsy, the stage for this patient is IA (see Table 1.5).

12. C Currently, breast cancer is most commonly diagnosed through screening mammography. It has replaced, breast self-examination as the most common detection method.

13. A A lucent mass (oil cyst) is imaged on the spot tangential view corresponding to the "lump" described by the patient. Fat-containing masses are benign and require no additional evaluation, intervention, or short-term interval follow-up. The patient needs to be reassured that what she is feeling is benign (e.g., not cancer) and not going to turn into cancer. Annual screening mammography is indicated.

14. D All the lesions listed are associated with an increased risk for breast cancer; however, lobular carcinoma in situ imparts the greatest lifetime risk for breast cancer and the risk does not decrease with advancing age.

15. C Less than 25% of patients with screen detected breast cancers should be node positive at the time of diagnosis. Greater than 50% of patients with screen-detected tumors should have stage 0 or I disease and more than 30% should be diagnosed with minimal breast cancer. The cancer detection rate is expected to be 6 to 10 cancers per 1,000 women undergoing their first screening mammography (prevalent) and 2 to 4 cancers per 1,000 women with prior screening mammographies (incident). Although a recall rate of less than 10% is considered ideal, keep in mind that this should be monitored over time; one's personal recall rate (and positive predictive values for biopsy recommendations) should improve with experience.

16. B Mammography facilities must be inspected annually by the FDA or its designee and certified by the FDA every 3 years. Mammography facilities are accredited every 3 years by an FDA-approved accredited body (e.g., American College of Radiology; States of Arkansas, Iowa and Texas).

17. A A fat-containing mass with indistinct margins and dystrophic calcifications is imaged at the anterior edge of the left pectoral muscle. The findings are consistent with fat necrosis and require no additional evaluation, intervention, or short-interval follow-up. This is a BI-RADS 2 lesion. In this patient, a screening mammogram is recommended in 1 year.

18. B Sentinel lymph node (SLN) biopsy cannot be done after a mastectomy. Patients with extensive DCIS are often most effectively treated with a mastectomy. In these patients, if a SLN biopsy is not done at the time of the mastectomy and invasive disease is found on the mastectomy specimen, a full axillary dissection would need to be done. The adequacy of histological evaluation is an additional consideration in patients with extensive DCIS. In these patients, representative sections are done through the breast such that invasive disease may go undetected histologically. Consequently, many surgeons advocate SLN biopsies in patients with extensive DCIS undergoing mastectomy. Patients with inflammatory carcinoma, those with clinically abnormal lymph nodes, and those with known distant metastatic disease undergo axillary dissections and not SLN biopsies.

19. D Currently, no stage is provided for patients with a complete pathological response following neo-adjuvant therapy (ypT0ypN0cM0).

20. B The image demonstrates collimator misalignment—artifact noted along the upper edge of the image. Given its degree, no additional patient images should be done until a service engineer is contacted and the misalignment is correct.

21. C Zuska disease refers to the spontaneous development of fistulas along the periareolar margin in patients with subareolar abscesses.

22. D The spot paddle is used at this point so that the hub of the needle is readily accessible. Having free and easy access to the needle hub facilities adjustments in the position of the needle and deployment of the wire. If a full sized compression paddle is used at this point, it can be difficult for the radiologist to get their hands in between the paddle and the detector to make fine adjustments and deploy the wire without inadvertently advancing or pulling the entire system out of the breast.

23. A Rim calcifications commonly develop in oil cysts.

24. C The presence of myoepithelial cells can be established using a p63 stain. It can be used to distinguish tubular carcinomas (lacking myoepithelial cells) from sclerosing adenosis (benign proliferative process). Analogously, in papillary lesions, the presence of myoepithelial cells is used to classify the lesion as benign, while those lacking myoepithelial cells are considered malignant. E-cadherin is a cell adhesion molecule that is helpful in distinguishing lobular processes (LCIS, ALH) that do not typically stain from proliferative processes in the duct (DCIS) that demonstrate E-cadherin. Polarizing microscopy is useful in identifying calcium oxalate crystals that may not be readily apparent on hematoxylin and eosin (H&E) stained tissue. Calcium oxalate is commonly identified in benign processes (fibrocystic changes). Calcium phosphate is easily seen on H&E and is the type of calcium found in DCIS. The presence or absence of estrogen receptors is used in the management of patients with invasive lesions. Rarely, in patients with metastatic disease and an unknown primary, the presence of estrogen receptors may be used to suggest the possibility of a breast primary; however, some non-breast primaries can demonstrate estrogen receptors.

25. A The images demonstrate an isodense mass with circumscribed margins and calcifications. The calcifications change in configuration between the two projections. On the craniocaudal view, they are discrete, dense, round calcifications that layer in the dependent portion of the mass on the oblique view. The findings are consistent with "milk of calcium" in a macrocyst. This is a BI-RADS 2 finding requiring no additional evaluation, intervention, or short-interval follow-up. As illustrated in this patient, the change in the appearance of milk of calcium calcifications is often apparent on the standard views (CC and MLO) such that no additional views are indicated. In some patients, the change is suggested on the MLO view; however, a 90-degree lateral view is needed for confirmation. In this patient, annual screening mammography is indicated.

26. C Breast imaging reports should be accurate and provide clinically relevant information. This is particularly applicable to the measurement of lesions. Terms such as large, medium, and small are useless and should not be used when describing breast lesions. Although relied upon by surgeons, clinical measurements are consistently inaccurate and can only be approximated in two planes; they should not be used. In fact, one of the characteristics of invasive ductal carcinomas is that they are often larger on palpation that what is seen on any imaging modality; this is thought to reflect reactive fibrotic changes in the tissue surrounding the lesion. Conversely, the size of invasive lobular carcinoma may be grossly underestimated on physical examination.

27. D The descriptors for the margins of a mass on mammography include circumscribed, indistinct, spiculated, and obscured. *Stellate* is not a term used in the American College of Radiology lexicon. *Irregular* refers to the shape of a mass and *angular* is a descriptor for the margins of some masses on ultrasound. The term *obscured* is used when glandular tissue is present and thought to obscure what are likely to be circumscribed margins. If the breast is predominantly fatty (e.g., if there is no glandular tissue in the area of the mass), the term *obscured* should not be used.

28. B The spot compression view demonstrates a high-density round mass with indistinct margins and associated calcifications. This mass in the lower central aspect of the right breast posteriorly is hypoechoic with no posterior acoustic enhancement or shadowing. Although subtle, an echogenic rim is noted and the margins are partially indistinct. Beware. Although you may initially think this might be a cyst, the mammographic and ultrasound features are not consistent with that diagnosis. This most likely represents an invasive ductal carcinoma, high nuclear grade, and biopsy is indicated. Invasive lobular carcinomas do not typically present as round (expansile) masses and are not usually associated with calcifications. The echotexture, orientation, and margins of the mass make a fibroadenoma less likely. Although not provided, when taking care of patients it is important to consider prior films and the age of the patient in the generating appropriate differentials. BI-RADS 4C, biopsy is indicated.

29. A In approximately 50% of patients presenting with spontaneous nipple discharge, a papilloma is identified as the underlying etiology. Fibrocystic changes and duct ectasia are less common representing approximately 35% and 5% of patients, respectively. Breast cancer is diagnosed in approximately 10% of patients presenting with spontaneous nipple discharge. In considering the imaging findings in the patients with cancer, consider three subgroups: (i) patients with papillomas associated with DCIS in whom the mammogram is often normal, an intraductal lesion may be identified on ultrasound and a filling defect, or obstructing lesion may be seen in a dilated duct on ductography; (ii) patients with DCIS only, in whom you may see some calcifications on the mammogram, no focal abnormality is readily apparent on ultrasound and the duct is diffusely abnormal but not usually dilated on ductography; and (iii) patients with an invasive ductal carcinoma in whom a mass possibly associated with calcifications may be seen on the mammogram and ultrasound, and a filling defect or obstructing lesion is identified on the ductogram. Make no assumptions in patients with nipple discharge and a mass that is likely to be cancer on their mammogram. It may be that the nipple discharge and mass are related; however, the patient may have two separate processes (see Fig. 12.9E-G).

30. B The diagnosis of inflammatory carcinoma is based on clinical findings (e.g., not based on imaging or histologic findings). It requires a history of rapidly developing peau d'orange changes, erythema, and an increased temperature of the involved breast. Histologically, most patients have nests of tumor cells plugging dilated dermal lymphatics; however, this is not required for the diagnosis. In a small percentage of patients who do not have the clinical signs and symptoms of inflammatory carcinoma, tumor-plugged dermal lymphatics are identified histologically; these patients should not be classified as having inflammatory carcinoma. Diffuse changes including increased density, decreased breast compression, skin thickening, and adenopathy are the most common mammographic findings (consider cm of breast compression, kVp needed for exposure, and resulting mAs compared with contralateral breast); however, these are nonspecific. The underlying tumor type is usually invasive ductal and not lobular.

31. D Gynecomastia is not considered a risk factor for breast cancer. It is commonly asymmetric and not usually associated with reactive adenopathy. By definition, glandular tissue "fans" or "flames" out symmetrically from the subareolar area. In men, parenchymal asymmetries that are not centered on the nipple should be considered and evaluated carefully.

32. C A predominantly hyperechoic macrolobulated mass with indistinct margins is imaged causing disruption of the ligaments in the lower central aspect of the left breast posteriorly. Initially, the hyperechogenicity of the mass with an internal area of hypoechogenicity may prompt a consideration of trauma; however, the location of the mass in the inferior aspect of the breast posteriorly makes trauma unlikely. A core biopsy of this lesion is indicated. Although hyperechogenicity is considered a benign feature of masses, assess hyperechoic lesions carefully: specifically focus on the margins, effect on surrounding tissue, and internal heterogeneity in deciding to follow or biopsy. BI-RADS 4B: Suspicious abnormality, biopsy is indicated.

33. A Under MQSA, the full name of the facility as well as the city, state, and zip code are required on mammography images. The initials of the technologist (not radiologist) are also required as is the room number of the equipment in facilities with more than one mammography machine. Technical factors are recommended but not required.

34. C Atypical ductal hyperplasia is considered a precursor to low-grade DCIS and invasive ductal carcinoma in a small percentage of patients. Multiple peripheral papillomas and lobular carcinoma in situ are considered marker lesions: they are associated with increased risk but the lesions themselves are not thought to progress to malignancy. Reportedly, other proliferative high-risk processes that include multiple peripheral papillomas, atypical ductal hyperplasia, LCIS as well as low-grade DCIS and low-grade invasive lesions including tubular carcinomas may be found associated with complex sclerosing lesions in as many as 33% of patients.

35. D An oval high-density mass possibly with indistinct margins is imaged in the upper outer quadrant of the right breast posteriorly. The size, density, and location of the mass correlate on the two projections. Given its location you may want to assume this is a lymph node: beware! No fatty hilum is readily apparent, no other lymph nodes are seen in the surrounding tissue and the density of the mass is such that additional evaluation is indicated. Comparison with prior films and the age of the patient are also considered. Short of this finding decreasing in size compared with prior studies, additional evaluation is indicated. BI-RADS 0: need additional imaging evaluation. Spot compression views are done to better assess margins and evaluate for a fatty hilum. Correlative physical examination, ultrasound, and biopsy are likely indicated.

36. B Following annual FDA inspection of mammography facilities: A level I noncompliance violation requires immediate action for remedy, reinspection, and sanctions if corrective actions are not taken (reportedly approximately 0.2% of facilities have level I violations). Level II violations require a written response with corrective actions within 30 days of the inspection (10.8% of facilities) and level III violations require corrective action before the next annual inspection (1% of facilities).

37. A Predominantly fatty tissue with low T2 signal linear bands and mounds of oval fatty tissue abutting the pectoral muscles bilaterally are consistent with TRAM flap reconstructions.

38. D Low nuclear grade DCIS and LCIS are found associated with tubular carcinomas in as many as 65% of patients. Tubular carcinomas are also often multifocal and centric, and have a higher likelihood of bilaterality. These types of tumors are more common in premenopausal women presenting as one or several small masses with spiculated margins.

39. C The MLO was selected as one of the two screening views to maximize the amount of tissue included on the image. It is actually harder to position an MLO view compared with 90-degree lateral views. However, when properly done, tissue is pulled out parallel to the underlying muscles fibers thereby maximizing the amount of posterior tissue included on the image.

40. B Fibroepithelial lesions require excisional biopsy. In these patients, a phyllodes tumor remains in the differential and as such excisional biopsy is indicated. Depending on the mammography/ultrasound finding, PASH, complex fibroadenomas, and apocrine metaplasia do not usually require excisional biopsy.

41. D This is an oval hyperechoic mass with central anechogenicity in the upper inner quadrant of the left breast. I would examine the patient for any bruising and ask the patient about trauma.

42. C Papillary carcinomas commonly present as complex cystic masses, particularly when they develop in the anterior aspect of the breast. Additional imaging features include round or oval shape, relatively circumscribed margins, and posterior acoustic enhancement.

43. A As part of the QA/QC program, phantom images are done weekly. At a minimum, the four largest fibers, three largest speck groups, and three largest masses should be seen (see Fig. 2.1). The image is also reviewed for artifacts and these are factored into the scoring. Regions of interest (ROI) are placed one over the disc and the other in an area adjacent to disc so that signal-to-noise (SNR) and contrast-to-noise (CNR) ratios can be calculated. The measured SNR must be equal to or greater than 40 and the CNR must be within ±15% of the value determined by the medical physicists when the image receptor was installed or after any major upgrade.

44. D Tubular carcinomas commonly present as one or multiple masses with spiculated margins under a centimeter in size. The malignant differential for masses with spiculated margins includes: invasive ductal carcinoma, not otherwise specified, tubular carcinoma, and invasive lobular carcinoma. Medullary carcinomas are usually expansile ("blow up") lesions and are more common in younger patients sometimes presenting as interval cancers. Mucinous and papillary carcinomas are likely to be round or oval and more common in postmenopausal women.

45. A A hypoechoic mass with indistinct margins and an echogenic rim is imaged in the lower inner quadrant of the left breast. Although a cyst with internal echoes may be fleetingly considered, the margins and echogenic rim make this unlikely. Likewise, given the eccentric focus of echogenicity, a reactive lymph node may be considered; however, the location of the lesion (less than 5% of all lymph nodes occur in the medial quadrants) and its overall appearance virtually eliminates this possibility. The most likely diagnosis is that of an invasive ductal carcinoma, high grade ("blow up" lesion); associated necrosis may also be present. BI-RADS 4C: Suspicious abnormality, biopsy is indicated.

46. C Quality control tests typically done weekly include DICOM printer quality control, detector flat-field calibration to assure the system is calibrated properly, artifact evaluation (for the detector), signal-to-noise and contrast-to-noise measurements to assure consistency of the digital image receptor, phantom image to assure overall image quality, compression thickness indicator to assure indicated compression thickness is accurate to ±0.5 cm from actual thickness, diagnostic review workstation QC, viewboxes, and viewing conditions. The visual checklist, repeat analysis, and compression QC test are done monthly, quarterly, and semiannually, respectively.

47. C Squamous metaplasia is a common pathologic finding in patients who undergo surgical treatment of subareolar abscesses.

48. A The palpable finding in this patient represents the valve of a saline implant ("angel"). This requires no additional imaging or short-interval follow-up. The patient needs to be re-assured that what she is feeling is not a "lump" in her breast but rather related to the implant. Biopsy or fine needle aspiration is not indicated (in fact, contraindicated).

49. D Granular cell tumors are thought to be neural in origin arising from Schwann cells.

50. D Extracapsular rupture is readily apparent mammographically. Although capsule formation can be inferred when the capsule calcifications, the capsule itself is not usually seen mammographically. Likewise, given the density of silicone, gel bleed, and intracapsular rupture are not apparent mammographically.

51. B The appropriate evaluation of this patient entails spotting the lesion in the projection in which it is seen and then determining its location on the orthogonal view. In this patient, a 90-degree LM view would help triangulate the location of the lesion on the CC view. If the lesion moves down on the 90-degree lateral view compared with the MLO, a spot compression view in the XCCL projection would be indicated. If the lesion moves up on the 90-degree lateral view, the lesion is medial in location and a spot cleavage view would be helpful. If the lesion does not shift very much between the MLO and the 90-degree lateral view, it is retroareolar in location and a spot from below (FB) view such that the detector is placed on the upper portion of the breast to image the lesion. Given the density of this mass, it is unlikely to represent a normal lymph node or a benign finding; additionally six-month follow-up recommendations should only be used following complete imaging evaluation. Without knowing the location of this lesion in orthogonal planes, ultrasound may be misleading. If a lesion is found in the lateral quadrants of the breast, does it correlate with the mammographic finding? Remember, make no assumptions, but rather follow a simple, logical, step wise approach in establishing the presence and exact location of lesions.

52. D Currently, the American Cancer Society (ACS) recommends annual screening MRI for women at high risk including: women with a BRCA mutation and their untested first-degree relatives, women who have had chest wall radiation between the ages of 10 and 30, women with syndromes (Li-Fraumeni, Cowden, and Bannayan–Riley–Ruvalcaba syndromes) associated with an increased breast cancer risk and those women with a lifetime risk of greater than 20% to 25% as determined by risk models (BRCAPRO, Tyrer-Cuzick).

53. C Following preoperative wire localizations, imaging the specimen serves several purposes including documentation that the localized lesion and the localization wire are excised. The specimen radiograph is also used to orient the pathologist to the location of the lesion in the specimen and the proximity of the lesion to the margins can sometimes be determined. Rarely, unsuspected lesions are identified in the specimen. In this image, the hook of the wire is not apparent. It may be the hook is being obscure by the wire so you can try to re-position the specimen, however, if it is not imaged this is communicated to the surgeon. A follow-up mammography may be appropriate if the return portion of the hook is not identified.

54. B Grouped, regional, and diffuse are neutral terms. Segmental distribution is suggestive of a malignant process.

55. B Patients with subareolar abscesses have a likelihood of recurrence after surgery. Bilateral disease and spontaneous fistula formation (Zuska disease) at the areolar margin are also common in these patients. Subareolar abscesses are not associated with nipple rings, do not usually develop as part of pregnancy or lactation and are more common in premenopausal women with a history of heavy smoking.

56. C A central beaded band of hyperechogenicity is imaged in a mass with angular margins. This is an air track from a prior core and not the needle. The beaded and somewhat curvilinear appearance of this echogenic line is what distinguishes this from the needle. During the real-time portion of the study, the echogenic "beads" can be seen moving as gentle pressure is applied over the lesion.

57. A Our approach to patients with complex cystic and solid masses characterized by a large fluid component is to aspirate as much of the fluid as possible and then core the remaining solid component. If the fluid in these lesions is inadvertently released into the surrounding tissue, a significant aseptic inflammatory reaction can develop: patients describe swelling, tenseness, redness, and tenderness that resolve slowly over several weeks. Antibiotic therapy is of limited usefulness since this is usually an aseptic inflammatory process. Concerns regarding the inability to identify a solid component after aspiration are not well founded; the solid component is readily identified following aspiration. Also, if there is a tumor, the fluid re-accumulates within days of the aspiration.

58. D Patients with diabetic fibrous mastopathy are managed conservatively. Development of multiple and bilateral lesions is common. The etiology of this process is unknown; however, an autoimmune component is thought to be likely. Patients have a long history of insulin-dependent, type I diabetes. Reactive lymphadenopathy is not a component of this process and patients do not require antibiotics.

59. B The shortest distance from the skin to the lesion is used to determine the approach for preoperative, mammographically guided wire localizations. Craniocaudal and oblique views are usually sufficient. Rarely, a 90-degree lateral view may be indicated to establish the approach. In this patient, the lesion is closest to lateral skin surface on the right CC view. Given its peripheral location, the lesion will drop in going from the MLO to the 90-degree lateral view but not so much that a from below approach would be appropriate. The starting position for the wire localization is a 90-degree LM—the needle will be advanced into the breast and through the mass from the lateral skin surface. The needle length is selected so that the tip of the needle will go beyond the lesion by at least 1 cm.

60. A Depending on the distance from the skin to lesion, a needle that will go beyond the lesion by at least 1 cm is selected. The needle can always be pulled back as needed, however, nothing, other than starting over can be done, if the needle is short of the lesion.

61. C Our imaging algorithm, in women presenting for diagnostic evaluation with focal signs and symptoms is to place a BB at the site of the focal finding, do CC and MLO views and a spot tangential view of the focal finding. In many patients, the lesion is partially or completely surrounded by subcutaneous fat on the tangential view enabling perception and characterization of the margins. Ultrasound is commonly indicated, unless the area of the finding is completely fatty and there is no chance the lesion has been excluded or "pushed" out of the image. MRI and fine-needle aspiration are not usually indicated unless concerns persist on physical examination, mammography, and ultrasound.

62. D Clusters and segmentally distributed fine, pleomorphic calcifications including linear forms are imaged on this spot compression magnification view of the left breast. These require biopsy and likely reflect the presence of ductal carcinoma in situ. BI-RADS 4C, Suspicious finding, biopsy is indicated. To histologically confirm the suspected extent of the disease in this patient, we would biopsy two suspicious sites as far apart as possible. Little is gained by doing more than the two biopsies in this patient.

63. C Mucinous carcinomas commonly develop in postmenopausal women and present mammographically as slowly growing round or oval masses. The margins may appear circumscribed; however, on close evaluation with spot compression views, they are often indistinct but not spiculated. On ultrasound, mucinous carcinomas may be difficult to identify because they are often isoechoic to slightly hyperechoic lesions. They may demonstrate posterior acoustic enhancement. On MRI, they are characterized by heterogeneous enhancement and components with a high T2 signal.

64. B Phantom images ed to be kept for 1 year. Some of these may be reviewed during FDA inspections.

65. D Excisional biopsy is recommended in patients with a diagnosis of atypical ductal hyperplasia on a core biopsy. This is usually diagnosed on cores done for calcifications, less commonly masses. In some patients, the diagnosis is confirmed at the time of the excision. In others, the lesion is upstaged to DCIS, less commonly an invasive lesion. Depending on how the imaging-guided biopsy is done, 15% to 45% (vacuum-assisted vs. 14G spring-loaded systems) of patients are upstaged on the excision biopsy.

66. A Regardless of the character (e.g., bloody), nipple discharge may be significant and requires further evaluation when it occurs spontaneously. Women should be discouraged from actively trying to express discharge; they should be encouraged to periodically check their bra cups and nightclothes for dark brown spots (reliable indicators of spontaneous discharge). Cytology of nipple discharge is useless. Normal results do not reliably exclude pathology and atypical cells are not necessarily indicators of significant pathology (and the location of the pathology in the duct is not established with cytology alone).

67. B Segmentally distributed, non-mass like clumped and linear enhancement as illustrated in this image requires biopsy. In this patient, we would biopsy the extremes so as to establish the extent of suspected disease histologically. Ultrasound is not helpful in evaluating patients with non-mass like enhancement. Establishing a diagnosis through needle biopsy is preferred to using surgical excision to establish a diagnosis (and for surgical excision, clips would need to be placed under MRI guidance). Without having a histological diagnosis, mastectomy would be grossly inappropriate.

68. C Papillomas (solitary or multiple) are characterized by the presence of a central fibrovascular core. Papillomatosis is a misleading term taken by some to mean multiple papillomas. However, papillomatosis is a term used by many pathologists to describe papillary epithelial hyperplasia (e.g., no fibrovascular core) and not papillomas. Solitary central papillomas typically present with spontaneous nipple discharge. Multiple peripheral papillomas are more commonly diagnosed on screening mammography as multiple small masses or clusters of round, punctate amorphous calcifications.

69. A Metaplastic carcinomas are a subtype of invasive ductal carcinoma representing less than 5% of all breast cancers. They are characterized by rapid growth and a poorer prognosis, and are typically estrogen and progesterone receptor and HER2/neu negative (e.g., triple negative). Although lymphatic metastases are reported in 8% to 40% of patients at the time of presentation, they can also metastasize hematogenously to lung and bone.

70. D Size is not a reliable criterion in evaluating axillary lymph nodes. The appearance of the fatty hilum (compressed, attenuated) or its absence is helpful. The echogenicity and relationship of the cortex to the fatty hilum are also helpful. Marked hypoechogenicity as well as thickening and bulging of the cortex are findings often associated with metastatic disease to axillary lymph nodes. Cysts are exceedingly rare in the axilla.

71. C Invasive lobular carcinoma is the usual underlying histology in patients presenting with a shrinking breast. Breast enlargement, decreased compressibility with skin thickening, and diffuse increases in density as well as axillary masses are typical mammographic findings in patients with inflammatory carcinoma. Decreases in breast size are coupled with increases in breast density (due to decreases in fatty tissue) in patients with weight loss. Although the size of the breast is usually asymmetrically decreased following lumpectomy and radiation therapy other associated findings in these patients include skin thickening, distortion, retraction, parenchymal distortion, and surgical clips. Skin thickening and diffuse prominence of the trabecular markings are seen acutely post-radiation therapy; these changes usually resolve within the first 2 years following treatment.

72. B Complex sclerosing lesions (CSL) are by definition greater than 1 cm in size (called radial scars when less than 1 cm in size). Distortion characterized by central fat and long curvilinear spicules that are better seen in one projection (planar lesions) compared with the orthogonal view characterize mammographic features of these lesions, associated round and punctate calcifications may be seen in approximately 30% of patients. These are idiopathic lesions not related to prior surgery or trauma. Association with high-risk lesions, including atypical ductal hyperplasia, lobular carcinoma in situ, multiple peripheral papillomas, low-grade ductal carcinoma in situ, and low-grade invasive lesions, has been reported in as many as 33% of these lesions; it is these associations that prompt some to recommend excisional biopsy when a CSL is diagnosed on core biopsy. Although they are often 2 to 3 cm in size on the mammogram, physical examination is usually normal and the ultrasound findings are normal or subtle distortion in one plane may be identified.

73. C Fatty tissue is imaged on this spot tangential view; however, given the axillary location of the symptom you need to consider the possibility that a lesion has been excluded (compressed out) from the field of view. Correlative physical examination and an ultrasound are indicated in patients in whom the clinical finding is close to the edge of the film. See Figure 3.2B for the ultrasound evaluation of this patient.

74. D By definition, focal parenchymal asymmetry needs to be seen in two projections: it should be at approximately the same location on CC and MLO views, and comparable in size and density. On spot compression views, the internal density is inhomogeneous related to presence of fat and the edges are scalloped. Normal tissue is palpated on physical examination and seen on ultrasound at the expected location of the asymmetry.

75. A These terms reflect genetic profiling of breast cancers. Luminal A tumors are typically ER+ and/or PR+, HER2 negative, and have a low Ki67 (<14%). These are usually lower histological grade tumors with low proliferation-related genes. Luminal B tumors can be subdivided into: (i) patients with ER+ and/or PR+, HER2-negative, and high Ki67 (>14%) tumors or (ii) those with ER+ and/or PR+ and HER2/neu +, also called the luminal-HER2 group. The HER2 tumors are ER−, PR−, HER2/neu-positive tumors, and higher histologic grade lesions with p53 mutations in younger patients. The basal-like profile is characterized by ER−, PR−, HER2/neu-negative tumors. Currently not much is known about the normal-like profile but it clusters with the HER2+ and basal-like tumors; however, they seem to have a better prognosis than basal-like lesions.

76. C The regionally distributed calcifications in the left breast warrant biopsy. Although stereotactic biopsy is technically not possibly secondary to the thickness of the breast, the density of the calcification suggests that they may be apparent and amenable to biopsy with ultrasound. If calcifications are not identified reliably on ultrasound, surgical excision would be appropriate to establish the diagnosis. In this patient, the diagnosis of DCIS and the suspected extent of disease are confirmed on ultrasound-guided core biopsies. The calcifications are not bilateral and their morphology is not consistent with the dystrophic stromal-type calcifications seen in patients with renal disease. Extensive, dense vascular calcifications in this patient are consistent with her long-standing history of diabetes. Shunt tubing is seen superimposed on the upper aspect of the right breast.

77. B The malignant cells of invasive lobular carcinoma are small, monomorphic, and morphologically similar to lymphocytes consequently, on touch preparations of lymph nodes metastatic disease may not be appreciated.

78. D Although smaller lesions may be amenable to lumpectomy, mastectomy is often indicated in patients presenting with larger malignant phyllodes tumors. The effectiveness of radiation therapy and chemotherapy in patients with phyllodes tumors is limited and as such these therapies are not used. These lesions metastasize hematogenously so axillary lymph node biopsies are not indicated. Even in patients with clinically enlarged lymph nodes, the nodes are usually found to be reactive if sampled.

79. A Endothelial cell stains are used in the evaluation of potential angiosarcomas. E-cadherin is a cell adhesion molecule used to distinguish lobular (with no E-cadherin) from ductal processes. Cytokeratin stains are used in the characterization of epithelial cells and are not usually expressed in angiosarcomas. The expression of p63 is typically associated with epithelial and myoepithelial cell differentiations and only rarely seen in endothelial cell lesions.

80. C In women who have implants in a subglandular location, CC and MLO views are often similar in appearance. The high location and triangular shape of the pectoral muscle on the MLO views is also commonly seen on the implant displaced MLO views. Better visualization and inclusion of the pectoral muscles on MLO views is expected in men as well as women following reduction mammoplasty and lumpectomies.

81. B Papillary lesions are characteristically friable tumors and seeding of epithelial cells following needle biopsies is a recognized phenomenon. Epithelial cells can seed the surrounding stroma and adjacent lymphatic channels rarely resulting in "transport" of cells into axillary lymph nodes compounding the accurate classification of these lesions. The history of recent needle instrumentation, altered red blood cells, inflammatory changes, and lack of a desmoplastic reaction surrounding the displaced cells can be used to recognize displacement from invasion. Evaluating the edge of the lesion away from areas of recent instrumentation is also recommended.

82. A Human epidermal growth factor receptor 2 gene (HER2/neu)-amplified tumors represent approximately 18% to 30% if breast cancers. HER2/neu-positive tumors are associated with higher recurrence rates and a poor prognosis.

83. D The image demonstrates a focally dilated duct with an intraductal lesion likely representing an intraductal papilloma.

84. C Fibromatosis requires wide surgical excision to minimize the likelihood of a local recurrence. Complex fibroadenomas, duct ectasia, and gynecomastia do not usually require surgical excision.

85. B Renal excretion of the gadolinium is dependent on glomerular filtration rates. Contrast administration is contraindicated in patients with GFRs lower than 30 mL/min/1.73 m². The dose of gadolinium (T1 shortening agents) used ranges from 0.1 to 0.2 mmol per kg of body weight and a power injector is used at a rate of 2 to 3 mL per second followed by a 20-mL saline flush. For breast MRI, a temporal resolution of 1 to 2 minutes (ideally closer to 1 minute) is optimal, and a magnetic field strength of 1.5 T is preferred.

86. A An irregular dense mass with spiculated margins, associated distortion, and fine pleomorphic calcifications that extend in a segmental distribution to the subareolar area is imaged in the retroareolar area of the right breast, zone B. These findings are consistent with an invasive ductal carcinoma, not otherwise specified (e.g., the mass) associated with extensive ductal carcinoma in situ (e.g., the calcifications). Although invasive lobular carcinomas commonly present as a mass with spiculated margins the associated calcifications are suggestive of a ductal process rather than a lobular one.

87. B Our management of this patient would entail a biopsy of the mass since this is likely to represent the invasive disease and a biopsy of a cluster of calcification at a maximal distance from the mass to document the extent of the disease. A mastectomy is indicated if the suspected extent of disease is confirmed histologically.

88. C Papillomas are common benign lesions that demonstrate rapid wash-in and wash-out kinetic curves (e.g., false positives). Although hormonally stimulated fibroadenomas in young women may enhance, in older postmenopausal patients they are hyalinized and do not usually enhance. The glandular tissue component of fibroadenolipomas may demonstrate persistent enhancement. Lobular carcinoma in situ is more commonly diagnosed in premenopausal women. In some patients with LCIS, non-mass like enhancement may be seen on MRI.

89. B The term *triple negative* refers to tumors that are estrogen and progesterone receptor as well as HER2/neu negative.

90. D This image demonstrates a complex cystic and solid mass. The differential includes postoperative/traumatic fluid collection, fat necrosis, papillary lesion, and necrotic tumor. Correlation with the patient's mammogram and her history are needed before doing anything further. The image shown in Question 13 is the spot tangential view for this patient. Given the mammogram findings, no further intervention or short-interval follow-up is indicated (in fact, given the mammogram findings, an ultrasound was NOT indicated).

91. C Injecting air into a cyst following aspiration reportedly decreases the likelihood of cyst recurrence—so it may be of therapeutic value. Injection of air is not associated with abscess formation. The injected air is absorbed over several days so it is not available to identify the cyst on subsequent mammograms. Rarely, in patients with a suspected intracystic lesion, spot compression magnification views can be done after the injection of air to assess for mural abnormalities (e.g., pneumocystogram); given current ultrasound technology, however, the indications for pneumocystography are almost completely obsolete.

92. B The wire is short of the lesion. A second wire needs to be placed to adequately localize the lesion.

93. A The amount of contrast used for a ductography is in the order of 0.2 to 0.4 mL.

94. D In patients with node-negative estrogen receptor-positive tumors, the use of the Oncotype DX assay reportedly provides prognostic information with respect to the likelihood of recurrence and response to chemotherapy. Oncotype DX is a reverse transcriptase/polymerase chain reaction assay based on the analysis of a 21-gene panel. It is used to calculate a recurrence score (RS) of 0 to 100. Patients with a low RS (RS < 18) have indolent tumors that are sensitive to hormonal therapy and chemotherapy adds little if any benefit. Patients with a high RS (RS ≥ 31) have aggressive tumors less likely to respond to hormone therapy and benefit significantly from adjuvant therapy with a decrease in the recurrence rate at 10 years of close to 30%. In patients with an intermediate recurrence score (RS ≥ 18 to 30), it is unclear if the benefits from chemotherapy exceed the associated risks.

95. C The images demonstrate a mass with indistinct margins in the left subareolar area. The only thing that should keep you from further evaluating this patient is a history of an excisional biopsy correlated to the site of the finding. Stability and a history of lactational mastitis should not keep you from further evaluating a lesion with this appearance. Similarly, a suspicious mammographic finding requires biopsy regardless of a lack of enhancement on MRI.

96. B Wire localization is combined with ductography when the lesion is more than 2 cm from the nipple or when it occurs in a side branch of a highly arborized duct (See Fig. 12.13B, C).

97. A The spot compression magnification view demonstrates regionally distributed predominantly amorphous calcifications; round and punctate forms are also present. Benign differential considerations for clusters of predominantly amorphous calcifications include: fibrocystic changes (sclerosing adenosis, columnar cell changes with apical snouts and secretions [CAPPS], focal fibrosis, hyperplasia, and atypical ductal hyperplasia), fibroadenomas, and papillomas. When more diffuse, as in this patient, the main considerations include sclerosing adenosis and focal fibrosis. In the malignant category, ductal carcinoma in situ, commonly low nuclear grade, is the primary consideration.

98. D Breast self-examination should be started late in adolescence or in the early 20s so patients become familiar with the consistency of their breasts. It should be done routinely 1 to 2 days after the menstrual cycle at which time breast tissue is least likely to be tender. After menopause, patients should select a specific day in the month to do their exam. Rather than having patients attempt to express nipple discharge, they should be encouraged to check their bra cups and nightclothes for dark brown spots (e.g., spontaneous discharge).

99. B An abnormal internal mammary lymph node is imaged high along the internal mammary chain on this patient. If it is on the same side as her cancer she would be N1.

100. C A false-negative mammogram is defined as a cancer diagnosis within a year of a "normal" screening mammogram.

101. D Cellular fibroadenomas are acceptable in young premenopausal women (e.g., women in their late teens, 20s, and early 30s). On a core biopsy of a new solid mass in a postmenopausal woman, however, a phyllodes tumor needs to be considered if a cellular fibroadenoma is described histologically. Excisional biopsy is indicated when "cellular fibroadenomas" are described in postmenopausal women.

102. A Triple-negative tumors commonly present as interval cancers in premenopausal African American women and represent approximately 15% to 20% of all breast cancers. Tumors developing in BRCA1-positive patients are often triple-negative tumors.

103. B An irregular collection of contrast is seen at the tip of the cannula. Additionally opacified tubular structures are seen. The findings are most consistent with contrast extravasation and opacification of lymphatic channels.

104. D Lesions in the retroareolar area do not shift much between MLO and 90-degree lateral views. The more peripheral in the breast (e.g., lateral or medial), the more it will shift between MLO and 90-degree lateral views.

105. A An irregular mass with spiculated margins is imaged. Regardless of stability, this is a BI-RADS 4C. The only thing that would keep me from evaluating this lesion aggressively is a history of a surgical biopsy correlated to this specific site.

106. C Mondor disease is a thrombophlebitis commonly affecting the lateral thoracic vein. It does not involve the nipple or areola and is not associated with fistula formation.

107. C Of the lesions listed, PASH can recur following surgical excision. Other benign lesions in the differential for recurrence following excision include multiple peripheral papillomas, fibromatosis, granular cell tumors, and phyllodes tumor.

108. D This ultrasound images demonstrates tubular hypoechogenicity as well as irregular areas of tissue disruption and hypoechogenicity within which echogenic foci are seen. Calcifications are likely apparent on the mammogram. See the image in Question 62 for this patient's mammogram.

109. B When postoperative changes occur, they often resolve in the first several months after the procedure. Unless a mammography is done in the first 6 months following a biopsy, mammograms are normal in over 50% of these women and, in those women in whom a change is seen, it is often recognizable as related to a biopsy particularly when correlated with the history and actual biopsy site. Postsurgical changes are often planar and as such often seen better in one of the two standard views as distortion. They typically resolve completely in more than half of the patients, rarely develop dystrophic calcifications.

110. A In patients without a history of surgery, skin calcifications commonly develop in the cleavage. They are also seen developing in a linear distribution along the incisions made as part of reduction mammoplasties.

111. C A high-density mass with circumscribed and indistinct margins is imaged on the spot tangential view corresponding to the "lump" described by the patient in the upper inner aspect of the right breast posteriorly (metallic BB used to mark the site of the palpable finding). On ultrasound, the mass is nearly anechoic with partially indistinct margins, an echogenic rim and minimal posterior acoustic enhancement. Without associated tenderness, an abscess is unlikely. Given the margins of this mass and the fact that it is a new *palpable* finding, it cannot be classified as probably benign; so a short-interval follow-up is not appropriate. The most likely diagnosis is that of an invasive ductal carcinoma, likely high grade (e.g., "blow-up" lesion), and an ultrasound-guided biopsy is indicated. Although the margins, echogenic rim, location, and minimal posterior enhancement relative to the size of the mass make a cyst unlikely, you can try to aspirate this prior to doing the core biopsy.

112. D Randomized controlled trials with blind randomization and mortality as the end-point are the gold standard in establishing the evidence needed to support the routine use of screening.

113. A Although in many patients exact causality is not established, drugs are probably the most common cause of gynecomastia. Testicular tumors, chest wall trauma, and HIV are rare causes of gynecomastia.

114. A The metastatic pattern for invasive lobular carcinomas may be distinctive. Unlike invasive ductal carcinomas that tend to metastasize to solid organs, including liver, lungs, bones, and brain, invasive lobular carcinomas often simulate ovarian carcinomas in their behavior. Seeding of peritoneal and pleural surfaces is seen with the development of ascites and pleural effusions; involvement of the leptomeninges, uterus, ovaries, and stomach can also occur.

115. B MQSA, passed in 1992, regulates mammographic modalities defined as technologies for radiography of the breast (e.g., mammography, tomosynthesis). Although radiography of the breast is used for stereotactic biopsies, needle localizations, and ductography, these procedures are exempt from the definition of mammographic modality and currently not regulated under MQSA. Ultrasound, magnetic resonance imaging, and breast-specific gamma imaging are not regulated under MQSA.

APPENDIX A

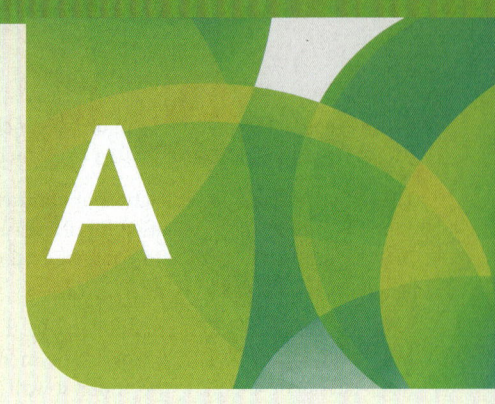

Table A.1 MAMMOGRAPHY: ACR BI-RADS® LEXICON (1)

Breast composition

- The breasts are almost entirely fatty
- There are scattered areas of fibroglandular density
- The breasts are heterogeneously dense, which may obscure small masses
- The breasts are extremely dense, which lowers the sensitivity of mammography

Findings

- Masses
  - Shape (oval, round, irregular)
  - Margin (circumscribed [at least 75% sharply demarcated], obscured [at least 25% not seen because of overlying or adjacent tissue], microlobulated, indistinct, spiculated)
  - Density (high density, equal density, low density, fat containing)
- Calcifications
  - Typically benign (skin, vascular, coarse or "popcorn-like," large rod-like, round, rim, dystrophic, milk of calcium, suture)
  - Suspicious morphology (amorphous, coarse heterogeneous, fine pleomorphic, fine linear, or fine-linear branching)
  - Distribution (diffuse, regional, grouped, linear, segmental)
- Architectural distortion
- Asymmetries
  - Asymmetry (fibroglandular tissue visible in one projection)
  - Global asymmetry (asymmetric tissue involving at least one quadrant)
  - Focal asymmetry (relatively small amount of asymmetric tissue seen in two projections; less than one quadrant)
  - Developing asymmetry (new or increasing in size)
- Intramammary lymph node
- Skin lesion
- Solitary-dilated duct
- Associated features (may see in the context of masses, calcifications or distortion, or alone)
  - Skin retraction
  - Nipple retraction
  - Skin thickening (>2 mm; may be focal or diffuse)
  - Trabecular thickening
  - Axillary adenopathy
  - Architectural distortion
  - Calcifications
- Location of lesion
  - Laterality
  - Quadrant and clock face
  - Depth
  - Distance from the nipple

Table A.2 BREAST ULTRASOUND: ACR BI-RADS® LEXICON (2)

Tissue composition (only for screening US)
    Homogeneous background echotexture—fat
    Homogenous background echotexture—fibroglandular
    Heterogeneous background echotexture

Findings

- Masses
  - Shape (oval, round, irregular)
  - Orientation (parallel [wider than tall or horizontal], not parallel [taller than wide or vertical])
  - Margin: circumscribed, not circumscribed (indistinct, angular, microlobulated, spiculated)
  - Echo pattern (anechoic, hyperechoic, complex cystic and solid, hypoechoic, isoechoic, heterogeneous [mixture of echogenic patterns in a solid mass])
  - Posterior features (no posterior features, enhancement, shadowing, combined pattern)
- Calcifications
  - Calcifications in a mass
  - Calcifications outside of a mass
  - Intraductal calcifications
- Associated features
  - Architectural distortion
  - Duct changes
  - Skin changes (thickening, retraction)
  - Edema
  - Vascularity (absent, internal vascularity, vessels in rim)
  - Elasticity assessment (soft, intermediate, hard)
- Special cases
  - Simple cyst
  - Clustered microcysts
  - Complicated cyst
  - Mass in or on skin
  - Foreign body including implants
  - Lymph nodes—intramammary
  - Lymph nodes—axillary
  - Vascular abnormalities (AVMs, Mondor disease)
  - Postsurgical fluid collection
  - Fat necrosis

Table A.3 BREAST MRI: ACR BI-RADS® LEXICON (3)

Amount of fibroglandular tissue

- Almost entirely fat
- Scattered fibroglandular tissue
- Heterogeneous fibroglandular tissue
- Extreme fibroglandular tissue

Background parenchymal enhancement

- Level (minimal, mild, moderate, marked)
- Symmetric or asymmetric

Findings

- Focus (<0.5 cm)
- Masses
  - Shape (oval, round, irregular)
  - Margin: circumscribed, not circumscribed (irregular, spiculated)
  - Internal enhancement characteristics (homogeneous, heterogeneous, rim enhancement, dark internal septations)

(continued)

Table A.3 BREAST MRI: ACR BI-RADS® LEXICON (3) (continued)

- Non-mass enhancement
  - Distribution (focal, linear, segmental, regional, multiple regions, diffuse)
  - Internal enhancement patterns (homogeneous, heterogeneous, clumped, clustered ring)
- Intramammary lymph node
- Skin lesion
- Nonenhancing findings
  - Ductal precontrast high signal on T1W
  - Cyst
  - Postoperative collections (hematoma/seroma)
  - Post therapy skin thickening and trabecular thickening
  - Non-enhancing mass
  - Architectural distortion
  - Signal void from foreign bodies, clips, etc.
- Associated features
  - Nipple retraction
  - Nipple invasion
  - Skin retraction
  - Skin thickening
  - Skin invasions (direct, inflammatory cancer)
  - Axillary adenopathy
  - Pectoralis muscle involvement
  - Chest wall invasion
  - Architectural distortion
- Fat-containing lesions
  - Lymph nodes (normal, abnormal)
  - Fat necrosis
  - Hamartoma
  - Postoperative seroma/hematoma with fat
- Location of lesion
  - Location
  - Depth
- Kinetic curve assessment—signal intensity (SI)/time curve description
  - Initial phase (slow, medium fast)
  - Delayed phase (persistent, plateau, washout)
- Implants
  - Implant material and lumen type: saline, silicone (intact, ruptured), other implant material, lumen type
  - Implant location (retroglandular, retropectoral)
  - Abnormal implant contour (focal bulge)
  - Intracapsular silicone findings: radial folds, subcapsular line, keyhole sign (teardrop, noose), linguine
  - Extracapsular silicone (breast, lymph nodes)
  - Water droplets
  - Peri-implant fluid

References

1. Sickles EA, D'Orsi CJ, Bassett LW, et al. ACR BI-RADS® mammography. In: *ACR BI-RADS® Atlas, Breast Imaging Reporting and Data System*. Reston, VA: American College of Radiology; 2013.
2. Mendelson EB, Böhm-Vélez M, Berg WA, et al. ACR BI-RADS® ultrasound. In: *ACR BI-RADS® Atlas, Breast Imaging Reporting and Data System*. Reston, VA: American College of Radiology; 2013.
3. Morris EA, Comstock CE, Lee CH, et al. ACR BI-RADS® magnetic resonance imaging. In: *ACR BI-RADS® Atlas, Breast Imaging Reporting and Data System*. Reston, VA: American College of Radiology; 2013.

INDEX

Note: Page numbers followed by *f* denote figures; those followed by *t* denote tables.

Abscess, 322*f*
   lactational, 201–202, 202*f*
   vs. mastitis, 106–107, 107*f*, 108*f*, 109
   peripheral, 203–205, 205*f*–206*f*
   subareolar, 202–203, 203*f*, 204*f*
Accordion effect, 411, 412*f*
Acini spaces, 152
Acute bacterial mastitis, 288*f*–289*f*
Acute hematoma, after excisional biopsy, 335*f*
Acute radiation therapy, lumpectomy, 444
Adenomas
   complex fibroadenoma, 210–211, 210*f*, 211*f*
   fibroadenomas, 206–208, 207*f*–210*f*
   lactational, 212, 212*f*
   phyllodes tumors, 212, 213*f*–215*f*, 216
   tubular, 211–212, 211*f*
Altered breast
   augmentation, 359, 361–365, 367
   conservative breast cancer treatment, 340–343, 350
   dacron central line cuff, 370, 371*f*, 372
   estrogen effect, 367–368, 369*f*
   excisional biopsy changes, 331–332, 331*f*–335*f*, 334–335, 336*f*, 337*f*
   foreign bodies, 368, 371*f*
   hormonal/aromatase inhibitor, as treatment for, 373, 374*f*
   mastectomy site, 350
   pacemakers, 372–373
   port-a-catheters, 372, 372*f*, 373*f*
   reconstruction after mastectomy, 350, 354–357, 354*f*–357*f*
   reduction mammoplasty, 357–359, 358*f*–359*f*, 360*f*, 361*f*
   transgender patients, 373, 374*f*
   trauma, 338, 339*f*–340*f*, 341*f*
   vacuum-assisted imaging-guided biopsy, 335–336, 337*f*–338*f*, 339*f*
   weight changes, 368, 370*f*
American Cancer Society (ACS), 3, 138
American College of Radiology (ACR)
   BI-RADS®, 173, 438*f*, 442, 445, 448, 451, 452–454
   lexicon for masses, 173*t*
   Mammography Accreditation Program (MAP), 4–5
Amorphous calcifications, 152–153, 157*f*, 167*f*
Anastrozole (Arimidex), 373
Angiolipoma, 230*f*
Angiomas, 230
Angiosarcomas, 225, 270*f*, 439, 449
Angle of obliquity, for MLO view, 16*f*
Angular descriptor, 446
Annual screening mammography, 431, 434*f*, 444, 445

Anterior compression views, use of, 26–29, 27*f*–32*f*
Antibiotic therapy, 448
Apocrine-lined cysts, 92, 199
Architectural distortion, 61*t*, 225
Arimidex. *See* Anastrozole
Aromasin. *See* Exemestane
Arterial calcifications, 150, 150*f*
Arteritis, 290, 290*f*
Artifacts
   bloom, from ferromagnetic objects, 115*f*
   breast magnetic resonance imaging, 115, 115*f*, 116*f*, 117–118, 117*f*
   breast within a breast, 35
   calcification, 166, 169*f*
   equipment-related, 33*t*
   mimicry, 166, 169*f*
   patient-related, 33*t*, 35
   post-biopsy needle, 116*f*
   reverberation, 92, 92*f*
   screening mammography, 31–35, 33*t*, 34*f*, 35*f*, 36*f*
   software processing, 33*t*
   vibration and electrical interference, 34*f*
Aspiration, 94, 95*f*
Atypical ductal hyperplasia (ADH), 2, 157, 218, 409, 435, 438, 446, 448
Atypical lobular hyperplasia (ALH), 2, 303, 409
Augmentation, 359, 361–365, 367
Autologous tissue transplantation, 354–355
Automated gun-needle combinations, 393–394, 394*f*
Axillary lymph nodes, 272, 275, 276, 276*f*–279*f*
Axillary lymphadenopathy, 188*t*
Axillary venous obstruction, 287

Background parenchymal enhancement, on breast MRI, 118, 122*f*
Benign breast calcifications, 147, 148*t*, 149*t*
Benign breast disease, 2
Benign breast masses
   abscess, 201–205, 202*f*, 203*f*, 204*f*, 205*f*–206*f*
   adenomas (fibroepithelial lesions), 206–212, 207*f*–215*f*, 216
   benign vascular lesions, 230, 230*f*, 231*f*
   complex sclerosing lesions (radial scar), 225, 225*f*–226*f*, 227
   cystic breast masses, 197–201, 198*f*, 199*f*, 200*f*, 201*f*
   diabetic mastopathy, 220–221, 223*f*
   evaluation and imaging features of, 172–176, 172*t*, 173*f*–175*f*, 173*t*, 174*t*
   extra-abdominal desmoid (fibromatosis), 227, 228*f*
   fat-containing masses, 180, 181*t*
   focal fibrosis, 220, 222*f*

   granular cell tumors, 227–228, 229*f*–230*f*, 230
   lipoma, 181, 182*f*, 183*f*, 184*f*
   in male, 320, 320*f*–322*f*, 323*f*
   mixed-density masses, 186, 186*f*–196*f*, 188, 191–192, 195–196
   multiple papillomas, 218, 220*f*, 221*f*
   oil cysts, 181, 184, 184*f*, 185*f*, 186, 186*f*
   other fluid collections, 205–206, 206*f*–207*f*
   pseudoangiomatous stromal hyperplasia, 221–222, 223*f*–224*f*, 225
   sclerosing adenosis, 227, 227*f*
   skin masses, 176, 176*f*–180*f*, 178–180, 181*f*
   solitary papilloma, 216–218, 216*f*–217*f*, 219*f*, 220*f*
   water density masses, 196–197, 197*t*
Benign complex cystic masses, 94
Benign vascular lesions, 230, 230*f*, 231*f*
BI-RADS®, 173, 438*f*, 442, 445, 448, 451, 452–454
Bilateral cancers, 238, 244*f*
Bloom artifact, from ferromagnetic objects, 115*f*
Bolus adequacy, 120*f*
BRCA, 113–114, 138
BRCAPRO risk models, 128
Breast. *See also* Altered breast; Calcifications, breast; Diffuse breast changes; Male breast
   FB projection for, 70, 71*f*, 72*f*
   hypertrophy, 357
   lateromedial oblique views, 70, 73, 73*f*
   lesion measurements in, 434, 445–446
   lymphoma, primary, 267
   masses, assessment of, 120*f*–121*f*, 125
   metastatic lung carcinoma to, 328*f*
   mobility, 16, 17*f*
   orthogonal views, 64
   radiography of, 451
   sagging of, 30*f*, 31*f*
   self-examination for, 442, 450
   structure of, 26–27
   superolateral to inferomedial oblique views, 73
   triangulation views, 73, 74*f*, 75–77, 75*f*, 76*f*–77*f*
   ultrasound scanning, 82*f*
Breast cancer
   conservative treatment, 340–343, 342, 342*f*–350*f*, 350, 351*f*
   diagnosis of, 432, 445
   hormonal/aromatase inhibitor for, 373, 374*f*
   increased risk of, 431, 444
   inflammatory, diagnosis of, 434, 446
   invasive, precursor to, 435, 446
   in male, 320, 323, 324*f*–326*f*, 326, 327*f*
   Mammography Accreditation Program (MAP), 4–5
   Mammography Quality Standards Act (MQSA), 4
   molecular profiling of, 439, 449
   mortality rates, decrease of, 443, 451

455

Breast cancer (*continued*)
    patient images of, 9–10
    risk factors, 1–3
    screening mammography and recommendations, 3–4
    staging of, 6–9
    treatment options, 5–6
Breast-conserving therapy, recurrence after, 293, 295*f*
Breast imaging. *See* Breast magnetic resonance imaging; Communication, in breast imaging; Diagnostic breast imaging; Magnetic resonance imaging
Breast Imaging and Reporting Data System (BI-RADS®), 173, 438*f*, 442, 445, 448, 451, 452–454
Breast magnetic resonance imaging, 113–114, 440, 450. *See also* Magnetic resonance imaging
    artifacts, 115, 115*f*, 116*f*, 117–118, 117*f*
    developing breast cancer, risk for, 138, 140*f*
    diagnosis of, 128, 130–133, 130*f*–133*f*
    indications for, 128
    lesion evaluation, 118, 119*f*–128*f*, 125, 126, 128, 129*f*
    of patients undergoing neoadjuvant therapy, 135, 135*f*–137*f*, 137
    patients with metastatic disease to axilla, 133, 134*f*, 135
    with positive margins, 137, 138*f*, 139*f*
    problem solving, 139, 141*f*, 142*f*, 143
    technical considerations, 114–115, 114*f*
    of women with implants, 138, 140*f*
Breast masses. *See* Benign breast masses; Malignant breast masses
Breast ultrasound. *See also* Ultrasound
    advantages of, 81
    breast anatomy on, 84–90, 85*f*, 86*f*–90*f*, 91*f*
    features of lesions to consider on, 82*t*
    masses with benign features on, 98*f*
Breast within a breast, 35, 35*f*, 189*f*
Burkitt non-Hodkins lymphoma, 296
Burkitt-type lymphoma, 269

Calcifications, breast, 145–147, 146*f*–147*f*, 147*t*, 148*t*, 148*f*
    artifacts, mimicry, 166, 169*f*
    associated with malignancy, 155–158, 160–164, 164*f*, 164*t*, 165*f*, 166, 166*f*, 167*f*–168*f*
    benign breast calcifications, 147, 148*t*, 149*t*
    benign-type calcifications in masses, 153–154, 158*f*, 159*f*, 160*f*, 161*f*, 162*f*
    ductal, 151, 154*f*
    lobular, 152–153, 155*f*, 156*f*, 156*t*, 157*f*
    parasites, 155, 163*f*, 164*f*
    skin (dermal) calcifications, 148–149, 149*f*
    stromal calcifications, 151, 151*f*, 152*f*, 153*f*
    sutures, 154–155, 162*f*
    ultrastructure, 168, 169*f*
    vascular calcifications, 150–151, 150*f*, 151*f*
Calcium oxalate (weddellite), 168, 169*f*, 445
Calcium phosphate crystals (hydroxyapatite), 168, 169*f*
Canadian National Breast Screening Study-1 (CNBSS-1), 3
Carcinoembryonic antigen (CEA), 230

Carcinoma. *See also* Breast cancer; Ductal carcinoma in situ
    ductal, 383*f*–384*f*
    inflammatory, 290–291, 291*f*–293*f*, 294*f*
    invasive ductal carcinoma NOS, 234–235, 235*f*–244*f*, 237–239, 241, 244, 245*f*
    invasive lobular, 261–262, 267, 294
    lobular carcinoma in situ (LCIS), 303, 432, 445, 446
    medullary, 249, 255
    metaplastic, 261
    metastatic, 326, 327*f*–328*f*
    mucinous, 125*f*, 248–249, 250*f*–255*f*, 294, 438, 448
    papillary, 255, 256*f*–260*f*, 260–261, 323
    tubular, 246, 248, 248*f*, 249*f*
Caudocranial projection, 70, 71*f*, 72*f*
CD68, 230
Cellular fibroadenoma, on core biopsy, 442, 450
Central venous obstruction, 287
Chemotherapy, 5–6
Chest wall involvement, 130, 132*f*, 133*f*
Chest wall sarcoma, radiation induced, 345*f*
Clinical regional lymph node classification, 7*t*
Clinical TNM (cTNM), 6
Clip placement, after imaging-guided biopsy, 407–409, 407*f*–409*f*
Closed capsulotomy, 365
Clustered microcysts, 199–200, 201*f*
Cocking mechanism, 393
Collimator misalignment, 34*f*
Comedo mastitis, 151
Communication, in breast imaging, 424–425
    benign concept, 425–428
    mammography report, 425, 426*t*, 427*t*
    medical audit, 428, 429*t*
    patient notification letters, 428
Complete pathologic response (cPR), 433, 445
Complex cystic masses, 92, 95*t*, 97*f*, 107, 108*f*, 200–201, 255, 256*f*
    and solid masses, 437, 441*f*, 448, 450
Complex fibroadenoma (CFA), 97*f*, 210–211, 210*f*, 211*f*
Complex sclerosing lesions (CSLs), 225, 225*f*–226*f*, 227, 439, 449
Complicated cysts, 197–198, 200*f*
Compression
    importance of, 26
    paddles, 15*f*
Congestive heart failure, 287*f*
Conservative breast cancer treatment, 340–343, 342, 342*f*–350*f*, 350, 351*f*
Contrast-to-noise ratios (CNR), 14
Cooper ligaments, 84–85, 86*f*–87*f*
Core biopsy, 435*f*, 446
    cellular fibroadenoma on, 442, 450
    necrotic invasive ductal carcinoma, 443, 451
Coronary artery disease, issue of, 368
Craniocaudal views, 19–25, 21*f*–22*f*, 21*t*, 23*f*
Curvilinear hyperechoic internal septations, 181, 182*f*
Cysts, 92, 94*f*, 118, 125, 126*f*
    aspiration and pneumocystography, 386, 387*f*–391*f*, 388–390
    breast mass, 197–201, 198*f*, 199*f*, 200*f*, 201*f*
    injecting air into, 441, 450
Cytokeratin stains, 449

Dacron central line cuff, 370, 371*f*, 372
Deep inferior epigastric perforator flap, 357
Dermal calcifications. *See* Skin, calcifications
Dermatofibrosarcoma protuberans, 271*f*–272*f*
Diabetic fibrous mastopathy, 223*f*
Diabetic mastopathy, 220–221, 223*f*, 437, 448
Diagnostic breast imaging
    approach to, 48–49
    from below, 70, 71*f*, 72*f*
    cleavage views, 69, 69*f*
    LMO and SIO views, 70, 73, 73*f*
    magnification views, 54, 56, 61*f*, 61*t*, 62*f*
    90-degree lateral views, 69–70, 70*f*, 71*f*
    rolled or change of angle views, 59–60, 62*f*–66*f*, 64
    spot compression views, 49–51, 52*f*, 53*f*, 54, 54*f*, 54*t*, 55*f*–57*f*, 58*f*, 59*f*, 60*f*
    symptomatic patients, 49, 49*t*, 50*f*, 51*f*
    tangential views, 64–65, 66*f*, 67*f*, 68*f*, 69*f*
    triangulation views, 73, 74*f*–77*f*, 75–77
Diffuse breast changes
    arteritis, 290, 290*f*
    axillary venous obstruction, 287
    breast-conserving therapy, recurrence after, 293, 295*f*
    central venous obstruction, 287
    ductal carcinoma in situ, 294, 296, 297*f*, 298*f*
    fluid overload, 284, 285*f*–286*f*, 286
    granulomatous mastitis, 287–288, 289*f*–290*f*
    inflammatory breast cancer, 290–291, 291*f*–293*f*, 294*f*
    invasive lobular carcinoma, 293–294, 295*f*–297*f*
    locally advanced breast cancer, 290–291, 291*f*–293*f*, 294*f*
    lymphoma, 296, 299*f*
    mastitis, 286–287, 288*f*, 289*f*
    radiation therapy effect, 283–284, 284*f*, 285*f*
    trauma, 286, 287*f*–288*f*
Diffuse glandular gynecomastia, 316
Diffuse skin thickening, 432, 444
Dilated vasculature, 306, 311, 311*f*
Directional vacuum-assisted biopsy probes, 393, 394*f*, 396
Draining sinus, development of, 95*f*
Duct ectasia, 383*f*
    focal, 311*f*
Duct extension, 99, 100*f*
Ductal calcification, 151, 154*f*
Ductal carcinoma in situ (DCIS), 61*f*, 155–156, 246, 246*f*, 247*f*, 294, 296, 297*f*, 298*f*
    calcifications suggestive of, 437, 448
    lesions, 128
    in male, 323
    screening mammography, 444
Ductography, 378–386, 378*t*, 379*f*–386*f*, 387*f*
    amount of contrast, 441, 450
    intraductal lesion on, 385, 441, 450
    in patients with papillomas, 432, 444
Dystrophic calcifications, 160*f*, 161*f*, 306. *See also* Stromal calcifications

E-cadherin, 304, 445, 449
Ecchymosis, 338
Eczema, 303
Eklund method, for location of lesion, 76*f*–77*f*
Endothelial cell stains, 439, 449
Enlarged axillary lymph nodes, 279*f*

INDEX

Epidermal inclusion cysts, 320
Epidermoid inclusion cyst, 176, 361f
Epithelial cells, displacement of, 440, 449
ERBB2 gene, 244
Estrogen effect, 367–368, 369f
Estrogen receptors (ER), 135
Exaggerated craniocaudal views (XCCL), 25, 25f–26f, 26t
Excisional biopsy
  acute hematoma after, 335f
  atypical ductal hyperplasia, 438, 448
  cellular fibroadenoma, on core biopsy, 442, 450
  changes, 331–332, 331f–335f, 334–335, 336f, 337f, 409
  fibroepithelial lesion, 436, 447
Exemestane (Aromasin), 373
Extensive ductal carcinoma in situ, invasive ductal carcinoma with, 440f, 450
Extensive intraductal component, 244, 246
Extra-abdominal desmoid, 227, 228f
Extracapsular rupture, 365, 366f, 367
  women with silicone implants, 437, 447

False-negative mammogram, 442, 450
Fat-containing masses, 180, 181t
Fat necrosis, 94, 98f, 191–192, 191f–196f, 195–196, 321f, 433, 445
  biopsy-related, 333f
  at lumpectomy, 341
Fat saturation, 117f
Fat suppression, 115
  homogeneous, 117
Fatty hilum, 272
Fatty tissue, 439f, 449
  and lobulation, 86f
Femara. See Letrozole
Fenestrated alphanumeric compression paddle, 64–65, 69f
Ferromagnetic materials, 115
FFDM. See Full field digital mammography
Fibroadenolipomas (FAL), 188, 189f, 190f
Fibroadenoma, 124f, 162f, 175f, 206–208, 207f–210f
  complex, 210–211, 210f, 211f
  hyalinizing, 173f
  and invasive ductal carcinoma, 189f
Fibroepithelial lesion. See also Adenomas; Phyllodes tumors
  excisional biopsy, 436, 447
Fibromatosis, wide surgical excision, 440, 450. See also Extra-abdominal desmoid
Filariasis (*Wuchereria bancrofti* and *Brugia malayi*), 155
Fine-needle aspiration (FNA), 391–393, 391f–392f
Flap necrosis, 357
FNA. See Fine-needle aspiration
Focal fibrosis, 220, 222f
Focal parenchymal asymmetry, 58f, 300f, 439, 449
Focal parenchymal enhancement, 118
Focal squamous metaplasia, 261
Focus enhancement, 128, 129f
Foreign bodies, in breast, 368, 371f
From below (FB) projection, 70, 71f, 72f
Full field digital mammography (FFDM), 4

Gadolinium, renal excretion of, 114, 440, 450
Galactoceles, 92, 94f, 206, 207f
Gamekeeper's thumb, 365
Gardner syndrome, 227
Gel bleed, 365
Genetic profiling, 8
Ghosting, 31, 117f
Giant cell arteritis, 290, 290f
Glandular gynecomastia, diffuse, 316
Global parenchymal asymmetry, 301f
Glomerular filtration rates (GFRs), 114
Granular cell tumors, 227–228, 229f–230f, 230, 437, 447
Granulomas, calcifying, 158f
Granulomatous mastitis, 106, 107f, 287–288, 289f–290f
Gurgling cyst, 93f
Gynecomastia, 318, 318f, 318t, 319f, 320f, 435, 446
  cause of, 443, 451
  diffuse glandular, 316
  unilateral dense, 323f

Halo sign, 173, 174f
Hamartoma. See Fibroadenolipomas
Hemangiomas, 230, 231f
Hematomas, 206, 206f
Hematopoietic lesion, 269
Hemorrhage, and postoperative fluid collection, 122f
Herceptin. See Trastuzumab
Heterogeneous calcifications, 148t
Hickman catheter placement, 370, 371f
Homogeneous enhancement, 118
Homogeneous fat suppression, 117
Hormonal/aromatase inhibitor, for breast cancer, 373, 374f
Hormone replacement therapy (HRT), 118, 367–368
Human epidermal growth factor receptor 2 gene (HER2/neu) amplified tumors, 440, 449
Hyalinized fibroadenomas, 42f, 84f
Hyperechogenicity, 97–98, 446
  central beaded band of, 437f, 448
Hyperechoic macrolobulated mass, 446
Hyperplasia, 157
Hypertrophy, breast, 357

Implant rupture, 365
Inflammatory breast cancer (IBC), 180, 290–291, 291f–293f, 294f
  diagnosis of, 434, 446
Inflammatory processes, 106–107, 107f, 108f, 109
Internal echogenic fibrous septations, 207
Internal mammary lymph node, 442, 450
Interventional procedures
  cyst aspiration and pneumocystography, 386, 387f–391f, 388–390
  ductography, 378–386, 378t, 379f–386f, 387f
  fine-needle aspiration, 391–393, 391f–392f
  needle biopsies, 393–394, 394f–396f
    magnetic resonance guidance, 402–404, 405f–406f, 407
    stereotactic guidance, 400–402, 403f, 404f
    ultrasound guidance, 396–398, 397f–400f, 400, 401f, 402f
  paraffin block radiography, 416, 420f
  preoperative wire localizations
    mammographic guidance, 411, 413, 413f–415f, 416f, 417f, 418f–420f
    ultrasound guidance, 409–411, 410f–411f, 412f
  specimen radiography, 415–416, 420f
  tumor location, clip placement to marking, 407–409, 407f–409f
Intracapsular implant rupture, 138, 365, 365f
Intracystic calcifications, 153
Intracystic papillary carcinoma, with invasive ductal carcinoma, 285f
Intracystic papilloma, 96
Intraductal papillomas, 303, 440, 450
Intramammary lymph node, 91f, 272, 275, 276, 276f–279f
  medial, 320f
Intramammary lymphadenopathy, 188t
Invasive breast cancer, precursor to, 435, 446
Invasive ductal carcinoma, 87f, 120f–121f, 327f
  anterior compression view, 28f
  chest wall involvement, 133f
  and DCIS, 62f, 167f, 174f
  diagnosis of, 431, 444
  with extensive ductal carcinoma in situ, 440f, 450
  high grade, 434f, 436f, 446, 447
  high nuclear grade with areas of necrosis, 124f–125f
  hyalinized fibroadenoma and, 42f
  intermediate nuclear grade, 57f
  intracystic papillary carcinoma with, 285f
  lateral tug for CC view, 22f
  with lobular features, 55f, 57f
  low nuclear grade, 57f
  low to intermediate grade, 56f
  metachronous lesions, 245f
  with metastatic disease to axilla, 123f
  multifocal, 174f
  non-mass-like enhancement, 127f–128f
  not otherwise specified, 234–235, 235f–244f, 237–239, 241, 244, 245f
  post-biopsy needle artifact, 116f
  XCCL view, 26f
Invasive lobular carcinoma, 59f, 261–262, 263f–267f, 267, 293–294, 295f–297f, 439, 449
  malignant cells of, 439, 449
  metastatic pattern with, 443, 451
  multicentric, 267f
Ipsilateral axillary lymph node, 267
Ipsilateral lymph nodes, with ultrasound, 439, 449
Ipsilateral reactive adenopathy, 202, 203f
Irregular descriptor, 446

Keloids, 178, 179f
Keratinocytes, 302

Lactational abscess, 201–202, 202f
Lactational adenoma, 212, 212f
Lateromedial oblique (LMO) views, for breast, 70, 73, 73f
Latissimus dorsi muscle flap reconstructions, 355, 355f
Leborgne sign, 225
Leiomyosarcoma, 269f
  metastatic to skin, 88
Letrozole (Femara), 373
Level I noncompliance violation, 435, 446
Lidocaine, 388–389, 392, 410, 413
Linear calcifications, 146, 146f, 147f, 167f–168f
Lipoma, 181, 182f, 183f, 184f
Liposarcoma, 270f
Lobular blushing, 380f

Lobular calcifications, 152–153, 155f, 156f, 156t, 157f
Lobular carcinoma in situ (LCIS), 303, 432, 445, 446
Lobular neoplasia (LN), 262, 303–304, 306, 409
Lobulocentric lesion, 227
Locally advanced breast cancer, 290–291, 291f–293f, 294f
Loiasis (*Loa loa*), 155
Lucent-centered calcifications, 158f
Lucent mass (oil cyst), 432, 445
Luminal A tumors, 8, 449
Luminal B tumors, 8
Luminal-HER2 group, 8, 449
Lumpectomy, and radiation therapy, 342f
Lymph nodes, 186–188, 186f–187f, 189f
Lymphatic opacification, extravasation with, 442, 451
Lymphoma, 267, 268f, 269, 296, 299f
Lymphoproliferative disorders, 277
Lymphoreticular lesion, 269

Magnetic resonance imaging (MRI). *See also* Breast magnetic resonance imaging
    conservative breast cancer treatment, 341
    extensive intraductal component, 244, 246
    fat necrosis on, 195
    of fibroadenomas, 207–208, 209f
    granular cell tumors, 228
    guided biopsies, 438, 448
    inflammatory carcinoma, 291
    invasive ductal carcinoma, 431, 444
    invasive lobular carcinoma, 294
    mucinous carcinomas, 249
    needle biopsies, 402–404, 405f–406f, 407
    in patient with BRCA mutation, 437, 447
    sebaceous cysts, 178, 179f
    of solitary papillomas, 217, 217f
    and ultrasound findings, 105–106
Magnification views, 54, 56, 61f, 61t, 62f
Male breast, 317f
    benign lesions, 320, 320f–322f, 323f
    breast cancer, 320, 323, 323t, 324f–326f, 326, 327f
    gynecomastia, 316, 318, 318f, 318t, 319f, 320f
    metastatic disease, 326, 327f–328f
Malignant breast masses
    ductal carcinoma in situ, 246, 246f, 247f
    extensive intraductal component, 244, 246
    imaging features and evaluation of, 234–279
    intramammary and axillary lymph nodes, metastatic disease to, 272, 275, 276, 276f–279f
    invasive ductal carcinoma NOS, 234–235, 235f–244f, 237–239, 241, 244, 245f
    invasive lobular carcinoma, 261–262, 263f–267f, 267
    lymphoma, 267, 268f, 269
    medullary carcinoma, 249, 255
    metaplastic carcinoma, 261, 261f, 262f
    metastatic disease to, 269, 272f–275f
    mucinous carcinoma, 248–249, 250f–255f
    papillary carcinoma, 255, 256f–260f, 260–261
    sarcomas, 269, 269f–272f
    tubular carcinoma, 246, 248, 248f, 249f
Malignant phyllodes tumors
    with liposarcomatous degeneration, 213f
    low grade, 213f–214f
    patients with, 439, 449
    recurrent at mastectomy site, 215f

Mammographically guided preoperative wire localization, 438, 448
Mammography
    facilities for, 432, 445
    FDA inspection of, 435, 446
    for invasive ductal carcinoma with extensive ductal carcinoma in situ, 440, 450
    lesion designation and longitudinal data, criteria for, 432, 444
    margins of mass on, 434, 446
    report outline, 426t
    screening, 3–4
Mammography Accreditation Program (MAP), ACR, 4
Mammography Quality Standards Act (MQSA), 4, 432, 435, 445, 446
    mammographic modalities, 443, 451
    phantom images, 438, 448
    quality control tests, 14
    repeat analysis for, 436, 447
Masses. *See also* Benign breast masses; Malignant breast masses; Solid masses
    benign-type calcifications in, 153–154, 158f, 159f, 160f, 161f, 162f
    complex cystic, 200–201
    cystic breast, 197–201, 198f, 199f, 200f, 201f
    mixed-density, 186, 186f–196f, 188, 195–196
    on skin, 176, 176f–180f, 178–180, 181f
    water density, 196–197, 197t
Mastectomy
    reconstruction following, 350, 354–357, 354f–357f
    single mediolateral oblique (MLO) view of, 350
Mastitis, 201–202, 286–287, 288f, 289f
    vs. abscess, 106–107, 107f, 108f, 109
    granulomatous, 107f
    obliterans, 151
Maximum intensity projection (MIP), 115
Medical audit, 428
    derived data for, 429t
    raw data needed for, 428t
Mediolateral oblique (MLO) view, 15–19, 16f, 17f, 18f, 18t, 19f, 20f–21f
    angle of obliquity for, 16f
    assessing positioning on, 18f, 18t
    pectoral muscle shape and, 19f
    projection, 435, 447
    single, 350
Medullary carcinomas, 249, 255f, 447
Metachronous invasive ductal carcinoma, 351f
Metaplastic carcinomas, 261, 261f, 262f, 439, 448–449
Metastatic disease, 326, 327f, 328f
    to breast, 269, 272f–275f
    chemotherapy for, 5–6
    to intramammary and axillary lymph nodes, 272, 275, 276, 276f–279f, 278f
Metastatic leukemia, 327f
Methicillin-resistant *Staphylococcus aureus* (MRSA) infection, 181f
Methotrexate, 288
Methysergide, 287
Microcysts, 93f, 153
Milk of calcium, 153, 159f, 160f
Mixed-density masses
    appropriate management for, 431, 444
    fat necrosis, 191–192, 191f–196f, 195–196
    fibroadenolipomas (hamartoma), 188, 189f, 190f
    lymph nodes, 186–188, 186f–187f, 189f

Mondor disease, 88, 90f, 311–312, 312f–313f, 312t, 443, 451
MRI. *See* Magnetic resonance imaging
Mucinous carcinomas, 125f, 248–249, 250f–255f, 438, 448
Mucopolysaccharides, 225
Multicentric cancers, 238, 241f
Multicentric invasive lobular carcinoma, 267f
Multifocal lesions, 238, 239f
Multiloculated lactational abscess, 202f
Multiple papillomas, 218, 220f, 221f
Multiple peripheral papillomas, 438, 446, 448
Mural calcifications, 158f

Necrotic breast, 238f
Necrotic cellular debris, calcifications in, 163–164, 164f
Necrotic invasive ductal carcinoma, core biopsy, 443, 451
Needle biopsies, 393–394, 394f–396f
    magnetic resonance guidance, 402–404, 405f–406f, 407
    stereotactic guidance, 400–402, 403f, 404f
    ultrasound guidance, 396–398, 397f–400f, 400, 401f, 402f
Neoadjuvant therapy, 6
    conservative breast cancer treatment, 340
    pathology stage, 431, 444
    tumor in patients on, 135, 135f–137f, 137
Nephrogenic systemic fibrosis (NSF), 114
Neurofibromatosis, 179–180, 180f
90-degree LM view
    for medial lesions, 69–70, 70f
    medial tissue against the imaging receptor, 444
90-degree ML view, for lateral lesions, 70, 71f
Nipple discharge, 88f, 306, 378t, 379f, 438, 448. *See also* Spontaneous nipple discharge
Nipple inversion and retraction, 235f
Non-mass-like enhancement, 126, 127f–128f, 128

Obscured descriptor, 446
Occult breast primary, 133
Oil cysts, 94, 97f, 181, 184, 184f, 185f, 186, 186f
    rim calcifications in, 433, 445
Onchocerciasis (*Onchocerca volvulus*), 155
Oncotype DX scores, 6, 441, 450
Opacified lymphatic channels, 385f
Open capsulotomy, 365
Optimal film quality, 145
Osteosarcoma, radiation induced, 344f
Oval hyperechoic mass, with central anechogenicity, 436f, 447

p63 stain, 433, 445
Pacemakers, 372–373
Paget cells, 302
Paget disease, 297–298, 302, 303, 305f
    of nipple, stages of, 432, 445
Papillary carcinoma, 255, 256f–260f, 260–261, 323, 436, 447
    thyroid, 431, 444
Papillary lesions
    of breast, 217
    displacement of epithelial cells with, 440, 449
    malignant, 260
    myoepithelial cells, 445
Papillomas
    ductography in patients with, 432, 444
    intracystic, 96

intraductal, 303
multiple, 218, 220, 221f
peripheral, multiple, 438, 448
solitary, 216–218, 216f–217f, 219f, 220f
spontaneous nipple discharge, cause of, 434, 446
wash-in and wash-out kinetics in postmenopausal woman, 440, 450
Paraffin block radiography, 416, 420f
Parasites calcifications, 155, 163f, 164f
Parenchyma, poor separation of, 27f
Parenchymal asymmetry, 296–297, 299f–300f, 301f, 302f, 303f, 304f
Parenchymal enhancement
background, 118, 122f
focal, 118
radiation and tamoxifen effect on, 123f
Parenchymal pattern descriptors, 2
Pathological lymph node classification, 7t
Pectoral fascia, 84
Pectoralis minor muscle, 18, 20f
medial insertion of, 23f
Periductal mastitis, 151
Peripheral abscess, 203–205, 205f–206f
Peritoneal seeding, 443, 451
Phantom images, 14, 14f, 438, 448
used to calculating SNR and CNR, 14, 436, 447
Phyllodes tumors, 212, 213f–215f, 216. *See also* Malignant phyllodes tumors
recurrent, 215f
Plasma cell mastitis, 151
Pleomorphic calcifications, 148t, 343
Pleomorphic liposarcoma, 328f
Pleomorphic lobular carcinoma in situ, 304
Pleomorphic nuclei, 160
Pneumothorax, 409
Poland syndrome, 19, 20f–21f
Popcorn calcifications, 153
Port-a-catheters, 372, 372f, 373f
Post-biopsy needle artifact, 116f
Posterior acoustic enhancement, 83–84, 207
Posterior nipple line (PNL), 23, 24f–25f, 25, 76–77
Postmenopausal woman
vs. premenopausal women, 368
wash-in and wash-out kinetics in, 440, 450
Postsurgical changes, 443, 451
Preoperative wire localizations
mammographic guidance, 411, 413, 413f–415f, 416f, 417f, 418f–420f
needle length for, 438, 448
ultrasound guidance, 409–411, 410f–411f, 412f
Primary breast lymphoma, 267
Progesterone receptors (PR), 135
Proliferative cellular processes, 156–157
Prostate cancer, 326
Psammoma bodies, 431, 444
Pseudoangiomatous stromal hyperplasia (PASH), 221–222, 223f–224f, 225, 443, 451
benign lesions, 320
complex cystic masses, 95t
for focal fibrosis, 220
unilateral dense gynecomastia and, 323f
Pseudolesions, 385
superimposed glandular tissue, 54f
pTNM, 6

Quirky calcifications, 151, 151f

Radial scar. *See* Complex sclerosing lesions
Radiation therapy
conservative breast cancer treatment, 340
effect of, 283–284, 284f, 285f
for extra-abdominal desmoid, 227
Radiography, specimen, 415–416, 420f
Radiologic–pathologic concordance, patient management after, 408–409, 408f–409f
Raloxifene, 3, 8
Randomization methodology, 3
Randomized controlled trials, 443, 451
Real-time scanning, 83
Recurrent invasive ductal carcinoma, 295f
Reduction mammoplasty, 357–359, 358f–359f, 360f, 361f
Region of interest (ROI) marker, 118
Renal excretion, of gadolinium, 440, 450
Renal failure, 432, 444
Residual disease, 135, 136f, 137f
Residual skin thickening, 341
Reverberation artifacts, 92, 92f
Rim calcifications, 433, 445
Rim enhancement, 125, 230
Rod-like calcifications, 146f
Rolled or change of angle views, 59–60, 62f–66f, 64
Round and punctate calcifications, 147f

S100, 230
Sagging breast, 30f, 31f
Sarcomas, 269, 269f–272f
Schwann cell origin, 227
Sclerosing adenosis, 227, 227f, 442, 450
Screening mammography, 435f, 446
anterior compression views, use of, 26–29, 27f–32f
artifacts, 31–35, 33t, 34f, 35f, 36f
benchmark for, 432, 445
for breast cancer, 432, 445
callbacks, 41–42, 44, 46, 46t
craniocaudal views, 19–25, 21f–22f, 21t, 23f
desired goals for, 429t
evaluation of images, 37, 38f–45f, 40–41
exaggerated craniocaudal views, 25, 25f–26f, 26t
film labeling, 14, 14t
imaging algorithm, 14–15
imaging women
with implants, 29–31, 31f, 32f
with large breasts, 15, 16f
with small breasts, 15, 15f
lump in right breast, 436f, 447
mediolateral oblique views, 15–19, 16f, 17f, 18f, 18t, 19f, 20f–21f
phantom images, 14, 14f
posterior nipple line, 23, 24f–25f, 25
programs, 156
purpose of, 35, 37
quality control tests, 14
report templates, 426t
viewing conditions, 37
Seat belt injury, 338, 341f
Sebaceous cysts, 69f, 87f, 176, 177f–178f, 179f
Seborrheic keratosis, 176
Secretory disease, 151
Sentinel lymph node (SLN) biopsy, 5, 431, 444
intraoperative evaluation of, 439, 449
for patients with extensive DCIS, 433, 445
Shrinking breast, 293, 439, 449

Signal flaring, 115f, 117
Signal-to-noise ratios (SNR), 14, 436, 447
Silicone fluid bleed, 365
Silicone implants, women with, 437, 447
Simple cysts, 92, 92f, 197–198, 198f, 199f
Single mediolateral oblique view, of mastectomy, 350
Skin
calcifications, 148–149, 149f, 443, 451
and developing skin lesion, 87f
leiomyosarcoma, metastatic to, 88
masses, 176, 176f–180f, 178–180, 181f
thickening
diffuse, 432, 444
and dilated subcutaneous lymphatics, 87f
and edema, 124f
residual, 341
ulceration, 236f, 237f
Solid masses
characterization of, 94, 97–99, 99f–103f, 101
complex cystic masses, 437, 441f, 448, 450
with cystic spaces, 200–201
Solitary central papillomas, 448
Solitary dilated duct, 306, 306f, 307f–311f
Solitary papillary carcinomas, 255
Solitary papillomas, 216–218, 216f–217f, 219f, 220f, 381, 381f
Spatial resolution, of lesion, 114
Specimen radiography, 415–416, 420f, 437f, 447
Spontaneous nipple discharge, 218
breast cancer, 382
cause of, 434, 446
ductography for, 379
with solitary papillomas, 216
Spot compression paddle, 53f
lesion inclusion, 52f
during mammographically guided wire localization, 416f
preoperative wire localizations, 433, 445
Spot compression views, 49–51, 54, 54f, 55f–57f, 58f, 59f, 60f, 434f, 446
cleavage, 432, 444
indication for, 54t
paddles for, 50, 52f–53f
Spot localization paddle, 413f
Spot tangential view
with focal pain, 439f, 449
on patient with lump, 432, 445
Spring-loaded mechanism, with 14G needle, 393
Squamous metaplasia, 203, 436, 447
Staphylococcus aureus, 202
Steatocystoma multiplex, 186
Stellate descriptor, 446
Stereotactically guided biopsy, 413
Sternalis muscle, 22, 23f, 316, 317f
Stromal calcifications, 151, 151f, 152f, 153f
Stromal fibrosis, 151, 222
Subareolar abscess, 202–203, 203f
pathologic finding in, 436, 447
patients with, 437, 448
with reactive lymphadenopathy, 204f
Suboptimal fat saturation, 117
Superolateral to inferomedial oblique (SIO) views, for breast imaging, 70, 73, 73f
Sutures calcifications, 154–155, 162f
Symptomatic patients, imaging algorithms for, 49, 49t
Synchronous bilateral disease, 131f

Tamoxifen, 3, 227, 368
Temporal arteritis, 290, 290f
Thoracoepigastric vein, 311
Thrombophlebitis, 443, 451
Tis (Paget), 445
TNM staging system, 6–7
Transgender patients, 373, 374f
Transverse rectus abdominis myocutaneous (TRAM) flap, 355
　appearance of, 356
　post mastectomy, reconstruction, 356f
　reconstructions, 435f, 446
Trastuzumab (Herceptin), 244
Trauma, 286, 287f–288f, 338, 339f–340f, 341f
Triangulation concepts, for breast, 73, 75–77, 76f–77f
　lesion localization, 74f, 75f
Trichinosis (*Trichinella spiralis*), 155
Trigger point, 379
Triple-negative cancers, 241, 440, 442, 450–451
Tubular adenoma, 211–212, 211f
Tubular carcinomas, 175f, 246, 248, 248f, 249f, 436, 447
　low nuclear grade DCIS and LCIS, 435, 447
　from sclerosing adenosis, 433, 445
Tubular hypoechogenicity, 443f, 451
Tumor
　granular cell, 227–228, 229f–230f, 230
　location, clip placement to marking, 407–409, 407f–409f
　luminal A and B, 8
　neoadjuvant therapy for, 135, 135f–137f, 137
　in patients on neoadjuvant therapy, 135, 135f–137f, 137
　phyllodes, 212, 213f–215f, 216
　sojourn time, 3
20G spinal needle, 389
Tyrer–Cuzick risk models, 128

Ultrasound. *See also* Breast ultrasound
　anatomy on, 84–90, 85f, 86f–90f, 91f
　for breast compression, 439f, 449
　clinical findings, 102–103, 104f, 105
　equipment and technical issues, 80, 81f, 81t
　for focal fibrosis, 220, 222f
　guided biopsies, 396
　indications for, 90–92
　mammographic and sonographic correlation, 108f–109f, 109, 110f
　masses with benign features on, 98f
　mastitis *vs.* abscess, 106–107, 107f, 108f, 109
　matrix determination, 92, 92f–94f, 94, 95f–96f, 97f–98f
　MRI-detected findings, 105–106, 106f
　nonspecific mammographic findings, 102, 103f
　scanning technique, 80–83, 82f–83f, 82t
　solid masses, characterization of, 94, 97–99, 99f–103f, 101
　terminology, 83–84, 84f
Underexposure effect, 34f
Unilateral dense gynecomastia, 323f
US Preventive Services Task Force (USPSTF), 3

Vacuum-assisted imaging-guided biopsy, 335–336, 337f–338f, 339f
Vascular calcifications, 28f, 90f, 150–151, 150f, 151f
Vascular lesions, benign, 230, 230f, 231f
Venous hemangiomas, 230
Venous obstruction, 287
Vimentin, 230

Water density masses, 196–197, 197t
Weight loss, 368
Wide surgical excision, 440, 450
Women
　abscess in, 201–205, 202f, 203f, 204f, 205f
　with breast lump, 438, 448
　developing breast cancer, risk for, 140f
　with implants, 138, 140f
　inflammatory symptoms in, 201–202
　lumpectomy for, 65
　with nipple discharge, 378t
　oil cysts in, 184, 186f
　with palpable abnormality, 64
　postmenopausal *vs.* premenopausal, 368
　preoperative breast MRI in, 130, 133f
　with sclerosing adenosis, 227, 227f
　with silicone implants, 437, 447
　with solitary papillomas, 216–218, 216f–217f, 219f, 220f
　subglandular location, with implants in, 31f–32f
　with tubular adenoma, 211–212, 211f
Wraparound artifact, 118

"yp" designation, 431, 444

Zuska disease, 202, 203f, 433, 445